NEW! FREE INTERNET DRUG UPDATES!

Your purchase of this book entitles you to receive our free online drug updates!

To help you keep pace with the constant changes in pharmacology, W.B. Saunders Company provides periodic drug information updates on our Web site. By visiting us at:

www.wbsaunders.com/SIMON/SaundersNDH

you'll be assured of receiving the most up-to-the-minute drug information, including*:

- New drug monographs
- Brief updates on other recently approved drugs
- Names and brief descriptions of new OTC drugs
- Drug alerts, including information about drugs taken off the market, significant new contraindications and dosage changes, and more
- Updated drug information, such as new uses and other information of interest to health care professionals
- Hyperlinks to additional useful drug information Web sites

Visit our Web site at **www.wbsaunders.com/SIMON/SaundersNDH** today to access this important information!

* Not every update will include each of these items. Information released by the FDA and other developments will determine the contents of each update.

COMMONLY USED ABBREVIATIONS

ac—before meals
ACE—angiotensin-converting enzyme
ANC—absolute neutrophil count
bid—twice daily
B/P—blood pressure
BSA—body surface area
CBC—complete blood count
Ccr—creatinine clearance
CHF—congestive heart failure
Cl—chloride
CNS—central nervous system
CO—cardiac output
COPD—chronic obstructive pulmonary disease
dl—deciliter
DNA—deoxyribonucleic acid
EEG—electroencephalogram
EKG—electrocardiogram
esp.—especially
g—gram
GI—gastrointestinal
gtt—drop
GU—genitourinary
h or hrs—hour(s)
Hct—hematocrit
Hgb—hemoglobin
hs—bedtime
HTN—hypertension
IM—intramuscular
IU—international unit
IV—intravenous
K—potassium
kg—kilogram
L—liter
lbs—pounds
LOC—level of consciousness
m²—meter squared
MAO—monoamine oxidase

mcg—microgram
mEq—milliequivalent
mg—milligram
MI—myocardial infarction
min—minute(s)
ml—milliliter
mo(s)—month(s)
Na—sodium
NaCl—sodium chloride
NSAIDs—nonsteroidal anti-inflammatory drugs
OD—right eye
OS—left eye
OU—both eyes
oz—ounce
pc—after meals
PO—orally, by mouth
prn—as needed
pt—patient
qd—daily
qid—four times daily
qOd—every other day
REM—rapid eye movements
RBC—red blood cell count
RNA—ribonucleic acid
sec(s)—second(s)
SL—sublingual
SubQ—subcutaneous
tbs—tablespoon
tid—three times daily
TPR—temperature, pulse, respirations
tsp—teaspoonful
w/—with
w/o—without
WBC—white blood cell count
wk(s)—week(s)
yr(s)—year(s)

SAUNDERS
NURSING
DRUG
HANDBOOK
2001

SAUNDERS NURSING DRUG HANDBOOK 2001

BARBARA B. HODGSON, RN, OCN

Cancer Institute
St. Joseph's Hospital
Tampa, Florida

Formerly, Drug Research Coordinator
Diabetes Center
University of South Florida
Tampa, Florida

ROBERT J. KIZIOR, BS, RPh

Education Coordinator
Department of Pharmacy
Alexian Brothers Medical Center
Elk Grove Village, Illinois

Formerly, Adjunct Faculty
William Rainey Harper College
Palatine, Illinois

W.B. SAUNDERS COMPANY

A Harcourt Health Sciences Company

Philadelphia / London / New York / St. Louis / Sydney / Toronto

W.B. SAUNDERS COMPANY
A Harcourt Health Sciences Company

The Curtis Center
Independence Square West
Philadelphia, Pennsylvania 19106

SAUNDERS NURSING DRUG HANDBOOK 2001   ISBN 0-7216-7400-3

ISSN 1098-8661

Printed in the United States of America.

Last digit is the print number: 9   8   7   6   5   4   3   2   1

CONSULTANT REVIEWERS

Susan deWit, MSN, RNCS
Santa Barbara, California

Elizabeth Gloss, EdD, RN
Associate Professor
State University of New York Health
  Science Center at Brooklyn
Brooklyn, New York

Mary Ann Haeuser, MSN, RN
Dominican College
School of Nursing
San Rafael, California

Barbara D. Horton, RN, MS
Arnot Ogden Medical Center
  School of Nursing Elmira
Elmira, New York

Brenda P. Johnson, MSN, RN
Assistant Professor
Southeast Missouri State University
Cape Girardeau, Missouri

Kelly W. Jones, PharmD, BCPS
Associate Professor of Family
  Medicine
McLeod Family Medicine Center
McLeod Regional Medical Center
Florence, South Carolina

Victoria Lagle, RN, MSN, FNP
Nurse Practitioner, Private Practice
Bedford, Kentucky

Linda Laskowski-Jones, RN, MS,
  CS, CCRN, CEN
Trauma Clinical Specialist
Trauma Service
Medical Center of Delaware
Newark, Delaware

Linda L. Lindeke, PhD, RN, CPNP
School of Nursing
University of Minnesota
Minneapolis, Minnesota

Elaine Negley, RNC, MS
VA Nursing Home Care Unit
Wilmington, Delaware

Patricia A. Lange-Otsuka, RN, CS,
  MSN, CCRN
Assistant Professor of Nursing
Academic Coordinator
Hawaii Pacific University
Kaneoha, Hawaii

Christine Smith, RNC, MSN
Neonatal Clinical Nurse
  Specialist
Intensive Care Nursery
Thomas Jefferson University
  Hospital
Philadelphia, Pennsylvania

Thomas J. Smith, RNC, PhD
Associate Professor
Nicholls State University
Thibodaux, Louisiana

STUDENT REVIEWER PANEL

Jeff Lung
Golden West College
Huntington Beach, California

Kristin Cornmack
Beth-El College of Nursing &
   Health Sciences
Colorado Springs, Colorado

Greg Marvin
Youngstown State University
Youngstown, Ohio

AutumnWilliams
Marian College
Indianapolis, Indiana

Jill Bennett
San Diego State University
San Diego, California

Rachel Winograd Bollenbecker
California State University
Los Angeles, California

Tina Rorick
California State University
Los Angeles, California

Rodger Jarabek
Dakota Wesleyn University
Mitchell, South Dakota

Marcelle Hayes
Pikes Peak Community College
Colorado Springs, Colorado

David Marshall
De Anza College
San Jose, California

Elaine Horton
Beth-El College of Nursing &
   Health Sciences
Colorado Springs, Colorado

PREFACE

Nurses and other health care providers face many challenges in today's environment, not the least of which is familiarity with the large number of medications available. New medications are being introduced, and new applications, dosage forms, and different routes of administration for existing medications are increasing at a rapid rate. This voluminous amount of drug information must be integrated into the patient care environment quickly.

Saunders Nursing Drug Handbook 2001 is designed as an easy-to-use source of the current drug information needed by the busy health care provider. What separates this book from others is that it guides the user through patient care to better practice, and to better care.

HOW TO USE THIS HANDBOOK

The main objective of **Saunders Nursing Drug Handbook 2001** is to provide essential drug information for thousands of medications in a user friendly format. The first major section of the handbook contains an alphabetical listing of drug monographs by generic name. Each drug monograph provides the following information:

Generic and Brand Names. The monographs begin with the generic and brand names for both the United States and Canada, followed by the pronunciation of the drug and the most common classification for the medications.

Fixed-Combination Drugs. Where appropriate, fixed-combinations, or drugs made up of two or more generic medications, are listed with the generic drug. Including this information in the drug monograph provides easy access to identify these combined medications.

Product Availability. New to this edition, each drug monograph gives the form and availability and indicates whether the drug is obtainable by prescription **(Rx)** or over the counter **(OTC).**

Pharmacokinetics. Pharmacokinetics describes what happens to the medication once it is administered to the patient. Each monograph gives the absorption, distribution, metabolism, excretion, and half-life of the medication.

Action/Therapeutic Effect. The action in each monograph concisely explains how the drug is expected to act, with the expected *therapeutic effect* given in italics. Listing of therapeutic effects is new to this edition of the handbook.

Uses/*Unlabeled Uses.* The listing of uses for each drug has been expanded to include both the common FDA uses and *unlabeled uses,* which appear in italics. Listing of unlabeled uses is new to this edition of the handbook.

Storage/Handling. Instructions on storage and handling are given for each drug monograph. Considerations include, "Does the medication need special storage requirements such as refrigeration?" and "How long is the medication stable once it is reconstituted?"

Administration. Instructions for administration are given for each route of administration, such as PO, Rectal, IM, and IV. For IV administration, each step is enumerated, and flow rates are provided. Other considerations include, "Should the medication be taken with food?" and "How fast should the IV medication be given?"

Indication/Dosage/Routes. Each monograph includes specific dosing guidelines for adults, the elderly, children, and patients with renal and/or hepatic impairment. Dosages are clearly indicated for each approved indication and route. Where appropriate, rates for creatinine clearance are provided for each dose.

Precautions. The drug monograph lists conditions in which use of the drug is contraindicated and should not be used. Also, the cautions warn the health care provider of specific situations when the drug should be closely monitored. Additional information on drug use during pregnancy and lactation is given, expanding on the FDA Pregnancy Category. Nurses and health care providers must ask patients about the possibility of pregnancy before any drug therapy is initiated. Ideally, no drug should be administered during pregnancy, but there are situations that may demand a risk/benefit decision by the physician and the patient.

Interactions. Drug interactions are important, especially as the number of medications a patient receives increases. The most clinically significant reactions are noted along with their results. The health care provider should ask the patient if he or she has any allergies to medications. Additionally, altered lab values are included with each monograph to show what effects the drug may have on lab results.

Side Effects. Side effects are defined as those responses that are usually predictable with the drug, are not life-threatening, and may or may not require discontinuation of the drug. Unique to this handbook, side effects are listed by frequency so the nurse can focus on patient care without wading through a myriad of signs and symptoms of side effects.

Adverse Reactions/Toxic Effects. Adverse reactions and toxic effects are very serious and often life-threatening, undesirable responses that require prompt intervention from a health care provider.

Nursing Implications. Nursing implications are organized as care is organized. That is, "What needs to be assessed or done before the first dose is administered?" "What interventions and evaluations are needed during drug therapy?" and "What explicit teaching is needed for the patient and family?" Nursing implications are given in color throughout the book for easy identification.

The second major section of **Saunders Nursing Drug Handbook 2001** is the Classification section. This section provides groups of medications frequently encountered in clinical practice. The content for each classification gives action; uses; precautions; interactions; side effects; adverse reactions/toxic effects; and nursing implications, which are in color and include patient/family teaching. Each classification includes an easy-to-use table, unique to this handbook, which compares all the drugs within the classification to help the practitioner distinguish the drugs according to dosages, routes of administration, and other characteristics. New classifications included in **Saunders Nursing Drug Handbook 2001** are *medications for the treatment of HIV, oral contraceptives, antiglaucoma agents, hormones, quinolone and macrolide antibiotics, antivirals, fertility agents, vitamins,* and *topical antifungals.* The total number of classifications listed in this section is 55.

Like the Classification section, the appendixes have been expanded. Important additions to the appendixes include information on the *dialysis of medication, therapeutic and toxic blood levels of medications, an atlas of medication administration techniques, components of a medication prescription, and herbal therapies.* As in previous editions, the appendixes also contain normal laboratory values, FDA pregnancy categories, review of dosage calculations, signs and symptoms of adverse reactions and toxic effects, rates of intermittent IV (piggyback) administration, and nomograms for body surface area. At the beginning of the handbook, a pull-out IV compatibility chart has been included. This chart lists compatibilities for over 80 drugs in an easy-to-use table format.

Finally, the *New Drug Supplement* includes the latest FDA-approved medications and several medications that are anticipated being available by the end of 2000. The Supplement provides information on the action, uses, dosage, and side effects for over 140 medications.

NEW COLOR MEDICATION CHART

New to **Saunders Nursing Drug Handbook 2001** is a color medication chart from the United States Pharmacopeial Convention, Inc. containing photographs of more than 100 of the most commonly used medications. The medications, both brand and generic, are shown in their different pill dosage forms. The medicine chart serves as an aid to help health care providers identify and distinguish different pills quickly.

NEW SOFTWARE INCLUDED

New to **Saunders Nursing Drug Handbook 2001** is the Windows-compatible mini CD-ROM packaged in the back of the book. The software features a drug information database consisting of more than 200 of the most commonly used medications. Users can select a drug by generic or brand name by typing the name of the drug or simply typing the first letter of the drug. The information will appear as it does in **Saunders Nursing Drug Handbook 2001.** Users can print the drug information in its entirety, or they can customize specific information to be printed on a one-page drug card or patient handout. Nursing students using this handbook and the accompanying software will find the pharmacology NCLEX review questions particularly useful. While working through the computerized NCLEX review, the student can access the drug database information immediately by clicking the mouse on the drug name in the question. This versatile software will be useful to all nurses, students, and other health care providers.

THE NURSE'S ROLE IN DRUG THERAPY

The new edition of this handbook features an introduction to the principles of pharmacology and the nurse's role in drug therapy. This section presents an overview of pharmacology, considerations for patients throughout the life span, guidelines for patient and family education, and much more. The introductory information offers both students and clinicians a refresher on pharmacology and the nursing process.

SUMMARY

After an intensive review by Consultant Reviewers and the Student Reviewer Panel, **Saunders Nursing Drug Handbook 2001** has undergone an extensive revision. Every drug entry and classification has been revised, new drugs and classifications have been added, and the appendixes have been expanded. Each drug monograph now contains additional information: *Product Availability, Therapeutic Effect,* and *Unlabeled Uses.* **Saunders Nursing Drug Handbook 2001** is an easy-to-use source of the current drug information for nurses, students, and other health care providers. It is our hope that this handbook will help you provide quality care to your patients.

Barbara B. Hodgson, RN, OCN
Robert J. Kizior, BS, RPh

ACKNOWLEDGMENTS

I offer a special heartfelt thank you to my co-author, Bob Kizior, for his continuing, superb work. Without Bob's effort in this major endeavor, this book would not have reached the *par excellence* it has achieved; to Linda Silvestri, MSN, RN, for contributing the NCLEX questions on the accompanying software; and especially to Jane and Mike Sperry, Greg Boyd, Carolyn Steele, and CI-3 for their unflagging support.

Barbara Hodgson

ILLUSTRATION CREDITS

Behrman RE (ed.): *Nelson Textbook of Pediatrics,* 15th ed. Philadelphia: WB Saunders Company, 1996.
Boothby WM, Sandiford RBL: *Boston Med Surg J* 185:337, 1921.
Kee JL, Hayes ER (eds.): *Pharmacology: A Nursing Process Approach,* 2nd ed. Philadelphia: WB Saunders Company, 1997.
Lehne RA: *Pharmacology for Nursing Care,* 2nd ed. Philadelphia: WB Saunders Company, 1994.
Micromedex, Inc., 2000.

NOTICE

Pharmacology is an ever-changing field. Standard safety precautions must be followed, but as new research and clinical experience broaden our knowledge, changes in treatment and drug therapy become necessary or appropriate. Readers are advised to check the product information currently provided by the manufacturer of each drug to be administered to verify the recommended dose, the method and duration of administration, and contraindications. It is the responsibility of the treating licensed health-care provider, relying on experience and knowledge of the patient, to determine dosages and the best treatment for the patient. Neither the Publisher nor the editor assumes any responsibility for any injury and/or damage to persons or property.

THE PUBLISHER

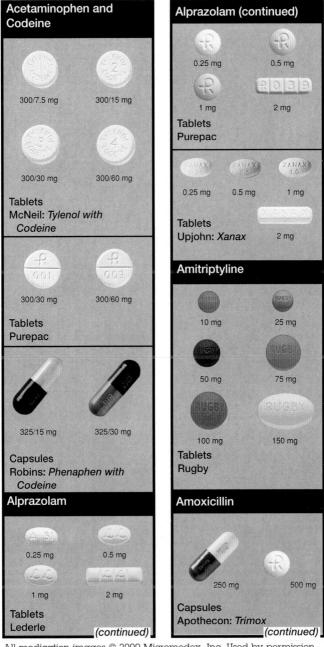

Acetaminophen and Codeine

300/7.5 mg   300/15 mg

300/30 mg   300/60 mg

Tablets
McNeil: *Tylenol with Codeine*

300/30 mg   300/60 mg

Tablets
Purepac

325/15 mg   325/30 mg

Capsules
Robins: *Phenaphen with Codeine*

Alprazolam

0.25 mg   0.5 mg

1 mg   2 mg

Tablets
Lederle

Alprazolam (continued)

0.25 mg   0.5 mg

1 mg   2 mg

Tablets
Purepac

0.25 mg   0.5 mg   1 mg

Tablets
Upjohn: *Xanax*   2 mg

Amitriptyline

10 mg   25 mg

50 mg   75 mg

100 mg   150 mg

Tablets
Rugby

Amoxicillin

250 mg   500 mg

Capsules
Apothecon: *Trimox*

(continued)

Amoxicillin (continued)

250 mg   500 mg

Capsules
SmithKline Beecham:
Amoxil

125 mg   250 mg

Tablets, Chewable
SmithKline Beecham:
Amoxil

250 mg   500 mg

Capsules
Wyeth-Ayerst: *Wymox*

Amoxicillin and Clavulanate

250/125 mg   500/125 mg

Tablets
SmithKline Beecham:
Augmentin

(continued)

Amoxicillin and Clavulanate (continued)

875/125 mg

Tablets
SmithKline Beecham:
Augmentin

Atenolol

50 mg   100 mg

Tablets
Geneva

25 mg   50 mg   100 mg

Tablets
Lederle

25 mg   50 mg   100 mg

Tablets
Zeneca: *Tenormin*

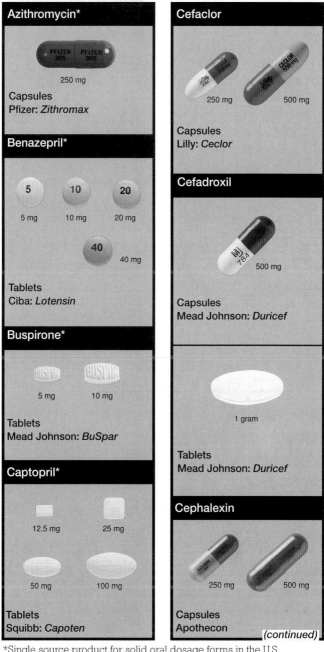

Azithromycin*

PFIZER 305 PFIZER 305

250 mg

Capsules
Pfizer: *Zithromax*

Benazepril*

5   10   20

5 mg   10 mg   20 mg

40   40 mg

Tablets
Ciba: *Lotensin*

Buspirone*

BUSPAR   BUSPAR

5 mg   10 mg

Tablets
Mead Johnson: *BuSpar*

Captopril*

12.5 mg   25 mg

50 mg   100 mg

Tablets
Squibb: *Capoten*

Cefaclor

250 mg   500 mg

Capsules
Lilly: *Ceclor*

Cefadroxil

500 mg

Capsules
Mead Johnson: *Duricef*

1 gram

Tablets
Mead Johnson: *Duricef*

Cephalexin

250 mg   500 mg

Capsules
Apothecon   *(continued)*

*Single source product for solid oral dosage forms in the U.S.

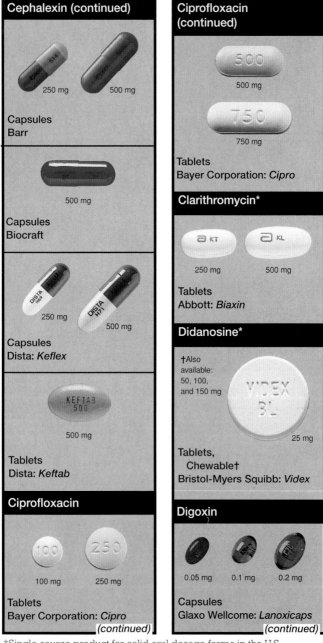

Cephalexin (continued)

250 mg   500 mg

Capsules
Barr

500 mg

Capsules
Biocraft

250 mg   500 mg

Capsules
Dista: *Keflex*

KEFTAB
500

500 mg

Tablets
Dista: *Keftab*

Ciprofloxacin

100 mg   250 mg

Tablets
Bayer Corporation: *Cipro*
(continued)

Ciprofloxacin (continued)

500

500 mg

750

750 mg

Tablets
Bayer Corporation: *Cipro*

Clarithromycin*

250 mg   500 mg

Tablets
Abbott: *Biaxin*

Didanosine*

†Also available: 50, 100, and 150 mg

VIDEX
BL

25 mg

Tablets, Chewable†
Bristol-Myers Squibb: *Videx*

Digoxin

0.05 mg   0.1 mg   0.2 mg

Capsules
Glaxo Wellcome: *Lanoxicaps*
(continued)

*Single source product for solid oral dosage forms in the U.S.

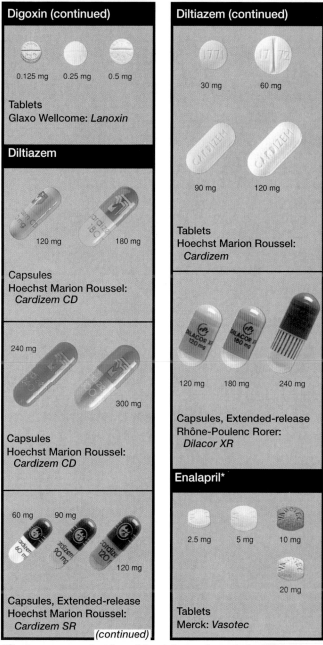

Digoxin (continued)

0.125 mg   0.25 mg   0.5 mg

Tablets
Glaxo Wellcome: *Lanoxin*

Diltiazem

120 mg   180 mg

Capsules
Hoechst Marion Roussel:
Cardizem CD

240 mg

300 mg

Capsules
Hoechst Marion Roussel:
Cardizem CD

60 mg   90 mg

120 mg

Capsules, Extended-release
Hoechst Marion Roussel:
Cardizem SR
(continued)

Diltiazem (continued)

30 mg   60 mg

90 mg   120 mg

Tablets
Hoechst Marion Roussel:
Cardizem

120 mg   180 mg   240 mg

Capsules, Extended-release
Rhône-Poulenc Rorer:
Dilacor XR

Enalapril*

2.5 mg   5 mg   10 mg

20 mg

Tablets
Merck: *Vasotec*

*Single source product for solid oral dosage forms in the U.S.

Erythromycin

250 mg

Capsules, Delayed-release
Abbott

250 mg   500 mg

Tablets
Abbott

333 mg   500 mg

Tablets
Abbott: *PCE*

250 mg   333 mg   500 mg

Tablets, Delayed-release
Abbott: *Ery-Tab*

250 mg

Capsules, Delayed-release
Barr

(continued)

Erythromycin (continued)

250 mg   333 mg

Tablets, Delayed-release
Knoll: *E-Mycin*

250 mg

Capsules, Delayed-release
PD: *Eryc*

250 mg

Capsules, Delayed-release
Purepac

Estradiol

0.5 mg   1 mg   2 mg

Tablets
Bristol-Myers Squibb:
Estrace

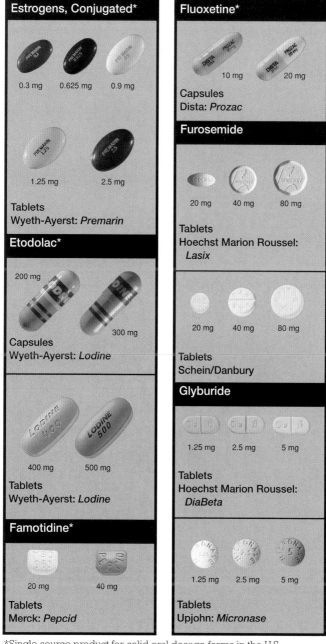

Estrogens, Conjugated*

0.3 mg   0.625 mg   0.9 mg

1.25 mg   2.5 mg

Tablets
Wyeth-Ayerst: *Premarin*

Etodolac*

200 mg

300 mg

Capsules
Wyeth-Ayerst: *Lodine*

400 mg   500 mg

Tablets
Wyeth-Ayerst: *Lodine*

Famotidine*

20 mg   40 mg

Tablets
Merck: *Pepcid*

Fluoxetine*

10 mg   20 mg

Capsules
Dista: *Prozac*

Furosemide

20 mg   40 mg   80 mg

Tablets
Hoechst Marion Roussel:
Lasix

20 mg   40 mg   80 mg

Tablets
Schein/Danbury

Glyburide

1.25 mg   2.5 mg   5 mg

Tablets
Hoechst Marion Roussel:
DiaBeta

1.25 mg   2.5 mg   5 mg

Tablets
Upjohn: *Micronase*

*Single source product for solid oral dosage forms in the U.S.

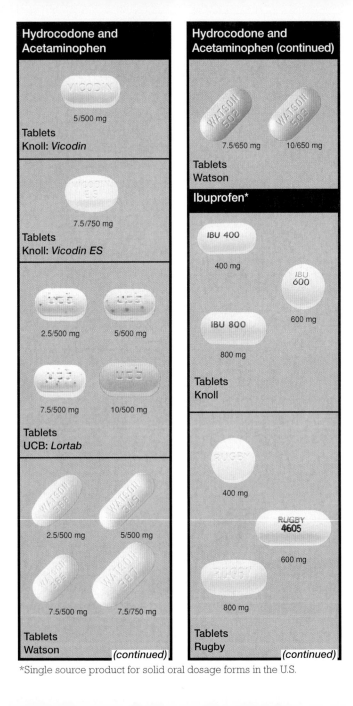

Hydrocodone and Acetaminophen

5/500 mg
Tablets
Knoll: *Vicodin*

7.5/750 mg
Tablets
Knoll: *Vicodin ES*

2.5/500 mg   5/500 mg

7.5/500 mg   10/500 mg
Tablets
UCB: *Lortab*

2.5/500 mg   5/500 mg

7.5/500 mg   7.5/750 mg
Tablets
Watson

Hydrocodone and Acetaminophen (continued)

7.5/650 mg   10/650 mg
Tablets
Watson

Ibuprofen*

IBU 400
400 mg

IBU 600
600 mg

IBU 800
800 mg
Tablets
Knoll

RUGBY
400 mg

RUGBY 4605
600 mg

RUGBY
800 mg
Tablets
Rugby

(continued)   *(continued)*

*Single source product for solid oral dosage forms in the U.S.

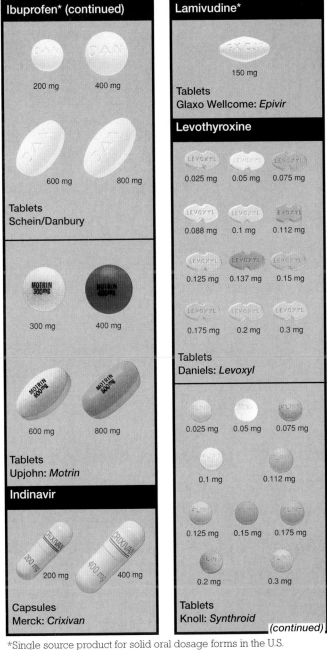

Ibuprofen* (continued)

200 mg   400 mg

600 mg   800 mg

Tablets
Schein/Danbury

300 mg   400 mg

600 mg   800 mg

Tablets
Upjohn: *Motrin*

Indinavir

200 mg   400 mg

Capsules
Merck: *Crixivan*

Lamivudine*

150 mg

Tablets
Glaxo Wellcome: *Epivir*

Levothyroxine

0.025 mg   0.05 mg   0.075 mg

0.088 mg   0.1 mg   0.112 mg

0.125 mg   0.137 mg   0.15 mg

0.175 mg   0.2 mg   0.3 mg

Tablets
Daniels: *Levoxyl*

0.025 mg   0.05 mg   0.075 mg

0.1 mg   0.112 mg

0.125 mg   0.15 mg   0.175 mg

0.2 mg   0.3 mg

Tablets
Knoll: *Synthroid*

(continued)

*Single source product for solid oral dosage forms in the U.S.

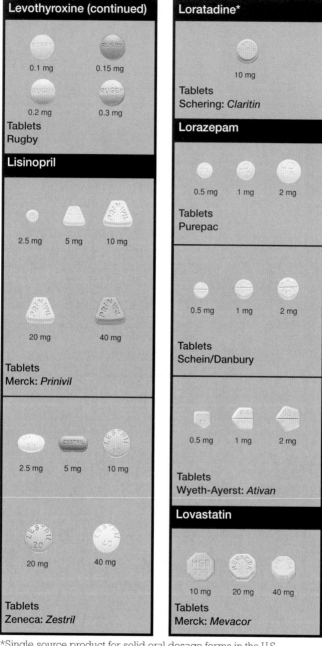

Levothyroxine (continued)

0.1 mg
0.15 mg
0.2 mg
0.3 mg

Tablets
Rugby

Lisinopril

2.5 mg
5 mg
10 mg

20 mg
40 mg

Tablets
Merck: *Prinivil*

2.5 mg
5 mg
10 mg

20 mg
40 mg

Tablets
Zeneca: *Zestril*

Loratadine*

10 mg

Tablets
Schering: *Claritin*

Lorazepam

0.5 mg
1 mg
2 mg

Tablets
Purepac

0.5 mg
1 mg
2 mg

Tablets
Schein/Danbury

0.5 mg
1 mg
2 mg

Tablets
Wyeth-Ayerst: *Ativan*

Lovastatin

10 mg
20 mg
40 mg

Tablets
Merck: *Mevacor*

*Single source product for solid oral dosage forms in the U.S.

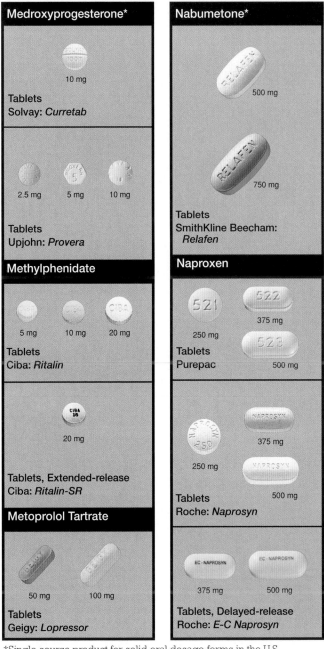

Medroxyprogesterone*

10 mg

Tablets
Solvay: *Curretab*

2.5 mg   5 mg   10 mg

Tablets
Upjohn: *Provera*

Methylphenidate

5 mg   10 mg   20 mg

Tablets
Ciba: *Ritalin*

20 mg

Tablets, Extended-release
Ciba: *Ritalin-SR*

Metoprolol Tartrate

50 mg   100 mg

Tablets
Geigy: *Lopressor*

Nabumetone*

500 mg

750 mg

Tablets
SmithKline Beecham:
Relafen

Naproxen

521   522
       375 mg
250 mg
523
Tablets   500 mg
Purepac

250 mg   375 mg
                500 mg
Tablets
Roche: *Naprosyn*

EC-NAPROSYN   EC-NAPROSYN
375 mg   500 mg

Tablets, Delayed-release
Roche: *E-C Naprosyn*

*Single source product for solid oral dosage forms in the U.S.

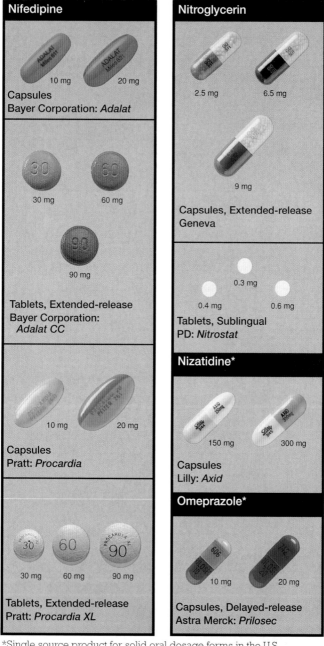

Nifedipine

10 mg **20 mg**
Capsules
Bayer Corporation: *Adalat*

30 mg **60 mg**

90 mg
Tablets, Extended-release
Bayer Corporation:
Adalat CC

10 mg **20 mg**
Capsules
Pratt: *Procardia*

30 mg **60 mg** **90 mg**
Tablets, Extended-release
Pratt: *Procardia XL*

Nitroglycerin

2.5 mg **6.5 mg**

9 mg

Capsules, Extended-release
Geneva

0.3 mg
0.4 mg **0.6 mg**
Tablets, Sublingual
PD: *Nitrostat*

Nizatidine*

150 mg **300 mg**
Capsules
Lilly: *Axid*

Omeprazole*

10 mg **20 mg**
Capsules, Delayed-release
Astra Merck: *Prilosec*

*Single source product for solid oral dosage forms in the U.S.

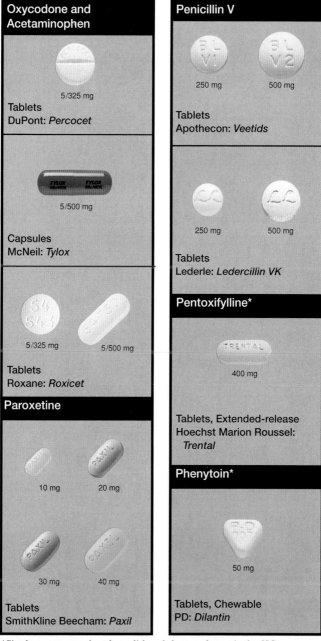

Oxycodone and Acetaminophen

5/325 mg

Tablets
DuPont: *Percocet*

TYLOX McNEIL   TYLOX McNEIL

5/500 mg

Capsules
McNeil: *Tylox*

54 543   5/500 mg

5/325 mg

Tablets
Roxane: *Roxicet*

Paroxetine

10 mg   20 mg

30 mg   40 mg

Tablets
SmithKline Beecham: *Paxil*

Penicillin V

B L V1   B L V2

250 mg   500 mg

Tablets
Apothecon: *Veetids*

250 mg   500 mg

Tablets
Lederle: *Ledercillin VK*

Pentoxifylline*

TRENTAL

400 mg

Tablets, Extended-release
Hoechst Marion Roussel:
Trental

Phenytoin*

50 mg

Tablets, Chewable
PD: *Dilantin*

*Single source product for solid oral dosage forms in the U.S.

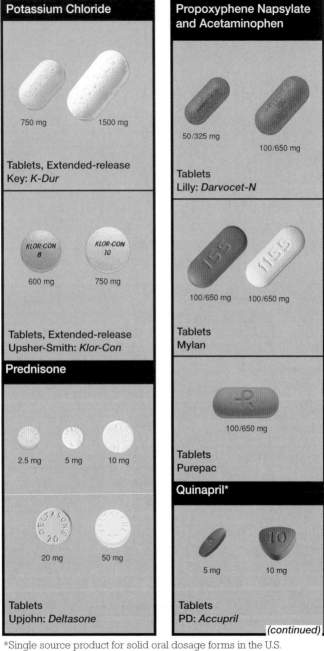

Potassium Chloride

750 mg 1500 mg

Tablets, Extended-release
Key: *K-Dur*

KLOR-CON 8 600 mg
KLOR-CON 10 750 mg

Tablets, Extended-release
Upsher-Smith: *Klor-Con*

Prednisone

2.5 mg 5 mg 10 mg

DELTASONE 20 — 20 mg
DELTASONE 50 — 50 mg

Tablets
Upjohn: *Deltasone*

Propoxyphene Napsylate and Acetaminophen

50/325 mg 100/650 mg

Tablets
Lilly: *Darvocet-N*

155 — 100/650 mg
1155 — 100/650 mg

Tablets
Mylan

100/650 mg

Tablets
Purepac

Quinapril*

5 mg 10 mg

Tablets
PD: *Accupril*

(continued)

*Single source product for solid oral dosage forms in the U.S.

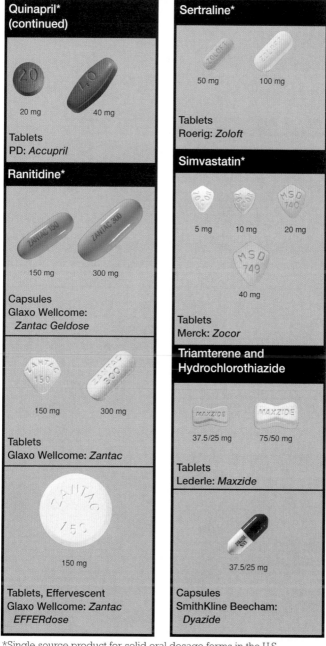

Quinapril*
(continued)

20 mg   40 mg

Tablets
PD: *Accupril*

Ranitidine*

ZANTAC 150   ZANTAC 300

150 mg   300 mg

Capsules
Glaxo Wellcome:
Zantac Geldose

ZANTAC 150   ZANTAC 300

150 mg   300 mg

Tablets
Glaxo Wellcome: *Zantac*

ZANTAC 150

150 mg

Tablets, Effervescent
Glaxo Wellcome: *Zantac
EFFERdose*

Sertraline*

ZOLOFT   ZOLOFT

50 mg   100 mg

Tablets
Roerig: *Zoloft*

Simvastatin*

MSD 726   MSD 735   MSD 740

5 mg   10 mg   20 mg

MSD 749

40 mg

Tablets
Merck: *Zocor*

Triamterene and
Hydrochlorothiazide

MAXZIDE   MAXZIDE

37.5/25 mg   75/50 mg

Tablets
Lederle: *Maxzide*

37.5/25 mg

Capsules
SmithKline Beecham:
Dyazide

*Single source product for solid oral dosage forms in the U.S.

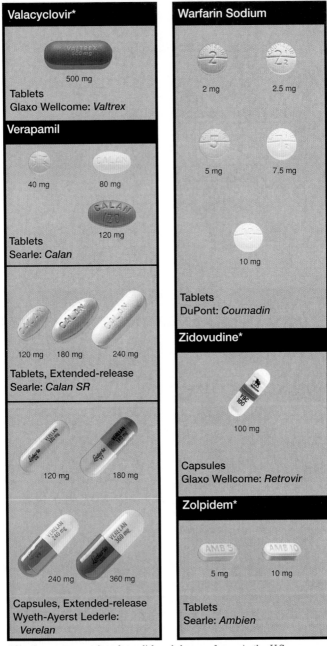

Valacyclovir*

500 mg

Tablets
Glaxo Wellcome: *Valtrex*

Verapamil

40 mg

80 mg

120 mg

Tablets
Searle: *Calan*

120 mg   180 mg   240 mg

Tablets, Extended-release
Searle: *Calan SR*

120 mg   180 mg

240 mg   360 mg

Capsules, Extended-release
Wyeth-Ayerst Lederle:
Verelan

Warfarin Sodium

2 mg   2.5 mg

5 mg   7.5 mg

10 mg

Tablets
DuPont: *Coumadin*

Zidovudine*

100 mg

Capsules
Glaxo Wellcome: *Retrovir*

Zolpidem*

5 mg   10 mg

Tablets
Searle: *Ambien*

*Single source product for solid oral dosage forms in the U.S.

CONTENTS

THE NURSE'S ROLE IN DRUG THERAPY

Drug therapy is an integral part of medical care in the treatment, prevention, and maintenance of acute and chronic conditions or diseases. One of the responsibilities of the nurse is to assess the client's response to drug therapy. The nurse must understand the basic principles of pharmacology to adequately care for the client undergoing drug therapy.

BASIC PRINCIPLES OF PHARMACOLOGY

The relationship between drug dosage and drug effect is described by two basic areas of pharmacology: pharmacokinetics and pharmacodynamics.

PHARMACOKINETICS

Pharmacokinetics refers to the movement of a drug throughout the body. The four processes involved in pharmacokinetics are absorption, distribution, metabolism, and excretion. Pharmacokinetics plus the dosage administered determines the drug concentration at its site of action and the intensity of its effect.

Absorption is the movement of a drug from the site of its administration into the blood. For oral medications, the site of absorption is the gastrointestinal tract. IM medications are absorbed in the muscles, and IV medications are absorbed immediately into the bloodstream. Absorption into the body's cells occurs in one of three ways. Passive absorption, or diffusion, is the movement of the drug from an area of higher concentration to an area of lower concentration. Active absorption occurs when the drug particles are carried by an enzyme or protein across the concentration gradient. Energy is required for active absorption to occur. Pinocytosis occurs when the drug particles are engulfed by the cell membrane and incorporated into the cell. Absorption is affected by the rate of dissolution, surface area, blood flow, lipid solubility, and pH. Some oral drugs are not absorbed in the stomach but instead are passed on to the liver. This is known as the first-pass effect or hepatic first-pass. Another category of absorption is bioavailability, the percentage of the drug that has been absorbed. For example, since IV medications are absorbed immediately into the bloodstream, they are 100% bioavailable.

Distribution is the movement of the drug throughout the body as it becomes available to fluids and body tissues. Distribution is influenced by the blood flow to the tissues, body tissue availability, and protein binding. As drugs flow through the body fluids, they form bonds with proteins, mainly albumin. The portion of the drug that is bound to the protein is inactive because it cannot react to other potential receptors. The portion of the drug that is not bound to the protein is active and will cause a pharmacologic response with receptor sites.

Metabolism, also known as biotransformation, is the conversion of the drug structure by enzymes. Drug metabolism occurs in the liver. The enzymes can either break a drug structure into substrate molecules or synthesize a larger molecule to create a pharmacologic effect. Patients with hepatic disease must be closely monitored for therapeutic effect and toxicity because the disease may cause drug metabolism to increase, decrease, or remain unchanged. Also, infants and elderly patients experience altered hepatic function and thus must be monitored closely as well.

Excretion, or elimination, is the removal of the drug from the body. The half-life of a drug, represented by the symbol t1/2, is the amount of time it takes one half of the concentration of the drug to be eliminated from the body. Most drugs are removed through urine, bile, or feces. The key organ involved in drug elimination is the kidney. If a patient experiences altered kidney function, then the drug dosage may need to be supplemented due to excessive elimination. See Appendix I in this handbook for a list of medications eliminated during dialysis.

PHARMACODYNAMICS

Pharmacodynamics deals with the drug's mechanism of action and the biochemical and physiologic effects of the drug. Drug actions can be classified into two categories: structurally nonspecific drugs and structurally specific drugs. Structurally nonspecific drugs produce physical or chemical changes in the cell's membrane or internal environment. They do not combine with cell receptors. Structurally specific drugs do combine with cell receptors or act through enzyme interactions. These drugs alter cellular function by affecting membrane transport or energy metabolism.

Factors that affect pharmacodynamics are efficacy and drug potency. *Efficacy* is the drug's ability to initiate biologic activity. *Drug potency* is the amount of drug required to produce the desired biologic response. As the dosage of the drug increases, the biologic response increases. The relationship between the drug dosage and the biologic response is called the dose-response curve. The *Therapeutic Index* is the dose range that provides therapeutic efficacy while producing minimum adverse effects. For example, if the difference between the dose that produces the desired effect and the dose that produces the lethal effect is great, the drug has a large therapeutic index.

THE NURSE AND DRUG THERAPY

The nurse must understand what the drug is supposed to do and its therapeutic effect. The nurse has many roles during drug therapy. Safe, effective administration of medications is an integral part of a nurse's responsibility that requires theoretical, clinical, and critical thinking skills. Appendix J in this handbook guides you through several administration techniques. The nurse also monitors the patient during drug therapy in order to prevent or minimize unwanted effects on the patient. An important role for the nurse is to teach the patient about the prescribed drug's purpose and to encourage patient compliance in self-administration.

In order to better understand the nurse's role in drug therapy in the complex and often bewildering field of pharmacology, use of the Classification Section in this handbook will assist the nurse by breaking down drug information according to its therapeutic classification or grouping of drugs. Each classification of drugs has common traits. Consider that even though bronchodilators have different actions in order to fit the patient's needs, their effect may be the same, which is to relax the bronchial smooth muscle, and thereby relieve bronchospasm. The physician, however, may have prescribed one bronchodilator to patient A and a different bronchodilator to patient B. One drug may be offered because oral inhalation is preferred for patient A, whereas the IV route of administration is necessary for patient B. In gaining knowledge of a specific drug's classification, a clearer understanding of the drug's purpose will be met since almost all drugs fit into a classification of drugs. The continuing introduction of new drugs into the patient care environment requires nurses to constantly review medications. Understanding the classifications of drugs assists the nurse to differentiate among drugs with similar clinical uses.

MEDICATION ADMINISTRATION

Using the *Five Rights of Drug Administration,* i.e., giving the *right* drug in the *right* dose to the *right* patient using the *right* route at the *right* time, assures that the nurse will administer safe and accurate drug therapy as prescribed. This can occur only if the nurse has sufficient drug knowledge to be able to question or to recognize errors. Correct administration will ensure quality patient care, permitting maximum beneficial drug treatment.

Knowledge of the patient's condition, the disease being treated, age, and medication history as well as medical history will assist the nurse in anticipating untoward drug reactions as well as the therapeutic results of drug therapy. Knowledge of the drug's potential effects permits the nurse to anticipate possible reactions the drug may cause and to respond effectively in order to prevent patient harm, rather than just to react to the drug's untoward effects.

ASSESSMENT

Besides a health history, a clear medication history should be obtained. The nurse should ask the patient specific questions:

What are the current medications you are taking (strength, frequency, route)?

For what reason has each drug been prescribed?

Have you been compliant (following faithfully) with your drug regimen?

Is there a history of hypersensitivity (allergic reaction) to drugs previously taken?

Have you experienced any food or dye intolerance?

What symptoms have you experienced (difficulty breathing or swallowing, numbness in fingers or face, hives, itching, or skin erythema)?

What are the names of all the drugs you are taking regularly or on an as-needed basis, including oral contraceptives, vitamins, etc.?

How much nicotine and caffeine do you consume daily (coffee, tea, chocolate)?

What are the names of all over-the-counter (OTC) products you have recently taken or are now taking?

Since many OTC drugs interact with medication prescribed by the health care provider, the nurse must ask which OTC drugs are taken for colds, hay fever, headache or general aches, diarrhea or constipation—eye drops, antacids, or laxatives. The patient may not consider these preparations as drugs. Many

OTC drugs are of the fixed-combination type, particularly cold preparations. A tablet or capsule may contain an antipyretic to reduce fever, an analgesic for muscle aches, an antihistamine for itchy eyes, a sympathomimetic to reduce nasal secretion. Some narcotic preparations contain either acetaminophen or aspirin. A patient taking an anticoagulant cannot take aspirin owing to its additive effects. Careful questioning of the patient prior to drug administration will alert the nurse to potential problems.

PROMOTING PATIENT COMPLIANCE

Patient compliance during drug therapy is essential in order to prevent a recurrence or an exacerbation of a condition or disease or prevent possible future ineffectiveness of the drug. The nurse must inform the patient to take the prescribed medication as ordered and not to adjust the dosage or the frequency or timing of the dosage. Some patients may have a tendency to believe that a double dose promotes a quicker drug response.

The nurse teaches the patient the proper techniques of drug administration for home care, i.e., eye drops or ointment, ear instillation, nose drops, or sprays, inhalation, sublingual, topical, transdermal, subcutaneous, vaginal, or rectal. If possible, instruct more than one person, such as a spouse, parent, or friend. Including the family or caregiver during patient education aids in the reinforcement and retention of the information, and ultimately the patient's compliance with the drug therapy regimen.

SIDE EFFECTS AND ADVERSE REACTIONS

The patient should report any unusual symptoms while taking medications. The nurse may instruct the patient of expected side effects. For example, a drug may change urine to a reddish, brown color, or feces may turn yellowish. In some cases, an unusual taste sensation may occur, or sun-protective clothing and sunscreens may be required to protect against a photosensitivity reaction. If postural hypotension occurs frequently with a certain drug, the patient should be advised to rise slowly from a sitting to a standing position. Many drugs produce a transient drowsiness, fatigue, or a hypotensive effect, especially during early therapy. Advise the patient to avoid tasks that require alertness or motor skills until a response to the drug is established. Be specific when informing the patient whether the medication should be taken with food or on an empty stomach. If applicable, inform the patient *before* an IM or IV medication is given if burning or stinging is an expected result of administration. For example, phenytoin, which is given for anticonvulsant therapy, causes a chemical irritation of the vein and produces an intense burning when given IV push. If the vein is not flushed with sterile saline after the IV injection, the patient continues to feel the pain far longer than is necessary. The drug entries in this handbook list side effects according to frequency, which the nurse will find helpful while teaching patients what to expect during drug therapy.

LIFE-SPAN CONSIDERATIONS DURING DRUG THERAPY

PREGNANCY AND LACTATION

Women of childbearing years should be asked about the possibility of pregnancy before any drug therapy is initiated. Advise a woman who is either planning a pregnancy or believes she may be pregnant to inform her physician immediately. During pregnancy, medications given to the mother pass to the fetus via the placenta. Teratogenic (fetal abnormalities) effects may occur. Breast-feeding while the mother is taking certain medications may not be recommended due to the potential for adverse effects on the newborn. The choice of drug ordered for the pregnant woman by the physician is based on the stage of pregnancy, since the organs of the fetus are developed during the first trimester. Cautious use of drugs in women of reproductive age who are sexually active and who are not using contraceptives is essential to prevent the potential for teratogenic or embryotoxic effects.

The drug entries in this handbook include dosages, where appropriate, for pregnant women and precautions during pregnancy and lactation. Appendix E describes the different pregnancy categories.

CHILDREN

In pediatric drug therapy, drug administration is guided by the child's age, weight, level of growth and development, and height. The dosage ordered is depicted in the amount of the drug to be given by either the kilogram of body weight or the square meter of body surface area, which is based on height and weight. Calculations based on body surface area are considered more accurate than those based on age or weight. Many dosages based on these calculations must be individualized based on pediatric response. The drug entries in this handbook provide dosages for children in different age ranges.

If oral route of administration is used, syrup or chewable tablets are given. Sometimes medicine can be added to liquids or mixed in foods. Never force a child to take oral medications because choking or emotional trauma may ensue. If IM injection is ordered, the vastus lateralis muscle in the mid-lateral thigh is used, since the gluteus maximus is not developed until walking occurs and the deltoid muscle is too small. Administer IV injections very slowly in children. An IV push that is administered too rapidly may produce high serum drug levels with a potential for toxicity. Never refer to medicine as candy in front of children.

ELDERLY

Adverse drug reactions are more likely to occur in this population owing to physiologic changes (aging or disease) and cognitive changes (short-term memory loss or alteration in thought processing) that may lead to multiple drug dosing. In chronic disease states such as hypertension, glaucoma, asthma, or arthritis, the daily taking of multiple drugs increases the incidence of adverse reaction and toxic effects. Decreased liver or renal function impairment may also lead to lower metabolism of drugs in the liver and reduced excretion of medications, thus prolonging the half-life of drugs. To reduce the potential for toxicity, the dosage should initially be smaller than for the general adult population, and then slowly increased or decreased, based on patient response and the therapeutic effect of the drug. The drug entries in this handbook include dosages for elderly patients.

CONCLUSION

As we enter the new millennium, excellent drug therapy treatment by the nurse should be given to the patient. This nursing goal is based on knowledge of drugs, anticipation of patient needs, and continued education of new drugs approved for market use. The nurse's role in drug therapy becomes an even more essential part of attaining the goal of quality medical care.

abacavir

(Ziagen)
See Supplement
*See Classification section under:
Human immunodeficiency virus
(HIV) infection*

abciximab

ab-**six**-ih-mab
(ReoPro, c7E3 Fab)
CANADIAN AVAILABILITY:
ReoPro

CLASSIFICATION

Antiplatelet; antithrombotic

AVAILABILITY (Rx)

Injection: 2 mg per ml (single-use vial)

PHARMACOKINETICS

Clears rapidly from plasma. Following IV bolus administration, half-life decreases <10 min, second phase of half-life within 30 min. Platelet function recovers after 48 hrs. At end of infusion, bleeding time returns to <12 min within 12 hrs in 75% of pts, within 24 hrs in 90% of pts.

ACTION/*THERAPEUTIC EFFECT*

Produces rapid inhibition of platelet aggregation by preventing the binding on fibrinogen to receptor sites on platelets. *Prevents closure of treated coronary arteries. Prevents acute cardiac ischemic complications.*

USES

Adjunct therapy to prevent cardiac ischemic complications in pts undergoing percutaneous coronary intervention (PCI) and those with unstable angina not responding to conventional medical therapy when PCI is planned within 24 hrs.

STORAGE/HANDLING

Store vials in refrigerator. Do not shake. Discard any unused portion left in vial.

IV ADMINISTRATION

1. Give in separate IV line; do not add any other medication to infusion.
2. Discard any abciximab preparation containing *any* opaque particles.
3. Use care when attempting vascular access so only the anterior wall of femoral artery is punctured.
4. For bolus injection and continuous infusion, use sterile, non-pyrogenic, low protein-binding 0.2 or 0.22 micron filter.
5. While vascular sheath is in position, maintain pt on complete bed rest w/head of bed elevated at 30°.
6. Maintain affected limb in straight position.
7. Following sheath removal, apply femoral pressure for 30 min, either manually or mechanically, then apply pressure dressing.

INDICATIONS/DOSAGE/ROUTES

PCI:
IV Bolus: Adults: 0.25 mg/kg given 10–60 min before the PCI, then 12 hr IV infusion of 0.125 mcg/kg/min. **Maximum:** 10 mcg/min.

PCI (unstable angina):
IV Bolus: Adults: 0.25 mg/kg, followed by 18–24 hr infusion of 10 mcg/min, concluding 1 hr after procedure.

PRECAUTIONS

CONTRAINDICATIONS: Active internal bleeding, recent (within 6 wks) GI or GU bleeding, history of CVA <2 yrs or CVA w/residual neurologic defect, oral anticoagulants <7 days unless prothrombin time <1.2 × control, thrombocytopenia (<100,000 cells/mcl), recent surgery or trauma (within 6 wks), intracranial neoplasm, arteriovenous malformation or aneurysm, severe uncontrolled hypertension, history of vasculitis, prior IV dextran use before or during PTCA. **CAUTIONS:** Pts who weigh <75 kg, those >65 yrs, those with history of GI disease, those receiving thrombolytics, heparin, aspirin, PTCA <12 hrs of onset of symptoms for acute MI, prolonged PTCA (>70 min), failed PTCA. **PREGNANCY/ LACTATION:** Unknown if drug causes fetal harm or can affect reproduction capacity. Unknown if distributed in breast milk. **Pregnancy Category C**.

INTERACTIONS

DRUG INTERACTIONS: Anticoagulants, heparin may increase risk of hemorrhage. Platelet aggregation inhibitors (e.g., aspirin, dextran, thrombolytic agents) may increase risk of bleeding. **ALTERED LAB VALUES:** Increases clotting time (ACT), prothrombin time (PT), activated partial thromboplastin time (APTT), platelet count.

SIDE EFFECTS

FREQUENT: Hypotension, nausea. **OCCASIONAL:** Vomiting, bradycardia, pain in extremities. **RARE:** Abnormal thinking, pain, peripheral edema, UTI, abnormal vision, dizziness.

ADVERSE REACTIONS/TOXIC EFFECTS

Anticipate a hypersensitivity reaction when medication is given. If symptoms occur, stop infusion immediately. An increase in both major (intracranial hemorrhage, decrease in hemoglobin >5 g/dl) and minor bleeding (spontaneous hematuria, hgb decrease of >4 g/dl).

NURSING IMPLICATIONS
BASELINE ASSESSMENT:

Heparin should be discontinued 4 hrs prior to arterial sheath removal. Maintain pt on bed rest for 6–8 hrs following sheath removal or drug discontinuation, whichever is later. Check platelet count, PT, APTT before med infusion (assess for preexisting blood abnormalities), 2–4 hrs after treatment, and at 24 hrs or before discharge, whichever is first. Check insertion site, distal pulse of affected limb while femoral artery sheath is in place, and then routinely for 6 hrs after femoral artery sheath removal. Minimize need for numerous injection sites, blood drawings, intubations, catheters.

INTERVENTION/EVALUATION:

Stop abciximab and/or heparin infusion if any serious bleeding occurs that is uncontrolled by pressure. Assess skin for bruises, petechiae, particularly femoral arterial access, also catheter insertion, arterial and venous puncture, cutdown, needle site, gastrointestinal sites. Assess clinical response, vital signs (pulse, temperature, respiratory rate, B/P) q4h or per protocol. Handle pt carefully and as infrequently as possible to prevent bleeding. Do not obtain B/P in lower extremities (possible deep vein thrombi). Check stool for occult blood. Assess for decrease in B/P, increase in pulse rate, complaint of abdominal/back pain, severe headache, evidence of hemorrhage, ACT, PT, APTT, platelet count. Question for increase in discharge during menses. Assess urine output for hematuria. Monitor for any occurring hematoma. Use care in removing any dressings.

---

acarbose

ah-**car**-bose
(Precose)

CANADIAN AVAILABILITY:
Prandase

CLASSIFICATION

Antidiabetic: Oral

AVAILABILITY (Rx)

Tablets: 25 mg, 50 mg, 100 mg

PHARMACOKINETICS

	ONSET	PEAK	DURATION
PO	—	1 hr	12–24 hrs

Absorption not necessary for therapeutic effect. Metabolized by intestinal digestive enzymes/microorganisms. Elimination occurs through renal and fecal route. Half-life: 2.7–9 hrs (increased in impaired renal function).

ACTION/*THERAPEUTIC EFFECT*

Delays glucose absorption and digestion of carbohydrates, *resulting in smaller rise in blood glucose concentration after meals, lowering postprandial hyperglycemia.* Does not enhance insulin secretion.

USES

Use as monotherapy or in combination with a sulfonylurea, insulin, or metformin to lower blood glucose in pts with type II diabetes mellitus when diet plus either acarbose or sulfonylurea do not give adequate control.

PO ADMINISTRATION

Give with the first bite of each main meal.

INDICATIONS/DOSAGE/ROUTES

Diabetes mellitus:

PO: Adults, elderly: Initially, 25 mg ($1/2$ a 50 mg tablet) 3 times/day at the start (w/first bite) of each main meal. **Range:** 50–100 mg 3 times/day. **Maximum: <60 kg:** 50 mg 3 times/day; **>60 kg:** 100 mg 3 times/day.

PRECAUTIONS

CONTRAINDICATIONS: Significant renal dysfunction (serum creatinine >2mg/dl), hypersensitivity to drug, diabetic ketoacidosis or cirrhosis, inflammatory bowel disease, colonic ulceration, partial intestinal obstruction or predisposition to intestinal obstruction, chronic intestinal diseases associated w/marked disorders of digestion or absorption, conditions that may deteriorate as result of increased gas formation in the intestine. **CAUTIONS:** Elderly, malnourished, or debilitated, those w/renal or hepatic dysfunction, cardiac disease. Increased risk for hypoglycemia when given in combination w/insulin. **PREGNANCY/ LACTATION:** Insulin is drug of choice during pregnancy. Unknown if drug crosses placenta or is distributed in breast milk. **Pregnancy Category B.**

INTERACTIONS

DRUG INTERACTIONS: Digestive enzymes, intestinal absorbents (e.g., charcoal) reduce acarbose effect. Do not use concurrently. Sulfonylureas may produce hypoglycemia. Diuretics, corticosteroids, phenytoin, sympathomimetics, phenothiazines, nicotinic acid, thyroid hormones, estrogens, oral contraceptives, calcium channel blockers, isoniazid may produce hyperglycemia. **ALTERED LAB VALUES:** May increase serum transaminase levels and slightly reduce hematocrit.

SIDE EFFECTS

FREQUENT: Transient GI disturbances: Flatulence (77%), diarrhea (33%), abdominal pain (21%). Symptoms tend to diminish in frequency and intensity over time.

ADVERSE REACTIONS/TOXIC EFFECTS

None significant.

NURSING IMPLICATIONS

BASELINE ASSESSMENT:

Question for hypersensitivity to acarbose. Check blood glucose level. Discuss lifestyle to determine extent of learning, emotional needs. Assure follow-up instruction if pt/family do not thoroughly understand diabetes management or glucose-testing technique.

INTERVENTION/EVALUATION:

Monitor blood glucose and food intake. Monitor liver function, glycosylated hemoglobin. Assess for hypoglycemia (cool wet skin, tremors, dizziness, anxiety, headache, tachycardia, numbness in mouth, hunger, diplopia) or hyperglycemia (polyuria, polyphagia, polydipsia, nausea, vomiting, dim vision, fatigue, deep rapid breathing). Check for adverse skin reactions, jaundice. Monitor hematology reports. Assess for bleeding or bruising. Be alert to conditions that alter glucose requirements: fever, increased activity or stress, surgical procedure.

PATIENT/FAMILY TEACHING:

Carry oral glucose (dextrose) instead of cane sugar (sucrose) for immediate response to hypoglycemic episode. Prescribed diet is principal part of treatment; do not skip or delay meals. Diabetes mellitus requires lifelong control. Check blood glucose/urine as ordered. Serum transaminase levels should be checked q3 months during first year of treatment and periodically thereafter. Wear medical alert identification. Check w/physician when glucose demands are altered (e.g., fever, infection, trauma, stress, heavy physical activity). Avoid alcoholic beverages. Do not take other medication w/o consulting physician. Weight control, exercise, hygiene (including foot care), and nonsmoking are an essential part of therapy. Protect skin, limit sun exposure. Avoid exposure to infections. Select clothing, positions that do not restrict blood flow. Notify physician promptly of skin eruptions, itching, bleeding, yellow skin, dark urine. Inform dentist, physician, or surgeon of this medication before any treatment.

---

acebutolol

ah-see-**beaut**-oh-lol
(Sectral)

CANADIAN AVAILABILITY:
Monitan, Sectral

CLASSIFICATION

Beta$_1$-adrenergic blocker

AVAILABILITY (Rx)

Capsules: 200 mg, 400 mg

PHARMACOKINETICS

	ONSET	PEAK	DURATION
PO (hypotensive)	1–1.5 hrs	2–8 hrs	24 hrs
PO (antiarrhythmic)	1 hr	4–6 hrs	10 hrs

Well absorbed from GI tract. Undergoes extensive first-pass

liver metabolism to active metabolite. Eliminated via bile, secreted into GI tract via intestine, excreted in urine. Removed by hemodialysis. Half-life: 3–4 hrs; metabolite: 8–13 hrs.

ACTION / *THERAPEUTIC EFFECT*

Predominantly blocks beta$_1$-adrenergic receptors in cardiac tissue, *slowing sinus heart rate, decreasing cardiac output, decreasing B/P*. Large doses may block beta$_2$ receptors, *increasing airway resistance*. Exhibits antiarrhythmic activity, slows AV conduction, reduces rate of spontaneous firing of sinus pacemaker.

USES / *UNLABELED*

Management of mild to moderate hypertension. Used alone or in combination w/diuretics, especially thiazide type. Management of cardiac arrhythmias (primarily PVCs). *Treatment of chronic angina, pectoris, hypertrophic cardiomyopathy, myocardial infarction, pheochromocytoma, tremors, anxiety, thyrotoxicosis, syndrome of mitral valve prolapse.*

PO ADMINISTRATION

May be given w/o regard to meals.

INDICATIONS / DOSAGE / ROUTES

Mild to moderate hypertension:
PO: Adults: Initially, 400 mg/day in 1–2 divided doses. **Maintenance:** 200–800 mg/day.

Severe hypertension:
PO: Adults: Up to 1,200 mg/day in 2 divided doses.

Ventricular arrhythmias:
PO: Adults: Initially, 200 mg q12h. Increase gradually up to 600–1,200 mg/day in 2 divided doses.

Usual elderly dosage:
PO: Initially, 200–400 mg/day.
Maximum: 800 mg/day.

Dosage in renal impairment:

CREATININE CLEARANCE	% OF NORMAL DOSAGE
<50 ml/min	50
<25 ml/min	25

PRECAUTIONS

CONTRAINDICATIONS: Overt cardiac failure, cardiogenic shock, heart block greater than first degree, severe bradycardia. **CAUTIONS:** Impaired renal or hepatic function, peripheral vascular disease, hyperthyroidism, diabetes, inadequate cardiac function, bronchospastic disease. **PREGNANCY/LACTATION:** Readily crosses placenta; distributed in breast milk. May produce bradycardia, apnea, hypoglycemia, hypothermia during delivery, small birth weight infants. **Pregnancy Category B**.

INTERACTIONS

DRUG INTERACTIONS: Diuretics, other hypotensives may increase hypotensive effect; sympathomimetics, xanthines may mutually inhibit effects; may mask symptoms of hypoglycemia, prolong hypoglycemic effect of insulin, oral hypoglycemics; NSAIDs may decrease antihypertensive effect; Cimetidine may increase concentration. **ALTERED LAB VALUES:** May increase ANA titer, SGOT (AST), SGPT (ALT), alkaline phosphatase, LDH, bilirubin, BUN, creatinine, K, uric acid, lipoproteins, triglycerides.

SIDE EFFECTS

Generally well tolerated, w/mild and transient effects. **FREQUENT:** Hypotension manifested as dizziness, nausea, diaphoresis, headache, cold extremities, fatigue, constipation/diarrhea. **OCCASIONAL:** Insomnia, flatulence, urinary frequency, impotence or decreased libido. **RARE:** Rash, arthralgia, myalgia, confusion (esp. elderly), change in taste.

ADVERSE REACTIONS/TOXIC EFFECTS

Overdosage may produce profound bradycardia, hypotension. Abrupt withdrawal may result in sweating, palpitations, headache, tremulousness. May precipitate CHF, MI in pts w/cardiac disease, thyroid storm in those w/thyrotoxicosis, peripheral ischemia in those w/existing peripheral vascular disease. Hypoglycemia may occur in previously controlled diabetics. Thrombocytopenia (unusual bruising, bleeding) occurs rarely.

NURSING IMPLICATIONS
BASELINE ASSESSMENT:

Assess baseline renal/liver function tests. Assess B/P, apical pulse immediately before drug is administered. (If pulse is 60/min or below, or systolic B/P is below 90 mm Hg, withhold medication, contact physician.)

INTERVENTION/EVALUATION:

Monitor B/P for hypotension, respiration for shortness of breath. Assess pulse for strength/weakness, irregular rate, bradycardia. Monitor EKG for cardiac arrhythmias, particularly shortening of QT interval, prolongation of PR interval. Assess frequency and consistency of stools. Assist w/ambulation if dizziness occurs. Assess for evidence of CHF: dyspnea (particularly on exertion or lying down), night cough, peripheral edema, distended neck veins, decreased urine output, weight gain. Monitor I&O, daily weight. Assess for nausea, diaphoresis, headache, fatigue.

PATIENT/FAMILY TEACHING:

Do not abruptly discontinue medication. Compliance w/therapy regimen is essential to control hypertension, arrhythmias. To avoid hypotensive effect, rise slowly from lying to sitting position; wait momentarily before standing. Avoid tasks that require alertness, motor skills until response to drug is established. Report shortness of breath, excessive fatigue, weight gain, prolonged dizziness or headache. Do not use nasal decongestants, over-the-counter cold preparations (stimulants) w/o physician approval. Take B/P, pulse before taking medication. (Instruct on proper technique, when to contact physician.) Avoid smoking; follow physician's instructions for weight loss, exercise. Restrict salt, alcohol intake.

acetaminophen
ah-see-tah-**min**-oh-fen
(Datril, Tempra, Tylenol)

FIXED-COMBINATION(S):

W/butabarbital, a sedative-hypnotic; w/ caffeine, a stimulant (**Fioricet**); codeine, a narcotic analgesic (**Tylenol w/codeine**); w/hydrocodone, a narcotic analgesic (**Vicodin, Zydone**); w/oxycodone, a narcotic analgesic (**Percocet, Tylox**); w/propoxyphene, an analgesic (**Darvocet**).

CANADIAN AVAILABILITY:
Abenol, Apo-Acetaminophen, Atasol, Tempra, Tylenol

CLASSIFICATION

Nonnarcotic analgesic, antipyretic

AVAILABILITY (OTC)

Capsules: 500 mg. **Elixir:** 120 mg/5 ml, 160 mg/5 ml, 325 mg/5 ml. **Liquid:** 160 mg/5 ml. **Solution:** 100 mg/ml, 120 mg/2.5 ml. **Suppository:** 120 mg, 325 mg, 650 mg. **Tablets (chewable):** 80 mg. **Tablets:** 160 mg, 325 mg, 500 mg, 650 mg.

PHARMACOKINETICS

	ONSET	PEAK	DURATION
PO	15–30 min	1–1.5 hrs	4–6 hrs

Rapid, completely absorbed from GI tract; rectal absorption variable. Widely distributed to most body tissues. Metabolized in liver; excreted in urine. Half-life: 1–4 hrs (increased in hepatic disease, elderly, neonates; decreased in children).

ACTION/ *THERAPEUTIC EFFECT*

Exact mechanism unknown, but appears to inhibit prostaglandin synthesis in CNS and, to a lesser extent, by blocking pain impulse through peripheral action, *resulting in analgesia.* Acts centrally on hypothalamic heat-regulating center, producing peripheral vasodilation (skin erythema, sweating, heat loss), *resulting in antipyresis.*

USES

Relief of mild to moderate pain, fever.

PO/RECTAL ADMINISTRATION

PO:

1. Give w/o regard to meals.
2. Tablets may be crushed.

RECTAL:

Moisten suppository w/cold water before inserting well up into rectum.

INDICATIONS/DOSAGE/ROUTES

Analgesia, antipyresis:
Note: Children may repeat doses 4–5 times/day; maximum of 5 doses/24 hrs.

PO: Adults, elderly: 325–650 mg q4–6h. **Maximum:** 4 g/day. **Children (11 yrs):** 480 mg/dose; **(9–10 yrs):** 400 mg/dose; **(6–8 yrs):** 320 mg/dose; **(4–5 yrs):** 240 mg/dose; **(2–3 yrs):** 160 mg/dose; **(1–2 yrs):** 120 mg/dose; **(4–11 months):** 80 mg/dose; **(0–3 months):** 40 mg/dose.

Rectal: Adults: 650 mg q4–6h. **Maximum:** 6 doses/24 hrs. **Children (6–12 yrs):** 325 mg q4–6h. **Maximum:** 2.6 g/24 hrs. **Children (3–6 yrs):** 120 mg q4–6h. **Maximum:** 720 mg/24 hrs. **Children (<3 months):** Consult physician.

PRECAUTIONS

CONTRAINDICATIONS: Hypersensitivity to acetaminophen. **CAUTIONS:** Impaired hepatic function, anemia. **PREGNANCY/LACTATION:** Crosses placenta; distributed in breast milk. Routinely used in all stages of pregnancy, appears safe for short-term use. **Pregnancy Category B.**

INTERACTIONS

DRUG INTERACTIONS: Alcohol (chronic use), liver enzymes inducers (e.g., cimetidine), hepatotoxic medications (e.g., phenytoin) may increase risk of hepatotoxicity w/prolonged high dose or single toxic dose. May increase risk of bleeding w/warfarin w/regular use. **ALTERED LAB VALUES:** May increase SGOT (AST), SGPT (ALT), bilirubin, prothrombin levels (may indicate hepatotoxicity).

SIDE EFFECTS

Well tolerated. **RARE:** Hypersensitivity reaction.

ADVERSE REACTIONS/TOXIC EFFECTS

Early signs of acetaminophen toxicity: anorexia, nausea, diaphoresis, generalized weakness within first 12–24 hrs. Later signs of toxicity: vomiting, right upper quadrant tenderness, elevated liver function tests within 48 to 72 hrs after ingestion. *Antidote:* Acetylcysteine.

NURSING IMPLICATIONS
BASELINE ASSESSMENT:

Question for sensitivity to acetaminophen. Assess onset, type, location, and duration of pain. Effect of medication is reduced if full pain recurs before next dose. *Fixed combination:* Obtain vital signs before giving medication. If respirations are 12/min or lower (20/min or lower in children), withhold medication, contact physician.

INTERVENTION/EVALUATION:

Assess for clinical improvement and relief of pain, fever.

PATIENT/FAMILY TEACHING:

Do not exceed dosage. Consult physician for use in children <3 yrs, oral use >5 days (children), >10 days (adults), or fever >3 day duration. Severe/recurrent pain or high/continuous fever may indicate serious illness. *Fixed-combination:* Avoid tasks that require alertness, motor skills until response to drug is estab-lished. **Tolerance/dependence may occur w/prolonged use.**

---

acetazolamide

ah-seat-ah-**zole**-ah-myd
(Dazamide, Diamox, AK-Zol)

acetazolamide sodium

(Diamox) [injection]

CANADIAN AVAILABILITY:
Apo-Acetazolamide, Diamox

CLASSIFICATION

Carbonic anhydrase inhibitor

AVAILABILITY (Rx)

Capsules (sustained release): 500 mg. **Tablets:** 125 mg, 250 mg. **Powder for Injection:** 500 mg.

PHARMACOKINETICS

	ONSET	PEAK	DURATION
PO			
(tablets)			
	60–90 min	2–4 hrs	8–12 hrs
(capsules)			
	2 hrs	8–18 hrs	18–24 hrs
IV	2 min	15 min	4–5 hrs

Well absorbed from GI tract. Primarily excreted unchanged in urine. Half-life: 10–15 hrs.

ACTION/ *THERAPEUTIC EFFECT*

Reduces formation of hydrogen and bicarbonate ions from carbon dioxide and water by inhibiting, in proximal renal tubule, the enzyme carbonic anhydrase, thereby promoting renal excretion of sodium, potassium, bicarbonate, water. **Ocular:** Reduces rate of aqueous humor formation, *lowers intraocular pressure.* **Diamox only:** Exact mechanism unknown, but may increase CO_2 tension, *producing anticonvulsant activity by retarding neuronal conduction.*

USES/*UNLABELED*

Treatment of open-angle, secondary or angle closure glaucoma, adjunct in managing absence seizures (e.g., petit mal), tonic-clonic, simple partial and myoclonic seizures. *Lowers intraocular pressure in treatment of malignant glaucoma, treatment of toxicity of weakly acidic medications, prevents uric acid/cystine renal calculi by alkalinizing the urine.*

STORAGE/HANDLING

Store tablets, capsules, parenteral form at room temperature. Syrup suspension mixed w/acetazolamide is stable for 1 week at room temperature. After reconstitution, IV solution is stable for 24 hrs.

PO/IV ADMINISTRATION

PO:

1. When oral liquid is needed, tablet may be crushed and mixed w/5 ml cherry, chocolate, raspberry, or other highly flavored carbohydrate syrup. Each tablet may be softened in 2 tsp hot water, then added to 2 tsp honey or syrup (mix just prior to administration). Drug will not dissolve in fruit juice.

2. Scored tablets may be crushed; do not crush or break extended-release capsules.

3. May give w/food if GI upset occurs.

IV:

Note: IM injection painful due to alkaline pH. IV preferred.

Reconstitute 500 mg vial w/5 ml sterile water for injection to provide solution containing 100 mg/ml.

INDICATIONS/DOSAGE/ROUTES

Glaucoma:
PO: Adults: 250 mg 1–4 times/day. **Extended-Release:** 500 mg 1–2 times/day usually given in morning and evening.

Secondary glaucoma, preop treatment of acute congestive glaucoma:
PO/IV: Adults: 250 mg q4h, 250 mg q12h; or 500 mg, then 125–250 mg q4h. **PO: Children:** 10–15 mg/kg/day in divided doses. **IV: Children:** 5–10 mg/kg q6h.

Epilepsy:
PO: Adults, children: 375–1,000 mg/day in 1–4 divided doses.

Acute mountain sickness:
PO: Adults: 500–1,000 mg/day in divided doses. If possible, begin 24–48 hrs before ascent, continue at least 48 hrs at high altitude.

Usual elderly dosage:
PO: Initially, 250 mg 2 times/day; use lowest effective dose.

PRECAUTIONS

CONTRAINDICATIONS: Hypersensitivity to sulfonamides, severe renal disease, adrenal insufficiency, hypochloremic acidosis. **CAUTIONS:** History of hypercalcemia, diabetes mellitus, gout, digitalized patients, obstructive pulmonary disease. **PREGNANCY/LACTATION:** Drug crosses placenta, unknown if distributed in breast milk. May produce skeletal anomalies, embryocidal effects at high doses. **Pregnancy Category C.**

INTERACTIONS

DRUG INTERACTIONS: May increase digoxin toxicity (due to hypokalemia). May increase effects/toxicity of amphetamines; may decrease effects of methenamine. **ALTERED LAB VALUES:** May increase ammonia, bilirubin, glucose, chloride, uric acid, calcium; may decrease bicarbonate, potassium.

SIDE EFFECTS

FREQUENT: Unusually tired/weak, diarrhea, increased urination/frequency, decreased appetite/weight, altered taste (metallic), nausea, vomiting, numbness in extremities, lips, mouth. **OCCASIONAL:** Depression, drowsiness. **RARE:** Headache, photosensitivity, confusion, tinnitus, severe muscle weakness, loss of taste.

ADVERSE REACTION/TOXIC EFFECTS

Long-term therapy may result in acidotic state. Nephrotoxicity/hepatotoxicity occurs occasionally, manifested as dark urine/stools, pain in lower back, jaundice, dysuria, crystalluria, renal colic/calculi. Bone marrow depression may be manifested as aplastic anemia, thrombocytopenia, thrombocytopenic purpura, leukopenia, agranulocytosis, hemolytic anemia.

NURSING IMPLICATIONS

BASELINE ASSESSMENT:

Glaucoma: **Assess peripheral vision, acuity. Assess affected pupil for dilation, response to light.** *Epilepsy:* **Take history of seizure disorders (length, intensity, duration of seizures, presence of auras, LOC).**

INTERVENTION/EVALUATION:

Monitor I&O, BUN, electrolytes (particularly serum potassium). Monitor pattern of daily bowel activity and stool consistency. **Observe for signs of infection (fever, sore throat, unusual bleeding/bruising, fatigue) due to bone marrow depression. Monitor for acidosis (headache, lethargy progressing to drowsiness, CNS depression, Kussmaul's respiration).**

PATIENT/FAMILY TEACHING:

Report presence of tingling or tremor in hands or feet, unusual bleeding/bruising, unexplained fever, sore throat, flank pain. Avoid tasks that require alertness, motor skills until response to drug is established.

---

acetohexamide
(Dymelor)
See Classification section under: Antidiabetic

---

acetylcysteine (*N*-acetylcysteine)

ah-sea-tyl-**sis**-teen
(Mucomyst, Mucosil)

CANADIAN AVAILABILITY:
Mucomyst, Parvolex

CLASSIFICATION

Antidote, mucolytic

AVAILABILITY (Rx)

Solution: 10%, 20%

PHARMACOKINETICS

	ONSET	PEAK	DURATION
Inhalant	1 min	5 min	—

After oral inhalation/intratracheal instillation, most of drug involved in sulfhydryl-disulfide reaction. Remainder absorbed from pulmonary epithelium. After oral administration, readily absorbed from GI tract. Metabolized in liver.

ACTION/*THERAPEUTIC EFFECT*

Splits linkage of mucoproteins, *reducing viscosity of pulmonary secretions, facilitates removal by coughing, postural drainage, mechanical means. Maintains/ restores hepatic concentration of glutathione* (necessary for inactivation of hepatotoxic acetaminophen toxicity).

USES

Adjunctive treatment for abnormally viscid mucous secretions present in acute and chronic bronchopulmonary disease and pulmonary complication of cystic fibrosis, tracheostomy care; treatment of acetaminophen overdose.

STORAGE/HANDLING

A light purple color may occur in opened bottle (does not impair safety or effectiveness of medication). After exposure to air, refrigerate solution and use within 96 hrs.

PO/NEBULIZATION ADMINISTRATION

Note: A slight, disagreeable odor from solution may be noticed during initial administration but disappears quickly.

NEBULIZATION:

1. 20% solution may be diluted w/0.9% NaCl or sterile water for injection; 10% solution may be used undiluted.

2. Avoid contact w/iron, copper, rubber (reacts w/acetylcysteine).

3. Use parts made of glass, plastic, aluminum, chromed metal, sterling silver, or stainless steel.

ORAL SOLUTION:

1. Give as 5% solution; dilute 1:3 w/cola, soft drink, or juice.

2. Prepare fresh; use within 1 hr.

3. May give via duodenal tube.

INDICATIONS/DOSAGE/ROUTES

Note: Use 20% solution for oral inhalation or intratracheal instillation.

Bronchopulmonary, tracheostomy: **Nebulization: Adults, elderly: (20% solution):** 3–5 ml 3–4 times daily. **Range:** 1–10 ml q2–6h. **Adults, elderly: (10% solution):** 6–10 ml 3–4 times daily. **Range:** 2–20 ml q2–6hr. **Intratracheal Instillation: Adults:** 1–2 ml of 10–20% solution instilled into tracheostomy q1–4h.

Acetaminophen overdose: **Oral Solution (5%): Adults, elderly:** Loading dose of 140 mg/kg, followed in 4 hrs by maintenance dose of 70 mg/kg q4h for 17 additional doses (unless acetaminophen assay reveals nontoxic level).

PRECAUTIONS

CONTRAINDICATIONS: None significant. **CAUTIONS:** Bronchial asthma, elderly, debilitated w/severe respiratory insufficiency. **PREGNANCY/LACTATION:** Unknown if drug crosses placenta or is distributed in breast milk. **Pregnancy Category B.**

INTERACTIONS

DRUG INTERACTIONS: None significant. **ALTERED LAB VALUES:** None significant.

SIDE EFFECTS

FREQUENT: *Inhalation:* Stickiness on face, transient unpleasant odor. **OCCASIONAL:** *Inhalation:* Increased bronchial secretions, irritated throat, nausea, vomiting, rhinorrhea. **RARE:** *Inhalation:* Skin rash. *Oral:* Facial edema, bronchospasm, wheezing.

ADVERSE REACTION/TOXIC EFFECTS

Large dosage may produce severe nausea, vomiting.

NURSING IMPLICATIONS

BASELINE ASSESSMENT:

Mucolytic: Assess pretreatment respirations for rate, depth, rhythm. Place tissue within easy reach of patient. *Antidote:* Assess acetaminophen plasma level. Determine baselines for AST, ALT, bilirubin, PT, creatinine, BUN, blood sugar, and electrolytes. Assure that the stomach is empty by lavaging or inducing emesis. If activated charcoal has been administered, lavage before administering acetylcysteine.

INTERVENTION/EVALUATION:

Mucolytic: Have suction equipment available in case pt cannot clear airway. If bronchospasm occurs, treatment should be discontinued and physician notified; bronchodilator may be added to therapy. Monitor rate, depth, rhythm, type of respiration (abdominal, thoracic). Assess for evidence of stomatitis (erythema of mucous membranes, dry mouth, burning of oral mucosa). Check sputum for color, consistency, amount. Assess lung sounds for rhonchi, wheezing, rales. *Antidote:* Continue to monitor lab test results (see Baseline Assessment)

daily. Monitor I&O. Assess pt for vomiting (potential is increased due to vomiting from acetaminophen). Treat hypoglycemia as necessary. Avoid diuretics. Vitamin K_1 may be administered if prothombin time ratio exceeds 1.5, fresh frozen plasma if ratio exceeds 3. Monitor vital signs.

PATIENT/FAMILY TEACHING:

Mucolytic: A slight, disagreeable odor from solution may be noticed during initial administration but disappears quickly. Explain importance of adequate hydration. Teach proper coughing and deep breathing. *Antidote:* Explain purpose of therapy. Report any bleeding at once.

---

acitretin

(Soriatane)
See Supplement

---

acyclovir

aye-**sigh**-klo-veer
(Zovirax)

CANADIAN AVAILABILITY:
Avirax, Zovirax

CLASSIFICATION

Antiviral

AVAILABILITY (Rx)

Tablets: 400 mg, 800 mg. **Capsules:** 200 mg. **Oral Suspension:** 200 mg/5 ml. **Powder for Injection:** 500 mg, 1,000 mg. **Ointment.**

PHARMACOKINETICS

Poorly absorbed from GI tract; minimal absorption following topical application. Widely distributed. Partially metabolized by cellular enzymes. Excreted primarily in urine. Removed by hemodialysis. Half-life: 2.5 hrs (increased in impaired renal function).

ACTION/THERAPEUTIC EFFECT

Converted to acyclovir triphosphate, becoming part of DNA chain, *interfering w/DNA synthesis and viral replication.* Virustatic.

USES

Parenteral: Initial treatment for severe herpes genitalis; herpes zoster ophthalmicus; initial/recurrent mucocutaneous herpes simplex; neonatal herpes simplex; herpes simplex encephalitis; herpes zoster caused by varicella zoster virus (VZV) in immunocompromised pts and disseminated herpes zoster in nonimmunocompromised pts. *Oral:* Initial treatment, management of recurrent and prophylaxis of frequently recurrent herpes genitalis; treatment of herpes zoster (shingles); herpes zoster ophthalmicus; varicella infections (chickenpox) in nonimmunocompromised pts. *Topical:* Initial episodes of genital herpes, immunocompromised pts w/limited nonthreatening herpes simplex infections.

STORAGE/HANDLING

Store capsules at room temperature. Solutions of 50 mg/ml stable for 12 hrs at room temperature; may form precipitate when refrigerated. Potency not affected by precipitate and redissolution. IV infusion (piggyback) stable for 24 hrs at room temperature. Yellow discoloration does not affect potency.

PO/IV ADMINISTRATION

PO:

1. Give w/o regard to food.

2. Do not crush or break capsules.

IV:

Note: Do not administer by IM, SubQ, or rapid IV infusion or rapid IV injection.

1. Infuse for at least 1 hr.
2. Maintain adequate hydration, especially during urine concentration that occurs 2 hrs following IV administration.
3. Alternating IV sites, use large veins to reduce risk of phlebitis.

INDICATIONS/DOSAGE/ROUTES

Initial genital herpes infections, intermittent treatment of recurrent episodes:
PO: **Adults, elderly:** 200 mg q4h while awake (5 times/day).

Prophylaxis of recurrent episodes:
PO: **Adults, elderly:** 400 mg 2 times/day up to 12 months.

Chickenpox:
PO: **Adults, elderly, children (2–12 yrs):** 20 mg/kg (maximum 800 mg) 4 times/day for 5 days.

Mucosal or cutaneous herpes simplex, severe genital herpes:
IV: **Adults, elderly:** 5 mg/kg q8h. **Children <12 yrs:** 250 mg/m^2 q8h. Continue for 7 days for herpes simplex; 5 days for genital herpes.

Herpes simplex encephalitis:
IV: **Adults, elderly:** 10 mg/kg q8h for 10 days. **Children, 6 months–12 yrs:** 500 mg/m^2 q8h for 10 days.

Neonatal herpes simplex:
IV: **Neonates:** 10 mg/kg q8h for 10 days.

Varicella zoster infections:
IV: **Adults, elderly:** 10 mg/kg q8h. **Children:** 500 mg/m^2 q8h. Continue for 7 days.

Herpes zoster (acute):
PO: Adults, elderly: 800 mg q4h (5 times/day) for 7–10 days.

Usual topical dosage:
Topical: Adults, elderly: 3–6 times/day for 7 days.

Dosage in renal impairment:
Dose/frequency is modified based on severity of infection, degree of renal impairment.
Oral: Creatinine clearance of 10 ml/1.73m^2 or less: 200 mg q12h.

IV:

CREATININE CLEARANCE	DOSAGE (ADULTS)	DOSAGE (CHILDREN)
>50 ml/min	5 mg/kg q8h	250 mg/m^2 q8h
25–50 ml/min	5 mg/kg q12h	250 mg/m^2 q12h
10–25 ml/min	5 mg/kg q24h	250 mg/m^2 q24h
0–10 ml/min	2.5 mg/kg q24h	125 mg/m^2 q24h

PRECAUTIONS

CONTRAINDICATIONS: Hypersensitivity to acyclovir or components of preparation. Acyclovir reconstituted w/bacteriostatic water containing benzyl alcohol should not be used in neonates. **CAUTIONS:** Renal or hepatic impairment, dehydration, fluid/electrolyte imbalance, concurrent use of nephrotoxic agents, neurologic abnormalities. **PREGNANCY/LACTATION:** Crosses placenta; distributed in breast milk. **Pregnancy Category C.**

INTERACTIONS

DRUG INTERACTIONS: Probenecid may increase half-life. Nephrotoxic medications (e.g., aminoglycosides) may increase nephrotoxicity. **ALTERED LAB VALUES:** May increase BUN, serum creatinine concentrations.

SIDE EFFECTS

FREQUENT: *Parenteral:* Phlebitis/ inflammation at IV site, anorexia, nausea, vomiting, lightheadedness. *Topical:* Burning, stinging. **OCCASIONAL:** *Parenteral:* Hypotension, diaphoresis. *Oral:* Nausea, diarrhea, vomiting, abdominal pain, headache, lightheadedness. *Topical:* Itching. **RARE:** *Parenteral:* Confusion, hallucinations, seizures, tremors. *Topical:* Skin rash.

ADVERSE REACTION/TOXIC EFFECTS

Rapid parenteral administration, excessively high doses, or fluid/ electrolyte imbalance may produce renal failure (abdominal pain, decreased urination, decreased appetite, increased thirst, nausea, vomiting). Toxicity not reported w/oral or topical use.

NURSING IMPLICATIONS
BASELINE ASSESSMENT:

Question history of allergies, particularly to acyclovir. Avoid nephrotoxic drugs if possible. Tissue cultures for HSV should be done before giving first dose (therapy may proceed before results are known).

INTERVENTION/EVALUATION:

Monitor I&O, renal function tests if ordered, electrolyte levels. Check food tolerance, vomiting. Assess IV site for phlebitis (heat, pain, red streaking over vein). Evaluate cutaneous lesions. Be alert to neurologic effects: headache, lethargy, confusion, agitation, hallucinations, seizures. Assure adequate ventilation. Manage chickenpox and disseminated herpes zoster with strict isolation. Provide analgesics and comfort measures; esp. exhausting to elderly. Encourage fluids. Keep pt's fingernails short, hands clean.

PATIENT/FAMILY TEACHING:

Drink adequate fluids. Notify physician if side effects develop. Do not touch lesions with fingers to avoid spreading infection to new site. *Genital herpes:* Continue therapy for full length of treatment. Space doses evenly. Use finger cot or rubber glove to apply topical ointment. Avoid sexual intercourse during duration of lesions to prevent infecting partner. Acyclovir does not cure herpes. Notify physician if lesions do not improve or recur. Avoid driving or operating machinery if dizziness is present. Pap smears should be done at least annually due to increased risk of cancer of cervix in women w/genital herpes. *Chickenpox:* Unknown whether treatment of childhood chickenpox will have effect on long-term immunity.

---

adapalene
(Differin)
See Supplement

---

adefovir
(Preveon)
See Supplement
See Classification section under: Human immunodeficiency virus (HIV) infection

---

adenosine
ah-**den**-oh-seen
(Adenocard)

CANADIAN AVAILABILITY:
Adenocard

CLASSIFICATION

Antiarrhythmic

AVAILABILITY (Rx)

Injection: 3 mg/ml

PHARMACOKINETICS

Immediate onset of action. Rapidly metabolized by enzymes and taken up by erythrocytes and vascular endothelial cells to inosine and adenosine monophosphate.

ACTION/*THERAPEUTIC EFFECT*

Slows impulse formation in SA node, slows conduction time through AV node, *depressing left ventricular function and restoring normal sinus rhythm.*

USES

Treatment of paroxysmal supraventricular tachycardia, including those associated w/accessory bypass tracts (Wolff-Parkinson-White syndrome). Adjunct in myocardial perfusion imaging or stress echocardiography as diagnostic aid.

STORAGE/HANDLING

Store at room temperature. Solution appears clear. Crystallization occurs if refrigerated; if crystallization occurs, dissolve crystals by warming to room temperature. Discard unused portion.

IV ADMINISTRATION

1. Administer directly into vein, or if using IV line, as proximal as possible. Follow by rapid saline flush.
2. Administer rapidly (over 1–2 sec).

INDICATIONS/DOSAGE/ROUTES

Usual adult dosage:
IV: Adults, elderly: Initially, 6 mg (over 1–2 sec). If 1st dose does not convert within 1–2 min, give 12 mg; may repeat 12 mg dose in 1–2 min if no response has occurred.

Diagnostic testing:
IV Infusion: Adults: 140 mcg/kg/min for 6 min.

PRECAUTIONS

CONTRAINDICATIONS: Second- or third-degree AV block or sick sinus syndrome (w/functioning pacemaker), atrial flutter or fibrillation, ventricular tachycardia. **CAUTIONS:** Heart block, arrhythmias at time of conversion, asthma, hepatic/renal failure. **PREGNANCY/LACTATION:** Unknown if drug crosses placenta or is excreted in breast milk. **Pregnancy Category C**.

INTERACTIONS

DRUG INTERACTIONS: Methylxanthines (e.g., caffeine, theophylline) may decrease effect. Dipyridamole may increase effect. Carbamazepine may increase degree of heart block caused by adenosine. **ALTERED LAB VALUES:** None significant.

SIDE EFFECTS

FREQUENT: Facial flushing, headache, new arrhythmias (e.g., PVCs, sinus bradycardia); pain in chest/arm/jaw/throat; shortness of breath. **OCCASIONAL:** Cough, dizziness, nausea, numbness/tingling in arms.

ADVERSE REACTION/THERAPEUTIC EFFECTS/TOXIC EFFECTS

May produce short-lasting heart block.

NURSING IMPLICATIONS

BASELINE ASSESSMENT:

Identify arrhythmia per cardiac monitor and apical pulse.

INTERVENTION/EVALUATION:

Assess cardiac performance per continuous EKG. Monitor B/P, apical pulse (rate, rhythm, and strength), and respirations. Monitor I&O; assess for fluid retention. Check electrolytes.

---

albendazole
(Albenza)
See Supplement

---

albumin, human

al-**byew**-min
(Albuminar, Albutein, Buminate, Plasbumin)

CANADIAN AVAILABILITY:
Plasbumin

CLASSIFICATION

Blood derivative

AVAILABILITY (Rx)

Injection: 5%, 25%

ACTION/*THERAPEUTIC EFFECT*

Regulates circulating blood volume, tissue fluid balance and maintains pressure, *restoring intravascular volume, plasma volume, and maintaining cardiac output.* Binds and functions as carrier of intermediate metabolites (hormones, enzymes, drugs) in transport and exchange of tissue products.

USES

Symptomatic/supportive treatment of shock due to burns, trauma, surgery, infections. Prevents hemoconcentration and combats water, protein, electrolyte losses in severely burned or hemorrhaging pt, hypoproteinemia, ARDS (adult respiratory distress syndrome), cardiopulmonary bypass surgery (preop blood dilution), acute nephrosis, renal dialysis (treat shock or hypotension), hyperbilirubinemia and erythroblastosis fetalis.

STORAGE/HANDLING

Store at room temperature. Clear, brownish, odorless, moderate viscous fluid. Do not use if solution has been frozen, solution appears turbid, or contains sediment, or if not used within 4 hrs of opening vial.

IV ADMINISTRATION

1. Give by IV infusion.
2. 5% administered undiluted; 25% may be administered undiluted or diluted w/0.9% NaCl or 5% dextrose.
3. May give w/o regard to pt blood group or Rh factor.

INDICATIONS/DOSAGE/ROUTES

Note: Dosage based on pt's condition; duration of administration based on pt's response.

Usual dosage:
IV: Adults, elderly: 25 g by infusion. May be repeated in 15–30 min. **Maximum:** 125 g/24 hrs or 250 g/48 hrs.

Shock (greatly reduced blood volume):
IV: Adults, elderly: Administer 5% or 25% fluid as rapidly as possible to improve condition and restore normal blood volume. May be repeated in 15–30 min. **Infants, neonates:** 10–20 ml/kg of 5% solution.

Shock (slightly reduced blood volume):
IV: Adults, elderly: 5%: Give 2–4 ml/min. **Children:** Give 0.5–2 ml/min.
IV: Adults, elderly: 25%: Give 1 ml/min.

Burns (5% or 25%):
IV: Adults, elderly, children: Maintain plasma albumin concentration of 2.5 ± 0.5 g/100 ml (or plasma protein level of 5.2 g/100 ml).

Hypoproteinemia:
IV: Adults, elderly: 50–75 g/day. **Children:** 25 g/day. Give at rate not to exceed 5–10 ml/min (5%) or 2–3 ml/min (25%). This minimizes circulatory overload, pulmonary edema.

Acute nephrosis:
IV: Adults, elderly: 25%: 100–200 ml (25–50 g) daily for 7–10 days.

Renal dialysis:
IV: Adults, elderly: 25%: 100 ml (25 g).

Hyperbilirubinemia, erythroblastosis fetalis:
IV: Infants: 1 g/kg 1–2 hrs before transfusion.

PRECAUTIONS

CONTRAINDICATIONS: Severe anemia, cardiac failure, history of allergic reaction to albumin, no albumin deficiency. **CAUTIONS:** Low cardiac reserve, pulmonary disease, hepatic or renal failure. **PREGNANCY/LACTATION:** Unknown if drug crosses placenta or is distributed in breast milk. **Pregnancy Category C.**

INTERACTIONS

DRUG INTERACTIONS: None significant. **ALTERED LAB VALUES:** May increase serum alkaline phosphatase concentrations.

SIDE EFFECTS

OCCASIONAL: Hypotension. **RARE:** High dose, repeated therapy may result in altered vital signs; chills, fever, increased salivation, nausea, vomiting, urticaria, tachycardia.

ADVERSE REACTION/TOXIC EFFECTS

Fluid overload (headache, weakness, blurred vision, behavioral changes, incoordination, isolated muscle twitching) and CHF (rapid breathing, rales, wheezing, coughing, increased B/P, distended neck veins) may occur.

NURSING IMPLICATIONS
BASELINE ASSESSMENT:

Obtain B/P, pulse, respirations immediately before administration. There should be adequate hydration before albumin is administered.

INTERVENTION/EVALUATION:

Monitor B/P for hypo/hypertension. Assess frequently for evidence of fluid overload, pulmonary edema (see Adverse Reaction/Toxic Effects). Check skin for flushing, urticaria. Monitor hemoglobin, hematocrit. Monitor I&O ratio (watch for decreased output). Assess for therapeutic response (increased B/P, decreased edema).

albuterol
ale-**beut**-er-all
(Proventil, Proventil HFA, Ventolin [inhalation])

albuterol sulfate
(Proventil, Ventolin [syrup, tablets, nebulization], Volmax)

FIXED-COMBINATION(S):
W/ipratropium, a bronchodilator (**Combivent**)

CANADIAN AVAILABILITY:
Airomir, Novosalmol, Ventolin

CLASSIFICATION

Bronchodilator

AVAILABILITY (Rx)

Tablets: 2 mg, 4 mg. **Tablets** (extended-release): 4 mg. **Syrup:** 2 mg/5 ml. **Aerosol:** Metered dose inhaler. **Solution for Inhalation:** 0.83 mg/ml, 5 mg/ml. **Capsules for Inhalation:** 200 mcg, 400 mcg.

PHARMACOKINETICS

	ONSET	PEAK	DURATION
Inhalation			
	5–15 min	0.5–2 hrs	3–6 hrs
Oral	<30 min	2–3 hrs	4–8 hrs

Rapid, well absorbed from GI tract; gradual absorption from bronchi following inhalation. Metabolized in liver. Primarily excreted in urine. Half-life: 3.8 hrs oral; 3.7–5 hrs inhalation.

ACTION/THERAPEUTIC EFFECT

Stimulates beta$_2$-adrenergic receptors in the lungs *resulting in relaxation of bronchial smooth muscle. Relieves bronchospasm, reduces airway resistance.*

USES

Relief of bronchospasm due to reversible obstructive airway disease, exercise-induced bronchospasm.

PO/INHALATION ADMINISTRATION

PO:
Do not crush or break extended-release tablets.

INHALATION:

1. Shake container well, exhale completely, then holding mouthpiece 1 inch away from lips, inhale and hold breath as long as possible before exhaling.
2. Wait 1–10 min before inhaling second dose (allows for deeper bronchial penetration).
3. Rinse mouth w/water immediately after inhalation (prevents mouth/throat dryness).

NEBULIZATION:

1. Dilute 0.5 ml of 0.5% solution to final volume of 3 ml w/0.9% NaCl to provide 2.5 mg.

2. Administer over 5–15 min.

3. Nebulizer should be used w/compressed air or oxygen at rate of 6–10 liters/min.

INDICATIONS/DOSAGE/ROUTES

Bronchospasm:

Inhalation (Aerosol): Adults, elderly, children >12 yrs: 2 inhalations q4–6h. One inhalation q4h may be sufficient in some pts. Wait 1–10 min before administering second inhalation.

Inhalation (Capsules): Adults, elderly, children >4 yrs: 200–400 mcg q4–6h.

Inhalation (Solution): Adults, elderly: 2.5 mg 3–4 times/day by nebulization.

Tablets: Adults, children >12 yrs: 2 or 4 mg 3–4 times/day. Gradually increased to maximum dose of 8 mg 4 times/day (32 mg/day). **Children 6–12 yrs:** Initially, 2 mg 3–4 times/day. Gradually increase to maximum dose of 24 mg/day in divided doses. **Elderly:** 2 mg 3–4 times/day. Gradually increased to maximum dose of 8 mg 3–4 times/day.

Syrup: Adults, children >14 yrs: 2–4 mg 3–4 times/day. Maximum: 32 mg/day. **Children 6–14 yrs:** 2 mg 3–4 times/day. Dosage may be gradually increased to 24 mg/day in divided doses. **Children 2–6 yrs:** Initially, 0.1 mg/kg 3 times/day (do not exceed 2 mg 3 times/day). Gradually increased to 0.2 mg/kg 3 times/day (do not exceed 4 mg 3 times/day).

Extended-Release: Adults, children >12 yrs: 4 or 8 mg q12h. May be gradually increased to 16 mg daily.

Exercise-induced bronchospasm:

Inhalation: Adults, elderly, children >12 yrs: 2 inhalations 30 min before exercise.

PRECAUTIONS

CONTRAINDICATIONS: History of hypersensitivity to sympathomimetics. **CAUTIONS:** Hypertension, cardiovascular disease, hyperthyroidism, diabetes mellitus. **PREGNANCY/LACTATION:** Appears to cross placenta; unknown if distributed in breast milk. May inhibit uterine contractility. **Pregnancy Category C**.

INTERACTIONS

DRUG INTERACTIONS: Beta-adrenergic blocking agents (beta blockers) antagonize effects. May increase risk of arrhythmias w/digoxin. MAO inhibitors, tricyclic antidepressants may potentiate cardiovascular effects. **ALTERED LAB VALUES:** May decrease serum potassium levels.

SIDE EFFECTS

FREQUENT: Headache (27%), nausea (15%), restlessness, nervousness, trembling (20%), dizziness (<7%), throat dryness/irritation, pharyngitis (<6%), B/P changes/hypertension (3–5%), heartburn, transient wheezing (<5%). **OCCASIONAL (2–3%):** Insomnia, weakness, unusual/bad taste or taste/smell change. *Inhalation:* Dry, irritated mouth or throat, coughing, bronchial irritation. **RARE:** Drowsiness, diarrhea, dry mouth, flushing, sweating, anorexia.

ADVERSE REACTIONS/TOXIC EFFECTS

Excessive sympathomimetic stimulation may produce palpitations, extrasystoles, tachycardia, chest pain, slight increase in B/P followed by substantial decrease, chills, sweating, blanching of skin. Too frequent or excessive use may lead to loss of bronchodilating effectiveness and/or severe, paradoxical bronchoconstriction.

NURSING IMPLICATIONS

BASELINE ASSESSMENT:

Offer emotional support (high incidence of anxiety due to difficulty in breathing and sympathomimetic response to drug).

INTERVENTION/EVALUATION:

Monitor rate, depth, rhythm, type of respiration; quality and rate of pulse. Assess lung sounds for wheezing (bronchoconstriction) and rales.

PATIENT/FAMILY TEACHING:

Instruct on proper use of inhaler. Increase fluid intake (decreases lung secretion viscosity). Do not take more than 2 inhalations at any one time (excessive use may produce paradoxical bronchoconstriction or a decreased bronchodilating effect). Rinsing mouth with water immediately after inhalation may prevent mouth/throat dryness. Avoid excessive use of caffeine derivatives (chocolate, coffee, tea, cola, cocoa). Do not take OTC medications w/o physician approval: may increase sympathetic stimulation. Avoid smoking, smoke-filled areas.

---

alclometasone
(Aclovate)
See Classification section under: Corticosteroid: topical

---

aldesleukin

all-des-**lyew**-kin
(Proleukin, Interleukin-2, IL-2)

CANADIAN AVAILABILITY:
Proleukin

CLASSIFICATION

Antineoplastic, biological response modifier

AVAILABILITY (Rx)

Powder for Injection: 22 million units (1.3 mg)

PHARMACOKINETICS

Distributed to extravascular, extracellular space. Metabolized in kidney (to amino acids in cells lining the proximal convoluted tubule). Excreted in urine. Half-life: 30–120 min.

ACTION/*THERAPEUTIC EFFECT*

A highly purified protein (lymphokine) is modified, *providing enhancement of lymphocyte mitogenesis, enhancement of lymphocyte cytotoxicity, induction of natural killer cells and interferon gamma production. Activates cellular immunity, inhibits tumor growth.*

USES

Treatment of metastatic renal cell carcinoma, metastatic melanoma.

STORAGE/HANDLING

Refrigerate vial before and after reconstitution. Reconstituted solutions stable for 48 hrs. Discard solution that does not appear clear, colorless to slightly yellow. Discard unused portion.

IV ADMINISTRATION

Note: Hold administration in those who develop moderate to severe lethargy or somnolence (continued administration may result in coma).

1. Reconstitute 22 million unit vial w/1.2 ml sterile water for injection to provide concentration of 18 million units/ml. Do not use bacteriostatic sterile water or NS.

2. During reconstitution, direct

the sterile water for injection at the side of vial. Swirl contents gently to avoid foaming. Do not shake.

3. Further dilute dose in 50 ml 5% dextrose and infuse over 15 min. Do not use an in-line filter.

4. Solution should be warmed to room temperature before pt infusion.

5. Monitor diligently for drop in mean arterial B/P (sign of capillary leak syndrome [CLS]). Continued treatment may result in significant hypotension (<90 mm Hg or a 20 mm Hg drop from baseline systolic pressure), edema, pleural effusion, mental status changes.

INDICATIONS/DOSAGE/ROUTES

Note: Restrict therapy to those w/normal cardiac and pulmonary functions as defined by thallium stress testing, pulmonary function testing. Dosage individualized based on clinical response, tolerance to adverse effects.

Metastatic melanoma, metastatic renal cell carcinoma:
IV: Adults >18: 600,000 IU/kg q8h for 14 doses; rest 9 days, repeat 14 doses. Total: 28 doses. May repeat treatment no sooner than 7 wks from date of hospital discharge.

PRECAUTIONS

CONTRAINDICATIONS: Abnormal thallium stress test or pulmonary function tests, organ allografts, retreatment in those who experience the following toxicities: sustained ventricular tachycardia, cardiac rhythm disturbances uncontrolled or unresponsive, recurrent chest pain w/EKG changes, angina, MI; intubation >72 hrs, pericardial tamponade, renal dysfunction requiring dialysis >72 hrs, coma or toxic psychosis >48 hrs, repetitive or difficult-to-control seizures, bowel ischemia/perforation, GI bleeding requiring surgery. **EXTREME CAUTION:** Those w/normal thallium stress tests and pulmonary function tests who have history of prior cardiac or pulmonary disease. **CAUTIONS:** Those w/fixed requirements for large volumes of fluid (e.g., those w/hypercalcemia), history of seizures. **PREGNANCY/LACTATION:** Avoid use in those of either sex not practicing effective contraception. **Pregnancy Category C**.

INTERACTIONS

DRUG INTERACTIONS: Antihypertensives may increase hypotensive effect. Glucocorticoids may decrease effects. Cardiotoxic, hepatotoxic, nephrotoxic, myelotoxic producing medications may increase toxicity. **ALTERED LAB VALUES:** May increase bilirubin, BUN, serum creatinine, transaminase, alkaline phosphatase. May decrease magnesium, calcium, phosphorus, potassium, sodium.

SIDE EFFECTS

Note: Side effects generally self-limiting and reversible within 2–3 days after discontinuation of therapy. **FREQUENT:** Fever, chills, nausea, vomiting, hypotension, diarrhea, oliguria/anuria, mental status changes, sinus tachycardia, pain (abdomen, chest, back), fatigue, dyspnea, pruritus. **OCCASIONAL:** Erythema, rash, edema, anorexia, headache, weight gain, infection (urinary tract, injection site, catheter tip), dizziness. **RARE:** Dry skin, sensory disorders (vision, speech, taste), dermatitis, arthralgia, myalgia, weight loss, conjunctivitis, hematuria, proteinuria.

ADVERSE REACTIONS/TOXIC EFFECTS

Anemia, thrombocytopenia, leukopenia occur commonly. GI bleeding, pulmonary edema occur occasionally. CLS results in hypotension (<90 mm Hg or a 20 mm Hg drop from baseline systolic pressure) and extravasation of plasma proteins and fluid into extravascular space and loss of vascular tone. May result in cardiac arrhythmias, angina, MI, respiratory insufficiency, deficiency in mental status. Fatal malignant hyperthermia, cardiac arrest or stroke, pulmonary emboli as well as bowel perforation/gangrene, severe depression leading to suicide have occurred in less than 1% of pts.

NURSING IMPLICATIONS

BASELINE ASSESSMENT:

Preexisting bacterial infections and those w/indwelling central lines should be treated w/antibiotic therapy before treatment begins. All pts should be neurologically stable with a negative CT scan before treatment begins. CBC, differential and platelet counts, blood chemistries including electrolytes, renal and hepatic function tests, chest x-ray should be performed before therapy begins and daily thereafter. Obtain baseline B/P, temperature, pulse, weight.

INTERVENTION/EVALUATION:

Determine serum amylase concentration frequently during therapy. Discontinue medication at first sign of hypotension and hold for moderate to severe lethargy (physician must decide whether therapy should continue). Assess B/P and pulse, temperature, mental status changes (irritability, confusion, depression), weight gain or loss. Maintain strict I&O. Check hypovolemia by catheterization and central pressure monitoring (correction may require IV fluid management). Assess for extravas-

cular fluid accumulation: rales in lungs, edema in dependent areas.

PATIENT/FAMILY TEACHING:

Nausea may decrease during therapy. Evaluation 4 wks after therapy and before each course of therapy to determine additional courses (given only if some tumor shrinkage). At home, increase fluid intake (protects against renal impairment). Do not have immunizations; avoid those who have recently taken live virus vaccine.

---

alendronate sodium

ah-**len**-drew-nate
(Fosamax)

CANADIAN AVAILABILITY:
Fosamax

CLASSIFICATION

Bone resorption inhibitor, calcium regulator

AVAILABILITY (Rx)

Tablets: 5 mg, 10 mg, 40 mg

PHARMACOKINETICS

Poorly absorbed following oral administration. After oral administration, rapidly taken into bone, w/uptake greatest at sites of active bone turnover. Excreted in urine. Terminal half-life: >10 yrs (reflects release from skeleton as bone is resorbed).

ACTION/THERAPEUTIC EFFECT

Inhibits normal and abnormal bone resorption, without retarding mineralization, *leading to significant increased bone mineral density, reversing the progression of osteoporosis.*

USES / *UNLABELED*

Treatment of osteoporosis, gluco-corticoid-induced osteoporosis, Paget's disease; prevention of osteoporosis, vertebral compression fractures in postmenopausal women. *Treatment of breast cancer.*

PO ADMINISTRATION

1. Give first thing in morning, at least 30 full minutes before first food, beverage, or medication of the day.

2. Give w/6–8 oz plain water only (mineral water, coffee, tea, juice will decrease absorption).

3. Instruct patient *not* to lie down for at least 30 minutes after administering medication and until eating first food of the day (plain water and not lying down allows medication to reach stomach quickly, minimizes esophageal irritation).

INDICATIONS / DOSAGE / ROUTES

Note: Take with full glass plain water only, 30 minutes before first food, beverage, or medication.

Treatment of osteoporosis, prevention of fractures:
PO: **Adults, elderly:** 10 mg once daily, in the morning.

Paget's disease:
PO: **Adults, elderly:** 40 mg once daily, in the morning.

Prevention of osteoporosis:
PO: **Adults, elderly:** 5 mg once daily, in the morning.

PRECAUTIONS

CONTRAINDICATIONS: Hypersensitivity to biphosphonates, renal impairment when serum creatinine clearance 5mg/dl, hypocalcemic. Concurrent use with hormone replacement therapy not recommended. **CAUTIONS:** Gastrointestinal diseases (duodenitis, dysphagia, esophagitis, gastritis, ulcers (drug may exacerbate these conditions), hypocalcemia, vitamin D deficiency. **PREGNANCY/LACTATION:** Possible incomplete fetal ossification, decreased maternal weight gain, delay in delivery. Excretion in breast milk unknown. Do not give to nursing women. **Pregnancy Category C**.

INTERACTIONS

DRUG INTERACTIONS: Concurrent dietary supplements, food, beverages may interfere with alendronate absorption. IV ranitidine may double drug bioavailability. Aspirin may increase GI disturbances. **ALTERED LAB VALUES:** Reduces serum calcium, phosphate concentrations. Significant decrease in serum alkaline phosphatase noted in those w/Paget's disease.

SIDE EFFECTS

FREQUENT (7–8%): Back pain, abdominal pain. **OCCASIONAL (2–3%):** Nausea, abdominal distension, constipation/diarrhea, flatulence. **RARE (<2%):** Skin rash, esophageal irritation.

ADVERSE REACTIONS / TOXIC EFFECTS

Hypocalcemia, hypophosphatemia, significant GI disturbances result from overdosage.

NURSING IMPLICATIONS

BASELINE ASSESSMENT:

Hypocalcemia, vitamin D deficiency must be corrected before therapy

INTERVENTION / EVALUATION:

Check electrolytes (esp. calcium and alkaline phosphatase serum levels).

PATIENT / FAMILY TEACHING:

Instruct pt that expected benefits

occur only when medication is taken w/full glass (6–8 oz) of plain water, first thing in the morning and at least 30 minutes before first food, beverage, or medication of the day is taken. Any other beverage (mineral water, orange juice, coffee) significantly reduces absorption of medication. Do not lie down for at least 30 minutes after taking medication (potentiates delivery to stomach, reduces risk of esophageal irritation). If chest pain occurs, discontinue therapy, contact physician. Consider weight-bearing exercises, modify behavioral factors (e.g., cigarette smoking, alcohol consumption).

alfentanil
(Alfenta)
See Classification section under: Opioid analgesics

alitretinoin
(Panretin)
See Supplement
See Classification section under: Antineoplastics

allopurinol
al-low-**pure**-ih-nawl
(Aloprim, Lopurin, Zyloprim)

CANADIAN AVAILABILITY:
Apo-Allopurinol, Purinol, Zyl+prim

CLASSIFICATION
Antigout

AVAILABILITY (Rx)
Tablets: 100 mg, 300 mg. **Powder for Injection:** 500 mg.

PHARMACOKINETICS
Well absorbed from GI tract. Widely distributed. Metabolized in liver to active metabolite. Excreted primarily in urine. Removed by hemodialysis. Half-life: 1–3 hrs; metabolite: 12–30 hrs.

ACTION/*THERAPEUTIC EFFECT*
Decreases uric acid production by inhibition of xanthine oxidase, an enzyme, *reducing uric acid concentrations in both serum and urine.*

USES/*UNLABELED*
Treatment of chronic gouty arthritis, uric acid nephropathy. Prevents or treats hyperuricemia secondary to blood dyscrasias, cancer chemotherapy. Prevents recurrence of uric acid or calcium stone formation. Aloprim: Management of elevated uric acid in cancer pts unable to tolerate oral therapy. *Used in mouthwash following fluorouracil therapy to prevent stomatitis.*

PO ADMINISTRATION
1. May give w/or immediately after meals or milk.
2. Instruct pt to drink at least 10–12 eight oz glasses of water/day.
3. Doses >300 mg/day to be administered in divided doses.

INDICATIONS/DOSAGE/ROUTES
Gout, hyperuricemia:
PO: Adults: 200–600 mg/day. **Range:** 100–800 mg/day. **Maximum:** 800 mg/day. **Children (6–10 yrs):** 300 mg/day. **Children (< 6 yrs):** 150 mg/day.

Prevention uric acid nephropathy during neoplastic disease therapy:
PO: Adults: 600–800 mg/day for 2–3 days (w/high fluid intake).

Reduction acute gouty attacks:
PO: Adults: Initially, 100 mg/day. May increase by 100 mg/day at weekly intervals (up to maximum of 800 mg/day) until serum uric acid ≤6 mg/dl attained.

Recurrent calcium oxalate stones:
PO: Adults: 200–300 mg/day.

Usual elderly dosage:
PO: Initially, 100 mg/day, gradually increased to optimal uric acid level.

Usual parenteral dosage:
IV infusion: Adults 200–400 mg/m^2/day. **Maximum:** 600 mg/m^2/day. **Children:** Initially, 200 mg/m^2/day.

Dosage in renal impairment:
Based on creatinine clearance using serum uric acid as index.

CREATININE CLEARANCE	DOSAGE
10–20 ml/min	200 mg/day
3–10 ml/min	100 mg/day maximum
<3 ml/min	100 mg at increased intervals

PRECAUTIONS

CONTRAINDICATIONS: Asymptomatic hyperuricemia. **CAUTIONS:** Impaired renal, hepatic function. **PREGNANCY/LACTATION:** Unknown if drug crosses placenta or is distributed in breast milk. **Pregnancy Category C**.

INTERACTIONS

DRUG INTERACTIONS: Thiazide diuretics may decrease effect. May increase effect of oral anticoagulants. May increase effect, toxicity of azathioprine, mercaptopurine. Ampicillin, amoxicillin may increase incidence of skin rash. **ALTERED LAB VALUES:** May increase alkaline phosphatase, SGOT (AST), SGPT (ALT), BUN, creatinine.

SIDE EFFECTS

OCCASIONAL: Drowsiness, unusual hair loss. **RARE:** Diarrhea, headache.

ADVERSE REACTIONS/TOXIC EFFECTS

Pruritic maculopapular rash should be considered a toxic reaction. May be accompanied by malaise, fever, chills, joint pain, nausea, vomiting. Severe hypersensitivity may follow appearance of rash. Bone marrow depression, hepatotoxicity, peripheral neuritis, or acute renal failure occurs rarely.

NURSING IMPLICATIONS
BASELINE ASSESSMENT:

Question pt for hypersensitivity to allopurinol. Instruct pt to drink 10–12 glasses (8 oz) of fluid daily while on medication.

INTERVENTION/EVALUATION:

Discontinue medication immediately if rash or other evidence of allergic reaction appears. Encourage high fluid intake (3,000 ml/day). Monitor I&O (output should be at least 2,000 ml/day). Assess CBC, serum uric acid levels. Assess urine for cloudiness, unusual color, odor. Assess for therapeutic response (reduced joint tenderness, swelling, redness, limitation of motion).

PATIENT/FAMILY TEACHING:

May take 1 or more wks for full therapeutic effect. Encourage low purine food intake, drinking 10–12 glasses (8 oz) of fluid daily while on medication. Avoid tasks that require alertness, motor skills until response to drug is established. Contact physician/nurse if rash, irritation of eyes, swelling of lips/mouth occurs.

alpha₁-proteinase inhibitor (human, alpha₁-PI)
(Prolastin)

CANADIAN AVAILABILITY:
Prolastin

CLASSIFICATION

Proteinase inhibitor

AVAILABILITY (Rx)

Powder for Injection: 500 mg, 1,000 mg

ACTION/*THERAPEUTIC EFFECT*

Protects alveolar epithelial lining of lower respiratory tract by alleviating imbalance between elastase (enzyme capable of degrading elastin tissue in lower respiratory tract) and alpha₁-proteinase inhibitor (inhibits neutrophil elastase), *allowing for subsequent protection from degradation of elastin tissue.*

USES

Chronic replacement therapy in patients w/clinically demonstrable panacinar emphysema. Do not use in patients w/PiMZ or PiMS phenotypes (small risk of panacinar emphysema).

STORAGE/HANDLING

Store parenteral form in refrigerator. After reconstitution, do not refrigerate. Use within 3 hrs. Discard unused portion.

IV ADMINISTRATION

1. Reconstitute each vial w/20 or 40 ml sterile water (total functional activity stated in mg is noted on label of each vial). 20 ml = about 500 mg; 40 ml = about 1,000 mg activity.

2. May use 0.9% NaCl as diluent.

3. Infuse at rate of at least 0.08 ml/kg.

INDICATIONS/DOSAGE/ROUTES

Replacement therapy:
IV Infusion: Adults, elderly: 60 mg/kg once weekly at rate of at least 0.08 ml/kg.

PRECAUTIONS

CONTRAINDICATIONS: Pts w/known antibody reaction against IgA (may experience severe reaction, including anaphylaxis). **CAUTIONS:** Those at risk for circulatory overload. Safety in children not established. **PREGNANCY/LACTATION:** Unknown if drug crosses placenta or is distributed in breast milk. **Pregnancy Category C**.

INTERACTIONS

DRUG INTERACTIONS: None significant. **ALTERED LAB VALUES:** None significant.

SIDE EFFECTS

RARE (<1%): Delayed fever (occurring 12 hrs after administration, resolves spontaneously), lightheadedness, dizziness.

ADVERSE REACTIONS/TOXIC EFFECTS

Mild leukocytosis occurs rarely.

NURSING IMPLICATIONS

BASELINE ASSESSMENT:

All patients should be immunized against hepatitis B before initial dose is given.

INTERVENTION/EVALUATION:

Maintain blood levels of alpha₁-PI at 80 mg/dl. Monitor respiratory status throughout therapy.

PATIENT/FAMILY TEACHING:

Explain purpose of medication, importance of hepatitis B vaccine, periodic pulmonary function tests. Avoid smoking. Notify physician of changes in respiratory condition.

alprazolam

ale-**praz**-oh-lam
(Xanax)

CANADIAN AVAILABILITY:
Apo-Alpraz, Novo-Alprazol, Xanax

CLASSIFICATION

Antianxiety: Benzodiazepine

AVAILABILITY (Rx)

Tablets: 0.25 mg, 0.5 mg, 1 mg, 2 mg. **Oral Solution:** 0.5 mg/5ml, 1 mg/ml

PHARMACOKINETICS

Well absorbed from GI tract. Metabolized in liver. Primarily excreted in urine. Minimal removed by hemodialysis. Half-life: 11–16 hrs.

ACTION/THERAPEUTIC EFFECT

Enhances action of inhibitory neurotransmitters in the brain, *producing anxiolytic effect due to CNS depressant action.*

USES/*UNLABELED*

Management of anxiety disorders associated w/depression, panic disorder. *Improves mood, relieves cramps, insomnia w/premenstrual syndrome.*

PO ADMINISTRATION

1. May be given w/o regard to meals.
2. Tablets may be crushed.

INDICATIONS/DOSAGE/ROUTES

Anxiety disorders:
PO: Adults >18 yrs: Initially, 0.25–0.5 mg 3 times daily. Titrate to maximum of 4 mg daily in divided doses. **Elderly/debilitated/liver disease/low serum albumin:** Initially, 0.25 mg 2–3 times daily. Gradually increase to optimum therapeutic response.

Panic disorder:
PO: Adults: Initially, 0.5 mg 3 times/day. May increase at 3–4 day intervals at no more than 1 mg/day. **Range:** 1–10 mg/day.

Usual elderly dosage:
PO: Initially, 0.125–0.25 mg 2 times/day; may increase in 0.125 mg increments until desired effect attained.

Premenstrual syndrome:
PO: Adults: 0.25 mg 3 times/day.

PRECAUTIONS

CONTRAINDICATIONS: Acute narrow-angle glaucoma, acute alcohol intoxication w/depressed vital signs, severe chronic obstructive pulmonary disease, myasthenia gravis, ketoconazole, itraconazole. **CAUTIONS:** Impaired renal/hepatic function. **PREGNANCY/LACTATION:** Crosses placenta; distributed in breast milk. Chronic ingestion during pregnancy may produce withdrawal symptoms, CNS depression in neonates. **Pregnancy Category D.**

INTERACTIONS

DRUG INTERACTIONS: Potentiated effects when used w/other CNS depressants (including alcohol). **ALTERED LAB VALUES:** May produce abnormal renal function tests, elevate SGOT (AST), SGPT (ALT), LDH, alkaline phosphatase, serum bilirubin.

SIDE EFFECTS

FREQUENT: Muscular incoordination (ataxia), lightheadedness, transient mild drowsiness, slurred speech (particularly in elderly, debilitated). **OCCASIONAL:** Confusion, depression, blurred vision, constipation/diarrhea, dry mouth, headache, nausea. **RARE:** Behavioral problems (e.g., anger), impaired memory, paradoxical reaction (insomnia, nervousness, irritability).

ADVERSE REACTIONS/TOXIC EFFECTS

Abrupt or too rapid withdrawal may result in pronounced restlessness, irritability, insomnia, hand tremors, abdominal/muscle cramps, sweating, vomiting, seizures. Overdosage results in somnolence, confusion, diminished reflexes, coma. Blood dyscrasias noted rarely.

NURSING IMPLICATIONS

BASELINE ASSESSMENT:

Offer emotional support to anxious pt. Assess motor responses (agitation, trembling, tension) and autonomic responses (cold, clammy hands, sweating).

INTERVENTION/EVALUATION:

For those on long-term therapy, liver/renal function tests, blood counts should be performed periodically. Assess for paradoxical reaction, particularly during early therapy. Assist w/ambulation if drowsiness, lightheadedness occur. Evaluate for therapeutic response: calm facial expression, decreased restlessness and/or insomnia.

PATIENT/FAMILY TEACHING:

Drowsiness usually disappears during continued therapy. If dizziness occurs, change positions slowly from recumbent to sitting position before standing. Avoid tasks that require alertness, motor skills until response to drug is established. Smoking reduces drug effectiveness. Sour hard candy, gum, or sips of tepid water may relieve dry mouth. Do not abruptly withdraw medication after long-term therapy. Avoid alcohol. Do not take other medications w/o consulting physician.

alprostadil (prostaglandin E₁; PGE₁)

ale-**pros**-tah-dill
(Caverject, Edex, Muse, Prostin VR Pediatric)

CANADIAN AVAILABILITY:
Caverject, Prostin VR

CLASSIFICATION

Prostaglandin

AVAILABILITY (Rx)

Injection: 500 mcg/ml. **Powder for Injection:** 5 mcg, 10 mcg, 20 mcg, 40 mcg. **Urethral Suppository (Muse):** 125 mcg, 250 mcg, 500 mcg, 1,000 mcg.

PHARMACOKINETICS

After IV administration, rapidly metabolized in lungs (oxidation). Excreted in urine. Half-life: 5–10 min.

ACTION/*THERAPEUTIC EFFECT*

Vasodilator having direct effect on vascular smooth muscle, ductus arteriosus. *Relaxes cavernous smooth muscle, dilates penile arteries, increases arterial blood flow to penis. Prevents closure of ductus arteriosus.*

USES/*UNLABELED*

Temporarily maintains patency of ductus arteriosus until surgery is performed in those w/congenital heart defects and dependent on patent ductus for survival (e.g., pulmonary atresia or stenosis). Treatment of erectile dysfunction due to neurogenic, vasculogenic, psychogenic causes, adjunct in diagnosis of erectile dysfunction. *Treatment of atherosclerosis, gan-*

grene, pain due to severe peripheral arterial occlusive disease.

STORAGE/HANDLING

Store parenteral form in refrigerator. Must dilute before use. Prepare fresh every 24 hrs. Discard unused portions. Refrigerate suppositories unless used within 14 days.

IV ADMINISTRATION

1. Infuse for shortest time, lowest dose possible.

2. If significant decrease in arterial pressure is noted via umbilical artery catheter, auscultation, or Doppler transducer, decrease infusion rate immediately.

3. Discontinue infusion immediately if apnea or bradycardia occurs (overdosage).

4. Dilute 500 mcg amp w/5% dextrose or 0.9% NaCl to volume appropriate for available pump delivery system.

INDICATIONS/DOSAGE/ROUTES

Note: Give by continuous IV infusion or through umbilical artery catheter placed at ductal opening.

Maintain patency ductus arteriosus:
IV Infusion: Neonate: Initially, 0.05–0.1 mcg/kg/min. After therapeutic response achieved, use lowest dose to maintain response. **Maximum:** 0.4 mcg/kg/min.

Impotence:
Suppository, Intracavernosal: Individualized.

PRECAUTIONS

CONTRAINDICATIONS: Respiratory distress syndrome (hyaline membrane disease). Conditions predisposing to priaprism, anatomical deformation of penis, penile implants. **CAUTIONS:** Severe liver disease, coagulation defects.

INTERACTIONS

DRUG INTERACTIONS: Anticoagulants, heparin, thrombolytics may increase risk of bleeding. Sympathomimetics may decrease effect. Vasodilators may increase risk of hypotension. **ALTERED LAB VALUES:** May increase bilirubin. May decrease calcium, glucose, potassium.

SIDE EFFECTS

FREQUENT: *Intracavernosal (1–4%):* Penile ipan (37%), prolonged erection, hypertension, local pain, penile fibrosis, injection site hematoma/ecchymosis, headache, respiratory infection, flulike symptoms. *Intraurethral (3%):* Penile pain (36%), urethral pain/burning, testicular pain, urethral bleeding, headache, dizziness, respiratory infection, flu-like symptoms. *Systemic (>1%):* Fever, seizures, flushing, bradycardia, hypotension, tachycardia, apnea, diarrhea, sepsis. **OCCASIONAL:** *Intracavernosal (<1%):* Hypotension, pelvic pain, back pain, dizziness, cough, nasal congestion. *Intraurethral (<3%):* Fainting, sinusitis, back/pelvic pain. *Systemic (<1%):* Jitteriness, lethargy, stiffness, arrhythmias, respiratory depression, anemia, bleeding, thrombocytopenia, hematuria.

ADVERSE REACTIONS/TOXIC EFFECTS

Overdosage manifested as apnea, flushing of face/arms, bradycardia. Cardiac arrest, sepsis occur rarely.

NURSING IMPLICATIONS

INTERVENTION/EVALUATION:

Monitor arterial pressure by umbilical artery catheter, auscultation, or Doppler transducer. If significant decrease in arterial pressure occurs, decrease infusion rate immediately. Maintain continuous cardiac monitoring. Assess heart sounds, femoral pulse (circulation to lower extremities), and respiratory status frequently. Monitor symptoms of hypotension, B/P, arterial blood gases, temperature. If apnea or bradycardia occurs, discontinue infusion and notify physician.

PATIENT/FAMILY TEACHING:

Explain purpose of this palliative therapy to parents. *Impotence:* Erection is to occur within 2–5 min. Do not use if female pregnant (unless using condom barrier). Inform physician if erection >4 hrs or becomes painful, or bleeding at injection site persists.

---

alteplase, recombinant

all-teh-place
(Activase)

CANADIAN AVAILABILITY: Activase rt-PA

CLASSIFICATION

Thrombolytic

AVAILABILITY (Rx)

Powder for Injection: 20 mg, 50 mg, 100 mg

PHARMACOKINETICS

Rapidly metabolized in liver. Primarily excreted in urine. Half-life: 35 min.

ACTION/*THERAPEUTIC EFFECT*

Activates fibrinolytic system by directly cleaving bond in plasminogen-producing plasmin, an enzyme that *degrades fibrin clots, fibrinogen, other plasma proteins.* Appears to be more readily clot selective binding within a clot than circulating fibrinogen.

USES

Management of acute myocardial infarction (AMI) for lysis of thrombi obstructing coronary arteries and management of acute massive pulmonary embolus for lysis of acute pulmonary emboli. Treatment acute ischemic stroke (within 5 hrs of symptoms).

STORAGE/HANDLING

Store vials at room temperature. After reconstitution, solutions are colorless to pale yellow. Solution is stable for 8 hrs after reconstitution. Discard unused portions.

IV ADMINISTRATION

1. Give by IV infusion via infusion pump.
2. Reconstitute immediately prior to use w/sterile water for injection.
3. Reconstitute 50 mg vial w/50 ml sterile water for injection without preservative (20 ml for 20 mg vial) to provide a concentration of 1 mg/ml. (May be further diluted w/50 ml 5% dextrose or 0.9% NaCl to provide a concentration of 0.5 mg/ml.)
4. Avoid excessive agitation; gently swirl or slowly invert vial to reconstitute.
5. If minor bleeding occurs at puncture sites, apply pressure for 30 sec; if unrelieved, apply pressure dressing.
6. If uncontrolled hemorrhage occurs, discontinue infusion immediately (slowing rate of infusion may produce worsening hemorrhage).
7. Avoid undue pressure when drug is injected into catheter (can

rupture catheter or expel clot into circulation).

INDICATIONS/DOSAGE/ROUTES

Acute myocardial infarction:
IV Infusion: Adults: 100 mg over 90 min; 15 mg bolus given over 1–2 min; then, 50 mg over 30 min; then, 35 mg over 60 min.

Acute pulmonary emboli:
IV Infusion: Adults: 100 mg over 2 hrs. Institute or reinstitute heparin near end or immediately after infusion (when PTT or thrombin time returns to twice normal or less).

Acute ischemic stroke:
IV Infusion: Adults: 0.9 mg/kg over 60 minutes (10% total dose as initial IV bolus over 1 min).

PRECAUTIONS

CONTRAINDICATIONS: Active internal bleeding, recent (within 2 months) cerebrovascular accident, intracranial or intraspinal surgery or trauma, intracranial neoplasm, arteriovenous malformation or aneurysm, bleeding diathesis, severe uncontrolled hypertension. **CAUTIONS:** Recent (10 days) major surgery or GI bleeding, OB delivery, organ biopsy, recent trauma (cardiopulmonary resuscitation, left heart thrombus, endocarditis, severe hepatic/renal disease, pregnancy, elderly, cerebrovascular disease, diabetic retinopathy, thrombophlebitis, occluded AV cannula at infected site). **PREGNANCY/LACTATION:** Use only when benefit outweighs potential risk to fetus. Unknown if drug crosses placenta or is distributed in breast milk. **Pregnancy Category C.**

INTERACTIONS

DRUG INTERACTIONS: Anticoagulants, heparin, cefotetan, plicamycin, valproic acid may increase risk of hemorrhage. Platelet aggregation inhibitors (e.g., aspirin), NSAIDs, ticlodipine may increase risk of bleeding. **ALTERED LAB VALUES:** Decreases plasminogen and fibrinogen level during infusion, decreasing clotting time (confirms presence of lysis).

SIDE EFFECTS

FREQUENT: Superficial bleeding at puncture sites, decreased B/P. **OCCASIONAL:** Allergic reaction (rash, wheezing), bruising.

ADVERSE REACTIONS/TOXIC EFFECTS

Severe internal hemorrhage may occur. Lysis of coronary thrombi may produce atrial or ventricular dysrhythmias, stroke.

NURSING IMPLICATIONS
BASELINE ASSESSMENT:

Obtain baseline B/P, apical pulse. Record weight. Evaluate 12-lead EKG, CPK, CPK-MB, electrolytes. Assess hematocrit, platelet count, thrombin (TT), activated thromboplastin (APTT), prothrombin time (PT), fibrinogen level, before therapy is instituted. Type and hold blood.

INTERVENTION/EVALUATION:

Continuous cardiac monitoring for arrhythmias, B/P, pulse and respirations q15 min until stable, then hourly. Check peripheral pulses, heart and lung sounds. Monitor chest pain relief and notify physician of continuation or recurrence (note location, type, and intensity). Assess for bleeding: overt blood, blood in any body substance. Monitor PTT per protocol. Maintain B/P; avoid any trauma that might increase risk of bleeding (injections, shaving, etc.). **Assess neurologic status.**

PATIENT/FAMILY TEACHING:

Report any bleeding.

altretamine (hexam-ethylmelamine)

all-**treh**-tih-meen
(Hexalen)

CANADIAN AVAILABILITY:
Hexalen

CLASSIFICATION

Antineoplastic

AVAILABILITY (Rx)

Capsules: 50 mg

PHARMACOKINETICS

Well absorbed from GI tract. Metabolized in liver to active metabolites (necessary for action). Primarily excreted in urine. Half-life: 4.7–10.2 hrs.

ACTION/ *THERAPEUTIC EFFECT*

Exact mechanism unknown. *May inhibit DNA, RNA synthesis.*

USES

Palliative treatment for persistent or recurrent ovarian cancer following therapy with a cisplatin or alkylating combination.

PO ADMINISTRATION

Give after meals and at bedtime.

INDICATIONS/DOSAGE/ROUTES

Ovarian cancer:
Note: Give total daily dose as 4 equally divided doses after meals and bedtime.
PO: Adults, elderly: 260 mg/m^2/day in 4 divided doses for 14 or 21 consecutive days in 28 day cycle. May be temporarily held or discontinued w/dose decreased to 200 mg/m^2/day if GI intolerance, WBC <2,000/mm^3 or granulocyte <1,000/mm^3, platelets <75,000/mm^3, progressive neurotoxicity.

PRECAUTIONS

CONTRAINDICATIONS: Severe bone marrow depression, severe neurologic toxicity. **CAUTIONS:** Decreased neurological function. **PREGNANCY/LACTATION:** Unknown if drug crosses placenta or is distributed in breast milk. **Pregnancy Category D.**

INTERACTIONS

DRUG INTERACTIONS: Bone marrow depressants may increase bone marrow depression. MAOIs may cause severe orthostatic hypotension. Live virus vaccines may potentiate virus replication, increase vaccine side effects, decrease pt's antibody response to vaccine. **ALTERED LAB VALUES:** May increase alkaline phosphatase, BUN, serum creatinine; reduce platelet, WBC count.

SIDE EFFECTS

FREQUENT: Mild to moderate nausea and vomiting, mild peripheral neuropathy, mild anemia, leukopenia, neurologic effects (confusion, mental depression), unusual bleeding, bruising. **OCCASIONAL:** Diarrhea, anorexia, abdominal cramps, skin rash, pruritus.

ADVERSE REACTIONS/TOXIC EFFECTS

Mild to moderate myelosuppression expected. Neurologic toxicity generally disappears when drug is discontinued.

NURSING IMPLICATIONS
BASELINE ASSESSMENT:

Give emotional support to patient and family. Perform neurologic function tests prior to chemotherapy. Check blood counts prior to each course of therapy, monthly or as clinically indicated.

INTERVENTION/EVALUATION:

Monitor for hematologic toxicity (fever, sore throat, signs of local infection, easy bruising, unusual bleeding), symptoms of anemia (excessive tiredness, weakness). Measure all vomitus (general guideline requiring immediate notification of physician: 750 ml/8 hrs, urinary output less than 100 ml/hr).

PATIENT/FAMILY TEACHING:

Nausea may decrease during therapy. Do not have immunizations w/o physician's approval (drug lowers body's resistance). Avoid contact w/those who have recently taken live virus vaccine. Report unusual bleeding/bruising, blood in urine/stools, red spots on skin; fever, chills, cough, hoarseness; painful/difficult urination.

aluminum acetate
(Burrow's Solution)

FIXED-COMBINATION(S):
Aluminum sulfate w/calcium acetate (**Domboro Powder, Domboro Tablets, Bluboro Powder, Pedi-Boro Soak Paks, Modified Burrow's Solution**)

CANADIAN AVAILABILITY:
Acid Mantle

CLASSIFICATION

Astringent

AVAILABILITY (OTC)

Solution. Powder packets

ACTION

Precipitates proteins; lowers pH w/increase in skin acidity; inhibits discharge by causing contraction (shrinkage of tissue). *Anti-inflammatory, antipruritic, mild antiseptic properties.*

USES

Relief of inflammation, irritation of the skin such as insect bites, poison ivy, diaper rash, acne, allergy, anal pruritus, eczema, bruises.

TOPICAL ADMINISTRATION

1. Mix 1 tablet or packet w/1 pint of water (warm or cool, as ordered).
2. Do not cover dressing w/ plastic or other occlusive covering.
3. Keep away from eyes.

INDICATIONS/DOSAGE/ROUTES

Usual topical dosage:
Topical: Adults, elderly: Apply for 15–30 min q4–8h.

PRECAUTIONS

CONTRAINDICATIONS: Sensitivity to aluminum. **CAUTIONS:** For external use only. **PREGNANCY/LACTATION:** Pregnancy Category N/A.

INTERACTIONS

DRUG INTERACTIONS: None significant. **ALTERED LAB VALUES:** None significant.

SIDE EFFECTS

RARE: Increased irritation, extension of inflammation.

NURSING IMPLICATIONS
BASELINE ASSESSMENT:

Determine extent of skin irritation, inflammation.

Intervention/Evaluation:

Assess therapeutic response, increased redness, irritation, discomfort.

Patient/Family Teaching:

Discontinue if increased irritation or inflammation occurs. Avoid using near eyes. Do not cover with plastic or other occlusive material.

aluminum carbonate
(Basaljel)

aluminum hydroxide
(Alternagel, Alu-Cap, Alu-Tab, Amphojel, Dialume)

FIXED-COMBINATION(S):
W/magnesium, an antacid (**Aludrox, Delcid, Gaviscon, Maalox**); w/magnesium and simethicone, an antiflatulent (**DiGel, Gelusil, Maalox Plus, Mylanta, Silain-Gel**); w/magnesium and calcium, an antacid (**Camalox**).

CANADIAN AVAILABILITY:
Amphojel, Basaljel

CLASSIFICATION

Antacid

AVAILABILITY (OTC)

Aluminum carbonate: **Tablets:** 500 mg. **Capsules:** 500 mg. **Suspension:** 400 mg/5 ml.

Aluminum hydroxide: **Tablets:** 300 mg, 500 mg, 600 mg. **Capsules:** 400 mg, 500 mg. **Suspension:** 320 mg/5 ml, 450 mg/5 ml, 675 mg/5 ml. **Liquid:** 600 mg/5 ml.

PHARMACOKINETICS

Small amount absorbed from intestine. Onset of action based on solubility in stomach and reaction w/hydrochloric acid. Duration of action based primarily on gastric emptying time (20 min when given ac, up to 3 hrs when given pc).

ACTION/THERAPEUTIC EFFECT

Reduces gastric acid, *thereby neutralizing or increasing gastric pH.* Binds w/phosphate in intestine, then excreted in feces *(reduces phosphates in urine, preventing formation of phosphate urinary stones; reduces serum phosphate levels).* May increase absorption of calcium (due to decreased serum phosphate levels). Astringent, adsorbent properties *(decreases fluidity of stools).*

USES

Symptomatic relief of upset stomach associated w/hyperacidity (heartburn, acid indigestion, sour stomach). Hyperacidity associated w/gastric, duodenal ulcers. Symptomatic treatment of gastroesophageal reflux disease. Prophylactic treatment of GI bleeding secondary to gastritis and stress ulceration. In conjunction w/low phosphate diet, prevents formation of phosphate urinary stones, reduces elevated phosphate levels.

PO ADMINISTRATION

1. Usually administered 1–3 hrs after meals.
2. Individualize dose (based on neutralizing capacity of antacids).
3. Chewable tablets: Thoroughly chew tablets before swallowing (follow w/glass of water or milk).
4. If administering suspension, shake well before use.

INDICATIONS/DOSAGE/ROUTES

Note: Usual dose is 30–60 ml.

Aluminum Carbonate:

Antacid:
PO: Adults, elderly: 2 capsules or 10 ml q2h up to 12 times/day.

Hyperphosphatemia:
PO: Adults, elderly: 2 capsules or 12.5 ml 3–4 times/day w/meals.

ALUMINUM HYDROXIDE:

Antacid:
PO: Adults, elderly: 500–1,800 mg 3–6 times/day between meals and bedtime.

Hyperphosphatemia:
PO: Children: 50–150 mg/kg/24 hrs in divided doses q4–6h.

PRECAUTIONS

CONTRAINDICATIONS: Intestinal obstruction. **CAUTIONS:** Impaired renal function, gastric outlet obstruction, elderly, dehydration, fluid restriction, Alzheimer's disease, symptoms of appendicitis, GI/rectal bleeding, constipation, fecal impaction, chronic diarrhea. **PREGNANCY/LACTATION:** May produce hypercalcemia, hypo/hypermagnesemia, increase tendon reflexes in neonate/fetus whose mother is a chronic, high-dose user. May be distributed in breast milk. **Pregnancy Category N/A.**

INTERACTIONS

DRUG INTERACTIONS: May decrease excretion of quinidine, anticholinergics. May decrease effects of methenamine. May increase salicylate excretion. May decrease absorption of quinolones, iron preparations, isoniazid, ketoconazole, tetracyclines. **ALTERED LAB VALUES:** May increase gastrin, systemic/urinary pH. May decrease serum phosphate.

SIDE EFFECTS

FREQUENT: Chalky taste, mild constipation, stomach cramps. **OCCASIONAL:** Nausea, vomiting, speckling/whitish discoloration of stools.

ADVERSE REACTIONS/TOXIC EFFECTS

Prolonged constipation may result in intestinal obstruction. Excessive or chronic use may produce hypophosphatemia (anorexia, malaise, muscle weakness, bone pain) resulting in osteomalacia, osteoporosis. Prolonged use may produce urinary calculi.

NURSING IMPLICATIONS
BASELINE ASSESSMENT:

Do not give other oral medication within 1–2 hrs of antacid administration.

INTERVENTION/EVALUATION:

Assess pattern of daily bowel activity and stool consistency. Monitor serum phosphate, calcium, uric acid levels. Assess for relief of gastric distress.

PATIENT/FAMILY TEACHING:

Chewable tablets: Chew tablets thoroughly before swallowing (may be followed by water or milk). Tablets may discolor stool. Maintain adequate fluid intake.

---

amantadine hydrochloride

ah-**man**-tih-deen
(Symadine, Symmetrel)

CANADIAN AVAILABILITY: Symmetrel

CLASSIFICATION

Antiviral, antiparkinson.

AVAILABILITY (Rx)

Tablets: 100 mg. **Syrup:** 50 mg/5 ml.

PHARMACOKINETICS

Rapid, completely absorbed from GI tract. Widely distributed. Primarily excreted in urine. Minimal removed by hemodialysis. Half-life: 11–15 hrs (increased in elderly, decreased renal function).

ACTION/*THERAPEUTIC EFFECT*

Antiviral action against influenza A virus believed *to prevent uncoating of virus, penetration of host cells, release of nucleic acid into host cells.* Antiparkinsonism *due to increased release of dopamine.* Virustatic.

USES/*UNLABELED*

Prevention, treatment of respiratory tract infections due to influenza virus, Parkinson's disease, drug-induced extrapyramidal reactions. *Treatment of fatigue associated w/multiple sclerosis.*

PO ADMINISTRATION

Administer nighttime dose several hours before bedtime (prevents insomnia).

INDICATIONS/DOSAGE/ROUTES

Prophylaxis, symptomatic treatment respiratory illness due to influenza A virus:
Note: Give as single or in 2 divided doses.
PO: Adults (10–64 yrs): 200 mg daily. **Adults (>64 yrs):** 100 mg daily. **Children (9–12 yrs):** 100 mg 2 times/day. **Children (1–9 yrs):** 4.4–8.8 mg/kg/day (up to 150 mg/day).

Parkinson's disease, extrapyramidal symptoms:
PO: Adults: 100 mg 2 times/day. May increase up to 400 mg/day in divided doses.

Usual elderly dosage:
PO: Based on renal function. Ccr 40–50 ml/min: 100 mg/day; Ccr 20 ml/min: 100 mg 3 times/wk.

Dosage in renal impairment:
Dose and/or frequency is modified based on creatinine clearance (Ccr).

CREATININE CLEARANCE	DOSAGE
30–50 ml/min	200 mg first day; 100 mg/day thereafter
15–29 ml/min	200 mg first day; 100 mg on alternate days
<15 ml/min	200 mg every 7 days

PRECAUTIONS

CONTRAINDICATIONS: None significant. **CAUTIONS:** History of seizures, orthostatic hypotension, CHF, peripheral edema, liver disease, recurrent eczematoid dermatitis, cerebrovascular disease, renal dysfunction, those receiving CNS stimulants. **PREGNANCY/LACTATION:** Unknown if drug crosses placenta; distributed in breast milk. **Pregnancy Category C**.

INTERACTIONS

DRUG INTERACTIONS: Tricyclic antidepressants, antihistamines, phenothiazine, anticholinergics may increase anticholinergic effects. Hydrochlorothiazide, triamterene may increase concentration, toxicity. **ALTERED LAB VALUES:** None significant.

SIDE EFFECTS

FREQUENT (5–10%): Nausea, dizziness, poor concentration, insomnia, nervousness. **OCCASIONAL (1–5%):** Orthostatic hypotension, anorexia, headache, livedo reticularis (reddish blue, netlike blotching of skin), blurred vision, urinary retention, dry mouth/nose. **RARE:** Vomiting, depression, irritation/swelling of eyes, skin rash.

ADVERSE REACTIONS/TOXIC EFFECTS

CHF, leukopenia, neutropenia occur rarely. Hyperexcitability, convulsions, ventricular arrhythmias may occur.

NURSING IMPLICATIONS
BASELINE ASSESSMENT:

Question history of allergies, especially to amantadine. When treating infections caused by influenza A virus, obtain specimens for viral diagnostic tests before giving first dose (therapy may begin before results are known).

INTERVENTION/EVALUATION:

Monitor I&O, renal function tests if ordered; check for peripheral edema. Evaluate food tolerance, vomiting. Assess skin for rash, blotching. Be alert to neurologic effects: headache, lethargy, confusion, agitation, blurred vision, seizures. Assess B/P at least twice daily. Determine bowel pattern, modify diet, or administer laxative as needed. Assess for dizziness. *Parkinsonism:* Assess for clinical reversal of symptoms (improvement of tremor of head/hands at rest, mask-like facial expression, shuffling gait, muscular rigidity).

PATIENT/FAMILY TEACHING:

Continue therapy for full length of treatment. Doses should be evenly spaced. Do not take any medications w/o consulting physician. Avoid alcoholic beverages. Do not drive, use machinery, or engage in other activities that require mental acuity if experiencing dizziness, confusion, blurred vision. Get up slowly from a sitting or lying position. Advise physician if no improvement in 2–3 days when taking for viral infection. Inform physician of new symptoms, especially blotching, rash, dizziness, blurred vision, nausea/vomiting. Take nighttime dose several hours before bedtime to prevent insomnia.

amcinonide
(Cyclocort)
See Classification section under: Corticosteroid: topical

amifostine
am-ih-**fos**-teen
(Ethyol)

CANADIAN AVAILABILITY:
Ethyol

CLASSIFICATION
Antineoplastic adjunct, cytoprotective agent

AVAILABILITY (Rx)
Powder for Injection: 500 mg, 500 mg mannitol (10 ml single-use vial)

PHARMACOKINETICS
Rapidly cleared from plasma. Converted in tissue to active free thiol metabolite. Tissue uptake highest in bone marrow, skin, GI mucosa, salivary glands. Following administration, distribution half-life <1 min. Less than 10% remains in plasma 6 min after drug administration.

ACTION/*THERAPEUTIC EFFECT*
Converted by alkaline phosphatase in tissues, allowing its ability to protect normal tissue rel-

ative to tumor tissue, *reducing the toxic effect of chemotherapeutic agent, cisplatin.*

USES / UNLABELED

Reduces cumulative renal toxicity associated w/repeated administration of cisplatin in those w/advanced ovarian cancer. Treatment of postoperative radiation-induced dry mouth in pts w/head or neck cancer. *Protects lung fibroblasts from damaging effects of chemotherapeutic agent paclitaxel.*

STORAGE / HANDLING

Reconstituted solution stable for 5 hrs at room temperature, 24 hrs under refrigeration. Do not use if discolored or contains particulate matter.

IV ADMINISTRATION

1. Reconstitute with 9.5 ml 0.9% NaCl.

2. Further dilute w/0.9% NaCl for a concentration of 5–40 mg/ml.

3. Administer over 15 min (30 min prior to chemotherapy).

4. If hypotension requires interruption of therapy, place pt in Trendelenburg position, give an infusion of normal saline using a separate IV line.

5. An antiemetic (dexamethasone 20 mg IV) and serotonin $5HT_3$ (receptor antagonist) should be given prior to and concurrently w/amifostine.

INDICATIONS / DOSAGE / ROUTES

Cytoprotective (chemotherapy):
IV Infusion: Adults: 910 mg/m^2 once daily as 15 min infusion, beginning 30 min prior to chemotherapy (15 min infusion is better tolerated than extended infusions). If full dose cannot be administered, dose for subsequent cycles should be 740 mg/m^2.

Treatment of dry mouth:
IV Infusion: Adults: 200 mg/m^2 once daily as 3-min infusion, starting 15–30 min before radiation therapy.

PRECAUTIONS

CONTRAINDICATIONS: Sensitivity to aminothiol compounds or mannitol. **EXTREME CAUTION:** Uncorrected dehydration or hypotensive pts, those receiving antihypertensive therapy that cannot be interrupted prior to 24 hrs before amifostine treatment, preexisting cardiovascular or cerebrovascular conditions, i.e., ischemic heart disease, arrhythmias, CHF, history of stroke or TIA, pts receiving chemotherapy for malignancies that are potentially curable (e.g., certain malignancies of germ cell origin). **CAUTIONS:** Safety not established in elderly >70 yrs. **PREGNANCY/LACTATION:** Unknown if drug causes fetal harm or can affect reproduction capacity. Unknown if distributed in breast milk. Recommended not to breast-feed during therapy. **Pregnancy Category C**.

INTERACTIONS

DRUG INTERACTIONS: Pts receiving antihypertensive medication or drugs that may potentiate hypotension. **ALTERED LAB VALUES:** May reduce calcium serum levels, esp. those w/nephrotic syndrome.

SIDE EFFECTS

FREQUENT: Transient reduction in B/P (62% of pts), w/onset 14 min into infusion, lasts about 6 min. B/P generally returns to normal in 5–15 min, severe nausea, vomiting. **OCCASIONAL (10–20%):** Flushing/feeling of warmth or chills/feeling of coldness, dizziness, hiccups, sneezing, somnolence. **RARE (<1%):** Clinically relevant hypocalcemia, mild skin rash.

ADVERSE REACTIONS/TOXIC EFFECTS

A pronounced drop in B/P may require temporary cessation of amifostine.

NURSING IMPLICATIONS

BASELINE ASSESSMENT:

Be sure pt is adequately hydrated prior to infusion. Pt should maintain supine position during the infusion. Monitor B/P q5 min during infusion. Interrupt infusion if systolic B/P decreases significantly from baseline (for baseline of <100, B/P drop by 20 mm Hg; for baseline of 100–119, a drop by 25 mm Hg; for baseline of 120–139, a drop by 30 mm Hg; for baseline of 140–179, a drop by 40 mm Hg; for baseline of >180, a drop by 50 mm Hg). If B/P returns to normal within 5 min and pt appears asymptomatic, begin infusion again so full dose can be administered.

INTERVENTION/EVALUATION:

Carefully monitor pt for fluid balance, adequate hydration. Monitor serum calcium levels in those at risk of hypocalcemia (nephrotic syndrome). Monitor B/P every 5 min during infusion.

amikacin sulfate

am-ih-**kay**-sin
(Amikin)

CANADIAN AVAILABILITY:
Amikin

CLASSIFICATION

Antibiotic: Aminoglycoside

AVAILABILITY (Rx)

Injection: 50 mg/ml, 250 mg/ml

PHARMACOKINETICS

Rapid, complete absorption after IM administration. Widely distributed (does not cross blood-brain barrier, low concentrations in CSF). Excreted unchanged in urine. Removed by hemodialysis. Half-life: 2–4 hrs (increased in decreased renal function, neonates; decreased in cystic fibrosis, burn or febrile pts).

ACTION/*THERAPEUTIC EFFECT*

Irreversibly binds to protein on bacterial ribosome, *interfering in protein synthesis of susceptible microorganisms.*

USES

Treatment of skin/skin structure, bone, joint, respiratory tract, intra-abdominal and complicated urinary tract infections; postop, burns, septicemia, meningitis.

STORAGE/HANDLING

Store vials at room temperature. Solutions appear clear but may become pale yellow (does not affect potency). Intermittent IV infusion (piggyback) stable for 24 hrs at room temperature. Discard if precipitate forms or dark discoloration occurs.

IM/IV ADMINISTRATION

Note: Coordinate peak and trough lab draws w/administration times.

IM:

To minimize discomfort, give deep IM slowly. Less painful if injected into gluteus maximus rather than lateral aspect of thigh.

IV:

1. Infuse over 30–60 min for adults, older children, and over 60–120 min for infants, young children.

2. Alternating IV sites, use

large veins to reduce risk of phlebitis.

INDICATIONS/DOSAGE/ROUTES

Note: Space doses evenly around the clock. Dosage based on ideal body weight. Peak, trough serum level is determined periodically to maintain desired serum concentrations (minimizes risk of toxicity). *Recommended peak level:* 15–30 mcg/ml; *trough level:* 5–10 mcg/ml.

Uncomplicated urinary tract infections:
IM/IV: Adults, elderly: 250 mg q12h.

Moderate to severe infections:
IM/IV: Adults, elderly, children: 15 mg/kg/day in divided doses q8–12h. Do not exceed 15 mg/kg or 1.5 g/day. **Neonates: Loading dose:** 10 mg/kg, then 7.5 mg/kg q12h.

Dosage in renal impairment:
Dose and/or frequency is modified based on degree of renal impairment, serum concentration of drug. After loading dose of 5–7.5 mg/kg, maintenance dose/frequency based on serum creatinine or creatinine clearance.

PRECAUTIONS

CONTRAINDICATIONS: Sulfite sensitivity (may result in anaphylaxis, especially in asthmatics). **CAUTIONS:** Possible cross-sensitivity to other aminoglycosides. Elderly, neonates (potential for renal insufficiency or immaturity); neuromuscular disorders (potential for respiratory depression), prior hearing loss, vertigo, renal impairment. **PREGNANCY/LACTATION:** Readily crosses placenta; unknown if distributed in breast milk. May produce fetal nephrotoxicity. **Pregnancy Category C.**

INTERACTIONS

DRUG INTERACTIONS: Other aminoglycosides, nephrotoxic- and ototoxic-producing medications may increase toxicity. May increase effects of neuromuscular blocking agents. **ALTERED LAB VALUES:** May increase BUN, SGPT (ALT), SGOT (AST), bilirubin, creatinine, LDH concentrations; may decrease serum calcium, magnesium, potassium, sodium concentrations.

SIDE EFFECTS

FREQUENT: Pain, induration at IM injection site; phlebitis, thrombophlebitis w/IV administration. **OCCASIONAL:** Hypersensitivity reactions (rash, fever, urticaria, pruritus). **RARE:** Neuromuscular blockade (difficulty breathing, drowsiness, weakness).

ADVERSE REACTIONS/TOXIC EFFECTS

Frequently occurring nephrotoxicity (evidenced by increased BUN and serum creatinine, decreased creatinine clearance) may be reversible if drug stopped at first sign of symptoms; irreversible ototoxicity (tinnitus, dizziness, ringing/roaring in ears, reduced hearing) and neurotoxicity (headache, dizziness, lethargy, tremors, visual disturbances) occur occasionally. Risk is greater w/higher dosages, prolonged therapy. Superinfections, particularly w/fungi, may result from bacterial imbalance.

NURSING IMPLICATIONS

BASELINE ASSESSMENT:

Dehydration must be treated before aminoglycoside therapy. Establish pt's baseline hearing acuity before beginning therapy. Question for history of allergies, especially to aminoglycosides and sulfite. Obtain specimen for culture, sensitivity before giving the first dose (therapy may begin before results are known).

INTERVENTION/EVALUATION:

Monitor I&O (maintain hydration), urinalysis (casts, RBC, WBC, decrease in specific gravity). Monitor results of peak/trough blood tests. Be alert to ototoxic and neurotoxic symptoms (see Adverse Reactions/Toxic Effects). Check IM injection site for pain, induration. Evaluate IV site for phlebitis (heat, pain, red streaking over vein). Assess for skin rash. Assess for superinfection, particularly genital/anal pruritus, changes of oral mucosa, diarrhea. When treating those w/neuromuscular disorders, assess respiratory response carefully.

PATIENT/FAMILY TEACHING:

Continue antibiotic for full length of treatment. Space doses evenly. Discomfort may occur w/IM injection. Notify physician in event of any hearing, visual, balance, urinary problems even after therapy is completed. Do not take other medication w/o consulting physician. Lab tests are essential part of therapy.

---

amiloride hydrochloride

ah-**mill**-or-ride
(Midamor)

FIXED-COMBINATION(S):
W/hydrochlorothiazide, a thiazide diuretic (**Moduretic**)

CANADIAN AVAILABILITY:
Midamor

CLASSIFICATION

Diuretic: Potassium-sparing

AVAILABILITY (Rx)

Tablets: 5 mg

PHARMACOKINETICS

	ONSET	PEAK	DURATION
PO	2 hrs	6–10 hrs	24 hrs

Incompletely absorbed from GI tract. Primarily excreted in urine; partially eliminated in feces. Half-life: 6–9 hrs.

ACTION/THERAPEUTIC EFFECT

Directly interferes w/sodium reabsorption in distal tubule, *increasing sodium and water excretion and decreasing potassium excretion.* Initial decrease in B/P occurs by decreasing plasma and extracellular fluid volume.

USES/UNLABELED

Adjunctive therapy in treatment of diuretic-induced hypokalemia in those w/CHF or hypertension. Used when maintenance of serum potassium levels is necessary (digitalized patients, cardiac arrhythmias). *Reduce lithium-induced polyuria; slow pulmonary function reduction in cystic fibrosis; treatment of edema associated w/CHF, hepatic cirrhosis, nephrotic syndrome; hypertension.*

PO ADMINISTRATION

Give w/food to avoid GI distress.

INDICATIONS/DOSAGE/ROUTES

PO: Adults: Initially, 5 mg daily. May be increased to 10 mg daily, as single dose or in divided doses. If hypokalemia persists, dose may be increased to 15 mg, then to 20 mg, w/electrolyte monitoring.

Usual elderly dosage:
PO: Initially, 5 mg/day or every other day.

PRECAUTIONS

CONTRAINDICATIONS: Serum potassium >5.5 mEq/L, pts on

other potassium-sparing diuretics, anuria, acute or chronic renal insufficiency, diabetic nephropathy. **CAUTIONS:** Those w/BUN >30 mg/dl or serum creatinine >1.5 mg/dl, elderly, debilitated, hepatic insufficiency, those w/cardiopulmonary disease, diabetes mellitus. **PREGNANCY/LACTATION:** Unknown if drug crosses placenta or is distributed in breast milk. **Pregnancy Category B**.

INTERACTIONS

DRUG INTERACTIONS: May decrease effect of anticoagulants, heparin. NSAIDs may decrease antihypertensive effect. ACE inhibitors (e.g., captopril), potassium-containing diuretics, potassium supplements may increase potassium. May decrease lithium clearance, increase toxicity. **ALTERED LAB VALUES:** May increase BUN, calcium excretion, creatinine, glucose, magnesium, potassium, uric acid. May decrease sodium.

SIDE EFFECTS

FREQUENT (3–8%): Headache, nausea, diarrhea, vomiting, decreased appetite. **OCCASIONAL (<3%):** Dizziness, constipation, abdominal pain, weakness, fatigue, cough, impotence. **RARE (<1%):** Tremors, vertigo, confusion, nervousness, insomnia, thirst, dry mouth, heartburn, shortness of breath, increased urination, hypotension, rash.

ADVERSE REACTIONS/TOXIC EFFECTS

Severe hyperkalemia may produce irritability, anxiety, heaviness of legs, paresthesia of hands/face/lips, hypotension, bradycardia, tented T waves, widening of QRS, ST depression.

NURSING IMPLICATIONS
BASELINE ASSESSMENT:

Assess baseline electrolytes, particularly for low potassium. Assess renal/hepatic functions. Assess edema (note location, extent), skin turgor, mucous membranes for hydration status. Assess muscle strength, mental status. Note skin temperature, moisture. Obtain baseline weight. Initiate strict I&O. Note pulse rate/regularity.

INTERVENTION/EVALUATION:

Monitor B/P, vital signs, electrolytes (particularly potassium), I&O, weight. Note extent of diuresis. Watch for changes from initial assessment; hyperkalemia may result in muscle strength changes, tremor, muscle cramps, change in mental status (orientation, alertness, confusion), cardiac arrhythmias. Monitor potassium level, particularly during initial therapy. Weigh daily. Assess lung sounds for rales, wheezing.

PATIENT/FAMILY TEACHING:

Expect increase in volume and frequency of urination. Therapeutic effect takes several days to begin and can last for several days when drug is discontinued. High potassium diet/potassium supplements can be dangerous, especially if pt has renal/hepatic problems. Avoid foods high in potassium such as whole grains (cereals), legumes, meat, bananas, apricots, orange juice, potatoes (white, sweet), raisins. Contact physician if confusion, irregular heartbeat, nervousness, numbness of hands/feet/lips, difficulty breathing, unusual tiredness, weakness in legs occurs (hyper-kalemia).

aminocaproic acid

ah-meen-oh-kah-**pro**-ick
(**Amicar**)

CANADIAN AVAILABILITY: Amicar

CLASSIFICATION

Antifibrinolytic, antihemorrhagic

AVAILABILITY (Rx)

Tablets: 500 mg. **Syrup:** 250 mg/5 ml. **Injection:** 250 mg/ml.

PHARMACOKINETICS

Rapidly absorbed. Primarily excreted in urine.

ACTION/ *THERAPEUTIC EFFECT*

Inhibits activation of plasminogen, preventing an enzyme (plasmin), *preventing fibrin clots from forming.*

USES/ *UNLABELED*

Treatment of excessive bleeding from hyperfibrinolysis or urinary fibrinolysis. Use only in acute life-threatening situations. *Prevents reoccurrence of subarachnoid hemorrhage. Prevents hemorrhage in hemophiliacs following dental surgery.*

PO/IV ADMINISTRATION

PO:

1. Scored tablets may be crushed.

2. May take w/o regard to food.
3. Syrup used by pts unable to take tablets.

IV:

1. Give only by IV infusion.
2. Dilute each 1 g with up to 50 ml 5% dextrose, 0.9% NaCl, or other compatible solution.
3. Monitor for hypotension during infusion. Rapid infusion may produce bradycardia, arrhythmias.

INDICATIONS/DOSAGE/ROUTES

Note: Reduce dosage in presence of cardiac, renal, or hepatic impairment.

Acute bleeding:
PO/IV Infusion: **Adults, elderly:** Initially, 4–5 g over 1 hr, then 1–1.25 g/hr. Continue for 8 hrs or until bleeding is controlled. **Maximum:** Up to 30 g/24 hrs.

Chronic bleeding:
PO: **Adults, elderly:** 5–30 g/day, in divided doses at 3–6 hr intervals.

PRECAUTIONS

CONTRAINDICATIONS: Evidence of active intravascular clotting process, disseminated intravascuar coagulation w/o concurrent heparin therapy, hematuria of upper urinary tract origin (unless benefits outweigh risk). *Parenteral:* Newborns. **EXTREME CAUTION:** Impaired cardiac, hepatic, or renal disease, those w/hyperfibrinolysis. **PREGNANCY/LACTATION:** Unknown if drug crosses placenta or is distributed in breast milk. **Pregnancy Category C.**

INTERACTIONS

DRUG INTERACTIONS: None significant. **ALTERED LAB VALUES:** May elevate serum potassium level.

SIDE EFFECTS

OCCASIONAL: Nausea, diarrhea, cramps, decreased urination, decreased B/P, dizziness, headache, muscle fatigue/weakness (myopathy), bloodshot eyes.

ADVERSE REACTIONS/TOXIC EFFECTS

Too rapid IV administration produces tinnitus, skin rash, arrhythmias, unusual tiredness, weakness. Rarely, grand mal seizure occurs, generally preceded by weakness, dizziness, headache.

NURSING IMPLICATIONS

INTERVENTION/EVALUATION:

Monitor serum creatine kinase in those undergoing long-term therapy. If increase is noted in serum creatine kinase test, drug should be discontinued. Question any change in skeletal strength as noted by pt (consider possibility of cardiac damage as a result). Skeletal myopathy characterized by increase in creatine kinase, aldolase, and SGOT (AST) serum levels. Monitor these lab results frequently. Monitor heart rhythm. Assess for decrease in B/P, increase in pulse rate, abdominal or back pain, severe headache (may be evidence of hemorrhage). Assess peripheral pulses, skin for bruises, petechiae. Question for increase in amount of discharge during menses. Check for excessive bleeding from minor cuts, scratches. Assess gums for erythema, gingival bleeding. Assess urine output for hematuria.

PATIENT/FAMILY TEACHING:

Use electric razor, soft toothbrush to prevent bleeding. Report any sign of red/dark urine, black/red stool, coffee-ground vomitus, red-speckled mucus from cough. Do not use any OTC medication w/o physician approval (may interfere w/platelet aggregation).

aminolevulinic acid
(Levulan)
See Supplement

aminophylline (theophylline ethylenediamine)
am-in-**ah**-phil-lin
(Aminophylline, Phyllocontin)

theophylline
Immediate-release: **Aerolate, Slo-Phyllin, Theolair.** Extended-release: **Slo-Bid, Theo-Dur, Theo-24, Uni-Dur, Uniphyl**

CANADIAN AVAILABILITY:
Aminophylline: **Phyllocontin;** theophylline: **Theo-Dur, Theolair, Uniphyl**

CLASSIFICATION

Bronchodilator

AVAILABILITY (Rx)

Capsules (immediate-release): 100 mg, 200 mg. **Capsules (extended-release):** 50 mg, 60 mg, 75 mg, 100 mg, 125 mg, 200 mg, 250 mg, 300 mg. **Tablets (immediate-release):** 100 mg, 125 mg, 200 mg, 250 mg, 300 mg. **Tablets (extended-release):** 100 mg, 200 mg, 250 mg, 300 mg, 400 mg, 450 mg, 500 mg. **Elixir:** 80

mg/15 ml. **Solution:** 80 mg/15 ml, 150 mg/15 ml. **Syrup:** 80 mg/15 ml, 150 mg/15 ml. **Injection:** 25 mg/ml.

PHARMACOKINETICS

Well absorbed from GI tract (absorption may vary w/dosage form used). Metabolized in liver. Excreted in urine. Half-life: dependent on age, liver, cardiac function, lung disease, smoking.

ACTION/THERAPEUTIC EFFECT

Directly relaxes smooth muscle of bronchial airway, pulmonary blood vessels, *relieving bronchospasm, increasing vital capacity. Produces cardiac, skeletal muscle stimulation.*

USES/UNLABELED

Symptomatic relief, prevention of bronchial asthma, reversible bronchospasm due to chronic bronchitis, emphysema, or COPD. *Treatment of apnea in neonates.*

STORAGE/HANDLING

Store solution, suppositories at room temperature. Discard if solution contains a precipitate.

PO/IV ADMINISTRATION

PO:

1. Give w/food to avoid GI distress.
2. Do not crush or break extended-release forms.

IV:

1. Give loading dose diluted in 100–200 ml of 5% dextrose or 0.9% NaCl. Maintenance dose in larger volume parenteral infusion.
2. Do not exceed flow rate of 1 ml/min (25 mg/min) for either piggyback or infusion.
3. Administer loading dose over 20–30 min.

4. Use infusion pump or microdrip to regulate IV administration.

INDICATIONS/DOSAGE/ROUTES

Note: Dosage calculated on basis of lean body weight. Dosage based on peak serum theophylline concentrations, clinical condition, presence of toxicity.

Chronic bronchospasm:
PO: Adults, elderly, children: Initially, 16 mg/kg or 400 mg/day (whichever is less) in 2–4 divided doses (6–12 hr intervals). May increase by 25% every 2–3 days up to maximum of 24 mg/kg/day **(1–9 yrs);** 20 mg/kg/day **(9–12 yrs);** 18 mg/kg/day **(12–16 yrs);** 13 mg/kg/day **(>16 yrs).** Doses above maximum based on serum theophylline concentrations, clinical condition, presence of toxicity.

Acute bronchospasm in pts not currently on theophylline:
IV Loading Dose: Adults, children (>1 yr): Initially, 6 mg/kg (aminophylline), then begin maintenance aminophylline dosage based on patient group.

PT GROUP	MAINTENANCE AMINOPHYLLINE DOSAGE
Neonates	0.2 mg/kg/hr
Children (1–12 mo)	0.2–0.9 mg/kg/hr
Children (1–9 yrs)	1–1.2 mg/kg/hr
Children (9–16 yrs), young adult smokers	0.8–1 mg/kg/hr
Older pts, pts w/cor pulmonale	0.3–0.6 mg/kg/hr
Pts w/CHF, liver disease	0.1–0.5 mg/kg/hr

PO/Loading Dose: Adults, children >1 yr: Initially, 5 mg/kg (theophylline), then begin maintenance theophylline dosage based on patient group.

PT GROUP	MAINTENANCE THEOPHYLLINE DOSAGE
Children (1–9 yrs)	4 mg/kg q6h
Children (9–16 yrs), young adult smokers	3 mg/kg q6h
Healthy, non-smoking adults	3 mg/kg q8h
Older pts, pts w/cor pulmonale	2 mg/kg q8h
Pts w/CHF, liver disease	1–2 mg/kg q12h

Acute bronchospasm in patients currently on theophylline:
IV/PO: Adults, children >1 yr: Obtain serum theophylline level. If not possible and pt in respiratory distress and not experiencing toxicity, may give 2.5 mg/kg dose. **Maintenance:** Dosage based on peak serum theophylline concentrations, clinical condition, presence of toxicity.

PRECAUTIONS

CONTRAINDICATIONS: History of hypersensitivity to xanthine, caffeine. **CAUTIONS:** Impaired cardiac, renal, or hepatic function, hypertension, hyperthyroidism, diabetes mellitus, peptic ulcer, glaucoma, severe hypoxemia, underlying seizure disorder. **PREGNANCY/LACTATION:** Readily crosses placenta; distributed in breast milk. May inhibit uterine contractions; produce irritability in nursing infants. **Pregnancy Category C**.

INTERACTIONS

DRUG INTERACTIONS: Glucocorticoids may produce hypernatremia. Phenytoin, primidone, rifampin may increase metabolism. Beta blockers may decrease effects. Cimetidine, ciprofloxacin, erythromycin, norfloxacin may increase concentration, toxicity. Smoking may decrease concentration. **ALTERED LAB VALUES:** None significant.

SIDE EFFECTS

FREQUENT: Momentary change in sense of smell during IV administration; shakiness, restlessness, tachycardia, trembling. **OCCASIONAL:** Heartburn, vomiting, headache, mild diuresis, insomnia, nausea.

ADVERSE REACTIONS/TOXIC EFFECTS

Too rapid rate of IV administration may produce marked fall in B/P w/accompanying faintness and lightheadedness, palpitations, tachycardia, hyperventilation, nausea, vomiting, angina-like pain, seizures, ventricular fibrillation, cardiac standstill.

NURSING IMPLICATIONS
BASELINE ASSESSMENT:

Offer emotional support (high incidence of anxiety due to difficulty in breathing and sympathomimetic response to drug). Peak serum concentration should be taken 1 hr after IV, 1–2 hrs following immediate-release dose, 3–8 hrs following extended-release. Take trough level just before next dose.

INTERVENTION/EVALUATION:

Monitor rate, depth, rhythm, type of respiration; quality and rate of pulse. Assess lung sounds for rhonchi, wheezing, rales. Monitor arterial blood gases. Observe lips, fingernails for blue or dusky color in light-skinned pts; gray in dark-skinned pts. Observe for clavicular retractions, hand tremor. Evaluate for clinical improvement (quieter, slower respirations, relaxed facial expression, cessation of clavicular retractions). Monitor theophylline blood serum levels (therapeutic serum level range: 10–20 mcg/ml).

PATIENT/FAMILY TEACHING:

Increase fluid intake (decreases lung secretion viscosity). Avoid excessive use of caffeine derivatives (chocolate, coffee, tea, cola, cocoa). Smoking, charcoal-broiled food, high-protein, low-carbohydrate diet may decrease theophylline level. Notify physician if nausea, vomiting, insomnia, nervousness, headache, rash, GI pain, seizures, irregular heartbeat occur.

amiodarone hydrochloride

ah-me-**oh**-dah-roan
(Cordarone, Pacerone)

CANADIAN AVAILABILITY:
Cordarone

CLASSIFICATION

Antiarrhythmic

AVAILABILITY (Rx)

Tablets: 200 mg. **Injection:** 50 mg/ml.

PHARMACOKINETICS

Slowly, variably absorbed from GI tract. Extensively metabolized in liver to active metabolite. Excreted via bile; not removed by hemodialysis. Half-life: 26–107 days; metabolite: 61 days.

ACTION/*THERAPEUTIC EFFECT*

Prolongs myocardial cell action potential duration and refractory period by direct action on all cardiac tissue, *decreasing AV conduction, sinus node function.*

USES/*UNLABELED*

Treatment of documented, life-threatening, recurrent ventricular fibrillation, and recurrent, hemodynamically unstable ventricular tachycardia in those who have not responded adequately to other antiarrhythmic agents. *Treatment/prophylaxis of supraventricular arrhythmias refractory to conventional treatment.*

PO/IV ADMINISTRATION

PO:

1. Give w/meals to reduce GI distress.
2. Tablets may be crushed.

IV:

1. Administer through central venous catheter (CVC) if possible, using in-line filter.
2. Use w/5% dextrose using polyolefin, glass container.
3. Infusions >1 hr, concentration not to exceed 2 mg/ml (unless CVC used).
4. Does not need protection from light during administration.

INDICATIONS/DOSAGE/ROUTES

Life-threatening ventricular arrhythmias:
PO: Adults, elderly: Initially, 800–1,600 mg/day in 1–2 divided doses for 1–3 wks. After arrhythmias controlled or side effects occur, reduce to 600–800 mg/day for about 4 wks. **Maintenance:** 200–600 mg/day.
IV Infusion: Adults: Initially, 1,050 mg over 24 hrs: 150 mg over 10 min, follow by 360 mg over 6 hrs, follow by 540 mg over 18 hrs. May continue at 0.5 mg/min up to 2–3

wks regardless of age, renal or left ventricular function.

PRECAUTIONS

CONTRAINDICATIONS: Severe sinus-node dysfunction, second- and third-degree AV block, bradycardia-induced syncope (except in presence of pacemaker), severe hepatic disease. **CAUTIONS:** Thyroid disease. **PREGNANCY/LACTATION:** Crosses placenta; distributed in breast milk. May adversely affect fetal development. **Pregnancy Category C.**

INTERACTIONS

DRUG INTERACTIONS: May increase cardiac effects w/other antiarrhythmics. May increase effect of beta-blockers, oral anticoagulants. May increase concentration, toxicity of digoxin, phenytoin. **ALTERED LAB VALUES:** May increase SGOT (AST), SGPT (ALT), alkaline phosphatase, ANA titer. May cause changes in EKG, thyroid function tests.

SIDE EFFECTS

Corneal microdeposits are noted in almost all pts treated for >6 months (can lead to blurry vision). **FREQUENT (>3%):** *Parenteral:* Hypotension, nausea, fever, bradycardia. *Oral:* Constipation, headache, decreased appetite, nausea, vomiting, numbness of fingers/toes, photosensitivity, muscular incoordination. **OCCASIONAL (<3%):** *Oral:* Bitter/metallic taste, decreased sexual ability/interest, dizziness, facial flushing, blue-gray coloring of skin of face, arms, neck, blurred vision, slow heartbeat, asymptomatic corneal deposits. **RARE (<1%):** *Oral:* Skin rash, vision loss, blindness.

ADVERSE REACTIONS/TOXIC EFFECTS

Serious, potentially fatal pulmonary toxicity (alveolitis, pulmonary fibrosis, pneumonitis, adult respiratory distress syndrome) may begin w/progressive dyspnea and cough w/rales, decreased breath sounds, pleurisy. CHF, hepatotoxicity may be noted. May worsen existing arrhythmias or produce new arrhythmias.

NURSING IMPLICATIONS

BASELINE ASSESSMENT:

Obtain baseline pulmonary function tests, chest x-ray, liver enzyme tests, SGOT (AST), SGPT (ALT), alkaline phosphatase. Assess B/P, apical pulse immediately before drug is administered (if pulse is 60/min or below, or systolic B/P is below 90 mm Hg, withhold medication, contact physician).

INTERVENTION/EVALUATION:

Monitor for symptoms of pulmonary toxicity (progressively worsening dyspnea, cough). Dosage should be discontinued or reduced if toxicity occurs. Assess pulse for strength/weakness, irregular rate, bradycardia. Monitor EKG for cardiac changes, particularly widening of QRS, prolongation of PR and QT intervals. Notify physician of any significant interval changes. Assess for nausea, fatigue, paresthesia, tremor. Monitor for signs of hypothyroidism (periorbital edema, lethargy, pudgy hands/feet, cool/pale skin, vertigo, night cramps) and hyperthyroidism (hot/dry skin, bulging eyes [exophthalmos], frequent urination, eyelid edema, weight loss, breathlessness). Monitor SGOT (AST), SGPT (ALT), alkaline phosphatase for evidence of liver toxicity. Assess skin, cornea for bluish discoloration in those who have been on drug therapy longer than 2 mos. Monitor liver function tests, thyroid test results. If elevated liver enzymes, dose reduction or discontinuation is evident. Monitor for therapeutic serum level (1.5–2.5 mcg/ml).

PATIENT/FAMILY TEACHING:

Protect against photosensitivity reaction on skin exposed to sunlight. Bluish skin discoloration gradually disappears when drug is discontinued. Report shortness of breath, cough. Outpatients should monitor pulse before taking medication. Do not abruptly discontinue medication. Compliance w/therapy regimen is essential to control arrhythmias. Do not use nasal decongestants, over-the-counter preparations (stimulants) w/o physician approval. Restrict salt, alcohol intake. Recommend ophthalmic exams every 6 months. Report any vision changes.

amitriptyline hydrochloride

a-me-**trip**-tih-leen
(Elavil, Endep)

FIXED-COMBINATION(S):
W/chlordiazepoxide, an antianxiety (**Limbitrol**); w/perphenazine, an antipsychotic (**Etrafon, Triavil**)

CANADIAN AVAILABILITY:
Apo-Amitriptyline, Elavil

CLASSIFICATION

Antidepressant: Tricyclic

AVAILABILITY (Rx)

Tablets: 10 mg, 25 mg, 50 mg, 75 mg, 100 mg, 150 mg. **Injection:** 10 mg/ml.

PHARMACOKINETICS

Rapid, well absorbed from GI tract. Metabolized in liver, undergoes first pass metabolism. Primarily excreted in urine. Minimal removal by hemodialysis. Half-life: 10–26 hrs.

ACTION/*THERAPEUTIC EFFECT*

Blocks reuptake of neurotransmitters (norepinephrine, serotonin) at presynaptic membranes, increasing synaptic concentration at postsynaptic receptor sites, *resulting in antidepressant effect.* Has strong anticholinergic activity.

USES/*UNLABELED*

Treatment of various forms of depression, exhibited as persistent, prominent dysphoria (occurring nearly every day for at least 2 wks) manifested by 4 of 8 symptoms: appetite change, sleep pattern change, increased fatigue, impaired concentration, feelings of guilt or worthlessness, loss of interest in usual activities, psychomotor agitation or retardation, suicidal tendencies. *Relieves neuropathic pain (e.g., diabetic neuropathy, postherpetic neuralgia, treatment of bulimia nervosa).*

STORAGE/HANDLING

Store parenteral form at room temperature. Protect from light (precipitate may form). Store tablets at room temperature.

PO/IM ADMINISTRATION

PO:
Give w/food or milk if GI distress occurs.

IM:
1. Give by IM only if oral administration is not feasible.
2. Crystals may form in injection. Redissolve by immersing ampule in hot water for 1 min.

3. Give deep IM slowly.

INDICATIONS/DOSAGE/ROUTES

Note: May give entire daily oral dose at one time (preferably bedtime).

Inpatient:
PO: Adults: Initially, 75–100 mg/day in 1–4 divided doses. Gradually increase by 25–50 mg increments to maximum of 300 mg/day, then reduce slowly to minimum therapeutic level. **Elderly, adolescents:** Initially, 10 mg 3 times/day, plus 20 mg at bedtime. **Maintenance:** 40–100 mg/day. **IM: Adults:** 20–30 mg 4 times/day.

Outpatient:
PO: Adults: Initially, 50–100 mg/day. May be gradually increased to 150 mg/day. **Elderly, adolescents:** 10 mg 3 times/day, plus 20 mg at bedtime. Dosage should be gradually reduced to minimum therapeutic level (therapeutic effect noted in 2–4 wks).

Usual elderly dosage:
PO: Initially, 10–25 mg at bedtime; increase at weekly intervals of 10–25 mg. **Range:** 25–150 mg/day.

PRECAUTIONS

CONTRAINDICATIONS: Acute recovery period following MI, within 14 days of MAO inhibitor ingestion. **CAUTIONS:** Prostatic hypertrophy, history of urinary retention or obstruction, glaucoma, diabetes mellitus, history of seizures, hyperthyroidism, cardiac/hepatic/renal disease, schizophrenia, increased intraocular pressure, hiatal hernia. **PREGNANCY/LACTATION:** Crosses placenta; minimally distributed in breast milk. **Pregnancy Category D**.

INTERACTIONS

DRUG INTERACTIONS: CNS depressants (including alcohol, barbiturates, phenothiazines, sedative-hypnotics, anticonvulsants). May increase sedation, respiratory depression, hypotensive effects. Antithyroid agents may increase risk of agranulocytosis. Phenothiazines may increase sedative, anticholinergic effects. Cimetidine, valproic acid may increase concentration, toxicity. May decrease effects of clonidine, guanadrel. May increase cardiac effects w/sympathomimetics. May increase risk of hypertensive crisis, hyperpyretic, convulsions w/MAO inhibitors. **ALTERED LAB VALUES:** May alter EKG readings (flattens T wave), glucose.

SIDE EFFECTS

FREQUENT: Dizziness, drowsiness, dry mouth, orthostatic hypotension, headache, increased appetite/weight, nausea, unusual tiredness, unpleasant taste. **OCCASIONAL:** Blurred vision, confusion, constipation, hallucinations, delayed micturation, eye pain, arrhythmias, fine muscle tremors, Parkinsonian syndrome, nervousness, diarrhea, increased sweating, heartburn, insomnia. **RARE:** Hypersensitivity, alopecia, tinnitus, breast enlargement.

ADVERSE REACTIONS/TOXIC EFFECTS

High dosage may produce confusion, seizures, severe drowsiness, fast/slow/irregular heartbeat, fever, hallucinations, agitation, shortness of breath, vomiting, unusual tiredness/weakness. Abrupt withdrawal from prolonged therapy may produce headache, malaise, nausea, vomiting, vivid dreams. Rarely, blood dyscrasias, cholestatic jaundice noted.

NURSING IMPLICATIONS
BASELINE ASSESSMENT:

Observe/record behavior. Assess psychological status,

thought content, sleep patterns, appearance, interest in environment. For those on long-term therapy, liver/renal function tests, blood counts should be performed periodically.

INTERVENTION/EVALUATION:

Supervise suicidal risk patient closely during early therapy (as depression lessens, energy level improves, increasing suicide potential). Assess appearance, behavior, speech pattern, level of interest, mood. Monitor pattern of daily bowel activity and stool consistency. Monitor B/P, pulse for hypotension, arrhythmias. Assess for urinary retention by bladder palpation.

PATIENT/FAMILY TEACHING:

Change positions slowly to avoid hypotensive effect. Tolerance to postural hypotension, sedative and anticholinergic effects usually develops during early therapy. Maximum therapeutic effect may be noted in 2–4 wks. Sensitivity to sun may occur. Dry mouth may be relieved by sugarless gum or sips of tepid water. Report visual disturbances. Do not abruptly discontinue medication. Avoid tasks that require alertness, motor skills until response to drug is established.

---

amlexanex
(Apthasol)
See Supplement

---

amlodipine
am-**low**-dih-peen
(Norvasc)

FIXED-COMBINATION(S)
W/benazepril, an angiotensin converting enzyme inhibitor (**Lotrel**)

CANADIAN AVAILABILITY:
Norvace

CLASSIFICATION

Calcium channel blocker

AVAILABILITY (Rx)

Tablets: 2.5 mg, 5 mg, 10 mg

PHARMACOKINETICS

	ONSET	PEAK	DURATION
PO	—	—	24 hrs

Slowly absorbed from GI tract. Undergoes first-pass metabolism in liver. Excreted primarily in urine. Half-life: 30–50 hrs (increased in elderly, pts w/hepatic cirrhosis).

ACTION/*THERAPEUTIC EFFECT*

Inhibits calcium movement across cell membranes of cardiac and vascular smooth muscle, *dilates coronary arteries, peripheral arteries/arterioles. Decreases total peripheral vascular resistance by vasodilation.*

USES

Management of hypertension, chronic stable angina, vasospastic (Prinzmetal's or variant) angina. May be used alone or w/other antihypertensives or antianginals.

PO ADMINISTRATION

May take w/o regard to food. Grapefruit juice may increase concentration.

INDICATIONS/DOSAGE/ROUTES

Note: Dosage should be titrated >7–14 days.

Hypertension:
PO: Adults: Initially, 5 mg/day as single dose. **Maximum:** 10 mg/day.

PO: Small frame, fragile, elderly: Initially, 2.5 mg/day as single dose.

Angina (chronic stable or vasospastic):
PO: Adults: 5–10 mg. **Elderly, hepatic insufficiency:** 5 mg.

PRECAUTIONS

CONTRAINDICATIONS: Hypersensitivity to amlodipine, severe hypotension. **CAUTIONS:** Impaired hepatic function, aortic stenosis, congestive heart failure. **PREGNANCY/LACTATION:** Unknown if drug crosses placenta or is distributed in breast milk. **Pregnancy Category C.**

INTERACTIONS

DRUG INTERACTIONS: None significant. **ALTERED LAB VALUES:** None significant.

SIDE EFFECTS

FREQUENT (>5%): Peripheral edema, headache, flushing. **OCCASIONAL (<5%):** Dizziness, palpitations, nausea, unusual tiredness/weakness. **RARE (<1%):** Chest pain, slow heartbeat, orthostatic hypotension.

ADVERSE REACTIONS/TOXIC EFFECTS

Overdosage may produce excessive peripheral vasodilation, marked hypotension w/reflex tachycardia.

NURSING IMPLICATIONS
BASELINE ASSESSMENT:

Assess baseline renal/liver function tests, B/P, and apical pulse.

INTERVENTION/EVALUATION:

Assess B/P (if systolic B/P is below 90 mm Hg, withhold medication, contact physician). Assist w/ambulation if lightheaded-ness, dizziness occurs. Assess for peripheral edema behind medial malleolus (sacral area in bedridden pts). Assess skin for flushing. Monitor liver enzyme tests. Question for headache, asthenia.

PATIENT/FAMILY TEACHING:

Do not abruptly discontinue medication. Compliance w/therapy regimen is essential to control hypertension. To avoid hypotensive effect, rise slowly from lying to sitting position, wait momentarily before standing. Avoid tasks that require alertness, motor skills until response to drug is established. Contact physician/nurse if irregular heartbeat, shortness of breath, pronounced dizziness, or nausea occurs. Avoid concomitant ingestion of grapefruit juice.

---

amoxapine
ah-**mocks**-ah-peen
(Asendin)

CANADIAN AVAILABILITY: Asendin

CLASSIFICATION

Antidepressant: Tricyclic

AVAILABILITY (Rx)

Tablets: 25 mg, 50 mg, 100 mg, 150 mg

PHARMACOKINETICS

Rapid, well absorbed from GI tract. Metabolized in liver, undergoes first-pass metabolism. Primarily excreted in urine. Minimal removal by hemodialysis. Half-life: 8–30 hrs.

ACTION/ *THERAPEUTIC EFFECT*

Blocks reuptake of neurotransmitters (norepinephrine, serotonin) at presynaptic membranes, increasing synaptic concentration at postsynaptic receptor sites, *resulting in antidepressant and antianxiety effect.* Has substantive neuroleptic activity.

USES

Treatment of endogenous depression and anxiety.

PO ADMINISTRATION

Give w/food or milk if GI distress occurs.

INDICATIONS/DOSAGE/ROUTES

Note: May give entire daily dose at one time (preferably bedtime).

PO: Adults: Initially, 50 mg 2–3 times/day. May gradually increase to 200–300 mg/day by end of first wk of therapy. If therapeutic response does not occur by end of 2 wks, may increase dose to maximum 400 mg/day for outpatients. Hospitalized pts w/no history of seizures may receive up to 600 mg/day in divided doses.

Usual elderly dosage:
PO: Initially, 25 mg 2–3 times/day, then increase at 25 mg increments q3days for hospitalized pts; q7days for outpts. **Range:** 50–150 mg/day. **Maximum:** 300 mg/day.

PRECAUTIONS

CONTRAINDICATIONS: Acute recovery period following MI, within 14 days of MAO inhibitor ingestion. **CAUTIONS:** Prostatic hypertrophy, history of urinary retention or obstruction, glaucoma, diabetes mellitus, history of seizures, hyperthyroidism, cardiac/hepatic/renal disease, schizophrenia, increased intraocular pressure, hiatal hernia. **PREGNANCY/LACTATION:** Crosses placenta; is distributed in breast milk. **Pregnancy Category C**.

INTERACTIONS

DRUG INTERACTIONS: CNS depressants (including alcohol, barbiturates, phenothiazines, sedative-hypnotics, anticonvulsants). May increase sedation, respiratory depression, hypotensive effects. Antithyroid agents may increase risk of agranulocytosis. Phenothiazines may increase sedative, anticholinergic effects. Cimetidine may increase concentration, toxicity. May decrease effects of clonidine, guanadrel. May increase cardiac effects w/sympathomimetics. May increase risk of hypertensive crisis, hyperpyretic, convulsions w/MAO inhibitors. **ALTERED LAB VALUES:** May alter EKG readings, glucose.

SIDE EFFECTS

FREQUENT: Dizziness, drowsiness, dry mouth, orthostatic hypotension, headache, increased appetite/weight, nausea, unusual tiredness, unpleasant taste. **OCCASIONAL:** Blurred vision, confusion, constipation, hallucinations, delayed micturation, eye pain, arrhythmias, fine muscle tremors, Parkinsonian syndrome, nervousness, diarrhea, increased sweating, heartburn, insomnia. **RARE:** Hypersensitivity, alopecia, tinnitus, neuroleptic malignant syndrome (convulsions, irregular pulse, fever, altered B/P, diaphoresis, severe muscle stiffness).

ADVERSE REACTIONS/TOXIC EFFECTS

High dosage may produce cardiovascular effects (severe postural hypotension, dizziness, tachycardia, palpitations, arrhythmias, altered temperature regulation).

Abrupt withdrawal from prolonged therapy may produce headache, malaise, nausea, vomiting, vivid dreams. Rarely, blood dyscrasias, cholestatic jaundice noted.

NURSING IMPLICATIONS

BASELINE ASSESSMENT:

For those on long-term therapy, liver/renal function tests, blood counts should be performed periodically.

INTERVENTION/EVALUATION:

Supervise suicidal risk patient closely during early therapy (as depression lessens, energy level improves, increasing suicide potential). Assess appearance, behavior, speech pattern, level of interest, mood. Monitor pattern of daily bowel activity and stool consistency. Monitor B/P, pulse for hypotension, arrhythmias. Assess for urinary retention by bladder palpation.

PATIENT/FAMILY TEACHING:

Change positions slowly to avoid hypotensive effect. Tolerance to postural hypotension, sedative and anticholinergic effects usually develops during early therapy. Therapeutic effect may be noted within 1–2 wks. Dry mouth may be relieved by sugarless gum or sips of tepid water. Report visual disturbances. Do not abruptly discontinue medication. Avoid tasks that require alertness, motor skills until response to drug is established.

---

amoxicillin

ah-**mocks**-ih-sill-in
(Amoxil, Polymox, Trimox, Wymox)

CANADIAN AVAILABILITY:
Amoxil, Apo-Amoxi, Novamoxin

CLASSIFICATION

Antibiotic: Penicillin

AVAILABILITY (Rx)

Tablets (chewable): 125 mg, 200 mg, 250 mg, 400 mg. **Tablets:** 500 mg, 875 mg. **Capsules:** 250 mg, 500 mg. **Powder for Oral Suspension:** 50 mg/ml, 125 mg/5 ml, 200 mg/ml, 250 mg/5 ml, 400 mg/5 ml.

PHARMACOKINETICS

Well absorbed from GI tract. Partially metabolized in liver. Primarily excreted in urine. Removed by hemodialysis. Half-life: 1–1.3 hrs (increased in reduced renal function).

ACTION/THERAPEUTIC EFFECT

Bactericidal in susceptible microorganisms by *inhibition of cell wall synthesis.*

USES/UNLABELED

Treatment of skin/skin structure, respiratory, GI, and genitourinary infections, otitis media, gonorrhea. Treatment of *H. pylori* associated w/peptic ulcer; *Lyme disease; typhoid fever.*

STORAGE/HANDLING

Store capsules, tablets at room temperature. Oral solution, after reconstitution, is stable for 14 days at either room temperature or refrigeration.

PO ADMINISTRATION

1. Give orally w/o regard to meals.
2. Instruct pt to chew or crush chewable tablets thoroughly before swallowing.

INDICATIONS/DOSAGE/ROUTES

Ear, nose, throat, genitourinary, skin/skin structure infections:
PO: **Adults, children >20 kg:** 250–500 mg q8h (or 500–875 mg tablets BID). **Children <20 kg:** 20–40 mg/kg/day in divided doses q8–12h.

Lower respiratory tract infections:
PO: **Adults, children >20 kg:** 500 mg q8h (or 875 mg tablets BID). **Children <20 kg:** 40 mg/kg/day in divided doses q8–12h.

Acute, uncomplicated gonorrhea, epididymo-orchitis:
PO: **Adults:** 3 g one time w/1 g probenecid. Follow w/tetracycline or erythromycin therapy.

Acute otitis media:
PO: **Children:** 80–90 mg/kg/day.

H. pylori:
PO: **Adults (in combination):** 1 g 2 times/day for 10 days.

PRECAUTIONS

CONTRAINDICATIONS: Infectious mononucleosis, hypersensitivity to any penicillin. **CAUTIONS:** History of allergies (especially cephalosporins), antibiotic-associated colitis. **PREGNANCY/LACTATION:** Crosses placenta, appears in cord blood, amniotic fluid. Distributed in breast milk in low concentrations. May lead to allergic sensitization, diarrhea, candidiasis, skin rash in infant. **Pregnancy Category B**.

INTERACTIONS

DRUG INTERACTIONS: Allopurinol may increase incidence of rash. Probenecid may increase concentration, toxicity risk. May decrease effects of oral contraceptives. **ALTERED LAB VALUES:** May increase SGOT (AST), SGPT (ALT), LDH, bilirubin, creatinine, BUN. May cause positive Coombs' test.

SIDE EFFECTS

FREQUENT: GI disturbances (mild diarrhea, nausea or vomiting), headache, oral/vaginal candidiasis. **OCCASIONAL:** Generalized rash, urticaria.

ADVERSE REACTIONS/TOXIC EFFECTS

Superinfections, potentially fatal antibiotic-associated colitis (abdominal cramps, watery severe diarrhea, fever) may result from altered bacterial balance. Severe hypersensitivity reactions including anaphylaxis, acute interstitial nephritis occur rarely.

NURSING IMPLICATIONS

BASELINE ASSESSMENT:

Question for history of allergies, especially penicillins, cephalosporins. Obtain specimen for culture and sensitivity before giving first dose (therapy may begin before results of test are known).

INTERVENTION/EVALUATION:

Hold medication and promptly report rash or diarrhea (w/fever, abdominal pain, mucus and blood in stool may indicate antibiotic-associated colitis). Assess food tolerance. Monitor I&O, urinalysis, renal function tests. Be alert for superinfection: increased fever, sore throat onset, vomiting, diarrhea, black/hairy tongue, ulceration or changes of oral mucosa, anal/genital pruritus.

PATIENT/FAMILY TEACHING:

Continue antibiotic for full length of treatment. Space doses evenly. Take w/meals if GI upset occurs. Thoroughly chew the chewable tablets before swallowing. Notify physician in event of rash, diarrhea, or other new symptom.

amoxicillin/ clavulanate potassium

a-**mocks**-ih-sill-in/klah-view-**lan**-ate

(Augmentin)

CANADIAN AVAILABILITY: Clavulin

CLASSIFICATION

Antibiotic: Penicillin

AVAILABILITY (Rx)

Tablets (chewable): 125 mg, 200 mg, 250 mg, 400 mg. **Tablets:** 250 mg, 500 mg, 875 mg. **Powder for Oral Suspension:** 125 mg/5 ml, 200 mg/5 ml, 250 mg/5 ml, 400 mg/5 ml.

PHARMACOKINETICS

Well absorbed from GI tract. Partially metabolized in liver. Primarily excreted in urine. Removed by hemodialysis. Half-life: 1–1.3 hrs (increased in decreased renal function).

ACTION/ *THERAPEUTIC EFFECT*

Amoxocillin is bactericidal in susceptible microorganisms *by inhibition of cell wall synthesis.* Clavulanate inhibits bacterial beta-lactamase, *protecting amoxicillin from enzymatic degradation.*

USES/ *UNLABELED*

Treatment of skin/skin structure, lower respiratory tract and urinary infections, otitis media, sinusitis. *Treatment of bronchitis, chancroid.*

STORAGE/HANDLING

Store tablets at room temperature. Oral suspension, after reconstitution, is stable for 10 days if refrigerated.

PO ADMINISTRATION

1. Give w/o regard to meals.
2. Instruct pt to chew or crush chewable tablets thoroughly before swallowing.

INDICATIONS/DOSAGE/ROUTES

Note: Dosage expressed in terms of amoxicillin. Alternative dosing in adults: 500–875 mg 2 times/day; in children: 200–400 mg 2 times/day.

Mild to moderate infections:
PO: Adults, elderly, children >40 kg: 250 mg q8h. **Children <40 kg:** 20 mg/kg/day in divided doses q8h.

Respiratory tract infections, severe infections:
PO: Adults, elderly, children >40 kg: 500 mg q8h. **Children <40 kg:** 40 mg/kg/day in divided doses q8h.

Otitis media, sinusitis, lower respiratory tract infections:
PO: Children <40 kg: 40 mg/kg/day in divided doses q8h.

PRECAUTIONS

CONTRAINDICATIONS: Infectious mononucleosis, hypersensitivity to any penicillin. **CAUTIONS:** History of allergies, especially cephalosporins, antibiotic-associated colitis. **PREGNANCY/LACTATION:** Crosses placenta, appears in cord blood, amniotic fluid. Distributed in breast milk in low concentrations. May lead to allergic sensitization, diarrhea, candidiasis, skin rash in infant. **Pregnancy Category B.**

INTERACTIONS

DRUG INTERACTIONS: Allopurinol may increase incidence of rash. Probenecid may increase concentration, toxicity risk. May decrease effects of oral contraceptive. **ALTERED LAB VALUES:** May increase SGOT (AST), SGPT (ALT). May cause positive Coombs' test.

SIDE EFFECTS

FREQUENT: GI disturbances (mild diarrhea, nausea or vomiting), headache, oral/vaginal candidiasis. **OCCASIONAL:** Generalized rash, urticaria.

ADVERSE REACTIONS/TOXIC EFFECTS

Superinfections, potentially fatal antibiotic-associated colitis (abdominal cramps, watery severe diarrhea, fever) may result from altered bacterial balance. Severe hypersensitivity reactions including anaphylaxis, acute interstitial nephritis occur rarely.

NURSING IMPLICATIONS
BASELINE ASSESSMENT:

Question for history of allergies, especially penicillins, cephalosporins. Obtain specimen for culture and sensitivity before giving first dose (therapy may begin before results of test are known).

INTERVENTION/EVALUATION:

Hold medication and promptly report rash (hypersensitivity) or diarrhea (w/fever, abdominal pain, blood and mucus in stool may indicate antibiotic-associated colitis). Assess food tolerance. Monitor I&O, urinalysis, renal function tests. Be alert for superinfection: increased fever, sore throat onset, vomiting, diar-

rhea, black/hairy tongue, ulceration or changes of oral mucosa, anal/genital pruritus.

PATIENT/FAMILY TEACHING:

Space doses evenly. Take antibiotic for full length of treatment. Take w/meals if GI upset occurs. Thoroughly chew the chewable tablets before swallowing. Notify physician in event of rash, diarrhea, or other new symptom.

amphotericin B

am-foe-**tear**-ih-sin
(Abelcet, AmBisome, Amphotec, Fungizone)

CANADIAN AVAILABILITY: Fungizone

CLASSIFICATION

Antifungal

AVAILABILITY (Rx)

Injection: 50 mg, 100 mg (Amphotec). **Suspension for Injection:** 5 mg/ml (lipid complex: Abelcet). **Cream, Lotion, Ointment. Oral Suspension:** 100 mg/ml.

PHARMACOKINETICS

Widely distributed. Metabolic fate unknown. Cleared by nonrenal pathways. Minimal removal by hemodialysis. Half-life: 24 hrs (increased in neonates, children).

ACTION/*THERAPEUTIC EFFECT*

Generally fungistatic but may be fungicidal w/high dosage or very susceptible microorganisms. Binds to sterols in fungal cell membrane, *increasing membrane permeability, allowing loss of potassium, other cellular components.*

USES

Parenteral: Treatment of severe systemic infections/meningitis due to susceptible fungi. Disseminated candidiasis, candidal prophylaxis during immunosuppressive therapy, aspergillosis, histoplasmosis, blastomycosis, coccidioidomycosis, cryptomycosis, sporotrichosis. *Topical:* Treatment of cutaneous/mucocutaneous infections caused by *Candida albicans* (paronychia, oral thrush, perleche, diaper rash, intertriginous candidiasis).

STORAGE/HANDLING

Refrigerate vials (store Amphotec at room temperature). Dilute with D_5W for IV infusion. Solution for IV infusion is stable for 48 hrs (Abelcet: 48 hrs when refrigerated, then 6 hrs at room temperature; AmBisome: 6 hrs). Not necessary to protect IV infusion from light. Discard if precipitate forms.

IV ADMINISTRATION

IV:

1. Give by slow IV infusion. Conventional amphoterecin over 1–6 hrs; Abelcet over 2 hrs (shake contents if infusion >2 hrs); Amphotec over 2–4 hrs; AmBisome over 1 hr.

2. Monitor B/P, temperature, pulse, respirations; assess for adverse reactions q15min ×2, then q30min for 4 hrs of initial infusion.

3. Potential for thrombophlebitis may be less w/use of pediatric scalp vein needles or (w/physician order) adding dilute heparin solution.

4. Observe strict aseptic technique, since no bacteriostatic agent or preservative is present in diluent.

INDICATIONS/DOSAGE/ROUTES

Usual parenteral dosage:

IV Infusion: Adults, elderly: Dosage based on pt tolerance, severity of infection. Initially, 1 mg test dose is given over 20–30 min. If test dose is tolerated, 5 mg dose may be given the same day. Subsequently, increases of 5 mg/dose are made q12–24h until desired daily dose is reached. Alternatively, if test dose is tolerated, a dose of 0.25 mg/kg is given same day; increased to 0.5 mg/kg the second day. Dose increased until desired daily dose reached. **Total Daily Dose:** 1 mg/kg/day up to 1.5 mg/kg every other day. Do not exceed maximum total daily dose of 1.5 mg/kg.

Usual AmBisome dosage:
IV Infusion: Adults, children: 1–5mg/kg over 1 hr.

Usual Amphotec dosage:
IV Infusion: Adults, children: 3–4 mg/kg over 2–4 hrs.

Usual Abelcet dosage:
IV Infusion: Adults, children: 5 mg/kg at rate of 2.5 mg/kg/hr.

Cutaneous infections:
Topical: Adults, elderly, children: Apply liberally and rub in 2–4 times/day.

PRECAUTIONS

CONTRAINDICATIONS: Hypersensitivity to amphotericin B, sulfite. **CAUTIONS:** Renal impairment, in combination w/antineoplastic therapy. Give only for progressive, potentially fatal fungal infection. **PREGNANCY/LACTATION:** Crosses placenta; unknown if distributed in breast milk. **Pregnancy Category B.**

INTERACTIONS

DRUG INTERACTIONS: Steroids may cause severe hypokalemia. Bone marrow depressants may increase anemia. May increase

digoxin toxicity (due to hypo-kalemia). Nephrotoxic medications may increase nephrotoxicity.
ALTERED LAB VALUES: May decrease magnesium, potassium; may increase CPK.

SIDE EFFECTS

Note: Less risk of reaction with Abelcet.
FREQUENT: *Parenteral:* Related reaction (spiking fever, severe chills/rigors, nausea, vomiting, headache, hypotension), indigestion, decreased appetite, diarrhea. **OCCASIONAL:** *Parenteral:* Blurred vision, arrhythmias, hypersensitivity reaction (rash, shortness of breath, wheezing, tightness in chest), numbness in hands/feet, seizures. *Topical:* Local irritation, dry skin. **RARE:** *Topical:* Skin rash.

ADVERSE REACTIONS/TOXIC EFFECTS

Each alternative formulation is less nephrotoxic than conventional amphotericin (Fungizone). Cardiovascular toxicity (hypotension, ventricular fibrillation), anaphylactic reaction occur rarely. Vision and hearing alterations, seizures, hepatic failure, coagulation defects may be noted.

NURSING IMPLICATIONS
BASELINE ASSESSMENT:

Question for history of allergies, especially to amphotericin B, sulfite. Avoid, if possible, other nephrotoxic medications. Confirm that a positive culture or histologic test was performed. Check for/obtain orders to reduce adverse reactions during IV therapy (antipyretics, antihistamines, antiemetics, or small doses of corticosteroids given before or dur-ing amphotericin administration may control reactions).

INTERVENTION/EVALUATION:

Monitor B/P, temperature, pulse, respirations; assess for adverse reactions q15min ×2, then q30min for 4 hrs of initial infusion (fever, shaking, chills, anorexia, nausea, vomiting, abdominal pain). Slow infusion and administer medication for symptomatic relief. For severe reactions or w/o symptomatic relief orders, stop infusion and notify physician immediately. Evaluate IV site for phlebitis (heat, pain, red streaking over vein). Determine pattern of bowel activity and stool consistency. Assess food intake, tolerance. Monitor I&O, renal function tests for nephrotoxicity. Check potassium and magnesium levels, hematologic and hepatic function test results. Assess for bleeding, bruising, soft tissue swelling. *Topical:* Assess for itching, irritation, burning.

PATIENT/FAMILY TEACHING:

Prolonged therapy (weeks or months) is usually necessary. Discomfort may occur at IV site. Notify physician of bleeding, bruising, soft tissue swelling, other new symptom. Fever reaction may decrease w/continued therapy. Muscle weakness may be noted during therapy (due to hypokalemia). *Topical:* Application may cause staining of skin or nails; soap and water or dry cleaning will remove fabric stains. Do not use other preparations or occlusive coverings w/o consulting physician. Keep areas clean, dry; wear light clothing. Separate personal items w/direct contact to area.

ampicillin sodium

amp-ih-**sill**-in
(Omnipen, Polycillin, Principen)

FIXED-COMBINATION(S):
W/probenecid, a uric acid inhibitor
(**Principen w/probenecid, Polycillin PRB, Proambicin**)

CANADIAN AVAILABILITY:
Apo-Ampi, Novo-Ampicillin,
Nu-Ampi

CLASSIFICATION

Antibiotic: Penicillin

AVAILABILITY (Rx)

Capsules: 250 mg, 500 mg.
Powder for Oral Suspension: 125 mg/5 ml, 250 mg/5 ml, 500 mg/5 ml. **Powder for Injection:** 125 mg, 250 mg, 500 mg, 1 g, 2 g.

PHARMACOKINETICS

Moderately absorbed from GI tract. Widely distributed. Partially metabolized in liver. Primarily excreted in urine. Removed by hemodialysis. Half-life: 1–1.5 hrs (increase in impaired renal function).

ACTION / THERAPEUTIC EFFECT

Bactericidal in susceptible microorganisms by *inhibition of cell wall synthesis.*

USES

Treatment of respiratory, GI and GU tract, skin/skin structure, bone and joint infections, otitis media, gonorrhea, endocarditis, meningitis, septicemia, mild to moderate typhoid fever, perioperative prophylaxis.

STORAGE/HANDLING

Store capsules at room temperature. Oral suspension, after reconstituted, is stable for 7 days at room temperature, 14 days if refrigerated. The IV solution, diluted w/0.9% NaCl, is stable for 3 days if refrigerated. If diluted w/5% dextrose, use immediately (drug inactivation). Discard if precipitate forms.

PO/IM/IV ADMINISTRATION

PO:
Give orally 1 hr before or 2 hrs after meals for maximum absorption.

IM:

1. Reconstitute each vial w/sterile water for injection or bacteriostatic water for injection (consult individual vial for specific volume of diluent).
2. Give deeply in large muscle mass.

IV:

1. For IV injection, dilute each vial w/5 ml sterile water for injection (10 ml for 1 and 2 g vials) and give over 3–5 min (10–15 min for 1–2 g dose).
2. For intermittent IV infusion (piggyback), further dilute w/50–100 ml 0.9% NaCl or 5% dextrose, infuse over 20–30 min.
3. Due to potential for hypersensitivity/anaphylaxis, start initial dose at few drops per minute, increase slowly to ordered rate; stay w/pt first 10–15 min, then check q10min.
4. Change to oral route as soon as possible.

INDICATIONS/DOSAGE/ROUTES

Respiratory tract, skin/skin structure infections:
PO: **Adults, elderly, children >20 kg:** 250 mg q6h. **Children <20 kg:** 50 mg/kg/day in divided doses q6h.

IM/IV: Adults, elderly, children >40 kg: 250–500 mg q6h. Children <40 kg: 25–50 mg/kg/day in divided doses q6–8h.

Bacterial meningitis, septicemia:
IM/IV: Adults, elderly: 2 g q4h or 3 g q6h. Children: 100–200 mg/kg/day in divided doses q4h.

Gonococcal infections:
PO: Adults: 3.5 g one time w/1 g probenecid plus tetracycline, erythromycin, or ampicillin.

Perioperative prophylaxis:
IM/IV: Adults, elderly: 2 g 30 min prior to procedure. May repeat in 8 hrs. Children: 50 mg/kg using same dosage regimen.

Usual dosage (neonates):
Note: Higher doses may be needed for neonatal meningitis.
IM/IV: Neonates 7–28 days: 75 mg/kg/day in divided doses q8h up to 200 mg/kg/day in divided doses q6h. Neonates 0–7 days: 50 mg/kg/day in divided doses q12h up to 150 mg/kg/day in divided doses q8h.

PRECAUTIONS

CONTRAINDICATIONS: Infectious mononucleosis, hypersensitivity to any penicillin. CAUTIONS: History of allergies, particularly cephalosporins, antibiotic-associated colitis. PREGNANCY/LACTATION: Readily crosses placenta; appears in cord blood, amniotic fluid. Distributed in breast milk in low concentrations. May lead to allergic sensitization, diarrhea, candidiasis, skin rash in infant. Pregnancy Category B.

INTERACTIONS

DRUG INTERACTIONS: Allopurinol may increase incidence of rash. Probenecid may increase concentration, toxicity risk. May decrease effects of oral contracep-

tive. ALTERED LAB VALUES: May increase SGOT (AST), SGPT (ALT). May cause positive Coombs' test.

SIDE EFFECTS

FREQUENT: Pain at IM injection site, GI disturbances (mild diarrhea, nausea or vomiting), oral/vaginal candidiasis. OCCASIONAL: Generalized rash, urticaria, phlebitis, thrombophlebitis w/IV administration, headache. RARE: Dizziness, seizures esp. w/IV therapy.

ADVERSE REACTIONS/TOXIC EFFECTS

Superinfections, potentially fatal antibiotic-associated colitis (abdominal cramps, watery severe diarrhea, fever) may result from altered bacterial balance. Severe hypersensitivity reactions including anaphylaxis, acute interstitial nephritis occur rarely.

NURSING IMPLICATIONS
BASELINE ASSESSMENT:

Question for history of allergies, esp. penicillins, cephalosporins. Obtain specimen for culture and sensitivity before giving first dose (therapy may begin before results are known).

INTERVENTION/EVALUATION:

Hold medication and promptly report rash (although common w/ampicillin, may indicate hypersensitivity) or diarrhea (w/fever, abdominal pain, mucus and blood in stool may indicate antibiotic-associated colitis). Assess food tolerance. Evaluate IV site for phlebitis (heat, pain, red streaking over vein). Check IM injection site for pain, induration. Monitor I&O, urinalysis, renal function tests. Assess for signs of superinfection: increased fever, sore throat onset, vomiting, diarrhea, anal/genital pruritus, changes in oral mucosa, black/hairy tongue.

PATIENT/FAMILY TEACHING:

Space doses evenly. Take antibiotic for full length of treatment. More effective if taken 1 hr before or 2 hrs after food/beverages. Discomfort may occur w/IM injection. Notify physician of rash, diarrhea, or other new symptom.

ampicillin/sulbactam sodium

amp-ih-**sill**-in/sull-**bak**-tam
(Unasyn)

CLASSIFICATION

Antibiotic: Penicillin

AVAILABILITY (Rx)

Powder for Injection: 1.5 g, 3 g

PHARMACOKINETICS

Moderately absorbed from GI tract. Widely distributed. Partially metabolized in liver. Primarily excreted in urine. Removed by hemodialysis. Half-life: 1 hr (increase in decreased renal function).

ACTION/ *THERAPEUTIC EFFECT*

Ampicillin is bactericidal in susceptible microorganisms *by inhibition of cell wall synthesis.* Sulbactam: inhibits bacterial beta-lactamase, protecting ampicillin from enzymatic degradation.

USES

Treatment of intra-abdominal, skin/skin structure, gynecologic infections.

STORAGE/HANDLING

When reconstituted w/0.9% NaCl, IV solution is stable for 8 hrs at room temperature, 48 hrs if refrigerated. Stability may be different w/other diluents. Discard if precipitate forms.

IM/IV ADMINISTRATION

IM:

1. Reconstitute each 1.5 g vial w/3.2 ml sterile water for injection to provide concentration of 250 mg ampicillin/125 mg sulbactam/ml.
2. Give deeply into large muscle mass within 1 hr after preparation.

IV:

1. For IV injection, dilute w/10–20 ml sterile water for injection. Give slowly over minimum of 10–15 min.
2. For intermittent IV infusion (piggyback) further dilute w/50–100 ml 5% dextrose, or NaCl, infuse over 15–30 min.
3. Alternating IV sites, use large veins to reduce risk of phlebitis.
4. Due to potential for hypersensitivity/anaphylaxis, start initial dose at few drops per min, increase slowly to ordered rate; stay w/pt first 10–15 min, then check q10min.
5. Change to oral antibiotic as soon as possible.

INDICATIONS/DOSAGE/ROUTES

Skin/skin structure, intra-abdominal, gynecologic infections:
IM/IV: Adults, elderly: 1.5 g (1 g ampicillin/500 mg sulbactam) to 3 g (2 g ampicillin/1 g sulbactam) q6h.

Skin/skin structure infections:
IV: Children 1–12 yrs: 300 mg/kg /day in divided doses q6 hrs.

Dosage in renal impairment:
Modification of dose and/or fre-

quency based on creatinine clearance and/or severity of infection.

CREATININE CLEARANCE	DOSAGE
≥30 ml/min	1.5–3 g q6–8h
15–29 ml/min	1.5–3 g q12h
5–14 ml/min	1.5–3 g q24h
<5 ml/min	Not recommended

PRECAUTIONS

CONTRAINDICATIONS: Infectious mononucleosis, hypersensitivity to any penicillin. **CAUTIONS:** History of allergies, particularly to cephalosporins, antibiotic-associated colitis. **PREGNANCY/LACTATION:** Readily crosses placenta; appears in cord blood, amniotic fluid. Distributed in breast milk in low concentrations. May lead to allergic sensitization, diarrhea, candidiasis, skin rash in infant. **Pregnancy Category B.**

INTERACTIONS

DRUG INTERACTIONS: Allopurinol may increase incidence of rash. Probenecid may increase concentration, toxicity risk. May decrease effects of oral contraceptive. **ALTERED LAB VALUES:** May increase SGOT (AST), SGPT (ALT), alkaline phosphatase, LDH, creatinine. May cause positive Coombs' test.

SIDE EFFECTS

FREQUENT: Diarrhea and rash (most common), urticaria, pain at IM injection site; thrombophlebitis w/IV administration; oral/vaginal candidiasis. **OCCASIONAL:** Nausea, vomiting, headache, malaise, urinary retention.

ADVERSE REACTIONS/TOXIC EFFECTS

Severe hypersensitivity reactions, including anaphylaxis, acute interstitial nephritis, blood dyscrasias may be noted. Superinfections, potentially fatal antibiotic-associated colitis (abdominal cramps, watery severe diarrhea, fever) may result from altered bacterial balance. Overdose may produce seizures.

NURSING IMPLICATIONS

BASELINE ASSESSMENT:

Question for history of allergies, esp. penicillins, cephalosporins. Obtain specimen for culture and sensitivity before giving first dose (therapy may begin before results are known).

INTERVENTION/EVALUATION:

Hold medication and promptly report rash (although common w/ampicillin, may indicate hypersensitivity) or diarrhea (w/fever, mucus and blood in stool, abdominal pain may indicate antibiotic-associated diarrhea). Assess food tolerance. Evaluate IV site for phlebitis (heat, pain, red streaking over vein). Check IM injection site for pain, induration. Monitor I&O, urinalysis, renal function tests. Assess for initial signs of superinfection: increased fever, sore throat onset, vomiting, diarrhea, anal/genital pruritus, ulceration or changes of oral mucosa.

PATIENT/FAMILY TEACHING:

Space doses evenly. Take antibiotic for full length of treatment. Discomfort may occur w/IM injection. Notify physician of rash, diarrhea, or other new symptom.

amprenavir
(Agenerase)
See Supplement
See Classification section under:
Human immunodeficiency virus (HIV) infection

anagrelide
(Agrylin)
See Supplement

anastrozole
ah-**nas**-trow-zole
(Arimidex)

CANADIAN AVAILABILITY:
Arimidex

CLASSIFICATION

Antineoplastic; hormone

AVAILABILITY (Rx)

Tablets: 1 mg

PHARMACOKINETICS

Well absorbed into systemic circulation. Food does not affect extent of absorption. Extensively metabolized. Eliminated by hepatic metabolism and, to a lesser extent, renal excretion. Mean half-life: 50 hrs in postmenopausal women. Plasma concentrations reach steady state levels at about 7 days.

ACTION/*THERAPEUTIC EFFECT*

Decreases circulating estrogen by inhibiting aromatase, an enzyme that catalyzes the final step in estrogen production. Since growth of many breast cancers are stimulated by estrogens, *drug significantly lowers serum estradiol (estrogen) concentration.*

USES

Treatment of advanced breast cancer in postmenopausal women who have developed progressive disease while receiving tamoxifen therapy.

INDICATIONS/DOSAGE/ROUTES

Breast cancer:
PO: Adults, elderly: 1 mg once daily.

PRECAUTIONS

CONTRAINDICATIONS: None significant. **CAUTIONS:** None significant. **PREGNANCY/LACTATION:** Crosses placenta, may cause fetal harm. Unknown if excreted in breast milk. **Pregnancy Category D.**

INTERACTIONS

DRUG INTERACTIONS: None significant. **ALTERED LAB VALUES:** May elevate serum GGT level in those w/liver metastases. May increase SGOT (AST), SGPT (ALT), alkaline phosphate, total cholesterol, LDL cholesterol.

SIDE EFFECTS

FREQUENT (8–16%): Asthenia (loss of strength/energy), nausea, headache, pain, hot flashes, dyspnea, vomiting, cough, diarrhea. **OCCASIONAL (2–8%):** Constipation, abdominal pain, decreased appetite, dizziness, rash, dry mouth, depression, peripheral edema.

ADVERSE REACTIONS/TOXIC EFFECTS

Thrombophlebitis, anemia, leukopenia occur rarely.

NURSING IMPLICATIONS
PATIENT/FAMILY TEACHING:

Notify physician if nausea, asthenia, hot flashes become unmanageable.

anistreplase
an-**is**-treh-place
(Eminase)

CANADIAN AVAILABILITY:
Eminase

CLASSIFICATION

Thrombolytic

AVAILABILITY (Rx)

Powder for Injection: 30 units

PHARMACOKINETICS

	ONSET	PEAK	DURATION
IV	—	—	4–6 hrs

Clearance of fibrinolytic activity due to tissue uptake, inactivation by inhibitors, and degradation by circulating antiplasmin. Half-life: 70–120 min.

ACTION/*THERAPEUTIC EFFECT*

Activates fibrinolytic system by cleaving bond in plasminogen-producing plasmin, an enzyme *that degrades fibrin clots, fibrinogen, other plasma proteins.* Acts indirectly by competing w/plasminogen. Converted to plasmin complex, which converts residual plasminogen to plasmin.

USES

Management of acute myocardial infarction (AMI) in adults, lysis of thrombi obstructing coronary arteries, reduces infarct size, improves ventricular function following AMI, reduces mortality associated w/AMI.

STORAGE/HANDLING

Refrigerate powder. Reconstituted solutions are colorless to pale yellow. Once reconstituted, discard solution if not used within 30 min.

IV ADMINISTRATION

1. Reconstitute 30 units vial w/5 ml sterile water for injection (direct fluid against side of vial).

2. Gently roll vial, mixing fluid and powder. Do not shake (minimizes foaming).

3. Give only by IV injection over 2–5 min into IV line or vein.

4. Do not dilute further w/any infusion fluid or add to other medications.

5. If minor bleeding occurs at puncture site, apply pressure for 30 min, then apply pressure dressing.

6. If uncontrolled hemorrhage occurs, discontinue infusion immediately (slowing rate of infusion may produce worsening hemorrhage).

7. Avoid undue pressure when drug is injected into catheter (can rupture catheter or expel clot into circulation).

INDICATIONS/DOSAGE/ROUTES

Management of acute myocardial infarction:
IV: Adults, elderly: 30 units over 2–5 min as soon as possible after onset of symptoms.

PRECAUTIONS

CONTRAINDICATIONS: Active internal bleeding, recent (within 2 mos) cerebrovascular accident, intracranial or intraspinal surgery or trauma, intracranial neoplasm, arteriovenous malformation or aneurysm, bleeding diathesis, severe uncontrolled hypertension. **CAUTIONS:** Recent (10 days) major surgery or GI bleeding, OB delivery, organ biopsy, recent trauma (cardiopulmonary resuscitation), left heart thrombus, endocarditis, severe hepatic or renal disease, pregnancy, elderly, cerebrovascular disease, diabetic retinopathy, thrombophlebitis, occluded AV cannula at infected site. **PREGNANCY/LACTATION:** Use only when benefit outweighs potential risk to fetus. Unknown if drug crosses placenta or is distributed in breast milk. **Pregnancy Category C.**

INTERACTIONS

DRUG INTERACTIONS: Anticoagulants, heparin, NSAIDs, aspirin, other platelet aggregation inhibitors may increase risk of bleeding. Antifibrinolytics (e.g., aminocaproic acid) may decrease effect. Valproic acid may increase risk of hemorrhage. **ALTERED LAB VALUES:** May increase activated partial thromboplastin time (APTT), prothrombin time (PT), thrombin time (TT). May decrease activity of alpha-2 antiplasmin, factor V, VIII, fibrinogen, plasminogen. May decrease hemoglobin, hematocrit.

SIDE EFFECTS

FREQUENT: Superficial or surface bleeding at puncture sites (venous cutdowns; arterial punctures; site of recent surgical intervention; IM, retroperitoneal, or intracerebral site). **OCCASIONAL:** Hypotension, allergic reaction (urticaria, flushing, rash), hematoma, internal bleeding (GI/GU tract, vagina). **RARE:** Severe allergic reactions or anaphylaxis.

ADVERSE REACTIONS/TOXIC EFFECTS

Severe internal hemorrhage (stroke, hemorrhagic, thromboembolic) may occur. Lysis of coronary thrombi may produce atrial or ventricular arrhythmias.

NURSING IMPLICATIONS

BASELINE ASSESSMENT:

Avoid arterial invasive technique before and during treatment. If arterial puncture is necessary, use upper extremity vessels. Assess hematocrit, platelet count, thrombin (TT), activated thromboplastin (APTT), prothrombin time (PT), fibrinogen level before therapy is instituted.

INTERVENTION/EVALUATION:

Handle pt carefully and infrequently as possible to prevent bleeding. Never give via IM injection route. Monitor clinical response, vital signs q4h. Do not obtain B/P in lower extremities (possible deep vein thrombi). Monitor TT, PT, APTT, fibrinogen level q4h after initiation of therapy, stool culture for occult blood. Assess for decrease in B/P, increase in pulse rate, complaint of abdominal or back pain, severe headache (may be evidence of hemorrhage). Question for increase in amount of discharge during menses. Assess area of thromboembolus for color, temperature. Assess peripheral pulses; skin for bruises, petechiae. Check for excessive bleeding from minor cuts, scratches. Assess urine output for hematuria.

antihemophilic factor (factor VIII, AHF)

(AlphaNine SD, Humate P, Koate, Monoclate, ReFacto)

CANADIAN AVAILABILITY: Koate-DVI, Koate-HP, Kogenate

CLASSIFICATION

Hemostatic

AVAILABILITY (Rx)

Injection: 200 IU, 250 IU, 500 IU, 1000 IU, 1250 IU, 1500 IU

PHARMACOKINETICS

Rapidly cleared from plasma. Half-life: 4–14 hrs.

ACTION/*THERAPEUTIC EFFECT*

Assists in conversion of prothrombin to thrombin (essential for blood coagulation), *increasing clotting time*. Replaces missing clotting factor, *correcting or preventing bleeding episodes.*

USES/UNLABELED

Treatment, prevention of bleeding in patients w/hemophilia A factor XIII deficiency, von Willebrand disease, hypofibrinogenemia. *Treatment of disseminated intravascular coagulation (DIC).*

STORAGE/HANDLING

Refrigerate, avoid freezing. After reconstitution, solution is clear, colorless, or yellow. Stable for 24 hrs at room temperature, but use within 1–3 hrs. Do not refrigerate reconstituted solution.

IV ADMINISTRATION

Note: May be given by slow IV injection or infusion.

1. Filter before administration. Use only plastic syringes for IV injection.

2. Warm concentrate and diluent to room temperature.

3. To dissolve, gently agitate or rotate. Do not shake vigorously. Complete dissolution may take 5–10 min.

4. Check pulse rate before and during administration. If pulse rate increases, reduce or stop administration.

5. After administration, apply prolonged pressure on venipuncture site.

6. Monitor IV site for oozing q5–15min for 1–2 hrs after administration.

INDICATIONS/DOSAGE/ROUTES

Note: Dosage is highly individualized, based on patient weight, severity of bleeding, coagulation studies.

Prophylaxis of spontaneous hemorrhage:
IV: **Adults, elderly, children:** 10 AHF/IU/kg as a single infusion.

Moderate hemorrhage, minor surgery:
IV: **Adults, elderly, children:** Initially, 15–25 AHF/IU/kg. **Maintenance:** 10–15 IU/kg q8–12h.

Severe hemorrhage (near vital organ):
IV: **Adults, elderly, children:** Initially, 40–50 AHF/IU/kg. **Maintenance:** 20–25 IU/kg q8–12h.

Major surgery:
IV: **Adults, elderly, children:** 40–50 AHF/IU/kg 1 hr prior to surgery, 20–25 IU/kg 5 hrs later, then 10–15 IU/kg/day for 10–14 days.

Von Willebrand disease:
IV: **Adults:** 40–80 IU/kg q8–12hrs.

PRECAUTIONS

CONTRAINDICATIONS: None significant. **CAUTIONS:** Hepatic disease, those w/blood type A, B, AB. **PREGNANCY/LACTATION:** Unknown if drug crosses placenta or is distributed in breast milk. **Pregnancy Category C**.

INTERACTIONS

DRUG INTERACTIONS: None significant. **ALTERED LAB VALUES:** None significant.

SIDE EFFECTS

OCCASIONAL: Allergic reaction (fever, chills, urticaria [hives], wheezing, slight hypotension, nausea, feeling of chest tightness), stinging at injection site, dizziness, dry mouth, headache, unpleasant taste.

ADVERSE REACTIONS/TOXIC EFFECTS

There is a risk of transmitting viral hepatitis and a slight risk of transmitting AIDS. Possibility of intravascular hemolysis is present if large or frequent doses used in those w/blood group A, B, or AB.

NURSING IMPLICATIONS
BASELINE ASSESSMENT:

When monitoring B/P, avoid overinflation of cuff. Remove adhesive tape from any pressure dressing very carefully and slowly.

INTERVENTION/EVALUATION:

After IV administration, apply prolonged pressure on venipuncture site. Monitor IV site for oozing q5–15min for 1–2 hrs after administration. Assess for allergic reaction (see Side Effects). Report any evidence of hematuria or change in vital signs immediately. Monitor hematocrit, direct antiglobulin (Coombs') test, CBC, urinalysis, PTT, thromboplastin/prothrombin, AHF test results. Assess for decrease in B/P, increase in pulse rate, complaint of abdominal or back pain, severe headache (may be evidence of hemorrhage). Question for increase in amount of discharge during menses. Assess peripheral pulses; skin for bruises, petechiae. Check for excessive bleeding from minor cuts, scratches. Assess gums for erythema, gingival bleeding. Assess urine for hematuria. Evaluate for therapeutic relief of pain, reduction of swelling, and restricted joint movement.

PATIENT/FAMILY TEACHING:

Use electric razor, soft toothbrush to prevent bleeding. Report any sign of red or dark urine, black or red stool, coffee-ground vomitus, red-speckled mucus from cough. Do not use any OTC medication w/o physician approval (may interfere w/platelet aggregation).

antithymocyte globulin
(Atgum)
See Supplement

apraclonidine
(Lopidine)
See Supplement
See Classification section under: Antiglaucoma agents

aprotinin
ah-**pro**-tih-nin
(Trasylol)

CANADIAN AVAILABILITY:
Trasylol

CLASSIFICATION

Antifibrinolytic; antihemorrhagic, natural proteinase inhibitor

AVAILABILITY (Rx)

Injection: 100 ml, 200 ml vial. Supplied as a solution containing 10,000 KIU/ml (equal to 1.4 mg/ml).

PHARMACOKINETICS

Rapidly distributed into extracellular space, primarily kidney. Actively reabsorbed and accumulated by proximal tubules in kidney. Initial half-life approx. 150 min. Five hrs after dosing, terminal elimination phase w/half-life about 10 hrs. Excreted in urine as inactive metabolite > 48 hrs.

ACTION/*THERAPEUTIC EFFECT*

Pts undergoing cardiac surgery w/use of a heart-lung machine normally develop adverse changes in blood components. These changes produce hemostatic defect, generally resulting in diffuse bleeding. Aprotinin inhibits coagulation, *directly preventing fibrinolysis, pre-*

serving platelet function, thereby decreasing bleeding.

USES/*UNLABELED*

For prophylactic, perioperative use to reduce blood loss and need for transfusions in pts undergoing cardiopulmonary bypass in repeat coronary artery bypass graft (CABG) surgery and in primary CABG surgery in pts w/high risk of bleeding (e.g., impaired hemostasis) or where access to blood is unavailable or unacceptable. *For reduction in bleeding and transfusion requirements in liver transplant, total hip replacement, colorectal surgery, peripheral vascular surgery, heart and heart-lung transplant.*

STORAGE/HANDLING

Store vials at room temperature. Discard if precipitate is present or contents appear cloudy. Discard any unused portion in vial.

IV ADMINISTRATION

1. Place pt in supine position.
2. Test dose is required before therapy begins. Give 1 ml test dose IV at least 10 min before loading dose.
3. Administer all aprotinin doses through central line (do not administer any other drug using the same IV line).
4. Give loading dose over 20–30 min after anesthesia induction but before sternotomy (rapid administration can produce fall in B/P). When loading dose is complete, follow by continuous IV infusion until surgery is completed and pt leaves operating room.
5. In those who have previously received aprotinin, after a successful test dose, IV diphenhydramine recommended shortly before loading dose of aprotinin.

INDICATIONS/DOSAGE/ROUTES

Note: Regimen A more effective than Regimen B in pts given aspirin operatively.

Regimen A (high dose):
IV: Adults, elderly: Initially, 2 million KIU loading dose, 2 million KIU into pump prime volume, then continuous IV infusion of 500,000 KIU/hr of operation.

Regimen B (low dose):
IV: Adults, elderly: Initially, 1 million KIU loading dose, 1 million KIU into pump prime volume, then continuous IV infusion of 250,000 KIU/hr of operation.

PRECAUTIONS

CONTRAINDICATIONS: Allergy to aprotinin. **EXTREME CAUTION:** History of allergies, previous aprotinin therapy, those undergoing deep hypothermic circulatory arrest, >65 yrs, surgery of aortic arch. **PREGNANCY/LACTATION:** Unknown if drug crosses placenta or is distributed in breast milk. **Pregnancy Category B.**

INTERACTIONS

DRUG INTERACTIONS: May block hypotensive effect of ACE inhibitors (e.g., captopril), inhibits effects of fibrinolytic agents (alteplase, anistreplase, streptokinase, urokinase), increases effect of heparin (prolonging activated clotting time). **ALTERED LAB VALUES:** Prolongs whole blood clotting time of heparinized blood, significantly prolongs activated clotting time (ACT) and partial thromboplastin time (PTT), increases serum creatine kinase (CK) levels, serum creatinine, serum transaminase.

SIDE EFFECTS

Side effects reported are frequently seen in open-heart surgery and not necessarily attributed to aprotinin.

ADVERSE REACTIONS/TOXIC EFFECTS

Even after uneventful test dose, loading dose may produce anaphylaxis. Stop infusion immediately and initiate emergency treatment for anaphylaxis. Reactions may range from skin eruptions, itching, dyspnea, nausea, tachycardia, hypotension, bronchospasm to full anaphylactic shock, circulatory failure. Treatment: parenteral epinephrine, O_2, parenteral antihistamines, IV corticosteroids, airway management (including intubation).

NURSING IMPLICATIONS

BASELINE ASSESSMENT:

Question pt regarding previous use of aprotinin (increased risk of anaphylactic reaction to drug).

INTERVENTION/EVALUATION:

Monitor lab results frequently. Assess for decrease in B/P, increase in pulse rate, abdominal or back pain, severe headache (may be evidence of hemorrhage). Assess peripheral pulses; skin for bruises, petechiae. Question for increase in amount of discharge during menses. Check for excessive bleeding from minor cuts, scratches. Assess gums for erythema, gingival bleeding. Assess urine output for hematuria.

---

ardeparin
(Normiflo)
See Supplement
See Classification section under: Anticoagulants, Antiplatelets, Thrombolytics

---

artificial tears
(Isopto Tears, Liquifilm Forte, Hypotears, Neo-Tears, Just Tears, Tears Naturale, Lacril, Murocel, Lyteers, Isopto Plain, Ultra Tears, Moisture Drops)

CANADIAN AVAILABILITY:
Tears Naturale

CLASSIFICATION

Tearlike lubricant

AVAILABILITY (OTC)

Ophthalmic Solution: Many strengths

ACTION/*THERAPEUTIC EFFECT*

Stabilizes/thickens precorneal tear film, lengthening tear film breakup time. *Protects and lubricates the eyes.*

USES/*UNLABELED*

Relief of dryness and irritation due to deficient tear production; ocular lubricant for artificial eyes; some products may be used w/hard contact lenses. *Treatment of recurrent corneal erosions, decreased corneal sensitivity.*

STORAGE/HANDLING

Store at room temperature.

INDICATIONS/DOSAGE/ROUTES

Ophthalmic Lubricant: Adults, elderly: 1–2 drops 3–4 times/day as needed.

PRECAUTIONS

CONTRAINDICATIONS: Hypersensitivity to any component of preparation. **PREGNANCY/LACTATION: Pregnancy Category C.**

INTERACTIONS

DRUG INTERACTIONS: None significant. **ALTERED LAB VALUES:** None significant.

SIDE EFFECTS

OCCASIONAL: Eye irritation, blurred vision, stickiness of eyelashes.

NURSING IMPLICATIONS

BASELINE ASSESSMENT:

Determine extent of dryness, irritation.

INTERVENTION/EVALUATION:

Assess therapeutic response, increased irritation or discomfort.

PATIENT/FAMILY TEACHING:

Wash hands thoroughly. Do not touch the tip of the dropper or container to any surface. Cover immediately after administration. Instruct patient on proper instillation. No one else should use the product. Notify physician if condition worsens or redness, irritation is not relieved within 3 days.

ascorbic acid (vitamin C)
(Cecon)

CANADIAN AVAILABILITY: Apo-C, Redoxon

CLASSIFICATION

Vitamin

AVAILABILITY (OTC)

Tablets: 100 mg, 250 mg, 500 mg, 1,000 mg. **Tablets (chewable):** 100 mg, 250 mg, 500 mg. **Tablets (time-release):** 500 mg, 1,000 mg, 1,500 mg. **Capsules (time-release):** 500 mg. **Solution:** 100 mg/ml. **Syrup:** 250 mg/ml. **Injection:** 250 mg/ml, 500 mg/ml.

PHARMACOKINETICS

Readily absorbed from GI tract. Metabolized in liver. Excreted in urine. Removed by hemodialysis.

ACTION/THERAPEUTIC EFFECT

Nutritional supplement necessary for collagen formation, tissue repair, oxidation-reduction reactions. *Involved in metabolism, carbohydrate utilization, synthesis of lipids, proteins, carnitine. Preserves blood vessel integrity.*

USES/UNLABELED

Prophylaxis, treatment of vitamin C deficiency. Increased requirement may be needed in GI disease, malignancy, peptic ulcer, tuberculosis, smokers, oral contraceptive users, hyperthyroidism, prolonged stress, burns, infection, chronic fever, parenteral hyperalimentation, hemodialysis. *Prevention of common cold, urinary acidifier, control idiopathic methemoglobinemia.*

PO/IV ADMINISTRATION

1. Give orally unless infeasible or malabsorption occurs. Incompatible w/potassium penicillin G.

2. Administer IV slowly to avoid dizziness.

INDICATIONS/DOSAGE/ROUTES

Dietary supplement:
PO: Adults, elderly: 45–60 mg/day. **Children >4 yrs:** 30–40 mg/day.

Deficiency:
PO/IM/IV: Adults, elderly: 75–150 mg/day.

Scurvy:
PO: Adults, elderly: 300 mg–1 g/day.

Burns:
PO: Adults, elderly: Up to 2 g/day.

Enhance wound healing:
PO: Adults, elderly: 300–500 mg/day for 7–10 days.

PRECAUTIONS

CONTRAINDICATIONS: None significant. CAUTIONS: Those on sodium restriction, daily salicylate treatment, warfarin therapy, pts w/diabetes mellitus, history of renal stones. PREGNANCY/LACTATION: Crosses placenta, excreted in breast milk. Large doses during pregnancy may produce scurvy in neonates. Pregnancy Category C.

INTERACTIONS

DRUG INTERACTIONS: May increase iron toxicity w/deferoxamine. ALTERED LAB VALUES: May decrease bilirubin, urinary pH. May increase uric acid, urine oxalate.

SIDE EFFECTS

RARE: Abdominal cramps, nausea, vomiting, diarrhea, increased urination with doses exceeding 1 g. *Parenteral:* Flushing, headache, dizziness, sleepiness or insomnia, soreness at injection site.

ADVERSE REACTIONS/TOXIC EFFECTS

May produce urine acidification leading to crystalluria. Large doses given IV may lead to deep vein thrombosis. Prolonged use of large doses may result in scurvy when dosage is reduced to normal.

NURSING IMPLICATIONS
INTERVENTION/EVALUATION:

Monitor lab values for improvement of megaloblastic anemia, increased serum ascorbic acid (0.4–1.5 mg/dl), urine acidity. Assess for clinical improvement (improved sense of well-being and sleep patterns). Observe for reversal of deficiency symptoms (gingivitis, bleeding gums, poor wound healing, digestive difficulties, joint pain).

PATIENT/FAMILY TEACHING:

Discomfort may occur w/parenteral administration. Report diarrhea (dosage adjustment may be needed). Abrupt vitamin C withdrawal may produce rebound deficiency. Reduce dosage gradually. Foods rich in vitamin C include rose hips, guava, black currant jelly, brussel sprouts, green peppers, spinach, watercress, strawberries, citrus fruits.

asparaginase
ah-spa-**raj**-in-ace
(Elspar)

CANADIAN AVAILABILITY:
Kidrolase

CLASSIFICATION
Antineoplastic

AVAILABILITY (Rx)
Powder for Injection: 10,000 IU

PHARMACOKINETICS
Metabolized via slow sequestration by reticuloendothelial system. Half-life: 39–49 hrs IM; 8–30 hrs IV.

ACTION/THERAPEUTIC EFFECT
Breaks down extracellular supplies of amino acid, asparagine

(necessary for survival of these cells), *interfering w/DNA, RNA, protein synthesis in leukemic cells.* Cell cycle-specific for G_1 phase of cell division.

USES / *UNLABELED*

Treatment of acute lymphocytic leukemia (in combination w/other agents). *Treatment of acute myelo-cytic leukemia, acute myelomono-cytic leukemia, chronic lymphocytic leukemia, Hodgkin's disease, lymphosarcoma, reticulum cell sarcoma, melanosarcoma.*

STORAGE / HANDLING

Note: May be carcinogenic, mutagenic, or teratogenic. Handle w/extreme care during preparation/administration. Handle voided urine as infectious waste.

Refrigerate powder for injection. Reconstituted solutions stable for 8 hrs if refrigerated. Discard solutions not clear, colorless. Gelatinous fiberlike particles may develop (remove via 5 micron filter during administration).

IM / IV ADMINISTRATION

Note: Powder, solution may irritate skin on contact. Wash area for 15 min if contact occurs.

IM:

1. Add 2 ml 0.9% NaCl injection to 10,000 IU vial to provide a concentration of 5,000 IU/ml.
2. Administer no more than 2 ml at any one site.

IV:

Note: Administer intradermal test dose (2 IU) prior to initiating therapy or when more than 1 wk has elapsed between doses. Observe pt for 1 hr for appearance of wheal or erythema. **Test Solution:**

Reconstitute 10,000 IU vial w/5 ml sterile water for injection or 0.9% NaCl injection. Shake to dissolve. Withdraw 0.1 ml, inject into vial containing 9.9 ml same diluent for concentration of 20 IU/ml.

1. Reconstitute 10,000 IU vial w/5 ml sterile water for injection or 0.9% NaCl injection to provide a concentration of 2,000 IU/ml.
2. Shake gently to assure complete dissolution (vigorous shaking produces foam, some loss of potency).
3. For IV injection, administer into tubing of freely running IV solution of 5% dextrose or 0.9% NaCl over at least 30 min.
4. For IV infusion, further dilute w/ up to 1,000 ml 5% dextrose or 0.9% NaCl.

INDICATIONS / DOSAGE / ROUTES

Note: Dosage individualized based on clinical response, tolerance to adverse effects. When used in combination therapy, consult specific protocols for optimum dosage, sequence of drug administration.

Acute lymphocytic leukemia:
IV: Adults, elderly, children: Single agent: 200 IU/kg/day for 28 days.
IV: Children: Combination (w/ prednisone, vincristine): 1,000 IU/kg/day for 10 days beginning day 22 of treatment period.
IM: Children: Combination (w/ prednisone, vincristine): 6,000 IU/m^2 on days 4, 7, 10, 13, 16, 19, 22, 25, 28.

PRECAUTIONS

CONTRAINDICATIONS: Previous anaphylactic reaction, pancreatitis, history of pancreatitis. **CAUTIONS:** None significant. **PREGNANCY/LACTATION:** If possible, avoid use during pregnancy, especially first trimester. Breast feeding not recommended. **Pregnancy Category C**.

INTERACTIONS

DRUG INTERACTIONS: Steroids, vincristine may increase hyperglycemia, risk of neuropathy, disturbances of erythropoiesis. May decrease effect of antigout medications. May block effects of methotrexate. Live virus vaccines may potentiate virus replication, increase vaccine side effects, decrease pt's antibody response to vaccine. **ALTERED LAB VALUES:** May increase blood ammonia, BUN, uric acid, glucose, partial thromboplastin time (PTT), platelet count, prothrombin time (PT), thrombin time (TT), SGOT (AST), SGPT (ALT), alkaline phosphatase, bilirubin. May decrease blood clotting factors (plasma fibrinogen, antithrombin, plasminogen), albumin, calcium, cholesterol.

SIDE EFFECTS

FREQUENT: Allergic reaction (rash, urticaria, arthralgia, facial edema, hypotension, respiratory distress), pancreatitis (severe stomach pain w/nausea/vomiting). **OCCASIONAL:** CNS effects (confusion, drowsiness, depression, nervousness, tiredness), stomatitis (sores in mouth/lips), hypoalbuminemia/uric acid nephropathy (swelling of feet or lower legs), hyperglycemia. **RARE:** Hyperthermia (fever or chills), thrombosis, seizures.

ADVERSE REACTIONS/TOXIC EFFECTS

Hepatotoxicity usually occurs within 2 weeks of initial treatment.

Increased risk of allergic reaction, including anaphylaxis, after repeated therapy, severe bone marrow depression.

NURSING IMPLICATIONS
BASELINE ASSESSMENT:

Before giving medication, agents for adequate airway and allergic reaction (antihistamine, epinephrine, oxygen, IV corticosteroid) should be readily available (an abrupt fall in serum asparaginase generally precedes allergic reaction). Skin testing, hepatic, renal, pancreatic (including blood glucose), CBC, differential, CNS functions should be performed before therapy begins and when a wk or more has elapsed between doses.

INTERVENTION/EVALUATION:

Determine serum amylase concentration frequently during therapy. Discontinue medication at first sign of renal failure, pancreatitis (abdominal pain, nausea, vomiting). Monitor for hematologic toxicity (fever, sore throat, signs of local infection, easy bruising, unusual bleeding), symptoms of anemia (excessive tiredness, weakness).

PATIENT/FAMILY TEACHING:

Increase fluid intake (protects against renal impairment). Nausea may decrease during therapy. Do not have immunizations w/o physician's approval (drug lowers body's resistance). Avoid contact w/those who have recently taken live virus vaccine. Contact physician if nausea/vomiting continues at home.

aspirin (acetylsalicylic acid, ASA)

ass-purr-in
(Ascriptin, Bayer, Bufferin, Ecotrin, Halfprin)

FIXED-COMBINATION(S):
W/butabarbital, a barbiturate, and codeine, a narcotic (**Fiorinal**); w/dipyridamole, an antiplatelet agent (**Aggrenox**); w/oxycodone, a narcotic (**Percodan**); w/pentazocine, an analgesic (**Talwin Cmpd**); w/caffeine, a stimulant (**Anacin, Midol**).

CANADIAN AVAILABILITY:
Entrophen, Novasen

CLASSIFICATION
Nonsteroidal anti-inflammatory: Salicylate

AVAILABILITY (OTC)
Tablets: 325 mg, 500 mg. **Tablets (chewable):** 81 mg. **Tablets (enteric coated):** 81 mg, 165 mg, 325 mg, 500 mg, 650 mg, 975 mg. **Tablets (controlled-release):** 650 mg, 800 mg. **Suppository:** 120 mg, 200 mg, 300 mg, 600 mg.

PHARMACOKINETICS
Rapidly, completely absorbed from GI tract; enteric coated absorption delayed; rectal absorption delayed, incomplete. Widely distributed. Rapidly hydrolyzed to salicylate. Half-life: 15–20 min (aspirin); salicylate: 2–3 hrs at low dose; >20 hrs at high dose.

ACTION/*THERAPEUTIC EFFECT*
Produces analgesic, anti-inflammatory effect by inhibiting prosta-glandin synthesis, *reducing inflammatory response and intensity of pain stimulus reaching sensory nerve endings.* Antipyresis produced by drug's effect on hypothalamus, producing vasodilation, *thereby decreasing elevated body temperature.* Inhibits platelet aggregation.

USES/*UNLABELED*
Treatment of mild to moderate pain, fever, inflammatory conditions. Treatment of transient ischemic attack, ischemic stroke, angina, acute myocardial infarction (MI), recurrent MI, specific revascularization procedures, rheumatologic diseases. *Prophylaxis against thromboembolism, treatment of Kawasaki disease.*

STORAGE/HANDLING
Refrigerate suppositories.

PO/RECTAL ADMINISTRATION
PO:
1. Do not crush or break enteric coated or sustained-release form.
2. May give w/water, milk, or meals if GI distress occurs.

RECTAL:
1. If suppository is too soft, chill for 30 min in refrigerator or run cold water over foil wrapper.
2. Moisten suppository w/cold water before inserting well up into rectum.

INDICATIONS/DOSAGE/ROUTES
Pain, fever:
PO/Rectal: Adults, elderly: 325–650 mg q4h as needed, up to 4 g/day.

Rheumatoid arthritis, osteoarthritis, other inflammatory conditions:
PO: Adults, elderly: 3.2–6 g/day in divided doses.

76 / aspirin (acetylsalicylic acid, ASA)

Juvenile arthritis:
PO: Children: 60–110 mg/kg/day in divided doses (q6–8h). May increase dose at 5–7 day intervals.

Acute rheumatic fever:
PO: Adults, elderly: 5–8 g/day. **Children:** 100 mg/kg/day, then decrease to 75 mg/kg/day for 4–6 wks.

Thrombosis (decrease TIAs):
PO: Adults, elderly: 1.3 g/day in 2–4 divided doses.

Thrombosis (decrease MI):
PO: Adults, elderly: 300–325 mg/day.

Usual pediatric dosage:
PO/Rectal: Children: 10–15 mg/kg/dose q4h up to 60–80 mg/kg/day.

PRECAUTIONS

CONTRAINDICATIONS: Chickenpox or flu in children/teenagers, GI bleeding or ulceration, bleeding disorders, history of hypersensitivity to aspirin or NSAIDs, allergy to tartrazine dye, impaired hepatic function. **CAUTIONS:** Vitamin K deficiency, chronic renal insufficiency, those w/"aspirin triad" (rhinitis, nasal polyps, asthma). **PREGNANCY/LACTATION:** Readily crosses placenta; distributed in breast milk. May prolong gestation and labor, decrease fetal birth weight, increase incidence of stillbirths, neonatal mortality, hemorrhage. Avoid use during last trimester (may adversely affect fetal cardiovascular system: premature closure of ductus arteriosus). **Pregnancy Category C.** (Category D if full dose used 3rd trimester.)

INTERACTIONS

DRUG INTERACTIONS: Alcohol, NSAIDs may increase risk of GI effects (e.g., ulceration). Urinary alkalinizers, antacids increase excretion. Anticoagulants, heparin, thrombolytics increase risk of bleeding. Large dose may increase effect of insulin, oral hypoglycemics. Valproic acid, platelet aggregation inhibitors may increase risk of bleeding. May increase toxicity of methotrexate, zidovudine. Ototoxic medications, vancomycin may increase ototoxicity. May decrease effect of probenecid, sulfinpyrazone. **ALTERED LAB VALUES:** May alter SGOT (AST), SGPT (ALT), alkaline phosphatase, uric acid; prolong prothrombin time, bleeding time. May decrease cholesterol, potassium, T_3, T_4.

SIDE EFFECTS

OCCASIONAL: GI distress (cramping, heartburn, abdominal distention, mild nausea), allergic reaction (pruritus, urticaria, bronchospasm).

ADVERSE REACTIONS/TOXIC EFFECTS

High doses may produce GI bleeding and/or gastric mucosal lesions. Low-grade toxicity characterized by ringing in ears, generalized pruritus (may be severe), headache, dizziness, flushing, tachycardia, hyperventilation, sweating, thirst. Febrile, dehydrated children can reach toxic levels quickly. Marked intoxication manifested by hyperthermia, restlessness, abnormal breathing pattern, convulsions, respiratory failure, coma.

NURSING IMPLICATIONS
BASELINE ASSESSMENT:

Do not give to children/teenagers who have flu or chickenpox (increases risk of Reye's syndrome). Do not use if vinegar-like odor is noted (indicates chemical breakdown). Assess type, location, duration of pain, inflammation. Inspect appearance of affected joints for immobility, deformities, skin condition. Therapeutic serum level for antiarthritic effect: 20–30 mg/dl (toxicity occurs if levels are over 30 mg/dl).

INTERVENTION/EVALUATION:

In long-term therapy, monitor plasma salicylic acid concentration. Monitor urinary pH (sudden acidification, pH from 6.5 to 5.5), may result in toxicity. Assess skin for evidence of bruising. If given as antipyretic, assess temperature directly before and 1 hr after giving medication. Evaluate for therapeutic response: relief of pain, stiffness, swelling, increase in joint mobility, reduced joint tenderness, improved grip strength.

PATIENT/FAMILY TEACHING:

Do not crush or chew sustained-release or enteric coated form. Take w/food or after meals; take w/full glass of water (reduces risk of lodging in esophagus). Report ringing in ears or persistent GI pain. Therapeutic anti-inflammatory effect noted in 1–3 wks.

astemizole

az-**tem**-ih-zole
(Hismanal)

CANADIAN AVAILABILITY:
Hismanal

CLASSIFICATION

Antihistamine

AVAILABILITY (Rx)

Tablets: 10 mg

PHARMACOKINETICS

	ONSET	PEAK	DURATION
PO	—	—	24 hrs

Well absorbed from GI tract. Metabolized in liver to active metabolite. Primarily eliminated in feces. Half-life: 0.9–2.3 days; metabolite: 11.6–14.6 days.

ACTION/*THERAPEUTIC EFFECT*

Competes w/histamine for receptor site *to prevent allergic responses mediated by histamine (urticaria, pruritus).* Minimal anticholinergic effect.

USES/*UNLABELED*

Treatment of seasonal allergic rhinitis, chronic idiopathic urticaria. *Treatment of bronchial asthma.*

PO ADMINISTRATION

Give on empty stomach (2 hrs after meal, no additional food intake for 1 hr postdosing).

INDICATIONS/DOSAGE/ROUTES

Allergic rhinitis, urticaria:
PO: Adults, children >12 yrs: 10 mg once/day.

Usual elderly dosage:
PO: 10 mg/day.

PRECAUTIONS

CONTRAINDICATIONS: Concomitant erythromycin, ketoconazole, itraconazole, significant liver dysfunction. **CAUTIONS:** Bladder neck obstruction, symptomatic prostatic hypertrophy, urinary retention, narrow-angle glaucoma, hypokalemia. **PREGNANCY/LACTATION:** Unknown if drug crosses placenta or is detected in breast milk. Increased risk of seizures in neonates, premature infants if used during third trimester of pregnancy. May inhibit lactation. **Pregnancy Category C**.

INTERACTIONS

DRUG INTERACTIONS: Alcohol, CNS depressants may increase CNS depressant effects. Anticholinergics may increase anticholinergic effects. Ketoconazole, fluconazole, itraconazole, miconazole, macrolide antibiotics (e.g., clarithromycin, erythromycin), fluoxetine, fluvoxamine, sertraline, paroxetine, zilenton, ritonavir, indinavir, saquinavir, nefazodone, nelfinavir, quinine may increase concentrations resulting in cardiotoxic effect. MAOIs may increase anticholinergic, CNS depressant effects. **ALTERED LAB VALUES:** May suppress wheal and flare reactions to antigen skin testing unless antihistamines are discontinued 4 days prior to testing.

SIDE EFFECTS

FREQUENT: Headache. **OCCASIONAL:** Appetite increase, weight gain, nausea, nervousness. **RARE:** Drowsiness, dizziness, disturbed coordination, diarrhea, pharyngitis, conjunctivitis, arthralgia, drowsiness, thick mucus.

ADVERSE REACTIONS/TOXIC EFFECTS

Overdosage may produce cardiac arrhythmias (prolonged QT interval, tachycardia, irregular beats, ventricular arrhythmias). Anticholinergic less likely (e.g., drowsiness, dry mouth, flushing, trouble breathing).

NURSING IMPLICATIONS

BASELINE ASSESSMENT:

If patient is undergoing allergic reaction, obtain history of recently ingested foods, drugs, environmental exposure, recent emotional stress. Monitor rate, depth, rhythm, type of respiration; quality and rate of pulse. Assess lung sounds for rhonchi, wheezing, rales.

INTERVENTION/EVALUATION:

Monitor B/P, especially in elderly (increased risk of hypotension). Monitor children closely for paradoxical reaction. Assess for therapeutic response from allergy: itching, red, watery eyes, relief from rhinorrhea, sneezing.

PATIENT/FAMILY TEACHING:

Tolerance to antihistaminic effect generally does not occur; tolerance to sedative effect may occur. Avoid tasks that require alertness, motor skills until response to drug is established. Dry mouth, drowsiness, dizziness may be an expected response of drug. Avoid alcoholic beverages during antihistamine therapy. Sugarless gum, sips of tepid water may relieve dry mouth. Coffee or tea may help reduce drowsiness.

atenolol
ay-**ten**-oh-lol
(Tenormin)

FIXED-COMBINATION(S):
W/chlorthalidone, a diuretic (Tenoretic)

CANADIAN AVAILABILITY:
Apo-Atenol, Tenormin

CLASSIFICATION

Beta$_1$-adrenergic blocker

AVAILABILITY (Rx)

Tablets: 25 mg, 50 mg, 100 mg.
Injection: 5 mg/10 ml.

PHARMACOKINETICS

	ONSET	PEAK	DURATION
PO (heart rate)			
	1 hr	2–4 hrs	24 hrs
PO (hypotensive)			
	—	—	24 hrs

Incompletely absorbed from GI tract. Minimal liver metabolism. Primarily excreted unchanged in urine. Removed by hemodialysis. Half-life: 6–7 hrs (increase in decreased renal function).

ACTION / *THERAPEUTIC EFFECT*

Blocks beta$_1$-adrenergic receptors in cardiac tissue, *slowing sinus heart rate, decreasing cardiac output, decreasing B/P.* Large doses may block beta$_2$-adrenergic receptors, increasing airway resistance. *Decreases myocardial oxygen demand.*

USES / *UNLABELED*

Management of mild to moderate hypertension. Used alone or in combination w/diuretics, especially thiazide type. Management of chronic stable angina pectoris. Reduces cardiovascular mortality in those w/definite or suspected acute MI. *Hypertrophic cardiomyopathy, pheochromocytoma, prophylaxis of migraine, tremors, thyrotoxicosis, syndrome of mitral valve prolapse. Improve survival in diabetics with heart disease.*

STORAGE / HANDLING

After reconstitution, parenteral form is stable for 48 hrs at room temperature.

PO / IV ADMINISTRATION

PO:

1. May be given w/o regard to meals.

2. Tablets may be crushed.

IV:

Dilutions w/5% dextrose or 0.9% NaCl may be used.

INDICATIONS / DOSAGE / ROUTES

Hypertension:
PO: Adults: Initially, 25–50 mg once/day. May increase up to 100 mg once/day.

Angina pectoris:
PO: Adults: Initially, 50 mg once daily. May increase up to 200 mg once daily.

Usual elderly dosage:
PO: Initially, 25 mg/day for angina/hypertension.

Acute myocardial infarction:
IV: Give 5 mg over 5 min, may repeat in 10 min. In those who tolerate full 10 mg IV dose, begin 50 mg tablets 10 min after last IV dose followed by another 50 mg oral dose 12 hrs later. Thereafter, give 100 mg once/day or 50 mg twice/day for 6–9 days. (Alternatively, for those who do not tolerate full IV dose, give 50 mg orally 2 times/day or 100 mg once/day for at least 7 days.)

Dosage in renal impairment:

CREATININE CLEARANCE	DOSAGE
15–35 ml/min	50 mg daily
<15 ml/min	50 mg q other day

PRECAUTIONS

CONTRAINDICATIONS: Overt cardiac failure, cardiogenic shock, heart block greater than first degree, severe bradycardia. **CAUTIONS:** Impaired renal or hepatic function, peripheral vascular disease, hyperthyroidism, diabetes, inadequate cardiac function, bronchospastic disease. **PREGNANCY/LACTATION:** Readily crosses placenta; distributed in breast milk.

Avoid use during first trimester. May produce bradycardia, apnea, hypoglycemia, hypothermia during delivery, small birth weight infants. **Pregnancy Category D.**

INTERACTIONS

DRUG INTERACTIONS: Diuretics, other hypotensives may increase hypotensive effect; sympathomimetics, xanthines may mutually inhibit effects; may mask symptoms of hypoglycemia, prolong hypoglycemic effect of insulin, oral hypoglycemics; NSAIDs may decrease antihypertensive effect; Cimetidine may increase concentration. **ALTERED LAB VALUES:** May increase ANA titer, BUN, creatinine, potassium, uric acid, lipoproteins, triglycerides.

SIDE EFFECTS

Generally well tolerated, w/mild and transient side effects. **FREQUENT:** Hypotension manifested as dizziness, nausea, diaphoresis, headache, cold extremities, fatigue, constipation/diarrhea. **OCCASIONAL:** Insomnia, flatulence, urinary frequency, impotence or decreased libido. **RARE:** rash, arthralgia, myalgia, confusion (esp. in elderly), change in taste.

ADVERSE REACTIONS/TOXIC EFFECTS

Overdosage may produce profound bradycardia, hypotension. Abrupt withdrawal may result in sweating, palpitations, headache, tremulousness. May precipitate CHF, MI in those w/cardiac disease, thyroid storm in those w/thyrotoxicosis, peripheral ischemia in those w/existing peripheral vascular disease. Hypoglycemia may occur in previously controlled diabetics. Thrombocytopenia (unusual bruising, bleeding) occurs rarely.

NURSING IMPLICATIONS
BASELINE ASSESSMENT:

Assess B/P, apical pulse immediately before drug is administered (if pulse is 60/min or below, or systolic B/P is below 90 mm Hg, withhold medication, contact physician). *Antianginal:* Record onset, type (sharp, dull, squeezing), radiation, location, intensity and duration of anginal pain, and precipitating factors (exertion, emotional stress). Assess baseline renal/liver function tests.

INTERVENTION/EVALUATION:

Monitor B/P for hypotension, pulse for bradycardia, respiration for shortness of breath. Assess pattern of daily bowel activity and stool consistency. Assess for evidence of CHF: dyspnea (particularly on exertion or lying down), night cough, peripheral edema, distended neck veins). Monitor I&O (increase in weight, decrease in urine output may indicate CHF). Assess extremities for coldness. Assist w/ambulation if dizziness occurs. Assess skin for rash, bruising.

PATIENT/FAMILY TEACHING:

Do not abruptly discontinue medication. Compliance w/therapy essential to control hypertension, angina. To reduce hypotensive effect, rise slowly from lying to sitting position and permit legs to dangle from bed momentarily before standing. Avoid tasks that require alertness, motor skills until drug reaction is established. Report dizziness, depression, confusion, rash, unusual bruising or bleeding. Do not use nasal decongestants, OTC cold preparations (stimulants) w/o physician approval. Outpatients should monitor B/P, pulse before taking medication (teach correct technique). Restrict salt, alcohol intake. Therapeutic antihypertensive effect noted in 1–2 wks. May change warning signs of hypoglycemia.

atorvastatin

(Lipitor)
See Supplement
See Classification section under:
Antihyperlipidemics

atovaquone

ah-**tow**-vah-quon
(Mepron)

CANADIAN AVAILABILITY:
Mepron

CLASSIFICATION

Antiprotozoal

AVAILABILITY (Rx)

Suspension: 750 mg/5 ml

PHARMACOKINETICS

Poorly absorbed from GI tract (increased when given w/food, esp. high-fat foods). Primarily eliminated unchanged in feces. Half-life: 50–77 hrs.

ACTION / THERAPEUTIC EFFECT

Inhibits mitochondrial electron-transport system at the cytochrome bc$_1$ complex (Complex III). Interrupts nucleic acid and ATP synthesis.

USES

Treatment or prevention of mild to moderate Pneumocystis carinii pneumonia (PCP) in those intoler-

ant to trimethoprim-sulfamethoxazole (TMP-SMZ).

PO ADMINISTRATION

Give w/food (esp. high-fat foods).

INDICATIONS/DOSAGE/ROUTES

Pneumocystis carinii pneumonia (PCP):
PO: Adults: 750 mg w/food 2 times/day for 21 days.
Prevention of PCP:
PO: Adults: 1,500 mg once daily w/food.

PRECAUTIONS

CONTRAINDICATIONS: Development or history of potentially life-threatening allergic reaction to drug. **CAUTIONS:** Elderly, pts w/severe PCP, chronic diarrhea, malabsorption syndromes. **PREGNANCY/LACTATION:** May produce maternal toxicity; body length and weight of fetus may be decreased. Unknown if distributed in breast milk. **Pregnancy Category C**.

INTERACTIONS

DRUG INTERACTIONS: Rifampin may decrease concentration, atovaquone may increase rifampin concentration. **ALTERED LAB VALUES:** May elevate SGOT (AST), SGPT (ALT), alkaline phosphatase, amylase. May decrease sodium.

SIDE EFFECTS

FREQUENT (>10%): Skin rash, nausea, diarrhea, headache, vomiting, fever, insomnia, cough. **OCCASIONAL (<10%):** Abdominal discomfort, thrush, asthenia (loss of strength, energy), anemia, neutropenia.

ADVERSE REACTIONS/TOXIC EFFECTS

None significant.

NURSING IMPLICATIONS
INTERVENTION/EVALUATION:

Assess for GI discomfort, nausea, vomiting. Check consistency and frequency of stools. Assess skin for rash. Monitor I&O, renal function tests, hemoglobin, neutrophil counts. Atovaquone has not been fully evaluated in pts >65 years of age; monitor elderly closely because of decreased hepatic, renal, and cardiac function.

PATIENT/FAMILY TEACHING:

Continue therapy for full length of treatment. Doses should be evenly spaced. Do not take any other medication unless approved by physician. Notify physician in event of rash, diarrhea, or other new symptom.

---

atracurium
(Tracrium)
See Classification section under: Neuromuscular blockers

---

atropine sulfate

ah-trow-peen
(Atropine Sulfate, Isopto Atropine, Ocu-Tropine)

FIXED-COMBINATION(S):
W/phenobarbital, a sedative-hypnotic (**Antrocol**); w/diphenoxylate, a constipating meperidine derivative (**Lomotil**); w/hyoscyamine, scopolamine, an anticholinergic, and phenobarbital, a sedative-hypnotic (**Donnatal**); w/prednisolone, a steroid (**Mydropred Ophthalmic**).

CANADIAN AVAILABILITY:
Atropine Minims, Atropisol, Isopto-Atropine

CLASSIFICATION

Anticholinergic

AVAILABILITY (Rx)

Injection: 0.05 mg/ml, 0.3 mg/ml, 0.4 mg/ml, 0.5 mg/ml, 0.8 mg/ml, 1 mg/ml. **Ophthalmic Ointment:** 1%. **Ophthalmic Solution:** 0.5%, 1%, 2%.

PHARMACOKINETICS

Mydriatic effect: Peak 30–40 min; recovery 7–12 days. *Cycloplegic effect:* Peak 60–180 min; recovery 6–12 days. Rapidly absorbed after IM, oral administration. Metabolized in liver. Primarily excreted in urine. Half-life: 2–3 hrs. After PO/IM administration, inhibits salivation within 30–60 min (peak 1–2 hrs), duration 4 hrs; increases heart rate within 2–4 min (IV), 5–40 min (IM), or 30–120 min (PO), peak in 0.5–1 hr (IM), 1–2 hrs (PO).

ACTION/THERAPEUTIC EFFECT

Inhibits action of acetylcholine on structures innervated by postganglionic sites (smooth/cardiac muscle, SA/AV nodes, exocrine glands). Larger doses may *decrease motility, secretory activity of GI system, tone of ureter, urinary bladder.* Blocks responses of sphincter muscle and accommodation muscle ciliary body *producing mydriasis, cycloplegia.*

USES

Adjunct in treatment of peptic ulcer disease. Treatment of functional disturbances of GI motility, hypermotility disorders of lower urinary tract, GI hypermotility, diarrhea. Preop medication to prevent or reduce salivation, excessive secretions of respiratory tract. May also prevent cholinergic effects during surgery: cardiac arrhythmias, hypotension, reflex bradycardia. Blocks adverse muscarinic effects of anticholinesterase agents (i.e., neostigmine). Management of sinus bradycardia in those w/acute MI who have hypotension and increased ventricular irritability. For cycloplegic refraction and to dilate pupil in inflammatory conditions of iris and uveal tract.

PO/IM/IV/OPHTHALMIC ADMINISTRATION

PO:
Administer 30 min before meals and at bedtime.
IM:
May be given SubQ or IM.
IV:
Generally given rapidly (prevents paradoxical slowing of heart rate).

Ophthalmic:

1. Place finger on lower eyelid and pull out until pocket is formed between eye and lower lid. Hold dropper above pocket and place prescribed number of drops ($^1/_4$–$^1/_2$-inch ointment) in pocket. Close eye gently. *Drops:* Apply digital pressure to lacrimal sac for 1–2 min (minimize drainage into nose and throat, reducing risk of systemic effects). *Ointment:* Close eye for 1–2 min, rolling eyeball (increases contact area of drug to eye). W/either method, remove excess solution or ointment around eye w/tissue.

2. Ophthalmic solutions not to be used for injection.

INDICATIONS/DOSAGE/ROUTES

Usual oral dosage:
PO: Adults, elderly: 0.4–0.6 mg q4–6h. **Range:** 0.1–1.2 mg. **Children:** 0.01 mg/kg, not to exceed 0.4 mg q4–6h.

Usual parenteral dose:
SubQ/IM/IV: Adults, elderly: 0.4–0.6 mg q4–6h. **Range:** 0.3–1.2 mg. **Children:** 0.01 mg/kg, not to exceed 0.4 mg q4–6h.

Bradycardia in advanced cardiac life support:
IV: Adults, elderly: 0.4–1 mg. Repeat at 1–2 hr intervals until desired rate achieved. **Maximum:** 2 mg total dose. **Children:** 0.01–0.03 mg/kg (minimum dose: 0.1 mg).

Preoperative:
SubQ/IM/IV: Adults, elderly, children >20 kg: 0.4 mg (range: 0.2–0.6 mg) 30–60 min prior to time of induction of anesthesia or other preanesthetic medications. **Children (3 kg):** 0.1 mg; **(7–9 kg):** 0.2 mg; **(12–16 kg):** 0.3 mg.

Usual ophthalmic dose (mydriasis, cycloplegia):
Ointment: Adults, elderly: 0.3–0.5 cm 1–3 times/day. **Children:** 0.3 cm 3 times/day. Administer for 1–3 days prior to procedure.
Solution: Adults, elderly: 1 drop 1% solution. **Children:** 1–2 drops 0.5% solution 2 times/day. Administer for 1–3 days prior to and 1 hr before procedure.

Treatment of acute inflammatory ophthalmic conditions:
Solution: Adults, elderly: 1–2 drops of 0.5–1% solution up to 3–4 times/day. **Children:** 1–2 drops of 0.5% solution up to 3–4 times/day.

PRECAUTIONS

CONTRAINDICATIONS: Narrow-angle glaucoma, severe ulcerative colitis, toxic megacolon, obstructive disease of GI tract, paralytic ileus, intestinal atony, bladder neck obstruction due to prostatic hypertrophy, myasthenia gravis in those not treated w/neostigmine, tachycardia secondary to cardiac insufficiency or thyrotoxicosis, cardiospasm, unstable cardiovascular status in acute hemorrhage. **EXTREME CAUTION:** Autonomic neuropathy, known or suspected GI infections, diarrhea, mild to moderate ulcerative colitis. **CAUTIONS:** Hyperthyroidism, hepatic or renal disease, hypertension, tachyarrhythmias, CHF, coronary artery disease, gastric ulcer, esophageal reflux or hiatal hernia associated w/reflux esophagitis, infants, elderly, systemic administration in those w/COPD. **PREGNANCY/LACTATION:** Crosses placenta; unknown if distributed in breast milk. May produce fetal tachycardia. **Pregnancy Category C.**

INTERACTIONS

DRUG INTERACTIONS: Antacids, antidiarrheals may decrease absorption. Anticholinergics may increase effects. May decrease absorption of ketoconazole. May increase severity of GI lesions with KCl (wax matrix). **ALTERED LAB VALUES:** None significant.

SIDE EFFECTS

Note: Discontinue medication immediately if dizziness, increased pulse, or blurring of vision occurs.
FREQUENT: Dry mouth/nose/throat (may be severe), decreased sweating, constipation, irritation at SubQ/IM injection site. **OCCASIONAL:** Swallowing difficulty, blurred vision, bloated feeling, impotence, urinary hesitancy. *Ophthalmic:* Blurred vision, eye irritation, eyelid swelling, intolerance to light, headache. **RARE:** Allergic reaction (rash, urticaria), mental confusion/excitement (particularly children), fatigue.

ADVERSE REACTIONS/TOXIC EFFECTS

Overdosage may produce tachycardia, palpitations, hot/dry/flushed skin, absence of bowel sounds, increased respiratory rate, nausea, vomiting, confusion, drowsiness, slurred speech, CNS stimulation, psychosis (agitation, restlessness, rambling speech, visual hallucinations, paranoid behavior, delusions), followed by depression.

NURSING IMPLICATIONS

BASELINE ASSESSMENT:

Before giving medication, instruct pt to void (reduces risk of urinary retention).

INTERVENTION/EVALUATION:

Monitor changes in B/P, pulse, temperature. Assess skin turgor, mucous membranes to evaluate hydration status (encourage adequate fluid intake unless NPO for surgery), bowel sounds for peristalsis. Be alert for fever (increased risk of hyperthermia). Monitor I&O, palpate bladder for urinary retention. Assess stool frequency and consistency.

PATIENT/FAMILY TEACHING:

Take oral form 30 min before meals (food decreases absorption of medication). Avoid becoming overheated during exercise in hot weather (may result in heat stroke). Avoid hot baths, saunas. Avoid tasks that require alertness, motor skills until response to drug is established. Sugarless gum, sips of tepid water relieve dry mouth. Do not take antacids or medicine for diarrhea within 1 hr of taking this medication (decreased effectiveness). For preop use, explain that warm, dry, flushing feeling may occur. Remind pt to remain in bed and not eat or drink anything.

auranofin

aur-an-**oh**-fin
(Ridaura)

CANADIAN AVAILABILITY:
Ridaura

CLASSIFICATION

Antirheumatic: Gold compound

AVAILABILITY (Rx)

Capsule: 3 mg

PHARMACOKINETICS

Moderately absorbed from GI tract. Rapidly metabolized. Primarily excreted in urine. Half-life: 21–31 days.

ACTION

Alters cellular mechanisms, enzyme systems, immune responses, collagen biosynthesis, *suppressing synovitis of the active stage of rheumatoid arthritis.*

USES/UNLABELED

Management of rheumatoid arthritis in those w/insufficient therapeutic response to NSAIDs. *Treatment of pemphigus, psoriatic arthritis.*

PO ADMINISTRATION

Give w/o regard to food.

INDICATIONS/DOSAGE/ROUTES

Rheumatoid arthritis:
PO: Adults, elderly: 6 mg/day in 1 or 2 divided doses. May increase to 9 mg/day (in 3 divided doses) if no response in 6 months. If response still inadequate, discontinue.

PRECAUTIONS

CONTRAINDICATIONS: History of gold-induced pathologies (necrotizing enterocolitis, exfoliative dermatitis, pulmonary fibrosis, blood dyscrasias), bone marrow aplasia, severe blood dyscrasias. **CAUTIONS:** Renal/hepatic disease, marked hypertension, compromised cerebral or cardiovascular circulation. **PREGNANCY/LACTATION:** Crosses placenta; distributed in breast milk. Use only when benefits outweigh hazard to fetus. **Pregnancy Category C**.

INTERACTIONS

DRUG INTERACTIONS: Bone marrow depressants, hepatotoxic, nephrotoxic medications may increase toxicity. Penicillamine may increase risk of hematologic or renal adverse effects. **ALTERED LAB VALUES:** May decrease hemoglobin, hematocrit, platelets, WBCs. May alter liver function tests. May increase urine protein.

SIDE EFFECTS

FREQUENT: Diarrhea/loose stools, rash, pruritus, abdominal pain, nausea. **OCCASIONAL:** Vomiting, anorexia, flatulence, dyspepsia. **RARE:** Constipation, change in sense of taste, glossitis (irritation/soreness of tongue).

ADVERSE REACTIONS/TOXIC EFFECTS

Signs of gold toxicity: decreased hemoglobin, leukopenia (WBC below 4,000/mm³), reduced granulocyte counts (below 150,000/

mm^3), proteinuria, hematuria, stomatitis (ulcers, sores, white spots in mouth, throat), blood dyscrasias (anemia, leukopenia, thrombocytopenia, eosinophilia), glomerulonephritis, nephrotic syndrome, cholestatic jaundice.

NURSING IMPLICATIONS
BASELINE ASSESSMENT:

Rule out pregnancy before beginning treatment. CBC, urinalysis, platelet and differential, renal and liver function tests should be performed before therapy begins.

INTERVENTION/EVALUATION:

Monitor daily bowel activity and stool consistency. Assess urine tests for proteinuria or hematuria. Monitor WBC, hemoglobin, differential, platelet count, renal and hepatic function studies. Question for pruritus (may be first sign of impending rash). Assess skin daily for rash, purpura or ecchymoses. Assess oral mucous membranes, borders of tongue, palate, pharynx for ulceration, complaint of metallic taste sensation (sign of stomatitis). Evaluate for therapeutic response: relief of pain, stiffness, swelling, increase in joint mobility, reduced joint tenderness, improved grip strength.

PATIENT/FAMILY TEACHING:

Therapeutic response may be expected in 3–6 mos. Avoid exposure to sunlight (gray to blue pigment may appear). Contact physician if pruritus, rash, sore mouth, indigestion, or metallic taste occurs. Maintain diligent oral hygiene.

aurothioglucose
ah-row-thigh-oh-**glue**-cose
(Solganal)

CANADIAN AVAILABILITY:
Solganal

CLASSIFICATION
Antirheumatic: Gold compound

AVAILABILITY (Rx)
Injection: 50 mg/ml suspension

PHARMACOKINETICS
Slow, erratic absorption after IM administration. Metabolic fate unknown. Primarily excreted in urine. Half-life: 3–27 days (increased w/ increased number of doses).

ACTION/THERAPEUTIC EFFECT
Alters cellular mechanisms, enzyme systems, immune responses, collagen biosynthesis, *suppressing synovitis of the active stage of rheumatoid arthritis.*

USES
Management of rheumatoid arthritis in those w/insufficient therapeutic response to NSAIDs.

IM ADMINISTRATION
Give in upper outer quadrant of gluteus.

INDICATIONS/DOSAGE/ROUTES
Rheumatoid arthritis:
Note: Give as weekly injections.
IM: Adults, elderly: Initially, 10 mg, then 25 mg for 2 doses, then 50 mg weekly thereafter until total dose of 0.8–1 g given. If pt improved and no signs of toxicity, give 50 mg at 3–4 wk intervals for many months.

PRECAUTIONS

CONTRAINDICATIONS: History of gold-induced pathologies (necrotizing enterocolitis, exfoliative dermatitis, pulmonary fibrosis, blood dyscrasias), bone marrow aplasia, severe blood dyscrasias. **CAUTIONS:** Renal/hepatic disease, inflammatory bowel disease. **PREGNANCY/LACTATION:** Crosses placenta, distributed in breast milk. Use only when benefits outweigh hazard to fetus. **Pregnancy Category C**.

INTERACTIONS

DRUG INTERACTIONS: Bone marrow depressants, hepatotoxic, nephrotoxic medications may increase toxicity. Penicillamine may increase risk of hematologic or renal adverse effects. **ALTERED LAB VALUES:** May decrease hemoglobin, hematocrit, platelets, WBCs. May alter liver function tests. May increase urine protein.

SIDE EFFECTS

OCCASIONAL: Rash, pruritus, gingivitis, reddened skin, glossitis (soreness of tongue), metallic taste, stomatitis (ulcers, sores, white spots in mouth/throat). **RARE:** Proteinuria (cloudy urine), joint pain (esp. 1–2 days after injection), allergic reaction, abdominal cramping, diarrhea, conjunctivitis, anorexia.

ADVERSE REACTIONS/TOXIC EFFECTS

Signs of gold toxicity: decreased hemoglobin, leukopenia (WBC below 4,000/mm³), reduced granulocyte counts (below 150,000/mm³), proteinuria, hematuria, stomatitis, blood dyscrasias (anemia, leukopenia, thrombocytopenia, eosinophilia), glomerulonephritis, nephrotic syndrome, cholestatic jaundice.

NURSING IMPLICATIONS

BASELINE ASSESSMENT:

Rule out pregnancy before beginning treatment. CBC, urinalysis, platelet and differential, renal and liver function tests should be performed before therapy begins.

INTERVENTION/EVALUATION:

Monitor skin for color, rash. Check mouth for sores, white spots, reddened gums. Assess urine tests for proteinuria or hematuria. Monitor WBC, hemoglobin, differential, platelet count, renal, and hepatic function studies. Question for pruritus (may be first sign of impending rash). Assess skin daily for rash, purpura, or ecchymoses. Assess oral mucous membranes, borders of tongue, palate, pharynx for ulceration, complaint of metallic taste sensation (signs of stomatitis). Evaluate for therapeutic response: relief of pain, stiffness, swelling, increase in joint mobility, reduced joint tenderness, improved grip strength.

PATIENT/FAMILY TEACHING:

Therapeutic response may take 6 months or longer. Avoid exposure to sunlight (gray to blue pigment may appear). Contact physician/nurse if pruritus, rash, sore mouth, indigestion, or metallic taste occurs. Maintain diligent oral hygiene. Increased joint pain may continue 1–2 days after injection.

azathioprine

asia-**thigh**-oh-preen
(Imuran Oral)

azathioprine sodium

(Imuran Parenteral)

CANADIAN AVAILABILITY:
Imuran

CLASSIFICATION

Immunosuppressant

AVAILABILITY (Rx)

Tablet: 50 mg. **Injection:** 100 mg vial.

PHARMACOKINETICS

Well absorbed from GI tract. Converted to active metabolite. Further metabolized in liver and erythrocytes. Eliminated via biliary system. Minimal removal by hemodialysis. Half-life: 5 hrs.

ACTION

Antagonizes metabolism, inhibits RNA, DNA and protein synthesis, *suppressing cell-mediated hypersensitivities, alters antibody production, immune response in transplant recipients. Reduces arthritis severity.*

USES/*UNLABELED*

Adjunct in prevention of rejection in kidney transplantation; treatment of rheumatoid arthritis in those unresponsive to conventional therapy. *Treatment of inflammatory bowel disease, chronic active hepatitis, biliary cirrhosis, systemic lupus erythematosus, glomerulonephritis, nephrotic syndrome, inflammatory myopathy, myasthenia gravis, polymyositis, pemphigus, pemphigoid.*

STORAGE/HANDLING

Store oral, parenteral form at room temperature. After reconstitution, IV solution stable for 24 hrs.

PO/IV ADMINISTRATION

PO:
Give during or after meal to reduce potential for GI disturbances.

IV:
1. Reconstitute 100 mg vial w/10 ml sterile water for injection to provide concentration of 10 mg/ml.
2. Further dilute w/5% dextrose or 0.9% NaCl; infuse over 30–60 min.

INDICATIONS/DOSAGE/ROUTES

Note: May give in divided doses if GI disturbance occurs.

Kidney transplantation:
PO/IV: Adults, elderly, children: Initially, 3–5 mg/kg/day as single dose on day of transplant. **Maintenance:** 1–3 mg/kg/day.

Rheumatoid arthritis:
PO/IV: Adults: Initially, 1 mg/kg/day as single or in 2 divided doses. May increase by 0.5 mg/kg/day after 6–8 wks at 4 wk intervals up to maximum dose of 2.5 mg/kg/day. **Maintenance:** Lowest effective dose. May decrease dose by 0.5 mg/kg or 25 mg/day q4wks (other therapy maintained). **Elderly:** Initially, 1 mg/kg/day (50–100 mg); may increase by 25 mg/day until response or toxicity.

PRECAUTIONS

CONTRAINDICATIONS: Pregnant rheumatoid arthritis pts. **CAUTIONS:** Immunosuppressed pts, those previously treated for rheumatoid arthritis w/alkylating agents (cyclophosphamide, chlorambucil, melphalan), chickenpox (current or recent), herpes zoster, gout, decreased liver/renal function, infection.

INTERACTIONS

DRUG INTERACTIONS: Allourinol may increase activity, toxicity. Bone marrow depressants may increase bone marrow depression. Other immunosuppressants may increase risk of infection or development of neoplasms. Live virus vaccines may potentiate virus replication, increase vaccine side effects, decrease pt's antibody response to vaccine. **ALTERED LAB VALUES:** May decrease hemoglobin, albumin, uric acid. May increase SGPT (ALT), SGOT (AST), alkaline phosphatase, amylase, bilirubin.

SIDE EFFECTS

FREQUENT: Nausea, vomiting, anorexia, particularly during early treatment and w/large doses. **OCCASIONAL:** Rash. **RARE:** Severe nausea, vomiting w/diarrhea, stomach pain, hypersensitivity reaction.

ADVERSE REACTIONS/TOXIC EFFECTS

There is an increased risk of neoplasia (new, abnormal growth tumors). Significant leukopenia, thrombocytopenia may occur, particularly in those undergoing kidney rejection. Hepatotoxicity occurs rarely.

NURSING IMPLICATIONS
BASELINE ASSESSMENT:

Arthritis: Assess onset, type, location and duration of pain, fever, or inflammation. Inspect appearance of affected joints for immobility, deformities, and skin condition.

INTERVENTION/EVALUATION:

CBC, platelet count, liver function studies should be performed weekly during first month of therapy, twice monthly during second and third months of treatment, then monthly thereafter. If rapid fall in WBC occurs, dosage should be reduced or discontinued. Assess particularly for delayed bone marrow suppression. Report any major change in assessment of pt. Routinely watch for any change from normal. *Arthritis:* Evaluate for therapeutic response: relief of pain, stiffness, swelling, increase in joint mobility, reduced joint tenderness, improved grip strength.

PATIENT/FAMILY TEACHING:

Contact physician if unusual bleeding or bruising, sore throat, mouth sores, abdominal pain, or fever occurs. Therapeutic response in rheumatoid arthritis may take up to 12 wks. Women of childbearing age must avoid pregnancy (assure pt has adequate information and resources to comply).

azelaic acid
aye-zeh-**lay**-ick acid
(Azelex)

CLASSIFICATION
Antiacne, hypopigmentation agent

AVAILABILITY (Rx)
Cream: 20%

PHARMOKOKINETICS:

Dietary component (whole grain cereals, animal products). Following application, azelaic acid penetrates into stratum corneum and other viable skin layers; 4% absorbed systemically, which is excreted unchanged in urine.

ACTION/*THERAPEUTIC EFFECT*

Possesses antimicrobial action by inhibiting cellular protein synthesis in aerobic and anaerobic microorganisms, *improving acne vulgaris, normalizing keritin process.* Interrupts hyperactivity of normal melanocytes and their resulting growth in melasma, *reducing macular hyperpigmentation of facial or nuchal (back of neck) hair.*

USES/*UNLABELED*

Treatment of mild to moderate acne vulgaris. *Treatment of melasma (hyperfunctioning melanocytes).*

TOPICAL ADMINISTRATION

1. Apply thin coating to clean, dry skin, gently but thoroughly rubbing into affected area.
2. Wash hands thoroughly following application.
3. For external use only.
4. Avoid occlusive dressings and wrappings.

INDICATIONS/DOSAGE/ROUTES

Antiacne, hypopigmentation:
Topical: Adults, adolescents: Apply topically to affected area 2 times/day (morning and evening).

PRECAUTIONS

CONTRAINDICATIONS: None significant. **CAUTIONS:** None significant. **PREGNANCY/LACTATION:** Crosses placenta. Appears to be distributed in breast milk. **Pregnancy Category B.**

INTERACTIONS

DRUG INTERACTIONS: None significant. **ALTERED LAB VALUES:** None significant.

SIDE EFFECTS

OCCASIONAL (1–5%): Pruritus, stinging, burning, tingling. **RARE (<1%):** Erythema, dryness, rash, peeling, irritation, contact dermatitis.

ADVERSE REACTIONS/TOXIC EFFECTS

None significant.

NURSING IMPLICATIONS
INTERVENTION/EVALUATION:

Assess skin for erythema, dryness. Question pt regarding possible inflammatory reaction (burning, stinging, tingling of skin).

PATIENT/FAMILY TEACHING:

Inform pt mild burning, stinging, tingling of skin, and itching may occur at beginning of each treatment, may last 5–20 min but lessens w/continued use.Contact physician if acne worsens, does not improve in first 4 wks or if medication produces excessive redness, dryness, or peeling of skin. Avoid occlusive dressings. Keep away from mouth, eyes, other mucus membranes. Report abnormal changes in skin color or if skin irritation persists. Therapeutic improvement noted in about 4 wks.

azelastine
(Astelin)
See Supplement

azithromycin

aye-**zith**-row-my-sin
(Zithromax)

CANADIAN AVAILABILITY:
Zithromax

CLASSIFICATION

Antibiotic: Macrolide

AVAILABILITY (Rx)

Tablet: 250 mg. **Injection:** 500 mg. **Oral Suspension:** 100 mg/5 ml, 200 mg/5 ml.

PHARMACOKINETICS

Rapidly absorbed from GI tract. Widely distributed. Eliminated primarily unchanged via biliary excretion. Half-life: 68 hrs.

ACTION / *THERAPEUTIC EFFECT*

Binds to ribosomal receptor sites of susceptible organisms, *inhibiting protein synthesis.*

USES / *UNLABELED*

Treatment of mild to moderate infections of upper respiratory tract (pharyngitis, tonsillitis), lower respiratory tract (acute bacterial exacerbations, COPD, pneumonia), uncomplicated skin/skin structure infections, and sexually transmitted diseases (nongonococcal urethritis, cervicitis due to *Chlamydia trachomatis*), gonorrhea, chancroid. Prevents disseminated mycobacterium avium complex (MAC). Treatment of mycoplasma pneumonia. **Injection:** Community acquired pneumonia, PID, acne.

PO / IV ADMINISTRATION

PO:

1. May take tablets w/o regard to food.

2. May store suspension at room temperature.

IV:

Infuse over 60 minutes.

INDICATIONS / DOSAGE / ROUTES

Lower/upper respiratory tract, skin/skin structure infections:
PO: Adults, elderly: Initially, 500 mg on first day, then 250 mg on days 2–5 (total dose 1.5 g).

Prevention of MAC:
PO: Adults: 1,200 mg once/week.

Nongonococcal urethritis, cervicitis due to C. trachomatis:
PO: Adult: 1 g as a single dose.

Usual parenteral dosage:
IV: Adults: 500 mg/day followed by oral therapy.

Usual pediatric dosage:
PO: 10 mg/kg on day 1; then 5 mg/kg on days 2–5.

PRECAUTIONS

CONTRAINDICATIONS: Hypersensitivity to azithromycin, erythromycins, any macrolide antibiotic. **CAUTIONS:** Hepatic/renal dysfunction. **PREGNANCY/LACTATION:** Unknown if distributed in breast milk. **Pregnancy Category B.**

INTERACTIONS

DRUG INTERACTIONS: May increase serum concentrations of carbamazepine, cyclosporine, theophylline, warfarin. Aluminum/magnesium-containing antacids may decrease concentration (give 1 hr before or 2 hrs after antacid). **ALTERED LAB VALUES:** May increase serum CPK, SGOT (AST), SGPT (ALT).

SIDE EFFECTS

OCCASIONAL: Nausea, vomiting, diarrhea, abdominal pain. **RARE:** Headache, dizziness, allergic reaction.

ADVERSE REACTIONS/TOXIC EFFECTS

Superinfections, esp. antibiotic-associated colitis (abdominal cramps, watery severe diarrhea, fever) may result from altered bacterial balance.

NURSING IMPLICATIONS

BASELINE ASSESSMENT:

Question patient for history of allergies to azithromycin, erythromycins, hepatitis. Obtain specimens for culture, sensitivity before giving first dose (therapy may begin before results are known).

INTERVENTION/EVALUATION:

Check for GI discomfort, nausea, vomiting. Determine pattern of bowel activity and stool consistency. Assess skin for rash. Monitor hepatic function tests, assess for hepatotoxicity: malaise, fever, abdominal pain, GI disturbances. Evaluate for superinfection: genital/anal pruritus, sore mouth or tongue, moderate to severe diarrhea.

PATIENT/FAMILY TEACHING:

Continue therapy for full length of treatment. Doses should be evenly spaced. Take medication w/8 oz water at least 1 hr before or 2 hrs after food/beverage. Notify physician in event of GI upset, rash, diarrhea, or other new symptom.

aztreonam

az-**tree**-oh-nam
(Azactam)

CLASSIFICATION

Antibiotic: Monobactam

AVAILABILITY (Rx)

Injection: 500 mg, 1 g, 2 g

PHARMACOKINETICS

Completely absorbed following IM administration. Partially metabolized by hydrolysis. Primarily excreted unchanged in urine. Removed by hemodialysis. Half-life: 1.4–2.2 hrs (increase in decreased renal, liver function).

ACTION/*THERAPEUTIC EFFECT*

Bactericidal effects due to inhibition of cell wall synthesis, *producing cell lysis, death.*

USES/*UNLABELED*

Lower respiratory tract, skin/skin structure, intra-abdominal, gynecologic, complicated/uncomplicated urinary tract infections; septicemia. *Treatment of bone/joint infections.*

STORAGE/HANDLING

Solution appears colorless to light yellow. Following reconstitution for IM injection or IV use, solution stable for 48 hrs at room temperature, or 7 days if refrigerated. Discard if precipitate forms. Discard unused portions.

IM/IV ADMINISTRATION

Note: Give by deep IM injection, IV injection, intermittent IV infusion (piggyback).

IM:

1. Shake immediately, vigorously after adding diluent.
2. Inject deeply into large muscle mass.

IV:

1. For IV injection, dilute each g w/6–10 ml sterile water, give over 3–5 min.
2. For intermittent IV infusion, further dilute w/50–100 ml 5% dextrose or 0.9% NaCl, infuse over 20–60 min.

3. Alternating IV sites, use large veins to reduce risk of phlebitis.

INDICATIONS/DOSAGE/ROUTES

Urinary tract infections:
IM/IV: Adults, elderly: 500 mg to 1 g q8–12h.

Moderate to severe systemic infections:
IM/IV: Adults, elderly: 1–2 g q8–12h.

Severe or life-threatening infections:
IV: Adults, elderly: 2 g q6–8h.

Usual pediatric dosage:
IV: 30 mg/kg q6–8hrs. **Maximum:** 120 mg/kg/day.

Dosage in renal impairment:
Dose and/or frequency is modified based on creatinine clearance, severity of infection:

CREATININE CLEARANCE	DOSAGE
10–30ml/min	1–2 g initially; then $1/2$ usual dose at usual intervals
<10ml/min	1–2 g initially; then $1/4$ usual dose at usual intervals

PRECAUTIONS

CONTRAINDICATIONS: Hypersensitivity to aztreonam. **CAUTIONS:** History of allergy, especially antibiotics, hepatic or renal impairment. **PREGNANCY/LACTATION:** Crosses placenta, distributed in amniotic fluid; low concentration in breast milk. **Pregnancy Category B**.

INTERACTIONS

DRUG INTERACTIONS: None significant. **ALTERED LAB VALUES:** Positive Coombs' test. May increase SGOT (AST), SGPT (ALT), LDH, alkaline phosphatase, creatinine.

SIDE EFFECTS

OCCASIONAL (<3%): Discomfort/swelling at IM injection site, nausea, vomiting, diarrhea, rash. **RARE (<1%):** Phlebitis/thrombophlebitis at IV injection site, abdominal cramps, headache, hypotension.

ADVERSE REACTIONS/TOXIC EFFECTS

Superinfection, antibiotic-associated colitis (abdominal cramps, watery severe diarrhea, fever) may result from altered bacterial balance. Severe hypersensitivity reactions including anaphylaxis occur rarely.

NURSING IMPLICATIONS

BASELINE ASSESSMENT:

Question pt for history of allergies, especially to aztreonam, other antibiotics. Obtain culture and sensitivity tests prior to giving first dose (therapy may begin before results are known).

INTERVENTION/EVALUATION:

Evaluate for phlebitis (heat, pain, red streaking over vein), pain at IM injection site. Assess for GI discomfort, nausea, vomiting. Monitor stool frequency and consistency. Assess skin for rash. Monitor vital signs. B/P twice daily. Assess mental status; be alert to tremors, possible seizures. Monitor I&O, renal function tests if indicated. Be alert to superinfection: increased temperature, changes in oral mucosa, sore throat, anal/genital pruritus.

PATIENT/FAMILY TEACHING:

Continue therapy for full length of treatment. Doses should be evenly spaced. Notify physician in event of tremors, seizures, rash, diarrhea, other new symptom.

bacampicillin

(Spectrobid)
See Classification section under:
Antibiotic: penicillins

bacitracin

bah-cih-**tray**-sin
(Baciguent, Bacitracin, Baci-IM)

FIXED-COMBINATION(S):
W/polymixin B, an antibiotic (**Polysporin**); w/polymyxin B and neomycin, antibiotics (**Mycitracin, Neosporin**).

CANADIAN AVAILABILITY:
Baciguent

CLASSIFICATION

Anti-infective

AVAILABILITY (Rx)

Powder for Injection: 50,000 U.
Ophthalmic Ointment. (OTC)
Topical Ointment.

ACTION/ THERAPEUTIC EFFECT

Interferes w/plasma membrane permeability in susceptible microorganisms, *inhibiting cell wall synthesis.* Bacteriostatic.

USES

Ophthalmic: Superficial ocular infections (conjunctivitis, keratitis, corneal ulcers, blepharitis). *Topical:* Minor skin abrasions, superficial infections. *Irrigation:* Treatment, prophylaxis of surgical procedures.

OPHTHALMIC ADMINISTRATION

1. Place finger on lower eyelid and pull out until a pocket is formed between eye and lower lid. Place $1/4$–$1/2$ inch ointment in pocket.

2. Close eye gently for 1–2 min, rolling eyeball (increases contact area of drug to eye). Remove excess ointment around eye w/tissue.

INDICATIONS/DOSAGE/ROUTES

Usual ophthalmic dosage:
Adults: $1/2$-inch ribbon in conjunctival sac q3–4h.

Usual topical dosage:
Adults, children: Apply 1–5 times/day to affected area.

Irrigation:
Adults, elderly: 50,000–150,000 units, as needed.

PRECAUTIONS

CONTRAINDICATIONS: Hypersensitivity. **CAUTIONS:** None significant.
PREGNANCY/LACTATION: Avoid parenteral use during pregnancy.
Pregnancy Category C.

INTERACTIONS

DRUG INTERACTIONS: None significant. **ALTERED LAB VALUES:** None significant.

SIDE EFFECTS

Note: It is important to know side effects of components when bacitracin is used in fixed-combination. **RARE:** *Topical:* Hypersensitivity reaction (itching, burning, inflammation), allergic contact dermatitis. *Ophthalmic:* Burning, itching, redness, swelling, pain.

ADVERSE REACTIONS/TOXIC EFFECTS

Severe hypersensitivity reaction (hypotension, apnea) occurs rarely.

NURSING IMPLICATIONS
BASELINE ASSESSMENT:

Question pt for history of allergies, particularly to bacitracin, neomycin.

INTERVENTION/EVALUATION:

Topical: Evaluate for hypersensitivity: itching, burning, inflammation. W/preparations containing corticosteroids, consider masking effect on clinical signs. *Ophthalmic:* Assess eye for therapeutic response or increased redness, swelling, burning, itching.

PATIENT/FAMILY TEACHING:

Continue therapy for full length of treatment. Doses should be evenly spaced. Report burning, itching, rash, or increased irritation. Ophthalmic application may cause temporary blurred vision; check w/physician before using eye makeup.

baclofen

back-low-fin
(Lioresal)

CANADIAN AVAILABILITY:
Apo-Baclofen, Lioresal, Liotec

CLASSIFICATION

Skeletal muscle relaxant

AVAILABILITY (Rx)

Tablets: 10 mg, 20 mg

PHARMACOKINETICS

Well absorbed from GI tract. Partially metabolized in liver. Primarily excreted in urine. Half-life: 2.5–4 hrs.

ACTION/THERAPEUTIC EFFECT

Acts at spinal cord level *(decreases frequency/amplitude of muscle spasms in patients w/spinal cord lesions).*

USES/UNLABELED

Relief of signs and symptoms of spasticity due to spinal cord injuries or diseases and multiple sclerosis, especially flexor spasms, concomitant pain, clonus, and muscular rigidity. *Treatment of trigeminal neuralgia.*

PO ADMINISTRATION

1. Give w/o regard to meals.
2. Tablets may be crushed.

INDICATIONS/DOSAGE/ROUTES

Musculoskeletal spasm:
PO: Adults: Initially, 5 mg 3 times/day. May increase by 15 mg/day at 3 day intervals. **Range:** 40–80 mg/day. Total dose not to exceed 80 mg/day.

Usual elderly dosage:
PO: Initially, 5 mg 2–3 times/day. May gradually increase dose.

PRECAUTIONS

CONTRAINDICATIONS: Skeletal muscle spasm due to rheumatic disorders, stroke, cerebral palsy, Parkinson's disease. **CAUTIONS:** Impaired renal function, CVA, diabetes mellitus, epilepsy, pre-existing psychiatric disorders. **PREGNANCY/LACTATION:** Unknown if drug crosses placenta or is distributed in breast milk. **Pregnancy Category C.**

INTERACTIONS

DRUG INTERACTIONS: Potentiated effects when used w/other CNS depressants (including alcohol). **ALTERED LAB VALUES:** May increase SGOT (AST), alkaline phosphatase, blood sugar.

SIDE EFFECTS

FREQUENT (>10%): Transient drowsiness, weakness, dizziness, lightheadedness, nausea, vomiting. **OCCASIONAL (2–10%):** Headache, paresthesia of hands/feet, constipation, anorexia, hypotension, confusion, nasal congestion. **RARE (<1%):** Paradoxical CNS excitement/restlessness, slurred speech, tremor, dry mouth, diarrhea, nocturia, impotence.

ADVERSE REACTIONS/TOXIC EFFECTS

Abrupt withdrawal may produce hallucinations, seizures. Overdosage results in blurred vision, convulsions, myosis, mydriasis, severe muscle weakness, strabismus, respiratory depression, vomiting.

NURSING IMPLICATIONS
BASELINE ASSESSMENT:

Record onset, type, location, and duration of muscular spasm. Check for immobility, stiffness, swelling.

INTERVENTION/EVALUATION:

Assess for paradoxical reaction. Assist with ambulation at all times. For those on long-term therapy, liver/renal function tests, blood counts should be performed periodically. Evaluate for therapeutic response: decreased intensity of skeletal muscle pain. Be alert to signs of infection. *Intrathecal:* After bolus in screening phase, observe pt closely for decreased muscle spasm (frequency or severity). After implant, monitor carefully for side effects w/resuscitative equipment immediately available. Check pump function and catheter patency.

PATIENT/FAMILY TEACHING:

Drowsiness usually diminishes w/continued therapy. Avoid tasks that require alertness, motor skills until response to drug is established. Do not abruptly withdraw medication after long-term therapy. Avoid alcohol and CNS depressants. Notify physician of frequency or painful urination, constipation, headache, nausea, confusion, or insomnia.

balsalazide
(Colazide)
See Supplement

basiliximab
(Simulect)
See Supplement

BCG, intravesical
(TheraCys, Tice BCG)

CANADIAN AVAILABILITY:
Immu Cyst

CLASSIFICATION
Antineoplastic

AVAILABILITY (Rx)
Vials for Reconstitution: 27 mg (TheraCys), 50 mg (Tice BCG)

ACTION/*THERAPEUTIC EFFECT*
Promotes local inflammation reaction w/histiocytic and leukocytic infiltration in urinary bladder. *Inflammatory effects associated w/apparent elimination/reduction of superficial cancerous lesions of urinary bladder.*

USES
Treatment of carcinoma in situ w/or w/o associated papillary tumors; therapy for pts w/carcinoma in situ of bladder following failure to respond to other treatment regimens. *TheraCys:* Treatment of primary and relapsed carcinoma in situ of urinary bladder (eliminates residual tumor cells, reduces frequency of tumor recurrence). *Tice BCG:* Primary or secondary treatment in

absence of invasive cancer in pts w/contraindication to radical surgery.

STORAGE/HANDLING

Store in refrigerator. Use immediately after reconstitution; avoid exposure to sunlight, direct or indirect. Handle as infectious; use aseptic technique.

INTRAVESICAL ADMINISTRATION

TheraCys:

1. Do not remove rubber stopper from vial; prepare immediately prior to use.
2. Use mask, gloves while preparing solution.
3. Reconstitute only w/diluent provided by manufacturer.
4. After reconstitution, further dilute w/50 ml sterile, preservative-free saline to final volume of 53 ml for intravesical instillation.

Tice BCG:

1. Draw 1 ml sterile, preservative-free saline into syringe (3 ml); add to 1 ampule Tice BCG.
2. Draw mixture into syringe/ gently expel back into ampule 3 times (ensures mixing; decreased clumping).
3. Dispense BCG suspension into top end of catheter-tip syringe containing 49 ml saline.
4. Gently rotate syringe; do not filter.

INDICATIONS/DOSAGE/ROUTES

Intravesical treatment and prophylaxis for carcinoma in situ of urinary bladder:

TheraCys:

Intravesical: Adults, elderly: Vials (in 50 ml saline) once weekly for 6 wks, then one treatment at 3, 6, 12, 18, 24 mos after initial treatment. Begin 7–14 days after biopsy or transurethral resection.

Tice BCG:

Intravesical: Adults, elderly: One amp in 50 ml preservative-free saline/wk for 6 wks. May repeat once. Thereafter, continue monthly for 6–12 mos.

PRECAUTIONS

CONTRAINDICATIONS: Those on immunosuppressive or corticosteroid therapy, those who have compromised immune system, positive HIV virus, undetermined fever or fever due to infection, urinary tract infection, positive Mantoux test, as immunizing agent for tuberculosis prevention, within 1–2 wks following transurethral resection. **CAUTIONS:** None significant. **PREGNANCY/LACTATION:** If possible, avoid use during pregnancy. Breast-feeding not recommended. **Pregnancy Category C**.

INTERACTIONS

DRUG INTERACTIONS: Bone marrow depressants, immunosuppressants may decrease immune response, increase risk of osteomyelitis of disseminated BCG infection. Live virus vaccines may potentiate virus replication, increase vaccine side effects, decrease pt's antibody response to vaccine. **ALTERED LAB VALUES:** None significant.

SIDE EFFECTS

FREQUENT: Dysuria, urinary frequency, hematuria, hypersensitivity reaction manifested as malaise, fever, chills. **OCCASIONAL:** Cystitis, urinary urgency, anemia, nausea, vomiting, anorexia, diarrhea, myalgia/arthralgia. **RARE:** Urinary tract infection, urinary incontinence, cramping.

ADVERSE REACTIONS/TOXIC EFFECTS

Systemic BCG infection manifested as fever >103° F or persistent fever >101° F for more than 2 days or severe malaise has produced deaths. Infectious disease specialist should be notified and fast-acting antituberculosis therapy begun immediately.

NURSING IMPLICATIONS
BASELINE ASSESSMENT:

Use aseptic technique when administering drug (handle as infectious) and avoid introducing contaminants into urinary tract. Pt symptoms usually begin 2–4 hrs after instillation and last 24–72 hrs. Hepatic and renal tests should be performed before therapy begins and when a wk or more has elapsed between doses.

INTERVENTION/EVALUATION:

Have pt sit to void after instillation. For 6 hrs postinstillation, urine should be disinfected w/equal volume 5% hypochlorite solution (undiluted household bleach) before flushing. Diligently monitor renal status (assess for hematuria, urinary frequency, dysuria, urinalysis for bacterial urinary tract infection). Inform physician immediately if any urinary difficulties arise. Monitor closely for BCG systemic infection (see Adverse Reactions/Toxic Effects) and contact physician immediately if such occur.

PATIENT/FAMILY TEACHING:

Notify physician/nurse immediately if cough develops. Check w/physician if symptoms persist or increase or if any of the following occur: blood in urine, fever, chills, a frequent urge to urinate, joint pain, nausea and vomiting, or painful urination. Do not have immunizations w/o physician's approval (drug low-ers body's resistance). Avoid contact w/those who have recently taken live virus vaccine.

---

becaplermin
(Regranex)
See Supplement

---

beclomethasone dipropionate

beck-low-**meth**-ah-sewn
(Beclovent, Vanceril, Beconase, Vancenase, Beconase AQ, Vancenase AQ)

CANADIAN AVAILABILITY:
Beclovent, Beclodisk, Beconase, Becloforte inhaler, Vancenase, Vanceril

CLASSIFICATION
Corticosteroid

AVAILABILITY (Rx)
Aerosol for oral, intranasal

PHARMACOKINETICS
Rapidly absorbed from pulmonary, nasal, and GI tissue. Metabolized in liver, undergoes extensive first-pass effect. Primarily eliminated in feces. Half-life: 15 hrs.

ACTION/*THERAPEUTIC EFFECT*
Inhalation: Decreases number, activity of inflammatory cells into bronchial wall, *inhibits bronchoconstriction, produces smooth muscle relaxation, decreases mucus secretion.* **Intranasal:** Inhibits early phase allergic reaction, migration of inflammatory cells into nasal tissue, *decreasing response to seasonal and perennial rhinitis.*

USES/*UNLABELED*

Inhalation: Control of bronchial asthma in those requiring chronic steroid therapy. *Intranasal:* Relief of seasonal/perennial rhinitis; prevention of nasal polyps from recurring after surgical removal; treatment of nonallergic rhinitis. *Nasal: Prophylaxis of seasonal rhinitis.*

INHALATION ADMINISTRATION

Shake container well, exhale completely, then holding mouthpiece 1 inch away from lips, inhale and hold breath as long as possible before exhaling.

INDICATIONS/DOSAGE/ROUTES

Usual inhalation dosage:
Inhalation: Adults, elderly: 2 inhalations 3–4 times/day. **Maximum:** 20 inhalations/day. **Children 6–12 yrs:** 1–2 inhalations 3–4 times/day. **Maximum:** 10 inhalations/day. **Vanceril DS:** 2 inhalations 2 times/day. **Maximum:** 5 inhalations/day.

Usual intranasal dosage:
Intranasal: Adults, elderly, children >12 yrs: 1 inhalation each nostril 2–4 times/day. **Children 6–12 yrs:** 1 inhalation 3 times/day. **Vancenase AQ Forte:** 1 inhalation each nostril once daily.

PRECAUTIONS

CONTRAINDICATIONS: Hypersensitivity to any corticosteroid or components, primary treatment of status asthmaticus, systemic fungal infections, persistently positive sputum cultures for *Candida albicans*, untreated localized infection involving nasal mucosa. **CAUTIONS:** Adrenal insufficiency. **PREGNANCY/LACTATION:** Unknown if drug crosses placenta or is distributed in breast milk. **Pregnancy Category C.**

INTERACTIONS

DRUG INTERACTIONS: None significant. **ALTERED LAB VALUES:** None significant.

SIDE EFFECTS

FREQUENT: *Inhalation (4–14%):* Throat irritation, dry mouth, hoarseness, cough. *Intranasal:* Burning, dryness inside nose. **OCCASIONAL:** *Inhalation (2–3%):* Localized fungal infection (thrush). *Intranasal:* Nasal crusting nosebleed, sore throat, ulceration nasal mucosa. **RARE:** *Inhalation:* Transient bronchospasm, esophageal candidiasis. *Intranasal:* Nasal/pharyngeal candidiasis, eye pain.

ADVERSE REACTIONS/TOXIC EFFECTS

Acute hypersensitivity reaction (urticaria, angioedema, severe bronchospasm) occurs rarely. Transfer from systemic to local steroid therapy may unmask previously suppressed bronchial asthma condition.

NURSING IMPLICATIONS
BASELINE ASSESSMENT:

Question for hypersensitivity to any corticosteroids, components.

INTERVENTION/EVALUATION:

In those receiving bronchodilators by inhalation concomitantly with inhalation of steroid therapy, advise pt to use bronchodilator several minutes before corticosteroid aerosol (enhances penetration of steroid into bronchial tree).

PATIENT/FAMILY TEACHING:

Do not change dose schedule or stop taking drug; must taper off gradually under medical supervision. *Inhalation:* Maintain careful mouth hygiene. **Rinse mouth w/water immediately after inhalation (prevents mouth/throat dryness, fungal infection of mouth). Contact physician/nurse if sore throat or mouth occurs.** *Intranasal:* **Contact physician if no improvement in symptoms, sneezing or nasal irritation occur. Clear nasal passages prior to use. Improvement seen in several days.**

benazepril

ben-**ayz**-ah-prill
(Lotensin)

FIXED-COMBINATION(S):
W/hydrochlorothiazide, a diuretic (**Lotensin-HCT**); w/amlodipine, a calcium channel blocker (**Lotrel**)

CANADIAN AVAILABILITY:
Lotensin

CLASSIFICATION

Angiotensin-converting enzyme (ACE) inhibitor; antihypertensive

AVAILABILITY (Rx)

Tablets: 5 mg, 10 mg, 20 mg, 40 mg

PHARMACOKINETICS

	ONSET	PEAK	DURATION
PO	1 hr	2–4 hrs	24 hrs

Partially absorbed from GI tract. Metabolized in liver to active metabolite. Primarily excreted in urine. Minimal removal by hemodialysis. Half-life: 35 min; metabolite: 10–11 hrs.

ACTION/ *THERAPEUTIC EFFECT*

Decreases rate of conversion of angiotensin I to angiotensin II, a potent vasoconstrictor. Reduces peripheral arterial resistance, *lowers B/P.*

USES/ *UNLABELED*

Treatment of hypertension. Used alone or in combination w/other antihypertensives. *Treatment of CHF.*

ADMINISTRATION

May give w/o regard to food.

INDICATIONS/DOSAGE/ROUTES

Hypertension (used alone):
PO: Adults: Initially, 10 mg/day. **Maintenance:** 20–40 mg/day as single dose. **Maximum:** 80 mg/day.

Usual elderly dosage:
PO: Initially, 10 mg/day. **Range:** 20–40 mg/day.

Hypertension (combination therapy):
Note: Discontinue diuretic 2–3 days prior to initiating benazepril therapy.
PO: Adults: Initially, 5 mg/day titrated to pt's needs.

Dosage in renal impairment (Ccr <30 ml/min):
Initially, 5 mg/day titrated up to maximum of 40 mg/day.

PRECAUTIONS

CONTRAINDICATIONS: History of angioedema w/previous treatment w/ACE inhibitors. **CAUTIONS:** Renal impairment, those w/sodium depletion or on diuretic therapy, dialysis, hypovolemia, coronary or cerebrovascular insufficiency, liver impairment, diabetes mellitus. **PREGNANCY/LACTATION:** Crosses placenta; unknown if distributed in breast milk. May cause fetal-neonatal mortality/morbidity. **First Trimester: Pregnancy Category C; Second and Third Trimester: Pregnancy Category D.**

INTERACTIONS

DRUG INTERACTIONS: Alcohol, diuretics, hypotensive agents may increase effects. NSAIDs may decrease effect. Potassium-sparing diuretics, potassium supplements may cause hyperkalemia. May increase lithium concentration, toxicity. **ALTERED LAB VALUES:** May increase potassium, SGOT (AST), SGPT (ALT), alkaline phosphatase, bilirubin, BUN, creatinine. May decrease sodium. May cause positive ANA titer.

SIDE EFFECTS

FREQUENT (3–6%): Cough, headache, dizziness. **OCCASIONAL (2%):** Fatigue, somnolence/drowsiness, nausea. **RARE (<1%):** Skin rash, fever, joint pain, diarrhea, loss of taste.

ADVERSE REACTIONS/TOXIC EFFECTS

Excessive hypotension ("first-dose syncope") may occur in those w/CHF, severe salt/volume depletion. Angioedema (swelling of face/lips), hyperkalemia occur rarely. Agranulocytosis, neutropenia may be noted in those w/impaired renal function or collagen vascular disease (systemic lupus erythematosus, scleroderma). Nephrotic syndrome may be noted in those w/history of renal disease.

NURSING IMPLICATIONS
BASELINE ASSESSMENT:

Obtain B/P immediately before each dose, in addition to regular monitoring (be alert to fluctuations). If excessive reduction in B/P occurs, place pt in supine position w/legs elevated. Renal function tests should be performed before therapy begins. In those w/renal impairment, auto- immune disease, or taking drugs that affect leukocytes or immune response, CBC and differential count should be performed before therapy begins and q2wks for 3 mos, then periodically thereafter.

INTERVENTION/EVALUATION:

Monitor pattern of daily bowel activity and stool consistency. Assist w/ambulation if dizziness occurs. Monitor B/P, renal function, urinary protein, leukocyte count.

PATIENT/FAMILY TEACHING:

To reduce hypotensive effect, rise slowly from lying to sitting position and permit legs to dangle from bed momentarily before standing. Cola, unsalted crackers, dry toast may relieve nausea. Full therapeutic effect may take 2–4 wks. Report any sign of infection (sore throat, fever). Skipping doses or voluntarily discontinuing drug may produce severe, rebound hypertension.

---

benzocaine
(Americaine, Anbesol, Orajel, Cetacaine, Chloroseptic Lozenges, Dermoplast, Hurricane)
See Classification section under: Anesthetics: local

---

benzonatate
ben-**zow**-nah-tate
(Tessalon Perles)

CLASSIFICATION

Antitussive

AVAILABILITY (Rx)

Capsules: 100 mg

PHARMACOKINETICS

	ONSET	PEAK	DURATION
PO	15–20 min	—	3–8 hrs

ACTION/*THERAPEUTIC EFFECT*

Anesthetizes stretch receptors in respiratory passages, lungs, pleura, *thereby reducing cough production.*

USES

Relief of nonproductive cough including acute cough of minor throat/bronchial irritation.

PO ADMINISTRATION

1. Give w/o regard to meals.
2. Swallow whole, do not chew/dissolve in mouth (may produce temporary local anesthesia/choking).

INDICATIONS/DOSAGE/ROUTES

Antitussive:
PO: **Adults, elderly, children >10 yrs:** 100 mg 3 times/day, up to 600 mg/day.

PRECAUTIONS

CONTRAINDICATIONS: None significant. **CAUTIONS:** Productive cough. **PREGNANCY/LACTATION:** Unknown if drug crosses placenta or is distributed in breast milk. **Pregnancy Category C.**

INTERACTIONS

DRUG INTERACTIONS: CNS depressants may increase effect. **ALTERED LAB VALUES:** None significant.

SIDE EFFECTS

OCCASIONAL: Mild drowsiness, mild dizziness, constipation, GI upset, skin eruptions, nasal congestion.

ADVERSE REACTIONS/TOXIC EFFECTS

Paradoxical reaction (restlessness, insomnia, euphoria, nervousness, tremors) has been noted.

NURSING IMPLICATIONS

BASELINE ASSESSMENT:

Assess type, severity, frequency of cough, and production.

INTERVENTION/EVALUATION:

Initiate deep breathing and coughing exercises, particularly in those with impaired pulmonary function. Monitor for paradoxical reaction. Increase fluid intake and environmental humidity to lower viscosity of lung secretions. Assess for clinical improvement and record onset of relief of cough.

PATIENT/FAMILY TEACHING:

Avoid tasks that require alertness, motor skills until response to drug is established. Dry mouth, drowsiness, dizziness may be an expected response of drug. Coffee or tea may help reduce drowsiness.

---

benztropine mesylate

benz-**trow**-peen
(Cogentin)

CANADIAN AVAILABILITY:
Apo-Benztropine, Cogentin

CLASSIFICATION

Anticholinergic; antiparkinson

AVAILABILITY (Rx)

Tablets: 0.5 mg, 1 mg, 2 mg. **Injection:** 1 mg/ml.

PHARMACOKINETICS

	ONSET	PEAK	DURATION
PO	1 hr	—	24 hrs
IM	15 min	—	24 hrs

Well absorbed from GI tract.

ACTION/THERAPEUTIC EFFECT

Selectively blocks central cholinergic receptors, assists in balancing cholinergic/dopaminergic activity. *Reduces incidence, severity of akinesia, rigidity, and tremor.*

USES

Treatment of Parkinson's disease, drug-induced extrapyramidal reactions, except tardive dyskinesia.

INDICATIONS/DOSAGE/ROUTES

Idiopathic Parkinsonism:
PO/IM: Adults: Initially, 0.5–1 mg/day at bedtime up to 6 mg/day.

Postencephalitic Parkinsonism:
PO/IM: Adults: 2 mg/day as single or divided dose.

Drug-induced extrapyramidal symptoms:
PO/IM: Adults: 1–4 mg 1–2 times/day.

Acute dystonic reactions:
IM/IV: Adults: 1–2 mg, then 1–2 mg orally 2 times/day to prevent recurrence.

Usual elderly dosage:
PO: Initially, 0.5 mg 1–2 times/day, may increase by 0.5 mg every 5–6 days. **Maximum:** 6 mg/day.

PRECAUTIONS

CONTRAINDICATIONS: Angle closure glaucoma, GI obstruction, paralytic ileus, intestinal atony, severe ulcerative colitis, prostatic hypertrophy, myasthenia gravis, megacolon, children <3 yrs. **CAUTIONS:** Treated open-angle glaucoma, heart disease, hyperten-sion, pts w/tachycardia, arrhythmias, prostatic hypertrophy, liver/renal impairment, obstructive diseases of the GI or genitourinary tract, urinary retention. **PREGNANCY/LACTATION:** Unknown if drug crosses placenta; distributed in breast milk. **Pregnancy Category C.**

INTERACTIONS

DRUG INTERACTIONS: Alcohol, CNS depressants may increase sedation. Amantadine, anticholinergics, MAO inhibitors may increase effects. Antacids, antidiarrheals may decrease absorption, effects. **ALTERED LAB VALUES:** None significant.

SIDE EFFECTS

Note: Elderly (>60 yrs) tend to develop mental confusion, disorientation, agitation, psychotic-like symptoms. **FREQUENT:** Drowsiness, dry mouth, blurred vision, constipation, decreased sweating/urination, GI upset, photosensitivity. **OCCASIONAL:** Headache, memory loss, muscle cramping, nervousness, peripheral paresthesia, orthostatic hypotension, abdominal cramping. **RARE:** Rash, confusion, eye pain.

ADVERSE REACTIONS/TOXIC EFFECTS

Overdosage may vary from severe anticholinergic effects (unsteadiness, severe drowsiness, severe dryness of mouth/nose/throat, tachycardia, SOB, skin flushing). Also produces severe paradoxical reaction (hallucinations, tremor, seizures, toxic psychosis).

NURSING IMPLICATIONS
BASELINE ASSESSMENT:

Assess mental status for confusion, disorientation, agitation, psychotic-like symptoms (medication frequently produces such side effects in those >60 yrs). Monitor rate, depth, rhythm, type of respiration; quality and rate of pulse. Assess lung sounds for rhonchi, wheezing, rales.

INTERVENTION/EVALUATION:

Be alert to neurologic effects: headache, lethargy, mental confusion, agitation. Assess for clinical reversal of symptoms (improvement of tremor of head/hands at rest, mask-like facial expression, shuffling gait, muscular rigidity). Monitor intraocular pressure.

PATIENT/FAMILY TEACHING:

Avoid tasks that require alertness, motor skills until response to drug is established. Dry mouth, drowsiness, dizziness may be an expected response of drug. Avoid alcoholic beverages during therapy. Sugarless gum, sips of tepid water may relieve dry mouth. Coffee or tea may help reduce drowsiness. Drowsiness tends to diminish or disappear w/continued therapy.

bepridil hydrochloride

beh-prih-dill
(Bepadin, Vascor)

CLASSIFICATION

Calcium channel blocker; antianginal

AVAILABILITY (Rx)

Tablets: 200 mg, 300 mg, 400 mg

PHARMACOKINETICS

Rapid, completely absorbed from GI tract. Undergoes first-pass metabolism in liver. Metabolized in liver to active metabolite. Primarily excreted in urine. Not removed by hemodialysis. Half-life: <24 hrs.

ACTION/*THERAPEUTIC EFFECT*

Inhibits calcium ion entry across cell membranes of cardiac and vascular smooth muscle *(dilates coronary arteries, peripheral arteries/arterioles)*; decreases heart rate, myocardial contractility, slows SA and AV conduction.

USES

Treatment of chronic stable angina (effort-associated angina) in those who have failed to respond or are intolerant to other antianginal drugs. May be used alone or concurrent w/beta blockers, nitrates.

PO ADMINISTRATION

1. Do not crush or break film-coated tablets.
2. May give w/o regard to food. May give w/meals and at bedtime (decreases nausea).

INDICATIONS/DOSAGE/ROUTES

Chronic stable angina:
PO: Adults, elderly: Initially, 200 mg/day; after 10 days, dosage may be adjusted. **Maintenance:** 200–400 mg/day.

PRECAUTIONS

CONTRAINDICATIONS: Sick sinus syndrome/second- or third-degree AV block (except in presence of pacemaker), severe hypotension (<90 mm Hg, systolic), history of serious ventricular arrhythmias, uncompensated cardiac insufficiency, congenital QT interval prolongation, use w/other drugs prolonging QT interval. **CAUTIONS:** Impaired renal/hepatic function, CHF. **PREGNANCY/LACTATION:** Unknown if drug crosses placenta. Distributed in breast milk. **Pregnancy Category C**.

INTERACTIONS

DRUG INTERACTIONS: Beta blockers may have additive effect. May increase digoxin concentration. Procainamide, quinidine may increase risk of QT interval prolongation. Hypokalemia-producing agents may increase risk of arrhythmias. **ALTERED LAB VALUES:** QT interval may be increased.

SIDE EFFECTS

FREQUENT (>10%): Dizziness, lightheadedness, nervousness, headache, asthenia (loss of strength), nausea, diarrhea. **OCCASIONAL (2–10%):** Drowsiness, insomnia, tinnitus, tremors, constipation, abdominal discomfort, dry mouth, palpitations, shortness of breath, wheezing, anorexia. **RARE (<2%):** Peripheral edema, anxiety, flatulence, nasal congestion, paresthesia.

ADVERSE REACTIONS/TOXIC EFFECTS

Can induce serious arrhythmias. CHF, second- and third-degree AV block occur rarely. Overdosage produces nausea, drowsiness, confusion, slurred speech, profound bradycardia.

NURSING IMPLICATIONS
BASELINE ASSESSMENT:

Record onset, type (sharp, dull, squeezing), radiation, location, intensity, and duration of anginal pain, and precipitating factors (exertion, emotional stress). Assess baseline renal/liver function tests. Assess pulse rate, EKG for arrhythmias before drug is administered.

INTERVENTION/EVALUATION:

Assist w/ambulation if lightheadedness, dizziness, drowsiness occur. Question for asthenia, headache, ringing/roaring in ears. Monitor liver enzyme tests. Monitor daily bowel activity and stool consistency. Assess EKG for arrhythmias, lung sounds for rales, wheezing.

PATIENT/FAMILY TEACHING:

Do not abruptly discontinue medication. Compliance w/therapy regimen is essential to control anginal pain. To avoid hypotensive effect, rise slowly from lying to sitting position, wait momentarily before standing. Avoid tasks that require alertness, motor skills until response to drug is established. Contact physician/nurse if irregular heartbeat, shortness of breath, pronounced dizziness, nausea, dyspepsia, ringing/roaring in ears, or constipation occurs.

beractant
burr-**act**-tant
(Survanta)

CANADIAN AVAILABILITY:
Survanta

CLASSIFICATION

Lung surfactant

AVAILABILITY (Rx)

Suspension: 25 mg/ml vials

ACTION/ *THERAPEUTIC EFFECT*

Lowers surface tension on alveolar surfaces during respiration, stabilizes alveoli vs. collapse that may occur at resting transpulmonary pressures. *Replenishes surfactant, restores surface activity to lungs.*

USES

Prevention/treatment (rescue) of respiratory distress syndrome (RDS—hyaline membrane disease) in premature infants. Oxygenation improves within minutes of administration.

STORAGE/HANDLING

Refrigerate vials. Warm by standing vial at room temperature for 20 min or warm in hand 8 min. If settling occurs, gently swirl vial (do not shake) to redisperse. After warming, may return to refrigerator within 8 hrs. Each vial should be injected w/a needle only one time; discard unused portions. Color is off-white to light brown.

INTRATRACHEAL ADMINISTRATION

1. Instill through catheter inserted into infant's endotracheal tube. Do not instill into main stem bronchus.
2. Monitor for bradycardia, decreased oxygen saturation during administration. Stop dosing procedure if these effects occur; begin appropriate measures before reinstituting therapy.

INDICATIONS/DOSAGE/ROUTES

Usual dosage:
Intratracheal: Infants: 100 mg of phospholipids/kg birth weight (4 ml/kg). Give within 15 min of birth if infant <1,250 g w/evidence of surfactant deficiency; give within 8 hrs when RDS confirmed by x-ray and requiring mechanical ventilation. May repeat no sooner than 6 hrs after preceding dose.

PRECAUTIONS

CONTRAINDICATIONS: None significant. CAUTIONS: Those at risk for circulatory overload.

INTERACTIONS

DRUG INTERACTIONS: None significant. ALTERED LAB VALUES: None significant.

SIDE EFFECTS

FREQUENT: Transient bradycardia, oxygen desaturation; increased CO_2 tension. OCCASIONAL: Endotracheal tube reflux. RARE: Apnea, endotracheal tube blockage, hypo/hypertension, pallor, vasoconstriction.

ADVERSE REACTIONS/TOXIC EFFECTS

Nosocomial sepsis may occur (not associated w/increased mortality).

NURSING IMPLICATIONS
BASELINE ASSESSMENT:

Drug must be administered in highly supervised setting. Clinicians in care of neonate must be experienced w/intubation, ventilator management. Give emotional support to parents.

INTERVENTION/EVALUATION:

Monitor infant w/arterial or transcutaneous measurement of systemic O_2 and CO_2. Assess lung sounds for rales and moist breath sounds.

betamethasone

bay-tah-**meth**-a-sone
(Celestone)

betamethasone benzoate

(Uticort)

betamethasone sodium phosphate

(Cel-U-Jec, Selestoject)

betamethasone dipropionate

(Alphatrex, Diprolene, Diprosone)

betamethasone valerate

(Luxiq Foam, Valisone, Beta-Val, Betatrex)

FIXED-COMBINATION(S):
Betamethasone sodium phosphate w/betamethasone acetate (**Celestone Soluspan**). Betamethasone dipropionate w/clotrimazole, an antifungal (**Lotrisone**)

CANADIAN AVAILABILITY:
Beben, Betaderm, Betnesol, Celestone, Diprolene, Diprosone

CLASSIFICATION

Corticosteroid

AVAILABILITY (Rx)

Tablets: 0.6 mg. **Syrup:** 0.6 mg/5 ml. **Injection, Cream:** 0.025%, 0.05%, 0.01%, 0.1%. **Lotion:** 0.025%, 0.05%, 0.1%. **Gel:** 0.025%. **Ointment:** 0.05%, 0.1%. **Aerosol:** 0.1%.

PHARMACOKINETICS

Rapid, complete absorption after oral, IM administration. Metabolized in liver, kidneys, tissue. Primarily excreted in urine. Half-life: 3–5 hrs.

ACTION / *THERAPEUTIC EFFECT*

Systemic: Inhibits accumulation of inflammatory cells at inflammation sites, inhibits synthesis of mediators of inflammation, *decreases tissue response to inflammatory process.* **Topical:** Forms complexes that enter cell nucleus stimulating formation of enzymes, *reducing inflammatory effect.*

USES

Substitution therapy in *deficiency states:* acute/chronic adrenal insufficiency, congenital adrenal hyperplasia, adrenal insufficiency secondary to pituitary insufficiency. *Nonendocrine disorders:* arthritis, rheumatic carditis, allergic, collagen, intestinal tract, liver, ocular, renal, and skin diseases, bronchial asthma, cerebral edema, malignancies. *Topical:* Relief of inflammatory and pruritic dermatoses. *Foam:* Relief of inflammation, itching associated w/dermatosis.

PO / IM / TOPICAL ADMINISTRATION

PO:

1. Give w/milk or food (decreases GI upset).

2. Single doses given prior to 9 AM; multiple doses at evenly spaced intervals.

Topical:

1. Gently cleanse area prior to application.

2. Use occlusive dressings only as ordered.

3. Apply sparingly and rub into area thoroughly.

4. When using aerosol, spray

area 3 sec from 15 cm distance; avoid inhalation.

IM:

Celestone Soluspan should not be mixed w/diluent or anesthetics containing preservatives.

INDICATIONS/DOSAGE/ROUTES

Usual dosage:
PO: Adults, elderly: 0.6–7.2 mg/day.
IM/IV: Adults, elderly: Up to 9 mg/day.

Usual topical dosage:
Adults, elderly: 2–4 times/day.
Foam: Apply twice daily.

PRECAUTIONS

CONTRAINDICATIONS: Hypersensitivity to any corticosteroid or sulfite, systemic fungal infection, peptic ulcers (except life-threatening situations). Avoid live virus vaccine such as smallpox. *Topical:* marked circulation impairment. **CAUTIONS:** Hypothyroidism, cirrhosis, ocular herpes simplex, history of tuberculosis (may reactivate disease), nonspecific ulcerative colitis, CHF, hypertension, psychosis, renal insufficiency. Prolonged therapy should be discontinued slowly. *Topical:* Do not apply to extensive areas. **PREGNANCY/ LACTATION:** Drug crosses placenta, distributed in breast milk. May cause cleft palate (chronic use first trimester). Nursing contraindicated. **Pregnancy Category C**.

INTERACTIONS

DRUG INTERACTIONS: Amphotericin may increase hypokalemia. May decrease effect of oral hypoglycemics, insulin, diuretics, potassium supplements. May increase digoxin toxicity (due to hypokalemia). Hepatic enzyme inducers may decrease effect. Live virus vaccines may potentiate virus replication, increase vaccine side effects, decrease pt's antibody response to vaccine. **ALTERED LAB VALUES:** May decrease calcium, potassium, thyroxine. May increase cholesterol, lipids, glucose, sodium, amylase.

SIDE EFFECTS

FREQUENT: *Systemic:* Increased appetite, abdominal distension, nervousness, insomnia, false sense of well-being. *Foam:* Burning, stinging, pruritus. **OCCASIONAL:** *Systemic:* Dizziness, facial flushing, diaphoresis, decreased/blurred vision, mood swings. *Topical:* Allergic contact dermatitis, purpura (blood-containing blisters, thinning of skin w/easy bruising), telangiectasis (raised dark red spots on skin). **RARE:** *Systemic:* General allergic reaction (rash, hives), pain/redness/swelling at injection site, hallucinations, mental depression.

ADVERSE REACTIONS/TOXIC EFFECTS

High dose or long-term therapy: acne, Cushing syndrome (moon face), muscle wasting (esp. arms, legs), osteoporosis, bone fractures, cataracts, glaucoma, psychosis, diabetes mellitus, pancreatitis, peptic ulcer, amenorrhea, poor healing, hypercalcemia, hypokalemia. Abrupt withdrawal following long-term therapy: anorexia, nausea, fever, headache, joint pain, rebound inflammation, fatigue, weakness, lethargy, dizziness, orthostatic hypotension.

NURSING IMPLICATIONS
BASELINE ASSESSMENT:

Question for hypersensitivity to any of the corticosteroids, sulfite. Obtain baselines for height, weight, B/P, glucose, electrolytes.

Check results of initial tests, e.g., TB skin test, x-rays, EKG.

INTERVENTION/EVALUATION:

Monitor I&O, daily weight; assess for edema. Check lab results for blood coagulability and clinical evidence of thromboembolism. Evaluate food tolerance and bowel activity; report hyperacidity promptly. Check B/P, temperature, pulse, respiration at least 2 times/day. Be alert to infection: sore throat, fever, or vague symptoms. Monitor electrolytes. Watch for hypocalcemia (muscle twitching, cramps, positive Trousseau's or Chvostek's signs) or hypokalemia (weakness and muscle cramps, numbness/tingling esp. lower extremities, nausea and vomiting, irritability, EKG changes). Assess emotional status, ability to sleep. Provide assistance w/ambulation.

PATIENT/FAMILY TEACHING:

Take w/food or milk. Carry identification of drug and dose, physician's name and phone number. Do not change dose/schedule or stop taking drug; must taper off gradually under medical supervision. Notify physician of fever, sore throat, muscle aches, sudden weight gain/swelling. W/dietician give instructions for prescribed diet (usually sodium restricted w/high vitamin D, protein, and potassium). Maintain careful personal hygiene, avoid exposure to disease or trauma. Severe stress (serious infection, surgery, or trauma) may require increased dosage. Do not take aspirin or any other medication w/o consulting physician. Follow-up visits, lab tests are necessary; children must be assessed for growth retardation. Inform dentist or other physicians of betamethasone therapy now or within past 12 mos. Caution against overuse of joints injected for symptomatic relief. Topical: Apply after shower or bath for best absorption. Do not cover unless physician orders; do not use tight diapers, plastic pants or coverings. Avoid contact w/eyes. Do not expose treated area to sunlight.

betaxolol

beh-**tax**-oh-lol
(Kerlone, Betopic)

CANADIAN AVAILABILITY:
Betoptic

CLASSIFICATION

Beta-adrenergic blocker; antihypertensive; antiglaucoma

AVAILABILITY (Rx)

Tablets: 10 mg, 20 mg. **Ophthalmic Solution:** 0.5%. **Ophthalmic Suspension:** 0.25%.

PHARMACOKINETICS

ONSET	PEAK	DURATION
Eyedrops		
30 min	2 hrs	12 hrs

Completely absorbed from GI tract. Metabolized in liver. Primarily excreted unchanged in urine. Not removed by hemodialysis. Half-life: 14–22 hrs (increase in decreased renal function).

ACTION/THERAPEUTIC EFFECT

Systemic: Predominantly blocks beta₁-adrenergic receptors in cardiac tissue by binding to receptor sites, *slowing sinus heart rate,* *decreasing cardiac output, decreasing B/P.* Large doses may block beta$_2$ receptors, *increasing airway resistance.* **Ophthalmic:** Reduces aqueous humor production, *decreasing intraocular pressure.*

USES / *UNLABELED*

Management of mild to moderate hypertension. Used alone or in combination w/diuretics, especially thiazide type. Reduces intraocular pressure in management of chronic open-angle glaucoma, ocular hypertension. *W/miotics decreases IOP in acute/chronic angle closure glaucoma, treatment of secondary glaucoma, malignant glaucoma, angle closure glaucoma during/after iridectomy.*

STORAGE / HANDLING

Store oral form, ophthalmic solution at room temperature.

PO / OPHTHALMIC ADMINISTRATION

PO:

May be given w/o regard to meals.

OPHTHALMIC:

1. Place finger on lower eyelid and pull out until pocket is formed between eye and lower lid. Hold dropper above pocket and place prescribed number of drops in pocket. Instruct pt to close eyes gently so medication will not be squeezed out of sac.

2. Apply gentle finger pressure to the lacrimal sac at inner canthus for 1 min following installation (lessens risk of systemic absorption).

INDICATIONS / DOSAGE / ROUTES

Hypertension:
PO: Adults: Initially, 10 mg/day alone or added to diuretic therapy. Dose may be doubled if no response in 7–14 days. If used alone, addition of another antihypertensive to be considered.

Usual elderly dosage:
PO: Initially, 5 mg/day.

Glaucoma:
Eyedrops: Adults, elderly: 1 drop 2 times/day.

Dosage in renal impairment (dialysis):
Initially 5 mg/day, increase by 5 mg/day q2wks. **Maximum:** 20 mg/day.

PRECAUTIONS

CONTRAINDICATIONS: Sinus bradycardia, overt cardiac failure, cardiogenic shock, heart block greater than first degree. **CAUTIONS:** Impaired renal or hepatic function, peripheral vascular disease, hyperthyroidism, diabetes, inadequate cardiac function. **PREGNANCY/LACTATION:** Unknown if drug crosses placenta or is distributed in breast milk. May produce bradycardia, apnea, hypoglycemia, hypothermia during delivery, small birth weight infants. **Pregnancy Category C**.

INTERACTIONS

DRUG INTERACTIONS: Diuretics, other hypotensives may increase hypotensive effect; sympathomimetics, xanthines may mutually inhibit effect; may mask symptoms of hypoglycemia, prolong hypoglycemic effect of insulin, oral hypoglycemics; NSAIDs may decrease antihypertensive effect; cimetidine may increase concentration. **ALTERED LAB VALUES:** May increase ANA titer, BUN, creatinine, potassium, uric acid, lipoproteins, triglycerides.

SIDE EFFECTS

Generally well tolerated, w/mild and transient side effects. **FREQUENT:** *Systemic:* Hypotension manifested as dizziness, nausea, diaphoresis, headache, fatigue, constipation/diarrhea; SOB. *Ophthalmic:* Eye irritation, visual disturbances. **OCCASIONAL:** *Systemic:* Insomnia, flatulence, urinary frequency, impotence or decreased libido. *Ophthalmic:* Increased light sensitivity, watering of eye. **RARE:** *Systemic:* Rash, arrhythmias, arthralgia, myalgia, confusion, change in taste, increased urination. *Ophthalmic:* Dry eye, conjunctivitis, eye pain.

ADVERSE REACTIONS/TOXIC EFFECTS

Oral form may produce profound bradycardia, hypotension, bronchospasm. Abrupt withdrawal may result in sweating, palpitations, headache, tremulousness. May precipitate CHF, MI in those w/cardiac disease, thyroid storm in those w/thyrotoxicosis, peripheral ischemia in those w/existing peripheral vascular disease. Hypoglycemia may occur in previously controlled diabetics. Ophthalmic overdosage may produce bradycardia, hypotension, bronchospasm, acute cardiac failure.

NURSING IMPLICATIONS

BASELINE ASSESSMENT:

Oral: Assess baseline renal/liver function tests. Assess B/P, apical pulse immediately before drug is administered (if pulse is 60/min or below, or systolic B/P is below 90 mm Hg, withhold medication, contact physician).

INTERVENTION/EVALUATION:

Monitor B/P for hypotension, respiration for shortness of breath. Assess pulse for strength/weakness, irregular rate, bradycardia. Monitor EKG for cardiac arrhythmias. Monitor daily bowel activity and stool activity. Assist w/ambulation if dizziness occurs. Assess for evidence of CHF: dyspnea (particularly on exertion or lying down), night cough, peripheral edema, distended neck veins. Monitor I&O (increase in weight, decrease in urine output may indicate CHF). Assess for nausea, diaphoresis, headache, fatigue.

PATIENT/FAMILY TEACHING:

Do not abruptly discontinue medication. Compliance w/therapy regimen is essential to control glaucoma, hypertension, angina, arrhythmias. To avoid hypotensive effect, rise slowly from lying to sitting position, wait momentarily before standing. Avoid tasks that require alertness, motor skills until response to drug is established. Report shortness of breath, excessive fatigue, prolonged dizziness, or headache. Do not use nasal decongestants, OTC cold preparations (stimulants) w/o physician approval. Monitor B/P, pulse before taking medication. Restrict salt, alcohol intake.

bethanechol chloride

be-**than**-eh-coal
(Duvoid, Urecholine)

CANADIAN AVAILABILITY:
Duvoid, Myotonachol, Urecholine

CLASSIFICATION

Cholinergic

AVAILABILITY (Rx)

Tablets: 5 mg, 10 mg, 25 mg, 50 mg. **Injection:** 5 mg/ml.

PHARMACOKINETICS

	ONSET	PEAK	DURATION
PO	>30 min	60–90 min	1 hr
SubQ	5–15 min	15–30 min	2 hrs

Large oral doses (300–400 mg) may give up to 6 hrs duration of action. Poorly absorbed from GI tract.

ACTION/ THERAPEUTIC EFFECT

Acts directly at cholinergic receptors of smooth muscle of urinary bladder and GI tract. Increases tone of detrusor muscle, *may initiate micturition, bladder emptying. Stimulates gastric, intestinal motility.*

USES/ UNLABELED

Treatment of acute postop and postpartum nonobstructive urinary retention, neurogenic atony of bladder w/retention. *Treatment of postop gastric atony, congenital megacolon, gastroesophageal reflux.*

STORAGE/HANDLING

Store parenteral form at room temperature. Discard if particulate matter, discoloration occurs.

PO/SUBQ ADMINISTRATION

PO:
Give on an empty stomach (minimizes risk of GI upset).
SubQ:
Note: Violent cholinergic reaction if given IM or IV (circulatory collapse, severe hypotension, bloody diarrhea, shock, cardiac arrest). *Antidote:* 0.6–1.2 mg atropine sulfate.

Aspirate syringe before injecting (avoid intra-arterial administration).

INDICATIONS/DOSAGE/ROUTES

Postop/postpartum urinary retention, atony of bladder:
PO: Adults, elderly: 10–50 mg 3–4 times/day. Minimum effective dose determined by initially giving 5–10 mg, and repeating same amount at 1 hr intervals until desired response achieved, or maximum of 50 mg reached.
SubQ: Adults, elderly: Initially, 2.5–5 mg. Minimum effective dose determined by giving 2.5 mg (0.5 ml), repeating same amount at 15–30 min intervals up to a maximum of 4 doses. Minimum dose repeated 3–4 times/day.

PRECAUTIONS

CONTRAINDICATIONS: Hyperthyroidism, peptic ulcer, latent or active bronchial asthma, mechanical GI and urinary obstruction or recent GI resection, acute inflammatory GI tract conditions, anastomosis, bladder wall instability, pronounced bradycardia, hypotension, hypertension, cardiac disease, coronary artery disease, vasomotor instability, epilepsy, Parkinsonism. **CAUTIONS:** None significant. **PREGNANCY/LACTATION:** Unknown if drug crosses placenta or is distributed in breast milk. **Pregnancy Category C.**

INTERACTIONS

DRUG INTERACTIONS: Cholinesterase inhibitors may increase effects/toxicity. Procainamide, quinidine may decrease effect. **ALTERED LAB VALUES:** May increase amylase, lipase, SGOT (AST).

SIDE EFFECTS

Note: Effects more noticeable w/SubQ. **OCCASIONAL:** Belching, change in vision, blurred vision, diarrhea, frequent urinary urgency. **RARE:** (SubQ): Shortness of breath, tight chest, bronchospasm.

ADVERSE REACTIONS/TOXIC EFFECTS

Overdosage produces CNS stimulation (insomnia, nervousness,

orthostatic hypotension), cholinergic stimulation (headache, increased salivation/sweating, nausea, vomiting, flushed skin, stomach pain, seizures). Cholinergic overstimulation manifested as circulatory collapse, hypotension, bloody diarrhea, sudden cardiac arrest.

NURSING IMPLICATIONS

INTERVENTION/EVALUATION:

Assess for cholinergic reaction: GI discomfort/cramping, feeling of facial warmth, excessive salivation and sweating, lacrimation, pallor, urinary urgency, blurred vision. Assess eyes for pupillary contraction. Question for complaints of difficulty chewing, swallowing, progressive muscle weakness (see Adverse Reactions/Toxic Effects).

PATIENT/FAMILY TEACHING:

Report nausea, vomiting, diarrhea, sweating, increased salivary secretions, irregular heartbeat, muscle weakness, severe abdominal pain, or difficulty in breathing. Rise slowly from lying to sitting position and sitting to standing position (avoid orthostatic hypotension).

---

bexarotene
(Targretin)
See Supplement
See Classification section under:
Antineoplastics

---

bicalutamide
by-kale-**yew**-tah-myd
(Casodex)

CANADIAN AVAILABILITY:
Casodex

CLASSIFICATION

Antineoplastic: hormone

PHARMACOKINETICS

Well absorbed from GI tract. Metabolized in liver to inactive metabolite. Excreted in urine and feces. Half-life: 5.8 days.

ACTION/*THERAPEUTIC EFFECT*

Competitively inhibits androgen action by binding to androgen receptors in target tissue. *Decreases growth of prostatic carcinoma.*

USES

Treatment of advanced metastatic prostatic carcinoma (in combination w/LHRH agonist analogues—i.e., leuprolide). Treatment w/both drugs must be started at same time.

PO ADMINISTRATION

1. May be given with or without food.
2. Take at same time each day.

INDICATONS/DOSAGE/ROUTES

Prostatic carcinoma:
PO: Adults, elderly: 50 mg once daily (morning or evening).

PRECAUTIONS

CONTRAINDICATIONS: None significant. **CAUTIONS:** None significant. **PREGNANCY/LACTATION: Pregnancy Category X.**

INTERACTIONS

DRUG INTERACTIONS: May displace warfarin from protein-binding sites, increase warfarin effect. **ALTERED LAB VALUES:** May increase SGOT (AST), SGPT (ALT), alkaline phosphatase, serum creatinine, bilirubin, BUN. May increase WBC, hgb.

SIDE EFFECTS

FREQUENT: Hot flashes (49%), breast pain (38%), muscle pain (27%), constipation (17%), diarrhea (10%), asthenia (15%), nausea

(11%). **OCCASIONAL:** Nocturia, abdominal pain, peripheral edema. **RARE:** Vomiting, weight loss, dizziness, insomnia, rash, impotence, iron deficiency anemia, gynecomastia.

ADVERSE REACTIONS/TOXIC EFFECTS

Sepsis, CHF, hypertension may be noted.

NURSING IMPLICATIONS
INTERVENTION/EVALUATION:

Monitor B/P periodically and hepatic function tests in long-term therapy. Check for diarrhea, nausea, and vomiting.

PATIENT/FAMILY TEACHING:

Do not stop taking medication (both drugs must be continued). Take medications at same time each day. Explain possible expectancy of frequent side effects. Contact physician if vomiting continues at home.

---

bisacodyl

bise-ah-**co**-dahl
(Dacody, Dulcolax)

CANADIAN AVAILABILITY:
Apo-Bisacodyl, Dulcolax

CLASSIFICATION

Laxative: Stimulant

AVAILABILITY (OTC)

Tablets (enteric coated): 5 mg.
Suppository: 10 mg.

PHARMACOKINETICS

	ONSET	PEAK	DURATION
PO	6–12 hrs	—	—
Rectal	15–60 min	—	—

Minimal absorption following oral, rectal administration. Absorbed drug excreted in urine; remainder eliminated in feces.

ACTION/ *THERAPEUTIC EFFECT*

Increases peristalsis by direct effect on colonic smooth musculature (stimulates intramural nerve plexi). *Promotes fluid and ion accumulation in colon to increase laxative effect.*

USES

Facilitates defecation in those w/diminished colonic motor response; for evacuation of colon for rectal, bowel examination, elective colon surgery.

PO/RECTAL ADMINISTRATION

PO:

1. Give on empty stomach (faster action).
2. Offer 6–8 glasses of water/day (aids stool softening).
3. Administer tablets whole; do not chew or crush.
4. Avoid giving within 1 hr of antacids, milk, other oral medication.

RECTAL:

1. If suppository is too soft, chill for 30 min in refrigerator or run cold water over foil wrapper.
2. Moisten suppository w/cold water before inserting well up into rectum.

INDICATIONS/DOSAGE/ROUTES

Laxative:
PO: Adults: 10–15 mg as needed. **Children >6 yrs:** 5–10 mg (0.3 mg/kg) at bedtime or after breakfast.
Rectal: Adults, children >2 yrs:

10 mg to induce bowel movement. **Children <2 yrs:** 5 mg.

Usual elderly dosage:
PO: Initially 5 mg/day.
Rectal: 5–10 mg/day.

PRECAUTIONS

CONTRAINDICATIONS: Abdominal pain, nausea, vomiting, appendicitis, intestinal obstruction, undiagnosed rectal bleeding. **CAUTIONS:** None significant. **PREGNANCY/LACTATION:** Unknown if drug crosses placenta or is distributed in breast milk. **Pregnancy Category C**.

INTERACTIONS

DRUG INTERACTIONS: Antacids, cimetidine, ranitidine, famotidine; milk may cause rapid dissolution of bisacodyl (produces abdominal cramping, vomiting). May decrease transit time of concurrently administered oral medication, decreasing absorption. **ALTERED LAB VALUES:** None significant.

SIDE EFFECTS

FREQUENT: Some degree of abdominal discomfort, nausea, mild cramps, griping, faintness. **OCCASIONAL:** Rectal administration may produce burning of rectal mucosa, mild proctitis.

ADVERSE REACTIONS/TOXIC EFFECTS

Long-term use may result in laxative dependence, chronic constipation, loss of normal bowel function. Chronic use or overdosage may result in electrolyte disturbances (hypokalemia, hypocalcemia, metabolic acidosis, or alkalosis), persistent diarrhea, malabsorption, weight loss. Electrolyte disturbance may produce vomiting, muscle weakness.

NURSING IMPLICATIONS
INTERVENTION/EVALUATION:

Encourage adequate fluid intake. Assess bowel sounds for peristalsis. Monitor daily bowel activity and stool consistency (watery, loose, soft, semisolid, solid) and record time of evacuation. Assess for abdominal disturbances. Monitor serum electrolytes in those exposed to prolonged, frequent, or excessive use of medication.

PATIENT/FAMILY TEACHING:

Cola, unsalted crackers, dry toast may relieve nausea. Institute measures to promote defecation: increase fluid intake, exercise, high-fiber diet. Do not take antacids, milk, or other medication within 1 hr of taking medication (decreased effectiveness). Report unrelieved constipation, rectal bleeding, muscle pain or cramps, dizziness, weakness.

bismuth subsalicylate

bis-muth sub-sal-**ih**-sah-**late**
(Pepto-Bismol)

FIXED-COMBINATION(S):
W/ranitidine, an H-2 antagonist **(Tritec)**; kit w/metronidazole and tetracycline, anti-infectives **(Helidac)**

CANADIAN AVAILABILITY:
Bismed, PeptoBismol

CLASSIFICATION

Antidiarrheal, antinauseant

AVAILABILITY (OTC)

Tablets: 262 mg. **Suspension:** 262 mg/5 ml, 525 mg/5 ml.

PHARMACOKINETICS

Hydrolyzed in stomach; nondissociated bismuth subsalicylate reacts to form insoluble bismuth salt; salicylate component rapidly, extensively absorbed from small intestine; bismuth poorly absorbed. Salicylate primarily excreted in urine; bismuth eliminated in feces.

ACTION/ THERAPEUTIC EFFECT

Inhibits synthesis of prostaglandins responsible for intestinal inflammation and hypermotility. Binds toxins produced by *Escherichia coli.* Absorbs fluid and electrolytes across intestinal wall, *preventing diarrhea.*

USES/ UNLABELED

Control of diarrhea. Treatment of indigestion, nausea; relieves gas pain/abdominal cramps, *Helicobacter pylori*–associated duodenal ulcer, gastritis. *Prevents traveler's diarrhea.*

PO ADMINISTRATION

1. Shake suspension before administering.

2. Tablets may be chewed or dissolved in mouth.

INDICATIONS/DOSAGE/ROUTES

Diarrhea, gastric distress:
PO: Adults, elderly: 2 tablets (30 ml) q30–60 min up to 8 doses/24 hrs. **Children 9–12 yrs:** 1 tablet or 15 ml q30–60 min up to 8 doses/24 hrs. **Children 6–9 yrs:** $2/3$ tablet or 10 ml q30–60 min up to 8 doses/24 hrs. **Children 3–6 yrs:** $1/3$ tablet or 5 ml q30–60 min up to 8 doses/24 hrs.

H. pylori–associated duodenal ulcer, gastritis:
PO: Adults, elderly: 525 mg 3 times/day 1 hr before meals (w/500 mg amoxicillin and 500 mg metronidazole 3 times/day after meals) for 7–14 days.

PRECAUTIONS

CONTRAINDICATIONS: Bleeding ulcers, hemorrhagic states, gout, hemophilia, renal function impairment. **CAUTIONS:** Elderly, diabetic pts. **PREGNANCY/LACTATION:** Readily crosses placenta. May increase risk of birth defects. Chronic, high-dose therapy during late pregnancy increases risk of long labor, complicated delivery, maternal or fetal hemorrhage. Excreted in breast milk. **Pregnancy Category C (Pregnancy Category D** during third trimester).

INTERACTIONS

DRUG INTERACTIONS: Anticoagulants, heparin, thrombolytics may increase risk of bleeding. Large dose may increase oral hypoglycemic, insulin effects. Other salicylates may increase toxicity. May decrease absorption of tetracyclines. **ALTERED LAB VALUES:** May alter SGPT (ALT), SGOT (AST), alkaline phosphatase, uric acid. May decrease potassium. May prolong prothrombin time.

SIDE EFFECTS

FREQUENT: Darkening of tongue, grayish black stools. **RARE:** Constipation.

ADVERSE REACTIONS/TOXIC EFFECTS

Debilitated pts and infants may develop impaction.

NURSING IMPLICATIONS
INTERVENTION/EVALUATION:

Encourage adequate fluid intake. Assess bowel sounds for peristaltic activity. Monitor stool frequency and consistency (watery, loose, soft, semisolid, solid).

PATIENT/FAMILY TEACHING:

Stool may appear gray/black. If high fever accompanies diarrhea or if diarrhea continues longer than 2 days, contact physician. Dry crackers, cola may help relieve nausea. Chew tablets thoroughly before swallowing

---

bisoprolol fumarate
bye-**sew**-prow-lol
(Zebeta)

FIXED-COMBINATION(S):
W/hydrochlorothiazide, a diuretic
(Ziac)

CLASSIFICATION

Beta-adrenergic blocker; antihypertensive

AVAILABILITY (Rx)

Tablets: 5 mg, 10 mg

PHARMACOKINETICS

Well absorbed from GI tract. Metabolized in liver. Primarily excreted in urine. Half-life: 9–12 hrs (increased in decreased renal function).

ACTION/ *THERAPEUTIC EFFECT*

Predominantly blocks beta$_1$-adrenergic receptors in cardiac tissue by binding to receptor sites, *slowing sinus heart rate, decreasing cardiac output, decreasing B/P.* Large doses may block beta$_2$ receptors, *increasing airway resistance.*

USES

Management of hypertension, alone or in combination w/diuretics, other medications.

PO ADMINISTRATION

1. May give w/o regard to food.
2. Scored tablet may be crushed.

INDICATIONS/DOSAGE/ROUTES

Hypertension:
PO: Adults, elderly: Initially, 2.5–5 mg/day as single dose either alone or in combination w/diuretic. May increase gradually up to 20 mg/day.
PO: Renal impairment (<40 ml/min), hepatic impairment (cirrhosis, hepatitis): Initially, 2.5 mg.

PRECAUTIONS

CONTRAINDICATIONS: Overt cardiac failure, cardiogenic shock, heart block greater than first degree. **CAUTIONS:** Impaired renal or hepatic function, peripheral vascular disease, hyperthyroidism, diabetes, inadequate cardiac function, bronchospastic disease. **PREGNANCY/LACTATION:** Readily crosses placenta; distributed in breast milk. Avoid use during first trimester. May produce bradycardia, apnea, hypoglycemia, hypothermia during delivery, small birth weight infants. **Pregnancy Category C.**

INTERACTIONS

DRUG INTERACTIONS: Diuretics, other hypotensives may increase hypotensive effect; sympathomimetics, xanthines may mutually inhibit effects; may mask symptoms of hypoglycemia, prolong hypoglycemic effect of insulin, oral hypoglycemics; NSAIDs may decrease antihypertensive effect; cimetidine may increase concentration. **ALTERED LAB VALUES:** May increase ANA titer, BUN, creatinine, potassium, uric acid, lipoproteins, triglycerides.

SIDE EFFECTS

Generally well tolerated, w/mild and transient side effects. **FREQUENT:** Hypotension manifested as dizziness, nausea, diaphoresis, headache, cold extremities, fatigue, constipation/diarrhea. **OCCASIONAL:** Insomnia, flatulence, urinary frequency, impotence or decreased libido. **RARE:** Rash, arthralgia, myalgia, confusion (esp. elderly), change in taste.

ADVERSE REACTIONS/TOXIC EFFECTS

Overdosage may produce profound bradycardia, hypotension. Abrupt withdrawal may result in sweating, palpitations, headache, tremulousness. May precipitate CHF, MI in those w/cardiac disease, thyroid storm in those w/thyrotoxicosis, peripheral ischemia in those w/existing peripheral vascular disease. Hypoglycemia may occur in previously controlled diabetics. Thrombocytopenia (unusual bruising, bleeding) occurs rarely.

NURSING IMPLICATIONS
BASELINE ASSESSMENT:

Assess baseline renal/liver function tests. Assess B/P, apical pulse immediately before drug is administered (if pulse is 60/min or below, or systolic B/P is below 90 mm Hg, withhold medications, contact physician).

INTERVENTION/EVALUATION:

Assess pulse for strength/weakness, irregular rate, bradycardia. Monitor EKG for cardiac changes. Assist w/ambulation if dizziness occurs. Assess for peripheral edema of hands, feet (usually, first area of lower extremity swelling is behind medial malleolus in ambulatory, sacral area in bedridden). Monitor stool frequency and consistency. Assess skin for development of rash. Monitor any unusual changes in pt.

PATIENT/FAMILY TEACHING:

Do not abruptly discontinue medication. Compliance w/therapy regimen is essential to control hypertension. If dizziness occurs, sit or lie down immediately. Avoid tasks that require alertness, motor skills until response to drug is established. Teach pts how to take pulse properly before each dose and to report excessively slow pulse rate (<60 beats/min), peripheral numbness, dizziness. Do not use nasal decongestants, OTC cold preparations (stimulants) w/o physician approval. Restrict salt, alcohol intake.

bitolterol mesylate
by-**toll**-ter-all
(Tornalate)

CLASSIFICATION
Bronchodilator

AVAILABILITY (Rx)
Aerosol

PHARMACOKINETICS

	ONSET	PEAK	DURATION
Inhalation			
	3–4 min	0.5–2 hrs	5–8 hrs
			2.5–5 hrs
			(corticosteroid
			dependent)

Hydrolyzed in tissue/blood to active compound. Excreted in urine, eliminated in feces. Half-life: 3 hrs.

ACTION/ *THERAPEUTIC EFFECT*

Stimulates beta$_2$-adrenergic receptors in lungs, *relaxing bronchial smooth muscle. Relieves bronchospasm, reduces airway resistance.*

USES

Prophylaxis, symptomatic treatment of bronchial asthma, acute bronchitis, reversible obstructive airway disease.

INHALATION ADMINISTRATION

1. Shake container well, exhale completely, then holding mouthpiece 1 inch away from lips, inhale and hold breath as long as possible before exhaling.

2. Wait 1–10 min before inhaling second dose (allows for deeper bronchial penetration).

3. Rinse mouth w/water immediately after inhalation (prevents mouth/throat dryness).

INDICATIONS/DOSAGE/ROUTES

Symptomatic relief:
Inhalation: **Adults, elderly, children >12 yrs:** 2 inhalations, separated by 1–3 min interval. Third inhalation may be needed.

Prophylaxis:
Inhalation: **Adults, elderly, children >12 yrs:** 2 inhalations q8h. Do not exceed 3 inhalations q6h, or 2 inhalations q4h.

PRECAUTIONS

CONTRAINDICATIONS: History of hypersensitivity to sympathomimetics. **CAUTIONS:** Hypertension, cardiovascular disorders, hyperthyroidism, seizure disorders, diabetes mellitus. **PREGNANCY/LACTATION:** Unknown if drug crosses placenta or is distributed in breast milk. May inhibit uterine contractility. **Pregnancy Category C.**

INTERACTIONS

DRUG INTERACTIONS: May decrease effects of beta blockers. May increase risk of arrhythmias w/digoxin. **ALTERED LAB VALUES:** May decrease potassium.

SIDE EFFECTS

FREQUENT (9–14%): Tremor. **OCCASIONAL (3–5%):** Cough, dry or irritated mouth/throat, headache, nausea, vomiting. **RARE (<1%):** Dizziness, vertigo, palpitations, insomnia.

ADVERSE REACTIONS/TOXIC EFFECTS

Although tolerance to the bronchodilating effect has not been observed, prolonged or too frequent use may lead to tolerance. Severe paradoxical bronchoconstriction may occur w/excessive use.

NURSING IMPLICATIONS

BASELINE ASSESSMENT:

Offer emotional support (high incidence of anxiety due to difficulty in breathing and sympathomimetic response to drug).

INTERVENTION/EVALUATION:

Monitor rate, depth, rhythm, type of respiration; quality and rate of pulse. Assess lung sounds for wheezing. Monitor arterial blood gases. Observe lips, fingernails for blue or dusky color in light-skinned patients; gray in dark-skinned patients. Observe for clavicular retractions, hand tremor. Evaluate for clinical improvement (quieter, slower respirations, relaxed facial expression, cessation of clavicular retractions).

PATIENT/FAMILY TEACHING:

Increase fluid intake (decreases lung secretion viscosity). Instruct pt on proper administration technique. Do not exceed recommended dosage (excessive use may produce paradoxical bronchoconstriction or a decreased bronchodilating effect). Rinsing mouth with water immediately after inhalation may prevent mouth/throat dryness. Avoid excessive use of caffeine derivatives (chocolate, coffee, tea, cola, cocoa). Do not take OTC medications w/o consulting physician. Avoid smoking, smoke-filled environment. Notify physician of dizziness, palpitations/chest pain or lack of therapeutic response.

bleomycin sulfate

blee-oh-**my**-sin
(Blenoxane)

CANADIAN AVAILABILITY:
Blenoxane

CLASSIFICATION

Antineoplastic

AVAILABILITY (Rx)

Powder for Injection: 15 units

PHARMACOKINETICS

Well absorbed after IM, SubQ administration; moderately absorbed following intrapleural or intraperitoneal administration. Metabolized by enzyme degradation in tissues. Primarily excreted in urine. Half-life: 2 hrs (increased in decreased renal function).

ACTION/*THERAPEUTIC EFFECT*

Exact mechanism unknown. Most effective in G_2 phase of cell division. May bind to DNA; *decreases DNA, RNA, protein synthesis.*

USES/*UNLABELED*

Palliative treatment of lymphomas: Hodgkin's disease, reticulum cell sarcoma, lymphosarcoma. Squamous cell carcinomas: head and neck, including mouth, tongue, tonsil, nasopharynx, oropharynx, sinus, palate, lip, buccal mucosa, gingiva, epiglottis, larynx). Testicular carcinoma, choriocarcinoma. Treatment of malignant pleural effusions, prevention of recurrent pleural effusions. *Treatment of renal carcinoma, soft tissue sarcoma, osteosarcoma, ovarian tumors, mycosis fungoides.*

STORAGE/HANDLING

Note: May be carcinogenic, mutagenic, or teratogenic. Handle w/extreme care during preparation/administration.

Refrigerate powder. After reconstitution with 5% dextrose or 0.9% NaCl injection, solution stable for 24 h at room temperature.

SUBQ/IM/IV ADMINISTRATION

SubQ/IM:

Reconstitute 15 unit vial w/1–5 ml sterile water for injection, 0.9% NaCl injection, 5% dextrose or bacteriostatic water for injection to provide concentration of 3–15 units/ml.

IV:

Reconstitute 15 unit vial w/at least 5 ml 0.9% NaCl injection, 5% dextrose and administer over at least 10 min.

INDICATIONS/DOSAGE/ROUTES

Note: Dosage individualized based on clinical response, tolerance to adverse effects. When used in combination therapy, consult specific protocols for optimum dosage, sequence of drug administration. Cumulative doses >400 units increase risk of pulmonary toxicity. Test doses of 2 units or less for first 2 doses recommended, due to increased possibility of anaphylactoid reaction in lymphoma pts.

Squamous cell carcinoma, lymphosarcoma, reticulum cell sarcoma, testicular carcinoma, Hodgkin's disease:
SubQ/IM/IV: Adults, elderly: 0.25–0.50 units/kg (10–20 units/m^2) 1–2 times/wk.

Hodgkin's disease (maintenance dose after 50% response):
IM/IV: Adults, elderly: 1 unit/day (or 5 units/wk).

Pleural effusion:
Adults: 60 units as single dose.

PRECAUTIONS

CONTRAINDICATIONS: Previous allergic reaction. **EXTREMECAUTION:** Severe renal/pulmonary impairment. **PREGNANCY/LACTATION:** If possible, avoid use during pregnancy, especially first trimester. Breast feeding not recommended. **Pregnancy Category D**.

INTERACTIONS

DRUG INTERACTIONS: Other antineoplastics may increase toxicity. Cisplatin-induced renal impairment may decrease clearance, increase toxicity. **ALTERED LAB VALUES:** None significant.

SIDE EFFECTS

FREQUENT: Anorexia, weight loss, erythematous skin swelling, urticaria, rash, striae (streaking), vesiculation (small blisters), hyperpigmentation (particularly at areas of pressure, skin folds, nail cuticles, IM injection sites, scars), mucosal lesions of lips, tongue. Usually evident 1–3 wks after initial therapy. May also be accompanied by decreased skin sensitivity followed by hypersensitivity of skin, nausea, vomiting, alopecia, fever/chills w/parenteral form (particularly noted few hrs after large single dose, lasts 4–12 hrs). **OCCASIONAL:** Pain at tumor site, stomatitis, thrombophlebitis w/IV administration.

ADVERSE REACTIONS/TOXIC EFFECTS

Interstitial pneumonitis occurs in 10% of pts, occasionally progressing to pulmonary fibrosis. Appears to be dose/age related (over 70 years, those receiving total dose more than 400 units). Renal, hepatic toxicity occur infrequently.

NURSING IMPLICATIONS
BASELINE ASSESSMENT:

Obtain chest x-rays q1–2 wks.

INTERVENTION/EVALUATION:

Discontinue drug immediately if pulmonary toxicity occurs (increased risk of toxicity if oxygen administered concurrently during therapy). Monitor lung sounds for pulmonary toxicity (dyspnea, fine lung rales). Monitor hematologic, pulmonary function studies, hepatic, renal function tests. Assess skin daily for cutaneous toxicity. Monitor for stomatitis (burning/erythema of oral mucosa at inner margin of lips), hematologic toxicity (fever, sore throat, signs of local infection, easy bruising, unusual bleeding), symptoms of anemia (excessive tiredness, weakness).

PATIENT/FAMILY TEACHING:

Fever/chills reaction occurs less frequently w/continued therapy. Improvement of Hodgkin's disease, testicular tumors noted within 2 wks, squamous cell carcinoma within 3 weeks. Do not have immunizations w/o doctor's approval (drug lowers body's resistance). Avoid contact w/those who have recently taken live virus vaccine. Contact physician if nausea/vomiting continues at home.

bretylium tosylate

bre-**till**-ee-um
(Bretylol)

CANADIAN AVAILABILITY:
Bretylate

CLASSIFICATION

Antiarrhythmic

AVAILABILITY (Rx)

Injection: 50 mg/ml, 100 mg/ml

PHARMACOKINETICS

	ONSET	PEAK	DURATION
IM	20 min–6 hrs	6–9 hrs	6–24 hrs
IV	20 min–6 hrs	6–9 hrs	6–24 hrs

Well absorbed after IM administration. Primarily excreted in urine. Removed by hemodialysis. Half-life: 4–17 hrs (increased in decreased renal function).

ACTION/THERAPEUTIC EFFECT

Directly affects myocardial cell membrane. Initially, releases norepinephrine, then inhibits its release, *contributing to suppression of ventricular tachycardia.*

USES

Prophylaxis and treatment of ventricular fibrillation in those w/life-threatening ventricular tachyarrhythmias who have not responded to conventional antiarrhythmic therapy.

STORAGE/HANDLING

Solution should appear clear after reconstitution. Discard if precipitate forms. Slight discoloration does not indicate loss of potency. Solution is stable for 48 hrs at room temperature, or 7 days if refrigerated.

IM/IV ADMINISTRATION

IM:

1. Do not dilute.
2. Do not give more than 5 ml into one site (over 3 ml may cause pain at injection site).
3. Rotate injection sites (same-site injection may cause muscular atrophy and necrosis).

IV:

1. For injection, give undiluted over 1 min.
2. For intermittent IV infusion (piggyback), dilute w/at least 50 ml 5% dextrose or 0.9% NaCl to provide concentration of 10 mg/ml.
3. Infuse over at least 8 min (too rapid IV produces nausea, vomiting).

INDICATIONS/DOSAGE/ROUTES

Ventricular arrhythmias, immediate, life threatening:

IV: **Adults, elderly:** 5 mg/kg undiluted by rapid IV injection. May increase to 10 mg/kg, repeat as needed. **Maintenance:** 5–10 mg/kg diluted over >8 min, q6h or IV infusion at 1–2 mg/min. **Children:** 5 mg/kg, then 10 mg/kg at 15–30 min interval. **Maximum:** 30 mg/kg total dose. **Maintenance:** 5–10 mg/kg q6h.

Ventricular arrhythmias, other:
IM: **Adults, elderly:** 5–10 mg/kg undiluted, may repeat at 1–2 hr intervals. **Maintenance:** 5–10 mg/kg q6–8h.
IV: **Adults, elderly:** 5–10 mg/kg diluted over >8 min, may repeat at 1–2 hr intervals. **Maintenance:** 5–10 mg/kg q6h or IV infusion at 1–2 mg/min. **Children:** 5–10 mg/kg/dose diluted q6h.

PRECAUTIONS

CONTRAINDICATIONS: None significant. **EXTREME CAUTION:** Digitalis-induced arrhythmias, fixed cardiac output (severe pulmonary hypertension, aortic stenosis). **CAUTIONS:** Impaired renal function, sinus bradycardia. Risk of orthostatic hypotension in the elderly. **PREGNANCY/LACTATION:** Unknown if drug crosses placenta. May decrease uterine blood flow, produce bradycardia in fetus. **Pregnancy Category C**.

INTERACTIONS

DRUG INTERACTIONS: May increase digoxin toxicity (due to initial norepinephrine release). Procainamide, quinidine may decrease inotropic effect, increase hypotension. **ALTERED LAB VALUES:** None significant.

SIDE EFFECTS

FREQUENT: Transitory hypertension followed by postural and supine hypotension in 50% of pts observed as dizziness, lightheadedness, faintness, vertigo. **OCCASIONAL (1–3%):** Diarrhea, loose stools, nausea, vomiting. **RARE (<1%):** Angina, bradycardia.

ADVERSE REACTIONS/TOXIC EFFECTS

Respiratory depression from possible neuromuscular blockade.

NURSING IMPLICATIONS
BASELINE ASSESSMENT:

Have pt in area w/equipment and personnel for constant cardiac and B/P monitoring.

INTERVENTION/EVALUATION:

Assess for conversion of ventricular arrhythmias and absence of new arrhythmias. Constantly monitor B/P, pulse. Notify physician of systolic B/P <75 mm Hg (dopamine or norepinephrine may be needed, or blood, plasma, or volume correction). Keep pt supine (risk of hypotension) during life-threatening therapy and during infusion until tolerance develops. When permitted, assist w/slow position change and ambulation. Put infusions on continuous infusion pumps. Monitor I&O. Provide emotional support to pt and family.

PATIENT/FAMILY TEACHING:

Tolerance to hypotensive effect usually occurs within several days after initial therapy. One hr after dose administration, may rise slowly from lying to sitting position and permit legs to dangle from bed for at least 5 min before standing.

brimonidine
(Alphagen)
See Supplement
See Classification section under:
Antiglaucoma agents

brinzolamide
(Azopt)
See Supplement
See Classification section under:
Antiglaucoma agents

bromocriptine

brom-oh-**crip**-teen
(Parlodel)

CANADIAN AVAILABILITY:
Apo-Bromocriptine, Parlodel

CLASSIFICATION

Anti-Parkinson, prolactin inhibitor

AVAILABILITY (Rx)

Tablets: 2.5 mg. **Capsules:** 5 mg.

PHARMACOKINETICS

	ONSET	PEAK	DURATION
PO	1–2 hrs	—	4–5 hrs
(growth hormone decrease)			
PO	2 hrs	8 hrs	24 hrs
(prolactin decrease)			

Minimal absorption from GI tract. Metabolized in liver. Excreted in feces via biliary secretion. Half-life: 15 hrs.

ACTION / THERAPEUTIC EFFECT

Directly inhibits prolactin release from anterior pituitary. Stimulates presynaptic and postsynaptic dopamine receptors. *Suppresses secretion, reduction of elevated growth hormone concentration.*

USES / UNLABELED

Treatment of hyperprolactinemia conditions (amenorrhea w/or w/o galactorrhea, prolactin secreting adenomas, infertility). Treatment of Parkinson's disease, acromegaly. *Treatment of neuroleptic malignant syndrome, cocaine addiction, hyperprolactemia associated w/pituitary adenomas.*

PO ADMINISTRATION

1. Pt should be lying down before administering first dose.
2. Give after food intake (decreases incidence of nausea).

INDICATIONS / DOSAGE / ROUTES

Hyperprolactinemia:
PO: Adults, elderly: Initially, 1.25–2.5 mg/day. May increase by 2.5 mg/day at 3–7 day intervals. **Range:** 2.5–15 mg/day.

Parkinson's disease:
PO: Adults, elderly: Initially, 1.25 mg 2 times/day. Increase by 2.5 mg/day every 14–28 days. **Range:** 10–40 mg/day.

Acromegaly:
PO: Adults, elderly: Initially, 1.25–2.5 mg/day at bedtime for 3 days. May increase by 1.25–2.5 mg/day every 3–7 days. **Range:** 20–30 mg/day. **Maximum:** 100 mg/day.

PRECAUTIONS

CONTRAINDICATIONS: Pregnancy, peripheral vascular disease, severe ischemic heart disease, uncontrolled hypertension, hypersensitivity to ergot alkaloids. **CAUTIONS:** Impaired hepatic/cardiac function, hypertension, psychiatric disorders. **PREGNANCY/LACTATION: Pregnancy Category B.**

INTERACTIONS

DRUG INTERACTIONS: Disulfiram reaction may occur w/alcohol. Estrogens, progestins may decrease effects. Phenothiazines, haloperidol, MAO inhibitors may decrease prolactin effect. Hypotensive agents may increase hypotension. Levodopa may increase effects. **ALTERED LAB VALUES:** May elevate BUN, SGOT (AST), SGPT (ALT), CPK, alkaline phosphatase, uric acid.

SIDE EFFECTS

Note: Incidence of side effects is high, especially at beginning of therapy or w/high dosage. **FREQUENT (>10%):** Nausea, headache, dizziness. **OCCASIONAL (4–10%):** Fatigue, lightheadedness, vomiting, abdominal cramps, diarrhea, constipation, nasal congestion, drowsiness, dry mouth. **RARE:** Muscle cramping, urinary hesitancy.

ADVERSE REACTIONS/TOXIC EFFECTS

Visual or auditory hallucinations noted in Parkinsonism syndrome. Long-term, high-dose therapy may produce continuing runny nose, fainting, GI hemorrhage, peptic ulcer, severe abdominal/stomach pain.

NURSING IMPLICATIONS
BASELINE ASSESSMENT:

Determine baseline, stability of vital signs. Evaluation of pituitary (R/O tumor) should be done prior to treatment for hyperprolactinemia w/amenorrhea/galactorrhea and infertility. Obtain pregnancy test.

INTERVENTION/EVALUATION:

Assist w/ambulation if dizziness is noted after administration. Monitor B/P for evidence of hypotension, particularly during early therapy. Assess for therapeutic response (decrease in engorgement, decreases in

Parkinsonism symptoms). Monitor for constipation.

PATIENT/FAMILY TEACHING:

Take w/food. To reduce lightheadedness, rise slowly from lying to sitting position and permit legs to dangle momentarily before standing. Avoid sudden posture changes. Avoid tasks that require alertness, motor skills until response to drug is established. Must use contraceptive measures (other than oral) during treatment. Report any watery nasal discharge to physician. Do not suddenly discontinue the drug. Avoid alcohol.

---

brompheniramine
(Bromphen, Dimetane)
See Classification section under: Antihistamines

---

budesonide
byew-**des**-oh-nyd
(Pulmicort, Rhinocort, Rhinocort Aqua)

CANADIAN AVAILABILITY:
Entocort, Pulmicort, Rhinocort Aqua

CLASSIFICATION

Corticosteroid: nasal

AVAILABILITY (Rx)

Aerosol for Intranasal: 32 mcg/activation. **Dry Powder for Oral Inhalation:** 200 mcg. **Suspension for Nebulization. Nasal Spray:** 32 mcg.

PHARMACOKINETICS

Minimally absorbed from nasal tissue. Primarily metabolized in liver. Half-life: 2 hrs.

ACTION/ *THERAPEUTIC EFFECT*

Decreases/prevents tissue response to inflammatory process, *inhibits accumulation of inflammatory cells.*

USES/ *UNLABELED*

Management of symptoms of seasonal or perennial allergic rhinitis in adults and children and nonallergic perennial rhinitis in adults. Maintenance treatment of asthma. *Treatment of vasomotor rhinitis.*

INTRANASAL ADMINISTRATION

1. Clear nasal passages before use (topical nasal decongestants may be needed 5–15 min before use).

2. Tilt head slightly forward.

3. Insert spray tip up in 1 nostril, pointing toward inflamed nasal turbinates, away from nasal septum.

4. Pump medication into 1 nostril while holding other nostril closed and concurrently inspire through nose.

5. Discard used nasal solution after 6 mos.

INDICATIONS/DOSAGE/ROUTES

Usual intranasal dosage:
Note: 32 mcg/spray.
Adults, children >6 yrs: Initially, 2 sprays each nostril 2 times/day (morning and evening), or 4 sprays in each nostril in morning. **Maximum:** 4 sprays each nostril/day.

Usual inhalation dosage:
Note: May give 200–400 mcg once daily in pts w/mild-moderate asthma well controlled on inhaled corticosteroids.
Adults: 200–800 mcg 2 times/day.
Children >6 yrs: 200 mcg 2 times/day. **Maximum:** 400 mcg 2 times/day.

PRECAUTIONS

CONTRAINDICATIONS: Hypersensitivity to any corticosteroid or components, primary treatment of status asthmaticus, systemic fungal infections, persistently positive sputum cultures for *Candida albicans.* Untreated localized infections involving nasal mucosa. **CAUTIONS:** Glaucoma, ocular herpes simplex, latent/active tuberculosis, recent nasal trauma or surgery. **PREGNANCY/LACTATION:** Not known whether drug crosses placenta or is distributed in breast milk. **Pregnancy Category C.**

INTERACTIONS

DRUG INTERACTIONS: None significant. **ALTERED LAB VALUES:** None significant.

SIDE EFFECTS

FREQUENT (>3%): *Nasal:* Mild nasopharyngeal irritation, burning, stinging, dryness, headache, cough. *Inhalation:* Flulike syndrome, headache, pharyngitis. **OCCASIONAL (1–3%):** *Nasal:* Dry mouth, dyspepsia, rebound congestion, rhinorrhea, loss of sense of taste, *Inhalation:* Back pain, vomiting, altered taste/voice, abdominal pain, nausea, dyspepsia.

ADVERSE REACTIONS/TOXIC EFFECTS

Acute hypersensitivity reaction (urticaria, angioedema, severe bronchospasm) occurs rarely.

NURSING IMPLICATIONS

BASELINE ASSESSMENT:

Question for hypersensitivity to any corticosteroids, components.

PATIENT/FAMILY TEACHING:

Contact physician if no improvement in symptoms, sneezing or nasal irritation occurs. Clear nasal passages prior to use. Improvement seen 24 hrs; but full effect may take 3–7 days.

bumetanide

byew-**met**-ah-nide
(Bumex)

CANADIAN AVAILABILITY:
Burinex

CLASSIFICATION

Diuretic: Loop

AVAILABILITY (Rx)

Tablets: 0.5 mg, 1 mg, 2 mg.
Injection: 0.25 mg/ml.

PHARMACOKINETICS

	ONSET	PEAK	DURATION
PO	30–60 min	60–120 min	4–6 hrs
IM	40 min	60–120 min	4–6 hrs
IV	Rapid	15–30 min	2–3 hrs

Completely absorbed from GI tract (decreased in CHF, nephrotic syndrome). Partially metabolized in liver. Primarily excreted in urine. Half-life: 1–1.5 hrs.

ACTION/ *THERAPEUTIC EFFECT*

Enhances excretion of sodium, chloride, and, to lesser degree, potassium, by direct action at ascending limb of loop of Henle and in the proximal tubule, *producing diuresis.*

USES/ *UNLABELED*

Treatment of edema associated w/CHF, chronic renal failure including nephrotic syndrome, hepatic cirrhosis w/ascites; treatment of acute pulmonary edema. *Treatment of hypertension, hypercalcemia.*

STORAGE/HANDLING

Store oral, parenteral form at room temperature.

PO/IM/IV ADMINISTRATION

PO:

Give w/food to avoid GI upset, preferably w/breakfast (may prevent nocturia).

IV:

1. May give undiluted but is compatible w/5% dextrose in water, 0.9% sodium chloride or lactated Ringer's.
2. Administer direct IV >1–2 min.
3. May give through Y tube or 3-way stopcock.

INDICATIONS/DOSAGE/ROUTES

Edema:
PO: Adults >18 yrs: 0.5–2 mg given as single dose in AM. May repeat at 4–5 hr intervals. **Elderly:** 0.5 mg/day, increase as needed.
IM/IV: Adults, elderly: 0.5–1 mg given as single dose. May be repeated at 2–3 hr intervals.

PRECAUTIONS

CONTRAINDICATIONS: Anuria, hepatic coma, severe electrolyte depletion. **EXTREME CAUTION:** Hypersensitivity to sulfonamides. **CAUTIONS:** Impaired renal or hepatic function, diabetes mellitus, elderly/debilitated. **PREGNANCY/LACTATION:** Unknown if drug is distributed in breast milk. **Pregnancy Category C.**

INTERACTIONS

DRUG INTERACTIONS: Amphotericin, ototoxic, nephrotoxic agents may increase toxicity. May decrease effect of anticoagulants, heparin. Hypokalemia-causing agents may increase risk hypokalemia. May increase risk of lithium toxicity. **ALTERED LAB VALUES:** May increase glucose, BUN, uric acid, urinary phosphate. May decrease calcium, chloride, magnesium, potassium, sodium.

SIDE EFFECTS

EXPECTED: Increase in urine frequency/volume. **FREQUENT:** Orthostatic hypotension, dizziness. **OCCASIONAL:** Blurred vision, diarrhea, headache, anorexia, premature ejaculation, impotence, GI upset. **RARE:** Rash, urticaria, pruritus, weakness, muscle cramps, nipple tenderness.

ADVERSE REACTIONS/TOXIC EFFECTS

Vigorous diuresis may lead to profound water/electrolyte depletion, resulting in hypokalemia, hyponatremia, dehydration, coma, circulatory collapse. Acute hypotensive episodes may occur. Ototoxicity manifested as deafness, vertigo, tinnitus (ringing/roaring in ears) may occur, esp. in pts w/severe renal impairment or who are on other ototoxic drugs. Blood dyscrasias have been reported.

NURSING IMPLICATIONS

BASELINE ASSESSMENT:

Check vital signs, esp. B/P for hypotension prior to administration. Assess baseline electrolytes; particularly check for low potassium. Assess edema, skin turgor, mucous membranes for hydration status. Assess muscle strength, mental status. Note skin temperature, moisture. Obtain baseline weight. Initiate I&O.

INTERVENTION/EVALUATION:

Continue to monitor B/P, vital signs, electrolytes, I&O, weight. Note extent of diuresis. Watch for changes from initial assessment (hypokalemia may result in muscle strength changes, tremor, muscle cramps, change in mental status, cardiac arrhythmias; hyponatremia may result in confusion, thirst, cold/clammy skin).

PATIENT/FAMILY TEACHING:

Expect increased frequency and volume of urination. Report irregular heartbeat, signs of electrolyte imbalances (see Adverse Reactions/Toxic Effects), hearing abnormalities (such as sense of fullness in ears, ringing/roaring in ears). Eat foods high in potassium such as whole grains (cereals), legumes, meat, bananas, apricots, orange juice, potatoes (white, sweet), raisins. Avoid sun/sunlamps. Get up slowly from sitting/lying position. Report continued nausea, diarrhea, vomiting

bupivacaine
(Marcaine, Sensorcaine)
See Classification section under: Anesthetics: local

buprenorphine hydrochloride
byew-**pren**-or-phen
(Buprenex)

CLASSIFICATION
Opioid analgesic **(Schedule V)**

AVAILABILITY (Rx)
Injection: 0.3 mg/ml

PHARMACOKINETICS

	ONSET	PEAK	DURATION
IM	15 min	1 hr	<6 hrs
IV	Rapid	Rapid	<6 hrs

Rapidly absorbed from IM injection. Metabolized in liver, undergoes extensive first-pass metabolism. Primarily eliminated in feces via bile. Half-life: 2–3 hrs.

B

ACTION/*THERAPEUTIC EFFECT*

Binds w/opioid receptors within CNS, *altering pain perception, emotional response to pain.* May displace opioid agonists and competitively inhibit their action (may precipitate withdrawal symptoms).

USES

Relief of moderate to severe pain.

INDICATIONS/DOSAGE/ROUTES

Note: May be given IM or slow IV injection. Do not mix w/diazepam or lorazepam in same syringe.

Analgesia:
IM/IV: Adults, children >13 yrs: 0.3 mg q6h as needed; may repeat 30–60 min after initial dose. May increase to 0.6 mg and/or reduce dosing interval to q4h if necessary. **Children 2–12 yrs:** 2–6 mcg/kg q4–6h.

Usual elderly dosage:
IM/IV: 0.15 mg q6h prn.

PRECAUTIONS

CONTRAINDICATIONS: None significant. **CAUTIONS:** Impaired hepatic/renal function, elderly, debilitated, head injury, respiratory disease, hypertension, hypothyroidism, Addison's disease, acute alcoholism, urethral stricture. **PREGNANCY/LACTATION:** Crosses placenta; unknown if distributed in breast milk (breast feeding not recommended). Prolonged use during pregnancy may produce withdrawal symptoms (irritability, excessive crying, tremors, hyperactive reflexes, fever, vomiting, diarrhea, yawning, sneezing, seizures) in neonate. **Pregnancy Category C.**

INTERACTIONS

DRUG INTERACTIONS: CNS depressants, MAO inhibitors may increase CNS or respiratory depression, hypotension. May decrease effects of other opioid analgesics. **ALTERED LAB VALUES:** May increase amylase, lipase.

SIDE EFFECTS

FREQUENT: Sedation (66%), dizziness (5–10%). **OCCASIONAL:** Headache (1–5%), hypotension (1–5%), nausea/vomiting (1–5%), hypoventilation (1–5%), miosis (1–5%), sweating (1–5%). **RARE:** Dry mouth, pallor, visual abnormalities, injection site reaction.

ADVERSE REACTIONS/TOXIC EFFECTS

Overdosage results in cold, clammy skin, weakness, confusion, severe respiratory depression, cyanosis, pinpoint pupils, extreme somnolence progressing to convulsions, stupor, coma.

NURSING IMPLICATIONS

BASELINE ASSESSMENT:

Obtain vital signs before giving medication. If respirations are 12/min or lower (20/min or lower in children), withhold medication, contact physician. Assess onset, type, location, duration of pain. Effect of medication is reduced if full pain recurs before next dose.

INTERVENTION/EVALUATION:

Monitor for change in respirations, B/P, change in rate/quality of pulse. Monitor stool frequency, consistency. Initiate deep breathing, coughing exercises, particularly in those w/impaired pulmonary function. Change pt's position q2–4h. Assess for clinical improvement and record onset of relief of pain.

PATIENT/FAMILY TEACHING:

Change positions slowly to avoid dizziness. Avoid tasks that require alertness, motor skills until response to drug is established. Avoid alcohol and benzodiazapines. Do not exceed prescribed dosage.

bupropion

byew-**pro**-peon
(Wellbutrin, Zyban)

CANADIAN AVAILABILITY:
Wellbutrin SR

CLASSIFICATION

Antidepressant, smoking cessation aid

AVAILABILITY (Rx)

Tablets: 75 mg, 100 mg. **Tablets (sustained-release):** 50 mg, 100 mg, 150 mg.

PHARMACOKINETICS

Rapidly absorbed from GI tract. Crosses blood-brain barrier. Extensive first-pass metabolism in liver to active metabolite. Primarily excreted in urine. Half-life: 14 hrs.

ACTION/*THERAPEUTIC EFFECT*

Blocks reuptake of neurotransmitters (serotonin, norepinephrine) at CNS presynaptic membranes, increasing availability at postsynaptic receptor sites. Resulting enhancement of synaptic activity *produces antidepressant effect.*

USES

Treatment of depression, particularly endogenous depression, exhibited as persistent and prominent dysphoria (occurring nearly every day for at least 2 wks) manifested by 4 of 8 symptoms: change in appetite, change in sleep pattern, increased fatigue, impaired concentration, feelings of guilt/worthlessness, loss of interest in usual activities, psychomotor agitation/retardation, or suicidal tendencies. Smoking cessation.

PO ADMINISTRATION

1. Avoid bedtime dosage (decreases risk of insomnia).
2. Do not crush sustained-release preparations.

INDICATIONS/DOSAGE/ROUTES

Note: Reduce dosage in renal/hepatic impairment, elderly.
PO: Adults: Initially, 75 mg 3 times/day or 100 mg 2 times/day. May increase to 100 mg 3 times/day no sooner than 3 days after initial dosage. Do not exceed dose increase of 100 mg/day in 3 day period. **Maximum daily dose:** 150 mg 3 times/day. Do not exceed any single dose of 150 mg.

Usual elderly dosage:
PO: Initially, 50–100 mg/day. May increase by 50–100 mg/day every 3–4 days.

Smoking cessation:
PO: Adults: Initially, 150 mg daily for 3 days; then 150 mg 2 times/day.

PRECAUTIONS

CONTRAINDICATIONS: Pts w/seizure disorder, current or prior diagnosis of bulimia or anorexia nervosa, concurrent use of MAO inhibitor. **EXTREME CAUTION:** History of seizure, cranial trauma; those currently taking antipsychotics, antidepressants. **CAUTIONS:** Impaired renal, hepatic function. **PREGNANCY/LACTATION:** Unknown if drug crosses placenta or is distributed in breast milk. **Pregnancy Category B.**

INTERACTIONS

DRUG INTERACTIONS: Alcohol, tricyclic antidepressants, lithium, trazodone may increase risk of seizures.

May increase risk of acute toxicity w/MAO inhibitors. **ALTERED LAB VALUES:** May decrease WBCs.

SIDE EFFECTS

FREQUENT (>10%): Constipation, weight gain or loss, nausea, vomiting, anorexia, dry mouth, headache, increased sweating, tremor, sedation, insomnia, altered hearing, dizziness, agitation. **OCCASIONAL (5–9%):** Diarrhea, akinesia, blurred vision, tachycardia, confusion, hostility, fatigue.

ADVERSE REACTIONS/TOXIC EFFECTS

Increased risk of seizures w/increase in dosage greater than 150 mg/dose, in pts w/history of bulimia or seizure disorders, of discontinuing agents that may lower seizure threshold.

NURSING IMPLICATIONS

BASELINE ASSESSMENT:

For those on long-term therapy, liver/renal function tests should be performed periodically.

INTERVENTION/EVALUATION:

Supervise suicidal risk patient closely during early therapy (as depression lessens, energy level improves, increasing suicide potential). Assess appearance, behavior, speech pattern, level of interest, mood. Monitor pattern of daily bowel activity, stool consistency. Monitor B/P, pulse for hypotension, arrhythmias.

PATIENT/FAMILY TEACHING:

Full therapeutic effect may be noted in 4 wks. Avoid alcohol (increases risk of seizure). Avoid tasks that require alertness, motor skills until response to drug is established. Dry mouth may be relieved by sugarless gum/sips of tepid water.

buspirone hydrochloride

byew-spear-own
(BuSpar)

CANADIAN AVAILABILITY:
Buspar, Buspirex, Bustab

CLASSIFICATION

Antianxiety

AVAILABILITY (Rx)

Tablets: 5 mg, 10 mg, 15 mg

PHARMACOKINETICS

Rapidly completely absorbed from GI tract. Undergoes extensive first-pass metabolism. Metabolized in liver to active metabolite. Primarily excreted in urine. Half-life: 2–3 hrs.

ACTION/*THERAPEUTIC EFFECT*

Binds to serotonin, dopamine at presynaptic neurotransmitter receptors in the CNS, *producing antianxiety effect.*

USES

Short-term relief (up to 4 wks), management of anxiety disorders.

PO ADMINISTRATION

1. Give w/o regard to meals.
2. Tablets may be crushed.
3. Avoid concomitant administration of grapefruit juice.

INDICATIONS/DOSAGE/ROUTES

PO: Adults: 5 mg 2–3 times daily. May increase in 5 mg increments/day at intervals of 2–4 days. **Maintenance:** 15–30 mg/day in 2–3 divided doses. Do not exceed 60 mg/day.

Usual elderly dosage:
PO: Initially, 5 mg 2 times/day. May increase by 5 mg every 2–3 days. **Maximum:** 60 mg/day.

PRECAUTIONS

CONTRAINDICATIONS: Severe renal/hepatic impairment, MAO inhibitor therapy. **CAUTIONS:** Renal/hepatic impairment. **PREGNANCY/LACTATION:** Unknown if drug crosses placenta or is distributed in breast milk. **Pregnancy Category B.**

INTERACTIONS

DRUG INTERACTIONS: Alcohol, CNS depressants may increase sedation. MAO inhibitors may increase B/P. **ALTERED LAB VALUES:** May increase SGOT (AST), SGPT (ALT).

SIDE EFFECTS

FREQUENT: Dizziness (12%), drowsiness (10%), nausea (8%), headache (6%). **OCCASIONAL:** Nervousness (5%), fatigue (4%), insomnia (3%), dry mouth (3%), lightheadedness (3%), mood swings (2%), blurred vision (2%), poor concentration (2%), diarrhea (2%), numbness in hands/feet (2%). **RARE:** Muscle pain/stiffness, nightmares, chest pain, involuntary movements.

ADVERSE REACTIONS/TOXIC EFFECTS

No evidence of tolerance or psychologic and/or physical dependence, no withdrawal syndrome. Overdosage may produce severe nausea, vomiting, dizziness, drowsiness, abdominal distension, excessive pupil contraction.

NURSING IMPLICATIONS
BASELINE ASSESSMENT:

Offer emotional support to anxious pt. Assess motor responses (agitation, trembling, tension) and autonomic responses (cold, clammy hands; sweating).

INTERVENTION/EVALUATION:

For pts on long-term therapy, liver/renal function tests, blood counts should be performed periodically. Assist w/ambulation if drowsiness, lightheadedness occur. Evaluate for therapeutic response: calm, facial expression, decreased restlessness and/or insomnia.

PATIENT/FAMILY TEACHING:

Improvement may be noted in 7–10 days, but optimum therapeutic effect generally takes 3–4 wks. Drowsiness usually disappears during continued therapy. If dizziness occurs, change position slowly from recumbent to sitting position before standing. Avoid tasks that require alertness, motor skills until response to drug is established. Avoid alcohol. Do not take other CNS depressants (unless ordered by physician). Do not discontinue drug abruptly. Report any chronic abnormal movements (e.g., motor restlessness).

busulfan
bew-**sull**-fan
(Busulfex, Myleran)

CANADIAN AVAILABILITY: Myleran

CLASSIFICATION

Antineoplastic

AVAILABILITY (Rx)

Tablets: 2 mg. **Injection:** 60 mg ampoule.

PHARMACOKINETICS

Completely absorbed from GI

tract. Metabolized in liver. Primarily excreted in urine. Half-life: 2.5 hrs.

ACTION/ *THERAPEUTIC EFFECT*

Cell cycle-phase nonspecific. Interferes w/DNA replication, RNA synthesis, *disrupting nucleic acid function. Myelosuppressant.*

USES/ *UNLABELED*

Palliative treatment of chronic myelogenous leukemia (CML). *Injection:* Combined w/cyclophosphamide as conditioning regimen before allogeneic hematopoietic progenitor cell transplantation in pts w/CML. *Treatment of acute myelocytic leukemia.*

PO ADMINISTRATION

Note: May be carcinogenic, mutagenic, or teratogenic. Handle w/extreme care during administration.

1. Give at same time each day.
2. Give on empty stomach if nausea/vomiting occur.

INDICATIONS/DOSAGE/ROUTES

Note: Dosage individualized based on clinical response, tolerance to adverse effects. When used in combination therapy, consult specific protocols for optimum dosage, sequence of drug administration.

Remission induction:
PO: Adults: 4–8 mg/day. Withdraw drug when WBC falls below 15,000/ mm³.

Maintenance therapy:
PO: Adults: Induction dose (4–8 mg/day) when total leukocyte count reaches 50,000/mm³. If remission occurs <3 mos, 1–3 mg/day may produce satisfactory response.

Usual elderly dosage:
PO: Initially, lowest dose for adults.

Usual parenteral dosage:
Note: Premedicate w/phenytoin to decrease risk of seizures.

IV Infusion: Adults: 0.8 mg/kg q6hrs (as 2 hr infusion) for total of 16 doses.

PRECAUTIONS

CONTRAINDICATIONS: Disease resistance to previous therapy w/drug. **EXTREME CAUTION:** Compromised bone marrow reserve. **CAUTION:** Chickenpox, herpes zoster, infection, history of gout. **PREGNANCY/LACTATION:** If possible, avoid use during pregnancy, esp. first trimester. May cause fetal harm. Unknown if distributed in breast milk. Breast feeding not recommended. **Pregnancy Category D**.

INTERACTIONS

DRUG INTERACTIONS: May decrease effect of antigout medications. Bone marrow depressant may increase risk of bone marrow depression. Live virus vaccines may potentiate virus replication, increase vaccine side effects, decrease antibody response to vaccine. **ALTERED LAB VALUES:** May increase blood/urine uric acid.

SIDE EFFECTS

FREQUENT: Hyperpigmentation (darkening) of skin (5–10%). *Intravenous:* Myelosuppression, nausea, stomatitis, vomiting. **OCCASIONAL:** Nausea, vomiting, anorexia, weight loss, diarrhea, stomatitis (redness/burning/ulceration of oral mucosa, gum/tongue inflammation, difficulty swallowing), confusion. **RARE:** Cataracts (prolonged administration).

ADVERSE REACTIONS/TOXIC EFFECTS

Major toxic effect is bone marrow depression resulting in hematologic toxicity (severe leukopenia, anemia, severe thrombocytopenia). Agranulocytosis occurs generally w/overdosage, may progress to pancytopenia. Very high doses may produce dizziness, blurred vision, muscle twitching, tonic-clonic seizures. Long-term therapy (>4 yrs) may produce pulmonary syndrome ("busulfan lung") characterized by persistent cough, congestion, rales, dyspnea. Hyperuricemia may produce uric acid nephropathy, renal stones, acute renal failure.

NURSING IMPLICATIONS
BASELINE ASSESSMENT:

Hgb, Hct, WBC, differential, platelet count, hepatic and renal functions studies should be performed weekly (dosage based on hematologic values).

INTERVENTION/EVALUATION:

Monitor WBC, differential, platelet count for evidence of bone marrow depression. Monitor for hematologic toxicity (fever, sore throat, easy bruising or unusual bleeding from any site), symptoms of anemia (excessive tiredness, weakness). Monitor lung sounds for pulmonary toxicity (dyspnea, fine lung rales).

PATIENT/FAMILY TEACHING:

Maintain adequate daily fluid intake (may protect against renal impairment). Report consistent cough, congestion, difficulty breathing. Promptly report fever, sore throat, signs of local infection, easy bruising or unusual bleeding from any site. Do not have immunizations w/o physician's approval (drug lowers body's resistance). Avoid contact w/those who have recently taken live virus vaccine. Contact physician if nausea/vomiting continues at home. Take on empty stomach if nausea or vomiting occurs. Take at same time each day. Contra-

ception is recommended during therapy. Medication may cause darkening of skin.

butenafine
(Mentax)
See Supplement

butorphanol tartrate
byew-**tore**-phen-awl
(Stadol, Stadol NS)

CANADIAN AVAILABILITY:
Stadol

CLASSIFICATION
Opioid analgesic (**Schedule IV**)

AVAILABILITY (Rx)
Injection: 1 mg/ml, 2 mg/ml. Nasal Spray: 10 mg/ml.

PHARMACOKINETICS

	ONSET	PEAK	DURATION
IM	10–30 min	30–60 min	3–4 hrs
IV	<1 min	4–5 min	2–4 hrs
Nasal	15 min	1–2 hrs	4–5 hrs

Rapidly absorbed from IM injection. Extensively metabolized in liver. Primarily excreted in urine. Half-life: 2.5–4 hrs.

ACTION/*THERAPEUTIC EFFECT*
Binds w/opioid receptors within CNS, *altering pain perception, emotional response to pain.* May displace opioid agonists and competitively inhibit their action (may precipitate withdrawal symptoms).

USES
Management of pain (including postop pain). *Nasal only:* Migraine

headache pain. *Parenteral only:* Preop, preanesthetic medication, supplement balanced anesthesia, relief of pain during labor.

INDICATIONS/DOSAGE/ROUTES

Note: May be given by IM or IV injection.

Analgesia:
IM: Adults: 1–4 mg q3–4h as needed.
IV: Adults: 0.5–2 mg q3–4h as needed.
Nasal: Adults: 1 mg (1 spray in one nostril). May repeat in 60–90 min. May repeat 2 dose sequence q3–4h as needed. Alternatively, 2 mg (1 spray each nostril if pt remains recumbent), may repeat in 3–4h.

Usual elderly dosage:
IM/IV: 1 mg q4–6h prn.

PRECAUTIONS

CONTRAINDICATIONS: None significant. **CAUTIONS:** Impaired hepatic/renal function, elderly, debilitated, head injury, respiratory disease, hypertension, prior to biliary tract surgery (produces spasm of sphincter of Oddi), MI w/nausea, vomiting. Not recommended for children <18 yrs. **PREGNANCY/LACTATION:** Readily crosses placenta; distributed in breast milk (breast feeding not recommended). **Pregnancy Category B**. (Category D if used for prolonged time, high dose at term.)

INTERACTIONS

DRUG INTERACTIONS: Alcohol, CNS depressants may increase CNS or respiratory depression, hypotension. MAO inhibitors may produce severe, fatal reaction (reduce dose to $1/4$ usual dose). Effects may be decreased w/buprenorphine. **ALTERED LAB VALUES:** None significant.

SIDE EFFECTS

FREQUENT: *Parenteral:* Drowsiness (43%), dizziness (19%). *Nasal:* Nasal congestion (13%), insomnia (11%). **OCCASIONAL:** *Parenteral* (3–9%): Confusion, sweating/clammy skin, lethargy, headache, nausea, vomiting, dry mouth. *Nasal* (3–9%): Vasodilation, constipation, unpleasant taste, dyspnea, epistaxis, nasal irritation, upper respiratory infection, tinnitus. **RARE:** *Parenteral:* Hypotension, pruritus, blurred vision, sensation of heat, CNS stimulation, insomnia. *Nasal:* Hypertension, tremor, ear pain, paresthesia, depression, sinusitis.

ADVERSE REACTIONS/TOXIC EFFECTS

Abrupt withdrawal after prolonged use may produce symptoms of narcotic withdrawal (abdominal cramping, rhinorrhea, lacrimation, anxiety, increased temperature, piloerection [goose bumps]). Overdosage results in severe respiratory depression, skeletal muscle flaccidity, cyanosis, extreme somnolence progressing to convulsions, stupor, coma. Tolerance to analgesic effect, physical dependence may occur w/chronic use.

NURSING IMPLICATIONS
BASELINE ASSESSMENT:

Obtain vital signs before giving medication. If respirations are 12/min or lower (20/min or lower in children), withhold medication, contact physician. Assess onset, type, location, duration of pain. Effect of medication is reduced if full pain recurs before next dose. Protect from falls. During labor, assess fetal heart tones, uterine contractions.

INTERVENTION/EVALUATION:

Increase fluid intake and environmental humidity to improve viscosity of lung secretions. Monitor for change in respirations, B/P, change in rate/quality of pulse. Monitor pattern of daily bowel activity, stool consistency. Initiate deep breathing and coughing exercises, particularly in those w/ impaired pulmonary function. Change pt's position q2–4h. Assess for clinical improvement and record onset of relief of pain.

PATIENT/FAMILY TEACHING:

Change positions slowly to avoid dizziness. Avoid tasks that require alertness, motor skills until response to drug is established. Instruct pt on proper use of nasal spray. Avoid use of alcohol or CNS depressants.

---

cabergoline
(Dostinex)
See Supplement

---

calcipotriene
kal-sih-**poe**-tree-in
(Dovonex)

CANADIAN AVAILABILITY:
Dovonex

CLASSIFICATION

Antipsoriatic

AVAILABILITY (Rx)

Cream: 0.005%. **Ointment:** 0.005%. **Scalp solution:** 0.005%.

PHARMACOKINETICS

Absorbed systemically. Rapid metabolism. Excreted in bile.

ACTION/*THERAPEUTIC EFFECT*

A synthetic vitamin D_3 analogue. Regulates skin cell (keratinocyte) production and development, *preventing abnormal growth and production of psoriasis (abnormal keratinocyte growth)*.

USES

Treatment of mild to moderate plaque psoriasis. **Solution:** Treatment of chronic, moderately severe scalp psoriasis.

INDICATIONS/DOSAGE/ROUTES

Psoriasis:
Topical: **Adults, elderly, children >12 yrs:** Apply thin layer to affected skin twice daily (morning and evening); rub in gently and completely. **Solution:** Apply to lesions after combing hair.

PRECAUTIONS

CONTRAINDICATIONS: Hypersensitivity to components of preparation, hypercalcemia or evidence of vitamin D toxicity, use on face. **CAUTIONS:** History of nephrolithiasis. **PREGNANCY/LACTATION:** May enter fetal circulation. Unknown if distributed in breast milk. **Pregnancy Category C**.

INTERACTIONS

DRUG INTERACTIONS: None significant. **ALTERED LAB VALUES:** Excessive use may increase serum calcium level.

SIDE EFFECTS

FREQUENT: Burning, itching, skin irritation (10–15%). **OCCASIONAL:** Erythema, dry skin, peeling, rash, worsening of psoriasis dermatititis (1–10%). **RARE:** Skin atrophy, hyperpigmentation, folliculitis (<1%).

ADVERSE REACTIONS/TOXIC EFFECTS

Potential for hypercalcemia (abdominal pain, depression, easy fatigability, high B/P, anorexia, nausea, thirst) may occur.

NURSING IMPLICATIONS

BASELINE ASSESSMENT:

Establish baseline electrolytes, particularly serum and urine calcium.

INTERVENTION/EVALUATION:

Monitor serum calcium. Assess skin for irritation, erythema, worsening of psoriasis (children, those >65 are at greater risk of reactions than adults). If irritation of lesions or surrounding uninvolved skin develops or if serum calcium level increases outside normal range, medication should be discontinued.

PATIENT/FAMILY TEACHING:

Avoid contact w/face or eyes. Wash hands after application. Report any signs of local reactions. Improvement noted usually beginning after 2 wks of therapy, marked improvement after 8 wks of therapy. Follow-up lab tests, office visits are necessary.

---

calcitonin-salmon

kal-sih-**toe**-nin
(Calcimar, Miacalcin)

CANADIAN AVAILABILITY:
Calcimar, Caltine

CLASSIFICATION

Calcium regulator

AVAILABILITY (Rx)

Injection: 200 IU/ml. **Nasal Spray:** 200 IU/activation.

PHARMACOKINETICS

Rapidly metabolized (primarily in kidney). Primarily excreted in urine. Half-life: 70–90 min.

ACTION/THERAPEUTIC EFFECT

Reduces bone turnover by blocking bone resorption in Paget's disease; directly inhibits bone resorption, decreasing the number/function of osteoclasts in osteoporosis. *Reduces bone turnover, lowers serum calcium concentration.*

USES/UNLABELED

Management of moderate to severe Paget's disease of bone, early treatment of hypercalcemic emergencies. Management of postmenopausal osteoporosis to prevent progressive loss of bone mass (w/calcium, vitamin D). *Treatment of secondary osteoporosis due to hormone disturbance, drug therapy.*

STORAGE/HANDLING

Refrigerate. Nasal preparation can be stored at room temperature once pump is activated.

SUBQ/IM ADMINISTRATION

1. May be administered SubQ or IM. No more than 2 ml dose should be given IM.
2. Skin test should be performed before therapy.
3. Bedtime administration may reduce nausea, flushing.

INDICATIONS/DOSAGE/ROUTES

Skin testing:
Prepare a 10 units/ml dilution; withdraw 0.05 ml from 200 IU/ml vial solution in tuberculin syringe; fill up to 1 ml w/0.9% NaCl. Take 0.1 ml and inject intracutaneously on inner aspect of forearm.

Observe after 15 min (positive response: appearance of more than mild erythema or wheal).

Paget's disease:
IM/SubQ: Adults, elderly: Initially, 100 IU/day (improvement in biochemical abnormalities, bone pain seen in first few months; in neurologic lesion, often longer than 1 yr). **Maintenance:** 50 IU/day or every other day.

Postmenopausal osteoporosis:
IM/SubQ: Adults, elderly: 100 IU/day (w/adequate calcium and vitamin D intake).
Intranasal: 200 IU as single daily spray, alternating nostrils daily.

Hypercalcemia:
IM/SubQ: Adults, elderly: Initially, 4 IU/kg q12h; may increase to 8 IU/kg q12h if no response in 2 days; may further increase to 8 IU/kg q6h if no response in 2 days.

PRECAUTIONS

CONTRAINDICATIONS: Hypersensitivity to calcitonin. Data does not support use in children. **CAUTIONS:** History of allergy, renal dysfunction. **PREGNANCY/LACTATION:** Drug does not cross placenta; unknown if distributed in breast milk. Safe usage during lactation not established (inhibits lactation in animals). **Pregnancy Category B**.

INTERACTIONS

DRUG INTERACTIONS: None significant. **ALTERED LAB VALUES:** None significant.

SIDE EFFECTS

FREQUENT: *IM/SubQ:* Nausea may occur in 30 min after injection, usually diminishes w/continued therapy. Anorexia, vomiting, diarrhea, flushing of face, ears, hands, feet. *Nasal:* Rhinitis, rhinorrhea, facial flushing, nasal dryness, headache, arthralgia, epistaxis, back pain. **OCCASIONAL:** *IM/SubQ:* Tenderness/tingling of palms/soles, local inflammation at injection site, diuresis, unusual taste. *Nasal:* Fatigue, rash, hypertension, diarrhea, abdominal pain, angina, cystitis, conjunctivitis. **RARE:** *IM/SubQ:* Headache, chest pressure, nasal congestion, hypersensitivity (including rash, urticaria).

ADVERSE REACTIONS/TOXIC EFFECTS

Potential for hypocalcemic tetany or anaphylaxis w/protein allergy.

NURSING IMPLICATIONS
BASELINE ASSESSMENT:

Question for allergies, hypersensitivity to fish, calcitonin. Establish baseline electrolytes.

INTERVENTION/EVALUATION:

Assess for allergic response: rash, urticaria, swelling, shortness of breath, tachycardia, hypotension. Assure rotation of injection sites; check for inflammation. Monitor electrolytes. Periodic nasal exam. Assess vertebral bone mass (document stabilization/improvement).

PATIENT/FAMILY TEACHING:

Instruct pt/family on aseptic technique, proper injection of medication, including rotation of sites. Do not take any other medications w/o consulting physician. Nausea and flushing are transient; nausea and diuresis usually decrease w/continued therapy. Notify physician immediately if rash, urticaria, shortness of breath, significant nasal irritation occur. Follow-up lab tests, office visits are necessary.

calcium acetate
(Phos-Ex, PhosLo)

calcium carbonate
(Dicarbasil, OsCal, Titralac, Tums)

calcium chloride

calcium citrate
(Citracal)

calcium glubionate
(NeoCalglucon)

calcium gluconate

CANADIAN AVAILABILITY:
Apo-Cal, Calcijex, Calsan, Caltrate

CLASSIFICATION

Antacid, antihypocalcemic, nutritional supplement

AVAILABILITY (OTC)

Calcium acetate: **Tablets:** 250 mg, 667 mg, 1,000 mg. **Capsules:** 500 mg.

Calcium carbonate: **Tablets:** 500 mg, 650 mg, 1,250 mg, 1,500 mg. **Chewable tablets:** 350 mg, 500 mg, 750 mg, 1,250 mg. **Capsules:** 1,250 mg.

Calcium chloride (Rx): **Injection:** 10%

Calcium citrate: **Tablets:** 950 mg.

Calcium glubionate: **Syrup.**

Calcium gluconate: **Tablets:** 500 mg, 650 mg, 975 mg, 1,000 mg. **Injection: (Rx):** 10%.

PHARMACOKINETICS

Moderately absorbed from small intestine (dependent on presence of vitamin D metabolites, pH). Primarily eliminated in feces.

ACTION/*THERAPEUTIC EFFECT*

Calcium is essential for function, integrity of nervous, muscular, skeletal systems. Important role in normal cardiac, renal function, respiration, blood coagulation, and cell membrane and capillary permeability. Assists in regulating release/storage of neurotransmitter/hormones. Neutralizes or reduces gastric acid (increase pH). *Calcium acetate:* Combines w/dietary phosphate, forming insoluble calcium phosphate. *Replaces calcium in deficiency states, controls hyperphosphatemia in end-stage renal disease.*

USES/*UNLABELED*

Parenteral: Acute hypocalcemia (e.g., neonatal hypocalcemic tetany, alkalosis), electrolyte depletion, cardiac arrest (strengthens myocardial contractions), hyperkalemia (reverses EKG, cardiac depression), hypermagnesemia (aids in reversing CNS depression). *Oral:* Chronic hypocalcemia, calcium deficiency, antacid. *Calcium acetate:* Controls hyperphosphatemia in end-stage renal disease. *Calcium carbonate: Treatment of hyperphosphatemia.*

PO/IV ADMINISTRATION

PO:

1. Take tablets w/full glass of water 0.5–1 hr after meals. Give syrup before meals (increases absorption), diluted in juice or water.

2. Chew chewable tablets well before swallowing.

IV:

1. Give by slow IV injection (0.5–1 ml/min for calcium chloride; 1.5–3 ml/min for calcium gluconate).

2. Maximum rate for intermittent infusion is 200 mg/min of calcium gluconate (e.g., 10 ml/min when 1 g diluted w/50 ml diluent).

INDICATIONS/DOSAGE/ROUTES

CALCIUM ACETATE

Hypophosphatemia:
PO: Adults, elderly: 2 tablets 3 times/day w/meals.

CALCIUM CARBONATE

Antihypocalcemic, nutritional supplement:
PO: Adults, elderly: 0.5–1.25 g (500 mg calcium) 1–3 times/day.

Antacid:
PO: Adults, elderly: 0.5–1.25 g as needed.

CALCIUM CITRATE

Antihypocalcemic:
PO: Adults, elderly: 1–2 tablets 2–4 times/day.

Nutritional supplement:
PO: Adults, elderly: 4–8 tablets/ day in 3–4 divided doses.

CALCIUM GLUBIONATE

Antihypocalcemic:
PO: Adults, elderly: 15 ml 3–4 times/day. Children 1–4 yrs: 10 ml 3 times/day. Children <1 yr: 5 ml 5 times/day.

CALCIUM CHLORIDE

CALCIUM GLUCONATE

Emergency increase of calcium:
IV: Adults, elderly: 7–14 mEq. Children: 1–7 mEq. Infants: <1 mEq. May repeat dose q1–3 days.

Hypocalcemic tetany:
IV: Adults, elderly: 4.5–16 mEq. May repeat until therapeutic response. Children: 0.5–0.7 mEq/kg 3–4 times/day. Neonates: 2.4 mEq/kg/day in divided doses.

Cardiopulmonary resuscitation:
IV: Adults, elderly: *Calcium gluconate:* 2.3–3.7 mEq. May repeat as needed. *Calcium chloride:* 2.7 mEq. May repeat as needed. Children: *Calcium chloride:* 0.27 mEq/kg. May repeat in 10 min if needed.

Hyperkalemia:
IV: Adults, elderly: 2.25–14 mEq. Monitor EKG. May repeat after 1–2 min if needed.

Magnesium intoxication:
IV: Adults, elderly: 7 mEq. May repeat based on pt response.

PRECAUTIONS

CONTRAINDICATIONS: Ventricular fibrillation, hypercalcemia, hypercalciuria, calcium renal calculi, sarcoidosis, digoxin toxicity. *Calcium acetate:* Hypoparathyroidism, decreased renal function. CAUTIONS: Dehydration, history of renal calculi, chronic renal impairment, decreased cardiac function, ventricular fibrillation during cardiac resuscitation. PREGNANCY/LACTATION: Distributed in breast milk. Unknown whether calcium chloride or gluconate is distributed in breast milk. Pregnancy Category C.

INTERACTIONS

DRUG INTERACTIONS: May antagonize etidronate, gallium effects. May decrease absorption of ketoconazole, phenytoin, tetracyclines. May decrease effects of methenamine, parenteral magnesium. May increase risk of arrhythmias w/digoxin. ALTERED LAB VALUES: May increase calcium gastrin, pH. May decrease phosphate, potassium.

SIDE EFFECTS

FREQUENT: *Parenteral:* Hypotension, flushing, feeling of warmth, nausea, vomiting; pain, rash, redness, burning at injection site; sweating, decreased B/P. *Oral:* Chalky taste. **OCCASIONAL:** *Oral:* Mild constipation, fecal impaction, swelling of hands/feet, metabolic alkalosis (muscle pain, restlessness, slow breathing, poor taste). *Calcium carbonate:* Milk-alkali syndrome (headache, decreased appetite, nausea, vomiting, unusual tiredness). **RARE:** *Oral:* Difficult or painful urination.

ADVERSE REACTIONS/TOXIC EFFECTS

Hypercalcemia: Early signs: Constipation, headache, dry mouth, increased thirst, irritability, decreased appetite, metallic taste, fatigue, weakness, depression. Later signs: Confusion, drowsiness, increased B/P, increased light sensitivity, irregular heartbeat, nausea, vomiting, increased urination.

NURSING IMPLICATIONS

BASELINE ASSESSMENT:

Assess B/P, EKG readings, renal function, magnesium, phosphate, potassium concentrations.

INTERVENTION/EVALUATION:

Monitor B/P, EKG, renal function, magnesium, phosphate, potassium, serum and urine calcium concentrations. Monitor for signs of hypercalcemia.

PATIENT/FAMILY TEACHING:

Stress importance of diet. Take tablets w/full glass of water, ½–1 hr after meals. Give liquid before meals. Do not take within 1–2 hrs of other oral medications, fiber-containing foods. Avoid excessive alcohol, tobacco, caffeine.

calfactant
(Infasurf)
See Supplement

candesartan
(Atacand)
See Supplement

capecitabine
(Xeloda)
See Supplement
See Classification section under:
Antineoplastics

capsaicin

cap-**say**-sin
(Zostrix)

CANADIAN AVAILABILITY:
Zostrix

CLASSIFICATION

Topical analgesic

AVAILABILITY (OTC)

Cream: 0.025%, 0.075%

ACTION/*THERAPEUTIC EFFECT*

Depletes and prevents reaccumulation of the chemomediator of pain impulses (substance P) from peripheral sensory neurons to CNS, *relieving pain.*

USES/*UNLABELED*

Treatment of neuralgia (e.g., pain following shingles, painful diabetic neuropathy), osteoarthritis, rheumatoid arthritis. *Treatment of neurogenic pain.*

INDICATIONS/DOSAGE/ROUTES

Usual topical dosage:
Topical: Adults, elderly, children >2 yrs: Apply directly to affected area 3–4 times/day. Continue for 14–28 days for optimal clinical response.

PRECAUTIONS

CONTRAINDICATIONS: Hypersensitivity to any component of the preparation. **CAUTIONS:** For external use only. **PREGNANCY/LACTATION: Pregnancy Category C**.

INTERACTIONS

DRUG INTERACTIONS: None significant. **ALTERED LAB VALUES:** None significant.

SIDE EFFECTS

FREQUENT: Burning, stinging, erythema at site of application.

NURSING IMPLICATIONS
PATIENT/FAMILY TEACHING:

For external use only. Avoid contact w/eyes, broken/irritated skin. Transient burning may occur on application, usually disappears after 72 hrs. Wash hands immediately after application. If there is no improvement or condition deteriorates after 28 days, discontinue use and consult physician.

captopril

cap-toe-prill
(Capoten)

FIXED-COMBINATION(S):
W/hydrochlorothiazide, a diuretic (Capozide)

CANADIAN AVAILABILITY:
Capoten, Novo-Captoril

CLASSIFICATION

Angiotensin-converting enzyme (ACE) inhibitor; antihypertensive

AVAILABILITY (Rx)

Tablets: 12.5 mg, 25 mg, 50 mg, 100 mg

PHARMACOKINETICS

	ONSET	PEAK	DURATION
PO	0.25 hrs	0.5–1.5 hrs	dose related

Rapid, well absorbed from GI tract (decreased in presence of food). Metabolized in liver. Primarily excreted in urine. Removed by hemodialysis. Half-life: <3 hrs (increased in decreased renal function).

ACTION/*THERAPEUTIC EFFECT*

Suppresses renin-angiotensin-aldosterone system (prevents conversion of angiotensin I to angiotensin II, a potent vasoconstrictor; may also inhibit angiotensin II at local vascular and renal sites). Decreases plasma angiotensin II, increases plasma renin activity, decreases aldosterone secretion. *Reduces peripheral arterial resistance, pulmonary capillary wedge pressure, improves cardiac output, exercise tolerance.*

USES/*UNLABELED*

Treatment of hypertension alone or in combination w/other antihypertensives. Adjunctive therapy for CHF (in combination w/cardiac glycosides, diuretics). Reduces development of severe heart failure following MI in pts w/impaired left ventricular (LV) function. Treats nephropathy/prevents kidney failure in type I diabetes. *Treatment of hypertension/ renal crises in scleroderma.*

PO ADMINISTRATION

1. Best taken 1 hr before

meals for maximum absorption (food significantly decreases drug absorption).

2. Tablets may be crushed.

INDICATIONS/DOSAGE/ROUTES

Hypertension:
PO: Adults, elderly: Initially, 12.5–25 mg 2–3 times/day. After 1–2 weeks, may increase to 50 mg 2–3 times/day. Diuretic may be added if no response in additional 1–2 wks. If taken in combination w/diuretic, may increase to 100–150 mg 2–3 times/day after 1–2 wks. **Maintenance:** 25–150 mg 2–3 times/day. **Maximum:** 450 mg/day.

CHF:
PO: Adults, elderly: Initially, 6.25–25 mg 3 times/day. Increase to 50 mg 3 times/day. After at least 2 wks, may increase to 50–100 mg 3 times/day. **Maximum:** 450 mg/day.

Post MI, impaired liver function:
PO: Adults, elderly: 6.25 mg once, then 12.5 mg 3 times/day. Increase to 25 mg 3 times/day over several days up to 50 mg 3 times/day over several weeks.

Nephropathy/prevention of kidney failure:
PO: Adults, elderly: 25 mg 3 times/day.

PRECAUTIONS

CONTRAINDICATIONS: History of angioedema w/previous treatment w/ACE inhibitors. **CAUTIONS:** Renal impairment, those w/sodium depletion or on diuretic therapy, dialysis, hypovolemia, coronary/cerebrovascular insufficiency. **PREGNANCY/LACTATION:** Crosses placenta; distributed in breast milk. May cause fetal/neonatal mortality/morbidity. **Pregnancy Category D**.

INTERACTIONS

DRUG INTERACTIONS: Alcohol, diuretics, hypotensive agents may increase effect. NSAIDs may decrease effect. Potassium-sparing diuretics, potassium supplements may cause hyperkalemia. May increase lithium concentration, toxicity. **ALTERED LAB VALUES:** May increase potassium, SGOT (AST), SGPT (ALT), alkaline phosphatase, bilirubin, BUN, creatinine. May decrease sodium. May cause positive ANA titer.

SIDE EFFECTS

FREQUENT (4–7%): Rash. **OCCASIONAL (2–4%):** Pruritus, dysgeusia (change in sense of taste). **RARE (0.5–<2%):** Headache, cough, insomnia, dizziness, fatigue, paresthesia, malaise, nausea, diarrhea/constipation, dry mouth, tachycardia.

ADVERSE REACTIONS/TOXIC EFFECTS

Excessive hypotension ("first-dose syncope") may occur in those w/CHF, severely salt/volume depleted. Angioedema (swelling of face/lips), hyperkalemia occur rarely. Agranulocytosis, neutropenia may be noted in those w/impaired renal function or collagen vascular disease (systemic lupus erythematosus, scleroderma). Nephrotic syndrome may be noted in those w/history of renal disease.

NURSING IMPLICATIONS
BASELINE ASSESSMENT:

Obtain B/P immediately before each dose, in addition to regular monitoring (be alert to fluctuations). If excessive reduction in B/P occurs, place pt in supine position w/legs elevated. Renal function tests should be performed before therapy begins. In pts w/prior renal disease or receiving dosages higher than 150 mg/day, urine test for protein by dipstick method should be made w/first urine of day before therapy begins and periodically thereafter. In those w/renal impairment, autoimmune disease, or taking drugs that affect leukocytes or immune response, CBC and differential count should be performed before therapy begins and q2wks for 3 mos, then periodically thereafter.

INTERVENTION/EVALUATION:

Assess skin for rash, hives. Assist w/ambulation if dizziness occurs. Check for urinary frequency. Assess lung sounds for rales, wheezing in those w/CHF. Monitor urinalysis for proteinuria. Assess for anorexia secondary to decreased taste perception. Monitor serum potassium levels in those on concurrent diuretic therapy.

PATIENT/FAMILY TEACHING:

To reduce hypotensive effect, rise slowly from lying to sitting position and permit legs to dangle from bed momentarily before standing. Report peripheral edema or any sign of infection (sore throat, fever). Several weeks may be needed for full therapeutic effect of B/P reduction. Skipping doses or voluntarily discontinuing drug may produce severe, rebound hypertension. Avoid alcohol.

carbachol
(Isopto-Carbachol)
See Classification section under: Antiglaucoma

carbamazepine
car-bah-**may**-zeh-peen
(Carbatrol, Epitol, Tegretol)

CANADIAN AVAILABILITY:
Apo-Carbamazepine, Tegretol

CLASSIFICATION
Anticonvulsant

AVAILABILITY (Rx)
Tablets (chewable): 100 mg. **Tablets:** 200 mg. **Tablets (extended-release):** 100 mg, 200 mg, 300 mg, 400 mg. **Oral Suspension:** 100 mg/5ml.

PHARMACOKINETICS
Slowly, completely absorbed from GI tract. Metabolized in liver to active metabolite. Primarily excreted in urine. Half-life: 25–65 hrs (decreased w/chronic use).

ACTION/*THERAPEUTIC EFFECT*
Decreases sodium, calcium ion influx into neuronal membranes, reducing posttetanic potentiation at synapse; *prevents repetitive discharge.*

USES/*UNLABELED*
Management of generalized tonic-clonic seizures (grand mal), complex partial seizures (temporal lobe, psychomotor), mixed seizures; treatment of trigeminal neuralgia (tic douloureux). *Treatment of neurogenic pain, bipolar disorder, diabetes insipidus, alcohol withdrawal, psychotic disorders.*

STORAGE/HANDLING
Store oral suspension, tablets at room temperature.

PO ADMINISTRATION
1. Give w/meals to reduce risk of GI distress.
2. Shake oral suspension well.

Do not administer simultaneously w/other liquid medicine.

3. Do not crush extended-release tablets.

INDICATIONS/DOSAGE/ROUTES

Note: When replacement by another anticonvulsant is necessary, decrease carbamazepine gradually as therapy begins w/low replacement dose. When transferring from tablets to suspension, divide total tablet daily dose into smaller, more frequent doses of suspension. Administer extended-release tablets in 2 divided doses.

Seizure control:
PO: Adults, elderly, children >12 yrs: Initially, 200 mg 2 times/day. Increase dosage up to 200 mg/day at weekly intervals until response is attained. **Maintenance:** 800–1,200 mg/day. Do not exceed 1,000 mg/day in children 12–15 yrs, 1,200 mg/day in pts >15 yrs. **Children 6–12 yrs:** Initially, 100 mg 2 times/day. Increase by 100 mg/day until response is attained. **Maintenance:** 400–800 mg/day. Give dosage 200 mg or greater/day in 3–4 equally divided doses. **Syrup: Children 6–12 yrs:** Initially, 50 mg 4 times/day. Increase dosage slowly (reduces sedation risk). **Children <6 yrs:** 10–20 mg/kg/day in 2–4 divided doses.

Trigeminal neuralgia:
PO: Adults, elderly: 100 mg 2 times/day on day 1. Increase by 100 mg q12h until pain is relieved. **Maintenance:** 200–1,200 mg/day. Do not exceed 1,200 mg/day.

PRECAUTIONS

CONTRAINDICATIONS: History of bone marrow depression, history of hypersensitivity to tricyclic antidepressants, concomitant use of MAO inhibitors. **CAUTIONS:** Impaired cardiac, hepatic, renal function. **PREGNANCY/LACTATION:** Crosses placenta; distributed in breast milk. Accumulates in fetal tissue. **Pregnancy Category C**.

INTERACTIONS

DRUG INTERACTIONS: May decrease effect of steroids, anticoagulants. May increase metabolism of anticonvulsants, barbiturates, benzodiazepines, valproic acid. Tricyclic antidepressants, haloperidol, antipsychotics may increase CNS depressant effects. Cimetidine may increase concentration, toxicity. May decrease effects of estrogens, quinidine, clarithromycin, diltiazem, erythromycin, propoxyphene. Verapamil may increase toxicity. May increase metabolism of isoniazid (hepatotoxicity). Isoniazid may increase concentration, toxicity. MAO inhibitors may cause hypertensive crises, convulsions. **ALTERED LAB VALUES:** May increase BUN, glucose, protein, SGOT (AST), SGPT (ALT), alkaline phosphatase, bilirubin, cholesterol, HDL, triglycerides. May decrease calcium, T_3, T_4, T_4 index.

SIDE EFFECTS

OCCASIONAL: Drowsiness, dizziness, nausea, vomiting, visual abnormalities (spots before eyes, difficulty focusing, blurred vision), dry mouth/pharynx, tongue irritation, headache, water retention, increased sweating, constipation/diarrhea.

ADVERSE REACTIONS/TOXIC EFFECTS

Toxic reactions appear as blood dyscrasias (aplastic anemia, agranulocytosis, thrombocytopenia, leukopenia, leukocytosis, eosinophilia), cardiovascular disturbances (CHF, hypo/hypertension, thrombophlebitis, arrhythmias), dermatologic effects (rash, urticaria, pruritus, photosensitivity). Abrupt withdrawal may precipitate status epilepticus.

NURSING IMPLICATIONS
BASELINE ASSESSMENT:

Seizures: Review history of seizure disorder (intensity, frequency, duration, LOC). Provide safety precautions, quiet, dark environment. CBC, platelet count, serum iron determinations, urinalysis, BUN should be performed before therapy begins and periodically during therapy.

INTERVENTION/EVALUATION:

Seizures: Observe frequently for recurrence of seizure activity. Assess for clinical improvement (decrease in intensity/frequency of seizures). Monitor for therapeutic serum level (3–14 mcg/ml). Assess for clinical evidence of early toxic signs (fever, sore throat, mouth ulcerations, easy bruising, unusual bleeding, joint pain). *Neuralgia:* Avoid triggering tic douloureux (draft, talking, washing face, jarring bed, hot/warm/cold food or liquids).

PATIENT/FAMILY TEACHING:

Do not abruptly withdraw medication following long-term use (may precipitate seizures). Strict maintenance of drug therapy is essential for seizure control. Drowsiness usually disappears during continued therapy. Avoid tasks that require alertness, motor skills until response to drug is established. Report visual abnormalities. Blood tests should be repeated frequently during first 3 mos of therapy and at monthly intervals thereafter for 2–3 yrs. Do not take liquid simultaneously w/other liquid medicine. Report unusual bleeding/bruising, fever, sore throat, rash, ulcers in mouth. Do not give with grapefruit juice.

carbenicillin
(Geocillin)
See Classification section under: Antibiotic: penicillins

carbidopa/levodopa
car-bih-dope-ah/**lev**-oh-dope-ah
(Sinemet)

CANADIAN AVAILABILITY:
Sinemet

CLASSIFICATION
Antiparkinson

AVAILABILITY (Rx)

Tablets (expressed as carbidopa/levodopa): 10 mg/100 mg, 25 mg/100 mg, 25 mg/250 mg. **Tablets (extended-release):** 50 mg/200 mg.

PHARMACOKINETICS

Carbidopa: Rapidly, completely absorbed from GI tract. Widely distributed. Excreted primarily in urine. Half-life: 1–2 hrs. *Levodopa:* Converted to dopamine. Excreted primarily in urine. Half-life: 1–3 hrs.

ACTION/*THERAPEUTIC EFFECT*

Converted to dopamine in basal ganglia. Increases dopamine concentration in brain, inhibiting hyperactive cholinergic activity, *reducing tremor.* Carbidopa prevents peripheral breakdown of levodopa, allowing more levodopa to be available for transport into brain.

USES

Treatment of idiopathic Parkinson's disease (paralysis agitans), postencephalitic parkinsonism, symptomatic parkinsonism following injury to nervous system by carbon monoxide poisoning, manganese intoxication.

PO ADMINISTRATION

1. Scored tablets may be crushed.

2. May be given w/o regard to meals.

3. Do not crush sustained-release tablet; may cut in half.

INDICATIONS/DOSAGE/ROUTES
PARKINSONISM:

Not receiving levodopa:
PO: Adults: 25/100 mg tablet 3 times/day or 10/100 mg tablet 3–4 times/day. May increase by 1 tablet every 1–2 days up to 8 tablets/day.

Usual elderly dosage:
PO: Initially, 25/100 mg tablet 2 times/day, gradually increased as necessary.

Sustained-release:
Adults: 1 tablet 2 times/day no closer than 6 hrs between doses. **Range:** 2–8 tablets at 4–8 hr intervals. May increase dose at intervals not less than 3 days.

Receiving only levodopa:
Note: Discontinue levodopa at least 8 hrs prior to carbidopa/levodopa. Initiate w/dose providing at least 25% of previous levodopa dosage.
PO: Adults (<1,500 mg levodopa/day): 1 tablet (25/100 mg) 3–4 times/day. **PO: Adults (>1,500 mg levodopa/day):** 1 tablet (25/250 mg) 3–4 times/day.

Sustained-release:
Adults: 1 tablet 2 times/day.

Receiving carbidopa/levodopa:
Sustained-release:
Adults: Provide about 10% more levodopa; may increase up to 30% more at 4–8 hr dosing intervals.

PRECAUTIONS

CONTRAINDICATIONS: Narrow-angle glaucoma, those on MAO inhibitor therapy. **CAUTIONS:** History of MI, bronchial asthma (tartrazine sensitivity), emphysema; severe cardiac, pulmonary, renal, hepatic, endocrine disease; active peptic ulcer; treated open-angle glaucoma. **PREGNANCY/LACTATION:** Unknown if drug crosses placenta or is distributed in breast milk. May inhibit lactation. Do not nurse. **Pregnancy Category C.**

INTERACTIONS

DRUG INTERACTIONS: Anticonvulsants, benzodiazepines, haloperidol, phenothiazines may decrease effect. MAO inhibitors may increase risk of hypertensive crises. Selegiline may increase dyskinesias, nausea, orthostatic hypotension, confusion, hallucinations. **ALTERED LAB VALUES:** May increase alkaline phosphatase, SGOT (AST), SGPT (ALT), LDH, bilirubin, BUN.

SIDE EFFECTS

FREQUENT (10–90%): Uncontrolled body movements (including face, tongue, arms, upper body), nausea and vomiting **(80%)**, anorexia **(50%)**. **OCCASIONAL:** Depression, anxiety, confusion, nervousness, difficulty urinating, irregular heartbeats, dizziness, lightheadedness, decreased appetite, blurred vision, constipation, dry mouth, flushed skin, headache, insomnia, diarrhea, unusual tiredness, darkening of urine. **RARE:** Hypertension, ulcer, hemolytic anemia (tiredness/weakness).

ADVERSE REACTIONS/TOXIC EFFECTS

High incidence of involuntary choreiform, dystonic, dyskinetic movements may be noted in pts on long-term therapy. Mental changes (paranoid ideation, psychotic episodes, depression) may be noted. Numerous mild to severe CNS, psychiatric disturbances may include reduced attention span, anxiety, nightmares, daytime somnolence, euphoria, fatigue, paranoia, hallucinations.

NURSING IMPLICATIONS
BASELINE ASSESSMENT:

Instruct pt to void before giving medication (reduces risk of urinary retention).

INTERVENTION/EVALUATION:

Be alert to neurologic effects: headache, lethargy, mental confusion, agitation. Monitor for evidence of dyskinesia (difficulty w/movement). Assess for clinical reversal of symptoms (improvement of tremor of head/hands at rest, mask-like facial expression, shuffling gait, muscular rigidity).

PATIENT/FAMILY TEACHING:

Avoid tasks that require alertness, motor skills until response to drug is established. Dry mouth, drowsiness, dizziness may be an expected response to drug. Avoid alcoholic beverages during therapy. Sugarless gum, sips of tepid water may relieve dry mouth. Coffee/tea may help reduce drowsiness. Take w/food to minimize GI upset. Effects may be delayed from several wks to months. May cause darkening in urine/sweat (not harmful). Report any uncontrolled movement of face, eyelids, mouth, tongue, arms, hands, legs, mental changes, palpitations, irregular heartbeats, severe or continuing nausea/vomiting, difficulty in urinating.

carboplatin
car-bow-**play**-tin
(Paraplatin)

CANADIAN AVAILABILITY:
Paraplatin

CLASSIFICATION

Antineoplastic

AVAILABILITY (Rx)

Powder for Injection: 50 mg, 150 mg, 450 mg

PHARMACOKINETICS

Hydrolyzed in solution to active form. Primarily excreted in urine. Half-life: 2.6–5.9 hrs.

ACTION/*THERAPEUTIC EFFECT*

Inhibits DNA synthesis by cross-linking w/DNA strands, *preventing cellular division, interfering w/DNA function.* Cell cycle-phase nonspecific.

USES/*UNLABELED*

Treatment of recurrent ovarian carcinoma in those previously treated w/chemotherapy, including cisplatin. Initial treatment of advanced ovarian carcinoma. *Treatment of small cell, non small cell carcinoma of lung, head/neck carcinoma, testicular carcinoma.*

STORAGE/HANDLING

Note: May be carcinogenic, mutagenic, or teratogenic. Handle w/extreme care during preparation/administration. Store vials at room temperature. Reconstitute immediately before use. After reconstitution, solution stable for 8 hrs. Discard unused portions after 8 hrs.

IV ADMINISTRATION

1. Do not use aluminum needles or administration sets that come in contact w/drug (may produce black precipitate, loss of potency).

2. Reconstitute each 50 mg w/5 ml sterile water for injection, 5% dextrose, or 0.9% NaCl to provide concentration of 10 mg/ml.

3. May be further diluted w/5% dextrose or 0.9% NaCl to provide concentration as low as 0.5 mg/ml.

4. Infuse over 15–60 min.

5. Rarely, anaphylactic reaction occurs minutes after administration. Use of epinephrine, corticosteroids alleviates symptoms.

INDICATIONS/DOSAGE/ROUTES

Note: Dosage individualized based on clinical response, tolerance to adverse effects.

Ovarian carcinoma (single agent):
IV: Adults: 360 mg/m² on day 1; q4wks. Do not repeat dose until neutrophil, platelet counts are within acceptable levels. Adjust dose in those previously treated based on lowest posttreatment platelet or neutrophil value.
Note: Make only one escalation, not >125% of starting dose.

Ovarian carcinoma (combination therapy):
IV: Adults: 300 mg/m² (w/cyclophosphamide) on day 1; q4wks. Do not repeat dose until neutrophil, platelet counts are within acceptable levels.

Dosage in renal impairment:
Initial dose based on creatinine clearance; subsequent doses based on pt's tolerance, degree of myelosuppression.

CREATININE CLEARANCE	DOSAGE DAY 1
>60 ml/min	360 mg/m²
41–59 ml/min	250 mg/m²
16–40 ml/min	200 mg/m²

PRECAUTIONS

CONTRAINDICATIONS: History of severe allergic reaction to cisplatin, platinum compounds, mannitol; severe myelosuppression, severe bleeding. **PREGNANCY/LACTATION:** If possible, avoid use during pregnancy, esp. first trimester. May cause fetal harm. Unknown if distributed in breast milk. Breast feeding not recommended. **Pregnancy Category D**.

INTERACTIONS

DRUG INTERACTIONS: Bone marrow depressants may increase bone marrow depression. Nephrotoxic-, ototoxic-producing agents may increase toxicity. Live virus vaccines may potentiate virus replication, increase vaccine side effects, decrease antibody response to vaccine. **ALTERED LAB VALUES:** May decrease electrolytes (sodium, magnesium, calcium, potassium). High doses (above 4 times recommended dose) may elevate alkaline phosphatase, SGOT (AST), total bilirubin, BUN, serum creatinine concentrations.

SIDE EFFECTS

FREQUENT: Vomiting, generalized pain, asthenia (loss of energy, strength). **OCCASIONAL:** Nausea, constipation/diarrhea, anorexia, peripheral neuropathies. **RARE:** Alopecia, visual disturbances, ototoxicity, allergic reaction.

ADVERSE REACTIONS/TOXIC EFFECTS

Bone marrow suppression may be severe, resulting in anemia,

infection, bleeding (GI bleeding, sepsis, pneumonia). Prolonged treatment may result in peripheral neurotoxicity.

NURSING IMPLICATIONS

BASELINE ASSESSMENT:

Offer emotional support. Treatment should not be repeated until WBC, neutrophil, platelet count recovers from previous therapy. Transfusions may be needed in those receiving prolonged therapy (myelosuppression increased in those w/previous therapy, impaired kidney function).

INTERVENTION/EVALUATION:

Monitor lung sounds for pulmonary toxicity (dyspnea, fine lung rales). Monitor hematologic status, pulmonary function studies, hepatic and renal function tests. Monitor for fever, sore throat, signs of local infection, easy bruising or unusual bleeding from any site, symptoms of anemia (excessive tiredness, weakness).

PATIENT/FAMILY TEACHING:

Nausea, vomiting generally abates <24 hrs. Contact physician if nausea/vomiting continues at home. Do not have immunizations w/o physician's approval (drug lowers body's resistance). Avoid contact w/those who have recently received live virus vaccine. Teach signs of peripheral neuropathy.

---

carboprost

kar-boe-prost
(Hemabate)

CLASSIFICATION

Prostaglandin

AVAILABILITY (Rx)

Injection: 250 mcg/ml

PHARMACOKINETICS

Metabolized in liver and by enzymes in maternal lung tissues. Mean abortion time: 16 hrs. Primarily excreted in urine.

ACTION/*THERAPEUTIC EFFECT*

Direct action on myometrium. Stimulates contraction in gravid uterus, *produces cervical dilation and softening.*

USES/*UNLABELED*

To induce abortion between the 13th and 20th wk of pregnancy (as calculated from the first day of the last menstrual period), to treat postpartum hemorrhage related to uterine atony not responsive to conventional therapy. *Treatment of incomplete abortion, benign hydatiform mole, induction of labor, ripen cervix prior to abortion.*

STORAGE/HANDLING

Refrigerate.

IM ADMINISTRATION

1. Administer only in hospital setting w/emergency equipment available.
2. Give deep IM and rotate sites if subsequent doses necessary.
3. Avoid skin contact w/carboprost; if spilled on skin, wash thoroughly w/soap and water.

INDICATIONS/DOSAGE/ROUTES

Abortion:
IM: Adults: Initially, 100–250 mcg, may repeat at 1.5–3.5 hr intervals. May increase up to 500 mcg if uterine contractility inadequate. **Maximum:** 12 mg total dose or continuous administration >2 days.

Postpartum hemorrhage:
IM: Adults: Initially, 250 mcg, may repeat at 15–90 min intervals. **Maximum:** 2 mg total dose.

PRECAUTIONS

CONTRAINDICATIONS: Hypersensitivity to carboprost or other prostaglandins; acute pelvic inflammatory disease; active cardiac, pulmonary, renal, or hepatic disease. **CAUTIONS:** History of asthma, hypo/hypertension, anemia, jaundice, diabetes, epilepsy, compromised (scarred) uterus, cardiovascular, adrenal, or hepatic disease. **PREGNANCY/LACTATION:** Teratogenic, therefore abortion must be complete.

INTERACTIONS

DRUG INTERACTIONS: Oxytocin, oxytocics may cause uterine hypertonus, leading to uterine rupture or cervical lacerations. **ALTERED LAB VALUES:** None significant.

SIDE EFFECTS

FREQUENT: Nausea, vomiting, diarrhea. **OCCASIONAL:** Fever, chills, facial flushing, headache, hyper/hypotension. **RARE:** Wheezing, troubled breathing, tightness in chest (esp. asthmatic pts). Stomach cramps/pain, increased uterine bleeding, foul-smelling lochia may indicate postabortion complications.

ADVERSE REACTIONS/TOXIC EFFECTS

Excessive dosage may cause uterine hypertonicity w/spasm and tetanic contraction, leading to cervical laceration/perforation, uterine rupture/hemorrhage.

NURSING IMPLICATIONS
BASELINE ASSESSMENT:

Question for hypersensitivity to carboprost or other prostaglandins. Establish baseline B/P, temperature, pulse, respiration. Obtain orders for antiemetics and antidiarrheals, meperidine or other pain medication for abdominal cramps. Assess any uterine activity/vaginal bleeding.

INTERVENTION/EVALUATION:

Check strength, duration, frequency of contractions and monitor vital signs every 15 min until stable, then hourly until abortion complete. Check resting uterine tone. Administer medications for relief of GI effects if indicated, abdominal cramps. Provide emotional support as necessary.

PATIENT/FAMILY TEACHING:

Report fever, chills, foul-smelling/increased vaginal discharge, uterine cramps/pain promptly.

carisoprodol
(Soma, Rela)
See Classification section under: Skeletal muscle relaxants

carmustine
car-**muss**-teen
(BiCNU, Gliadel Wafer)

CANADIAN AVAILABILITY: BiCNU

CLASSIFICATION
Antineoplastic

AVAILABILITY (Rx)
Powder for Injection: 100 mg

PHARMACOKINETICS

Widely distributed (crosses blood-brain barrier, readily penetrates CSF). Metabolized in liver to active metabolite. Primarily excreted in urine.

ACTION / THERAPEUTIC EFFECT

Inhibits DNA, RNA synthesis by cross-linking w/DNA, RNA strands, preventing cellular division, *interfering w/DNA/RNA function.* Cell cycle-phase nonspecific.

USES / UNLABELED

Palliative treatment of primary and metastatic brain tumors, multiple myeloma, disseminated Hodgkin's disease, non-Hodgkin's lymphoma. *Gliadel Wafer:* Adjunct to surgery to prolong survival in recurrent glioblastoma multiforme. *Treatment of hepatic, GI carcinoma, malignant melanoma, mycosis fungoides.*

STORAGE / HANDLING

Note: May be carcinogenic, mutagenic, or teratogenic. Wear protective gloves during preparation of drug; may cause transient burning, brown staining of skin.

Refrigerate unopened vials of dry powder. Reconstituted vials are stable for 8 hrs at room temperature or 24 hrs if refrigerated. Solutions further diluted to 0.2 mg/ml w/5% dextrose or 0.9% NaCl are stable for 48 hrs if refrigerated or an additional 8 hrs at room temperature. Solutions are clear, colorless to yellow. Discard if precipitate forms, color change occurs, or oily film develops on bottom of vial.

IV ADMINISTRATION

1. Reconstitute 100 mg vial w/3 ml sterile dehydrated (absolute) alcohol, followed by 27 ml sterile water for injection to provide concentration of 3.3 mg/ml.

2. Further dilute w/50–250 ml 5% dextrose or 0.9% NaCl. Infuse over 1–2 hrs (shorter duration may produce intense pain, burning at injection site).

3. Flush IV line w/5–10 ml 0.9% NaCl injection or 5% dextrose before and after administration to prevent irritation at injection site.

4. Rapid IV may produce intense burning, pain, flushing of skin, conjunctiva.

INDICATIONS / DOSAGE / ROUTES

Note: Dosage individualized based on clinical response, tolerance to adverse effects. When used in combination therapy, consult specific protocols for optimum dosage, sequence of drug administration.

Single agent in previously untreated pt:
IV: Adults, elderly, children: 150–200 mg/m² as single dose or 75–100 mg/m² on 2 successive days. Alternatively, give 40 mg/m² daily on 5 successive days. Repeat doses q6–8wks. Reduce dose if given in combination w/myelosuppressive drugs or if pt has compromised bone marrow function. Repeat courses not given until circulating blood elements return to acceptable levels and adequate number of neutrophils present on peripheral blood smear. Adjust dose based upon hematologic response to previous doses.

PRECAUTIONS

CONTRAINDICATIONS: None significant. **CAUTIONS:** Pts w/decreased platelet, leukocyte, erythrocyte counts. **PREGNAN-**

CY/LACTATION: If possible, avoid use during pregnancy, esp. first trimester. May cause fetal harm. Unknown if distributed in breast milk. Breast feeding not recommended. **Pregnancy Category D.**

INTERACTIONS

DRUG INTERACTIONS: Bone marrow depressants, cimetidine may enhance myelosuppressive effect. Hepatotoxic, nephrotoxic drugs may enhance respective toxicities. Live virus vaccines may potentiate virus replication, increase vaccine side effects, decrease antibody response to vaccine. **ALTERED LAB VALUES:** May increase BUN, SGOT (AST), SGPT (ALT), alkaline phosphatase, bilirubin.

SIDE EFFECTS

FREQUENT: Pain at IV injection site, skin discoloration along course of vein; nausea and vomiting within minutes to 2 hrs (may last up to 6 hrs after administration). **OCCASIONAL:** Diarrhea, esophagitis, anorexia, dysphagia. **RARE:** Thrombophlebitis.

ADVERSE REACTIONS/TOXIC EFFECTS

Hematologic toxicity, due to bone marrow depression, occurs frequently. Thrombocytopenia occurs at about 4 wks, lasts 1–2 wks; leukopenia evident at about 5–6 wks, lasts 1–2 wks. Anemia occurs less frequently, is less severe. Mild, reversible hepatotoxicity also occurs frequently. Prolonged therapy w/high dosage may produce impaired renal function, pulmonary toxicity (pulmonary infiltrate and/or fibrosis).

NURSING IMPLICATIONS
BASELINE ASSESSMENT:

Perform pulmonary function tests before therapy begins and periodically during therapy. Perform liver function studies periodically during therapy. Perform blood counts weekly during and for at least 6 wks after therapy ends.

INTERVENTION/EVALUATION:

Monitor WBC, platelet count, BUN, Hct, serum transaminase, alkaline phosphatase, bilirubin; pulmonary, liver, renal function tests. Monitor for hematologic toxicity (fever, sore throat, signs of local infection, easy bruising, unusual bleeding from any site) or symptoms of anemia (excessive tiredness, weakness). Monitor lung sounds for pulmonary toxicity (dyspnea, fine lung rales).

PATIENT/FAMILY TEACHING:

Pain may occur w/IV administration. Maintain adequate daily fluid intake (may protect against renal impairment). Do not have immunizations w/o doctor's approval (drug lowers body's resistance). Avoid contact w/those who have recently received live virus vaccine. Contact physician if nausea/vomiting continues at home.

carteolol hydrochloride
cart-**hee**-oh-lol
(Cartrol, Ocupress)

CLASSIFICATION
Beta-adrenergic blocker

AVAILABILITY (Rx)

Tablets: 2.5 mg, 5 mg. **Ophthalmic Solution:** 1%.

PHARMACOKINETICS

Well absorbed from GI tract. Minimally metabolized in liver. Primarily excreted unchanged in urine. Half-life: 6 hrs (increased in decreased renal function).

ACTION/ *THERAPEUTIC EFFECT*

Blocks effects of adrenergic transmitter by competitive binding to receptor site. Predominantly blocks beta$_1$-adrenergic receptors in cardiac tissue, *slowing sinus heart rate, decreasing cardiac output, decreasing B/P.* Large doses may block beta$_2$-adrenergic receptors, *increasing airway resistance. Ophthalmic:* Reduces aqueous humor production, *decreasing intraocular pressure.*

USES/ *UNLABELED*

Oral: Management of mild to moderate hypertension. Used alone or in combination w/diuretics, especially thiazide type. *Ophthalmic:* Reduces intraocular pressure in management of chronic open-angle glaucoma, ocular hypertension. *W/miotics decreases IOP in acute/chronic angle closure glaucoma, treatment of secondary glaucoma, malignant glaucoma, angle closure glaucoma during/after iridectomy.*

PO/OPHTHALMIC ADMINISTRATION

PO:

May give w/o regard to food.

OPHTHALMIC:

1. Place finger on lower eyelid and pull out until pocket is formed between eye and lower lid. Hold dropper above pocket and place prescribed number of drops in pocket.

2. Close eye gently. Apply digital pressure to lacrimal sac for 1–2 min (minimized drainage into nose and throat, reducing risk of systemic effects).

3. Remove excess solution w/tissue.

INDICATIONS/DOSAGE/ROUTES

Hypertension:
PO: Adults, elderly: Initially, 2.5 mg/day as single dose either alone or in combination w/diuretic. May increase gradually to 5–10 mg/day as single dose. **Maintenance:** 2.5–5 mg/day.

Dosage in renal impairment:

CREATININE CLEARANCE	DOSAGE INTERVAL
>60 ml/min	24 hrs
20–60 ml/min	48 hrs
<20 ml/min	72 hrs

Usual ophthalmic dosage:
Adults, elderly: 1 drop 2 times/day.

PRECAUTIONS

CONTRAINDICATIONS: Bronchial asthma, COPD, bronchospasm, overt cardiac failure, cardiogenic shock, heart block greater than first degree, persistently severe bradycardia. **CAUTIONS:** Impaired renal/hepatic function, peripheral vascular disease, hyperthyroidism, diabetes, inadequate cardiac function. **PREGNANCY/LACTATION:** Readily crosses placenta; distributed in breast milk. Avoid use during first trimester. May produce bradycardia, apnea, hypoglycemia, hypothermia during delivery, small birth weight infants. **Pregnancy Category C**. (Category D if used in 2nd or 3rd trimester.)

INTERACTIONS

DRUG INTERACTIONS: Diuretics,

other hypotensives may increase hypotensive effect; sympathomimetics, xanthines may mutually inhibit effects; may mask symptoms of hypoglycemia, prolong hypoglycemic effect of insulin, oral hypoglycemics; NSAIDs may decrease antihypertensive effect; cimetidine may increase concentration. **ALTERED LAB VALUES:** May increase ANA titer, SGOT (AST), SGPT (ALT), alkaline phosphatase, LDH, bilirubin, BUN, creatinine, potassium, uric acid, lipoproteins, triglycerides.

SIDE EFFECTS

Generally well tolerated, w/mild and transient effects. **FREQUENT:** *Oral:* Hypotension manifested as dizziness, nausea, diaphoresis, headache, cold extremities, fatigue, constipation/diarrhea. *Ophthalmic:* Redness of eye or inside of eyelids, decreased night vision. **OCCASIONAL:** *Oral:* Insomnia, flatulence, urinary frequency, impotence or decreased libido. *Ophthalmic:* Blepharoconjunctivitis, edema, droopy eyelid, staining of cornea, blurred vision, brow ache, increased light sensitivity, burning, stinging. **RARE:** Rash, arthralgia, myalgia, confusion (especially elderly), change in taste.

ADVERSE REACTIONS/TOXIC EFFECTS

Abrupt withdrawal (particularly in those w/coronary artery disease) may produce angina or precipitate MI. May precipitate thyroid crisis in those w/thyrotoxicosis.

NURSING IMPLICATIONS
BASELINE ASSESSMENT:

Assess baseline renal/liver function tests. Assess B/P, apical pulse immediately before drug is administered (if pulse is 60/min or below, or systolic B/P is below 90 mm Hg, withhold medication, contact physician).

INTERVENTION/EVALUATION:

Assess pulse for strength/weakness, irregular rate, bradycardia. Monitor EKG for cardiac changes. Assist w/ambulation if dizziness occurs. Assess for peripheral edema of hands, feet (usually, first area of low extremity swelling is behind medial malleolus in ambulatory, sacral area in bedridden). Monitor pattern of daily bowel activity and stool consistency. Assess skin for development of rash. Monitor any unusual changes in pt. *Ophthalmic:* Monitor for potential systemic reaction.

PATIENT/FAMILY TEACHING:

Do not abruptly discontinue medication (compliance w/therapy regimen is essential to control hypertension). If dizziness occurs, sit or lie down immediately. Full therapeutic response may not occur for up to 2 wks. Avoid tasks that require alertness, motor skills until response to drug is established. Report excessively slow pulse rate (<60 beats/min), peripheral numbness, dizziness. Do not use nasal decongestants, OTC cold preparations (stimulants) w/o physician approval. Outpatients should monitor B/P, pulse before taking medication. Restrict salt, alcohol intake. *Ophthalmic:* Instruct pt on proper administration of drops. Do not use after expiration date. Transient stinging or discomfort is common; notify physician of severe or continued discomfort.

carvedilol

car-**veh**-dih-lol
(Coreg)

CANADIAN AVAILABILITY:
Coreg

CLASSIFICATION

Beta-adrenergic blocker; antihypertensive

AVAILABILITY (Rx)

Tablets: 3.125 mg, 6.25 mg, 12.5 mg, 25 mg

PHARMACOKINETICS

	ONSET	PEAK	DURATION
PO	30 min	1–2 hrs	24 hrs

Rapidly and extensively absorbed from GI tract. Metabolized in liver. Excreted primarily via bile into feces. Half-life: 7–10 hrs. Food delays rate of absorption.

ACTION/*THERAPEUTIC EFFECT*

Possesses nonselective beta-blocking and alpha-adrenergic blocking activity. *Reduces cardiac output, exercise-induced tachycardia, and reflex orthostatic tachycardia;* causes vasodilation; *reduces peripheral vascular resistance.*

USES/*UNLABELED*

Management of essential hypertension. Used alone or in combination w/diuretics, especially thiazide type. Treatment of CHF. *Treatment of angina pectoris, idiopathic cardiomyopathy.*

PO ADMINISTRATION

1. Give w/food (slows rate of absorption, reduces risk of orthostatic effects).
2. Take standing systolic B/P 1 hr after dosing as guide for tolerance.

INDICATIONS/DOSAGE/ROUTES

Hypertension:
PO: Adults, elderly: Initially, 6.25 mg twice daily. May double at 7–14 day intervals to highest tolerated dose. **Maximum:** 50 mg/day.
CHF:
PO: Adults, elderly: Initially, 3.125 mg twice daily. May double at 2 wk intervals to highest tolerated dose. **Maximum: <85 kg:** 25 mg twice daily; **>85 kg:** 50 mg twice daily.

PRECAUTIONS

CONTRAINDICATIONS: Class IV decompensated cardiac failure, bronchial asthma or related bronchospastic conditions, second- or third-degree AV block, cardiogenic shock, severe bradycardia. **CAUTIONS:** CHF controlled w/digitalis, diuretics, or angiotensin-converting enzyme inhibitor, peripheral vascular disease, anesthesia, diabetes mellitus, hypoglycemia, thyrotoxicosis, impaired hepatic function. **PREGNANCY/LACTATION:** Unknown if drug crosses placenta or is distributed in breast milk. May produce bradycardia, apnea, hypoglycemia, hypothermia during delivery, small birth weight infants. **Pregnancy Category C.**

INTERACTIONS

DRUG INTERACTIONS: Diuretics, other hypotensives may increase hypotensive effect; may mask symptoms of hypoglycemia, prolong hypoglycemic effect of insulin, oral hypoglycemics. Catapres may potentiate B/P effects, calcium blockers increase risk of conduction disturbances, increases digoxin concentrations. Cimetidine may increase concentration, rifampin decreases concentration. **ALTERED LAB VALUES:** None significant.

SIDE EFFECTS

Generally well tolerated, w/mild and transient side effects. **FREQUENT (4–6%):** Fatigue, dizziness. **OCCASIONAL (2%):** Diarrhea, bradycardia, rhinitis, back pain. **RARE (<2%):** Postural hypotension, somnolence, urinary tract infection, viral infection.

ADVERSE REACTIONS/TOXIC EFFECTS

Overdosage may produce profound bradycardia, hypotension, bronchospasm, cardiac insufficiency, cardiogenic shock, cardiac arrest. Abrupt withdrawal may result in sweating, palpitations, headache, tremulousness. May precipitate CHF, MI in those w/cardiac disease, thyroid storm in those w/thyrotoxicosis, peripheral ischemia in those w/existing peripheral vascular disease. Hypoglycemia may occur in previously controlled diabetics.

NURSING IMPLICATIONS
BASELINE ASSESSMENT:

Assess B/P, apical pulse immediately before drug is administered (if pulse is 60/min or below, or systolic B/P is below 90 mm Hg, withhold medication, contact physician).

INTERVENTION/EVALUATION:

Monitor B/P for hypotension, respiration for shortness of breath. Assess pulse for strength/weakness, irregular rate, bradycardia. Monitor EKG for cardiac arrhythmias. Assist w/ambulation if dizziness occurs. Assess for evidence of CHF: dyspnea (particularly on exertion or lying down), night cough, peripheral edema, distended neck veins. Monitor I&O

(increase in weight, decrease in urine output may indicate CHF).

PATIENT/FAMILY TEACHING:

Full antihypertensive effect noted 1–2 wks. Contact lens wearers may experience decreased lacrimation. Take w/food. Do not abruptly discontinue medication. Compliance w/therapy regimen is essential to control hypertension. Avoid tasks that require alertness, motor skills until response to drug is established. Report excessive fatigue, prolonged dizziness. Do not use nasal decongestants, OTC cold preparations (stimulants) w/o physician approval. Monitor B/P, pulse before taking medication. Restrict salt, alcohol intake.

cascara sagrada

cass-**care**-ah sah-**graud**-ah
(Cascara Sagrada)

FIXED-COMBINATION(S): W/milk of magnesia, a saline laxative (Same)

CANADIAN AVAILABILITY: Cascara Sagrada

CLASSIFICATION
Laxative: Stimulant

AVAILABILITY (OTC)
Tablets: 325 mg. **Liquid** (18% alcohol).

PHARMACOKINETICS

	ONSET	PEAK	DURATION
PO	6–12 hrs	—	—

Minimal absorption after oral administration. Hydrolyzed by enzymes of colonic flora to active form. Absorbed drug metabolized in liver, eliminated in feces via biliary system.

ACTION/*THERAPEUTIC EFFECT*

Increases peristalsis by direct effect on colonic smooth musculature (stimulates intramural nerve plexi). *Promotes fluid and ion accumulation in colon to increase laxative effect.*

USES

Facilitates defecation in those w/diminished colonic motor response, for evacuation of colon for rectal, bowel examination, elective colon surgery.

PO ADMINISTRATION

1. Give on empty stomach (faster results).
2. Offer 6–8 glasses water/day (aids softening stools).
3. Avoid giving within 1 hr of other oral medication (decreases drug absorption).

INDICATIONS/DOSAGE/ROUTES

Laxative:
PO: Adults, elderly: 1 tablet (or 5 ml) at bedtime.

PRECAUTIONS

CONTRAINDICATIONS: Abdominal pain, nausea, vomiting, appendicitis, intestinal obstruction. CAUTIONS: None significant. PREGNANCY/LACTATION: Distributed in breast milk (may produce loose stools in infant). Pregnancy Category C.

INTERACTIONS

DRUG INTERACTIONS: May decrease transit time of concurrently administered oral medication, decreasing absorption. ALTERED LAB VALUES: May increase blood glucose. May decrease potassium, calcium.

SIDE EFFECTS

FREQUENT: Pink-red, red-violet, red-brown, or yellow-brown discoloration of urine. OCCASIONAL: Some degree of abdominal discomfort, nausea, mild cramps, griping; faintness.

ADVERSE REACTIONS/TOXIC EFFECTS

Long-term use may result in laxative dependence, chronic constipation, loss of normal bowel function. Chronic use or overdosage may result in electrolyte disturbances (hypokalemia, hypocalcemia, metabolic acidosis or alkalosis), persistent diarrhea, malabsorption, weight loss. Electrolyte disturbance may produce vomiting, muscle weakness.

NURSING IMPLICATIONS
INTERVENTION/EVALUATION:

Encourage adequate fluid intake. Assess bowel sounds for peristalsis. Monitor daily bowel activity and stool consistency (watery, loose, soft, semisolid, solid) and record time of evacuation. Assess for abdominal disturbances. Monitor serum electrolytes in those exposed to prolonged, frequent, or excessive use of medication.

PATIENT/FAMILY TEACHING:

Urine may turn pink-red, red-violet, red-brown, or yellow-brown (only temporary and not harmful). Institute measures to promote defecation: increase fluid intake, exercise, high-fiber diet. Laxative effect generally occurs in 6–12 hrs, but may take 24 hrs. Do not use in presence of nausea, vomiting, abdominal pain longer than 1 wk. Do not take other oral medication within 1 hr of taking this medicine (decreased effectiveness due to increased peristalsis).

castor oil
(Neoloid)

CANADIAN AVAILABILITY:
Castor Oil

CLASSIFICATION

Laxative: Stimulant

AVAILABILITY (OTC)

Liquid. Emulsion.

PHARMACOKINETICS

	ONSET	PEAK	DURATION
PO	2–3 hrs	—	—

Minimal absorption. Converted to ricinoleic acid (active component) in GI tract.

ACTION / *THERAPEUTIC EFFECT*

Increases peristalsis by direct effect on small-bowel musculature (stimulates intramural nerve plexi). *Promotes fluid and ion accumulation in colon to increase laxative effect.*

USES

Facilitates defecation in those w/diminished colonic motor response, for evacuation of colon for rectal, bowel examination, elective colon surgery.

PO ADMINISTRATION

1. Do not give late in day (acts in 2–6 hrs).
2. Chill, mix w/juice (improves taste).
3. Give on empty stomach (faster action).
4. Offer 6–8 glasses of water/day (aids stool softening).
5. Avoid giving within 1 hr of other oral medication (decreases drug absorption).

INDICATIONS / DOSAGE / ROUTES

Laxative:
PO: **Adults, elderly:** (liquid): 15–60 ml; (emulsion): 30–60 ml. **Children 6–12 yrs:** (liquid): 5–15 ml; (emulsion): 7.5–30 ml. **Infants:** (emulsion): 2.5–5 ml.

PRECAUTIONS

CONTRAINDICATIONS: Menstruating/pregnant women, abdominal pain, nausea, vomiting, appendicitis, intestinal obstruction. **CAUTIONS:** None significant. **PREGNANCY/LACTATION:** Contraindicated in pregnancy (may cause pelvic area engorgement, may initiate reflex stimulation of gravid uterus, inducing premature labor). **Pregnancy Category X.**

INTERACTIONS

DRUG INTERACTIONS: May decrease transit time of concurrently administered oral medication, decreasing absorption. **ALTERED LAB VALUES:** May increase blood glucose. May decrease potassium, calcium.

SIDE EFFECTS

FREQUENT: Some degree of abdominal discomfort, nausea, mild cramps, griping, faintness. **OCCASIONAL:** Excessive colon irritation producing violent purgation. **RARE:** Pelvic congestion.

ADVERSE REACTIONS / TOXIC EFFECTS

Long-term use may result in laxative dependence, chronic constipation, loss of normal bowel function. Chronic use or overdosage may result in electrolyte disturbances (hypokalemia, hypocalcemia, metabolic acidosis or alkalosis), persistent diarrhea, malabsorption, weight loss. Electrolyte disturbance may produce vomiting, muscle weakness.

NURSING IMPLICATIONS
BASELINE ASSESSMENT:

Question for possibility of

pregnancy before initiating therapy (Pregnancy Category X).

INTERVENTION/EVALUATION:

Encourage adequate fluid intake. Assess bowel sounds for peristalsis. Monitor daily bowel activity and stool consistency (watery, loose, soft, semisolid, solid) and record time of evacuation. Assess for abdominal disturbances. Monitor serum electrolytes in those exposed to prolonged, frequent, or excessive use of medication.

PATIENT/FAMILY TEACHING:

Cola, unsalted crackers, dry toast may relieve nausea. Institute measures to promote defecation: increase fluid intake, exercise, high-fiber diet. Do not take other oral medication within 1 hr of taking this medicine (decreased effectiveness due to increased peristalsis). Do not use in presence of nausea, vomiting, abdominal pain longer than 1 wk. Effect usually occurs in 6–12 hrs, but may take up to 24 hrs.

cefaclor
sef-ah-klor
(Ceclor, Ceclor CD)

CANADIAN AVAILABILITY:
Apo-Cefaclor, Ceclor

CLASSIFICATION

Antibiotic: Second-generation cephalosporin

AVAILABILITY (Rx)

Capsules: 250 mg, 500 mg. **Tablets (extended-release):** 375 mg, 500 mg. **Oral Suspension:** 125 mg/5 ml, 187 mg/5 ml, 250 mg/5 ml, 375 mg/5 ml.

PHARMACOKINETICS

Well absorbed from GI tract. Widely distributed. Primarily excreted unchanged in urine. Moderately removed by hemodialysis. Half-life: 0.6–0.9 hrs (increased in decreased renal function).

ACTION/ *THERAPEUTIC EFFECT*

Bactericidal. Binds to bacterial membranes, *inhibiting bacterial cell wall synthesis.*

USES

Treatment of respiratory, skin/skin structure infections, otitis media, UTI. *Extended Release:* Bacterial infections of acute, chronic bronchitis, skin/skin structure, pharyngitis, tonsillitis.

STORAGE/HANDLING

Oral suspension: after reconstitution, stable for 14 days if refrigerated.

PO ADMINISTRATION

1. Shake oral suspension well before using.
2. Give w/o regard to meals; if GI upset occurs, give w/food or milk.
3. Do not cut, crush, or chew extended-release tablets.

INDICATIONS/DOSAGE/ROUTES

Mild to moderate infections:
PO: Adults, elderly: 250 mg q8h. **Children >1 mo:** 20 mg/kg/day in divided doses q8h.

Severe infections:
PO: Adults, elderly: 500 mg q8h. **Maximum:** 4 g/day. **Children >1 mo:** 40 mg/kg/day in divided doses q8h. **Maximum:** 1 g/day.

C

Usual dosage for extended-release tablets:
PO: Adults, children >16 yrs: 375–500 mg q12hrs.

Otitis media:
PO: Children >1 mo: 40 mg/kg/day in divided doses q8h. **Maximum:** 1 g/day.

Dosage in renal impairment:
Reduced dosage may be necessary in those w/creatinine clearance <40 ml/min.

PRECAUTIONS

CONTRAINDICATIONS: History of hypersensitivity to cephalosporins, anaphylactic reaction to penicillins. **CAUTIONS:** Renal impairment, history of allergies or GI disease (especially ulcerative colitis, antibiotic-associated colitis), concurrent use of nephrotoxic medications. **PREGNANCY/LACTATION:** Readily crosses placenta. Distributed in breast milk. **Pregnancy Category B**.

INTERACTIONS

DRUG INTERACTIONS: Probenecid may increase serum concentrations of cefaclor. **ALTERED LAB VALUES:** Positive direct/indirect Coombs' test. May increase BUN, serum creatinine, SGPT (ALT), SGOT (AST), alkaline phosphatase, bilirubin, LDH concentrations.

SIDE EFFECTS

FREQUENT: Oral candidiasis (sore mouth/tongue), mild diarrhea, mild abdominal cramping, vaginal candidiasis (itching, discharge). **OCCASIONAL:** Nausea, serum sickness reaction [joint pain, fever] (usually occurs following second course of therapy, resolves after drug discontinuation). **RARE:** Allergic reaction (rash, pruritus, urticaria).

ADVERSE REACTIONS/TOXIC EFFECTS

Antibiotic-associated colitis (severe abdominal pain and tenderness, fever, watery and severe diarrhea), other superinfections may result from altered bacterial balance. Nephrotoxicity may occur, esp. w/preexisting renal disease. Severe hypersensitivity reaction (severe pruritus, angioedema, bronchospasm, anaphylaxis), particularly those w/history of allergies, esp. penicillin.

NURSING IMPLICATIONS
BASELINE ASSESSMENT:

Question for history of allergies, particularly cephalosporins, penicillins. Obtain culture and sensitivity test before giving first dose (therapy may begin before results are known).

INTERVENTION/EVALUATION:

Check mouth for white patches on mucous membranes, tongue. Monitor bowel activity and stool consistency carefully; mild GI effects may be tolerable, but increasing severity may indicate onset of antibiotic-associated colitis. Assess skin for rash. Monitor I&O, urinalysis, renal function reports for nephrotoxicity. Be alert for superinfection: severe genital/anal pruritus, abdominal pain, severe mouth soreness, moderate to severe diarrhea.

PATIENT/FAMILY TEACHING:

Continue therapy for full length of treatment. Doses should be evenly spaced. May cause GI upset (may take w/food or milk).

cefadroxil

sef-ah-**drocks**-ill
(Duricef, Ultracef)

CANADIAN AVAILABILITY:
Duricef

CLASSIFICATION

Antibiotic: First-generation cephalosporin

AVAILABILITY (Rx)

Capsules: 500 mg. **Tablets:** 1,000 mg. **Oral Suspension:** 125 mg/5 ml, 250 mg/5 ml, 500 mg/5 ml.

PHARMACOKINETICS

Well absorbed from GI tract. Widely distributed. Primarily excreted unchanged in urine. Removed by hemodialysis. Half-life: 1.2–1.5 hrs (increased in decreased renal function).

ACTION / *THERAPEUTIC EFFECT*

Bactericidal. Binds to bacterial membranes, *inhibiting bacterial cell wall synthesis*.

USES

Treatment of respiratory and GU tract, skin and soft tissue infections; follow-up to parenteral therapy.

STORAGE / HANDLING

Oral suspension: after reconstitution, stable for 14 days if refrigerated.

PO ADMINISTRATION

1. Shake oral suspension well before using.
2. Give w/o regard to meals; if GI upset occurs, give w/food or milk.

INDICATIONS/DOSAGE/ROUTES

Note: Space doses evenly around the clock.

Urinary tract infections:
PO: Adults, elderly: 1–2 g/day in 1–2 divided doses.
Skin/skin structure infections, group A beta-hemolytic streptococcal pharyngitis, tonsillitis:
PO: Adults, elderly: 500 mg–1 g/day as single or 2 divided doses.

Usual dosage for children:
PO: Children: 30 mg/kg/day as single or 2 divided doses.

Dosage in renal impairment:
Dose and/or frequency is based on degree of renal impairment and/or severity of infection. After initial 1 g dose:

CREATININE CLEARANCE	DOSAGE INTERVAL
25–50 ml/min	500 mg q12h
10–25 ml/min	500 mg q24h
0–10 ml/min	500 mg q36h

PRECAUTIONS

CONTRAINDICATIONS: History of hypersensitivity to cephalosporins, anaphylactic reaction to penicillins. **CAUTIONS:** Renal impairment, history of allergies or GI disease (especially ulcerative colitis, antibiotic-associated colitis), concurrent use of nephrotoxic medications. **PREGNANCY/LACTATION:** Readily crosses placenta. Distributed in breast milk. **Pregnancy Category B.**

INTERACTIONS

DRUG INTERACTIONS: Probenecid increases serum concentrations of cefadroxil. **ALTERED LAB VALUES:** Positive direct/indirect Coombs' test. May increase BUN, serum creatinine, SGPT (ALT), SGOT (AST), alkaline phosphatase, bilirubin, LDH concentrations.

SIDE EFFECTS

FREQUENT: Oral candidiasis (sore mouth/tongue), mild diarrhea, nausea, vaginal candidiasis (itching, discharge). **OCCASIONAL:** Serum sickness reaction (skin rash, joint pain, fever), vomiting. **RARE:** Hemolytic anemia (unusual tiredness), erythema multiforme (blistering, peeling, loosening of skin).

ADVERSE REACTIONS/TOXIC EFFECTS

Antibiotic-associated colitis, (severe abdominal pain and tenderness, fever, watery and severe diarrhea), other superinfections may result from altered bacterial balance. Nephrotoxicity may occur, esp. w/preexisting renal disease. Severe hypersensitivity reaction (severe pruritus, angioedema, bronchospasm, anaphylaxis), particularly those w/history of allergies, esp. penicillin.

NURSING IMPLICATIONS
BASELINE ASSESSMENT:

Question history of allergies, particularly cephalosporins, penicillins. Obtain culture and sensitivity test before giving first dose (therapy may begin before results are known).

INTERVENTION/EVALUATION:

Check mouth for white patches on mucous membranes, tongue. Monitor bowel activity and stool consistency carefully; mild GI effects may be tolerable, but increasing severity may indicate onset of antibiotic-associated colitis. Assess skin for rash. Monitor I&O, urinalysis, renal function reports for nephrotoxicity. Be alert

for superinfection: genital/anal pruritus, moniliasis, abdominal pain, sore mouth or tongue, moderate to severe diarrhea.

PATIENT/FAMILY TEACHING:

Continue therapy for full length of treatment. Doses should be evenly spaced. May cause GI upset (may take w/food or milk).

cefamandole
(Mandol)
See Classification section under: Antibiotic: cephalosporins

cefazolin sodium
cef-ah-**zoe**-lin
(Ancef, Kefzol, Zolicef)

CANADIAN AVAILABILITY:
Ancef, Kefzol

CLASSIFICATION

Antibiotic: First-generation cephalosporin

AVAILABILITY (Rx)

Injection: 500 mg, 1 g. **Ready-to-Hang Infusion:** 1 g/50 ml.

PHARMACOKINETICS

Widely distributed. Primarily excreted unchanged in urine. Moderately removed by hemodialysis. Half-life: 1.4–1.8 hrs (increased in decreased renal function).

ACTION/THERAPEUTIC EFFECT

Bactericidal. Binds to bacterial membranes, *inhibiting bacterial cell wall synthesis.*

USES

Treatment of respiratory tract, skin, soft tissue, bone and joint, GU tract, serious intra-abdominal, biliary infections; septicemia. Preferred first-generation cephalosporin for perioperative prophylaxis.

STORAGE/HANDLING

Solutions appear light yellow to yellow. IV infusion (piggyback) stable for 24 hrs at room temperature, 96 hrs if refrigerated. Discard if precipitate forms.

IM/IV ADMINISTRATION

Note: Give by IM injection, direct IV injection, intermittent IV infusion (piggyback).
IM:

To minimize discomfort, inject deep IM slowly. Less painful if injected into gluteus maximus rather than lateral aspect of thigh.

IV:

1. For direct IV injection, administer over 3–5 min.
2. For intermittent IV infusion (piggyback), infuse over 20–40 min.
3. Alternating IV sites, use large veins to reduce risk of phlebitis.

INDICATIONS/DOSAGE/ROUTES

Note: Space doses evenly around the clock.

Uncomplicated UTI:
IM/IV: Adults, elderly: 1 g q12h.

Mild to moderate infections:
IM/IV: Adults, elderly: 250–500 mg q8–12h.

Severe infections:
IM/IV: Adults, elderly: 0.5–1 g q6–8h.

Life-threatening infections:
IM/IV: Adults, elderly: 1–1.5 g q6h. **Maximum:** 12 g/day.

Perioperative prophylaxis:
IM/IV: Adults, elderly: 1 g 30–60 min before surgery, 0.5–1 g during surger, and q6–8h for up to 24 hrs postop.

Usual dosage for children:
IM/IV: Children >1 mo: 25–100 mg/kg/day in 3–4 divided doses.

Dosage in renal impairment:
After initial loading dose of 500 mg, dose and/or frequency modified on basis of creatinine clearance and/or severity of infection.

CREATININE CLEARANCE	CHILDREN'S DOSAGE
40–70 ml/min	60% normal dose q12h
20–40 ml/min	25% normal dose q12h
5–20 ml/min	10% normal dose q24h

	ADULT DOSAGE
55 ml/min	250–1,000 mg q6–8h
35–54 ml/min	250–1,000 mg q8h
11–34 ml/min	125–500 mg q12h
10 ml/min	125–500 mg q24h

PRECAUTIONS

CONTRAINDICATIONS: History of hypersensitivity to cephalosporins, anaphylactic reaction to penicillins. **CAUTIONS:** Renal impairment, history of allergies or GI disease (especially ulcerative colitis, antibiotic-associated colitis), concurrent use of nephrotoxic medications. **PREGNANCY/LACTATION:** Readily crosses placenta; distributed in breast milk. **Pregnancy Category B.**

INTERACTIONS

DRUG INTERACTIONS: Probenecid increases serum concentrations of cefazolin. **ALTERED LAB VALUES:** Positive direct/indirect Coombs' test. May increase BUN, serum creatinine, SGPT (ALT), SGOT (AST), alkaline phosphatase, bilirubin, LDH concentrations.

SIDE EFFECTS

FREQUENT: Discomfort w/IM administration, oral candidiasis (sore mouth/tongue), mild diarrhea, mild abdominal cramping, vaginal candidiasis (itching, discharge). **OCCASIONAL:** Nausea, serum sickness reaction [joint pain, fever] (usually occurs following second course of therapy, resolves after drug discontinuation). **RARE:** Allergic reaction (rash, pruritus, urticaria), thrombophlebitis (pain, redness, swelling at injection site).

ADVERSE REACTIONS/TOXIC EFFECTS

Antibiotic-associated colitis (severe abdominal pain and tenderness, fever, watery and severe diarrhea), other superinfections may result from altered bacterial balance. Nephrotoxicity may occur, esp. w/preexisting renal disease. Severe hypersensitivity reaction (severe pruritus, angioedema, bronchospasm, anaphylaxis), particularly those w/history of allergies, esp. penicillin.

NURSING IMPLICATIONS

BASELINE ASSESSMENT:

Question for history of allergies, particularly cephalosporins, penicillins. Obtain culture and sensitivity test before giving first dose (therapy may begin before results are known).

INTERVENTION/EVALUATION:

Evaluate IV site for phlebitis (heat, pain, red streaking over vein). Check IM injection sites for induration, tenderness. Check mouth for white patches on mucous membranes, tongue.

Monitor bowel activity and stool consistency carefully; mild GI effects may be tolerable, but increasing severity may indicate onset of antibiotic-associated colitis. Assess skin for rash. Monitor I&O, urinalysis, renal function reports for nephrotoxicity. Be alert for superinfection: severe genital/anal pruritus, abdominal pain, severe mouth soreness, moderate to severe diarrhea.

PATIENT/FAMILY TEACHING:

Discomfort may occur w/IM injection. Doses should be evenly spaced. Continue antibiotic therapy for full length of treatment.

---

cefdinir
(Omnicef)
See Supplement
See Classification section under:
Antibiotic: cephalosporins

---

cefepime
sef-eh-**peem**
(Maxipime)

CANADIAN AVAILABILITY:
Maxipime

CLASSIFICATION

Antibiotic: Fourth-generation cephalosporin

AVAILABILITY (Rx)

Powder for Injection: 500 mg, 1 g, 2 g

PHARMACOKINETICS

Well absorbed after IM administration. Widely distributed. Primarily excreted unchanged in urine. Removed by hemodialysis. Half-life: 2–2.3 hrs (increased in decreased renal function, elderly).

ACTION/*THERAPEUTIC EFFECT*

Bactericidal. Binds to bacterial membrane, *inhibiting bacterial cell wall synthesis.*

USES

Treatment of pneumonia, bronchitis, urinary tract, skin and skin structure, intra-abdominal infections, bacteremia, septicemia, fever and neutropenia in cancer pts, complicated intra-abdominal infections (w/metronidazole).

STORAGE/HANDLING

Solutions stable for 24 hrs at room temperature or 7 days refrigerated.

IM/IV ADMINISTRATION

Note: May give by IM injection, IV injection, intermittent IV infusion (piggyback).

1. For IM injection, inject into a large muscle mass (e.g., upper gluteus maximus).

2. For direct IV injection, administer over 3–5 min.

3. For intermittent IV infusion, infuse over 15–30 min.

4. Alternating IV sites, use large veins to reduce risk of phlebitis.

INDICATIONS/DOSAGE/ROUTES

Note: Space doses evenly around the clock.

Complicated, uncomplicated UTI:
IM/IV: Adults, elderly: 0.5–1.0 g q12h.

Moderate to severe infections:
IM/IV: Adults, elderly: 1 g q12h.

Severe infections:
IV: Adults, elderly: 2 g q12h.

Life-threatening infections:
IV: Adults, elderly: 2 g q8h.

Usual pediatric dosage:
IM/IV: Children (2 mos–16 yrs): 50 mg/kg q8–12hrs. Do not exceed maximum adult dose.

Dosage in renal impairment:
Dose and/or frequency is based on degree of renal impairment (creatinine clearance) and/or severity of infection.

	CREATININE CLEARANCE	
	11–30 ML/MIN	**<10 ML/MIN**
Moderately severe infection	0.5 g q24h	0.25 g q24h
Severe infection	1 g q24h	0.5 g q24h
Life-threatening infection	1 g q12h	1 g q24h

PRECAUTIONS

CONTRAINDICATIONS: History of hypersensitivity to cephalosporins, anaphylactic reaction to penicillins. **CAUTIONS:** Renal impairment, history of allergies. **PREGNANCY/LACTATION:** Unknown whether distributed in breast milk. **Pregnancy Category B**.

INTERACTIONS

DRUG INTERACTIONS: Probenecid may increase concentration of cefepime. **ALTERED LAB VALUES:** Positive direct/indirect Coombs' test may occur. May increase SGOT (AST), SGPT (ALT), alkaline phosphatase, LDH, bilirubin.

SIDE EFFECTS

FREQUENT: Discomfort w/IM administration, oral candidiasis (sore mouth/tongue), mild diarrhea, mild abdominal cramping, vaginal candidiasis (itching, discharge). **OCCASIONAL:** Nausea, serum sickness reaction [joint pain, fever] (usually occurs following second course of therapy, resolves after drug discontinuation). **RARE:** Allergic reaction (rash, pruritus, urticaria), thrombophlebitis (pain, redness, swelling at injection site).

ADVERSE REACTIONS/TOXIC EFFECTS

Antibiotic-associated colitis (severe abdominal pain and tenderness, fever, watery and severe diarrhea), other superinfections may result from altered bacterial balance. Nephrotoxicity may occur, esp. w/preexisting renal disease. Severe hypersensitivity reaction (severe pruritus, angioedema, bronchospasm, anaphylaxis), particularly those w/history of allergies, esp. penicillin.

NURSING IMPLICATIONS

BASELINE ASSESSMENT:

Question history of allergies, particularly cephalosporins, penicillins. Obtain culture and sensitivity test before giving first dose (therapy may begin before results are known).

INTERVENTION/EVALUATION:

Monitor IV site for phlebitis (heat, pain, red streaking over vein). Check IM injection sites for induration, tenderness. Check mouth for white patches on mucous membranes, tongue. Monitor bowel activity and stool consistency carefully; mild GI effects may be tolerable, but increasing severity may indicate onset of antibiotic-associated colitis. Assess skin for rash. Monitor I&O, urinalysis, renal function reports for nephrotoxicity. Be alert for superinfection: severe genital/anal pruritus, abdominal pain, severe mouth soreness, moderate to severe diarrhea.

PATIENT/FAMILY TEACHING:

Discomfort may occur w/IM injection. Continue therapy for full length of treatment. Doses should be evenly spaced.

cefixime
sef-ih-zeem
(Suprax)

CANADIAN AVAILABILITY
Suprax

CLASSIFICATION

Antibiotic: Third-generation cephalosporin

AVAILABILITY (Rx)

Tablets: 200 mg, 400 mg. **Oral Suspension:** 100 mg/5 ml.

PHARMACOKINETICS

Moderately absorbed from GI tract. Widely distributed. Primarily excreted unchanged in urine. Minimally removed by hemodialysis. Half-life: 3–4 hrs (increased in decreased renal function).

ACTION/THERAPEUTIC EFFECT

Bactericidal. Binds to bacterial membranes, *inhibiting bacterial cell wall synthesis.*

USES

Otitis media, acute bronchitis and acute exacerbations of chronic bronchitis, pharyngitis, tonsillitis, uncomplicated UTI, uncomplicated gonorrhea.

STORAGE/HANDLING

Oral suspension: after reconstitution, stable for 14 days at room temperature. Do not refrigerate.

PO ADMINISTRATION

1. Give w/o regard to meals.
2. Shake oral suspension well before administering.

INDICATIONS/DOSAGE/RESULTS

Note: Use oral suspension to treat

otitis media (achieves higher peak blood level).

Usual oral dosage:
PO: Adults, elderly, children >50 kg: 400 mg/day as single or 2 divided doses. **Children <50 kg:** 8 mg/kg/day as single or 2 divided doses.

Uncomplicated gonorrhea:
PO: Adults: 400 mg as single dose.

Dosage in renal impairment:
Creatinine clearance 21–60 ml/min, pt on renal dialysis: 300 mg/day as single or 2 divided doses.
Creatinine clearance <20 ml/min, pt on continuous ambulatory peritoneal dialysis: 200 mg/day as single or 2 divided doses.

PRECAUTIONS

CONTRAINDICATIONS: Hypersensitivity to cephalosporins. **CAUTIONS:** Hypersensitivity to penicillins or other drugs; allergies; history of GI disease (e.g., colitis); renal impairment. **PREGNANCY/LACTATION:** Not recommended during labor and delivery. Excretion in breast milk not known. **Pregnancy Category B.**

INTERACTIONS

DRUG INTERACTIONS: Probenecid increases serum concentrations of cefixime. **ALTERED LAB VALUES:** Positive direct/indirect Coombs' test. May increase BUN, serum creatinine, SGPT (ALT), SGOT (AST), alkaline phosphatase, bilirubin, LDH concentrations.

SIDE EFFECTS

FREQUENT: Oral candidiasis (sore mouth/tongue), mild diarrhea, mild abdominal cramping, vaginal candidiasis (itching, discharge). **OCCASIONAL:** Nausea, serum sickness reaction [joint pain, fever] (usually occurs following second course of therapy, resolves after drug discontinuation). **RARE:** Allergic reaction (rash, pruritus, urticaria).

ADVERSE REACTIONS/TOXIC EFFECTS

Antibiotic-associated colitis (severe abdominal pain and tenderness, fever, watery and severe diarrhea), other superinfections may result from altered bacterial balance. Nephrotoxicity may occur, esp. w/preexisting renal disease. Severe hypersensitivity reaction (severe pruritus, angioedema, bronchospasm, anaphylaxis), particularly those w/history of allergies, esp. penicillin.

NURSING IMPLICATIONS
BASELINE ASSESSMENT:

Question for hypersensitivity to cefixime or other cephalosporins, penicillins, other drugs. Obtain specimens for culture and sensitivity test (therapy may begin before results are known).

INTERVENTION/EVALUATION:

Check mouth for white patches on mucous membranes, tongue. Monitor bowel activity and stool consistency carefully; mild GI effects may be tolerable, but increasing severity may indicate onset of antibiotic-associated colitis. Assess skin for rash. Monitor I&O, urinalysis, renal function reports for nephrotoxicity. Be alert for superinfection: severe genital/anal pruritus, abdominal pain, severe mouth soreness, moderate to severe diarrhea.

C

PATIENT/FAMILY TEACHING:

Continue medication for full length of treatment; do not skip doses. Doses should be evenly spaced. May cause GI upset (may take w/food or milk).

cefmetazole sodium

cef-**met**-ah-zole
(Zefazone)

CLASSIFICATION

Antibiotic: Second-generation cephalosporin

AVAILABILITY (Rx)

Powder for Injection: 1 g, 2 g

PHARMACOKINETICS

Widely distributed. Primarily excreted unchanged in urine. Moderately removed by hemodialysis. Half-life: 0.8–1.8 hrs (increased in decreased renal function).

ACTION/THERAPEUTIC EFFECT

Bactericidal. Binds to bacterial membranes, *inhibiting bacterial cell wall synthesis.*

USES

Treatment of GU, lower respiratory tract, skin and skin structure and intra-abdominal infections. Preop prophylaxis for certain clean, contaminated, or potentially contaminated surgical procedures (cesarean section, abdominal or vaginal hysterectomy, high-risk cholecystectomy, colorectal surgery).

STORAGE/HANDLING

After reconstitution, IV solution stable for 24 hrs at room temperature or 7 days if refrigerated.

IV ADMINISTRATION

1. Do not use if solution cloudy or insoluble precipitate noted.
2. For IV injection, administer over 3–5 min.
3. For IV infusion, infuse over 10–60 min.
4. Because of potential for hypersensitivity/anaphylaxis, start initial dose at few drops per minute, increase slowly to ordered rate; stay w/pt first 10–15 min, then check every 10 min for 1st hr.
5. Alternating IV sites, use large veins to reduce risk of phlebitis.

INDICATIONS/DOSAGE/ROUTES

Urinary tract infections:
IV: Adults, elderly: 2 g q12h.

Mild to moderate infections:
IV: Adults, elderly: 2 g q8h.

Severe infections:
IV: Adults, elderly: 2 g q6h.

Surgical prophylaxis:
IV: Adults, elderly: 2 g as single dose 30–90 min before surgery or after cord is clamped, or 1–2 g 30–90 min before surgery or after cord is clamped, and repeat 8 and 16 hrs later.

Dosage in renal impairment:
After loading dose of 1–2 g, dosage and/or frequency is modified on basis of creatinine clearance and/or severity of infection.

CREATININE CLEARANCE	DOSAGE
50–90 ml/min	1–2 g q12h
30–49 ml/min	1–2 g q16h
10–29 ml/min	1–2 g q24h
<10 ml/min	1–2 g q48h

PRECAUTIONS

CONTRAINDICATIONS: History of hypersensitivity to cefmetazole or cephalosporins. **CAUTIONS:** If given to penicillin-sensitive pt, use extreme caution; cross-sensitivity among beta-lactam antibiotics occurs in up to 10% of pts w/history of penicillin allergy. Concurrent use of nephrotoxic medications, history of allergies or GI disease (esp. colitis), renal impairment. Safety and effectiveness in children not established. **PREGNANCY/LACTATION:** Small amounts excreted in breast milk. **Pregnancy Category B**.

INTERACTIONS

DRUG INTERACTIONS: Disulfiram reaction (facial flushing, nausea, sweating, headache, tachycardia) occurs if alcohol is ingested within 48–72 hrs after dose. Probenecid increases half-life, duration of action. May increase bleeding risk w/anticoagulants, heparin, thrombolytics. **ALTERED LAB VALUES:** Positive direct/indirect Coombs' test may occur (interferes w/hematologic tests, cross-matching procedures). May prolong prothrombin times. May increase SGOT (AST), SGPT (ALT), alkaline phosphatase, bilirubin, LDH, BUN, serum creatinine.

SIDE EFFECTS

FREQUENT: Oral candidiasis (sore mouth/tongue), mild diarrhea, mild abdominal cramping, vaginal candidiasis (itching, discharge). **OCCASIONAL:** Nausea, serum sickness reaction [joint pain, fever] (usually occurs following second course of therapy, resolves after drug discontinuation). **RARE:** Allergic reaction (rash, pruritus, urticaria), thrombophlebitis (pain, redness, swelling at injection site).

ADVERSE REACTIONS/TOXIC EFFECTS

Antibiotic-associated colitis (severe abdominal pain and tenderness, fever, watery and severe diarrhea), other superinfections may result from altered bacterial balance. Nephrotoxicity may occur, esp. w/preexisting renal disease. Severe hypersensitivity reaction (severe pruritus, angioedema, bronchospasm, anaphylaxis), particularly those w/history of allergies, esp. penicillin.

NURSING IMPLICATIONS
BASELINE ASSESSMENT:

Question for history of allergies, esp. cefmetazole, cephalosporins, penicillins. Obtain culture and sensitivity test before giving first dose (therapy may begin before results are known).

INTERVENTION/EVALUATION:

Evaluate IV site for phlebitis (heat, pain, red streaking over vein). Check mouth for white patches on mucous membranes, tongue. Monitor bowel activity and stool consistency carefully; mild GI effects may be tolerable, but increasing severity may indicate onset of antibiotic-associated colitis. Assess skin for rash. Monitor I&O, urinalysis, renal function reports for nephrotoxicity. Be alert for superinfection: severe genital/anal pruritus, abdominal pain, severe mouth soreness, moderate to severe diarrhea. Monitor PT levels and be alert for signs of bleeding: overt bleeding, bruising or swelling of soft tissue. Check temperature and B/P at least 2 times/day.

PATIENT/FAMILY TEACHING:

Doses should be evenly spaced. Continue antibiotic therapy for full length of treatment. Do not take other medications w/o consulting physician. Avoid alcohol and alcohol-containing preparations (salad dressings, sauces, cough syrups—read all labels carefully) during and for 72 hrs after last dose of cefmetazole.

cefonicid sodium

ce-**fon**-oh-sid
(Monocid)

CLASSIFICATION

Antibiotic: Second-generation cephalosporin

AVAILABILITY (Rx)

Powder for Injection: 500 mg, 1 g

PHARMACOKINETICS

Widely distributed. Primarily excreted unchanged in urine. Moderately removed by hemodialysis. Half-life: 4.5 hrs (increased in decreased renal function).

ACTION/*THERAPEUTIC EFFECT*

Bactericidal. Binds to bacterial membranes, *inhibiting bacterial cell wall synthesis.*

USES

Treatment of respiratory, GU tract, skin and bone infections, septicemia, perioperative prophylaxis.

STORAGE/HANDLING

Solutions appear colorless to light amber. Solutions may darken (slight yellow color change does not indicate loss of potency). IV infusion (piggyback) stable for 24 hrs at room temperature, 72 hrs if refrigerated. Discard if precipitate forms.

IM/IV ADMINISTRATION

Note: Give IM, direct IV injection, intermittent IV infusion (piggyback).
IM:
Inject deep IM into gluteus maximus or lateral aspect of thigh. For 2 g dose, use 2 separate injection sites.

IV:

1. For direct IV injection, administer over 3–5 min.
2. For intermittent IV infusion (piggyback), infuse over 20–30 min.
3. Alternating IV sites, use large veins to reduce risk of phlebitis.

INDICATIONS/DOSAGE/ROUTES

Uncomplicated UTI:
IM/IV: Adults, elderly: 500 mg q24h.

Mild to moderate infections:
IM/IV: Adults, elderly: 1 g q24h.

Severe or life-threatening infections:
IM/IV: Adults, elderly: 2 g q24h.

Perioperative prophylaxis:
IM/IV: Adults, elderly: 1 g before surgery (in pts undergoing cesarean section, only after umbilical cord is clamped) up to 1 g daily for 2 days postop.

Dosage in renal impairment:
After loading dose of 7.5 mg/kg, dose and/or frequency based on creatinine clearance and/or severity of infection.

CREATINE CLEARANCE	MILD TO MODERATE INFECTIONS	SEVERE INFECTIONS
60–79 ml/min	10 mg/kg q24h	25 mg/kg q24h
40–59 ml/min	8 mg/kg q24h	20 mg/kg q24h
20–39 ml/min	4 mg/kg q24h	15 mg/kg q24h
10–19 ml/min	4 mg/kg q48h	15 mg/kg q48h
5–9 ml/min	4 mg/kg q3–5 days	15 mg/kg q3–5 days
<5 ml/min	3 mg/kg q3–5 days	4 mg/kg q3–5 days

PRECAUTIONS

CONTRAINDICATIONS: History of hypersensitivity to cephalosporins, anaphylactic reaction to penicillins. **CAUTIONS:** Renal impairment, history of allergies or GI disease (especially ulcerative colitis, antibiotic-associated colitis), concurrent use of nephrotoxic medications. **PREGNANCY/LACTATION:** Readily crosses placenta; distributed in breast milk. **Pregnancy Category B.**

INTERACTIONS

DRUG INTERACTIONS: Probenecid increases serum concentrations of cefonicid. **ALTERED LAB VALUES:** Positive direct/indirect Coombs' test may occur (interferes w/hematologic tests, cross-matching procedures). May increase SGOT (AST), SGPT (ALT), alkaline phosphatase, bilirubin, LDH, BUN, serum creatinine concentrations.

SIDE EFFECTS

FREQUENT: Oral candidiasis (sore mouth/tongue), mild diarrhea, nausea, vaginal candidiasis, discomfort w/IM administration. **OCCASIONAL:** Serum sickness reaction (skin rash, joint pain, fever), vomiting. **RARE:** Hemolytic anemia (unusual-

ly tired), erythema multiforme (blistering, peeling, loosening of skin), thrombophlebitis (pain, redness, swelling at injection site).

ADVERSE REACTIONS/TOXIC EFFECTS

Nephrotoxicity has occurred w/high dosages or preexisting renal impairment. Antibiotic-associated colitis, other superinfections may result from altered bacterial balance. Hypersensitivity reactions (ranging from rash, urticaria, fever to anaphylaxis) may occur, particularly those w/history of allergies, esp. penicillin.

NURSING IMPLICATIONS

BASELINE ASSESSMENT:

Question for history of allergies, particularly cephalosporins, penicillins. Obtain culture and sensitivity test before giving first dose (therapy may begin before results are known).

INTERVENTION/EVALUATION:

Evaluate IV site for phlebitis (heat, pain, red streaking over vein). Check IM injection sites for induration, tenderness. Monitor bowel activity and stool consistency carefully; mild GI effects may be tolerable, but increasing severity may indicate onset of antibiotic-associated colitis. Assess skin for rash. Monitor I&O, urinalysis, renal function reports for nephrotoxicity. Be alert for superinfection: nausea, diarrhea, vaginal discharge, genital/anal pruritus, ulceration or changes in oral mucosa.

PATIENT/FAMILY TEACHING:

Discomfort may occur w/IM injection. Doses should be evenly spaced. Continue antibiotic therapy for full length of treatment.

cefoperazone sodium

sef-o-**pear**-a-zone
(Cefobid)

CLASSIFICATION

Antibiotic: Third-generation cephalosporin

AVAILABILITY (Rx)

Powder for Injection: 1 g, 2 g

PHARMACOKINETICS

Widely distributed. Achieves high biliary concentration. Primarily excreted unchanged in bile (excreted primarily in urine in pts w/severe liver impairment). Minimally removed by hemodialysis. Half-life: 1.6–2.6 hrs (increased in decreased liver and/or biliary function).

ACTION / THERAPEUTIC EFFECT

Bactericidal. Binds to bacterial membranes, *inhibiting bacterial cell wall synthesis.*

USES

Treatment of intra-abdominal, biliary, pelvic inflammatory infections; respiratory, GU tract, skin and bone infections; septicemia.

STORAGE / HANDLING

Solutions appear colorless to light yellow. IV infusion (piggyback) stable for 24 hrs at room temperature, 5 days if refrigerated. Discard if precipitate forms.

IM / IV ADMINISTRATION

Note: Give by IM injection or intermittent IV infusion (piggyback).
IM:
To minimize discomfort, inject deep IM slowly. Less painful if injected into gluteus maximus rather than lateral aspect of thigh.

IV:
1. For intermittent IV infusion (piggyback), infuse over 15–30 min.
2. Alternating IV sites, use large veins to reduce risk of phlebitis.

INDICATIONS / DOSAGE / ROUTES

Note: Space doses evenly around the clock.

Mild to moderate infections:
IM/IV: Adults, elderly: 2–4 g/day in divided doses q12h.

Severe or life-threatening infections:
IM/IV: Adults, elderly: Total daily dose and/or frequency may be increased to 6–12 g/day divided into 2, 3, or 4 equal doses of 1.5–4 g per dose.

Dosage in renal and/or hepatic impairment:
Do not exceed 4 g/day in those w/liver disease and/or biliary obstruction. Modification of dose usually not necessary in those w/renal impairment. Dose should not exceed 1–2 g/day in those w/both hepatic and substantial renal impairment.

PRECAUTIONS

CONTRAINDICATIONS: History of hypersensitivity to cephalosporins, anaphylactic reaction to penicillins. **CAUTIONS:** History of allergies, GI disease (especially ulcerative colitis, antibiotic-associated colitis), hepatic or renal impairment. **PREGNANCY/LACTATION:** Readily crosses placenta. Distributed in breast milk. **Pregnancy Category B.**

INTERACTIONS

DRUG INTERACTIONS: Disulfiram reaction (facial flushing, nausea, sweating, headache, tachycardia) may occur when alcohol is ingested. May increase bleeding risk w/anticoagulants, heparin, thrombolytics. **ALTERED LAB VALUES:** Positive direct/indirect Coombs' test may occur (interferes w/hematologic tests, cross-matching procedures). Prothrombin times may be increased. May increase BUN, serum creatinine, SGOT (AST), SGPT (ALT), alkaline phosphatase concentrations.

SIDE EFFECTS

FREQUENT: Discomfort w/IM administration, oral candidiasis (sore mouth/tongue), mild diarrhea, mild abdominal cramping, vaginal candidiasis (itching, discharge). **OCCASIONAL:** Nausea, unusual bruising/bleeding, serum sickness reaction [joint pain, fever] (usually occurs following second course of therapy, resolves after drug discontinuation). **RARE:** Allergic reaction (rash, pruritus, urticaria), thrombophlebitis (pain, redness, swelling at injection site).

ADVERSE REACTIONS/TOXIC EFFECTS

Antibiotic-associated colitis (severe abdominal pain and tenderness, fever, watery and severe diarrhea), other superinfections may result from altered bacterial balance. Nephrotoxicity may occur, esp. w/preexisting renal disease. Severe hypersensitivity reaction (severe pruritus, angioedema, bronchospasm, anaphylaxis), particularly those w/history of allergies, esp. penicillin.

NURSING IMPLICATIONS
Baseline Assessment:

Question for history of allergies, particularly cephalosporins, penicillins. Obtain culture and sensitivity test before giving first dose (therapy may begin before results are known).

Intervention/Evaluation:

Evaluate IV site for phlebitis (heat, pain, red streaking over vein). Check IM injection sites for induration, tenderness. Check mouth for white patches on mucous membranes, tongue. Monitor bowel activity and stool consistency carefully; mild GI effects may be tolerable, but increasing severity may indicate onset of antibiotic-associated colitis. Assess skin for rash. Monitor I&O, urinalysis, renal function reports for nephrotoxicity. Be alert for superinfection: severe genital/anal pruritus, abdominal pain, severe mouth soreness, moderate to severe diarrhea.

Patient/Family Teaching:

Discomfort may occur w/IM injection. Doses should be evenly spaced. Continue antibiotic therapy for full length of treatment. Avoid alcohol and alcohol-containing preparations (salad dressings, sauces, cough syrups—read all labels carefully) during and for 72 hrs after last dose of cefoperazone.

cefotaxime sodium
seh-fo-**tax**-eem
(Claforan)

CANADIAN AVAILABILITY:
Claforan

CLASSIFICATION

Antibiotic: Third-generation cephalosporin

AVAILABILITY (Rx)

Powder for Injection: 1 g, 2 g

PHARMACOKINETICS

Widely distributed (including CSF). Partially metabolized in liver to active metabolite. Primarily excreted in urine. Moderately removed by hemodialysis. Half-life: 1 hr (increased in decreased renal function).

ACTION/THERAPEUTIC EFFECT

Bactericidal. Binds to bacterial membranes, *inhibiting bacterial cell wall synthesis.*

USES/UNLABELED

Treatment of respiratory, GU tract, skin and bone infections; septicemia, gonorrhea; gynecologic, intra-abdominal, biliary infections; meningitis; perioperative prophylaxis. *Treatment of Lyme disease.*

STORAGE/HANDLING

Solutions appear light yellow to amber. IV infusion (piggyback) may darken in color (does not indicate loss of potency). IV infusion (piggyback) stable for 24 hrs at room temperature, 5 days if refrigerated. Discard if precipitate forms.

IM/IV ADMINISTRATION

Note: Give by IM injection, direct IV injection, intermittent IV infusion (piggyback).
IM:

To minimize discomfort, inject deep IM slowly. Less painful if injected into gluteus maximus rather than lateral aspect of thigh. For 2 g IM dose, give at 2 separate sites.

IV:

1. For direct IV injection, administer over 3–5 min.

2. For intermittent IV infusion (piggyback), infuse over 20–30 min.

3. Alternating IV sites, use large veins to reduce risk of phlebitis.

INDICATIONS/DOSAGE/ROUTES

Note: Space doses evenly around the clock.

Uncomplicated infections:
IM/IV: Adults, elderly: 1 g q12h.

Mild to moderate infections:
IM/IV: Adults, elderly: 1–2 g q8h.

Severe infections:
IM/IV: Adults, elderly: 2 g q6–8h.

Life-threatening infections:
IM/IV: Adults, elderly: 2 g q4h.

Uncomplicated gonorrhea:
IM: Adults: 1 g one time.

Perioperative prophylaxis:
IM/IV: Adults, elderly: 1 g 30–90 min before surgery.

Cesarean section:
IV: Adults: 1 g as soon as umbilical cord is clamped, then 1 g 6 and 12 hrs after first dose.

Usual dosage for children:
IM/IV: Children >1 mo: 50–180 mg/kg/day in 4 to 6 divided doses. **Neonates 1–4 wks:** 25–50 mg/kg q8h. **Neonates 0–7 days:** 25–50 mg/kg q12h.

Dosage in renal impairment:
Creatinine clearance <20 ml/min: Give $1/2$ dose at usual dosage intervals.

PRECAUTIONS

CONTRAINDICATIONS: History of hypersensitivity to cephalosporins, anaphylactic reaction to penicillins. **CAUTIONS:** Concurrent use of nephrotoxic medications, history of allergies or GI disease (especially ulcerative colitis, antibiotic-associated colitis), renal impairment w/creatinine clearance <20 ml/min. **PREGNANCY/LACTATION:** Readily crosses placenta; distributed in breast milk. Pregnancy Category B.

INTERACTIONS

DRUG INTERACTIONS: Probenecid increases serum concentration of cefotaxime. **ALTERED LAB VALUES:** Positive direct/indirect Coombs' test may occur. May increase liver function tests.

SIDE EFFECTS

FREQUENT: Discomfort w/IM administration, oral candidiasis (sore mouth/tongue), mild diarrhea, mild abdominal cramping, vaginal candidiasis (itching, discharge). **OCCASIONAL:** Nausea, serum sickness reaction [joint pain, fever] (usually occurs following second course of therapy, resolves after drug discontinuation). **RARE:** Allergic reaction (rash, pruritus, urticaria), thrombophlebitis (pain, redness, swelling at injection site).

ADVERSE REACTIONS/TOXIC EFFECTS

Antibiotic-associated colitis (severe abdominal pain and tenderness, fever, watery and severe diarrhea), other superinfections may result from altered bacterial balance. Nephrotoxicity may occur, esp. w/preexisting renal disease. Severe hypersensitivity reaction (severe pruritus, angioedema, bronchospasm, anaphylaxis), particularly those w/history of allergies, esp. penicillin.

NURSING IMPLICATIONS
BASELINE ASSESSMENT:

Question for history of allergies, particularly cephalosporins, penicillins. Obtain culture and sensitivity test before giving first dose (therapy may begin before results are known).

INTERVENTION/EVALUATION:

Evaluate IV site for phlebitis (heat, pain, red streaking over vein). Check IM injection sites for induration, tenderness. Check mouth for white patches on mucous membranes, tongue. Monitor bowel activity and stool consistency carefully; mild GI effects may be tolerable, but increasing severity may indicate onset of antibiotic-associated colitis. Assess skin for rash. Monitor I&O, urinalysis, renal function reports for nephrotoxicity. Be alert for superinfection: severe genital/anal pruritus, abdominal pain, severe mouth soreness, moderate to severe diarrhea.

PATIENT/FAMILY TEACHING:

Discomfort may occur w/IM injection. Doses should be evenly spaced. Continue antibiotic therapy for full length of treatment.

cefotetan disodium

seh-fo-**teh**-tan
(Cefotan)

CANADIAN AVAILABILITY:
Cefotan

CLASSIFICATION

Antibiotic: Second-generation cephalosporin

AVAILABILITY (Rx)

Powder for Injection: 1 g, 2 g

PHARMACOKINETICS

Widely distributed. Primarily excreted unchanged in urine. Minimally removed by hemodialysis. Half-life: 3–4.6 hrs (increased in decreased renal function).

ACTION/*THERAPEUTIC EFFECT*

Bactericidal. Binds to bacterial membranes, *inhibiting bacterial cell wall synthesis.*

USES

Treatment of respiratory, GU tract, skin, bone, gynecologic, intra-abdominal infections; perioperative prophylaxis.

STORAGE/HANDLING

Solutions appear colorless to light yellow. Color change to deep yellow does not indicate loss of potency. IV infusion (piggyback) stable for 24 hrs at room temperature, 96 hrs if refrigerated. Discard if precipitate forms.

IM/IV ADMINISTRATION

Note: Give by IM injection, direct IV injection, intermittent IV infusion (piggyback).
IM:

To minimize discomfort, inject deep IM slowly. Less painful if injected into gluteus maximus rather than lateral aspect of thigh.

IV:

1. For direct IV injection, administer over 3–5 min.
2. For intermittent IV infusion (piggyback), infuse over 20–30 min.
3. Alternating IV sites, use large veins to reduce risk of phlebitis.

INDICATIONS/DOSAGE/ROUTES

Note: Space doses evenly around the clock.

Urinary tract infections:
IM/IV: Adults, elderly: 500 mg q12h, or 1–2 g q12–24h.

Mild to moderate infections:
IM/IV: Adults, elderly: 1–2 g q12h.

Severe infections:
IM/IV: Adults, elderly: 2 g q12h.

Life-threatening infections:
IM/IV: Adults, elderly: 3 g q12h.

Perioperative prophylaxis:
IV: Adults, elderly: 1–2 g 30–60 min before surgery.

Cesarean section:
IV: Adults: 1–2 g as soon as umbilical cord is clamped.

Dosage in renal impairment:
Dose and/or frequency modified on basis of creatinine clearance and/or severity of infection.

CREATININE CLEARANCE	DOSAGE INTERVAL
10–30 ml/min	Usual dose q24h
<10 ml/min	Usual dose q48h

PRECAUTIONS

CONTRAINDICATIONS: History of hypersensitivity to cephalosporins, anaphylactic reaction to penicillins. **CAUTIONS:** Renal impairment, history of allergies or GI disease (especially ulcerative colitis, antibiotic-associated colitis), concurrent use of nephrotoxic medications. **PREGNANCY/LACTATION:** Readily crosses placenta. Distributed in breast milk. **Pregnancy Category B.**

INTERACTIONS

DRUG INTERACTIONS: Disulfiram reaction (facial flushing, nausea, sweating, headache, tachycardia) may occur when alcohol is ingested. May increase bleeding risk w/anticoagulants, heparin, thrombolytics. **ALTERED LAB VALUES:** Positive direct/indirect Coombs' test may occur (interferes w/hematologic tests, crossmatching procedures). Prothrombin times may be increased. May increase BUN, serum creatinine, SGOT (AST), SGPT (ALT), alkaline phosphatase concentrations.

SIDE EFFECTS

FREQUENT: Discomfort w/IM administration, oral candidiasis (sore mouth/tongue), mild diarrhea, mild abdominal cramping, vaginal candidiasis (itching, discharge). **OCCASIONAL:** Nausea, unusual bruising/bleeding, serum sickness reaction [joint pain, fever] (usually occurs following second course of therapy, resolves after drug discontinuation). **RARE:** Allergic reaction (rash, pruritus, urticaria), thrombophlebitis (pain, redness, swelling at injection site).

ADVERSE REACTIONS/TOXIC EFFECTS

Antibiotic-associated colitis (severe abdominal pain and tenderness, fever, watery and severe diarrhea), other superinfections may result from altered bacterial balance. Nephrotoxicity may occur, esp. w/preexisting renal disease. Severe hypersensitivity reaction (severe pruritus, angioedema, bronchospasm, anaphylaxis), particularly those w/history of allergies, esp. penicillin.

NURSING IMPLICATIONS
BASELINE ASSESSMENT:

Question for history of allergies, particularly cephalosporins,

penicillins. Obtain culture and sensitivity test before giving first dose (therapy may begin before results are known).

INTERVENTION/EVALUATION:

Evaluate IV site for phlebitis (heat, pain, red streaking over vein). Check IM injection sites for induration, tenderness. Check mouth for white patches on mucous membranes, tongue. Monitor bowel activity and stool consistency carefully; mild GI effects may be tolerable, but increasing severity may indicate onset of antibiotic-associated colitis. Assess skin for rash. Monitor I&O, urinalysis, renal function reports for nephrotoxicity. Be alert for superinfection: severe genital/anal pruritus, abdominal pain, severe mouth soreness, moderate to severe diarrhea.

PATIENT/FAMILY TEACHING:

Discomfort may occur w/IM injection. Doses should be evenly spaced. Continue antibiotic therapy for full length of treatment. Avoid alcohol and alcohol-containing preparations (salad dressings, sauces, cough syrups—read all labels carefully) during and for 72 hrs after last dose of cefotetan.

cefoxitin sodium
seh-**fox**-ih-tin
(Mefoxin)

CANADIAN AVAILABILITY:
Mefoxin

CLASSIFICATION

Antibiotic: Second-generation cephalosporin

AVAILABILITY (Rx)

Powder for Injection: 1 g, 2 g

PHARMACOKINETICS

Widely distributed. Primarily excreted unchanged in urine. Moderately removed by hemodialysis. Half-life: 0.7–1.1 hrs (increased in decreased renal function).

ACTION/*THERAPEUTIC EFFECT*

Bactericidal. Binds to bacterial membranes, *inhibiting bacterial cell wall synthesis*.

USES

Treatment of respiratory, GU tract, skin, bone, intra-abdominal, gynecologic infections; gonorrhea, septicemia, perioperative prophylaxis.

STORAGE/HANDLING

Solutions appear colorless to light amber but may darken (does not indicate loss of potency). IV infusion (piggyback) stable for 24 hrs at room temperature, 48 hrs if refrigerated. Discard if precipitate forms.

IM/IV ADMINISTRATION

Note: Give IM, direct IV injection, or intermittent IV infusion (piggyback). **IM:**

To minimize discomfort, inject deep IM slowly. Less painful if injected into gluteus maximus rather than lateral aspect of thigh.

IV:

1. For direct IV injection, administer over 3–5 min.

2. For intermittent IV infusion (piggyback), infuse over 30 min.

3. Alternating IV sites, use large veins to reduce potential for phlebitis.

INDICATIONS/DOSAGE/ROUTES

Note: Space doses evenly around the clock.

Mild to moderate infections:
IM/IV: Adults, elderly: 1–2 g q6–8h.

Severe infections:
IM/IV: Adults, elderly: 1 g q4h or 2 g q6–8h up to 2 g q4h.

Uncomplicated gonorrhea:
IM: Adults: 2 g one time w/1 g probenecid.

Perioperative prophylaxis:
IM/IV: Adults, elderly: 2 g 30–60 min before surgery and q6h up to 24 hrs postop. **Children >3 mos:** 30–40 mg/kg 30–60 min before surgery and q6h postop for no more than 24 hrs.

Cesarean section:
IV: Adults: 2 g as soon as umbilical cord is clamped, then 2 g 4 and 8 hrs after first dose, then q6h for no more than 24 hrs.

Usual dosage for children:
IM/IV: Children >3 mos: 80–160 mg/kg/day in 4–6 divided doses. **Maximum:** 12 g/day.

Dosage in renal impairment:
After loading dose of 1–2 g, dosage and/or frequency is modified on basis of creatinine clearance and/or severity of infection.

CREATININE CLEARANCE	DOSAGE
30–50 ml/min	1–2 g q8–12h
10–29 ml/min	1–2 g q12–24h
5–9 ml/min	500 mg–1 g q12–24h
<5 ml/min	500 mg–1 g q24–48h

PRECAUTIONS

CONTRAINDICATIONS: History of hypersensitivity to cephalosporins, anaphylactic reaction to penicillins. **CAUTIONS:** Renal impairment, history of allergies or GI disease (especially ulcerative colitis, antibiotic-associated colitis), concurrent use of nephrotoxic medications. **PREGNANCY/LACTATION:** Readily crosses placenta. Distributed in breast milk. **Pregnancy Category B**.

INTERACTIONS

DRUG INTERACTIONS: Probenecid increases serum concentrations of cefoxitin. **ALTERED LAB VALUES:** Positive direct/indirect Coombs' test may occur (interferes w/hematologic tests, cross-matching procedures). May increase BUN, serum creatinine, SGOT (AST), SGPT (ALT), alkaline phosphatase concentrations.

SIDE EFFECTS

FREQUENT: Discomfort w/IM administration, oral candidiasis (sore mouth/tongue), mild diarrhea, mild abdominal cramping, vaginal candidiasis (itching, discharge). **OCCASIONAL:** Nausea, serum sickness reaction [joint pain, fever] (usually occurs following second course of therapy, resolves after drug discontinuation). **RARE:** Allergic reaction (rash, pruritus, urticaria), thrombophlebitis (pain, redness, swelling at injection site).

ADVERSE REACTIONS/TOXIC EFFECTS

Antibiotic-associated colitis (severe abdominal pain and tenderness, fever, watery and severe diarrhea), other superinfections may result from altered bacterial balance. Nephrotoxicity may occur, esp. w/preexisting renal disease. Severe hypersensitivity reaction (severe pruritus, angioedema, bronchospasm, anaphylaxis), particularly those w/history of allergies, esp. penicillin.

NURSING IMPLICATIONS

BASELINE ASSESSMENT:

Question for history of allergies, particularly cephalosporins, penicillins. Obtain culture and sensitivity test before giving first dose (therapy may begin before results are known).

INTERVENTION/EVALUATION:

Evaluate IV site for phlebitis (heat, pain, red streaking over vein). Check IM injection sites for induration, tenderness. Check mouth for white patches on mucous membranes, tongue. Monitor bowel activity and stool consistency carefully; mild GI effects may be tolerable, but increasing severity may indicate onset of antibiotic-associated colitis. Assess skin for rash. Monitor I&O, urinalysis, renal function reports for nephrotoxicity. Be alert for superinfection: severe genital/anal pruritus, abdominal pain, severe mouth soreness, moderate to severe diarrhea.

PATIENT/FAMILY TEACHING:

Discomfort may occur w/IM injection. Doses should be evenly spaced. Continue antibiotic therapy for full length of treatment.

cefpodoxime proxetil

sef-poe-**docks**-em
(Vantin)

CLASSIFICATION

Antibiotic: Second-generation cephalosporin

AVAILABILITY (Rx)

Tablets: 100 mg, 200 mg. **Oral Suspension:** 50 mg/5 ml, 100 mg/ 5 ml.

PHARMACOKINETICS

Well absorbed from GI tract (food increases absorption). Widely distributed. Primarily excreted unchanged in urine. Partially removed by hemodialysis. Half-life: 2.3 hrs (increased in decreased renal function, elderly).

ACTION/*THERAPEUTIC EFFECT*

Bactericidal. Binds to bacterial membrane, *inhibiting bacterial cell wall synthesis.*

USES

Treatment of lower respiratory tract infections (pneumonia, chronic bronchitis), upper respiratory tract (otitis media, pharyngitis/tonsillitis), acute maxillary sinusitis, sexually transmitted diseases (urethral and cervical gonorrhea, anorectal infection), skin and skin structure, urinary tract infections.

STORAGE/HANDLING

Oral suspension: after reconstitution, stable for 14 days if refrigerated.

PO ADMINISTRATION

Administer w/food to enhance absorption.

INDICATIONS/DOSAGE/ROUTES

Pneumonia, chronic bronchitis:
PO: Adults, elderly, children >13 yrs: 200 mg q12h for 10–14 days.

Gonorrhea, rectal gonococcal infection (women only):

PO: Adults, children >13 yrs: 200 mg as single dose.

Skin/skin structure infections:
PO: Adults, elderly, children >13 yrs: 400 mg q12h for 7–14 days.

Pharyngitis/tonsillitis:
PO: Adults, elderly, children >13 yrs: 100 mg q12h for 5–10 days. **Children 6 mos–12 yrs:** 5 mg/kg q12h for 5–10 days. **Maximum:** 100 mg/dose.

Acute maxillary sinusitis:
PO: Adults, children >13 yrs: 200 mg twice daily for 10 days. **Children 2 mos–12 yrs:** 5 mg/kg q12hrs for 10 days.

Urinary tract infection:
PO: Adults, elderly, children >13 yrs: 100 mg q12h for 7 days.

Acute otitis media:
PO: Children 6 mos–12 yrs: 5 mg/kg q12h for 5 days. **Maximum:** 400 mg/dose).

Dosage in renal impairment:
Dose and/or frequency is based on degree of renal impairment (creatinine clearance). Creatinine clearance <30 ml/min: dose q24h; on hemodialysis: 3 times/wk after dialysis.

PRECAUTIONS

CONTRAINDICATIONS: History of hypersensitivity to cephalosporins, anaphylactic reaction to penicillins. **CAUTIONS:** Renal impairment, history of allergies or GI disease (especially ulcerative colitis, antibiotic-associated colitis), concurrent use of nephrotoxic medications. **PREGNANCY/LACTATION:** Readily crosses placenta. Distributed in breast milk. **Pregnancy Category B.**

INTERACTIONS

DRUG INTERACTIONS: Antacids, H_2 antagonists may decrease absorption. Probenecid may increase concentration. **ALTERED LAB VALUES:** Positive direct/indirect Coombs' test may occur. May increase SGOT (AST), SGPT (ALT), alkaline phosphatase, LDH, bilirubin, BUN, serum creatinine.

SIDE EFFECTS

FREQUENT: Oral candidiasis (sore mouth/tongue), mild diarrhea, mild abdominal cramping, vaginal candidiasis (itching, discharge). **OCCASIONAL:** Nausea, serum sickness reaction [joint pain, fever] (usually occurs following second course of therapy, resolves after drug discontinuation). **RARE:** Allergic reaction (rash, pruritus, urticaria).

ADVERSE REACTIONS/TOXIC EFFECTS

Antibiotic-associated colitis (severe abdominal pain and tenderness, fever, watery and severe diarrhea), other superinfections may result from altered bacterial balance. Nephrotoxicity may occur, esp. w/preexisting renal disease. Severe hypersensitivity reaction (severe pruritus, angioedema, bronchospasm, anaphylaxis), particularly those w/history of allergies, esp. penicillin.

NURSING IMPLICATIONS
BASELINE ASSESSMENT:

Shake oral suspension well before using. Question history of allergies, particularly cephalosporins, penicillins. Obtain culture and sensitivity test before giving first dose (therapy may begin before results are known).

INTERVENTION/EVALUATION:

Check mouth for white patches on mucous membranes, tongue. Monitor bowel activity and stool consistency carefully; mild GI effects may be tolerable, but increasing severity may indicate onset of antibiotic-associated colitis. Assess skin for rash. Monitor I&O, urinalysis, renal function reports for nephrotoxicity. Be alert for superinfection: severe genital/anal pruritus, abdominal pain, severe mouth soreness, moderate to severe diarrhea.

PATIENT/FAMILY TEACHING:

Doses should be evenly spaced. Continue antibiotic therapy for full length of treatment. Take w/food.

---

cefprozil

sef-**proz**-ill
(Cefzil)

CANADIAN AVAILABILITY: Cefzil

CLASSIFICATION

Antibiotic: Second-generation cephalosporin

AVAILABILITY (Rx)

Tablets: 250 mg, 500 mg. **Oral Suspension:** 125 mg/5 ml, 250 mg/5 ml.

PHARMACOKINETICS

Well absorbed from GI tract. Widely distributed. Primarily excreted unchanged in urine. Moderately removed by hemodialysis. Half-life: 1.3 hrs (increased in decreased renal function).

ACTION/*THERAPEUTIC EFFECT*

Bactericidal. Binds to bacterial membranes, *inhibiting bacterial cell wall synthesis.*

USES

Treatment of pharyngitis/tonsillitis, otitis media, secondary bacterial infection of acute bronchitis and acute bacterial exacerbation of chronic bronchitis, uncomplicated skin/skin structure infections, acute sinusitis.

STORAGE/HANDLING

Oral suspension: after reconstitution, stable for 14 days if refrigerated.

PO ADMINISTRATION

1. Shake oral suspension well before using.
2. Give w/o regard to meals; if GI upset occurs, give w/food or milk.

INDICATIONS/DOSAGE/ROUTES

Note: Space doses evenly around the clock.

Pharyngitis, tonsillitis:
PO: Adults, elderly: 500 mg q24h for 10 days. **Children: (2–12 yrs):** 7.5 mg/kg q12h for 10 days.

Secondary bacterial infection of acute bronchitis; acute bacterial exacerbation of chronic bronchitis:
PO: Adults, elderly: 500 mg q12h for 10 days.

Skin/skin structure infections:
PO: Adults, elderly: 250–500 mg q12h for 10 days. **Children:** 20 mg/kg q24h.

Acute sinusitis:
PO: Adults, elderly: 250–500 mg q12h. **Children (6 mo–12 yrs):** 7.5–15 mg/kg q12h.

Otitis media:
PO: Children (6 mos–12 yrs): 15 mg/kg q12h for 10 days.

Dosage in renal impairment:
Dose and/or frequency is based on degree of renal impairment (creatinine clearance). Creatinine clearance <30 ml/min: 50% dosage at usual interval.

PRECAUTIONS

CONTRAINDICATIONS: History of hypersensitivity to cephalosporins, anaphylactic reaction to penicillins. **CAUTIONS:** Renal impairment, history of allergies or GI disease (especially ulcerative colitis, antibiotic-associated colitis), concurrent use of nephrotoxic medications. **PREGNANCY/LACTATION:** Readily crosses placenta. Distributed in breast milk. **Pregnancy Category B.**

INTERACTIONS

DRUG INTERACTIONS: Probenecid increases serum concentrations of cefprozil. **ALTERED LAB VALUES:** Positive direct/indirect Coombs' test may occur (interferes w/hematologic tests, crossmatching procedures). May increase liver function tests.

SIDE EFFECTS

FREQUENT: Oral candidiasis (sore mouth/tongue), mild diarrhea, mild abdominal cramping, vaginal candidiasis (itching, discharge). **OCCASIONAL:** Nausea, serum sickness reaction [joint pain, fever] (usually occurs following second course of therapy, resolves after drug discontinuation). **RARE:** Allergic reaction (rash, pruritus, urticaria).

ADVERSE REACTIONS/TOXIC EFFECTS

Antibiotic-associated colitis (severe abdominal pain and tenderness, fever, watery and severe diarrhea), other superinfections may result from altered bacterial balance. Nephrotoxicity may occur, esp. w/preexisting renal disease. Severe hypersensitivity reaction (severe pruritus, angioedema, bronchospasm, anaphylaxis), particularly those w/history of allergies, esp. penicillin.

NURSING IMPLICATIONS
BASELINE ASSESSMENT:

Question history of allergies, particularly cephalosporins, penicillins. Obtain culture and sensitivity test before giving first dose (therapy may begin before results are known).

INTERVENTION/EVALUATION:

Check mouth for white patches on mucous membranes, tongue. Monitor bowel activity and stool consistency carefully; mild GI effects may be tolerable, but increasing severity may indicate onset of antibiotic-associated colitis. Assess skin for rash. Monitor I&O, urinalysis, renal function reports for nephrotoxicity. Be alert for superinfection: severe genital/anal pruritus, abdominal pain, severe mouth soreness, moderate to severe diarrhea.

PATIENT/FAMILY TEACHING:

Doses should be evenly spaced. Continue antibiotic therapy for full length of treatment. May cause GI upset (may take w/food or milk).

ceftazidime
sef-**taz**-ih-deem
(Ceptaz, Fortaz, Tazicef, Tazidime)

CANADIAN AVAILABILITY:
Ceptaz, Fortaz, Tazidime

CLASSIFICATION

Antibiotic: Third-generation cephalosporin

AVAILABILITY (Rx)

Powder for Injection: 500 mg, 1 g, 2 g

PHARMACOKINETICS

Widely distributed (including CSF). Primarily excreted unchanged in urine. Removed by hemodialysis. Half-life: 2 hrs (increased in decreased renal function).

ACTION/*THERAPEUTIC EFFECT*

Bactericidal. Binds to bacterial membranes, *inhibiting bacterial cell wall synthesis.*

USES

Treatment of intra-abdominal, biliary tract infections, respiratory, GU tract, skin, bone infections; meningitis, septicemia.

STORAGE/HANDLING

Solutions appear light yellow to amber, tend to darken (color change does not indicate loss of potency). IV infusion (piggyback) stable for 18 hrs at room temperature, 7 days if refrigerated. Discard if precipitate forms.

IM/IV ADMINISTRATION

Note: Give by IM injection, direct IV injection, intermittent IV infusion (piggyback).
IM:
To minimize discomfort, inject deep IM slowly. Less painful if injected into gluteus maximus rather than lateral aspect of thigh.

IV:
1. For direct IV injection, administer over 3–5 min.
2. For intermittent IV infusion (piggyback), infuse over 15–30 min.
3. Alternating IV sites, use large veins to reduce risk of phlebitis.

INDICATIONS/DOSAGE/ROUTES

Note: Space doses evenly around the clock.

Urinary tract infections:
IM/IV: Adults: 250–500 mg q8–12h.

Mild to moderate infections:
IM/IV: Adults: 1 g q8–12h.

Uncomplicated pneumonia, skin or skin structure infection:
IM/IV: Adults: 0.5–1 g q8h.

Bone and joint infection:
IM/IV: Adults: 2 g q12h.

Meningitis, serious gynecologic, intra-abdominal infections:
IM/IV: Adults: 2 g q8h.

Pseudomonal pulmonary infections in pts w/cystic fibrosis:
IV: Adults: 30–50 mg/kg q8h. **Maximum:** 6 g/day.

Usual elderly dosage:
IM/IV: Normal renal function q12h.

Usual dosage for children:
IV: Children >1 mo: 30–50 mg/kg q8h. **Children <1 mo:** 30 mg/kg q12h (increase to 50 mg/kg for meningitis).

Dosage in renal impairment:
After initial 1 g dose, dose and/or frequency is modified on basis of creatinine clearance and/or severity of infection.

CREATININE CLEARANCE	DOSAGE
31–50 ml/min	1 g q12h
16–30 ml/min	1 g q24h
6–15 ml/min	500 mg q24h
<5 ml/min	500 mg q48h

PRECAUTIONS

CONTRAINDICATIONS: History of hypersensitivity to cephalosporins, anaphylactic reactions to penicillins. **CAUTIONS:** Renal impairment, history of GI disease (especially ulcerative colitis, antibiotic-associated colitis) or allergies, concurrent use of nephrotoxic medications. **PREGNANCY/LACTATION:** Readily crosses placenta. Distributed in breast milk. **Pregnancy Category B**.

INTERACTIONS

DRUG INTERACTIONS: None significant. **ALTERED LAB VALUES:** Positive direct/indirect Coombs' test may occur (interferes w/hematologic tests, crossmatching procedures). May increase BUN, serum creatinine, SGOT (AST), SGPT (ALT), alkaline phosphatase, LDH concentrations.

SIDE EFFECTS

FREQUENT: Discomfort w/IM administration, oral candidiasis (sore mouth/tongue), mild diarrhea, mild abdominal cramping, vaginal candidiasis (itching, discharge). **OCCASIONAL:** Nausea, serum sickness reaction [joint pain, fever] (usually occurs following second course of therapy, resolves after drug discontinuation). **RARE:** Allergic reaction (rash, pruritus, urticaria), thrombophlebitis (pain, redness, swelling at injection site).

ADVERSE REACTIONS/TOXIC EFFECTS

Antibiotic-associated colitis (severe abdominal pain and tenderness, fever, watery and severe diarrhea), other superinfections may result from altered bacterial balance. Nephrotoxicity may occur, esp. w/preexisting renal disease. Severe hypersensitivity reaction (severe pruritus, angioedema, bronchospasm, anaphylaxis), particularly those w/history of allergies, esp. penicillin.

NURSING IMPLICATIONS

Baseline Assessment:

Question for history of allergies, particularly cephalosporins, penicillins. Obtain culture and sensitivity test before giving first dose (therapy may begin before results are known).

INTERVENTION/EVALUATION:

Evaluate IV site for phlebitis (heat, pain, red streaking over vein). Check IM injection sites for induration, tenderness. Check mouth for white patches on mucous membranes, tongue. Monitor bowel activity and stool consistency carefully; mild GI effects may be tolerable, but increasing severity may indicate onset of antibiotic-associated colitis. Assess skin for rash. Monitor I&O, urinalysis, renal function reports for nephrotoxicity. Be alert for superinfection: severe genital/anal pruritus, abdominal pain, severe mouth soreness, moderate to severe diarrhea.

PATIENT/FAMILY TEACHING:

Discomfort may occur w/IM injection. Doses should be evenly spaced. Continue antibiotic therapy for full length of treatment.

ceftibuten

sef-tih-**byew**-ten
(Cedax)

CLASSIFICATION

Antibiotic: Third-generation cephalosporin

AVAILABILITY (Rx)

Capsules: 400 mg. **Oral Suspension:** 90 mg/5 ml, 180 mg/5 ml.

PHARMACOKINETICS

Moderately absorbed from GI tract. Widely distributed to most tissues and fluids. Primarily excreted unchanged in urine. Minimally removed by hemodialysis. Half-life: 2–3 hrs (increased in impaired renal function).

ACTION/THERAPEUTIC EFFECT

Bactericidal. Binds to bacterial cell membranes, *inhibiting bacterial cell wall synthesis.*

USES

Acute bacterial exacerbations of chronic bronchitis, acute bacterial otitis media, pharyngitis, tonsillitis.

STORAGE/HANDLING

After reconstitution, refrigerate oral suspension. Stable for 14 days. Discard unused portion after 14 days.

PO ADMINISTRATION

Capsule:
Give capsules w/o regard to meals.

Oral suspension:

1. Shake oral suspension well before administering.
2. Administer suspension at least 2 hrs before or 1 hr after a meal.

INDICATIONS/DOSAGE/RESULTS

Note: Use oral suspension to treat otitis media (achieves higher peak blood level).

Usual oral dosage:
PO: Adults, elderly, children ≥12 yrs: 400 mg/day as single daily dose for 10 days. **Children <12 yrs:** 9 mg/kg/day as single dose for 10 days. **Maximum:** 400 mg/day.

Dosage in renal impairment:
Based on creatinine clearance.

CREATININE CLEARANCE	DOSAGE
>50 ml/min	400 mg or 9 mg/kg q24h
30–49 ml/min	200 mg or 4.5 mg/kg q24h
<30 ml/min	100 mg or 2.25 mg/kg q24h

PRECAUTIONS

CONTRAINDICATIONS: Hypersensitivity to cephalosporins. **CAUTIONS:** Hypersensitivity to penicillins or other drugs; allergies; history of GI disease (e.g., colitis); renal impairment. **PREGNANCY/LACTATION:** Crosses placenta. Excreted in breast milk. **Pregnancy Category B.**

INTERACTIONS

DRUG INTERACTIONS: Probenecid increases cephalosporin serum levels. Increased risk of nephrotoxicity w/concurrent use of aminoglycosides. **ALTERED LAB VALUES:** Positive direct/indirect Coombs' test. May increase BUN, serum creatinine, SGPT (ALT), SGOT (AST), alkaline phosphatase, bilirubin, LDH concentrations.

SIDE EFFECTS

FREQUENT: Oral candidiasis (sore mouth/tongue), mild diarrhea, nausea, vaginal candidiasis. **OCCASIONAL:** Serum sickness reaction (skin rash, joint pain, fever), vomiting. **RARE:** Hemolytic anemia (unusual tiredness), erythema multiforme (blistering, peeling, loosening of skin).

ADVERSE REACTIONS/TOXIC EFFECTS

Antibiotic-associated colitis, other superinfections may result from altered bacterial balance. Hypersensitivity reactions (ranging from rash, urticaria, fever to anaphylaxis) may occur, particularly those w/history of allergies, esp. penicillin.

NURSING IMPLICATIONS

BASELINE ASSESSMENT:

Question for hypersensitivity to ceftibuten or other cephalosporins, penicillins, other drugs. Obtain specimens for culture and sensitivity test (therapy may begin before results are known).

INTERVENTION/EVALUATION:

Monitor bowel activity and stool consistency carefully; mild GI effects may be tolerable, but increasing severity may indicate onset of antibiotic-associated colitis. Report hypersensitivity reaction: skin rash, urticaria, pruritus, fever promptly. Be alert for superinfection (e.g., genital/anal pruritus, ulceration or changes in oral mucosa, moderate to severe diarrhea, new or increased fever). Provide symptomatic relief for nausea, flatulence. Monitor hematology reports.

PATIENT/FAMILY TEACHING:

Continue medication for full length of treatment; do not skip doses. Doses should be evenly spaced. Take w/meals if GI upset occurs. Notify physician promptly of onset of diarrhea, rash, bleeding or bruising, or other symptom.

ceftizoxime sodium

cef-tih-**zox**-eem
(Cefizox)

CANADIAN AVAILABILITY:
Cefizox

CLASSIFICATION

Antibiotic: Third-generation cephalosporin

AVAILABILITY (Rx)

Powder for Injection: 1 g, 2 g

PHARMACOKINETICS

Widely distributed (including CSF). Primarily excreted unchanged in urine. Moderately removed by hemodialysis. Half-life: 1.7 hrs (increased in decreased renal function).

ACTION/ *THERAPEUTIC EFFECT*

Bactericidal. Binds to bacterial membranes, *inhibiting bacterial cell wall synthesis.*

USES

Treatment of intra-abdominal, biliary tract, respiratory, GU tract, skin, bone infections; gonorrhea, meningitis, septicemia, pelvic inflammatory disease (PID).

STORAGE/HANDLING

Solutions appear clear to pale yellow. Color change from yellow to amber does not indicate loss of potency. IV infusion (piggyback) stable for 24 hrs at room temperature, 96 hrs if refrigerated. Discard if precipitate forms.

IM/IV ADMINISTRATION

Note: Give by IM injection, direct IV injection, intermittent IV infusion (piggyback).
IM:
   1. Inject deep IM slowly to minimize discomfort.
   2. When giving 2 g dose, divide dose, give in different large muscle masses.
IV:
   1. For direct IV injection, administer over 3–5 min.

   2. For intermittent IV infusion (piggyback), infuse over 15–30 min.
   3. Alternating IV sites, use large veins to reduce risk of phlebitis.

INDICATIONS/DOSAGE/ROUTES

Uncomplicated UTI:
IM/IV: Adults, elderly: 500 mg q12h.

Mild to moderate to severe infection:
IM/IV: Adults, elderly: 1–2 g q8–12h.

PID:
IV: Adults: 2 g q4–8h.

Life-threatening infections:
IV: Adults, elderly: 3–4 g q8h, up to 2 g q4h.

Uncomplicated gonorrhea:
IM: Adults: 1 g one time.

Usual dosage for children:
IM/IV: Children >6 mos: 50 mg/kg q6–8h.

Dosage in renal impairment:
   After loading dose of 0.5–1 g, dose and/or frequency is modified on basis of creatinine clearance and/or severity of infection.

CREATININE CLEARANCE	DOSAGE
50–79 ml/min	500 mg–1.5 g q8h
5–49 ml/min	250 mg–1 g q12h
<5 ml/min	250–500 mg q24h

PRECAUTIONS

CONTRAINDICATIONS: History of hypersensitivity to cephalosporins, anaphylactic reaction to penicillins. **CAUTIONS:** History of allergies, GI disease (especially ulcerative colitis, antibiotic-associated colitis), hepatic and renal impairment. **PREGNANCY/LACTATION:** Readily crosses placenta;

distributed in breast milk. **Pregnancy Category B**.

INTERACTIONS

DRUG INTERACTIONS: Probenecid increases serum concentration of ceftizoxime. **ALTERED LAB VALUES:** Positive direct/indirect Coombs' test may occur. May increase BUN, serum creatinine, SGOT (AST), SGPT (ALT), alkaline phosphatase concentrations.

SIDE EFFECTS

FREQUENT: Discomfort w/IM administration, oral candidiasis (sore mouth/tongue), mild diarrhea, mild abdominal cramping, vaginal candidiasis (itching, discharge). **OCCASIONAL:** Nausea, serum sickness reaction [joint pain, fever] (usually occurs following second course of therapy, resolves after drug discontinuation). **RARE:** Allergic reaction (rash, pruritus, urticaria), thrombophlebitis (pain, redness, swelling at injection site).

ADVERSE REACTIONS/TOXIC EFFECTS

Antibiotic-associated colitis (severe abdominal pain and tenderness, fever, watery and severe diarrhea), other superinfections may result from altered bacterial balance. Nephrotoxicity may occur, esp. w/preexisting renal disease. Severe hypersensitivity reaction (severe pruritus, angioedema, bronchospasm, anaphylaxis) particularly those w/history of allergies, esp. penicillin.

NURSING IMPLICATIONS

BASELINE ASSESSMENT:

Question for history of allergies, particularly cephalosporins, penicillins. Obtain culture and sensitivity test before giving first dose (therapy may begin before results are known).

INTERVENTION/EVALUATION:

Evaluate IV site for phlebitis (heat, pain, red streaking over vein). Check IM injection sites for induration, tenderness. Check mouth for white patches on mucous membranes, tongue. Monitor bowel activity and stool consistency carefully; mild GI effects may be tolerable, but increasing severity may indicate onset of antibiotic-associated colitis. Assess skin for rash. Monitor I&O, urinalysis, renal function reports for nephrotoxicity. Be alert for superinfection: severe genital/anal pruritus, abdominal pain, severe mouth soreness, moderate to severe diarrhea.

PATIENT/FAMILY TEACHING:

Discomfort may occur w/IM injection. Doses should be evenly spaced. Continue antibiotic therapy for full length of treatment.

ceftriaxone sodium

cef-try-**ox**-zone
(Rocephin)

CANADIAN AVAILABILITY:
Rocephin

CLASSIFICATION

Antibiotic: Third-generation cephalosporin

AVAILABILITY (Rx)

Powder for Injection: 1 g, 2 g

PHARMACOKINETICS

Widely distributed (including CSF). Primarily excreted unchanged in urine. Not removed by hemodialysis. Half-life: 4.3–4.6 hrs IV; 5.8–8.7 hrs IM (increased in decreased renal function).

ACTION/THERAPEUTIC EFFECT

Bactericidal. Binds to bacterial membranes, *inhibiting bacterial cell wall synthesis*.

USES

Treatment of respiratory, GU tract, skin, bone, intra-abdominal, biliary tract infections; septicemia, meningitis, gonorrhea, Lyme disease, acute bacterial otitis media.

STORAGE/HANDLING

Solution appears light yellow to amber. IV infusion (piggyback) stable for 3 days at room temperature, 10 days if refrigerated. Discard if precipitate forms.

IM/IV ADMINISTRATION

Note: Give by IM injection, intermittent IV infusion (piggyback).
IM:
To minimize discomfort, inject deep IM slowly. Less painful if injected into gluteus maximus rather than lateral aspect of thigh.

IV:

1. Administer over 2–4 min.
2. For intermittent IV infusion (piggyback), infuse over 15–30 min for adults, 10–30 min in children, neonates.
3. Alternating IV sites, use large veins to reduce potential for phlebitis.

INDICATIONS/DOSAGE/ROUTES

Mild to moderate infections:
IM/IV: **Adults, elderly:** 1–2 g given as single dose or 2 divided doses.

Serious infections:
IM/IV: **Adults, elderly:** Up to 4 g/day in 2 divided doses. **Chil-**dren: 50–75 mg/kg/day in divided doses q12h. **Maximum:** 2 g/day.

Skin/skin structure infections:
IM/IV: **Children:** 50–75 mg/kg/day as single or 2 divided doses. **Maximum:** 2 g/day.

Meningitis:
IV: **Children:** Initially, 75 mg/kg, then 100 mg/kg/day as single or in divided doses q12h. **Maximum:** 4 g/day.

Lyme's disease:
IV: **Adults, elderly:** 2–4 g daily for 10–14 days.

Acute bacterial otits media:
IM: **Children:** 50 mg/kg as single dose. **Maximum:** 1g.

Perioperative prophylaxis:
IM/IV: **Adults, elderly:** 1 g 0.5–2 hrs before surgery.

Uncomplicated gonorrhea:
IM: **Adults:** 250 mg one time plus doxycycline.

Dosage in renal impairment:
Dosage modification usually unnecessary, but should be monitored in those w/both renal and hepatic impairment or severe renal impairment.

PRECAUTIONS

CONTRAINDICATIONS: History of hypersensitivity to cephalosporins, anaphylactic reactions to penicillins. **CAUTIONS:** Renal or hepatic impairment, history of GI disease (especially ulcerative colitis, antibiotic-associated colitis), concurrent administration of nephrotoxic medications. **PREGNANCY/LACTATION:** Readily crosses placenta; distributed in breast milk. **Pregnancy Category B.**

INTERACTIONS

DRUG INTERACTIONS: None significant. **ALTERED LAB VALUES:**

Positive direct/indirect Coombs' test may occur (interferes w/hematologic tests, cross-matching procedures). May increase BUN, serum creatinine, SGOT (AST), SGPT (ALT), alkaline phosphatase, bilirubin concentrations.

SIDE EFFECTS

FREQUENT: Discomfort w/IM administration, oral candidiasis (sore mouth/tongue), mild diarrhea, mild abdominal cramping, vaginal candidiasis (itching, discharge). **OCCASIONAL:** Nausea, serum sickness reaction [joint pain, fever] (usually occurs following second course of therapy, resolves after drug discontinuation). **RARE:** Allergic reaction (rash, pruritus, urticaria), thrombophlebitis (pain, redness, swelling at injection site).

ADVERSE REACTIONS/TOXIC EFFECTS

Antibiotic-associated colitis (severe abdominal pain and tenderness, fever, watery and severe diarrhea), other superinfections may result from altered bacterial balance. Nephrotoxicity may occur, esp. w/preexisting renal disease. Severe hypersensitivity reaction (severe pruritus, angioedema, bronchospasm, anaphylaxis), particularly those w/history of allergies, esp. penicillin.

NURSING IMPLICATIONS

BASELINE ASSESSMENT:

Question for history of allergies, particularly cephalosporins, penicillins. Obtain culture and sensitivity test before giving first dose (therapy may begin before results are known).

INTERVENTION/EVALUATION:

Evaluate IV site for phlebitis (heat, pain, red streaking over vein). Check IM injection sites for induration, tenderness. Check mouth for white patches on mucous membranes, tongue. Monitor bowel activity and stool consistency carefully; mild GI effects may be tolerable, but increasing severity may indicate onset of antibiotic-associated colitis. Assess skin for rash. Monitor I&O, urinalysis, renal function reports for nephrotoxicity. Be alert for superinfection: severe genital/anal pruritus, abdominal pain, severe mouth soreness, moderate to severe diarrhea.

PATIENT/FAMILY TEACHING:

Discomfort may occur w/IM injection. Doses should be evenly spaced. Continue antibiotic therapy for full length of treatment.

cefuroxime axetil
sef-yur-**ox**-ime
(Ceftin)

cefuroxime sodium
(Kefurox, Zinacef)

CANADIAN AVAILABILITY:
Ceftin, Kefurox, Zinacef

CLASSIFICATION

Antibiotic: Second-generation cephalosporin

AVAILABILITY (Rx)

Tablets: 125 mg, 250 mg, 500 mg.
Oral Suspension: 125 mg/5 ml.
Powder for Injection: 750 mg, 1.5 g.

PHARMACOKINETICS

Rapidly absorbed from GI tract.

Oral form rapidly hydrolyzed to cefuroxime. Widely distributed (including CSF). Primarily excreted unchanged in urine. Moderately removed by hemodialysis. Half-life: 1.3 hrs (increased in decreased renal function).

ACTION/*THERAPEUTIC EFFECT*

Bactericidal. Binds to bacterial membranes, *inhibiting bacterial cell wall synthesis.*

USES

Treatment of otitis media, respiratory, GU tract, gynecologic, skin, bone infections; septicemia, bacterial meningitis, gonorrhea and other gonococcal infections; ampicillin-resistant influenza, perioperative prophylaxis, impetigo, acute bacterial maxillary sinusitis, early Lyme disease.

STORAGE/HANDLING

Solutions appear light yellow to amber; may darken, but color change does not indicate loss of potency. IV infusion (piggyback) stable for 24 hrs at room temperature, 7 days if refrigerated. Discard if precipitate forms.

PO/IM/IV ADMINISTRATION

Note: Give orally, IM, direct IV injection, intermittent IV infusion (piggyback).

PO:

1. Give w/o regard to meals. If GI upset occurs, give w/food or milk.
2. Tablets may be crushed, mixed w/food.
3. Suspension must be given w/food.

IM:

To minimize discomfort, inject deep IM slowly. Less painful if injected into gluteus maximus rather than lateral aspect of thigh.

IV:

1. For direct IV injection, dilute 750 mg in 8 ml (1.5 g in 14 ml) sterile water for injection to provide a concentration of 100 mg/ml. Administer over 3–5 min.
2. For intermittent IV infusion (piggyback), further dilute w/50–100 ml 5% dextrose or 0.9% NaCl, infuse over 15–60 min.
3. Alternating IV sites, use large veins to reduce risk of phlebitis.

INDICATIONS/DOSAGE/ROUTES

Pharyngitis/tonsillitis:
PO: Adults, elderly: 250 mg 2 times/day. **Children:** 125 mg 2 times/day or 20 mg/kg/day in 2 divided doses.

Acute otitis media:
PO: Children: 250 mg 2 times/day or 30 mg/kg/day in 2 divided doses.

Acute/chronic bronchitis:
PO: Adults: 250–500 mg 2 times/day.

Acute bacterial maxillary sinusitis:
PO: Adults, children >13 yrs: 250 mg 2 times/day for 10 days. **Children 3 mos–12 yrs:** 30 mg/kg in 2 divided doses.

Impetigo:
PO: Children: 30 mg/kg/day in 2 divided doses.

Skin/skin structure infections:
PO: Adults: 250–500 mg 2 times/day.
IM/IV: Adults: 750 mg-1.5 g q8h.

Early Lyme disease:
PO: Adults: 500 mg 2 times/day.

Urinary tract infections:
PO: Adults: 125–250 mg 2 times/day.
IM/IV: Adults: 750 mg–1.5 g q8h.

Pneumonia:
IM/IV: Adults: 750 mg–1.5 g q8h.

Uncomplicated gonorrhea:
PO: Adults: 1 g as single dose.
IM: Adults: 1.5 g as single dose.

Disseminated gonococcal infection:
IM/IV: Adults: 750 mg to 1.5 g q8h.

Bone/joint infections:
IM/IV: Adults, elderly: 1.5 g q8h.

Life-threatening infections:
IV: Adults, elderly: 1.5 g q8h.
Children: 150 mg/kg/day in 3 divided doses.

Bacterial meningitis:
IV: Adults: Up to 3 g q8h. **Children:** Initially, 200–240 mg/kg/day in 3–4 divided doses; then, 100 mg/kg/day w/clinical improvement.

Perioperative prophylaxis:
IV: Adults, elderly: 1.5 g 30–60 min before surgery and 750 mg q8h postop.

Dosage in renal impairment:
Adult dosage is modified on basis of creatinine clearance and/or severity of infection.

CREATININE CLEARANCE	DOSAGE
10–20 ml/min	750 mg q12h
<10 ml/min	750 mg q24h

PRECAUTIONS

CONTRAINDICATIONS: History of hypersensitivity to cephalosporins, anaphylactic reaction to penicillins. **CAUTIONS:** Renal impairment, history of allergies or GI disease (especially ulcerative colitis, antibiotic-associated colitis), concurrent use of nephrotoxic medications. **PREGNANCY/LACTATION:** Readily crosses placenta. Distributed in breast milk. **Pregnancy Category B**.

INTERACTIONS

DRUG INTERACTIONS: Probenecid increases serum concentration of cefuroxime. **ALTERED LAB VALUES:** Positive direct/indirect Coombs' test may occur (interferes w/hematologic tests, cross-matching procedures). May increase SGOT (AST), SGPT (ALT), alkaline phosphatase, bilirubin, LDH concentrations.

SIDE EFFECTS

FREQUENT: Discomfort w/IM administration, oral candidiasis (sore mouth/tongue), mild diarrhea, mild abdominal cramping, vaginal candidiasis (itching, discharge). **OCCASIONAL:** Nausea, serum sickness reaction [joint pain, fever] (usually occurs following second course of therapy, resolves after drug discontinuation). **RARE:** Allergic reaction (rash, pruritus, urticaria), thrombophlebitis (pain, redness, swelling at injection site).

ADVERSE REACTIONS/TOXIC EFFECTS

Antibiotic-associated colitis (severe abdominal pain and tenderness, fever, watery and severe diarrhea), other superinfections may result from altered bacterial balance. Nephrotoxicity may occur, esp. w/preexisting renal disease. Severe hypersensitivity reaction (severe pruritus, angioedema, bronchospasm, anaphylaxis), particularly those w/history of allergies, esp. penicillin.

NURSING IMPLICATIONS
BASELINE ASSESSMENT:

Question for history of allergies, particularly cephalosporins, penicillins. Obtain culture and sensitivity test before giving first dose (therapy may begin before results are known).

INTERVENTION/EVALUATION:

Evaluate IV site for phlebitis (heat, pain, red streaking over vein). Check IM injection sites for induration, tenderness. Check mouth for white patches on mucous membranes, tongue. Monitor bowel activity and stool consistency carefully; mild GI effects may be tolerable, but increasing severity may indicate onset of antibiotic-associated colitis. Assess skin for rash. Monitor I&O, urinalysis, renal function reports for nephrotoxicity. Be alert for superinfection: severe genital/anal pruritus, abdominal pain, severe mouth soreness, moderate to severe diarrhea.

PATIENT/FAMILY TEACHING:

Discomfort may occur w/IM injection. Doses should be evenly spaced. Continue antibiotic therapy for full length of treatment. May cause GI upset (may take w/food or milk).

---

celecoxib
(Celebrex)
See Supplement

---

cephalexin
cef-ah-**lex**-in
(Keflet, Keflex)

cephalexin hydrochloride
(Keftab)

CANADIAN AVAILABILITY:
Apo-Cephalex, Keflex, Novolexin

CLASSIFICATION

Antibiotic: First-generation cephalosporin

AVAILABILITY (Rx)

Capsules: 250 mg, 500 mg.
Tablets: 250 mg, 500 mg, 1 g.
Oral Suspension: 125 mg/5 ml, 250 mg/5 ml.

PHARMACOKINETICS

Rapidly absorbed from GI tract. Widely distributed. Primarily excreted unchanged in urine. Moderately removed by hemodialysis. Half-life: 0.9–1.2 hrs (increased in decreased renal function).

ACTION/*THERAPEUTIC EFFECT*

Bactericidal. Binds to bacterial membranes, *inhibiting bacterial cell wall synthesis.*

USES

Treatment of respiratory tract, GU tract, skin, soft tissue, bone infections; otitis media, rheumatic fever prophylaxis; follow-up to parenteral therapy.

STORAGE/HANDLING

Oral suspension: after reconstitution, stable for 14 days if refrigerated.

PO ADMINISTRATION

1. Shake oral suspension well before using.
2. Give w/o regard to meals. If GI upset occurs, give w/food or milk.

INDICATIONS/DOSAGE/ROUTES

Note: Space doses evenly around the clock.

Usual dosage for adults:
PO: Adults, elderly: 250–500 mg q6h up to 4 g/day.

Streptococcal pharyngitis, skin/skin structure infections, uncomplicated cystitis:
PO: Adults, elderly: 500 mg q12h.

Usual dosage for children:
PO: Children: 25–100 mg/kg/day in 2–4 divided doses.

Otitis media:
PO: Children: 75–100 mg/kg/day in 4 divided doses.

Dosage in renal impairment:
After usual initial dose, dose and/or frequency is modified on basis of creatinine clearance and/or severity of infection.

CREATININE CLEARANCE	DOSAGE
11–40 ml/min	500 mg q8–12h
5–10 ml/min	250 mg q12h
<5 ml/min	250 mg q12–24h

PRECAUTIONS

CONTRAINDICATIONS: History of hypersensitivity to cephalosporins, anaphylactic reaction to penicillins. **CAUTIONS:** Renal impairment, history of allergies or GI disease (especially ulcerative colitis, antibiotic-associated colitis), concurrent use of nephrotoxic medications. **PREGNANCY/LACTATION:** Readily crosses placenta; distributed in breast milk. **Pregnancy Category B**.

INTERACTIONS

DRUG INTERACTIONS: Probenecid increases serum concentration of cephalexin. **ALTERED LAB VALUES:** Positive direct/indirect Coombs' test may occur (interferes w/hematologic test, cross-matching procedures). May increase SGOT (AST), SGPT (ALT), alkaline phosphatase concentrations.

SIDE EFFECTS

FREQUENT: Oral candidiasis (sore mouth/tongue), mild diarrhea, nausea, vaginal candidiasis. **OCCASIONAL:** Serum sickness reaction (skin rash, joint pain, fever), vomiting. **RARE:** Hemolytic anemia (unusual tiredness), erythema multiforme (blistering, peeling, loosening of skin).

ADVERSE REACTIONS/TOXIC EFFECTS

Antibiotic-associated colitis, other superinfections may result from altered bacterial balance. Nephrotoxicity may occur, esp. w/preexisting renal disease. Hypersensitivity reactions (ranging from rash, urticaria, fever to anaphylaxis) occur in those w/history of allergies, esp. penicillin.

NURSING IMPLICATIONS
BASELINE ASSESSMENT:

Question history of allergies, particularly cephalosporins, penicillins. Obtain culture and sensitivity test before giving first dose (therapy may begin before results are known).

INTERVENTION/EVALUATION:

Check mouth for white patches on mucous membranes, tongue. Monitor bowel activity and stool consistency carefully; mild GI effects may be tolerable, but increasing severity may indicate onset of antibiotic-associated colitis. Assess skin for rash. Monitor I&O, urinalysis, renal function reports for nephrotoxicity. Be alert for superinfection: genital/anal pruritus, moniliasis, abdominal pain, sore mouth or tongue, moderate to severe diarrhea.

PATIENT/FAMILY TEACHING:

Continue therapy for full length of treatment. Doses should be evenly spaced. May cause GI upset (may take w/ food or milk).

cephalothin
(Keflin)
*See Classification section under:
Antibiotic: cephalosporins*

cerivastatin
(Baycol)
*See Supplement
See Classification section under:
Antihyperlipidemics*

cetirizine
sih-**tier**-eh-zeen
(Zyrtec)

CANADIAN AVAILABILITY:
Reactine, Zyrtec

CLASSIFICATION

Antihistamine

AVAILABILITY (Rx)

Tablets: 5 mg, 10 mg. **Syrup:** 5 mg/5ml.

PHARMACOKINETICS

	ONSET	PEAK	DURATION
PO	<1 hr	4–8 hr	<24 hrs

Rapidly, almost completely absorbed from GI tract. Food has no effect on absorption. Undergoes low first-pass metabolism; not extensively metabolized. Primarily excreted in urine (>80% as unchanged drug). Half-life: 6.5–10 hrs.

ACTION

Competes w/histamine at histaminic receptor sites on effector cells, *preventing allergic response (urticaria, pruritus). Also produces mild bronchodilation, blocks histamine-induced bronchoconstriction in asthmatic patients.* Minimal anticholinergic effects.

USES/ *UNLABELED*

Relief of symptoms (sneezing, rhinorrhea, postnasal discharge, nasal pruritus, ocular pruritus, tearing) of seasonal and perennial allergic rhinitis (hay fever). Treatment of chronic urticaria (hives). *Treatment of bronchial asthma.*

PO ADMINISTRATION

May give w/o regard to meals.

INDICATIONS/DOSAGE/ROUTES

Allergic rhinitis, hives:
PO: Adults, elderly, 5–10 mg /day. May increase up to 20 mg/day. **Children 2–5 yrs:** Initially, 2.5 mg once daily. **Maximum:** 5 mg once daily or 2.5 mg q12h. **Children 6–11 yrs:** 5–10 mg once daily.

Renal impairment (creatinine clearance 11–31 ml/min), hemodialysis (creatinine clearance <7 ml/min), hepatic impairment:
PO: Adults, elderly: 5 mg once daily.

PRECAUTIONS

CONTRAINDICATIONS: None significant. **CAUTIONS:** Impaired hepatic impairment, symptomatic prostatic hypertrophy, urinary retention, angle-closure glaucoma. **PREGNANCY/LACTATION:** Not recommended during early months of pregnancy. Unknown if excreted in breast milk (breast feeding not recommended). **Pregnancy Category B.**

INTERACTIONS

DRUG INTERACTIONS: Alcohol, CNS depressants may increase CNS depression. **ALTERED LAB VALUES:** May suppress wheal and flare reactions to antigen skin testing, unless antihistamines are discontinued 4 days before testing.

SIDE EFFECTS

Minimal anticholinergic effects.

OCCASIONAL (2–10%): Pharyngitis, dry mouth, nose, throat, nausea, vomiting, abdominal pain, headache, dizziness, fatigue, thickening mucus, drowsiness, increased sensitivity of skin to sun.

ADVERSE REACTIONS/TOXIC EFFECTS

Children may experience dominant paradoxical reaction (restlessness, insomnia, euphoria, nervousness, tremors). Dizziness, sedation, confusion more likely to occur in elderly pts.

NURSING IMPLICATIONS
BASELINE ASSESSMENT:

Assess lung sound, rhinitis, urticaria, or other symptoms, liver function tests.

INTERVENTION/EVALUATION:

For upper respiratory allergies, increase fluids to maintain thin secretions and offset thirst, loss of fluids from increased sweating. Monitor symptoms for therapeutic response.

PATIENT/FAMILY TEACHING:

Generally does not cause drowsiness; however, if blurred vision or eye pain occurs, do not drive or perform activities requiring visual acuity. Avoid alcohol during antihistamine therapy. May take w/food. Avoid prolonged exposure to sunlight.

charcoal, activated
(Actidose, Charcocaps)

CANADIAN AVAILABILITY:
Aqueous Charcodote

CLASSIFICATION

Antidote

AVAILABILITY (OTC)

Tablets: 260 mg, 325 mg, 650 mg. **Capsules:** 250 mg, 260 mg. **Suspension:** 12.5 g, 15 g, 25 g, 30 g, 50 g.

PHARMACOKINETICS

Not absorbed or metabolized. Eliminated via intestinal tract.

ACTION

Adsorbs (detoxifies) ingested toxic substances, irritants, intestinal gas.

USES

Emergency antidote in treatment of poisoning. Reduces volume of intestinal gas, diarrhea.

PO ADMINISTRATION

1. Give 2 hrs before or 1 hr after other oral medication.
2. Shake suspension well before using.

INDICATIONS/DOSAGE/ROUTES

Antidote:
PO: Adults, elderly: Can give 30–100 g as slurry (30 g in at least 8 oz H_2O) or 12.5–50 g in aqueous or sorbitol suspension. Usually given as single dose.

Antidiarrheal:
PO: Adults, elderly: 520 mg, repeat q30 min–1h up to 4.16 g/day.

Antiflatulent:
PO: Adults, elderly: 1.04–3.9 g 3 times/day after meals.

PRECAUTIONS

CONTRAINDICATIONS: None significant. **CAUTIONS:** None significant. **PREGNANCY/LACTATION:** Unknown whether drug crosses placenta or is distributed in breast milk. **Pregnancy Category C.**

INTERACTIONS

DRUG INTERACTIONS: May decrease absorption, effects of orally administered medications. **ALTERED LAB VALUES:** None significant.

SIDE EFFECTS

OCCASSIONAL: Diarrhea, GI discomfort, intestinal gas.

ADVERSE REACTIONS/TOXIC EFFECTS

None significant.

NURSING IMPLICATIONS

INTERVENTION/EVALUATION:

Monitor bowel pattern, stool consistency. Assess bowel sounds for peristalsis. When using activated charcoal as an antidote, monitor vital signs, level of consciousness, and other clinical signs related to specific drug ingested.

chloral hydrate

klor-al high-drate
(Noctec, Aquachloral Supprettes)

CANADIAN AVAILABILITY:
PMS-Chloral Hydrate

CLASSIFICATION

Sedative, hypnotic

AVAILABILITY (Rx)

Capsules: 250 mg, 500 mg.
Syrup: 250 mg/5 ml, 500 mg/5 ml.
Suppository: 324 mg, 500 mg, 648 mg.

PHARMACOKINETICS

	ONSET	PEAK	DURATION
PO	30–60 min	—	4–8 hrs
Rectal			
	30–60 min	—	4–8 hrs

Readily absorbed from GI tract. Metabolized in liver, erythrocytes to active metabolite. Excreted in urine. Half-life: 7–10 hrs.

ACTION/*THERAPEUTIC EFFECT*

Produces CNS depression (mechanism unknown). *Induces quiet, deep sleep, w/only slight decrease in respiration, B/P.*

USES

Treatment of insomnia (replaced by other medications), adjunct to anesthesia preoperatively to produce sedation/relieve anxiety.

PO/RECTAL ADMINISTRATION

PO:

1. May be given w/o regard to meals.
2. Capsules may be emptied and mixed w/food.
3. Mix syrup form with ½ glass (4 oz) water, fruit juice, ginger ale.

RECTAL:

1. If suppository is too soft, chill for 30 min in refrigerator or run cold water over foil wrapper.
2. Moisten suppository w/cold water before inserting well up into rectum.

INDICATIONS/DOSAGE/ROUTES

Premedication for dental/medical procedures:
PO/Rectal: Adults: 0.5–1 g.
Children: 75 mg/kg up to 1 g total.

Premedication for EEG:
PO/Rectal: Adults: 0.5–1.5 g.
Children: 25 mg/kg.

PRECAUTIONS

CONTRAINDICATIONS: Marked hepatic, renal impairment, severe cardiac disease, presence of gastritis. *Oral form:* Esophagitis, gastritis, gastric/duodenal ulcer. **CAUTIONS:** History of drug abuse, mental depression. **PREGNANCY/LACTATION:** Crosses placenta; small amount distributed in breast milk. Withdrawal symptoms may occur in neonates born to women who receive chloral hydrate during pregnancy. May produce sedation in nursing infants. **Pregnancy Category C**.

INTERACTIONS

DRUG INTERACTIONS: Alcohol, CNS depressants may increase effects. May increase effect of warfarin. IV furosemide given within 24 hrs following chloral hydrate may alter B/P, cause diaphoresis. **ALTERED LAB VALUES:** None significant.

SIDE EFFECTS

Generally well tolerated w/only mild and transient effects. **OCCASIONAL:** Gastric irritation (nausea, vomiting, flatulence, diarrhea), rash, sleepwalking, disorientation, paranoid behavior. **RARE:** Confusion, paradoxical excitement, residual hangover, headache, paradoxical CNS hyperactivity/nervousness in children, excitement/restlessness in elderly (particularly noted when given in presence of pain).

ADVERSE REACTIONS/TOXIC EFFECTS

Overdosage may produce somnolence, confusion, slurred speech, severe incoordination, respiratory depression, coma. Tolerance and psychological dependence may occur by second week of therapy. Abrupt withdrawal of drug after long-term use may produce weakness, facial flushing, sweating, vomiting, tremor.

NURSING IMPLICATIONS

BASELINE ASSESSMENT:

Assess B/P, pulse, respirations immediately before administration. Raise bed rails. Provide environment conducive to sleep (back rub, quiet environment, low lighting).

INTERVENTION/EVALUATION:

Assess sleep pattern of pt. Assess elderly/children for paradoxical reaction. Evaluate for therapeutic response to insomnia: a decrease in number of nocturnal awakenings, increase in length of sleep.

PATIENT/FAMILY TEACHING:

Do not abruptly withdraw medication after long-term use. Avoid tasks that require alertness, motor skills until response to drug is established. Tolerance/dependence may occur w/prolonged use of high doses.

chlorambucil

klor-**am**-bew-sill
(Leukeran)

CANADIAN AVAILABILITY:
Leukeran

CLASSIFICATION

Antineoplastic

AVAILABILITY (Rx)

Tablet: 2 mg

PHARMACOKINETICS

Rapidly, completely absorbed from GI tract. Rapidly metabolized in liver to active metabolite. Half-life: 1.5 hrs; metabolite: 2.5 hrs.

ACTION/ *THERAPEUTIC EFFECT*

Inhibits DNA, RNA synthesis by cross-linking w/DNA and RNA strands, *interfering w/nucleic acid function.* Cell cycle-phase nonspecific. Has immunosuppressive activity.

USES/ *UNLABELED*

Palliative treatment of chronic lymphocytic leukemia, advanced malignant (non-Hodgkin's) lymphomas, lymphosarcoma, giant follicular lymphomas, advanced Hodgkin's disease. *Treatment of ovarian, testicular carcinoma, hairy cell leukemia, polycythemia vera, nephrotic syndrome.*

INDICATIONS/DOSAGE/ROUTES

Note: May be carcinogenic, mutagenic, or teratogenic. Handle w/extreme care during administration. Dosage individualized on basis of clinical response, tolerance to adverse effects. When used in combination therapy, consult specific protocols for optimum dosage, sequence of drug administration.

Usual dosage (initial or short-course therapy):
PO: Adults, elderly, children: 0.1–0.2 mg/kg/day as single or divided dose for 3–6 wks. **Average dose:** 4–10 mg/day. **Single daily dose q2wks:** 0.4 mg/kg initially. Increase by 0.1 mg/kg q2wks until response and/or myelosuppression.

Usual dosage (maintenance):
PO: Adults, elderly, children: 0.03–0.1 mg/kg/day. **Average dose:** 2–4 mg/day.

PRECAUTIONS:

CONTRAINDICATIONS: Previous allergic reaction, disease resistance to previous therapy w/drug. **EXTREME CAUTION:** Within 4 weeks after full-course radiation therapy or myelosuppressive drug regimen. **PREGNANCY/LACTATION:** If possible, avoid use during pregnancy, especially first trimester. Breast feeding not recommended. **Pregnancy Category D.**

INTERACTIONS

DRUG INTERACTIONS: May decrease effect of antigout medications. Bone marrow depressants may increase bone marrow depression. Other immunosuppressants (e.g., steroids) may increase risk of infection or development of neoplasms. Live virus vaccines may potentiate virus replication, increase vaccine side effects, decrease antibody response to vaccine. **ALTERED LAB VALUES:** May increase SGOT (AST), alkaline phosphatase, uric acid.

SIDE EFFECTS

GI effects (nausea, vomiting, anorexia, diarrhea, abdominal distress) are generally mild, last less that 24 hrs, and occur only if single dose exceeds 20 mg. **OCCASIONAL:** Rash or dermatitis, pruritus, cold sores. **RARE:** Alopecia, urticaria (hives), erythema, hyperuricemia.

ADVERSE REACTIONS/TOXIC EFFECTS

Bone marrow depression manifested as hematologic toxicity (neutropenia, leukopenia, progressive lymphopenia, anemia, thrombocytopenia). After discontinuation of therapy, thrombocytopenia, leukopenia usually occur at 1–3 wks and lasts 1–4 wks. Neutrophil count decreases up to 10 days after last dose. Toxicity appears to be less severe w/intermittent rather than continuous drug administration. Overdosage may produce seizures in children. Excessive uric acid level, hepatotoxicity occurs rarely.

NURSING IMPLICATIONS
BASELINE ASSESSMENT:

CBC should be performed each week during therapy, WBC count performed 3–4 days after each weekly CBC during first 3–6 wks of therapy (4–6 wks if pt on intermittent dosing schedule).

INTERVENTION/EVALUATION:

Monitor serum uric acid concentration. Monitor for hematologic toxicity (fever, sore throat, signs of local infection, easy bruising, or unusual bleeding from any site), symptoms of anemia (excessive tiredness, weakness). Assess skin for rash, pruritus, urticaria. If there is abrupt fall in WBC count, or if WBC, platelet count are less than normal value, consult physician (dosage may be reduced). Dosage should be temporarily discontinued if further bone marrow depression occurs.

PATIENT/FAMILY TEACHING:

Increase fluid intake (may protect against hyperuricemia). Do not have immunizations w/o doctor's approval (drug lowers body's resistance). Avoid contact w/those who have recently received live virus vaccine. Promptly report fever, sore throat, signs of local infection, easy bruising, or unusual bleeding from any site. Contact physician if nausea/vomiting continues at home.

chloramphenicol
klor-am-**fen**-ih-call
(Chloromycetin, Chloroptic)

chloramphenicol palmitate
(Chloromycetin oral suspension)

chloramphenicol sodium succinate
(Chloromycetin)

FIXED-COMBINATION(S):
W/polymyxin B, an antibiotic, and hydrocortisone, acetate (**Ophthocort**)

CANADIAN AVAILABILITY:
Chloromycetin

CLASSIFICATION
Antibiotic

AVAILABILITY (Rx)
Capsule: 250 mg. **Oral Suspension:** 150 mg/5 ml. **Powder for Injection:** 100 mg/ml. **Ophthalmic Solution:** 5 mg/ml. **Ophthalmic Ointment:** 10 mg/g. **Otic Solution:** 0.5%.

PHARMACOKINETICS
Rapidly, completely absorbed after oral, IM administration. Widely distributed (including CSF). Metabolized in liver. Primarily excreted in urine. Minimally

removed by hemodialysis. Half-life: 1.5–3.5 hrs (increased in decreased renal, liver function, children, neonates).

ACTION/ THERAPEUTIC EFFECT

Bacteriostatic (may be bactericidal in high concentrations). Binds to ribosomal receptor sites, *inhibiting protein synthesis.*

USES

Intra-abdominal, soft tissue, or orificial infections, typhoid fever, osteomyelitis, septic arthritis, cellulitis, septicemia, meningitis; adjunctive therapy for cerebral abscesses or other CNS infections, rickettsial infections when tetracyclines are contraindicated. Treatment of superficial ocular infections, superficial infections of external auditory canal.

STORAGE/HANDLING

Store capsules, oral suspension at room temperature. Solution for injection is stable for 30 days at room temperature. Discard if cloudy or precipitate forms.

PO/IV/OPHTHALMIC ADMINIS-TRATION

PO:

1. Change therapy from IV to oral as soon as possible.
2. Administer oral doses on empty stomach 1 hr before or 2 hrs after meals (may give w/food if GI upset occurs).

IV:

Note: Give by IV injection or intermittent IV infusion (piggyback).
1. For IV injection, administer dose over at least 1 min.
2. Dosage adjusted to maintain plasma concentration at 5–20 mcg/ml.

3. For intermittent IV infusion (piggyback), infuse >30 min.
4. Pts should be hospitalized during chloramphenicol therapy for close observation, adequate blood studies.

OPHTHALMIC:

1. Place finger on lower eyelid and pull out until a pocket is formed between eye and lower lid.
2. Hold dropper above pocket and place correct number of drops ($^1/_4$–$^1/_2$ inch ointment) into pocket. Close eye gently.
3. *Solution:* Apply digital pressure to lacrimal sac for 1–2 min (minimizes drainage into nose and throat, reducing risk of systemic effects).
4. *Ointment:* Close eye for 1–2 min, rolling eyeball (increases contact area of drug to eye).
5. Remove excess solution or ointment around eye w/tissue.

INDICATIONS/DOSAGE/ROUTES

Mild to moderate infections:
PO/IV: Adults, elderly, children: 50 mg/kg/day in divided doses q6h.

Severe infections, infections due to moderately resistant organisms:
PO/IV: Adults, elderly, children: 50–100 mg/kg/day in divided doses q6h.

Dosage in renal or hepatic impairment:
Dosage is reduced on basis of degree of renal impairment, plasma concentration of drug. Initially, 1 g, then 500 mg q6h.

Usual dosage for neonates:
IV/PO: Newborn infants: 25 mg/kg/day in 4 doses q6h. **Infants >2 wks:** 50 mg/kg/day in 4 doses q6h. **Neonates <2 kg:** 25 mg/kg once daily. **Neonates <7days, >2 kg:**

25 mg/kg once daily. **Neonates >7 days, >2 kg:** 50 mg/kg/day in divided doses q12h.

Usual ophthalmic dosage:
Ointment: Adults, elderly, children: Apply thin strip to conjunctiva q3–4h.
Drops: Adults, elderly, children: 1–2 drops 4–6 times/day.

Usual otic dosage:
Otic: Adults, elderly, children: 2–3 drops into ear 3 times/day.

PRECAUTIONS

CONTRAINDICATIONS: Hypersensitivity to chloramphenicol or other components in fixed combination. Not for use in infections when less toxic drugs can be used. Prolonged treatment or frequent application should be avoided w/topical application. **CAUTIONS:** Bone marrow depression, previous cytotoxic drug therapy, radiation therapy, hepatic or renal impairment, infants/children <2 yr. **PREGNANCY/LACTATION:** Crosses placenta; distributed in breast milk. Not recommended at term or during labor (potential "gray baby" syndrome, bone marrow depression). **Pregnancy Category C**.

INTERACTIONS

DRUG INTERACTIONS: Anticonvulsants, bone marrow depressants may increase bone marrow depression. May increase effect of oral hypoglycemics. May antagonize effects of clindamycin, erythromycin. May increase concentration of phenobarbital, phenytoin, warfarin. **ALTERED LAB VALUES:** None significant.

SIDE EFFECTS

OCCASIONAL: *Systemic:* Nausea, vomiting, diarrhea. *Ophthalmic:* Blurred vision, burning, stinging, hypersensitivity reaction. *Otic:* Hypersensitivity reaction. **RARE:** "Gray baby" syndrome [neonates]: (abdominal distension, blue gray skin color, cardiovascular collapse, unresponsiveness), rash, shortness of breath, confusion, headache, optic neuritis (eye pain, blurred vision), peripheral neuritis (numbness/weakness in hands/feet).

ADVERSE REACTIONS/TOXIC EFFECTS

Superinfection due to bacterial or fungal overgrowth. Narrow margin between effective therapy and toxic levels producing blood dyscrasias: Bone marrow depression w/resulting aplastic anemia, hypoplastic anemia, pancytopenia (may occur weeks or months later).

NURSING IMPLICATIONS

BASELINE ASSESSMENT:

Question pt for history of allergies, particularly to chloramphenicol. Avoid, if possible, other drugs that cause bone marrow depression. Obtain specimens for culture and sensitivity test before giving first dose (therapy may begin before results are known). Establish baseline blood studies before therapy.

INTERVENTION/EVALUATION:

Monitor hematology reports carefully. Coordinate w/lab for drawing of chloramphenicol plasma levels. Assess for appetite, vomiting. Evaluate mental status. Check for visual disturbances. Assess skin for rash. Determine pattern of bowel activity and stool consistency. Monitor I&O, renal function tests if indicated. Watch for superinfection: diarrhea, anal/genital pruritus, change in oral mucosa, increased fever.

PATIENT/FAMILY TEACHING:

Continue therapy for full length of treatment; ophthalmic treatment should continue at least 48 hrs after eye returns to normal appearance. Doses should be evenly spaced. Take oral doses on empty stomach, 1 hr before or 2 hrs after meals (may take w/food if GI upset occurs, but not w/iron or vitamins). Notify physician in event of unusual bleeding or bruising, blurred vision, tired/weak feeling, or other new symptom; w/ophthalmic use report any increased irritation, burning, itching.

chlordiazepoxide

klor-dye-az-eh-**pox**-eyd
(**Libritabs**)

chlordiazepoxide hydrochloride

(Librium, Lipoxide)

FIXED-COMBINATION(S):
W/clidinium bromide, an anticholinergic (**Librax**); w/estrogen (**Menrium**); w/amitriptyline hydrochloride, an antidepressant (**Limbitrol**).

CANADIAN AVAILABILITY:
Apo-Chlordiazepoxide, Novopoxide

CLASSIFICATION

Antianxiety: Benzodiazepine

AVAILABILITY (Rx)

Capsules: 5 mg, 10 mg, 25 mg.
Tablets: 5 mg, 10 mg, 25 mg.
Injection: 100 mg ampul.

PHARMACOKINETICS

	ONSET	PEAK	DURATION
IV	1–5 min	—	15 min-1 hr

Well absorbed from GI tract; slow, erratic after IM administration. Metabolized in liver to active metabolite. Excreted in urine. Half-life: 5–30 hrs.

ACTION/*THERAPEUTIC EFFECT*

Enhances action of gamma aminobutyric acid (GABA) neurotransmission at CNS, *producing anxiolytic effect.*

USES/*UNLABELED*

Management of anxiety disorders, acute alcohol withdrawal symptoms; short-term relief of symptoms of anxiety, preop anxiety, tension. *Treatment of panic disorder, tension headache, tremors.*

STORAGE/HANDLING

Store unreconstituted parenteral form at room temperature. Refrigerate diluent; do not use if hazy or opalescent. Prepare immediately before administration; discard unused portions. Do not mix w/infusion fluids.

PO/IM/IV ADMINISTRATION

PO:

1. Give w/o regard to meals.
2. Tablets may be crushed (do not crush combination form).
3. Capsules may be emptied and mixed w/food.

IM:

1. Do not use IV preparation for IM injection (produces pain at injection site).

2. Add 2 ml of diluent provided to 100 mg ampule to yield 50 mg/ml. Add diluent carefully to minimize air bubbles. Agitate gently to dissolve.

3. Inject deep IM slowly into upper outer quadrant of gluteus maximus.

IV:

1. Do not use IM diluent solution for IV injection (air bubbles form during reconstitution of diluent).

2. Dilute each 100 mg ampule w/5 ml of 0.9% NaCl or sterile water for injection administration to yield 20 mg/ml. Agitate gently until dissolved.

3. Use Y tube or 3-way stopcock to control infusion rate.

4. Administer 100 mg or fraction thereof over at least 1 min.

5. A too rapid IV may produce hypotension, respiratory depression.

INDICATIONS/DOSAGE/ROUTES

Note: Use smallest effective dose in elderly or debilitated, those w/liver disease, low serum albumin.
Parenteral Form: Do not exceed 300 mg/24 hrs.

Mild to moderate anxiety:
PO: Adults: 5–10 mg 3–4 times/day. **Elderly/debilitated:** 5 mg 2–4 times/day. Do not exceed 10 mg/day initially. **Children >6 yrs:** 5 mg 2–4 times/day. Do not exceed 10 mg/day initially.

Severe anxiety:
PO: Adults: 20–25 mg 3–4 times/day.

IM/IV: Adults: Initially, 50–100 mg, then 25–50 mg 3–4 times/day. **Elderly:** 25–50 mg 3–4 times/day.

Preoperative:
IM/IV: Adults: 50–100 mg 1 hr before surgery. **Elderly/debilitated, children 12–18 yrs:** 25–50 mg 1 hr before surgery.

Alcohol withdrawal:
PO: Adults: 50–100 mg followed by repeated doses until agitation is controlled. Do not exceed 300 mg/day.
IM/IV: Adults: Initially, 50–100 mg. May repeat in 2–4 hrs, if necessary.

PRECAUTIONS

CONTRAINDICATIONS: Acute narrow-angle glaucoma, acute alcohol intoxication. **CAUTIONS:** Impaired kidney/liver function. **PREGNANCY/LACTATION:** Crosses placenta; distributed in breast milk. May increase risk of fetal abnormalities if administered during first trimester of pregnancy. Chronic ingestion during pregnancy may produce withdrawal symptoms, CNS depression in neonates. **Pregnancy Category D.**

INTERACTIONS

DRUG INTERACTIONS: Alcohol, CNS depressants may increase CNS depressant effect. **ALTERED LAB VALUES:** None significant.

SIDE EFFECTS

FREQUENT: Pain w/IM injection; drowsiness, ataxia, dizziness, confusion w/oral dose, particularly in elderly, debilitated. **OCCASIONAL:** Rash, peripheral edema, GI disturbances. **RARE:** Paradoxical CNS hyperactivity/nervousness in children, excitement/restlessness in elderly (generally noted during first 2 wks of therapy, particularly noted in presence of uncontrolled pain).

ADVERSE REACTIONS/TOXIC EFFECTS

IV route may produce pain, swelling, thrombophlebitis, carpal tunnel syndrome. Abrupt or too rapid withdrawal may result in pronounced restlessness, irritability, insomnia, hand tremors, abdominal/muscle cramps, sweating, vomiting, seizures. Overdosage results in somnolence, confusion, diminished reflexes, coma.

NURSING IMPLICATIONS

BASELINE ASSESSMENT:

Assess B/P, pulse, respirations immediately before administration. Pt must remain recumbent for up to 3 hrs (individualized) after parenteral administration to reduce hypotensive effect. Assess autonomic response (cold, clammy hands, sweating) and motor response (agitation, trembling, tension). Offer emotional support to anxious pt.

INTERVENTION/EVALUATION:

Assess motor responses (agitation, trembling, tension) and autonomic responses (cold, clammy hands, sweating). Assess children, elderly for paradoxical reaction, particularly during early therapy. Assist w/ambulation if drowsiness, ataxia occur. For those on long-term therapy, liver/renal function tests, blood counts should be performed periodically.

PATIENT/FAMILY TEACHING:

Discomfort may occur w/IM injection. Drowsiness usually disappears during continued therapy. If dizziness occurs, change positions slowly from recumbent to sitting before standing. Avoid tasks that require alertness, motor skills until response to drug is established. Smoking reduces drug effectiveness. Do not abruptly withdraw medication after long-term therapy.

chloroprocaine
(Nesacaine)
See Classification section under: Anesthetics: local

chloroquine hydrochloride

klor-oh-kwin
(Aralen hydrochloride)

chloroquine phosphate
(Aralen phosphate)

CANADIAN AVAILABILITY:
Aralen

CLASSIFICATION

Antimalarial, amebecide

AVAILABILITY (Rx)

Tablet: 500 mg. **Injection:** 50 mg/ml.

PHARMACOKINETICS

Readily absorbed from GI tract. Widely distributed. Partially metabolized in liver to active metabolite. Excreted slowly in urine. Removed by hemodialysis. Half-life: 1–2 mos.

ACTION/ *THERAPEUTIC EFFECT*

Concentrates in parasite acid vesicles, *increases pH (inhibits parasite growth)*. May interfere w/parasite protein synthesis.

USES/ *UNLABELED*

Treatment of *Plasmodium falciparum* malaria (terminates acute attacks, cures nonresistant strains), suppression of acute attacks, prolongation of interval between treatment/relapse in *P. vivax, P. ovale, P. malariae* malaria. Adjunctive therapy for extraintestinal amebiasis (including liver abscess). In combination w/primaquine cure for *P. vivax* and *P. ovale* malaria. *Treatment of sarcoid-associated hypercalcemia, juvenile arthritis, rheumatoid arthritis, systemic lupus erythematosus, solar urticaria, chronic cutaneous vasculitis.*

PO ADMINISTRATION

1. Administer w/meals to reduce adverse GI effects.
2. Tablets have bitter taste; may be crushed and mixed w/food or encased in gelatin capsule.

INDICATIONS/DOSAGE/ROUTES

Note: Chloroquine PO_4 500 mg = 300 mg base; chloroquine HCl 50 mg = 40 mg base.

CHLOROQUINE PHOSPHATE:

Treatment of malaria (acute attack): Dose (mg base)

DOSE	TIME	ADULTS	CHILDREN
Initial	Day 1	600 mg	10 mg/kg
Second	6 hrs later	300 mg	5 mg/kg
Third	Day 2	300 mg	5 mg/kg
Fourth	Day 3	300 mg	5 mg/kg

Suppression of malaria:
PO: Adults: 300 mg (base)/wk on same day each week beginning 2 wks before exposure; continue for 6–8 wks after leaving endemic area. **Children:** 5 mg base/kg/wk. If therapy is not begun prior to exposure, then: **PO: Adults:** 600 mg base initially given in 2 divided doses 6 hrs apart. **Children:** 10 mg base/kg.

Amebiasis:
PO: Adults: 1 g (600 mg base) daily for 2 days; then, 500 mg (300 mg base)/day for at least 2–3 wks.

CHLOROQUINE HCL:

Treatment of malaria:
IM: Adults: Initially, 160–200 mg base (4–5 ml), repeat in 6 hrs. **Maximum:** 800 mg base in first 24 hrs. Begin oral therapy as soon as possible and continue for 3 days until approximately 1.5 g base given. **Children:** Initially, 5 mg base/kg, repeat in 6 hrs. Do not exceed 10 mg base/kg/24 hrs.

Amebiasis:
IM: Adults: 160–200 mg base (4–5 ml) daily for 10–12 days. Change to oral therapy as soon as possible.

PRECAUTIONS

CONTRAINDICATIONS: Hypersensitivity to 4-aminoquinolones, retinal or visual field changes, psoriasis, porphyria. **CAUTIONS:** Alcoholism, severe blood disorders, liver disease, neurologic disorders, G-6-PD deficiency. Children are esp. susceptible to chloroquine fatalities. **PREGNANCY/LACTATION:** Unknown if drug crosses placenta; small amount excreted in breast milk. Vestibular apparatus teratogenicity may occur. **Pregnancy Category C**.

INTERACTIONS

DRUG INTERACTIONS: May increase concentration of penicillamine, increase risk of hematologic/renal or severe skin reaction. **ALTERED LAB VALUES:** Acute decrease in Hct, Hgb, RBC count may occur.

SIDE EFFECTS

FREQUENT: Discomfort w/IM administration, mild transient headache, anorexia, nausea, vomiting. **OCCASIONAL:** Visual disturbances (blurring, difficulty focusing); nervousness, fatigue, pruritus esp. of palms, soles, scalp; bleaching of hair, irritability, personality changes, diarrhea, skin eruptions. **RARE:** Stomatitis (redness/burning of oral mucosa, gingivitis, glossitis), exfoliative dermatitis.

ADVERSE REACTIONS/TOXIC EFFECTS

Ocular toxicity (tinnitus), ototoxicity (reduced hearing). Prolonged therapy: peripheral neuritis and neuromyopathy, hypotension, ECG changes, agranulocytosis, aplastic anemia, thrombocytopenia, convulsions, psychosis. Overdosage: headache, vomiting, visual disturbance, drowsiness, convulsions, hypokalemia followed by cardiovascular collapse, death.

NURSING IMPLICATIONS
BASELINE ASSESSMENT:

Question for hypersensitivity to chloroquine or hydroxychloroquine sulfate. Evaluate CBC, hepatic function results.

INTERVENTION/EVALUATION:

Check for and promptly report any visual disturbances. Evaluate for GI distress: give dose w/food, discuss w/physician dividing dose into separate days during week. Monitor hepatic function tests and check for fatigue, jaundice, or other signs of hepatic effects. Assess skin and buccal mucosa, inquire about pruritus. Check vital signs and be alert to signs/symptoms of overdosage (esp. w/parental administration, children). Monitor CBC results for adverse hematologic effects. Notify physician of tinnitus, reduced hearing. W/prolonged therapy, test for muscle weakness. Parenteral therapy should be converted to oral therapy as soon as possible.

PATIENT/FAMILY TEACHING:

IM administration may cause local pain. Continue drug for full length of treatment. Notify physician of *any* new symptom, visual difficulties or decreased hearing, tinnitus immediately. Do not take any other medication w/o consulting physician. Periodic lab and visual tests are important part of therapy. Keep out of reach of children (small amount can cause serious effects, death). Report blurred vision or any other change in vision.

chlorothiazide
(Diuril)
*See Classification section under:
Diuretics*

chlorotrianisene

klor-oh-trye-**an**-ih-seen
(TACE)

CLASSIFICATION

Antineoplastic, estrogen

AVAILABILITY (Rx)

Capsule: 12 mg, 25 mg

PHARMACOKINETICS

Well absorbed from GI tract. Widely distributed. Metabolized in liver. Primarily excreted in urine.

ACTION/THERAPEUTIC EFFECT

Increases synthesis of DNA, RNA, and various proteins in responsive tissues. *Reduces release of gonadotropin-releasing hormone, reducing follicle-stimulating hormone (FSH) and leuteinizing hormone (LH) levels; decreases serum concentration of testosterone.*

USES

Management of moderate to severe vasomotor symptoms associated w/menopause. Treatment of atrophic vaginitis, kraurosis vulvae, female hypogonadism. Palliative therapy for inoperable cancer of the prostate.

PO ADMINISTRATION

Give at the same time each day.

INDICATIONS/DOSAGE/ROUTES

Moderate to severe vasomotor symptoms associated w/menopause, atrophic vaginitis, kraurosis vulvae:
PO: Adults: 12–25 mg/day for 21 days; rest 7 days; repeat.

Female hypogonadism:
PO: Adults: 12–25 mg/day for 21 days (may follow immediately w/100 mg progesterone IM or oral progestin during last 5 days of therapy). Further therapy begun on fifth day of induced uterine bleeding.

Cancer of prostate:
PO: Adults, elderly: 12–25 mg/day.

PRECAUTIONS

CONTRAINDICATIONS: Known or suspected breast cancer, estrogen-dependent neoplasia; undiagnosed abnormal genital bleeding; active thrombophlebitis or thromboembolic disorders; history of thrombophlebitis, thrombosis, or thromboembolic disorders w/previous estrogen use, hypersensitivity to estrogen. **CAUTIONS:** Conditions that may be aggravated by fluid retention: cardiac, renal, or hepatic dysfunction, epilepsy, migraine. Metabolic bone disease w/potential hypercalcemia, mental depression, history of jaundice during pregnancy or strong family history of breast cancer, fibrocystic disease, or breast nodules, young pts in whom bone growth is not complete. **PREGNANCY/LACTATION:** Distributed in breast milk. May be harmful to fetus. Not for use during lactation. **Pregnancy Category X.**

INTERACTIONS

DRUG INTERACTIONS: May interfere w/effects of bromocriptine. May increase concentration of cyclosporine, increase hepatic nephrotoxicity. Hepatotoxic medications may increase hepatotoxicity. **ALTERED LAB VALUES:** May affect metapyrone, thyroid function tests. May decrease cholesterol,

LDL. May increase calcium, glucose, HDL, triglycerides.

SIDE EFFECTS

FREQUENT: Anorexia, nausea, swelling of breasts, edema. **OCCASIONAL:** Vomiting (esp. w/high dosages), intolerance to contact lenses, headache or migraine, increased B/P, changes in vaginal bleeding (spotting breakthrough or prolonged bleeding), glucose intolerance, brown spots on exposed skin, libido changes. **RARE:** Chorea, cholestatic jaundice, hirsutism, loss of scalp hair, depression.

ADVERSE REACTIONS/TOXIC EFFECTS

Prolonged administration increases risk of gallbladder, thromboembolic disease, and breast, cervical, vaginal, endometrial, and liver carcinoma.

NURSING IMPLICATIONS
BASELINE ASSESSMENT:

Question hypersensitivity to estrogen or tartrazine, previous jaundice or thromboembolic disorders associated w/pregnancy or estrogen therapy. Establish baseline B/P, blood glucose.

INTERVENTION/EVALUATION:

Assess B/P at least daily. Monitor blood glucose 4 times/day in diabetic pts. Check for edema, weigh daily. Promptly report signs and symptoms of thromboembolic or thrombotic disorders: sudden severe headache, shortness of breath, vision or speech disturbance, weakness or numbness of an extremity, loss of coordination, pain in chest, groin, or leg. Estrogen therapy should be noted on specimens.

PATIENT/FAMILY TEACHING:

Importance of medical supervision. Avoid smoking because of increased risk of heart attack or blood clots. Do not take other medications w/o physician approval. Teach how to perform Homan's test, signs and symptoms of blood clots (report these to physician immediately). Notify physician of vaginal discharge or bleeding. Teach female patients to perform self-breast exam. Avoid exposure to sun or ultraviolet light. Decreased libido, gynecomastia relieved when medication stopped. Check weight daily; report weekly gain of 5 lbs or more. Inform physician at once if pregnancy is suspected. Give labeling from drug package.

chlorpheniramine
(Teldrin, Chlor-Trimeton)
See Classification section under: Antihistamines

chlorpromazine
klor-**pro**-mah-zeen
(Thorazine)

chlorpromazine hydrochloride
(Thorazine)

CANADIAN AVAILABILITY:

Chlorpromanyl, Largactil

CLASSIFICATION

Antipsychotic

AVAILABILITY (Rx)

Tablets: 10 mg, 25 mg, 50 mg, 100 mg, 200 mg. **Capsules (sustained-release):** 30 mg, 75 mg, 150 mg, 200 mg, 300 mg. **Syrup:** 10 mg/5 ml. **Oral Concentrate:** 30 mg/ml, 100 mg/ml. **Injection:** 25 mg/ml. **Suppository:** 25 mg, 100 mg.

PHARMACOKINETICS

	ONSET	PEAK	DURATION
PO	30–60 min	—	4–6 hrs
Ext.-release			
	30–60 min	—	10–12 hrs
IM	Rapid	—	—
IV	Rapid	—	—
Rectal	>60 min	—	3–4 hrs

Variably absorbed after oral administration; well absorbed after IM administration. Metabolized in liver to some active metabolites. Excreted in urine, eliminated in feces. Half-life: 30 hrs.

ACTION/ *THERAPEUTIC EFFECT*

Blocks dopamine neurotransmission at postsynaptic dopamine receptor sites. Possesses strong anticholinergic, sedative, antiemetic effects, moderate extrapyramidal effects, slight antihistamine action. *Reduces psychosis, relieves nausea and vomiting, controls intractable hiccups, porphyria.*

USES/ *UNLABELED*

Management of psychotic disorders, manic phase of manic-depressive illness, severe nausea or vomiting, preop sedation, severe behavioral disturbances in children. Relief of intractable hiccups, acute intermittent porphyria. *Treatment of choreiform movement of Huntington's disease.*

STORAGE/HANDLING

Store at room temperature (including suppositories), protect from light (darkens on exposure). Yellow discoloration of solution does not affect potency, but discard if markedly discolored or if precipitate forms.

PO/IM/IV/RECTAL ADMINISTRATION

PO:

Dilute oral concentrate solution w/tomato, fruit juice, milk, orange syrup, carbonated beverages, coffee, tea, water. May also mix w/semisolid food.

IM:

Note: After parenteral administration, pt must remain recumbent for 30–60 min in head-low position w/legs raised to minimize hypotensive effect.

1. Inject slow, deep IM. If irritation occurs, further injections may be diluted w/0.9% NaCl or 2% procaine hydrochloride.

2. Massage IM injection site to reduce discomfort.

IV:

Note: Give by direct IV injection or IV infusion.

1. Direct IV used only during surgery to control nausea and vomiting.

2. For direct IV, dilute w/0.9% NaCl to concentration not exceeding 1 mg/ml.

3. Administer direct IV at rate not exceeding 1 mg/min for adults and 0.5 mg/min for children.

4. IV infusion used only for intractable hiccups.

5. For IV infusion, add chlorpromazine hydrochloride to 500–1,000 ml of 0.9% NaCl.

RECTAL:

1. If suppository is too soft, chill for 30 min in refrigerator or run cold water over foil wrapper.

2. Moisten suppository w/cold water before inserting well up into rectum.

INDICATIONS/DOSAGE/ROUTES

Outpatient: mild psychotic disorders, acute anxiety:
PO: Adults: 30–75 mg/day in 2–4 divided doses.
IM: Adults: 25 mg initially. May repeat in 1 hr.

Outpatient: moderate to severe psychotic disorders:
PO: Adults: 25 mg 3 times/day. Increase twice weekly by 20–25 mg until therapeutic response is achieved. Maintain dosage for 2 wks, then gradually reduce to maintenance level.

Hospitalized: acute psychotic disorders:
PO: Children: 0.55 mg/kg q4–6h.
IM: Adults: 25 mg. May give an additional 25–50 mg in 1 hr if needed. Gradually increase over several days to maximum 400 mg q4–6h.
Rectal: Adults: 50–100 mg 3–4 times/day. **Children:** 1.1 mg/kg q6–8h (severe cases).

Nausea, vomiting:
PO: Adults: 10–25 mg q4–6h.
Rectal: Adults: 50–100 mg q6–8h.
Children: 1.1 mg/kg q6–8h.

IM: Adults: 25 mg. Give additional 25–50 mg q3–4h if hypotension does not occur. **Children:** 0.55 mg/kg q6–8h.

Porphyria:
PO: Adults: 25–50 mg 3–4 times/day.
IM: Adults: 25 mg 3–4 times/day.

Intractable hiccups:
PO: Adults: 25–50 mg 3 times/day. If symptoms continue, administer by IM or slow IV infusion.

Preop:
PO: Adults: 25–50 mg 2–3 hrs before surgery. **Children:** 0.55 mg/kg.
IM: Adults: 12.5–25 mg 1–2 hrs before surgery. **Children:** 0.55 mg/kg.

Usual elderly dosage (nonpsychotic):
PO: Initially, 10–25 mg 1–2 times/day. May increase by 10–25 mg/day every 4–7 days. **Maximum:** 800 mg/day.

PRECAUTIONS

CONTRAINDICATIONS: Severe CNS depression, comatose states, severe cardiovascular disease, bone marrow depression, subcortical brain damage. **CAUTIONS:** Impaired respiratory/hepatic/renal/cardiac function, alcohol withdrawal, history of seizures, urinary retention, glaucoma, prostatic hypertrophy, hypocalcemia (increases susceptibility to dystonias). **PREGNANCY/LACTATION:** Crosses placenta; distributed in breast milk. **Pregnancy Category C.**

INTERACTIONS

DRUG INTERACTIONS: Alcohol, CNS depressants may increase CNS, respiratory depression, hypotensive effects. Tricyclic antidepressants, MAO inhibitors may increase sedative, anticholinergic effects. Antithyroid agents may increase risk of agranulocytosis. Increased risk of extrapyramidal symptoms (EPS) w/EPS-producing medications. Hypotensives may increase hypotension. May decrease levodopa effects. Lithium may decrease absorption, produce adverse neurologic effects. **ALTERED LAB VALUES:** May produce false-positive pregnancy test, phenylketonuria (PKU). EKG changes may occur, including Q and T wave disturbances.

SIDE EFFECTS

FREQUENT: Drowsiness, blurred vision, hypotension, defective color vision, difficulty in night vision, dizziness, decreased sweating, constipation, dry mouth, nasal congestion. **OCCASIONAL:** Difficulty urinating, increased skin sensivity to sun, skin rash, decreased sexual ability, swelling or pain in breasts, weight gain, nausea, vomiting, stomach pain, tremors.

ADVERSE REACTIONS/TOXIC EFFECTS

Extrapyramidal symptoms appear dose related (particularly high dosage), and divided into 3 categories: akathisia (inability to sit still, tapping of feet, urge to move around); parkinsonian symptoms (mask-like face, tremors, shuffling gait, hypersalivation); and acute dystonias: torticollis (neck muscle spasm), opisthotonos (rigidity of back muscles), and oculogyric crisis (rolling back of eyes). Dystonic reaction may also produce profuse sweating, pallor. Tardive dyskinesia (protrusion of tongue, puffing of cheeks, chewing/puckering of the mouth) occurs rarely (may be irreversible). Abrupt withdrawal after long-term therapy may precipitate nausea, vomiting, gastritis, dizziness, tremors. Blood dyscrasias, particularly agranulocytosis, mild leukopenia may occur. May lower seizure threshold.

NURSING IMPLICATIONS
BASELINE ASSESSMENT:

Avoid skin contact w/solution (contact dermatitis). *Antiemetic:* Assess for dehydration (poor skin turgor, dry mucous membranes, longitudinal furrows in tongue). *Antipsychotic:* Assess behavior, appearance, emotional status, response to environment, speech pattern, thought content.

INTERVENTION/EVALUATION:

Monitor B/P for hypotension. Assess for extrapyramidal symptoms. Monitor WBC, differential count for blood dyscrasias. Monitor for fine tongue movement (may be early sign of tardive dyskinesia). Supervise suicidal risk pt closely during early therapy (as depression lessens, energy level improves, increasing suicide potential). Assess for therapeutic response (interest in surroundings, improvement in self-care, increased ability to concentrate, relaxed facial expression).

PATIENT/FAMILY TEACHING:

Full therapeutic response may take up to 6 wks. Urine may darken. Do not abruptly withdraw from long-term drug therapy. Report visual disturbances. Sugarless gum or sips of tepid water may relieve dry mouth. Drowsiness generally subsides during continued therapy. Avoid tasks that require alertness, motor skills until response to drug is established. Avoid alcohol. Avoid exposure to sunlight. Report sore throat, fever, skin rash, impaired vision, involuntary muscle twitching/stiffness.

---

chlorpropamide
(Diabinese)
See Classification section under: Antidiabetic agents

---

chlorthalidone
klor-**thal**-ih-doan
(Hygroton, Thalitone)

FIXED-COMBINATION(S):
W/clonidine, an antihypertensive (**Combipres**); w/atenolol, an antihypertensive (**Tenoretic**); w/reserpine, an antihypertensive (**Demi-Regroton, Regroton**).

CANADIAN AVAILABILITY:
Apo-Chlorthalidone, Hygroton

CLASSIFICATION

Diuretic: Thiazide

AVAILABILITY (Rx)

Tablets: 15 mg, 25 mg, 50 mg, 100 mg

PHARMACOKINETICS

	ONSET	PEAK	DURATION
PO (diuretic)	2 hrs	2–6 hrs	Up to 36 hrs

Rapidly absorbed from GI tract. Excreted unchanged in urine.

Half-life: 35–50 hrs. Onset antihypertensive effect: 3–4 days; optimal therapeutic effect: 3–4 wks.

ACTION/ THERAPEUTIC EFFECT

Diuretic: Blocks reabsorption of sodium, potassium, chloride at distal convoluted tubule, *promoting renal excretion.* **Antihypertensive:** Reduces plasma, extracellular fluid volume, peripheral vascular resistance, *lowering B/P.*

USES

Adjunctive therapy in edema associated w/CHF, hepatic cirrhosis, corticoid or estrogen therapy, renal impairment. In treatment of hypertension, may be used alone or w/other antihypertensive agents.

PO ADMINISTRATION

Give w/food or milk if GI upset occurs, preferably w/breakfast (may prevent nocturia). Scored tablets may be crushed.

INDICATIONS/ DOSAGE/ ROUTES

Note: Fixed-combination medication should not be used for initial therapy but for maintenance therapy.

Edema:
PO: Adults: 50–100 mg 1 time/ day in morning or 100 mg every other day. May require 150–200 mg every day or every other day. Reduce dose to lowest maintenance level when dry weight is achieved (nonedematous state).

Hypertension:
PO: Adults: Initially, 25 mg/day. May increase to 50 mg/day. **Maintenance:** 25–50 mg/day.

Usual elderly dosage:
PO: Initially, 12.5–25 mg/day or every other day.

PRECAUTIONS

CONTRAINDICATIONS: History of hypersensitivity to sulfonamides or thiazide diuretics, renal decompensation, anuria. **CAUTIONS:** Severe renal disease, impaired hepatic function, diabetes mellitus, elderly/debilitated, gout, pts w/hypercholesterolemia. **PREGNANCY/LACTATION:** Crosses placenta; small amount distributed in breast milk—nursing not advised. **Pregnancy Category B**.

INTERACTIONS

DRUG INTERACTIONS: Cholestyramine, colestipol may decrease absorption, effects. May increase digoxin toxicity (due to hypokalemia). May increase lithium toxicity. **ALTERED LAB VALUES:** May increase bilirubin, serum calcium, LDL, cholesterol, triglycerides, creatinine, glucose, uric acid. May decrease urinary calcium, magnesium, potassium, sodium.

SIDE EFFECTS

EXPECTED: Increase in urine frequency/volume. **OCCASIONAL:** Anorexia, impotence, diarrhea, orthostatic hypotension, GI upset, photosensitivity. **RARE:** Rash.

ADVERSE REACTIONS/TOXIC EFFECTS

Vigorous diuresis may lead to profound water loss and electrolyte depletion, resulting in hypokalemia, hyponatremia, dehydration. Acute hypotensive episodes may occur. Hyperglycemia may be noted during prolonged therapy. Overdosage can lead to lethargy, coma w/o changes in electrolytes or hydration.

NURSING IMPLICATIONS

BASELINE ASSESSMENT:

Check vital signs, especially B/P for hypotension before administration. Assess baseline electrolytes, particularly check for low potassium. Assess edema, skin turgor, mucous membranes for hydration status. Evaluate muscle strength, mental status. Note skin temperature, moisture. Obtain baseline weight. Initiate I&O.

INTERVENTION/EVALUATION:

Continue to monitor B/P, vital signs, electrolytes, I&O, weight. Note extent of diuresis. Watch for electrolyte disturbances (hypokalemia may result in weakness, tremor, muscle cramps, nausea, vomiting, change in mental status, tachycardia; hyponatremia may result in confusion, thirst, cold/clammy skin). Periodically check blood sugar for hyperglycemia in prolonged therapy.

PATIENT/FAMILY TEACHING:

Expect increased frequency and volume of urination. To reduce hypotensive effect, rise slowly from lying to sitting position and permit legs to dangle momentarily before standing. Eat foods high in potassium such as whole grains (cereals), legumes, meat, bananas, apricots, orange juice, potatoes (white, sweet), raisins. May take w/food or milk. Avoid prolonged exposure to sunlight. Report muscle pain, weakness, cramps, nausea, vomiting, excessive thirst, tiredness, drowsiness, diarrhea, dizziness.

chlorzoxazone
(Paraflex, Parafon Forte DSC)
*See Classification section under:
Skeletal muscle relaxants*

cholestyramine resin

coal-es-**tie**-rah-mean
(Prevalite, Questran Lite)

CANADIAN AVAILABILITY:
Novo-Cholamine, Questran

CLASSIFICATION
Antihyperlipoproteinemic

AVAILABILITY (Rx)
Powder: 4 g

PHARMACOKINETICS
Not absorbed from GI tract. Decreases in LDL apparent in 5–7 days, serum cholesterol in 1 mo. Serum cholesterol returns to baseline levels about 1 mo after discontinuing drug.

ACTION/*THERAPEUTIC EFFECT*
Binds w/bile acids in intestine forming insoluble complex. Binding results in partial removal of bile acid from enterohepatic circulation, *removing low density lipoproteins (LDL) and cholesterol from plasma.*

USES/*UNLABELED*
Adjunct to dietary therapy to decrease elevated serum cholesterol levels in those w/primary hypercholesterolemia. Relief of pruritus associated w/partial biliary obstruction. *Treatment of diarrhea (due to bile acids); hyperoxaluria.*

PO ADMINISTRATION
1. Give other drugs at least 1 hr before or 4–6 hrs after cholestyramine (capable of binding drugs in GI tract).
2. Do not give in dry form (highly irritating). Mix w/3–6 oz water, milk, fruit juice, soup. Place powder on surface for 1–2 min (prevents lumping), then mix thoroughly. Excessive foaming w/carbonated beverages; use extra large glass and stir slowly.
3. Administer before meals.

INDICATIONS/DOSAGE/ROUTES
Primary hypercholesterolemia:
PO: Adults, elderly: Initially: 4 g 1–2 times/day before meals. **Maintenance:** 4 g 1–6 times/day before meals and at bedtime.

PRECAUTIONS
CONTRAINDICATIONS: Hypersensitivity to cholestyramine or tartrazine (frequently seen in aspirin hypersensitivity), complete biliary obstruction. **CAUTIONS:** GI dysfunction (especially constipation), hemorrhoids, bleeding disorders, osteoporosis. **PREGNANCY/LACTATION:** Not systemically absorbed. May interfere w/maternal absorption of fat-soluble vitamins. **Pregnancy Category B**.

INTERACTIONS
DRUG INTERACTIONS: May increase effects of anticoagulants by decreasing vitamin K. May decrease warfarin absorption. May bind, decrease absorption of digoxin, thiazides, penicillins, propranolol, tetracyclines, troglitazone, folic acid, thyroid hormones, other medications. Binds, decreases effect of oral vancomycin. **ALTERED LAB VALUES:** May

increase SGOT (AST), SGPT (ALT), alkaline phosphatase, magnesium. May decrease calcium, potassium, sodium. May prolong prothrombin time.

SIDE EFFECTS

FREQUENT: Constipation (may lead to fecal impaction), nausea, vomiting, stomach pain, indigestion. **OCCASIONAL:** Diarrhea, belching, bloating, headache, dizziness. **RARE:** Gallstones, peptic ulcer, malabsorption syndrome.

ADVERSE REACTIONS/TOXIC EFFECT

GI tract obstruction, hyperchloremic acidosis, osteoporosis secondary to calcium excretion. High dosage may interfere w/ fat absorption, resulting in steatorrhea.

NURSING IMPLICATIONS
BASELINE ASSESSMENT:

Question for history of hypersensitivity to cholestyramine, tartrazine, aspirin. Obtain specimens for baseline levels: serum cholesterol, serum triglyceride, electrolytes.

INTERVENTION/EVALUATION:

Determine pattern of bowel activity. Evaluate food tolerance, abdominal discomfort, and flatulence. Monitor lab results for electrolytes, serum cholesterol, and periodically serum triglyceride (may increase w/prolonged therapy). Assess skin and mucous membranes for rash/irritation. Encourage several glasses of water between meals.

PATIENT/FAMILY TEACHING:

Complete full course; do not omit or change doses. Take other drugs at least 1 hr before or 4–6 hrs after cholestyramine. Check w/physician before taking any other medication. Never take in dry form; mix w/3–6 oz water, milk, fruit juice, soup (place powder on surface for 1–2 min to prevent lumping, then mix well). Use extra large glass and stir slowly when mixing w/carbonated beverages due to foaming. Take before meals and drink several glasses of water between meals. Reduce fats, sugars, and cholesterol per diet determined by physician. Eat high-fiber foods (whole grain cereals, fruits, vegetables) to reduce potential for constipation. Notify physician immediately of bleeding, constipation, or development of new symptom.

chorionic gonadotropin, HCG

kore-ee-**on**-ik goe-**nad**-oh-troe-pin (Novarel, Pregnyl, APL, Profasai HP)

CANADIAN AVAILABILITY:
APL, Profasi HP

CLASSIFICATION

Gonadotropin

AVAILABILITY (Rx)

Powder for Injection: 5,000 unit, 10,000 unit, 20,000 unit vials

ACTION / THERAPEUTIC EFFECT

Stimulates production of gonadal steroid hormones by stimulating interstitial cells (Leydig cells) of the testes to produce androgen, and the corpus luteum of the ovary to produce progesterone. Androgen stimulation in the male *causes production of secondary sex characteristics and may stimulate descent of testes when no anatomic impediment exists.* In women of childbearing age w/normally functioning ovaries, *causes maturation of corpus luteum and triggers ovulation.*

USES / UNLABELED

Treatment of prepubertal cryptorchidism w/o obstruction, selected cases of hypogonadotropic hypogonadism. To induce ovulation and pregnancy in women w/secondary anovulation (after pretreatment w/menotropin). *Diagnosis of male hypogonadism, treatment of corpus luteum dysfunction.*

IM ADMINISTRATION

1. For IM use only.
2. Follow manufacturer's directions for reconstitution.
3. Use completely or refrigerate after reconstitution.

INDICATIONS / DOSAGE / ROUTES

Prepubertal cryptorchidism, hypogonadotropic hypogonadism:
IM: Adults: Dosage is individualized based on indication, age and weight of pt, and physician preference.

Induction of ovulation and pregnancy:
IM: Adults: (After pretreatment w/menotropins), 5,000–10,000 IU 1 day after last dose of menotropins.

PRECAUTIONS

CONTRAINDICATIONS: Prior allergic reaction to chorionic gonadotropin, precocious puberty, carcinoma of the prostate or other androgen-dependent neoplasia. Not for adjunctive therapy in obesity. **CAUTIONS:** Prepubertal males, conditions aggravated by fluid retention (cardiac or renal disease, epilepsy, migraine, asthma). **PREGNANCY/LACTATION:** Caution: excretion in breast milk unknown. **Pregnancy Category X.**

INTERACTIONS

DRUG INTERACTIONS: None significant. **ALTERED LAB VALUES:** None significant.

SIDE EFFECTS

FREQUENT: Pain at injection site. *Induction ovulation:* Ovarian cysts, uncomplicated ovarian enlargement. **OCCASIONAL:** Enlarged breasts, headache, irritability, fatigue, depression. *Induction ovulation:* Severe ovarian hyperstimulation, peripheral edema. *Cryptorchidism:* Precocious puberty (acne, deepening voice, penile growth, pubic/axillary hair).

ADVERSE REACTIONS / TOXIC EFFECTS

When used w/menotropins: increased risk of arterial thromboembolism, ovarian hyperstimulation w/high incidence (20%) of multiple births (premature deliveries and neonatal prematurity), ruptured ovarian cysts.

NURSING IMPLICATIONS
BASELINE ASSESSMENT:

Question for prior allergic reaction to drug. Obtain baseline weight, B/P.

INTERVENTION/EVALUATION:

Assess for edema: weigh every 2–3 days, report >5 lbs gain/wk; monitor B/P periodically during treatment; check for decreased urinary output, swelling of ankles, fingers.

PATIENT/FAMILY TEACHING:

Report promptly abdominal pain, vaginal bleeding, signs of precocious puberty in males (deepening of voice; axillary, facial, and pubic hair; acne, penile growth) or signs of edema. In anovulation treatment, proper method of taking/recording daily basal temperature; advise intercourse daily beginning the day preceding HCG treatment. Possibility of multiple births.

---

ciclopirox
(Loprox, Penlac)
See Classification section under: Antifungals: Topical

---

cidofovir
sid-dough-**foe**-vir
(Vistide)

CLASSIFICATION

Antiviral

AVAILABILITY (Rx)

Injection: 75 mg/ml (5 ml amp)

PHARMACOKINETICS

Excreted primarily unchanged in urine. Elimination half-life: 1.4–3.8 hrs.

ACTION/*THERAPEUTIC EFFECT*

Suppresses cytomegalovirus (CMV) replication *by inhibition of viral DNA synthesis*. Incorporation of cidofovir in growing viral DNA chain *results in reduction in rate of viral DNA synthesis*.

USES

Treatment of cytomegalovirus (CMV) retinitis in those w/ acquired immunodeficiency syndrome (AIDS).

STORAGE/HANDLING

Store at controlled room temperature (68°–77°F). Admixtures may be refrigerated for no more than 24 hrs. Allow refrigerated admixtures to warm to room temperature before use.

IV ADMINISTRATION

Note: Do not exceed the recommended dosage, frequency or infusion rate.

1. Dilute in 100 ml 0.9% saline solution prior to administration.

2. Infuse over 1 hr.

3. IV hydration with normal saline and probenecid therapy *must* be used w/each cidofovir infusion (minimizes risk of nephrotoxicity).

4. Ingestion of food before each dose of probenecid may reduce nausea and vomiting. An antiemetic may also reduce potential for nausea.

INDICATIONS/DOSAGE/ROUTES

Probenecid:
PO: Adults: Give 2 g 3 hrs prior to cidofovir dose, and 1 g given at 2 and again at 8 hrs after completion of the 1-hr cidofovir infusion (total of 4 g).

Hydration:
IV: Adults: 1 liter 0.9% NaCl given over 1–2 hrs immediately before cidofovir infusion. If tolerated, a 2nd liter may be given at start or immediately after cidofovir infusion and infused over 1–3 hrs.

Usual dosage:
IV Infusion: Adults: (Induction): 5 mg/kg at constant rate over 1 hr once weekly for 2 consecutive wks. **Maintenance:** 5 mg/kg at constant rate over 1 hr once every 2 wks.

Renal function impairment:
Dose based on creatinine clearance.

CREATININE CLEARANCE	INDUCTION DOSE	MAINTENANCE DOSE
(ml/min)		
41–55	2 mg/kg	2 mg/kg
30–40	1.5 mg/kg	1.5 mg/kg
20–29	1 mg/kg	1 mg/kg
≤19	0.5 mg/kg	0.5 mg/kg

PRECAUTIONS

CONTRAINDICATIONS: Hypersensitivity to cidofovir; history of clinically severe hypersensitivity to probenecid or other sulfa-containing medication; direct intraocular injection; renal function impairment (serum creatinine >1.5 mg/dl or creatinine clearance ≤55 ml/min or urine protein >100 mg/dl). **CAUTIONS:** Preexisting diabetes. **PREGNANCY/LACTATION:** Embryotoxic (reduced fetal body weight) in animals. Unknown if excreted in breast milk. Do not administer to nursing women. HIV-infected women not to breast feed. **Pregnancy Category C**.

INTERACTIONS

DRUG INTERACTIONS: Avoid concurrent administration of cidofovir and medication w/ nephrotoxic risk (amphotericin B, aminoglycosides, foscarnet, IV pentamidine). **ALTERED LAB VALUES:** May decrease neutrophil count, serum phosphate, uric acid, and bicarbonate; elevate serum creatinine.

SIDE EFFECTS

FREQUENT: Nausea, vomiting (65%), fever (57%), asthenia (46%), rash (30%), diarrhea (27%), headache (27%), alopecia (25%), chills (24%), anorexia (22%), dyspnea (22%), abdominal pain (17%).

ADVERSE REACTIONS/TOXIC EFFECTS

Proteinuria (80%), nephrotoxicity (53%), neutropenia (31%), serum creatinine elevations (29%), infection (24%), anemia (20%), ocular hypotony (12%) (decrease in intraocular pressure), pneumonia (9%). Probenecid may produce hypersensitivity reaction (rash, fever, chills, anaphylaxis). Acute renal failure.

NURSING IMPLICATIONS
BASELINE ASSESSMENT:

Establish baseline electrolytes. For those taking zidovudine, temporarily discontinue zidovudine administration or decrease zidovudine dose by 50% on days of infusion (probenecid reduces metabolic clearance of zidovudine). Emphasize need for close monitoring of renal function (urinalysis, serum creatinine) during therapy.

INTERVENTION/EVALUATION:

Monitor serum creatinine, urine protein, and WBC counts w/differential prior to each dose. In those w/proteinuria, give IV hydration and repeat test. Periodically monitor intraocular pressure (IOP), visual acuity, and ocular symptoms. Monitor for proteinuria (may be early indicator of dose-dependent nephrotoxicity).

PATIENT/FAMILY TEACHING:

Obtain regular follow-up ophthalmologic exams. Advise that cidofovir is not cure for CMV retinitis, and condition may progress in spite of treatment. Those of childbearing age should use effective contraception during and for 1 mo following treatment. Men should practice barrier contraceptive methods during and for 3 mos following treatment. Do not take any medications w/o physician approval. Must complete full course of probenecid with each cidofovir dose.

cilostazol
(Pletal)
See Supplement

cimetidine
sih-**met**-ih-deen
(Tagamet, Tagamet HB)

CANADIAN AVAILABILITY:
Apo-Cimetidine, Novocimetine, Peptol, Tagamet

CLASSIFICATION
H_2 receptor antagonist

AVAILABILITY (Rx)
Tablets: 100 mg **(OTC)**, 200 mg, 300 mg, 400 mg, 800 mg. **Oral Liquid:** 300 mg/5 ml. **Injection:** 300 mg/2 ml. **Suspension:** 200 mg/5 ml.

PHARMACOKINETICS
Well absorbed from GI tract. Widely distributed. Metabolized in liver. Primarily excreted in urine. Half-life: 2 hrs (increased in decreased renal function).

ACTION/*THERAPEUTIC EFFECT*
Inhibits histamine action at H_2 receptor sites of parietal cells, *inhibiting gastric acid secretion.*

USES/*UNLABELED*
Short-term treatment of active duodenal ulcer. Prevention of duodenal ulcer recurrence, upper GI bleeding in critically ill pts. Treatment of active benign gastric ulcer, pathologic GI hypersecretory conditions, gastroesophageal reflux disease (GERD). *Treatment of upper GI bleeding, prophylaxis of aspiration pneumonia, acute urticaria, chronic warts.*

STORAGE/HANDLING
Store tablets, liquid, parenteral form at room temperature. Reconstituted IV is stable for 48 hrs at room temperature.

PO/IM/IV ADMINISTRATION

PO:

1. Give w/o regard to meals. Best given with meals and at bedtime.

2. Do not administer within 1 hr of antacids.

IM:

1. Administer undiluted.

2. Inject deep into large muscle mass.

IV:

1. For direct IV injection, administer over not less than 2 mins (prevents arrhythmias, hypotension).

2. For intermittent IV (piggyback) administration, infuse over 15–20 mins.

3. For IV infusion, dilute w/100 to 1,000 ml 0.9% NaCl or 5% dextrose. Infuse over 24 hrs.

INDICATIONS/DOSAGE/ROUTES

Active duodenal ulcer:
PO: Adults, elderly: 300 mg 4 times/day, or 400 mg 2 times/day (morning and at bedtime), or 800 mg at bedtime.

Prophylaxis of recurrent duodenal ulcer:
PO: Adults, elderly: 400 mg at bedtime.

Benign active gastric ulcer:
PO: Adults, elderly: 300 mg 4 times/day or 800 mg at bedtime.

Pathologic gastric hypersecretory conditions:
PO: Adults, elderly: 300 mg 4 times/day up to 2,400 mg/day.

Gastroesophageal reflux disease:
PO: Adults, elderly: 1,600 mg/day in divided doses (800 mg 2 times/day or 400 mg 4 times/day) for 12 wks.

Usual parenteral dosage:
IM/IV: Adults, elderly: 300 mg q6–8h. Maximum: 2,400 mg/day.
IV Infusion: Adults, elderly: 900 mg/day.

Prevent upper GI bleeding:
IV Infusion: Adults, elderly: 1,200 mg/day (50 mg/hr).

Dosage in renal impairment:
PO/IM/IV: Adults, elderly: 300 mg q8–12h.

PRECAUTIONS

CONTRAINDICATIONS: None significant. **CAUTIONS:** Impaired renal/hepatic function, elderly. **PREGNANCY/LACTATION:** Crosses placenta; distributed in breast milk. In infants, may suppress gastric acidity, inhibit drug metabolism, produce CNS stimulation. **Pregnancy Category B**.

INTERACTIONS

DRUG INTERACTIONS: Antacids may decrease absorption (do not give within $1/2$–1 hr). May decrease absorption of ketoconazole (give at least 2 hrs after). May decrease metabolism, increase concentration of oral anticoagulants, tricyclic antidepressants, oral hypoglycemics, metoprolol, metronidazole, phenytoin, propranolol, theophylline, calcium channel blockers, cyclosporine, lidocaine. **ALTERED LAB VALUES:** Interferes w/skin tests using allergen extracts. May increase creatinine, prolactin, transaminase. May decrease parathyroid hormone concentration.

SIDE EFFECTS

OCCASIONAL (2–4%): Headache. *Elderly, severely ill, impaired renal function:* Confusion, agitation, psychosis, depression, anxiety, disorientation, hallucinations (effects reverse 3–4 days after discontinuance). **RARE (<2%):** Diarrhea, dizziness, drowsiness, headache, nausea, vomiting, gynecomastia, rash, impotence.

ADVERSE REACTIONS/TOXIC EFFECTS

Rapid IV may produce cardiac arrhythmias, hypotension.

NURSING IMPLICATIONS
BASELINE ASSESSMENT:

Do not administer antacids concurrently (separate by 1 hr).

INTERVENTION/EVALUATION:

Monitor B/P for hypotension during IV infusion. Assess for GI bleeding: Hematemesis, blood in stool. Check mental status in elderly, severely ill, those w/impaired renal function.

PATIENT/FAMILY TEACHING:

IM may produce transient discomfort at injection site. Do not take antacids within 1 hr of cimetidine administration. Avoid tasks that require alertness, motor skills until drug response is established. Avoid smoking. Report any blood in vomitus or stool, or dark, tarry stool.

ciprofloxacin hydrochloride

sip-row-**flocks**-ah-sin
(Ciloxan, Cipro)

FIXED COMBINATIONS:
W/hydrocortisone, a glucocorticoid **(Cipro HC Otic).**

CANADIAN AVAILABILITY:
Ciloxan, Cipro

CLASSIFICATION

Anti-infective: Quinolone

AVAILABILITY (Rx)

Tablets: 100 mg, 250 mg, 500 mg, 750 mg. **Oral Suspension. Injection:** 200 mg, 400 mg. **Ophthalmic Solution:** 3.5 mg/ml. **Ophthalmic Ointment:** 0.03%.

PHARMACOKINETICS

Well absorbed from GI tract (delayed by food). Widely distributed (including CSF). Metabolized in liver to active metabolite. Primarily excreted in urine. Minimal removal by hemodialysis. Half-life: 4–6 hrs (increased in decreased renal function, elderly).

ACTION/*THERAPEUTIC EFFECT*

Inhibits DNA enzyme in susceptible microorganisms, *interfering w/bacterial DNA replication.* Bactericidal.

USES/*UNLABELED*

Treatment of infections of urinary tract, chronic bacterial prostatitis skin/skin structure, GI tract, bone/joint, lower respiratory tract, infectious diarrhea, uncomplicated gonorrhea, empiric treatment of febrile neutropenia, acute sinusitis. *Ophthalmic:* Conjunctival keratitis, keratoconjunctivitis, corneal ulcers, blepharitis, dacryocystitis, blepharoconjunctivitis, acute meibomianitis. *Treatment of chancroid.*

C

PO/IV/OPHTHALMIC ADMINISTRATION

PO:

1. May be given w/o regard to meals (preferred dosing time: 2 hrs after meals).
2. Do not administer antacids (aluminum, magnesium) within 2 hrs of ciprofloxacin.
3. Encourage cranberry juice, citrus fruits (to acidify urine).
4. Suspension may be stored for 14 days at room temperature..

IV:

1. Use large vein to reduce venous irritation.
2. Infuse over 60 min.

OPHTHALMIC:

1. Tilt pt's head back; place solution in conjunctival sac.
2. Have pt close eyes; press gently on lacrimal sac for 1 min.
3. Do not use ophthalmic solutions for injection.
4. Unless infection very superficial, systemic administration generally accompanies ophthalmic.

INDICATIONS/DOSAGE/ROUTES

Mild to moderate urinary tract infections:
PO: Adults, elderly: 250 mg q12h.
IV: Adults, elderly: 200 mg q12h.

Complicated urinary tract, mild to moderate respiratory tract infections, skin/skin structure, bones and joint, infectious diarrhea:
PO: Adults, elderly: 500 mg q12h.
IV: Adults, elderly: 400 mg q12h.

Severe, complicated infections:
PO: Adults, elderly: 750 mg q12h.
IV: Adults, elderly: 400 mg q12h.

Prostatitis:
PO: Adults, elderly: 500 mg q12h × 28 days.

Uncomplicated bladder infection:
PO: Adults: 100 mg 2 times/day for 3 days.

Acute sinusitis:
PO: Adults: 500 mg q12 h.

Uncomplicated gonorrhea:
PO: Adults: 250 mg as single dose.

Dosage in renal impairment:
The dose and/or frequency is modified in pts based on severity of infection and degree of renal impairment.

CREATININE CLEARANCE	DOSAGE
>50 ml/min (PO); >30 ml/min (IV)	No change
30–50 ml/min	250–500 mg q12h
5–29 ml/min	250–500 mg PO q18h; 200–400 mg IV q18–24h
Hemodialysis, peritoneal dialysis	250–500 mg q24h (after dialysis)

Usual ophthalmic dosage:
Adults, elderly: Solution: 1–2 drops 4–6 times/day. **Ointment:** ½ inch ribbon 3 times/day for 2 days then 2 times/day for 5 days.

PRECAUTIONS

CONTRAINDICATIONS: Hypersensitivity to ciprofloxacin, quinolones, any component of the preparation. *Ophthalmic:* Vaccinia, varicella, epithelial herpes simplex, keratitis, mycobacterial infection, fungal disease of ocular structure. Not for use after uncomplicated removal of foreign body. **CAUTIONS:** Renal impairment, CNS disorders, seizures, those taking theophylline or caffeine. Suspension not for use in an NG tube. **PREGNANCY/LACTATION:** Unknown if distributed in breast milk. If possible, do not use during pregnancy/lactation (risk of arthropathy to fetus/infant). **Pregnancy Category C.**

INTERACTIONS

DRUG INTERACTIONS: Antacids, iron preparations, sucralfate may decrease absorption. Decreases clearance, may increase concentration, toxicity of theophylline. May increase effects of oral anticoagulants. **ALTERED LAB VALUES:** May increase SGOT (AST), SGPT (ALT), alkaline phosphatase, LDH, bilirubin, BUN, creatinine.

SIDE EFFECTS

FREQUENT (2–5%): Nausea, diarrhea, dyspepsia, vomiting, constipation, flatulence, confusion, crystalluria. *Ophthalmic:* Burning, crusting in corner of eye. **OCCASIONAL (<2%):** Abdominal pain/discomfort, headache, rash. *Ophthalmic:* Bad taste, sense of something in eye, redness of eyelids, eyelid itching. **RARE (<1%):** Dizziness, confusion, tremors, hallucinations, hypersensitivity reaction, insomnia, dry mouth, paresthesia.

ADVERSE REACTIONS/TOXIC EFFECTS

Superinfection (esp. enterococcal, fungal), nephropathy, cardiopulmonary arrest, cerebral thrombosis may occur. Arthropathy may occur if given to children <18 yrs. *Ophthalmic:* Sensitization may contraindicate later systemic use of ciprofloxacin.

NURSING IMPLICATIONS
BASELINE ASSESSMENT:

Question for history of hypersensitivity to ciprofloxacin, quinolones, any component of preparation. Obtain specimen for diagnostic tests before giving first dose (therapy may begin before results are known).

INTERVENTION/EVALUATION:

Evaluate food tolerance. Determine pattern of bowel activity; be alert to blood in feces. Check for dizziness, headache, visual difficulties, tremors. Monitor B/P at least twice daily. Assess for chest, joint pain. *Ophthalmic:* Check for therapeutic response, side effects (see Adverse Reactions/Toxic Effects).

PATIENT/FAMILY TEACHING:

Do not skip dose; take full course of therapy. Take w/8 oz water; drink several glasses of water between meals. Eat/drink high sources of ascorbic acid to prevent crystalluria (cranberry juice, citrus fruits). Do not take antacids (reduces/destroys effectiveness). Shake suspension well before using; do not chew microcapsules in suspension. Avoid tasks that require alertness, motor skills until response to drug is established. Avoid sunlight/ultraviolet exposure; wear sunscreen, protective clothing if photosensitivity develops. Sugarless gum or hard candy may relieve bad taste. Report inflammation or tendon pain. Notify nurse/physician if new symptoms occur. *Ophthalmic:* Explain possibility of crystal precipitate forming, and usual resolution. Report any increased burning, itching, or other discomfort promptly. Shake well before using suspension; do not chew microcapsules in suspension.

cisatracurium
(Nimbex)
*See Classification section under:
Neuromuscular blockers*

cisplatin

sis-**plah**-tin
(Platinol-AQ)

CANADIAN AVAILABILITY:
Platinol

CLASSIFICATION

Antineoplastic

AVAILABILITY (Rx)

Injection: 10 mg, 50 mg, 100 mg vials

PHARMACOKINETICS

Widely distributed. Undergoes rapid nonenzymatic conversion to inactive metabolite. Excreted in urine. Half-life: 58–73 hrs (increased in decreased renal function).

ACTION/*THERAPEUTIC EFFECT*

Inhibits DNA, and to lesser extent, RNA, protein synthesis by cross-linking w/DNA strands, *preventing cellular division.* Cell cycle-phase nonspecific.

USES/*UNLABELED*

Palliative treatment of metastatic testicular tumors, metastatic ovarian tumors, advanced bladder carcinoma. *Treatment of carcinoma of breast, cervical, endometrial, gastric, lung, prostate, head/neck, neuroblastoma, germ cell tumors, osteosarcoma.*

STORAGE/HANDLING

Note: May be carcinogenic, mutagenic, or teratogenic. Handle w/extreme care during preparation/administration.

Following reconstitution, solutions should be clear and colorless. Protect from direct bright sunlight; do not refrigerate (may precipitate). Discard if precipitate forms. Stable for 20 hrs at room temperature.

IV ADMINISTRATION

Note: Wear protective gloves during handling of cisplatin. Do not use aluminum needles or administration sets that may come in contact w/drug; may cause formation of black precipitate, loss of potency.

1. Reconstitute 10 mg vial w/10 ml sterile water for injection (50 ml for 50 mg vial) to provide concentration of 1 mg/ml.

2. For IV infusion, dilute desired dose in up to 1,000 ml 5% dextrose, 0.33 or 0.45% NaCl containing 18.75 g mannitol/L. Infuse over 2–24 hrs.

3. Avoid rapid IV injection over 1–5 min (increases risk of nephrotoxicity, ototoxicity).

4. Monitor for anaphylactic reaction during first few minutes of IV infusion.

INDICATIONS/DOSAGE/ROUTES

Note: Dosage individualized based on clinical response, tolerance to adverse effects. When used in combination therapy, consult specific protocols for optimum dosage, sequence of drug administration. Repeat courses should not be given more frequently than q 3–4 wks. Do not repeat unless auditory acuity within normal limits, serum creatinine below 1.5 mg/dl, BUN below 25 mg/dl, circulating blood elements (platelets, WBC) are within acceptable levels.

Metastatic testicular tumors:
IV: Adults: (Combined w/bleomycin, vinblastine): 20 mg/m^2/day for 5 days q 3 wks for 3–4 courses of therapy.

C

Metastatic ovarian tumors:
IV: Adults: (Combined w/doxorubicin): 50 mg/m^2 once q 3–4 wks. *Single:* 100 mg/m^2 once q 4 wks.

Advanced bladder cancer:
IV: Adults: Single: 50–70 mg/m^2 q 3–4 wks.

PRECAUTIONS

CONTRAINDICATIONS: Myelosuppression, hearing impairment. **CAUTIONS:** Previous therapy w/other antineoplastic agents, radiation. **PREGNANCY/LACTATION:** If possible, avoid use during pregnancy, esp. first trimester. Breast feeding not recommended. **Pregnancy Category D.**

INTERACTIONS

DRUG INTERACTIONS: May decrease effect of antigout medications. Bone marrow depressants may increase bone marrow depression. Nephrotoxic, ototoxic agents may increase toxicity. Live virus vaccines may potentiate virus replication, increase vaccine side effects, decrease pt's antibody response to vaccine. **ALTERED LAB VALUES:** May cause positive Coombs' test. May increase BUN, creatinine, uric acid, SGOT (AST). May decrease creatinine clearance, calcium, magnesium, phosphate, potassium, sodium.

SIDE EFFECTS

FREQUENT: Nausea, vomiting (begins 1–4 hrs after administration, generally last up to 24 hrs). Myelosuppression occurs in 25–30% of pts. Recovery can generally be expected in 18–23 days. **OCCASIONAL:** Peripheral neuropathy (numbness, tingling of fingers, toes, face) may occur w/prolonged therapy (4–7 mos), pain/redness at injection site, loss of taste/appetite. **RARE:** Hemolytic anemia, blurred vision, stomatitis.

ADVERSE REACTIONS/TOXIC EFFECTS

Anaphylactic reaction (facial edema, wheezing, tachycardia, hypotension) may occur in first few minutes of IV administration in those previously exposed to cisplatin. Nephrotoxicity in 28–36% of pts treated w/single dose of cisplatin, usually during 2nd week of therapy. Ototoxicity (tinnitus, hearing loss) in 31% of pts treated w/single dose of cisplatin (more severe in children). May become more frequent, severe with repeated doses.

NURSING IMPLICATIONS

BASELINE ASSESSMENT:

Pts should be well hydrated prior to and 24 hrs after medication to ensure good urinary output, decrease risk of nephrotoxicity. Give emotional support to pt and family.

INTERVENTION/EVALUATION:

Measure all vomitus (general guideline requiring immediate notification of physician: 750 ml/8 hrs, urinary output less than 100 ml/hr). Monitor I&O q1–2h beginning w/pretreatment hydration, continue for 48 hrs after cisplatin therapy. Assess vital signs q1–2h during infusion. Monitor urinalysis, renal function reports for nephrotoxicity.

PATIENT/FAMILY TEACHING:

Report signs of ototoxicity (ringing/roaring in ears, hearing loss). Do not have immunizations w/o physician's approval (drug lowers body's resistance). Avoid contact w/those who have recently taken oral polio vaccine. Contact physician if nausea/vomiting continues at home. Teach signs of peripheral neuropathy.

---

citalopram
(Celexa)
See Supplement'
See Classification section under: Antidepressants

---

citrates
potassium citrate
(Urocit K)

potassium citrate and citric acid
(Polycitra-K)

sodium citrate and citric acid
(Bicitra)

tricitrates
(Polycitra syrup)

CANADIAN AVAILABILITY:
Polycitra-K

CLASSIFICATION

Antiurolithic, alkalizer

AVAILABILITY (Rx)

Tablets: 5 mEq, 10 mEq. **Syrup.** Oral Solution.

PHARMACOKINETICS

Oxidized to form potassium or sodium bicarbonate. Primarily excreted in urine.

ACTION/*THERAPEUTIC EFFECT*

Increases urinary pH, increasing solubility of cystine in urine and ionization of uric acid to urate ion. Increasing urinary pH and urinary citrate decreases calcium ion activity and decreases saturation of calcium oxalate. Increases plasma bicarbonate, buffers excess hydrogen ion concentration, *increasing blood pH and reversing acidosis.*

USES

Treats/prevents uric acid/cystine lithiasis, prevents urate crystallization (increased urinary pH). Treats/prevents calcium phosphate, calcium oxalate or uric acid kidney stones (increase urinary citrate). Treats chronic metabolic acidosis. Neutralizes/buffers excess quantities of gastric hydrochloric acid.

PO ADMINISTRATION

1. Take after meals.
2. *Tablets:* Swallow whole; do not crush, chew; take w/full glass of water or juice.
3. *Liquid:* Dilute w/6 oz water or juice; chilling may increase palatability.

INDICATIONS/DOSAGE/ROUTES

POTASSIUM CITRATE

Antiurolithic, urinary alkalizer:
PO: **Adults, elderly:** 10 mEq 3 times/day up to 15 mEq 4 times/day or 20 mEq 3 times/day.

POTASSIUM CITRATE AND CITRIC ACID

Antiurolithic, urinary/systemic alkalizer:
PO: **Adults, elderly:** 20–30 mEq 4 times/day. **Children:** 10–30 mEq 4 times/day.

SODIUM CITRATE AND CITRIC ACID

Antiurolithic, urinary/systemic alkalizer:
PO: **Adults, elderly:** 10–30 mEq 4 times/day. **Maximum:** 150 mEq/day. **Children:** 5–15 mEq 4 times/day.

TRICITRATES

Antiurolithic, urinary alkalizer:
PO: Adults, elderly: 15–30 mEq 4 times/day. **Children:** 5–10 mEq 4 times/day.

PRECAUTIONS

CONTRAINDICATIONS: Aluminum toxicity, severe myocardial damage, heart failure, severe renal impairment, active urinary tract infection, hyperkalemia, peptic ulcer. **CAUTIONS:** Severe renal tubular acidosis. **PREGNANCY/LACTATION:** Unknown whether distributed in breast milk. **Pregnancy Category C.**

INTERACTIONS

DRUG INTERACTIONS: May increase quinidine excretion. Antacids may increase risk of systemic alkalosis. NSAIDs, angiotensin-converting enzyme inhibitors, potassium-sparing diuretics, potassium-containing medication may increase risk of hyperkalemia. May decrease effect of methenamine. ALTERED LAB VALUES: None significant.

SIDE EFFECTS

OCCASIONAL: Diarrhea, loose bowel movements, mild abdominal pain, nausea, vomiting. **RARE:** Metabolic alkalosis, bowel obstruction/perforation, hyperkalemia, hypernatremia.

ADVERSE REACTIONS/TOXIC EFFECTS

None significant.

NURSING IMPLICATIONS
BASELINE ASSESSMENT:

Assess urinary pH determination, EKG in pts w/cardiac disease, serum acid-base balance, CBC, hemoglobin, hematocrit, serum creatinine.

INTERVENTION/EVALUATION:

Monitor urinary pH, EKG in pts w/cardiac disease, serum acid-base balance, CBC, hemoglobin, hematocrit, serum creatinine.

PATIENT/FAMILY TEACHING:

Take after meals. Mix in water or juice and follow w/additional liquid if desired. Notify physician if diarrhea, nausea/vomiting, abdominal pain, or seizures occur. Check w/physician if black, tarry stools or other signs of GI bleeding are observed.

cladribine
clad-rih-bean
(Leustatin)

CANADIAN AVAILABILITY:
Leustatin

CLASSIFICATION

Antineoplastic

AVAILABILITY (Rx)

Injection: 1 mg/ml

PHARMACOKINETICS

Primarily excreted in urine. Half-life: 5.4 hrs.

ACTION/*THERAPEUTIC EFFECT*

Disrupts cellular metabolism by incorporating into DNA of dividing cells. Cytotoxic to both actively dividing and quiescent lymphocytes and monocytes, *preventing DNA synthesis.*

USES/*UNLABELED*

Treatment for active hairy cell leukemia defined by clinically significant anemia, neutropenia, thrombocytopenia. Chronic multiple sclerosis. *Treatment of chronic lymphocytic leukemia, non-Hodgkin's lymphomas.*

STORAGE/HANDLING

Refrigerate unopened vials. Use diluted solutions immediately or refrigerate for no more than 8 hrs before administration. Solutions stable for at least 24 hrs at room temperature. Wear gloves and protective clothing during handling; if contact w/skin, rinse with copious amounts of water. Discard unused portion.

IV ADMINISTRATION

Note: Must dilute before administration. Do not mix w/other IV drugs, additives, or infuse concurrently via a common IV line.

1. Add calculated dose (0.09 mg/kg) to 500 ml 0.9% NaCl. Avoid 5% dextrose (increases degradation of medication).

2. Monitor vital signs during infusion, especially during first hour. Observe for hypotension or bradycardia (usually both do not occur during same course).

3. Immediately discontinue administration if severe hypersensitivity reaction occurs.

INDICATIONS/DOSAGE/ROUTES

Hairy cell leukemia:
IV Infusion: Adults: 0.09 mg/kg/day as continuous infusion for 7 days.

PRECAUTIONS

CONTRAINDICATIONS: None significant. **CAUTIONS:** Renal/hepatic impairment, bone marrow suppression. **PREGNANCY/LACTATION:** May produce fetal harm; may be embryotoxic and fetotoxic; potential for serious reactions in nursing infants. **Pregnancy Category D.**

INTERACTIONS

DRUG INTERACTIONS: Bone marrow depressants may increase bone marrow depression. High doses w/cyclophosphamide and total body irradiation may cause severe, irreversible neurologic toxicity, acute renal dysfunction. Nephrotoxic, neurotoxic medications may increase toxicity. Live virus vaccines may potentiate virus replication, increase vaccine side effects, decrease pt's antibody response to vaccine. **ALTERED LAB VALUES:** None significant.

SIDE EFFECTS

FREQUENT: Fever (69%), injection site reactions (redness, swelling, pain), fatigue, mild nausea, headache, anorexia, rash, mild to moderate infection. **OCCASIONAL:** Chills, diaphoresis, asthenia, vomiting, diarrhea/constipation, purpura, insomnia, peripheral edema, cough. **RARE:** Dizziness, tachycardia, SOB, myalgia, arthralgia.

ADVERSE REACTIONS/TOXIC EFFECTS

Myelosuppression characterized as severe neutropenia (<500 cells/mm^3); severe anemia (hemoglobin <8.5 g/dl) and thrombocytopenia occur commonly. High-dose treatment may produce acute nephrotoxicity and/or neurotoxicity manifested as irreversible motor weakness of upper or lower extremities.

NURSING IMPLICATIONS
BASELINE ASSESSMENT:

Give emotional support to pt and family. Perform neurologic function tests before chemotherapy. Obtain baseline temperature. Use strict asepsis and protect pt from infection. Check blood counts, particularly neutrophil, platelet count before each course of therapy and as clinically indicated.

INTERVENTION/EVALUATION:

Monitor temperature and report fever promptly. Assess for signs of infection or anemia (excessive tiredness, weakness). Avoid unnecessary trauma (rectal temperature, IM injections) when platelet counts decreased. Pt may require transfusions of RBCs or platelets.

PATIENT/FAMILY TEACHING:

Narrow margin between therapeutic and toxic response. Avoid crowds, persons w/known infections; report signs of infection at once (fever, flulike symptoms). Do not have immunizations w/o physician's approval (drug lowers body's resistance). Avoid contact w/those who have recently received live virus vaccine. Women of childbearing potential should not become pregnant during treatment.

clarithromycin

clair-**rith**-row-my-sin
(Biaxin)

CANADIAN AVAILABILITY
Biaxin

CLASSIFICATION

Antibiotic: macrolide

AVAILABILITY (Rx)

Tablets: 250 mg, 500 mg. **Oral Suspension:** 125 mg/5 ml, 250 mg/5 ml.

PHARMACOKINETICS

Well absorbed from GI tract. Widely distributed. Metabolized in liver to active metabolite. Primarily excreted in urine. Half-life: 3–7 hrs; metabolite: 5–7 hrs (increased in decreased renal function).

ACTION/*THERAPEUTIC EFFECT*

Bacteriostatic. Binds to ribosomal receptor sites, *inhibiting protein synthesis.* May be bactericidal w/high dosage or very susceptible microorganisms.

USES/*UNLABELED*

Treatment of mild to moderate infections of upper respiratory tract (pharyngitis, tonsillitis, sinusitis), lower respiratory tract (acute exacerbation of chronic bronchitis, pneumonia), and uncomplicated skin/skin structure infections, disseminated mycobacterium complex in AIDS, *H. pylori*–associated peptic ulcer disease. Prevents disseminated Mycobacterium avium (MAC). *Treatment of Legionnaire's disease.*

PO ADMINISTRATION

1. May give w/o regard to food.
2. Do not crush/break tablets.

INDICATIONS/DOSAGE/ROUTES

Note: Space doses evenly around the clock.

Lower respiratory tract infections:
PO: Adults, elderly: 250–500 mg q12h for 7–14 days.

Upper respiratory tract infections:
PO: Adults, elderly: 250–500 mg q12h for 10–14 days.

Uncomplicated skin/skin structure infections:
PO: Adults, elderly: 250 mg q12h for 7–14 days.

H. pylori:
PO: Adults (in combination): 500 mg 2 times/day for 10–14 days.

Prevent MAC:
PO: Adults: 500 mg 2 times/day. **Children:** 7.5 mg/kg 2 times/day up to 500 mg 2 times/day.

Usual pediatric dosage:
PO: Children: (6 mos–12 yrs): 7.5–15 mg/kg q12h.

Disseminated mycobacterium complex:
PO: Adults: 500 mg q12h.

PRECAUTIONS

CONTRAINDICATIONS: Hypersensitivity to clarithromycin, erythromycins, any macrolide antibiotic. **CAUTIONS:** Hepatic and renal dysfunction, elderly w/severe renal impairment. **PREGNANCY/LACTATION:** Unknown if distributed in breast milk. **Pregnancy Category C**.

INTERACTIONS

DRUG INTERACTIONS: May increase concentration, toxicity of astemizole, carbamazepine, cisapride, digoxin, terfenadine, theophylline. May cause serious arrhythmias w/cisapride. May decrease concentration of zidovudine. May increase warfarin effects. Rifampin may decrease clarithromycin concentrations. **ALTERED LAB VALUES:** May rarely increase SGOT (AST), SGPT (ALT), BUN.

SIDE EFFECTS

FREQUENT (3–6%): Diarrhea, nausea, altered taste, vomiting, abdominal pain, rash. **OCCASIONAL (1–2%):** Headache, dyspepsia. **RARE (<1%):** Hypersensitivity reaction.

ADVERSE REACTIONS/TOXIC EFFECTS

Superinfections, esp. antibiotic-associated colitis may occur. Hepatotoxicity, thrombocytopenia occur rarely.

NURSING IMPLICATIONS

BASELINE ASSESSMENT:

Question pt for history of hepatitis or allergies to clarithromycin, erythromycins. Obtain specimens for culture and sensitivity before giving first dose (therapy may begin before results are known).

INTERVENTION/EVALUATION:

Check for GI discomfort, nausea. Determine pattern of bowel activity and stool consistency. Monitor hepatic function tests, assess for hepatotoxicity: malaise, fever, abdominal pain, GI disturbances. Evaluate for superinfection: genital/anal pruritus, sore mouth or tongue, moderate to severe diarrhea.

PATIENT/FAMILY TEACHING:

Continue therapy for full length of treatment. Doses should be evenly spaced. Take medication w/8 oz water w/o regard to food. Notify physician in event of GI upset, rash, diarrhea, or other new symptom.

clemastine fumarate
kleh-**mass**-teen
(Tavist, Tavist-1)

FIXED-COMBINATION(S): W/phenylpropanolamine, a nasal decongestant (**Tavist-D**)

Tavist

CLASSIFICATION

Antihistamine

AVAILABILITY (Rx)

Tablets: 1.34 mg, 2.68 mg.
Syrup: 0.67 mg/5 ml.

PHARMACOKINETICS

	ONSET	PEAK	DURATION
PO	15–60 min	5–7 hrs	10–12 hrs

Well absorbed from GI tract. Metabolized in liver. Excreted primarily in urine.

ACTION / *THERAPEUTIC EFFECT*

Competes w/histamine at histaminic receptor sites, *relieving allergic conditions (urticaria, pruritus).* Anticholinergic effects cause drying of nasal mucosa.

USES

Relief of allergic conditions (nasal allergies, allergic dermatitis), cold symptoms, hypersensitivity reaction.

PO ADMINISTRATION

1. Give w/o regard to meals.
2. Scored tablets may be crushed (do not crush extended-release or film-coated forms).

INDICATIONS / DOSAGE / ROUTES

Allergic rhinitis:
PO: Adults, children >12 yrs: 1.34 mg 2 times/day. May increase dose to maximum 8.04 mg/day, if needed. **Children 6–11 yrs:** 0.67 mg 2 times/day. May increase dose to maximum 4.02 mg/day, if needed.

Allergic urticaria, angioedema:
PO: Adults, children >12 yrs: 2.68 1–3 times/day. Do not exceed 8.04 mg/day. **Children 6–11 yrs:** 1.34 mg 2 times/day. Do not exceed 4.02 mg/day.

Usual elderly dosage:
PO: 1.34 mg 1–2 times/day.

PRECAUTIONS

CONTRAINDICATIONS: Acute asthmatic attack, those receiving MAO inhibitors. **CAUTIONS:** Narrow-angle glaucoma, peptic ulcer, prostatic hypertrophy, pyloroduodenal or bladder neck obstruction, asthma, COPD, increased intraocular pressure, cardiovascular disease, hyperthyroidism, hypertension, seizure disorders. **PREGNANCY/ LACTATION:** Crosses placenta; detected in breast milk (may produce irritability in nursing infants). Increased risk of seizures in neonates, premature infants if used during third trimester of pregnancy. May prohibit lactation. **Pregnancy Category B.**

INTERACTIONS

DRUG INTERACTIONS: Alcohol, CNS depressants may increase CNS depressant effects. MAO inhibitors may increase anticholinergic, CNS depressant effects. **ALTERED LAB VALUES:** May suppress wheal, flare reactions to antigen skin testing, unless antihistamines discontinued 4 days prior to testing.

SIDE EFFECTS

Note: Fixed-combination form (Tavist-D) may produce mild CNS stimulation.
FREQUENT: Drowsiness, dizziness, dry mouth/nose/throat, urinary retention, thickening of bronchial secretions. *Elderly:* Sedation, dizziness, hypotension. **OCCASIONAL:** Epigastric distress, flushing, blurred vision, tinnitus, paresthesia, sweating, chills.

ADVERSE REACTIONS/TOXIC EFFECTS

Children may experience dominant paradoxical reaction (restlessness, insomnia, euphoria, nervousness, tremors). Overdosage in children may result in hallucinations, convulsions, death. Hypersensitivity reaction (eczema, pruritus, rash, cardiac disturbances, angioedema, photosensitivity) may occur. Overdosage may vary from CNS depression (sedation, apnea, cardiovascular collapse, death) to severe paradoxical reaction (hallucinations, tremor, seizures).

NURSING IMPLICATIONS

BASELINE ASSESSMENT:

If pt is undergoing allergic reaction, obtain history of recently ingested foods, drugs, environmental exposure, recent emotional stress. Monitor rate, depth, rhythm, type of respiration; quality and rate of pulse. Assess lung sounds for rhonchi, wheezing, rales.

INTERVENTION/EVALUATION:

Monitor B/P, especially in elderly (increased risk of hypotension). Monitor children closely for paradoxical reaction.

PATIENT/FAMILY TEACHING:

Tolerance to antihistaminic effect generally does not occur; tolerance to sedative effect may occur. Avoid tasks that require alertness, motor skills until response to drug is established. Dry mouth, drowsiness, dizziness may be an expected response of drug. Avoid alcoholic beverages during antihistamine therapy. Sugarless gum, sips of tepid water may relieve dry mouth. Coffee or tea may help reduce drowsiness.

clindamycin hydrochloride

klin-da-**my**-sin
(Cleocin HCL)

clindamycin palmitate hydrochloride

(Cleocin Pediatric)

clindamycin phosphate

(Cleocin phosphate, Cleocin T)

CANADIAN AVAILABILITY:
Dalacin

CLASSIFICATION

Antibiotic

AVAILABILITY (Rx)

Capsules: 75 mg, 150 mg, 300 mg. **Oral Solution:** 75 mg/5 ml. **Injection:** 150 mg/ml. **Vaginal Cream:** 2%. Vaginal Suppository. Lotion. Topical Solution.

PHARMACOKINETICS

Rapidly absorbed from GI tract. Widely distributed. Metabolized in liver to some active metabolites. Primarily excreted in urine. Not removed by hemodialysis. Half-life: 2.4–3 hrs (increased in decreased renal function, premature infants).

ACTION/ *THERAPEUTIC EFFECT*

Bacteriostatic. Binds to ribosomal receptor sites, *inhibiting protein synthesis.* Topically, decreases fatty acid concentration on skin, preventing acne vulgaris breakout.

USES/ *UNLABELED*

Treatment of respiratory tract, skin/soft tissue, chronic bone/joint infections, septicemia, intra-abdominal, female genitourinary infections, bacterial vaginosis, endocarditis. *Topical:* Acne vulgaris. *Treatment of malaria, otitis media, PCP, toxoplasmosis.*

STORAGE/HANDLING

Store capsules at room temperature. After reconstitution, oral solution is stable for 2 wks at room temperature. Do not refrigerate oral solution (avoids thickening). IV infusion (piggyback) stable for 16 days at room temperature, 32 days if refrigerated.

PO/IM/IV ADMINISTRATION

Note: Space doses evenly around the clock. May be given by IM injection, intermittent IV infusion (piggyback).

PO:

Give w/8 oz water. May give w/o regard to food.

IM:

1. Do not exceed 600 mg/dose.
2. Administer deep IM.

IV:

1. Dilute 300–600 mg w/50 ml 5% dextrose or 0.9% NaCl (900–1,200 mg w/100 ml). 50 ml piggyback is infused >10–20 min; 100 ml piggyback is infused >30–40 min.
2. No more than 1.2 g should be given in 1 infusion.
3. Do not administer IV push.
4. Alternating IV sites, use large veins to reduce risk of phlebitis.
5. Avoid prolonged use of indwelling IV catheters.

INDICATIONS/DOSAGE/ROUTES

Mild to moderate infections:
PO: Adults, elderly: 150–300 mg q6h. **Children:** 8–16 mg/kg/day in 3–4 divided doses.
IM/IV: Adults, elderly: 600–1,200 mg/day in 2–4 divided doses. **Children >1 mo:** 15–25 mg/kg/day in 3-4 divided doses. **Children <1 mo:** 15–20 mg/kg/day in 3–4 divided doses.

Serious infections:
PO: Adults, elderly: 300–450 mg q6h. **Children:** 13–25 mg/kg/day in 3–4 divided doses. **Children <10 kg:** Minimum: 37.5 mg 3 times/day. **IM/IV: Adults, elderly:** 1.2–2.7 g/day in 2–4 divided doses. **Children:** 25–40 mg/kg/day in 3–4 divided doses.

Life-threatening infections:
IV: Adults, elderly: Up to 4.8 g/day in divided doses.

Bacterial vaginosis:
Intravaginal: Adults: One applicatorful at bedtime for 3–7 days or 1 suppository at bedtime for 3 days.

Acne vulgaris:
Topical: Adults: Apply thin film 2 times/day to affected area.

PRECAUTIONS

CONTRAINDICATIONS: Hypersensitivity to clindamycin or lincomycin, known allergy to tartrazine dye, history of ulcerative colitis, regional enteritis, or antibiotic-associated colitis. **CAUTIONS:** Severe renal or hepatic dysfunction, concomitant use of neuromuscular blocking agents, neonates. Topical preparations should not be applied to abraded areas or near eyes. **PREGNANCY/LACTATION:** Readily crosses placenta; distributed in breast milk. **Pregnancy Category B.** *Topical/vaginal:* Unknown if distributed in breast milk.

INTERACTIONS

DRUG INTERACTIONS: Adsorbent antidiarrheals may delay absorption. Chloramphenicol, erythromycin may antagonize effects. May increase effect of neuromuscular blockers. **ALTERED LAB VALUES:** May increase SGOT (AST), SGPT (ALT), alkaline phosphatase.

SIDE EFFECTS

FREQUENT: Abdominal pain, nausea, vomiting, diarrhea. *Vaginal:* Vaginitis, itching. *Topical:* Dry scaly skin. **OCCASIONAL:** Phlebitis, thrombophlebitis w/IV administration; pain, induration at IM injection site; allergic reaction, urticaria, pruritus. *Vaginal:* Headache, dizziness, nausea, vomiting, abdominal pain. *Topical:* Contact dermatitis, abdominal pain, mild diarrhea, stinging/burning. **RARE:** *Vaginal:* Hypersensitivity reaction.

ADVERSE REACTIONS/TOXIC EFFECTS

Antibiotic-associated colitis during and several weeks after therapy (including topical), superinfection (esp. fungal), due to bacterial imbalance may occur. Blood dyscrasias (leukopenia, thrombocytopenia), nephrotoxicity (proteinuria, azotemia, oliguria) occur rarely.

NURSING IMPLICATIONS

BASELINE ASSESSMENT:

Question pt for history of allergies, particularly to clindamycin, lincomycin, aspirin. Avoid, if possible, concurrent use of neuromuscular blocking agents. Obtain specimens for culture and sensitivity, Gram's stain for vaginitis, before giving first dose (therapy may begin before results are known).

INTERVENTION/EVALUATION:

Monitor bowel activity, stool consistency; report diarrhea promptly due to potential for serious colitis (even w/topical or vaginal). Monitor periodic renal, hepatic, blood cell reports. Assess for ability to swallow, vomiting. Check I&O. Assess skin for rash (dryness, irritation w/topical application). Observe for phlebitis: pain, heat, red streaking over vein. Check for pain, induration at IM sites. W/all routes of administration, assess for superinfection: severe diarrhea, anal/genital pruritus, increased fever, change of oral mucosa.

PATIENT/FAMILY TEACHING:

Continue therapy for full length of treatment. Doses should be evenly spaced. Take oral doses w/ 8 oz water. Caution should be used when applying topical clindamycin concurrently w/peeling, abrasive acne agents, soaps, or alcohol-containing cosmetics to avoid cumulative effect. Do not apply topical preparations near eyes or abraded areas. Notify physician immediately in event of diarrhea; report onset of new symptoms. *Vaginal:* Avoid contact w/eyes. In event of accidental contact w/eyes, rinse w/copious amounts of cool tap water. Do not engage in sexual intercourse during treatment. Instruct pt on correct application (manufacturer's insert).

clobetasol

(Temovate)
See Classification section under: Corticosteroids: topical

C

clofibrate
(Atromid-S)
See Classification section under:
Antihyperlipidemics

clomipramine hydrochloride

klow-**mih**-prah-meen
(Anafranil)

CANADIAN AVAILABILITY:
Anafranil

CLASSIFICATION

Antidepressant: tricyclic

AVAILABILITY (Rx)

Capsules: 25 mg, 50 mg, 75 mg

PHARMACOKINETICS

Well absorbed from GI tract. Metabolized in liver, undergoes first-pass metabolism. Primarily excreted in urine. Minimal removal by hemodialysis. Half-life: 21–31 hrs.

ACTION/*THERAPEUTIC EFFECT*

Blocks reuptake of neurotransmitters (norepinephrine, serotonin) at CNS presynaptic membranes, increasing availability at postsynaptic receptor sites, *reducing obsessive-compulsive behavior.* Strong anticholinergic activity.

USES/*UNLABELED*

Treatment of obsessive-compulsive disorder manifested as repetitive tasks producing marked distress, time-consuming, or significantly interfering w/social or occupational behavior. *Treatment of mental depression, panic disorder, neurogenic pain, cataplexy associated w/narcolepsy, bulimia.*

PO ADMINISTRATION

Give w/food or milk if GI distress occurs.

INDICATIONS/DOSAGE/ROUTES

Obsessive-compulsive disorder:
PO: Adults: Initially, 25 mg/day. Gradually increase over 2 wks to 100 mg/day in divided doses. May further increase over several weeks to 250 mg/day in divided doses. After titration, may give as single bedtime dose (reduces daytime sedation). **Children >10 yrs:** Initially, 25 mg/day. Gradually increase over 2 wks to 3 mg/kg or 100 mg/day in divided doses (whichever is less). May then increase over several weeks up to 3 mg/kg or 200 mg (whichever is less). **Maintenance:** Lowest effective dose.

PRECAUTIONS

CONTRAINDICATIONS: Acute recovery period following MI, within 14 days of MAO inhibitor ingestion. **CAUTIONS:** Prostatic hypertrophy, history of urinary retention or obstruction, glaucoma, diabetes mellitus, history of seizures, hyperthyroidism, cardiac/hepatic/renal disease, schizophrenia, increased intraocular pressure, hiatal hernia. **PREGNANCY/LACTATION:** Crosses placenta; minimally distributed in breast milk. May produce neonatal withdrawal. **Pregnancy Category C.**

INTERACTIONS

DRUG INTERACTIONS: Alcohol, CNS depressants may increase CNS, respiratory depression, hypotensive effects. Antithyroid agents may increase risk of agranulocytosis. Phenothiazines may increase sedative, anticholinergic effects. Cimetidine may increase concentration, toxicity. May decrease effects of clonidine, guanadrel. May increase cardiac effects w/sympathomimetics. May increase risk of hypertensive crisis, hyperpyretic, convulsions w/MAO inhibitors. **ALTERED LAB VALUES:** May alter EKG readings, glucose.

SIDE EFFECTS

FREQUENT: Drowsiness, fatigue, dry mouth, blurred vision, constipation, sexual dysfunction (42%), ejaculatory failure (20%), impotence; weight gain (18%), delayed micturition, postural hypotension, excessive sweating, disturbed concentration, increased appetite, urinary retention. **OCCASIONAL:** GI disturbances (nausea, GI distress, metallic taste), asthenia, aggressiveness, muscle weakness. **RARE:** Paradoxical reactions (agitation, restlessness, nightmares, insomnia, extrapyramidal symptoms, particularly fine hand tremor), laryngitis, seizures.

ADVERSE REACTIONS/TOXIC EFFECTS

High dosage may produce cardiovascular effects (severe postural hypotension, dizziness, tachycardia, palpitations, arrhythmias) and seizures. May also result in altered temperature regulation (hyperpyrexia or hypothermia). Abrupt withdrawal from prolonged therapy may produce headache, malaise, nausea, vomiting, vivid dreams. Anemia has been noted.

NURSING IMPLICATIONS
BASELINE ASSESSMENT:

For those on long-term therapy, liver/renal function tests, blood counts should be performed periodically.

INTERVENTION/EVALUATION:

Supervise suicidal risk pt closely during early therapy (as depression lessens, energy level improves, increasing suicide potential). Assess appearance, behavior, speech pattern, level of interest, mood. Monitor pattern of daily bowel activity and stool consistency. Monitor B/P, pulse for hypotension, arrhythmias. Assess for urinary retention by bladder palpation.

PATIENT/FAMILY TEACHING:

Change positions slowly to avoid hypotensive effect. Tolerance to postural hypotension, sedative, and anticholinergic effects usually develops during early therapy. Maximum therapeutic effect may be noted in 2–4 wks. Photosensitivity to sun may occur. Dry mouth may be relieved by sugarless gum, sips of tepid water. Report visual disturbances. Do not abruptly discontinue medication. Avoid tasks that require alertness, motor skills until response to drug is established. Avoid alcohol.

---

clonazepam
klon-**nah**-zih-pam
(Klonopin)

CANADIAN AVAILABILITY:
Rivotril

CLASSIFICATION
Anticonvulsant

AVAILABILITY (Rx)
Tablets: 0.125 mg, 0.25 mg, 0.5 mg, 1 mg, 2 mg

PHARMACOKINETICS

Well absorbed from GI tract. Metabolized in liver. Excreted in urine. Half-life: 18–50 hrs.

ACTION/*THERAPEUTIC EFFECT*

Elevates seizure threshold in response to electrical/chemical stimulation by enhancing presynaptic inhibition in CNS, *suppressing seizure activity.*

USES/*UNLABELED*

Adjunct in treatment of Lennox-Gastaut syndrome (petit mal variant epilepsy), akinetic, and myoclonic seizures, absence seizures (petit mal). Treatment of panic disorder. *Adjunct treatment of seizures, treatment of simple/complex partial seizures, tonic-clonic seizures.*

PO ADMINISTRATION

1. Give w/o regard to meals.
2. Tablets may be crushed.

INDICATIONS/DOSAGE/ROUTES

Anticonvulsant:

Note: When replacement by another anticonvulsant is necessary, decrease clonazepam gradually as therapy begins w/low replacement dose.

PO: Adults, elderly: 1.5 mg daily. Dosage may be increased in 0.5–1 mg increments at 3 day intervals until seizures are controlled. Do not exceed maintenance dose of 20 mg daily. **Infants, children <10 yrs, or <66 lbs:** 0.01–0.03 mg/kg daily in 2–3 divided doses. Dosage may be increased in up to 0.5 mg increments at 3 day intervals until seizures are controlled. Do not exceed maintenance dose of 0.2 mg/kg daily.

Panic disorder:

PO: Adults: Initially 0.25 mg 2 times/day. Increase up to target dose of 1 mg/day after 3 days.

PRECAUTIONS

CONTRAINDICATIONS: Significant liver disease, narrow-angle glaucoma. **CAUTIONS:** Impaired kidney/liver function, chronic respiratory disease. **PREGNANCY/ LACTATION:** Crosses placenta, may be distributed in breast milk. Chronic ingestion during pregnancy may produce withdrawal symptoms, CNS depression in neonates. **Pregnancy Category C**.

INTERACTIONS

DRUG INTERACTIONS: Alcohol, CNS depressants may increase CNS depressant effect. **ALTERED LAB VALUES:** None significant.

SIDE EFFECTS

FREQUENT: Mild, transient drowsiness, ataxia, behavioral disturbances (esp. in children) manifested as aggression, irritability, agitation. **OCCASIONAL:** Rash, ankle/facial edema, nocturia, dysuria, change in appetite/weight, dry mouth, sore gums, nausea, blurred vision. **RARE:** Paradoxical reaction (hyperactivity/nervousness in children, excitement/restlessness in elderly—particularly noted in presence of uncontrolled pain).

ADVERSE REACTIONS/TOXIC EFFECTS

Abrupt withdrawal may result in pronounced restlessness, irritability, insomnia, hand tremors, abdominal/muscle cramps, sweating, vomiting, status epilepticus. Overdosage results in somnolence, confusion, diminished reflexes, coma.

NURSING IMPLICATIONS

BASELINE ASSESSMENT:

Review history of seizure disorder (frequency, duration, intensity, level of consciousness). Implement safety measures and observe frequently for recurrence of seizure activity.

INTERVENTION/EVALUATION:

Assess children, elderly for paradoxical reaction, particularly during early therapy. Assist w/ambulation if drowsiness, ataxia occur. For those on long-term therapy, liver/renal function tests, blood counts should be performed periodically. Evaluate for therapeutic response: a decrease in intensity/frequency of seizures.

PATIENT/FAMILY TEACHING:

Drowsiness usually diminishes w/continued therapy. Avoid tasks that require alertness, motor skills until response to drug is established. Smoking reduces drug effectiveness. Do not abruptly withdraw medication after long-term therapy. Strict maintenance of drug therapy is essential for seizure control. Avoid alcohol.

clonidine
klon-ih-deen
(Catapres TTS)
clonidine hydrochloride
(Catapres, Duraclon)

FIXED-COMBINATION(S):
W/chlorthalidone, a diuretic (**Combipres**)

CANADIAN AVAILABILITY:
Catapres, Dixarit

CLASSIFICATION

Antihypertensive

AVAILABILITY (Rx)

Tablets: 0.1 mg, 0.2 mg, 0.3 mg. **Transdermal Patch:** 2.5 mg (release at 0.1 mg/24 hrs), 5 mg (release at 0.2 mg/24hrs, 7.5 mg (release at 0.3 mg/24 hrs).

PHARMACOKINETICS

	ONSET	PEAK	DURATION
PO	0.5–1 hr	2–4 hrs	up to 8 hrs

Well absorbed from GI tract. Transdermal best absorbed from chest, upper arm; least absorbed from thigh. Metabolized in liver. Primarily excreted in urine. Minimal removal by hemodialysis. Half-life: 12–16 hrs (increased in decreased renal function).

ACTION/*THERAPEUTIC EFFECT*

Stimulates alpha$_2$-adrenergic receptors in CNS (inhibits sympathetic cardioaccelerator and vasoconstrictor center); decreases sympathetic outflow from CNS. *Reduces peripheral resistance, decreases B/P, heart rate.*

USES/*UNLABELED*

Treatment of hypertension alone or in combination w/other antihypertensive agents. Treatment of severe pain in cancer pts. *Diagnosis of pheochromocytoma, prevents migraine headaches, treatment of dysmenorrhea/menopausal flushing, opioid withdrawal.*

PO/TRANSDERMAL ADMINISTRATION

PO:
1. May give w/o regard to food.
2. Tablets may be crushed.
3. Give last oral dose just before retiring.

TRANSDERMAL:
1. Apply transdermal system to dry, hairless area of intact skin on upper arm or chest.

2. Rotate sites (prevents skin irritation).

3. Do not trim patch to adjust dose.

INDICATIONS/DOSAGE/ROUTES

Hypertension:
PO: Adults: Initially, 0.1 mg 2 times/day. Increase by 0.1–0.2 mg q 2–4 days. **Maintenance:** 0.2–1.2 mg/day in 2–4 divided doses up to maximum of 2.4 mg/day. **Children:** 5–25 mcg/kg/day in divided doses q6h; increase at 5–7 day intervals.
Transdermal: Adults, elderly: System delivering 0.1 mg/24 hrs up to 0.6 mg/24 hrs every 7 days.

Usual elderly dosage:
PO: Initially, 0.1 mg at bedtime. May increase gradually.

Severe pain:
Epidural: Adults, elderly: 30 mcg/hr.

PRECAUTIONS

CONTRAINDICATIONS: None significant. **CAUTIONS:** Severe coronary insufficiency, recent MI, cerebrovascular disease, chronic renal failure, Raynaud's disease, thromboangiitis obliterans. **PREGNANCY/LACTATION:** Crosses placenta; distributed in breast milk. **Pregnancy Category C.**

INTERACTIONS

DRUG INTERACTIONS: Tricyclic antidepressants may decrease effect. Discontinuing concurrent beta blockers may increase risk of clonidine-withdrawal hypertensive crisis. **ALTERED LAB VALUES:** None significant.

SIDE EFFECTS

FREQUENT (10–40%): Dry mouth (40%), drowsiness (33%), dizziness (16%), sedation, constipation (10%). **OCCASIONAL (1–5%):** Depression, swelling of feet, loss of appetite, decreased sexual ability, itching eyes, dizziness, nausea, vomiting, nervousness. *Transdermal:* Itching, red skin, darkening of skin. **RARE (<1%):** Nightmares, vivid dreams, cold feeling in fingers/toes.

ADVERSE REACTIONS/TOXIC EFFECTS

Overdosage produces profound hypotension, irritability, bradycardia, respiratory depression, hypothermia, miosis (pupillary constriction), arrhythmias, apnea. Abrupt withdrawal may result in rebound hypertension associated w/nervousness, agitation, anxiety, insomnia, hand tingling, tremor, flushing, sweating.

NURSING IMPLICATIONS
BASELINE ASSESSMENT:

Obtain B/P immediately before each dose is administered, in addition to regular monitoring (be alert to B/P fluctuations).

INTERVENTION/EVALUATION:

Assist w/ambulation if dizziness occurs. Monitor pattern of daily bowel activity and stool consistency. If clonidine is to be withdrawn, discontinue concurrent beta-blocker therapy several days before discontinuing clonidine (prevents clonidine withdrawal hypertensive crisis). Slowly reduce clonidine dose over 2–4 days.

PATIENT/FAMILY TEACHING:

Sugarless gum, sips of tepid water may relieve dry mouth. If nausea occurs, unsalted crackers, noncola beverages, or dry toast may relieve effect. To reduce hypotensive effect, rise slowly from lying to sitting position and permit legs to dangle momentarily before standing. Skipping doses or voluntarily discontinuing drug may produce severe, rebound hypertension. Side effects tend to diminish during therapy.

clopidrogel
(Plavix)
See Supplement
See Classification section under:
Anticoagulants/Antiplatelets/Thrombolytics

clorazepate dipotassium

klor-**az**-eh-payt
(Tranxene)

CANADIAN AVAILABILITY:
Novoclopate, Tranxene

CLASSIFICATION

Antianxiety, anticonvulsant

AVAILABILITY (Rx)

Capsules: 3.75 mg, 7.5 mg, 15 mg. **Tablets:** 3.75 mg, 7.5 mg, 15 mg. **Tablets (single dose):** 11.25 mg, 22.5 mg.

PHARMACOKINETICS

Rapidly, well absorbed from GI tract. Widely distributed. Metabolized in stomach and liver (first-pass metabolism) to active metabolites. Excreted in urine. Half-life: metabolite: 48–96 hrs.

ACTION/*THERAPEUTIC EFFECT*

Enhances gamma-aminobutyric acid (GABA) neurotransmission at CNS, *producing anxiolytic effect.* Elevates seizure threshold in response to electrical/chemical stimulation by enhancing presynaptic inhibition in CNS, *suppressing seizure activity.*

USES

Management of anxiety disorders, short-term relief of anxiety symptoms, partial seizures, acute alcohol withdrawal symptoms.

PO ADMINISTRATION

1. Give w/o regard to meals.
2. Tablets may be crushed.
3. Capsules may be emptied and mixed w/food.

INDICATIONS/DOSAGE/ROUTES

Note: When replacement by another anticonvulsant is necessary, decrease clorazepate gradually as therapy begins w/low-replacement dose.

Anxiety:
PO: Adults: 30 mg daily in divided doses. **Elderly, debilitated:** 7.5–15 mg in divided doses or single bedtime dose. **Daily dose range:** 15–60 mg.

Partial seizures:
PO: Adults, children >12 yrs: Initially, up to 7.5 mg 3 times daily. Do not increase dosage more than 7.5 mg/wk or exceed 90 mg/day.

Alcohol withdrawal:
PO: Adults: Day 1: 30 mg followed by 30–60 mg in divided doses. **Day 2:** 45–90 mg in divided doses. **Day 3:** 22.5–45 mg in divided doses. **Day 4:** 15–30 mg in divided doses, then gradually reduce to 7.5–15 mg daily.

PRECAUTIONS

CONTRAINDICATIONS: Acute narrow-angle glaucoma. **CAUTIONS:** Impaired renal/hepatic function, acute alcohol intoxication. **PREGNANCY/LACTATION:** May cross placenta; distributed in breast milk. Chronic ingestion during pregnancy may produce withdrawal symptoms, CNS depression in neonates. **Pregnancy Category D**.

INTERACTIONS

DRUG INTERACTIONS: Alcohol, CNS depressants may increase CNS depressant effect. **ALTERED LAB VALUES:** None significant.

SIDE EFFECTS

FREQUENT: Drowsiness. **OCCASIONAL:** Dizziness, GI disturbances, nervousness, blurred vision, dry mouth, headache, confusion, ataxia, rash, irritability, slurred speech. **RARE:** Paradoxical CNS hyperactivity/nervousness in children, excitement/restlessness in elderly/debilitated (generally noted during first 2 wks of therapy, particularly noted in presence of uncontrolled pain).

ADVERSE REACTIONS/TOXIC EFFECTS

Abrupt or too rapid withdrawal may result in pronounced restlessness, irritability, insomnia, hand tremors, abdominal/muscle cramps, sweating, vomiting, seizures. Overdosage results in somnolence, confusion, diminished reflexes, coma.

NURSING IMPLICATIONS
BASELINE ASSESSMENT:

Anxiety: Assess autonomic response (cold, clammy hands, sweating) and motor response (agitation, trembling, tension). Offer emotional support to anxious pt. *Seizures:* Review history of seizure disorder (intensity, frequency, duration, LOC). Observe frequently for recurrence of seizure activity. Initiate seizure precautions.

INTERVENTION/EVALUATION:

For those on long-term therapy, liver/renal function tests, blood counts should be performed periodically. Assess for paradoxical reaction, particularly during early therapy. Assist w/ambulation if drowsiness, dizziness occur. Evaluate for therapeutic response: *Anxiety:* A calm facial expression; decreased restlessness. *Seizures:* A decrease in intensity or frequency of seizures.

PATIENT/FAMILY TEACHING:

Do not abruptly withdraw medication following long-term use (may precipitate seizures). Strict maintenance of drug therapy is essential for seizure control. Drowsiness usually disappears during continued therapy. If dizziness occurs, change positions slowly from recumbent to sitting position before standing. Avoid tasks that require alertness, motor skills until response to drug is established. Smoking reduces drug effectiveness. Avoid alcohol.

clotrimazole
kloe-**try**-mah-zole
(Mycelex, Mycelex-G, Lotrimin, Gyne-Lotrimin)

FIXED-COMBINATION(S):
W/betamethasone dipropionate, a corticosteroid (**Lotrisone**)

CANADIAN AVAILABILITY:
Canesten, Clotrimaderm

CLASSIFICATION

Antifungal

AVAILABILITY (Rx)

Troches: 10 mg. **Vaginal Tablets:** 100 mg, 500 mg. **Vaginal Cream:**

1%. **Topical Cream:** 1%. **Topical Solution:** 1%. **Lotion:** 1%.

PHARMACOKINETICS

Poorly, erratically absorbed from GI tract. Bound to oral mucosa. Absorbed portion metabolized in liver. Eliminated in feces. *Topical:* Minimal systemic absorption (highest concentration in stratum corneum). *Intravaginal:* Small amount systemically absorbed.

ACTION / *THERAPEUTIC EFFECT*

Binds w/phospholipids in fungal cell membrane. The altered cell membrane permeability *inhibits yeast growth.*

USES / *UNLABELED*

Oral lozenges: Treatment/prophylaxis oropharyngeal candidiasis due to *Candida* sp. *Topical:* Treatment of tinea pedis, tinea cruris, tinea corporis, tinea versicolor, cutaneous candidiasis (moniliasis) due to *Candida albicans. Intravaginally:* Treatment of vulvovaginal candidiasis (moniliasis) due to *Candida* sp. *Topical:* Treatment of paronychia, tinea barbae, tinea capitas.

PO / TOPICAL / VAGINAL / OROPHARYNGEAL ADMINISTRATION

PO:

1. Lozenges must be dissolved in mouth >15–30 min for oropharyngeal therapy.
2. Swallow saliva.

TOPICAL:

1. Rub well into affected, surrounding areas.
2. Do not apply occlusive covering or other preparations.

VAGINAL:

Use vaginal applicator; insert high in vagina.

INDICATIONS / DOSAGE / ROUTES

Oral-local/oropharyngeal:
PO: Adults, elderly: 10 mg 5 times/day for 14 days.

Prophylaxis vs. oropharyngeal candidiasis:
PO: Adults, elderly: 10 mg 3 times/day.

Usual topical dosage:
Topical: Adults, elderly: 2 times/day. Therapeutic effect may take up to 8 wks.

Vulvovaginal candidiasis:
Vaginal: (Tablets) Adults, elderly: 1 tablet (100 mg) at bedtime for 7 days; 2 tablets (200 mg) at bedtime for 3 days; or 500 mg tablet one time.

Vaginal: (Cream) Adults, elderly: 1 applicatorful at bedtime for 7–14 days.

PRECAUTIONS

CONTRAINDICATIONS: Hypersensitivity to clotrimazole or any ingredient in preparation, children <3 yrs. **CAUTIONS:** Hepatic disorder w/oral therapy. **PREGNANCY/LACTATION:** Pregnancy Category B.Distribution in breast milk unknown.

INTERACTIONS

DRUG INTERACTIONS: None significant. **ALTERED LAB VALUES:** May increase SGOT (AST).

SIDE EFFECTS

FREQUENT: *Oral:* Nausea, vomiting, diarrhea, abdominal pain. **OCCASIONAL:** *Topical:* Itching, burning, stinging, erythema, urticaria. *Vaginal:* Mild burning (tablets/cream); irritation, cystitis (cream). **RARE:** *Vaginal tablets:* Itching, rash, lower abdominal cramping, headache.

ADVERSE REACTIONS/TOXIC EFFECTS

None significant.

NURSING IMPLICATIONS

BASELINE ASSESSMENT:

Question for history of hypersensitivity to clotrimazole. Assess pt's ability to understand and follow directions regarding use of oral lozenges.

INTERVENTION/EVALUATION:

W/oral therapy, assess for nausea, vomiting; monitor hepatic function tests esp. w/preexisting hepatic disorder. Check skin for erythema, urticaria, blistering; inquire about itching, burning, stinging. W/vaginal therapy, evaluate for vulvovaginal irritation, abdominal cramping, urinary frequency, discomfort.

PATIENT/FAMILY TEACHING:

Continue for full length of therapy. Inform physician of increased irritation. Avoid contact w/eyes. *Topical:* Keep areas clean, dry; wear light clothing to promote ventilation. Separate personal items, linens. *Vaginal:* Continue use during menses. Refrain from sexual intercourse or advise partner to use condom during therapy.

cloxacillin sodium

clocks-ah-sill-in
(Cloxapen, Tegopen)

CANADIAN AVAILABILITY:
ApoCloxi, Novocloxin, Tegopen

CLASSIFICATION

Antibiotic: penicillin

AVAILABILITY (Rx)

Capsules: 250 mg, 500 mg.
Oral Solution: 125 mg/5 ml.

PHARMACOKINETICS

Moderately absorbed from GI tract. Partially metabolized in liver. Primarily excreted in urine. Not removed by hemodialysis. Half-life: 0.5–1.1 hrs (increased in decreased renal function).

ACTION/*THERAPEUTIC EFFECT*

Bactericidal in susceptible microorganisms by *inhibition of cell wall synthesis.*

USES

Treatment of mild to moderate infections of respiratory tract and skin/skin structure, chronic osteomyelitis, urinary tract infections; follow-up to parenteral therapy for acute, severe infections. Predominantly treatment of infections caused by penicillinase-producing staphylococci.

STORAGE/HANDLING

Store capsules at room temperature; oral solution, after reconstitution, is stable for 3 days at room temperature, 14 days if refrigerated.

PO ADMINISTRATION

1. Space doses evenly around clock.
2. Give 1 hr before or 2 hrs after meals.

INDICATIONS/DOSAGE/ROUTES

Mild to moderate upper respiratory, localized skin/skin structure infections:
PO: Adults, elderly, children >20 kg: 250 mg q6h. Children <20 kg:

50 mg/kg/day in divided doses q6h.

Severe infections, lower respiratory tract, disseminated infections: PO: Adults, elderly, children >20 kg: 500 mg q6h. **Children <20 kg:** 100 mg/kg/day in divided doses q6h.

PRECAUTIONS

CONTRAINDICATIONS: Hypersensitivity to any penicillin. **CAUTIONS:** History of allergies, particularly cephalosporins. **PREGNANCY/LACTATION:** Readily crosses placenta, appears in cord blood and amniotic fluid; distributed in breast milk in low concentrations. May lead to allergic sensitization, diarrhea, candidiasis, skin rash in infant. **Pregnancy Category B**.

INTERACTIONS

DRUG INTERACTIONS: Probenecid may increase concentration, toxicity risk. **ALTERED LAB VALUES:** May increase SGOT (AST), SGPT (ALT), alkaline phosphatase, LDH. May cause positive Coombs' test.

SIDE EFFECTS

FREQUENT: Mild diarrhea, nausea, vomiting, headache, oral/vaginal candidiasis. **OCCASIONAL:** Mild hypersensitivity reaction (fever, rash, pruritus).

ADVERSE REACTIONS/TOXIC EFFECTS

Superinfections, antibiotic-associated colitis (abdominal cramps, watery severe diarrhea, fever) may result from altered bacterial balance. Hematologic effects, severe hypersensitivity reactions, anaphylaxis occur rarely.

NURSING IMPLICATIONS

BASELINE ASSESSMENT:

Question for history of allergies, especially penicillins, cephalosporins. Obtain specimen for culture and sensitivity before giving first dose (therapy may begin before results are known).

INTERVENTION/EVALUATION:

Hold medication and promptly report rash (hypersensitivity) or diarrhea (w/fever, abdominal pain, mucus or blood in stool may indicate antibiotic-associated colitis). Assess food tolerance. Check hematology reports (esp. WBCs), periodic renal or hepatic reports in prolonged therapy. Be alert for superinfection: increased fever, onset sore throat, diarrhea, ulceration or changes of oral mucosa, vaginal discharge, anal/genital pruritus.

PATIENT/FAMILY TEACHING:

Space doses evenly. Continue antibiotic for full length of treatment. Notify physician in event of diarrhea, rash, other new symptom.

---

clozapine

klow-zah-peen
(Clozaril)

CANADIAN AVAILABILITY:
Clozaril

CLASSIFICATION

Antipsychotic

AVAILABILITY (Rx)

Tablets: 25 mg, 100 mg

PHARMACOKINETICS

Rapid, almost completely absorbed from GI tract. Widely distributed. Extensively metabolized by first-pass liver metabolism. Primarily excreted in urine. Half-life: 8–12 hrs.

ACTION/ *THERAPEUTIC EFFECT*

Interferes with the binding of dopamine at dopamine receptor sites (binds primarily at non-dopamine receptor sites), *diminishing schizophrenic behavior.* Unlike other antipsychotics, produces few extrapyramidal effects.

USES

Management of severely ill schizophrenic pts who fail to respond to other antipsychotic therapy.

PO ADMINISTRATION

May give w/o regard to meals.

INDICATIONS/DOSAGE/ROUTES

Schizophrenic disorders:
PO: Adults: Initially, 25 mg 1–2 times/day. May increase by 25–50 mg/day over 2 wks until dose of 300–450 mg/day achieved. May further increase dose by 50–100 mg/day no more frequently than 1–2 times/wk. **Range:** 200–600 mg/day. **Maximum:** 900 mg/day.

Usual elderly dosage:
PO: Initially, 25 mg/day. May increase by 25 mg/day. **Maximum:** 450 mg/day.

PRECAUTIONS

CONTRAINDICATIONS: Myeloproliferative disorders, history of clozapine-induced agranulocytosis or severe granulocytopenia, concurrent administration w/other drugs having potential to suppress bone marrow function, severe CNS depression, comatose state. **CAUTIONS:** History of seizures, cardiovascular disease, impaired respiratory, hepatic, renal function, alcohol withdrawal, urinary retention, glaucoma, prostatic hypertrophy. **PREGNANCY/LACTATION:** Crosses placenta; distributed in breast milk. **Pregnancy Category B.**

INTERACTIONS

DRUG INTERACTIONS: Alcohol, CNS depressants may increase CNS depressant effects. Bone marrow depressants may increase myelosuppression. Lithium may increase risk of seizures, confusion, dyskinesias. Phenobarbital decreases concentration. **ALTERED LAB VALUES:** None significant.

SIDE EFFECTS

FREQUENT: Drowsiness (39%), salivation (31%), tachycardia (25%), dizziness (19%), constipation (14%). **OCCASIONAL:** Hypotension (9%), headache (7%); tremor, syncope, sweating, dry mouth (6%); nausea, visual disturbances (5%); nightmares, restlessness, akinesia, agitation, hypertension, abdominal discomfort/heartburn, weight gain (4%). **RARE:** Rigidity, confusion, fatigue, insomnia, diarrhea, rash.

ADVERSE REACTIONS/TOXIC EFFECTS

Seizures occur occasionally (3%). Overdosage produces CNS depression (sedation, coma, delirium), respiratory depression, hypersalivation. Blood dyscrasias, particularly agranulocytosis, mild leukopenia may occur.

NURSING IMPLICATIONS
BASELINE ASSESSMENT:

Obtain baseline WBC and differential count before initiating treatment and WBC count every week for first 6 months of continuous therapy, then biweekly for those w/acceptable WBC counts. Assess behavior, appearance, emotional status, response to environment, speech pattern, thought content.

INTERVENTION/EVALUATION:

Monitor B/P for hyper/hypotension. Assess pulse for tachycardia (common side effect). Monitor WBC, differential count for blood dyscrasias. Question bowel activity for evidence of constipation. Supervise suicidal risk pt closely during early therapy (as depression lessens, energy level improves, increasing suicide potential). Assess for therapeutic response (interest in surroundings, improvement in self-care, increased ability to concentrate, relaxed facial expression).

PATIENT/FAMILY TEACHING:

Do not abruptly withdraw from long-term drug therapy. Report visual disturbances. Sugarless gum or sips of tepid water may relieve dry mouth. Drowsiness generally subsides during continued therapy. Avoid tasks that require alertness, motor skills until response to drug is established. Avoid alcohol.

cocaine

koe-**kane**
(Cocaine HCl)

CANADIAN AVAILABIILTY:
  Cocaine

CLASSIFICATION

Topical anesthetic

AVAILABILITY

Topical Solution: 4%, 10%

PHARMACOKINETICS

	ONSET	PEAK	DURATION
Topical			
	1 min	2–5 min	0.5–2 hrs

Readily absorbed from all mucous membranes. Hydrolyzed by plasma and liver cholinesterases to active metabolite. Primarily excreted in urine. Half-life: 1–1.5 hrs.

ACTION/*THERAPEUTIC EFFECT*

Blocks conduction of nerve impulses by decreasing membrane permeability, increases norepinephrine at postsynaptic receptor sites, producing intense vasoconstriction.

USES

Topical anesthesia for mucous membranes of oral laryngeal, nasal areas.

TOPICAL ADMINISTRATION

1. Avoid inhalation of any sprays. Do not puncture spray container or use near open flame.

2. Do not get preparations near eyes.

3. When used for anesthesia of throat, NPO until sensation returns (failure to protect from aspiration, difficulty w/swallowing).

INDICATIONS/DOSAGE/ROUTES

Usual topical dosage:
Topical: Adults, elderly: 1–10% solution. **Maximum single dose:** 1 mg/kg.

PRECAUTIONS

CONTRAINDICATIONS: Hypersensitivity to cocaine or local anesthetics. Systemic or ophthalmic use. **CAUTIONS:** History of drug sensitivities or drug abuse (can cause strong psychologic dependence and some tolerance); has been abused for cortical stimulant effect. Severe trauma or sepsis in area to be anesthetized. Limit to office and surgical procedures; prolonged use can cause ischemic damage to nasal mucosa. Safety in children not established. **PREGNANCY/LACTATION:** Safety during lactation not established. **Pregnancy Category C.** (Category X if nonmedical use.)

INTERACTIONS

DRUG INTERACTIONS: Tricyclic antidepressants, digoxin, methyldopa may increase arrhythmias. May decrease effects of beta blockers. Cholinesterase inhibitors may increase effects, risk of toxicity. CNS stimulation-producing agents may increase effects. Sympathomimetics increase CNS stimulation, risk of cardiovascular effects. **ALTERED LAB VALUES:** None significant.

SIDE EFFECTS

FREQUENT: Loss of sense of smell/taste. **OCCASIONAL:** Repeated nasal application: stuffy nose, chronic rhinitis.

ADVERSE REACTIONS/TOXIC EFFECTS

Nasal: None significant.
Systemic: Overdose, early signs: Increased B/P, increased pulse, irregular heartbeat, chills/fever, agitation, nervousness, confusion, inability to remain still, nausea, vomiting, abdominal pain, increased sweating, rapid breathing, large pupils.
Advanced: Arrhythmias, CNS hemorrhage, CHF, convulsions, delirium, hyperreflexia, loss of bladder/bowel control, respiratory weakness.
Late stage: Loss of reflexes, muscle paralysis, dilated pupils, LOC, cyanosis, pulmonary edema, cardiac/respiratory failure.

NURSING IMPLICATIONS
BASELINE ASSESSMENT:

Question for hypersensitivity to cocaine. Obtain baseline vital signs.

INTERVENTION/EVALUATION:

Monitor for anesthetic response. Be alert to CNS stimulation: assess for euphoria, restlessness, increased B/P, pulse, respirations. Be prepared to provide ventilatory support and emergency medications in event of progression of CNS response—death from overdose will occur within minutes, up to 3 hrs after initial reaction.

PATIENT/FAMILY TEACHING:

NPO until sensation returns when used for throat anesthesia. Onetime or infrequent use for procedures will not cause dependence. Report feelings of euphoria, restlessness, or rapid heartbeat if these develop during procedure.

codeine phosphate
koe-deen
codeine sulfate

FIXED-COMBINATION(S):
W/aspirin, butalbital, a barbiturate, and caffeine (**Fiorinal**); w/acetaminophen (**Phenaphen, Tylenol w/codeine**); w/aspirin (**Empirin w/codeine**)

CANADIAN AVAILABILITY:
Codeine Contin

CLASSIFICATION

Opioid analgesic: **Schedule II;** fixed-combination form: **Schedule III**

AVAILABILITY (Rx)

Tablets: 15 mg, 30 mg, 60 mg. **Soluble Tablets:** 15 mg, 30 mg, 60 mg. **Injection:** 30 mg, 60 mg.

PHARMACOKINETICS

	ONSET	PEAK	DURATION
PO	15–30 min	1–1.5 hrs	4–6 hrs
IM	15–30 min	30–60 min	4–6 hrs
SubQ	15–30 min	—	4–6 hrs

Moderately absorbed from GI tract; completely after IM administration. Widely distributed. Metabolized in liver. Excreted in urine. Half-life: 2.5–4 hrs.

ACTION / *THERAPEUTIC EFFECT*

Binds at opiate receptor sites in CNS. *Reduces intensity of pain stimuli incoming from sensory nerve endings, suppresses cough reflex, decreases intestinal motility.*

USES / *UNLABELED*

Relief of mild to moderate pain and/or nonproductive cough. *Treatment of diarrhea.*

STORAGE / HANDLING

Store oral, parenteral form at room temperature.

PO / SUBQ / IM ADMINISTRATION

PO:

1. Give w/o regard to meals.
2. Shake oral suspension well.

SubQ/IM:

1. Parenteral form incompatible w/aminophylline, ammonium chloride, amobarbital, chlorothiazide, heparin, methicillin, nitrofurantoin, pentobarbital, phenobarbital, sodium bicarbonate, sodium iodide, thiopental.
2. Pt should be recumbent before drug is administered.
3. Assess for wheals at injection site (sign of local tissue irritation, induration).
4. Those w/circulatory impairment may experience overdosage due to delayed absorption of repeated administration.

INDICATIONS / DOSAGE / ROUTES

Note: Reduce initial dosage in those w/hypothyroidism, concurrent CNS depressants, Addison's disease, renal insufficiency, elderly/debilitated.

Analgesia:
PO/SubQ/IM: Adults, elderly: 30 mg q4–6h. **Range:** 15–60 mg daily. **Children:** 0.5 mg/kg q4–6h.

Antitussive:
PO: Adults, elderly, children >12 yrs: 10–20 mg q4–6h. **Children 6–11 yrs:** 5–10 mg q4–6h. **Children 2–5 yrs:** 2.5–5 mg q4–6h.

PRECAUTIONS

CONTRAINDICATIONS: None significant. **EXTREME CAUTION:** CNS depression, anoxia, hypercapnia, respiratory depression, seizures, acute alcoholism, shock, untreated myxedema, respiratory dysfunction. **CAUTIONS:** Increased intracranial pressure, impaired hepatic function, acute abdominal conditions, hypothyroidism, prostatic hypertrophy, Addison's disease, urethral stricture, COPD. **PREGNANCY/LACTATION:** Readily crosses placenta;

distributed in breast milk. May prolong labor if administered in latent phase of first stage of labor or before cervical dilation of 4–5 cm has occurred. Respiratory depression may occur in neonate if mother received opiates during labor. Regular use of opiates during pregnancy may produce withdrawal symptoms in the neonate (irritability, excessive crying, tremors, hyperactive reflexes, fever, vomiting, diarrhea, yawning, sneezing, seizures). **Pregnancy Category C**. (Category D if used for prolonged periods or in high doses at term.)

INTERACTIONS

DRUG INTERACTIONS: Alcohol, CNS depressants may increase CNS or respiratory depression, hypotension. MAO inhibitors may produce severe, fatal reaction (reduce dose to 1/4 usual dose). **ALTERED LAB VALUES:** May increase amylase, lipase.

SIDE EFFECTS

Note: Ambulatory pts, those not in severe pain may experience dizziness, nausea, vomiting, hypotension more frequently than those in supine position or w/severe pain. **FREQUENT:** Constipation, drowsiness, nausea, vomiting. **OCCASIONAL:** Paradoxical excitement, confusion, pounding heartbeat, facial flushing, decreased urination, blurred vision, dizziness, dry mouth, headache, hypotension, decreased appetite, redness/burning/pain at injection site. **RARE:** Hallucinations, depression, stomach pain, insomnia.

ADVERSE REACTIONS/TOXIC EFFECTS

Too frequent use may result in paralytic ileus. Overdosage results in cold/clammy skin, confusion, convulsions, decreased B/P, restlessness, pinpoint pupils, bradycardia, respiratory depression, LOC, severe weakness. Tolerance to analgesic effect, physical dependence may occur w/repeated use.

NURSING IMPLICATIONS
BASELINE ASSESSMENT:

Obtain vital signs before giving medication. If respirations are 12/min or lower (20/min or lower in children), withhold medication, contact physician. *Analgesic:* Assess onset, type, location, and duration of pain. Effect of medication is reduced if full pain recurs before next dose. *Antitussive:* Assess type, severity, frequency of cough, and production. Increase fluid intake and environmental humidity to lower viscosity of lung secretions.

INTERVENTION/EVALUATION:

Monitor vital signs q15–30min after parenteral administration (monitor for decreased B/P, change in rate or quality of pulse). Increase fluid intake and environmental humidity to improve viscosity of lung secretions. Palpate bladder for urinary retention. Monitor pattern of daily bowel activity and stool consistency. Initiate deep breathing and coughing exercises, particularly in those w/impaired pulmonary function. Assess for clinical improvement; record onset of relief of pain or cough.

PATIENT/FAMILY TEACHING:

Discomfort may occur w/ injection. Change positions slowly to avoid orthostatic hypotension. Avoid tasks that require alertness, motor skills until response to drug is established. Tolerance/dependence may occur w/prolonged use of high doses. Avoid alcohol. Report shortness of breath or breathing difficulty.

---

colchicine

coal-cheh-seen
(Colchicine)

CANADIAN AVAILABILITY: Colchicine

CLASSIFICATION

Antigout

AVAILABILITY (Rx)

Tablets: 0.5 mg, 0.6 mg. **Injection:** 1 mg.

PHARMACOKINETICS

Rapidly absorbed from GI tract. Highest concentration in liver, spleen, kidney. Re-enters intestinal tract (biliary secretion), reabsorbed from intestines. Partially metabolized in liver. Eliminated primarily in feces.

ACTION/*THERAPEUTIC EFFECT*

Decreases leukocyte motility, phagocytosis, lactic acid production, *resulting in decreased urate crystal deposits, inflammatory process.*

USES/*UNLABELED*

Treatment of attacks of acute gouty arthritis, prophylaxis of recurrent gouty arthritis. *Reduce frequency of familial Mediterranean fever, treatment of acute attacks of calcium pyrophosphate, deposition, sarcoid arthritis, amyloidosis, biliary cirrhosis, recurrent pericarditis.*

PO/IV ADMINISTRATION

PO:
   May give w/o regard to meals.

IV:

Note: SubQ or IM administration produces severe local reaction. Use via IV route only.
   1. Administer over 2–5 min.
   2. May dilute w/0.9% NaCl or sterile water for injection.
   3. Do not dilute w/5% dextrose.

INDICATIONS/DOSAGE/ROUTES

Acute gouty arthritis:
PO: Adults, elderly: 0.5–1.2 mg, then 0.5–0.6 mg q1–2h or 1–1.2 mg q2h until pain relieved or nausea, vomiting, or diarrhea occurs. Total dose: 4–8 mg.
IV: Adults, elderly: Initially, 2 mg, then 0.5 mg q6h until satisfactory response. **Maximum:** 4 mg/24 hrs or 4 mg/one course of treatment. **Note:** If pain recurs, may give 1–2 mg/day for several days but no sooner than 7 days after a full course of IV therapy (4 mg).

Chronic gouty arthritis:
PO: Adults, elderly: 0.5–0.6 mg once weekly up to once daily (dependent on number of attacks per year).

PRECAUTIONS

CONTRAINDICATIONS: Severe gastrointestinal, renal, hepatic, or cardiac disorders; blood dyscrasias. **CAUTIONS:** Impaired hepatic function, elderly, debilitated. **PREGNANCY/LACTATION:** Unknown if drug crosses placenta or is distributed in breast milk. **Pregnancy Category D.**

INTERACTIONS

DRUG INTERACTIONS: NSAIDs may increase risk of neutropenia, thrombocytopenia, bone marrow depression. Bone marrow depressants may increase risk of blood dyscrasias. **ALTERED LAB VALUES:** May decrease platelet count. May increase SGOT (AST), alkaline phosphatase.

SIDE EFFECTS

Note: Those w/impaired renal function may exhibit myopathy and neuropathy manifested as generalized weakness. **FREQUENT:** *Oral:* Nausea, vomiting, abdominal discomfort. **OCCASIONAL:** *Oral:* Anorexia. **RARE:** Hypersensitivity reaction, including angioedema. *Parenteral only:* Nausea, vomiting, diarrhea, abdominal discomfort, pain/redness at injection site, neuritis in injected arm.

ADVERSE REACTIONS/TOXIC EFFECTS

Bone marrow depression (aplastic anemia, agranulocytosis, thrombocytopenia) may occur w/long-term therapy. Overdose: *Initially:* Burning feeling in throat/skin, severe diarrhea, abdominal pain. *Secondly:* Fever, seizures, delirium, renal damage (hematuria, oliguria). *Third stage:* Hair loss, leukocytosis, stomatitis.

NURSING IMPLICATIONS
BASELINE ASSESSMENT:

Instruct pt to drink 8–10 glasses (8 oz) of fluid daily while on medication. Medication should be discontinued if any GI symptoms occur. Periodic CBC should be performed routinely in those receiving long-term therapy.

INTERVENTION/EVALUATION:

Discontinue medication immediately if GI symptoms occur. Encourage high fluid intake (3,000 ml/day). Monitor I&O (output should be at least 2,000 ml/day). Assess CBC, serum uric acid levels. Assess for therapeutic response (reduced joint tenderness, swelling, redness, limitation of motion).

PATIENT/FAMILY TEACHING:

Encourage low-purine food intake, to drink 8–10 glasses (8 oz) of fluid daily while on medication. Report skin rash, sore throat, fever, unusual bruising/bleeding, weakness, tiredness, numbness. Stop medication as soon as gout pain is relieved or at first sign of nausea, vomiting, or diarrhea.

---

colestipol
(Cholestid)
See Classification section under: Antihyperlipidemics

---

colfosceril palmitate
kol-**foss**-er-ill
(Exosurf)

CANADIAN AVAILABILITY: Exosurf

CLASSIFICATION

Lung surfactant

AVAILABILITY (Rx)

Powder for Injection: 108 mg

ACTION/*THERAPEUTIC EFFECT*

Lowers surface tension on alveolar surfaces during respiration, stabilizes alveoli vs. collapse that may occur at resting pulmonary pressures. *Replenishes surfactant, restores surface activity to lungs.*

USES

Prophylactic use in infants <1,350 g at risk of developing RDS, infants >1,350 g w/evidence of pulmonary immaturity; treatment in infants w/RDS.

STORAGE/HANDLING

Store vials at room temperature. After reconstitution, stable for 12 hrs.

INTRATRACHEAL ADMINISTRATION

1. Reconstitute immediately prior to use w/8 ml preservative-free sterile water for injection. Refer to manufacturer's instructions.
2. Do not use if vacuum in vial not present.
3. Instill through catheter inserted into infant's endotracheal tube. Do not instill into main stem bronchus.
4. Stop administration if reflux into endotracheal tube occurs. If needed, increase peak inspiratory pressure on ventilator by 4–5 cm H_2O until tube clears.
5. Stop administration if transcutaneous oxygen saturation decreases. If needed, increase peak inspiratory pressure on ventilator by 4–5 cm H_2O for 1–2 min. May also need to increase FiO_2 for 1–2 min.

INDICATIONS/DOSAGE/ROUTES

Prophylaxis for RDS:
Intratracheal: Neonates: 5 ml/kg given as two 2.5 ml/kg doses as soon as possible after birth. May repeat 12 and 24 hrs later in infants remaining on mechanical ventilator.

RDS rescue:
Intratracheal: Neonates: 5 ml/kg given as two 2.5 ml/kg doses. Repeat in 12 hrs in all infants remaining on ventilator.

PRECAUTIONS

CONTRAINDICATIONS: None significant. **CAUTIONS:** Those at risk for circulatory overload.

INTERACTIONS

DRUG INTERACTIONS: None significant. **ALTERED LAB VALUES:** None significant.

SIDE EFFECTS

OCCASIONAL: Gagging. **RARE:** Apnea, bradycardia, tachycardia.

ADVERSE REACTIONS/TOXIC EFFECTS

Failure to reduce peak ventilator inspiratory pressures after chest expansion, after dosing, may result in lung overdistension and fatal pulmonary air leak. Failure to reduce transcutaneous oxygen saturation if in excess of 95% by decreasing FiO_2 in small but repeated steps until saturation is 90% to 95% may result in hyperoxia. Failure to reduce ventilator if arterial or transcutaneous CO_2 measurements are <30 may result in hypocarbia, reducing brain blood flow.

NURSING IMPLICATIONS
BASELINE ASSESSMENT:

Drug must be administered in highly supervised setting. Clinicians in care of neonate must be experienced w/intubation, ventilator management. Give emotional support to parents. Suctioning infant before dosing may decrease chance of mucous plugs obstructing endotracheal tube.

INTERVENTION/EVALUATION:

Monitor infant w/arterial or transcutaneous measurement of systemic O_2 and CO_2. Maintain vigilant clinical attention to neonate prior to, during, and after drug administration. Assess lung sounds for rales and moist breath sounds. If chest expansion improves dramatically after dosing, reduce peak ventilator inspiratory pressures immediately (failure to do so may result in lung overdistension and fatal pulmonary air leak). If transcutaneous oxygen saturation >95% and neonate appears pink, reduce FiO_2 in small but repeated steps until saturation is 90% to 95% (failure to do so may result in hyperoxia). If arterial or transcutaneous CO_2 measurements are <30, reduce ventilator immediately (failure to do so may result in hypocarbia, reducing brain blood flow).

conjugated estrogens

ess-troe-jenz
(Cenestin, Premarin)

FIXED-COMBINATION(S):

W/meprobamate, a tranquilizer (**Milprem**); Premarin w/methyltestosterone, an androgen, w/medroxyprogesterone, a progestin (**Premphase, Prempro**).

CANADIAN AVAILABILITY:
C.E.S., Congest, Premarin

CLASSIFICATION

Estrogen

AVAILABILITY (Rx)

Tablets: 0.3 mg, 0.625 mg, 0.9 mg, 1.25 mg, 2.5 mg. **Injection:** 25 mg. **Vaginal Cream.**

PHARMACOKINETICS

Well absorbed from GI tract. Widely distributed. Metabolized in liver. Primarily excreted in urine.

ACTION/*THERAPEUTIC EFFECT*

Increases synthesis of DNA, RNA, and various proteins in responsive tissues. Reduces release of gonadotropin-releasing hormone, reducing follicle-stimulating hormone (FSH) and luteinizing hormone (LH). *Promotes vasomotor stability, maintains genitourinary function, normal growth, development of female sex organs. Prevents accelerated bone loss by inhibiting bone resorption, restoring balance of bone resorption and formation. Inhibits LH, decreases serum concentration of testosterone.*

USES/*UNLABELED*

Management of moderate to severe vasomotor symptoms associated w/menopause. Treatment of atrophic vaginitis, kraurosis vulvae, female hypogonadism and castration, primary ovarian failure. Retardation of osteoporosis in postmenopausal women. Palliative treatment of inoperable, progressive cancer of the prostate in men and of the breast in postmenopausal women. *Prevents estrogen deficiency–induced premenopausal osteoporosis. Cream: Prevention of nosebleeds.*

STORAGE/HANDLING

Keep tablets at room temperature. Refrigerate vials for IV use. Reconstituted solution stable for 60 days refrigerated. Do not use if solution darkens or precipitate forms.

PO/IV ADMINISTRATION

PO:

1. Administer at the same time each day.
2. Give w/milk or food if nausea occurs.

IV:

1. Reconstitute w/5 ml sterile water for injection containing benzyl alcohol (diluent provided).
2. Slowly add diluent, shaking gently. Avoid vigorous shaking.
3. Give slowly to prevent flushing reaction.

INDICATIONS/DOSAGE/ROUTES

Vasomotor symptoms associated w/menopause, atrophic vaginitis, kraurosis vulvae:
PO: Adults, elderly: 0.3–1.25 mg/day cyclically (21 days on; 7 days off). If pt is menstruating, begin on 5th day of cycle; if pt not menstruating within previous 2 mos, start arbitrarily.
Intravaginal: Adults, elderly: 2–4 g/day cyclically.

Female hypogonadism:
PO: Adults: 2.5–7.5 mg/day in divided doses for 20 days; rest 10 days. If bleeding occurs prior to 10th drug-free day, a 20 day estrogen-progestin regimen given for 20 days, w/progestin given during last 5 days of estrogen therapy. If menstruation begins prior to completing the estrogen-progestin regimen, discontinue therapy, reinstitute on 5th day of menstruation.

Female castration, primary ovarian failure:
PO: Adults: Initially, 1.25 mg/day cyclically.

Osteoporosis:
PO: Adults, elderly: 0.3–0.625 mg/day, cyclically.

Breast cancer:
PO: Adults, elderly: 10 mg 3 times/day for at least 3 mos.

Prostate cancer:
PO: Adults, elderly: 1.25–2.5 mg 3 times/day.

Abnormal uterine bleeding:
IM/IV: Adults: 25 mg, may repeat once in 6–12 hrs.

PRECAUTIONS

CONTRAINDICATIONS: Known or suspected breast cancer (except select pts w/metastasis), estrogen-dependent neoplasia; undiagnosed abnormal genital bleeding; active thrombophlebitis or thromboembolic disorders; history of thrombophlebitis, thrombosis, or thromboembolic disorders w/previous estrogen use, hypersensitivity to estrogen. CAUTIONS: Conditions that may be aggravated by fluid retention: cardiac, renal, or hepatic dysfunction, epilepsy, migraine, mental depression, metabolic bone disease w/potential hypercalcemia, history of jaundice during pregnancy, strong family history of breast cancer, fibrocystic disease or breast nodules, children in whom bone growth is not complete. PREGNANCY/LACTATION: Distributed in breast milk. May be harmful to fetus. Not for use during lactation. Pregnancy Category X.

INTERACTIONS

DRUG INTERACTIONS: May interfere w/effects of bromocriptine. May increase concentration of cyclosporine, increase hepatic, nephrotoxicity. Hepatotoxic medications may increase hepatotoxicity. **ALTERED LAB VALUES:** May affect metapyrone, thyroid function tests. May decrease cholesterol, LDH. May increase calcium, glucose, HDL, triglycerides.

SIDE EFFECTS

FREQUENT: Change in vaginal bleeding (spotting, breakthrough), breast pain/tenderness, gynecomastia. **OCCASIONAL:** Headache, increased B/P, intolerance to contact lenses. *High-dose therapy:* Anorexia, nausea. **RARE:** Loss of scalp hair, clinical depression.

ADVERSE REACTIONS/TOXIC EFFECTS

Prolonged administration may increase risk of gallbladder, thromboembolic disease, and breast, cervical, vaginal, endometrial, and liver carcinoma.

NURSING IMPLICATIONS
BASELINE ASSESSMENT:

Question hypersensitivity to estrogen, previous jaundice, or thromboembolic disorders associated w/pregnancy or estrogen therapy. Establish baseline B/P, blood glucose.

INTERVENTION/EVALUATION:

Assess blood pressure periodically. Check for swelling, weigh daily. Monitor blood glucose q.i.d. for pts w/diabetes. Promptly report signs and symptoms of thromboembolic or thrombotic disorders: sudden severe headache, shortness of breath, vision or speech disturbance, weakness or numbness of an extremity, loss of coordination, pain in chest, groin, or leg. Note estrogen therapy on specimens.

PATIENT/FAMILY TEACHING:

Need for medical supervision. Avoid smoking due to increased risk of heart attack or blood clots. Explain importance of diet and exercise when taken to retard osteoporosis. Do not take other medications w/o physician approval. Teach how to perform Homan's test, signs and symptoms of blood clots (report these to physician immediately). Also notify physician of abnormal vaginal bleeding, depression, other symptoms. Teach female pts to perform breast self-exam. Avoid exposure to sun or ultraviolet light. Check weight daily; report weekly gain of >5 lbs. Stop taking medication and contact physician if suspect pregnancy. Give labeling from drug package.

corticorelin
(Acthrel)
See Supplement

corticotropin injection
kore-tih-koe-**troe**-pin
(ACTH, Acthar)

corticotropin repository
(Cortigel, Cortrophin-Gel, Acthar Gel)

CLASSIFICATION

Adrenocorticotropic hormone

AVAILABILITY (Rx)

Powder for Injection: 25 units,

40 units. **Repository Injection:** 40 units/ml, 80 units/ml.

PHARMACOKINETICS

Rapid absorption from IM/SubQ sites (respiratory forms have delayed absorption). Widely distributed.

ACTION/ *THERAPEUTIC EFFECT*

Stimulates adrenal cortex to secrete cortisol, corticosterone, aldosterone and androgenic substances. Acts to stimulate synthesis of adrenocortical hormones. *Suppresses immune response, inflammation.*

USES

Diagnostic testing of adrenocortical function. Limited therapeutic value in conditions responsive to corticosteroid therapy. May be used in hypercalcemia of cancer, acute exacerbations of multiple sclerosis, nonsuppurative thyroiditis.

STORAGE/HANDLING

Refrigerate repository dosage forms. After reconstitution, corticotropin injection is stable for 24 hrs if refrigerated.

IM/IV/SUBQ ADMINISTRATION

Assess for hypersensitivity reaction during first 15 minutes of IV administration or immediately following IM or SubQ injection.

IM/SubQ:

1. Repository corticotropin may be given SubQ or IM for prolonged effects.

2. Reconstitute in 0.9% sodium chloride solution or sterile water for injection to produce final volume of 1–2 ml.

IV:

1. Give IV only for diagnostic use or in adults w/idiopathic thrombocytopenic purpura.

2. For IV infusion, further dilute in 0.9% NaCl, 5% dextrose, or 5% dextrose in 0.9% NaCl solutions.

INDICATIONS/DOSAGE/ROUTES

Note: May give IM, SubQ. IV only for corticotropin injection; IM only for corticotropin zinc hydroxide.

Diagnostic testing:
IV: Adults: 10–25 units in 500 ml D_5W infused over 8 hrs.
IM/SubQ: Adults: 20 units 4 times/day.

Acute exacerbation of multiple sclerosis:
IM: Adults: 80–120 units/day for 2–3 wks.

Infantile spasms:
IM: Infants: 20–40 units/day or 80 units every other day for 3 mos (or 1 mo after cessation of seizures).

Usual repository injection dosage:
IM/SubQ: Adults: 40–80 units q24–72h.

PRECAUTIONS

CONTRAINDICATIONS: Hypersensitivity to any corticosteroid or porcine proteins, systemic fungal infection, peptic ulcers (except life-threatening situations), scleroderma, primary adrenocortical insufficiency. Avoid live virus vaccine; long-term therapy in children. **CAUTIONS:** Thromboembolic disorders, history of tuberculosis (may reactivate disease), hypothyroidism, cirrhosis, nonspecific ulcerative colitis, CHF, hypertension, psychosis, renal insufficiency, seizures. Prolonged therapy should be discontinued slowly. **PREGNANCY/LACTATION:** Unknown if distributed in breast milk. May have embryocidal effects. Nursing contraindicated. **Pregnancy Category C**.

INTERACTIONS

DRUG INTERACTIONS: Amphotericin may increase hypokalemia. May decrease effect of oral hypoglycemics, insulin, diuretics, potassium supplements. May increase digoxin toxicity (due to hypokalemia). Hepatic enzyme inducers may decrease effect. Live virus vaccines may potentiate virus replication, increase vaccine side effects, decrease pt's antibody response to vaccine. **ALTERED LAB VALUES:** May decrease calcium, potassium, thyroxine. May increase cholesterol, lipids, glucose, sodium, amylase.

SIDE EFFECTS

FREQUENT: Insomnia, heartburn, nervousness, abdominal distension, increased sweating, acne, mood swings, increased appetite, facial flushing, delayed wound healing, increased susceptibility to infection, diarrhea/constipation. **OCCASIONAL:** Headache, edema, change in skin color, frequent urination. **RARE:** Tachycardia, allergic reaction (rash, hives), pain, redness, swelling at injection site, psychic changes, hallucinations, depression.

ADVERSE REACTIONS/TOXIC EFFECTS

Long-term therapy: Hypocalcemia, hypokalemia, muscle wasting (esp. arms, legs), osteoporosis, spontaneous fractures, amenorrhea, cataracts, glaucoma, peptic ulcer, CHF. *Abrupt withdrawal following long-term therapy:* Anorexia, nausea, fever, headache, joint pain, rebound inflammation, fatigue, weakness, lethargy, dizziness, orthostatic hypertension.

NURSING IMPLICATIONS

BASELINE ASSESSMENT:

Question for hypersensitivity to any of the corticosteroids. Obtain baseline values for weight, B/P, glucose, cholesterol, electrolytes. Check results of initial tests, e.g., TB skin test, x-rays, EKG.

INTERVENTION/EVALUATION:

Monitor I&O, daily weight; assess for edema. Check B/P, temperature, respirations, pulse at least b.i.d. Be alert to infection (reduced immune response): sore throat, fever, or vague symptoms. Evaluate bowel activity. Monitor electrolytes. Watch for hypocalcemia (muscle twitching, cramps, positive Trousseau's or Chvostek's signs) or hypokalemia (weakness and muscle cramps, numbness/tingling esp. lower extremities, nausea and vomiting, irritability, EKG changes.) Assess emotional status, ability to sleep.

PATIENT/FAMILY TEACHING:

Carry identification of drug and dose, physician's name and phone number. Do not change dose/schedule or stop taking drug, *must* taper off under medical supervision. Notify physician of fever, sore throat, muscle aches, sudden weight gain/swelling. W/dietician, give instructions for prescribed diet (usually sodium restricted w/high vitamin D, protein, and potassium). Maintain careful personal hygiene, avoid exposure to disease or trauma. Severe stress (serious infection, surgery, or trauma) may require increased dosage. Do not take aspirin or any other medication w/o consulting physician. Follow-up visits, lab tests are necessary; children must be assessed for growth retardation. Inform dentist or other physicians of cortisone therapy now or within past 12 months.

cortisone acetate

kore-tih-zone
(Cortone Acetate)

CANADIAN AVAILABILITY:
Cortone

CLASSIFICATION

Corticosteroid

AVAILABILITY (Rx)

Tablets: 5 mg, 10 mg, 25 mg

PHARMACOKINETICS

Rapid, complete absorption from GI tract. Widely distributed. Primarily metabolized in liver to hydrocortisone. Primarily excreted in urine. Half-life: 30 min.

ACTION/*THERAPEUTIC EFFECT*

Inhibits accumulation of inflammatory cells at inflammation sites, phagocytosis, lysosomal enzyme release and synthesis and/or release of mediators of inflammation. *Prevents/suppresses cell-mediated immune reactions.*

Decreases/prevents tissue response to inflammatory process.

USES

Substitution therapy in deficiency states: acute/chronic adrenal insufficiency, congenital adrenal hyperplasia, adrenal insufficiency secondary to pituitary insufficiency.

Nonendocrine disorders: arthritis, rheumatic carditis, allergic, collagen, intestinal tract, liver, ocular, renal, and skin diseases, bronchial asthma, cerebral edema, malignancies.

PO ADMINISTRATION

1. Give w/milk or food (decreases GI upset).
2. Single doses given prior to 9 AM; multiple doses at evenly spaced intervals.

INDICATIONS/DOSAGE/ROUTES

Note: Individualize dose based on disease, pt, and response.

Usual oral dosage:
PO: Adults: Initially 25–300 mg/day. **Maintenance:** Lowest dosage that maintains adequate clinical response.

Usual elderly dosage:
PO: Use lowest effective dosage.

PRECAUTIONS

CONTRAINDICATIONS: Hypersensitivity to any corticosteroid, systemic fungal infection, peptic ulcers (except life-threatening situations). Avoid live virus vaccine. **CAUTIONS:** Thromboembolic disorders, history of tuberculosis (may reactivate disease), hypothyroidism, cirrhosis, nonspecific ulcerative colitis, CHF, hypertension, psychosis, renal insufficiency, seizure disorders. Prolonged therapy should be discontinued slowly. **PREGNANCY/LACTATION:** Drug crosses placenta, distributed in breast milk. May cause cleft palate (chronic use first trimester). Nursing contraindicated. **Pregnancy Category D.**

INTERACTIONS

DRUG INTERACTIONS: Amphotericin may increase hypokalemia. May decrease effect of oral hypoglycemics, insulin, diuretics, potassium supplements. May increase digoxin toxicity (due to hypokalemia). Hepatic enzyme inducers may decrease effect. Live virus vaccines may potentiate virus replication, increase vaccine side effects, decrease pt's antibody response to vaccine. **ALTERED LAB VALUES:** May decrease calcium, potassium, thyroxine. May increase cholesterol, lipids, glucose, sodium, amylase.

SIDE EFFECTS

FREQUENT: Insomnia, heartburn, nervousness, abdominal distension, increased sweating, acne, mood swings, increased appetite, facial flushing, delayed wound healing, increased susceptibility to infection, diarrhea/constipation. **OCCASIONAL:** Headache, edema, change in skin color, frequent urination. **RARE:** Tachycardia, allergic reaction (rash, hives), psychic changes, hallucinations, depression.

ADVERSE REACTIONS/TOXIC EFFECTS

Long-term therapy: Hypocalcemia, hypokalemia, muscle wasting (esp. arms, legs), osteoporosis, spontaneous fractures, amenorrhea, cataracts, glaucoma, peptic ulcer, CHF. *Abrupt withdrawal following long-term therapy:* Anorex-

ia, nausea, fever, headache, joint pain, rebound inflammation, fatigue, weakness, lethargy, dizziness, orthostatic hypertension.

NURSING IMPLICATIONS
BASELINE ASSESSMENT:

Question for hypersensitivity to any of the corticosteroids. Obtain baseline values for weight, B/P, glucose, cholesterol, electrolytes. Check results of initial tests, e.g., TB skin test, x-rays, EKG.

INTERVENTION/EVALUATION:

Monitor I&O, daily weight; assess for edema. Check B/P, temperature, respirations, pulse at least b.i.d. Be alert to infection (reduced immune response): sore throat, fever, or vague symptoms. Evaluate bowel activity. Monitor electrolytes. Watch for hypocalcemia (muscle twitching, cramps, positive Trousseau's or Chvostek's signs) or hypokalemia (weakness and muscle cramps, numbness/tingling esp. lower extremities, nausea and vomiting, irritability, EKG changes). Assess emotional status, ability to sleep.

PATIENT/FAMILY TEACHING:

Carry identification of drug and dose, physician's name and phone number. Do not change dose/schedule or stop taking drug, *must* taper off under medical supervision. Notify physician of fever, sore throat, muscle aches, sudden weight gain/swelling. W/dietician, give instructions for prescribed diet (usually sodium restricted w/high vitamin D, protein, and potassium). Maintain careful personal hygiene, avoid exposure to disease or trauma. Severe stress (serious infection, surgery, or trauma) may require increased dosage. Do not take aspirin or any other medication w/o consulting physician. Follow-up visits, lab tests are necessary; children must be assessed for growth retardation. Inform dentist or other physicians of cortisone therapy now or within past 12 months.

cosyntropin
koe-syn-**troe**-pin
(Cortrosyn)

CANADIAN AVAILABILITY:
Cortrosyn

CLASSIFICATION
Adrenocorticotropic hormone

AVAILABILITY (Rx)
Powder for Injection: 0.25 mg

PHARMACOKINETICS
Rapid absorption from IM/SubQ sites. Widely distributed.

ACTION
Increases endogenous corticoid synthesis. Stimulates initial reaction in synthesis of adrenal steroids from cholesterol. Other effects due to generated endogenous corticosteroids.

USES
Diagnostic testing of adrenocortical function.

IM/IV ADMINISTRATION
1. Reconstitute by adding 1 ml of 0.9% NaCl injection to a 0.25 mg vial of cosyntropin to produce solution of 0.25 mg/ml.

2. For IV infusion, dilute w/5% dextrose or 0.9% NaCl and infuse at rate of 0.04 mg/hr over 6 hrs.

INDICATIONS/DOSAGE/ROUTES
Screening test for adrenal function:
IM: Adults: 0.25–0.75 mg one time. **Children (<2 yrs):** 0.125 mg one time.
IV infusion: Adults: 0.25 mg in 5% dextrose or 0.9% NaCl, infuse at rate of 0.04 mg/hr.

PRECAUTIONS
CONTRAINDICATIONS: Hypersensitivity to cosyntropin or corticotropin. **CAUTIONS:** (Short duration for diagnostic use does not produce effects of long-term corticotropin therapy). **PREGNANCY/LACTATION:** Nursing not recommended. **Pregnancy Category C.**

INTERACTIONS
DRUG INTERACTIONS: None significant. **ALTERED LAB VALUES:** None significant.

SIDE EFFECTS
OCCASIONAL: Nausea, vomiting. **RARE:** Hypersensitivity reaction (fever, pruritus).

ADVERSE REACTIONS/TOXIC EFFECTS
None significant.

NURSING IMPLICATIONS
BASELINE ASSESSMENT:
Question for hypersensitivity to cosyntropin or corticotropin. Hold cortisone, hydrocortisone, or spironolactone on the test day. Assure that baseline plasma cortisol concentration has been

drawn prior to start of test, or 24 hour urine for 17-KS or 17-OHCS is initiated.

INTERVENTION/EVALUATION:

Assess for pruritus, rash, or other sign of hypersensitivity reaction. Adhere to time frame for blood draws; monitor collection of urine if indicated.

PATIENT/FAMILY TEACHING:

Explain the procedure and purpose of the test.

co-trimoxazole (sulfamethoxazole-trimethoprim)

koe-try-**mox**-oh-zole
(Bactrim, Cotrim, Septra, Sulfamethoprim)

FIXED-COMBINATION(S):

W/sulfamethoxazole, a sulfonamide and trimethoprim, a folate antagonist

CANADIAN AVAILABILITY:

Apo-Sulfatrim, Bactrim, Novotrimel, Septra

CLASSIFICATION

Anti-infective

AVAILABILITY (Rx)

Tablets: 80 mg trimethoprim/400 mg sulfamethoxazole; 160 mg/800 mg. **Oral Suspension:** 40 mg/200 mg. **Injection:** 80 mg/400 mg per 5 ml.

PHARMACOKINETICS

Rapid, well absorbed from GI tract. Widely distributed. Metabolized in liver. Excreted in urine. Half-life: 6–12 hrs (trimethoprim 8–10 hrs). Half-life increased in decreased renal function.

ACTION/*THERAPEUTIC EFFECT*

Blocks bacterial synthesis of essential nucleic acids, *producing bactericidal action in susceptible microorganisms.*

USES/*UNLABELED*

Acute/complicated and recurrent/chronic urinary tract infection, *Pneumocystis carinii* pneumonia, shigellosis, enteritis, otitis media, chronic bronchitis, traveler's diarrhea. Prophylaxis of *Pneumocystis carinii* pneumonia. *Treatment of biliary tract, bone/joint, chancroid, bacterial endocarditis, chlamydial infection, gonorrhea, intra-abdominal, meningitis, sinusitis, septicemia, skin/soft tissue.*

STORAGE/HANDLING

Store tablets, suspension at room temperature. IV infusion (piggyback) stable for 2–6 hrs (use immediately); discard if cloudy or precipitate forms.

PO/IV ADMINISTRATION

Note: Space doses evenly around the clock.

PO:

1. Administer on empty stomach w/8 oz water.
2. Give several extra glasses of water/day.

IV:

For IV infusion (piggyback), dilute each 5 ml w/75 –125 ml 5% dextrose.

1. Do not mix w/other drugs or solutions.
2. Infuse over 60–90 min. Must avoid bolus or rapid infusion.
3. Do not give IM.
4. Assure adequate hydration.

INDICATIONS/DOSAGE/ROUTES

Note: Potency expressed in terms of trimethoprim content.

UTI, enteritis, acute otitis media:
PO: Adults, elderly: 160 mg q12h for 7–14 days. **Children >2 mos:** 7.5–8 mg/kg/day q12h for 5–10 days.

Severe UTI, enteritis:
IV: Adults, elderly, children >2 mos: 8–10 mg/kg/day in 2–4 equally divided doses q6–12h for 5–14 days. **Maximum:** 960 mg/day.

Pneumocystis carinii pneumonia:
PO: Adults, elderly, children >2 mos: 20 mg/kg/day in 4 divided doses q6h.
IV: Adults, elderly, children >2 mos: 15–20 mg/kg/day in 3–4 divided doses q6–8h.

Prevention of Pneumocystis carinii pneumonia:
PO: Adults: 160 mg/day. **Children:** 150 mg/m²/day on 3 consecutive days/wk.

Traveler's diarrhea:
PO: Adults, elderly: 160 mg q12h for 5 days.

Acute exacerbation of chronic bronchitis:
PO: Adults, elderly: 160 mg q12h for 14 days.

Dosage in renal impairment:
The dose and/or frequency is modified based on severity of infection, degree of renal impairment, and serum concentration of drug. For those w/creatinine clearance of 15–30 ml/min, a reduction in dose of 50% is recommended.

PRECAUTIONS

CONTRAINDICATIONS: Hypersensitivity to trimethoprim or any sulfonamides, megaloblastic anemia due to folate deficiency, infants <2 mos. Not for treatment of streptococcal pharyngitis. **CAUTIONS:** Elderly, impaired renal or hepatic function, history of severe allergy or bronchial asthma (allergic reaction to metabisulfite in injection more likely), AIDS (higher incidence of adverse reactions). **PREGNANCY/LACTATION:** Contraindicated during pregnancy at term and lactation. Readily crosses placenta; distributed in breast milk. May produce kernicterus in newborns. **Pregnancy Category C**.

INTERACTIONS

DRUG INTERACTIONS: May increase, prolong effects, increase toxicity w/warfarin, hydantoin anticonvulsants, oral hypoglycemics. May increase risk of toxicity w/other hemolytics. Hepatotoxic medications may increase risk of hepatotoxicity. Methenamine may form precipitate. May increase effect of methotrexate. **ALTERED LAB VALUES:** May increase SGOT (AST), SGPT (ALT), alkaline phosphatase, BUN, creatinine, potassium.

SIDE EFFECTS

FREQUENT: Anorexia, nausea, vomiting, rash (generally 7–14 days after therapy begins), urticaria. **OCCASIONAL:** Diarrhea, abdominal pain, local pain/irritation at IV site. **RARE:** Headache, vertigo, insomnia, seizures, hallucinations, depression.

ADVERSE REACTIONS/TOXIC EFFECTS

Rash, fever, sore throat, pallor, purpura, cough, shortness of breath may be early signs of serious adverse reactions. Fatalities are rare but have occurred in sulfonamide therapy following Stevens-Johnson syndrome, toxic epidermal necrolysis, fulminant hepatic necrosis, agranulocytosis, aplastic anemia, other blood dyscrasias. Elderly are at increased risk of adverse reactions: bone marrow suppression, decreased platelets, severe dermatologic reactions.

NURSING IMPLICATIONS
BASELINE ASSESSMENT:

Check history for hypersensitivity to trimethoprim or any sulfonamide, sulfite sensitivity, severe allergy or bronchial asthma. Obtain specimens for diagnostic tests before giving first dose (therapy may begin before results are known). Determine renal, hepatic, hematologic baselines.

INTERVENTION/EVALUATION:

Evaluate food tolerance. Determine pattern of bowel activity. Assess skin for rash, pallor, purpura. Check IV site, flow rate. Monitor renal, hepatic, hematology reports. Assess I&O. Check for CNS symptoms: headache, vertigo, insomnia, hallucinations. Monitor vital signs at least twice a day. Watch for cough or shortness of breath. Assess for overt bleeding, bruising, or swelling.

PATIENT/FAMILY TEACHING:

Continue medication for full length of therapy. Space doses evenly around the clock. Take oral doses w/8 oz water and drink several extra glasses of water daily. Notify physician of new symptoms immediately, especially rash or other skin changes, bleeding or bruising, fever, sore throat.

cromolyn sodium
krom-oh-lin
(Crolom, Gastrocom, Intal, Nasalcrom, Opticrom)

CANADIAN AVAILABILITY:
Apo-Cromolyn, Intal, Nalcrom, Opticrom

CLASSIFICATION
Antiasthmatic, antiallergic, mast cell stabilizer

AVAILABILITY (Rx)
Oral Concentrate, Capsules for Inhalation: 20 mg. **Solution for Nebulization:** 20 mg amp. **Aerosol Spray:** 800 mcg/spray. **Nasal Spray (OTC):** 40 mg/ml. **Capsules (oral):** 100 mg. **Ophthalmic Solution:** 4%.

PHARMACOKINETICS
Minimal absorption following oral, inhalation, or nasal administration. Absorbed portion excreted in urine or via biliary elimination.

ACTION/*THERAPEUTIC EFFECT*
Possesses no direct antihistaminic, anti-inflammatory properties. *Prevents release of mast cells (e.g., histamine) after exposure to allergens that produces allergic reaction.*

USES
Prophylactic management of severe bronchial asthma, exercise-induced bronchospasm, perennial or seasonal allergic rhinitis, symptomatic treatment of systemic mastocytosis. *Ophthalmic:* conjunctivitis.

INHALATION/NASAL/ORAL/ OPHTHALMIC ADMINISTRATION

INHALATION:

1. Shake container well; exhale completely; then holding mouthpiece 1 inch away from lips, inhale and hold breath as long as possible before exhaling.

2. Wait 1–10 min before inhaling 2nd dose (allows for deeper bronchial penetration).

3. Rinse mouth w/water immediately after inhalation (prevents mouth/throat dryness).

NEBULIZATION, INHALATION CAPSULES: Inhalation capsules are not to be swallowed; instruct patient on use of Spinhaler.

OPHTHALMIC:

1. Place finger on lower eyelid and pull out until pocket is formed between eye and lower lid. Hold dropper above pocket and place prescribed number of drops in pocket. Instruct pt to close eyes gently so medication will not be squeezed out of sac.

2. Apply gentle finger pressure to the lacrimal sac at inner canthus for 1 min following installation (lessens risk of systemic absorption).

ORAL CAPSULES:

1. Give at least 30 min before meals.

2. Pour contents of capsule in hot water, stirring until completely dissolved; add equal amount cold water while stirring.

3. Do not mix w/fruit juice, milk, or food.

NASAL:

1. Nasal passages should be clear (may require nasal decongestant).

2. Inhale through nose.

INDICATIONS/DOSAGE/ROUTES

Asthma:
   Oral Inhalation: Adults, elderly, children >2 yrs (oral solution), children >5 yrs (oral powder): 20 mg 4 times/day.

Prevention of bronchospasm:
Oral Inhalation: Adults, elderly, children >2 yrs (oral solution), children >5 yrs (oral powder): 20 mg not longer than 1 hr before exercise or exposure to precipitating factor.

Allergic rhinitis:
Intranasal: Adults, elderly, children >6 yrs: 1 spray each nostril 3–4 times/day. May increase up to 6 times/day.

Systemic mastocytosis:
PO: Adults, elderly, children >12 yrs: 200 mg 4 times/day. **Children 2–12 yrs:** 100 mg 4 times/day. **Children <2 yrs:** 20 mg/kg/day in 4 divided doses.

Usual ophthalmic dose:
Ophthalmic: Adults, elderly: 1–2 drops in both eyes 4–6 times/day.

PRECAUTIONS

CONTRAINDICATIONS: None significant. **CAUTIONS:** Impaired renal or hepatic function. **PREGNANCY/LACTATION:** Unknown if drug crosses placenta or is distributed in breast milk. **Pregnancy Category B.**

INTERACTIONS

DRUG INTERACTIONS: None significant. **ALTERED LAB VALUES:** None significant.

SIDE EFFECTS

FREQUENT: *Inhalation:* Cough, dry mouth/throat, stuffy nose, throat irritation, unpleasant taste. *Nasal:* Burning, stinging, irritation of nose, increased sneezing. *Ophthalmic:* Burning, stinging of eye. *Oral:* Headache, diarrhea. **OCCASION-ALLY:** *Inhalation:* Bronchospasm, hoarseness, watering eyes. *Nasal:* Cough, headache, unpleasant taste, postnasal drip. *Ophthalmic:* Increased watering/itching of eye. *Oral:* Skin rash, abdominal pain, joint pain, nausea, insomnia. **RARE:** *Inhalation:* Dizziness, painful urination, muscle/joint pain, skin rash. *Nasal:* Nosebleeds, skin rash. *Ophthalmic:* Chemosis (edema of conjunctiva), eye irritation.

ADVERSE REACTIONS/TOXIC EFFECTS

Nasal, oral, inhalation: Anaphylaxis occurs rarely.

NURSING IMPLICATIONS
BASELINE ASSESSMENT:

Offer emotional support (high incidence of anxiety due to difficulty in breathing and sympathomimetic response to drug).

INTERVENTION/EVALUATION:

Monitor rate, depth, rhythm, type of respiration; quality and rate of pulse. Assess lung sounds for rhonchi, wheezing, rales. Monitor arterial blood gases. Observe lips, fingernails for blue or dusky color in light-skinned patients; gray in dark-skinned patients. Observe for clavicular retractions, hand tremor. Evaluate for clinical improvement (quieter, slower respirations, relaxed facial expression, cessation of clavicular retractions).

PATIENT/FAMILY TEACHING:

Increase fluid intake (decreases lung secretion viscosity). Do not take more than 2 inhalations at any one time (excessive use may produce paradoxical bronchoconstriction or a decreased bronchodilating effect). Rinsing mouth with water immediately after inhalation may prevent mouth/throat dryness. Effect of therapy dependent on administration at regular intervals.

---

cyanocobalamin (vitamin B$_{12}$)

sye-ah-no-koe-**bal**-a-min
(Rubramin PC, Crysti-12, Cyanoject, Cyomin, Nascobal)

hydroxocobalamin (vitamin B$_{12}$a)

(Hydrobexan, Hydro-Cobex)

FIXED-COMBINATION(S):

W/liver extract, 10 mcg/ml (**liver injection**); w/liver excrete crude, 2 mcg/ml; vitamin B$_{12}$ w/intrinsic factor (**Ciopar Forte**).

CANADIAN AVAILABILITY:
Rubramin

CLASSIFICATION

Vitamin, antianemic

AVAILABILITY (Rx)

Tablets: 25 mcg, 50 mcg, 100 mcg, 250 mcg, 500 mcg, 1,000 mcg. **Injection:** 100 mcg/ml, 1,000 mcg/ml. **Nasal Gel:** 500 mcg/spray.

PHARMACOKINETICS

Absorbed in lower half of ileum in presence of calcium. Initially bound to intrinsic factor; this complex passes down intestine, binding to receptor sites on ileal mucosa. In presence of calcium, absorbed systemically. Metabolized in liver. Eliminated via biliary excretion. Half-life: 6 days.

ACTION/THERAPEUTIC EFFECT

Coenzyme for metabolic functions (fat, carbohydrate metabolism, protein synthesis). *Necessary for growth, cell replication, hematopoiesis, and myelin synthesis.*

USES

Prophylaxis, treatment of pernicious anemia, vitamin B$_{12}$ deficiency due to inadequate diet or intestinal malabsorption, hemolytic anemia, hyperthyroidism, malignancy of pancreas, bowel, gastrectomy, GI lesions, neurologic damage, malabsorption syndrome, vegetarians, breast-fed infants, metabolic disorders, prolonged stress, chronic fever, renal disease. Deficiency generally occurs concurrently w/other B-vitamin deficiencies.

PO ADMINISTRATION

Give w/meals (increases absorption).

INDICATIONS/DOSAGE/ROUTES

Deficiency:
SubQ/IM: Adults, elderly: Initially, 100 mcg/day for 6–7 days, then every other day for 7 doses, then every 3–4 days for 2–3 wks. **Maintenance:** 100–200 mcg every month. **Children:** Initially, 30–50 mcg/day for at least 2 wks. **Maintenance:** 100 mcg every month.

Usual nasal dosage:
Adults, elderly: 500 mcg (1 spray) every week (after deficiency corrected).

Supplement:
PO: Adults, elderly: 1–25 mcg/day.

Children >1 yr: 1 mcg/day. **Children <1 yr:** 0.3 mcg/day.

PRECAUTIONS

CONTRAINDICATIONS: History of allergy to cobalamin, folate deficient anemia, hereditary optic nerve atrophy. **CAUTIONS:** None significant. **PREGNANCY/LACTATION:** Crosses placenta; excreted in breast milk. **Pregnancy Category A**. (Category C if used at doses greater than RDA.)

INTERACTIONS

DRUG INTERACTIONS: Alcohol, colchicine may decrease absorption. Ascorbic acid may destroy vitamin B$_{12}$. Folic acid (large doses) may decrease concentration. **ALTERED LAB VALUES:** None significant.

SIDE EFFECTS

OCCASIONAL: Diarrhea, itching.

ADVERSE REACTIONS/TOXIC EFFECTS

Rare allergic reaction generally due to impurities in preparation. May produce peripheral vascular thrombosis, pulmonary edema, hypokalemia, CHF.

NURSING IMPLICATIONS
INTERVENTION/EVALUATION:

Assess for CHF, pulmonary edema, hypokalemia in cardiac pts receiving SubQ/IM therapy. Monitor potassium levels (3.5–5 mEq/L), serum B$_{12}$ (200–800 pg/ml), rise in reticulocyte count (peaks in 5–8 days). Assess for reversal of deficiency symptoms: hyporeflexia, loss of positional sense, ataxia, fatigue, irritability, insomnia, anorexia, pallor, palpitation on exertion. Therapeutic response to treatment usually dramatic within 48 hrs.

C

PATIENT/FAMILY TEACHING:

Lifetime treatment may be necessary w/pernicious anemia. Report symptoms of infection. Foods rich in vitamin B$_{12}$ include organ meats, clams, oysters, herring, red snapper, muscle meats, fermented cheese, dairy products, egg yolks.

cyclobenzaprine hydrochloride

cy-klow-**benz**-ah-preen
(Flexeril)

CANADIAN AVAILABILITY:
Flexeril, Novo-Cycloprine

CLASSIFICATION

Skeletal muscle relaxant

AVAILABILITY (Rx)

Tablet: 10 mg

PHARMACOKINETICS

	ONSET	PEAK	DURATION
PO	1 hr	3–4 hrs	12–24 hrs

Well (slow) absorbed from GI tract. Metabolized in GI tract, liver. Primarily excreted in urine. Half-life: 1–3 days.

ACTION/*THERAPEUTIC EFFECT*

Acts within CNS at brain stem, *relieving local skeletal muscle spasm.*

USES/*UNLABELED*

For short-term (2–3 wks) use as adjunct to rest, physical therapy, other measures for relief of discomfort due to acute, painful musculoskeletal conditions. *Treatment of fibromyalgia.*

INDICATIONS/DOSAGE/ROUTES

Note: Do not use longer than 2–3 wks.

Acute, painful musculoskeletal conditions:
PO: Adults, elderly: 10 mg 3 times/day. **Range:** 20–40 mg/day in 2–4 divided doses. **Maximum:** 60 mg/day.

PRECAUTIONS

CONTRAINDICATIONS: Concurrent use of MAO inhibitors or within 14 days after their discontinuation, acute recovery phase of MI, those w/arrhythmias, heart blocks or conduction disturbances, CHF, hyperthyroidism. **CAUTIONS:** Impaired renal or hepatic function, history of urinary retention, angle-closure glaucoma, increased intraocular pressure. **PREGNANCY/LACTATION:** Unknown if drug crosses placenta or is distributed in breast milk. **Pregnancy Category B.**

INTERACTIONS

DRUG INTERACTIONS: Tricyclic antidepressants, CNS depression-producing medications may increase CNS depression. MAO inhibitors may increase risk of hypertensive crisis, severe seizures. **ALTERED LAB VALUES:** None significant.

SIDE EFFECTS

FREQUENT (>10%): Drowsiness (39%), dry mouth (27%), dizziness (11%). **RARE (1–3%):** Fatigue, tiredness, asthenia, blurred vision, headache, nervousness, confusion, nausea, constipation, dyspepsia, unpleasant taste.

ADVERSE REACTIONS/TOXIC EFFECTS

Overdosage may result in visual hallucinations, hyperactive reflexes, muscle rigidity, vomiting, hyperpyrexia.

NURSING IMPLICATIONS

BASELINE ASSESSMENT:

Record onset, type, location, and duration of muscular spasm. Check for immobility, stiffness, swelling.

INTERVENTION/EVALUATION:

Assist w/ambulation at all times. Evaluate for therapeutic response: decreased intensity of skeletal muscle pain/tenderness, improved mobility, decrease in stiffness.

PATIENT/FAMILY TEACHING:

Drowsiness usually diminishes w/continued therapy. Avoid tasks that require alertness, motor skills until response to drug is established. Avoid alcohol or other depressants while taking medication. Avoid sudden changes in posture. Sugarless gum, sips of water may relieve dry mouth.

cyclophosphamide

sigh-klo-**phos**-fah-mide
(Cytoxan, Neosar)

CANADIAN AVAILABILITY:
Cytoxan, Procytox

CLASSIFICATION

Antineoplastic

AVAILABILITY (Rx)

Tablets: 25 mg, 50 mg. **Powder for Injection:** 100 mg, 200 mg, 500 mg, 1 g, 2 g.

PHARMACOKINETICS

Well absorbed from GI tract. Crosses blood-brain barrier. Metabolized in liver to active metabolites. Primarily excreted in urine. Half-life: 3–12 hrs.

ACTION/ THERAPEUTIC EFFECT

Inhibits DNA, RNA protein synthesis by cross-linking w/DNA, RNA strands, *inhibiting protein synthesis, preventing cell growth.* Potent immunosuppressant.

USES/ UNLABELED

Treatment of Hodgkin's disease, non-Hodgkin's lymphomas, multiple myeloma, leukemia (acute lymphoblastic, acute myelogenous, acute monocytic, chronic granulocytic, chronic lymphocytic), mycosis fungoides, disseminated neuroblastoma, adenocarcinoma of ovary, retinoblastoma, carcinoma of breast. Biopsy-proven "minimal change" nephrotic syndrome in children. *Treatment of carcinoma of lung, cervix, endometrium, bladder, prostate, testicles, osteosarcoma, germ cell ovarian tumors, rheumatoid arthritis, systemic lupus erythematosus.*

STORAGE/HANDLING

Note: May be carcinogenic, mutagenic, or teratogenic. Handle w/extreme care during preparation/administration.

Solutions prepared w/bacteriostatic water for injection for IV use are stable for 24 hrs at room temperature, 6 days if refrigerated.

PO/IV ADMINISTRATION

PO: Give on an empty stomach. If GI upset occurs, give w/food.

IV:

   1. For IV injection, reconstitute each 100 mg w/5 ml sterile water for injection or bacteriostatic water for injection to provide concentration of 20 mg/ml.
   2. Shake to dissolve. Allow to stand until clear.
   3. May give by IV injection or further dilute w/5% dextrose, 0.9% NaCl, or other compatible fluid for IV infusion.
   4. IV may produce faintness, facial flushing, diaphoresis, oropharyngeal sensation.

INDICATIONS/DOSAGE/ROUTES

Note: Dosage individualized based on clinical response, tolerance to adverse effects. When used in combination therapy, consult specific protocols for optimum dosage, sequence of drug administration.

Malignant diseases:
PO: Adults, children: 1–5 mg/kg/day.
IV: Adults, children: 40–50 mg/kg in divided doses over 2–5 days; or 10–15 mg/kg q7–10 days or 3–5 mg/kg 2 times/wk.

Biopsy-proven "minimal change" nephrotic syndrome:
PO: Children: 2.5–3 mg/kg/day for 60–90 days.

PRECAUTIONS

CONTRAINDICATIONS: None significant. **CAUTIONS:** Severe leukopenia, thrombocytopenia, tumor infiltration of bone marrow, previous therapy w/other antineoplastic agents, radiation. **PREGNANCY/LACTATION:** If possible, avoid use during pregnancy. May cause malformations (limb abnormalities, cardiac anomalies, hernias). Distributed in breast milk. Breast-feeding not recommended. **Pregnancy Category D.**

INTERACTIONS

DRUG INTERACTIONS: May decrease effect of antigout medications. Allopurinol, bone marrow depressants may increase bone marrow depression. Cytarabine may increase cardiomyopathy. Immunosuppressants may increase risk of infection, development of neoplasms. Live virus vaccines may potentiate virus replication, increase vaccine side effects, decrease pt's antibody response to vaccine. **ALTERED LAB VALUES:** May increase uric acid.

SIDE EFFECTS

EXPECTED: Marked leukopenia 8–15 days after initial therapy. **FREQUENT:** Nausea, vomiting begins about 6 hrs after administration and lasts about 4 hrs; alopecia (33%). **OCCASIONAL:** Diarrhea, darkening of skin/fingernails, mucosal irritation, oral ulceration, headache, diaphoresis. **RARE:** Anaphylactic reaction, hemorrhagic colitis, pain/redness at injection site, stomatitis.

ADVERSE REACTIONS/TOXIC EFFECTS

   Major toxic effect is bone marrow depression resulting in hematologic toxicity (leukopenia, anemia, thrombocytopenia, hypoprothrombinemia). Thrombocytopenia may occur 10–15 days after drug initiation. Anemia generally occurs after large doses or prolonged therapy. Hemorrhagic cystitis occurs commonly in long-term therapy (esp. in children). Pulmonary fibrosis, cardiotoxicity noted w/high doses. Amenorrhea, azoospermia, hyperkalemia may also occur.

NURSING IMPLICATIONS
BASELINE ASSESSMENT:

Obtain WBC count weekly during therapy or until maintenance dose is established, then at intervals of 2–3 wks.

INTERVENTION/EVALUATION:

Monitor serum uric acid concentration, hematologic status. Monitor WBC closely during initial therapy (at least 3,000–4,000 cells/mm³ should be maintained). Assess urine output for hematuria (hemorrhagic cystitis). Assess pattern of daily bowel activity and stool consistency. Monitor for hematologic toxicity (fever, sore throat, signs of local infection, easy bruising or unusual bleeding from any site), symptoms of anemia (excessive tiredness, weakness). Recovery from marked leukopenia due to bone marrow depression can be expected in 17–28 days.

PATIENT/FAMILY TEACHING:

Encourage copious fluid intake and frequent voiding (assists in preventing cystitis) at least 24 hrs before, during, after therapy. Do not have immunizations w/o physician's approval (drug lowers body's resistance). Avoid contact w/those who have recently received live virus vaccine. Promptly report fever, sore throat, signs of local infection, easy bruising or unusual bleeding from any site. Alopecia is reversible, but new hair growth may have different color or texture. Contact physician if nausea/vomiting continue at home.

cyclosporine
sigh-klo-**spore**-in
(Neoral, Restasis, Sandimmune, Sang Cya)

CANADIAN AVAILABILITY:
Neoral, Sandimmune

CLASSIFICATION

Immunosuppressant

AVAILABILITY (Rx)

Capsules: 25 mg, 100 mg. **Oral Solution:** 100 mg/ml (in 50 ml calibrated liquid measuring device). **IV Solution:** 50 mg/ml (5 ml amps). **Ophthalmic Emulsion:** 0.05%.

PHARMACOKINETICS

Variably absorbed from GI tract. Widely distributed. Metabolized in liver. Eliminated primarily by biliary/fecal excretion. Half-life: adults 10–27 hrs, children 7–19 hrs.

ACTION/ THERAPEUTIC EFFECT

Inhibits interleukin-2, a proliferative factor needed for T cell activity. *Inhibits both cellular and humoral immune responses.*

USES/ UNLABELED

Prevents rejection of kidney, liver, heart in combination w/steroid therapy. Treatment of chronic allograft rejection in those previously treated w/other immunosuppressives. Capsules/solution: Treatment of severe, active rheumatoid arthritis, psoriasis. *Treatment of alopecia areata, aplastic anemia, atopic dermatitis, Behçet's disease, biliary cirrhosis, corneal transplantation.*

STORAGE/HANDLING

Store capsules, oral solution, parenteral form at room temperature. Protect IV solution from light. After diluted, stable for 24 hrs. Avoid refrigeration of oral solution (separation of solution may occur). Discard oral solution after 2 mos once bottle is opened.

PO/IV ADMINISTRATION

Note: Oral solution available in bottle form w/calibrated liquid measuring device. Oral form should replace IV administration as soon as possible.

PO:

1. Oral solution may be mixed in glass container w/milk, chocolate milk, or orange juice (preferably at room temperature). Stir well. Drink immediately. Grapefruit/grapefruit juice may interfere w/metabolism.

2. Add more diluent to glass container and mix w/remaining solution to ensure total amount is given.

3. Dry outside of calibrated liquid measuring device before replacing in cover. Do not rinse w/water.

IV:

1. Dilute each ml concentrate w/20–100 ml 0.9% NaCl or 5% dextrose.

2. Infuse over 2–6 hrs.

3. Monitor pt continuously for first 30 min after instituting infusion and frequently thereafter for hypersensitivity reaction (see Side Effects).

INDICATIONS/DOSAGE/ROUTES

Note: May be given w/adrenal corticosteroids, but not w/other immunosuppressive agents (increases susceptibility to infection, development of lymphoma).

Prevention of allograft rejection:
PO: Adults, elderly, children: Initially, 15 mg/kg as single dose 4–12 hrs prior to transplantation, continue daily dose of 10–14 mg/kg/day for 1–2 wks. Taper dose by 5%/wk over 6–8 wks. **Maintenance:** 5–10 mg/kg/day.

IV: Adults, elderly, children: Give about one-third of oral dose: 5–6 mg/kg as single dose 4–12 hrs prior to transplantation, continue this daily single dose until pt is able to take oral medication.

Psoriasis, rheumatoid arthritis:
PO: Adults: 2.5 mg/kg daily in 2 divided doses.

PRECAUTIONS

CONTRAINDICATIONS: History of hypersensitivity to cyclosporine or polyoxyethylated castor oil. **CAUTIONS:** Impaired hepatic, renal, cardiac function, malabsorption syndrome, pregnancy, chickenpox, herpes zoster, infection, hypokalemia. **PREGNANCY/LACTATION:** Readily crosses placenta, distributed in breast milk. Avoid nursing. **Pregnancy Category C.**

INTERACTIONS

DRUG INTERACTIONS: Cimetidine, danazol, diltiazem, erythromycin, ketoconazole may increase concentration, risk of hepatotoxicity, nephrotoxicity; ACE inhibitors, potassium-sparing diuretics, potassium supplements may cause hyperkalemia. Immunosuppressants may increase risk of infection, lymphoproliferative disorders. Lovastatin may increase risk of rhabdomyolysis, acute renal failure. Live virus vaccines may potentiate virus replication, increase vaccine side effects, decrease pt's antibody response to vaccine. **ALTERED LAB VALUES:** May increase BUN, creatinine, SGOT (AST), SGPT (ALT), alkaline phosphatase, amylase, bilirubin, uric acid, potassium. May decrease magnesium.

SIDE EFFECTS

FREQUENT (12–26%): Mild to moderate hypertension (26%), increased hair growth [hirsutism]

(21%), tremor (12%). **OCCASIONAL (2–4%):** Acne, cramping, gingival hyperplasia (bleeding, tender gums), paresthesia, diarrhea, nausea, vomiting, headache. **RARE (<1%):** Flushing, abdominal discomfort, gynecomastia, sinusitis.

ADVERSE REACTIONS/TOXIC EFFECTS

Mild nephrotoxicity occurs in 25% of renal transplants after transplantation, 38% in cardiac transplants, and 37% of liver transplants, respectively. Hepatotoxicity occurs in 4% of renal, 7% of cardiac, and 4% of liver transplants, respectively. Both toxicities usually responsive to dosage reduction. Severe hyperkalemia, hyperuricemia occur occasionally.

NURSING IMPLICATIONS
BASELINE ASSESSMENT:

Note that if nephrotoxicity occurs, mild toxicity is generally noted 2–3 mos after transplantation; more severe toxicity noted early after transplantation; hepatotoxicity may be noted during first month after transplantation.

INTERVENTION/EVALUATION:

Diligently monitor BUN, creatinine, bilirubin, SGOT (AST), SGPT (ALT), LDH blood serum levels for evidence of hepatotoxicity or nephrotoxicity (mild toxicity noted by slow rise in serum levels; more overt toxicity noted by rapid rise in levels; hematuria also noted). Assess potassium level for evidence of hyperkalemia. Encourage diligent oral hygiene (gum hyperplasia). Monitor B/P for evidence of hypertension.

PATIENT/FAMILY TEACHING:

Essential to repeat blood testing on a routine basis while receiving medication. Headache, tremor may occur as a response to medication. Avoid grapefruit, grapefruit juice (increases concentration, side effects).

---

cyproheptadine hydrochloride

sigh-pro-**hep**-tah-deen
(Periactin)

CANADIAN AVAILABILITY:
Periactin

CLASSIFICATION

Antihistamine

AVAILABILITY (Rx)

Tablets: 4 mg. **Syrup:** 2 mg/5 ml.

PHARMACOKINETICS

Well absorbed from GI tract. Metabolized in liver. Primarily eliminated in feces.

ACTION/*THERAPEUTIC EFFECT*

Competes w/histamine at histaminic receptor sites, *relieving allergic conditions (urticaria, pruritus)*. Anticholinergic effects cause drying of nasal mucosa.

USES/*UNLABELED*

Relief of nasal allergies, allergic dermatitis, cold urticaria, hypersensitivity reactions. *Stimulates appetite in underweight pts, those w/anorexia nervosa. Treatment of vascular cluster headaches.*

PO ADMINISTRATION

1. Give w/o regard to meals.
2. Scored tablets may be crushed.

INDICATIONS/DOSAGE/ROUTES

Allergic condition:
PO: Adults, children >15 yrs: 4 mg 3 times/day. May increase dose but do not exceed 0.5 mg/kg/day. **Children 7–14 yrs:** 4 mg 2–3 times/day, or 0.25 mg/kg daily in divided doses. **Children 2–6 yrs:** 2 mg 2-3 times/day, or 0.25 mg/kg daily in divided doses.

Usual elderly dosage:
PO: Initially, 4 mg 2 times/day.

PRECAUTIONS

CONTRAINDICATIONS: Acute asthmatic attack, pts receiving MAO inhibitors. **CAUTIONS:** Narrow-angle glaucoma, peptic ulcer, prostatic hypertrophy, pyloroduodenal or bladder neck obstruction, asthma, COPD, increased intraocular pressure, cardiovascular disease, hyperthyroidism, hypertension, seizure disorders. **PREGNANCY/LACTATION:** Unknown if drug crosses placenta or is distributed in breast milk. Increased risk of seizures in neonates, premature infants if used during third trimester of pregnancy. May prohibit lactation. **Pregnancy Category B**.

INTERACTIONS

DRUG INTERACTIONS: Alcohol, CNS depressants may increase CNS depressant effects. MAO inhibitors may increase anticholinergic, CNS depressant effects. **ALTERED LAB VALUES:** May suppress wheal, flare reactions to antigen skin testing, unless antihistamines discontinued 4 days prior to testing.

SIDE EFFECTS

FREQUENT: Drowsiness, dizziness, muscular weakness, dry mouth/nose/throat/lips, urinary retention, thickening of bronchial secretions. Sedation, dizziness, hypotension more likely noted in elderly. **OCCASIONAL:** Epigastric distress, flushing, visual disturbances, hearing disturbances, paresthesia, sweating, chills.

ADVERSE REACTIONS/TOXIC EFFECTS

Children may experience dominant paradoxical reaction (restlessness, insomnia, euphoria, nervousness, tremors). Overdosage in children may result in hallucinations, convulsions, death. Hypersensitivity reaction (eczema, pruritus, rash, cardiac disturbances, angioedema, photosensitivity) may occur. Overdosage may vary from CNS depression (sedation, apnea, cardiovascular collapse, death) to severe paradoxical reaction (hallucinations, tremor, seizures).

NURSING IMPLICATIONS

BASELINE ASSESSMENT:

If pt is undergoing allergic reaction, obtain history of recently ingested foods, drugs, environmental exposure, recent emotional stress. Monitor rate, depth, rhythm, type of respiration; quality and rate of pulse. Assess lung sounds for rhonchi, wheezing, rales.

INTERVENTION/EVALUATION:

Monitor B/P, especially in elderly (increased risk of hypotension). Monitor children closely for paradoxical reaction.

PATIENT/FAMILY TEACHING:

Tolerance to antihistaminic effect generally does not occur; tolerance to sedative effect may occur. Avoid tasks that require alertness, motor skills until response to drug is established. Dry mouth, drowsiness, dizziness may be an expected response of drug. Avoid alcoholic beverages during antihistamine therapy. Sugarless gum, sips of tepid water may relieve dry mouth. Coffee or tea may help reduce drowsiness.

---

cysteamine
(Cystagon)
See Supplement

---

cytarabine
sigh-**tar**-ah-bean
(Cytosar-U, Ara-C, DepoCyt)

CANADIAN AVAILABILITY:
Cytosar

CLASSIFICATION

Antineoplastic

AVAILABILITY (Rx)

Powder for Injection: 100 mg, 500 mg, 1 g, 2 g. **Injectable Sustained-release Formulation.**

PHARMACOKINETICS

Widely distributed, moderate amount crosses blood-brain barrier. Primarily excreted in urine. Half-life: 1–3 hrs.

ACTION/ *THERAPEUTIC EFFECT*

Converted intracellularly to nucleotide, *appears to inhibit DNA synthesis.* Cell cycle-specific for S phase of cell division. Potent immunosuppressive activity.

USES/ *UNLABELED*

Treatment of acute and chronic myelocytic leukemia, acute lymphocytic leukemia, meningeal leukemia, non-Hodgkin's lymphoma in children. *Treatment of Hodgkin's lymphoma, myelodysplastic syndrome.*

STORAGE/HANDLING

Note: May be carcinogenic, mutagenic, or teratogenic (embryonic deformity). Handle w/extreme care during preparation/administration.

Reconstituted solution stable for 48 hrs at room temperature. IV infusion solutions at concentration up to 0.5 mg/ml stable for 7 days at room temperature. Discard if slight haze develops.

SUBQ/IV/INTRATHECAL ADMINISTRATION

Note: May give SubQ, IV injection, IV infusion, or intrathecally.
1. Reconstitute 100 mg vial w/5 ml bacteriostatic water for injection w/benzyl alcohol (10 ml for 500 mg vial) to provide concentration of 20 mg/ml and 50 mg/ml, respectively.
2. Dose may be further diluted w/up to 1,000 ml 5% dextrose or 0.9% NaCl for IV infusion.
3. For intrathecal use, reconstitute vial w/preservative-free 0.9% NaCl or pt's spinal fluid. Dose usually administered in 5–15 ml of solution, after equivalent volume of CSF removed.

INDICATIONS/DOSAGE/ROUTES

Note: Dosage individualized based on clinical response, tolerance to adverse effects. When used in combination therapy, consult specific protocols for optimum dosage, sequence of drug administration. Modify dose when serious hematologic depression occurs.

Acute nonlymphocytic leukemia:
IV Infusion: Adults, children: (Combination): 100 mg/m²/day, days 1–7.
IV: Adults: 100 mg/m² q12h, days 1–7.

Acute lymphocytic leukemia:
Refer to specific protocol.

PRECAUTIONS

CONTRAINDICATIONS: None significant. **CAUTIONS:** Impaired hepatic function. **PREGNANCY/ LACTATION:** If possible, avoid use during pregnancy. May cause malformations. Unknown if distributed in breast milk. Breast feeding not recommended. **Pregnancy Category D.**

INTERACTIONS

DRUG INTERACTIONS: May decrease effect of antigout medications. Bone marrow depressants may increase bone marrow depression. Cyclophosphamide may increase cardiomyopathy risk. Live virus vaccines may potentiate virus replication, increase vaccine side effects, decrease pt's antibody response to vaccine. **ALTERED LAB VALUES:** May increase SGOT (AST), bilirubin, alkaline phosphatase, uric acid.

SIDE EFFECTS

FREQUENT: Nausea and vomiting, particularly after IV injection, rather than continuous IV infusion. **OCCASIONAL:** Diarrhea, anorexia, oral/anal inflammation, peripheral motor and sensory neuropathies w/high-dose therapy, abdominal pain, esophagitis, nausea, vomiting, fever, transient headache w/intrathecal administration.

ADVERSE REACTIONS/TOXIC EFFECTS

Major toxic effect is bone marrow depression resulting in hematologic toxicity (leukopenia, anemia, thrombocytopenia, megaloblastosis, reticulocytopenia), occurring minimally after single IV dose, but leukopenia, anemia, thrombocytopenia should be expected w/daily or continuous IV. Cytarabine syndrome (fever, myalgia, rash, conjunctivitis, malaise, chest pain), hyperuricemia may be noted. High-dose therapy may produce severe CNS, GI, pulmonary toxicity.

NURSING IMPLICATIONS
BASELINE ASSESSMENT:

Obtain WBC, platelet count before and periodically during therapy. Leukocyte count decreases within 24 hrs after initial dose, continues to decrease for 7–9 days followed by brief rise at 12 days, then decreases again at 15–24 days, then rises rapidly for next 10 days. Platelet count decreases 5 days after drug initiation to low count at 12–15 days, then rises rapidly for next 10 days.

INTERVENTION/EVALUATION:

Monitor WBC, differential, platelet count for evidence of bone marrow depression. Monitor for hematologic toxicity (fever, sore throat, signs of local infection, easy bruising, or unusual bleeding from any site), symptoms of anemia (excessive tiredness, weakness). Monitor for signs of neuropathy (gait disturbances, handwriting difficulties, numbness).

PATIENT/FAMILY TEACHING:

Increase fluid intake (may protect against hyperuricemia). Do not have immunizations w/o physician's approval (drug lowers body's resistance). Avoid contact w/those who have recently received live virus vaccine. Promptly report fever, sore throat, signs of local infection, easy bruising or unusual bleeding from any site. Contact physician if nausea/vomiting continue at home.

---

dacarbazine

day-**car**-bah-zeen
(DTIC-Dome)

CANADIAN AVAILABILITY:
DTIC

CLASSIFICATION

Antineoplastic

AVAILABILITY (Rx)

Powder for Injection: 10 mg/ml

PHARMACOKINETICS

Minimally crosses blood-brain barrier. Metabolized in liver. Excreted in urine. Half-life: 5 hrs (increased in decreased renal function).

ACTION/ THERAPEUTIC EFFECT

Cell cycle-phase nonspecific. Some activity and toxicity results from activation of drug by hepatic enzymes. Forms carbonium ions, *inhibiting DNA, RNA synthesis.*

USES/ UNLABELED

Treatment of metastatic malignant melanoma, 2nd line therapy of Hodgkin's disease. *Treatment of soft tissue sarcoma.*

STORAGE/HANDLING

Note: May be carcinogenic, mutagenic, or teratogenic. Handle w/

extreme care during preparation administration.

Protect from light; refrigerate vials. Color change from ivory to pink indicates decomposition; discard. Solutions containing 10 mg/ml stable for 8 hrs at room temperature or 72 hrs if refrigerated. Solutions diluted w/up to 500 ml 5% dextrose or 0.9% NaCl stable for at least 8 hrs at room temperature or 24 hrs if refrigerated.

IV ADMINISTRATION

Note: May give by IV injection or IV infusion.

1. Reconstitute 100 mg vial w/9.9 ml sterile water for injection (19.7 ml for 200 mg vial) to provide concentration of 10 mg/ml.

2. Give IV injection over 1–2 min.

3. For IV infusion, further dilute w/up to 250 ml 5% dextrose or 0.9% NaC1. Infuse over 15–30 min.

4. Apply hot packs to relieve local pain, burning sensation, irritation at injection site.

5. Avoid extravasation (stinging, swelling, coolness, slight or no blood return at injection site).

INDICATIONS/DOSAGE/ROUTES

Note: Dosage individualized based on clinical response, tolerance to adverse effects. When used in combination therapy, consult specific protocols for optimum dosage, sequence of drug administration.

Malignant melanoma:
IV: Adults, elderly: 2–4.5 mg/kg/day for 10 days, repeated at 4 wk intervals, or 250 mg/m^2 daily for 5 days, repeated q3wks.

Hodgkin's disease:
IV: Adults, elderly: Combination

therapy: 150 mg/m^2 daily for 5 days, repeated q4 wks, or 375 mg/m^2 once, repeated q15days.

PRECAUTIONS

CONTRAINDICATIONS: Demonstrated hypersensitivity to drug. **CAUTIONS:** Impaired hepatic function. **PREGNANCY/LACTATION:** If possible, avoid use during pregnancy, esp. first trimester. Breast-feeding not recommended. **Pregnancy Category C.**

INTERACTIONS

DRUG INTERACTIONS: Bone marrow depressants may enhance myelosuppression. Live virus vaccines may potentiate virus replication, increase vaccine side effects, decrease pt's antibody response to vaccine. **ALTERED LAB VALUES:** May increase SGOT (AST), SGPT (ALT), alkaline phosphatase, BUN.

SIDE EFFECTS

HIGH INCIDENCE: Nausea, vomiting, anorexia (occurs within 1 hr of initial dose, may last up to 12 hrs). **OCCASIONAL:** Facial flushing, paresthesia, alopecia, flulike syndrome (fever, myalgia, malaise), dermatologic reactions, CNS symptoms (confusion, blurred vision, headache, lethargy). **RARE:** Diarrhea, stomatitis (redness/burning of oral mucous membranes, gum/tongue inflammation), intractable nausea and vomiting, photosensitivity.

ADVERSE REACTIONS/TOXIC EFFECTS

Bone marrow depression resulting in hematologic toxicity (leukopenia, thrombocytopenia) generally appears 2–4 wks after last drug dose. Hepatotoxicity occurs rarely.

NURSING IMPLICATIONS

BASELINE ASSESSMENT:

Some clinicians recommend food/fluids be restricted 4–6 hrs before treatment; other clinicians believe good hydration to within 1 hr of treatment will avoid dehydration due to vomiting. Conflicting reports of effectiveness of administering antiemetics for nausea, vomiting.

INTERVENTION/EVALUATION

Monitor leukocyte, erythrocyte, platelet counts for evidence of bone marrow depression. Monitor for hematologic toxicity (fever, sore throat, signs of local infection, easy bruising, unusual bleeding from any site).

PATIENT/FAMILY TEACHING:

Tolerance to GI effects occurs rapidly (generally after 1–2 days treatment). Do not have immunizations w/o physician's approval (drug lowers body's resistance). Avoid contact w/those who have recently received live virus vaccine. Promptly report fever, sore throat, signs of local infection, easy bruising, unusual bleeding from any site. Contact physician if nausea/vomiting continues at home.

---

dacliximab
(Zenapax)
See Supplement

---

dactinomycin
dak-tin-oh-**my**-sin
(Cosmegen)

CANADIAN AVAILABILITY:
Cosmegen

CLASSIFICATION

Antineoplastic

AVAILABILITY (Rx)

Powder for Injection: 0.5 mg

PHARMACOKINETICS

Widely distributed. Does not cross blood-brain barrier. Extensive tissue binding. Primarily eliminated via biliary/fecal route. Half-life: 36 hrs.

ACTION / *THERAPEUTIC EFFECT*

Forms DNA complex, *inhibiting DNA-dependent RNA synthesis.* Actively growing cells are most sensitive to drug's action. Cell cycle-phase nonspecific.

USES / *UNLABELED*

Treatment of Wilms' tumor, rhabdomyosarcoma, Ewing's sarcoma, advanced nonseminomatous testicular carcinoma, sarcoma botryoides, metastatic and nonmetastatic choriocarcinoma. *Treatment of ovarian cancer, Kaposi's sarcoma, osteosarcoma, malignant melanoma.*

STORAGE / HANDLING

Note: May be carcinogenic, mutagenic, or teratogenic. Handle w/ extreme care during preparation/administration.

Prepare solution immediately before use. Discard unused portion. Solution should be clear, gold color.

IV ADMINISTRATION

Note: Give by IV injection or IV infusion. Wear protective gloves when handling drug.

1. Reconstitute 500 mcg vial w/1.1 ml sterile water for injection w/o preservative (avoids precipitate) to provide concentration of 500 mcg/ml.

2. For IV injection, administer over 1–3 min into tubing of running IV. Withdraw dose from vial w/one needle, use 2nd needle for injection.

3. For IV infusion, add up to 50 ml 5% dextrose or 0.9% NaCl and infuse over 20–30 min.

4. Extravasation usually produces immediate pain, severe local tissue damage. Aspirate as much infiltrated drug as possible; then infiltrate area w/hydrocortisone, sodium succinate injection (50–100 mg hydrocortisone), and/or isotonic sodium thiosulfate injection or ascorbic acid injection (1 ml of 5% injection). Apply cold compresses.

INDICATIONS / DOSAGE / ROUTES

Note: Dosage is individualized based on clinical response and tolerance to adverse effects. When used in combination therapy, consult specific protocols for optimum dosage and sequence of drug administration. Do not exceed 15 mcg/kg or 400–800 mcg/m²/day. Dosage for obese or edematous pts based on surface area. Repeat dosage at least at 3 wk intervals, provided all signs of toxicity have disappeared.

Usual dosage:
IV: Adults, elderly: 500 mcg/day for maximum of 5 days. **Children:** 15 mcg/kg/day (up to maximum of 500 mcg/day) for 5 days, or total dosage of 2.5 mg/m^2 in divided doses over 1 wk.

Isolation Perfusion: Adults, elderly: 50 mcg/kg for lower extremity or pelvis; 35 mcg/kg for upper extremity.

PRECAUTIONS

CONTRAINDICATIONS: Those w/chickenpox or herpes zoster. **CAUTIONS:** Within first 2 mos of radiation therapy. **PREGNANCY/ LACTATION:** If possible, avoid use during pregnancy, esp. first trimester. Breast-feeding not recommended. **Pregnancy Category C**.

INTERACTIONS

DRUG INTERACTIONS: May decrease effect of antigout medications. Bone marrow depressants may enhance myelosuppression. Live virus vaccines may potentiate virus replication, increase vaccine side effects, decrease pt's antibody response to vaccine. **ALTERED LAB VALUES:** May increase uric acid.

SIDE EFFECTS

FREQUENT: Nausea, vomiting, buccal/pharangeal/skin erythema, rash (particularly when combined w/radiation). **OCCASIONAL:** Anorexia, alopecia, abdominal distress.

ADVERSE REACTIONS/TOXIC EFFECTS

Bone marrow depression resulting in hematologic toxicity (leukopenia, thrombocytopenia, and to lesser extent, anemia, pancytopenia, reticulopenia, agranulocytosis, aplastic anemia). GI and oral mucosal toxicity may result in diarrhea, oral/GI ulceration, stomatitis, glossitis, esophagitis, pharyngitis.

NURSING IMPLICATIONS

BASELINE ASSESSMENT:

Obtain baseline hematologic results. Nausea/vomiting occurs a few hours after dosing, can last up to 24 hrs. Decrease in platelet count generally appears 1–7 days after last drug dose, reaches lowest count at 14–21 days, returns to normal within 21–25 days.

INTERVENTION/EVALUATION:

Monitor hematologic status, renal/hepatic function studies, serum uric acid level. Assess pattern of daily bowel activity and stool consistency. Monitor for hematologic toxicity (fever, sore throat, signs of local infection, easy bruising, or unusual bleeding from any site), symptoms of anemia (excessive tiredness, weakness). Assess skin for dermatologic effects.

PATIENT/FAMILY TEACHING:

Alopecia is reversible, but new hair growth may have different color or texture. Pain, redness may occur at injection site. Do not have immunizations w/o physician's approval (drug lowers body's resistance). Avoid contact w/those who have recently received live virus vaccine. Promptly report fever, sore throat, signs of local infection, easy bruising, unusual bleeding from any site. Increase fluid intake. Contact physician if nausea/vomiting continues at home.

dalteparin sodium

dawl-teh-pear-in
(Fragmin)

CANADIAN AVAILABILITY:
Fragmin

CLASSIFICATION

Anticoagulant

AVAILABILITY (Rx)

Solution: 2,500 anti-Factor Xa IU per 0.2 ml. **Single-Dose Syringe:** 5,000 IU single dose syringe **Multidose Vial:** 95,000 IU.

PHARMACOKINETICS

	ONSET	PEAK	DURATION
SubQ	—	4 hrs	—

Terminal half-life following SubQ administration: 3–5 hrs.

ACTION/ *THERAPEUTIC EFFECT*

Antithrombin; in presence of low molecular weight heparin, *produces anticoagulation* by inhibition of factor Xa and thrombin by antithrombin. Only slightly influences platelet aggregation, prothrombin time (PT), activated partial thromboplastin time (APTT).

USES

Treatment of unstable angina and non Q-wave myocardial infarction (MI) to prevent ischemic events. Prevention of deep vein thrombosis (DVT) in pts undergoing hip replacement or abdominal surgery who are at risk of thromboembolic complications. Those at risk are >40 yrs, obese, undergoing surgery under general anesthesia lasting >30 min, malignancy or history of DVT or pulmonary embolism.

STORAGE/HANDLING

Store at room temperature.

SubQ ADMINISTRATION

Note: Do not mix w/other injections or infusions. Do not give IM.

1. Instruct pt to lie down before administering by deep SubQ injection.

2. Inject in U-shaped area around the navel, upper outer side of thigh, or upper outer quadrangle of buttock.

3. Introduce entire length of needle ($^1/_2$ inch) into skin fold held between thumb and forefinger, holding skin fold during injection at a 45° to 90° angle.

4. Vary injection site daily.

INDICATIONS/DOSAGE/ROUTES

Prevent deep vein thrombosis:
SubQ: Adults: 2,500–5,000 IU each day, starting 1–2 hrs before surgery. Repeat once daily for 5–10 days postoperatively.

Prevention of ischemic events in unstable angina, non Q-wave MI:
SubQ: Adults, elderly: 120 IU/kg q12h (w/concurrent aspirin). **Maximum:** 10,000 IU.

PRECAUTIONS

CONTRAINDICATIONS: Active major bleeding, concurrent heparin therapy, thrombocytopenia associated w/positive in vitro test for antiplatelet antibody, hypersensitivity to dalteparin, heparin, or pork products. **CAUTIONS:** Conditions w/increased risk of hemorrhage, bacterial endocarditis, history of heparin-induced thrombocytopenia, impaired renal or hepatic function, uncontrolled arterial hypertension, history of recent GI ulceration and hemorrhage, hypertensive or diabetic retinopathy. **PREGNANCY/ LACTATION:** Use w/caution, particularly during last trimester, immediate postpartum period (increased risk of maternal hemorrhage). Unknown if distributed in breast milk. **Pregnancy Category B**.

INTERACTIONS

DRUG INTERACTIONS: Anticoagulants, platelet inhibitors may increase bleeding (use w/care). **ALTERED LAB VALUES:** Reversible increases in SGOT (AST), SGPT (ALT), alkaline phosphatase, lactate dehydrogenase (LDH).

SIDE EFFECTS

OCCASIONAL (3–7%): Hematoma at injection site. **RARE (<1%):** Hypersensitivity reaction (chills, fever, pruritus, urticaria, asthma, rhinitis, lacrimation, headache), mild, local skin irritation.

ADVERSE REACTIONS/TOXIC EFFECTS

Accidental overdosage may lead to bleeding complications ranging from local ecchymoses to major hemorrhage. Thrombocytopenia occurs rarely.

NURSING IMPLICATIONS
BASELINE ASSESSMENT:

Assess complete blood count, including platelet count. Determine initial B/P.

INTERVENTION/EVALUATION:

Periodically monitor CBC, platelet count, stool for occult blood (no need for daily monitoring in pts w/normal presurgical coagulation parameters). Assess for any sign of bleeding: bleeding at surgical site, hematuria, blood in stool, bleeding from gums, petechiae, bruising, bleeding from injection sites.

PATIENT/FAMILY TEACHING:

Usual length of therapy is 5–10 days. Report any sign of bleeding (as above). Do not take any OTC medication (esp. aspirin) w/o consulting physician. Report bleeding, bruising, dizziness or lightheadedness, rash, itching, fever, swelling, breathing difficulty. Rotate injection sites daily. Teach proper injection technique. Excessive bruising at injection site may be lessened by ice massage prior to injection.

---

danaparoid
(Orgaran)
See Supplement

---

danazol
dan-ah-zole
(Danocrine)

CANADIAN AVAILABILITY:
Cyclomen

CLASSIFICATION

Gonadotropin inhibitor

AVAILABILITY (Rx)

Capsules: 50 mg, 100 mg, 200 mg

PHARMACOKINETICS

Metabolized in liver. Excreted in urine. Half-life: 4.5 hrs.

ACTION/*THERAPEUTIC EFFECT*

As a gonadotropin inhibitor, suppresses the pituitary-ovarian axis *by inhibiting the output of pituitary gonadotropins.* In endometriosis, *causes atrophy of both normal and ectopic endometrial tissue, producing anovulation and amenorrhea.* For fibrocystic breast disease, follicle-stimulating hormone (FSH) and luteinizing hormone (LH) are depressed, *reducing the production of estrogen;* inhibits steroid synthesis and binding of steroids to their receptors in breast tissue. Increases serum levels of esterase inhibitor, *correcting biochemical deficiency as seen in hereditary angioedema.*

USES/*UNLABELED*

Palliative treatment of endometriosis, fibrocystic breast disease; prophylactic treatment of hereditary angioedema. *Treatment of gynecomastia, menorrhagia, precocious puberty.*

INDICATIONS/DOSAGE/ROUTES

Note: Initiate therapy during menstruation or when pt not pregnant.

Endometriosis:
PO: Adults: 200–800 mg/day in 2 divided doses for 3–9 mos.

Fibrocystic breast disease:
PO: Adults: 100–400 mg/day in 2 divided doses.

Hereditary angioedema:
PO: Adults: Initially, 200 mg 2–3 times/day. Decrease dose by 50% or less at 1–3 mo intervals. If attack occurs, increase dose by up to 200 mg/day.

PRECAUTIONS

CONTRAINDICATIONS: Hypersensitivity to danazol or ingredients. Undiagnosed abnormal genital bleeding; severe hepatic, renal, or cardiac impairment. **CAUTIONS:** Conditions aggravated by fluid retention (cardiac or renal disease, epilepsy, migraine, asthma). Possibility of carcinoma of the breast should be excluded prior to therapy. **PREGNANCY/LACTATION:** Contraindicated during pregnancy, breast-feeding. **Pregnancy Category X**.

INTERACTIONS

DRUG INTERACTIONS: May increase effect of oral anticoagulants. May decrease effect of insulin, oral hypoglycemics. May increase concentration, toxicity of cyclosporine. **ALTERED LAB VALUES:** May increase SGOT (AST), SGPT (ALT), glucose, LDL. May decrease HDL. May alter thyroid function tests.

SIDE EFFECTS

FREQUENT: *Females:* Amenorrhea, breakthrough bleeding/spotting, decreased breast size, increased weight, irregular menstrual period. **OCCASIONAL:** *Males/females:* Edema, rhabdomyolysis (muscle cramps, unusual fatigue), virilism (acne, oily skin), flushed skin, altered moods. **RARE:** *Males/females:* Hematuria, gingivitis, carpal tunnel syndrome, cataracts, severe headache, vomiting, rash, photosensitivity. *Females:* Enlarged clitoris, hoarseness, deepening voice, hair growth, monilial vaginitis. *Males:* Decreased testicle size.

ADVERSE REACTIONS/TOXIC EFFECTS

Jaundice may occur in those receiving 400 mg/day or more. Liver dysfunction, eosinophilia, thrombocytopenia, pancreatitis occur rarely.

NURSING IMPLICATIONS

BASELINE ASSESSMENT:

Inquire about menstrual cycle: Therapy should begin during menstruation. Establish baseline weight, B/P.

INTERVENTION/EVALUATION:

Weigh 2–3 times/week; report >5 lbs/wk gain or swelling of fingers or feet. Monitor B/P periodically. Check for jaundice (yellow eyes or skin, dark urine, clay-colored stools).

PATIENT/FAMILY TEACHING:

Patient should use nonhormonal contraceptive during therapy. Do not take drug, check w/physician if suspect pregnancy (risk to fetus). Importance of full length of therapy, regular visits to physician's office (hepatic function tests, etc.). Notify physician promptly of masculinizing effects (may not be reversible), weight gain, muscle cramps, or fatigue. Spotting or bleeding may occur in first months of therapy for endometriosis (does not mean lack of efficacy). In fibrocystic breast disease, irregular menstrual periods and amenorrhea may occur w/ or w/o ovulation.

dantrolene sodium

dan-trow-lean
(Dantrium)

CANADIAN AVAILABILITY:
Dantrium

CLASSIFICATION

Skeletal muscle relaxant

AVAILABILITY (Rx)

Capsules: 25 mg, 50 mg, 100 mg. **Powder for Injection:** 20 mg vial.

PHARMACOKINETICS

Poorly absorbed from GI tract. Metabolized in liver. Primarily excreted in urine. Half-life: IV 4–8 hrs; oral 8.7 hrs.

ACTION/*THERAPEUTIC EFFECT*

Reduces muscle contraction by interfering w/release of calcium ion, *dissociating excitation-contraction coupling.* Reduced calcium ion concentration, *interfering w/catabolic process associated w/malignant hyperthermic crisis.*

USES/*UNLABELED*

Oral: Relief of signs and symptoms of spasticity due to spiral cord injuries, stroke, cerebral palsy, multiple sclerosis, esp. flexor spasms, concomitant pain, clonus, and muscular rigidity. *Parenteral:* Management of fulminant hypermetabolism of skeletal muscle due to malignant hyperthermia crisis. *Treatment of neuroleptic malignant syndrome, relief of exercise-induced pain in patients w/muscular dystrophy, treatment of flexor spasms.*

STORAGE/HANDLING

Store oral, parenteral form at room temperature. Use within 6 hrs after reconstitution. Solution is clear, colorless. Discard if cloudy, precipitate formed.

PO/IV ADMINISTRATION

PO:

Give w/o regard to meals.

IV:

1. Diligently monitor for ex-travasation (high pH of IV preparation). May produce severe complications.

2. Reconstitute 20 mg vial w/60 ml sterile water for injection to provide concentration of 0.33 mg/ml.

3. For IV infusion, administer over 1 hr.

INDICATIONS/DOSAGE/ROUTES

Spasticity:
Note: Best to begin w/low-dose therapy, then increase gradually at 4–7 day intervals (reduces incidence of side effects).
PO: Adults, elderly: Initially, 25 mg/day. Increase to 25 mg 2–4 times/day, then by 25 mg increments up to 100 mg 2–4 times/day. **Children >5 yrs:** Initially, 0.5 mg/kg 2 times/day. Increase to 0.5 mg/kg 3–4 times/day, then increase by 0.5 mg/kg/day up to 3 mg/kg 2–4 times/day.

Prevention of malignant hyperthermia crisis:
PO: Adults, elderly, children: 4–8 mg/kg/day in 3–4 divided doses 1–2 days prior to surgery (last dose 3-4 hrs prior to surgery).
IV Infusion: Adults, elderly, children: 2.5 mg/kg about 1.25 hrs prior to surgery.

Management of hyperthermia crisis:
IV: Adults, elderly, children: Initially (minimum), 1 mg/kg rapid IV; may repeat up to total maximum dose of 10 mg/kg. May follow w/4–8 mg/kg/day orally in 4 divided doses up to 3 days after crisis.

PRECAUTIONS

CONTRAINDICATIONS: Oral: Active liver disease (i.e., hepatitis, cirrhosis), when spasticity is needed to maintain upright posture and balance when walking or to achieve or support increased function, severely impaired cardiac function, previous liver disease/dysfunction. **CAUTIONS:** Females, those >35 yrs of age, impaired liver, or pulmonary function. **PREGNANCY/LACTATION:** Readily crosses placenta; do not use in breast-feeding mothers. Pregnancy Category C.

INTERACTIONS

DRUG INTERACTIONS: CNS depressants may increase CNS depression (short-term use). Hepatotoxic medications may increase risk of hepatotoxicity (chronic use). **ALTERED LAB VALUES:** May alter liver function tests.

SIDE EFFECTS

Note: Effects are generally transient and appear during early treatment.
FREQUENT: Drowsiness, dizziness, weakness, general malaise, diarrhea. **OCCASIONAL:** Confusion, headache, insomnia, constipation, urinary frequency. **RARE:** Paradoxical CNS excitement/restlessness, paresthesia, tinnitus, slurred speech, tremor, blurred vision, dry mouth, diarrhea, nocturia, impotence.

ADVERSE REACTIONS/TOXIC EFFECTS

Risk of hepatotoxicity, most notably in females, those >35 yrs of age, those taking other medications concurrently. Overt hepatitis noted most frequently between 3rd and 12th mo of therapy. Overdosage results in vomiting, muscular hypotonia, muscle twitching, respiratory depression, seizures.

NURSING IMPLICATIONS
BASELINE ASSESSMENT:

Obtain baseline liver function

tests (SGOT [AST], SGPT [ALT], alkaline phosphatase, total bilirubin). Record onset, type, location, and duration of muscular spasm. Check for immobility, stiffness, swelling.

INTERVENTION/EVALUATION:

Assist w/ambulation at all times. For those on long-term therapy, liver/renal function tests, blood counts should be performed periodically. Evaluate for therapeutic response: decreased intensity of skeletal muscle pain.

PATIENT/FAMILY TEACHING:

Drowsiness usually diminishes w/continued therapy. Avoid tasks that require alertness, motor skills until response to drug is established. Avoid alcohol or other depressants while taking medication. Report continued weakness, fatigue, nausea or diarrhea, skin rash, itching, bloody/black stools.

daunorubicin
dawn-oh-**rue**-bih-sin
(Cerubidine, DaunoXome)

CANADIAN AVAILABILITY:
Cerubidine

CLASSIFICATION

Antineoplastic

AVAILABILITY (Rx)

Injection: 2 mg/ml

PHARMACOKINETICS

Widely distributed. Does not cross blood-brain barrier. Metabolized in liver to active metabolite. Excreted in urine, eliminated by biliary excretion. Half-life: 18.5 hrs; metabolite: 55 hrs.

ACTION/*THERAPEUTIC EFFECT*

Cell cycle-phase nonspecific. Most active in S phase of cell division. Appears to bind to DNA, *inhibiting DNA, DNA-dependent RNA synthesis.*

USES/*UNLABELED*

Remission induction in acute nonlymphocytic leukemia (myelogenous, monocytic, erythroid) of adults; acute lymphocytic leukemia of both children and adults. DaunoXome: Advanced HIV-related Kaposi's sarcoma. *Treatment of neuroblastoma, non-Hodgkin's lymphoma, Ewing's sarcoma, Wilms' tumor, chronic myelocytic leukemia.*

STORAGE/HANDLING

Note: May be carcinogenic, mutagenic, or teratogenic. Handle w/ extreme care during preparation/ administration.

Reconstituted solution stable for 24 hrs at room temperature or 48 hrs if refrigerated. Color change from red to blue-purple indicates decomposition; discard.

IV ADMINISTRATION

Note: Give by IV injection or IV infusion. IV infusion not recommended due to vein irritation, risk of thrombophlebitis. Avoid small veins, swollen or edematous extremities, areas overlying joints and tendons.

1. Reconstitute each 20 mg vial w/4 ml sterile water for injection to provide concentration of 5 mg/ml.

2. Gently agitate vial until completely dissolved.

3. For IV injection, withdraw desired dose into syringe containing 10–15 ml 0.9% NaCl. Inject over 2–3 min into tubing of running IV solution of 5% dextrose or 0.9% NaCl.

4. For IV infusion, further dilute w/100 ml 5% dextrose or 0.9% NaCl. Infuse over 30–45 min.

5. Extravasation produces immediate pain, severe local tissue damage. Aspirate as much infiltrated drug as possible, then infiltrate area w/hydrocortisone sodium succinate injection (50–100 mg hydrocortisone) and/or isotonic sodium thiosulfate injection or ascorbic acid injection (1 ml of 5% injection). Apply cold compresses.

INDICATIONS/DOSAGE/ROUTES

Note: Dosage individualized based on clinical response, tolerance to adverse effects. When used in combination therapy, consult specific protocols for optimum dosage, sequence of drug administration. Do not exceed total dosage of 500–600 mg/m^2 in adults, 400–450 mg/m^2 in those who received irradiation of cardiac region, 300 mg/m^2 in children >2 yrs, 10 mg/kg in children <2 yrs (increases risk of cardiotoxicity). Reduce dosage in those w/liver and/or renal impairment. Use body weight to calculate dose in children <2 yrs or surface area <0.5 m^2.

Acute nonlymphocytic leukemia (induction remission):

IV: Adults <60 yrs: Combined w/ cytosine: 45 mg/m^2/day for 3 successive days for first course of induction therapy. Give 45 mg/m^2/ day for 2 successive days on subsequent courses. **Adults >60 yrs:** 30 mg/m^2/day following same dosage regimen as above.

Acute lymphocytic leukemia (induction remission):

IV: Adults, elderly: Combination therapy: 45 mg/m^2/day first 3 days of induction therapy. **Children:** 25 mg/m^2 on day 1 once a week.

Kaposi's sarcoma (DaunoXome):
IV: Adults: 40 mg/m^2 over 1 hr. Repeat q2wks.

PRECAUTIONS

CONTRAINDICATIONS: None significant. **EXTREME CAUTION:** Preexisting bone marrow depression. **PREGNANCY/LACTATION:** If possible, avoid use during pregnancy, esp. first trimester. May cause fetal harm. Breast-feeding not recommended. **Pregnancy Category D.**

INTERACTIONS

DRUG INTERACTIONS: May decrease effect of antigout medications. Bone marrow depressants may enhance myelosuppression. Live virus vaccines may potentiate virus replication, increase vaccine side effects, decrease pt's antibody response to vaccine. **ALTERED LAB VALUES:** May increase serum bilirubin, SGOT (AST), and alkaline phosphatase levels. May raise blood uric acid level.

SIDE EFFECTS

FREQUENT: Complete alopecia (scalp, axillary, pubic hair), nausea, vomiting begins a few hours after administration, lasts 24–48 hrs. *DaunoXome:* Mild to moderate nausea, fatigue, fever. **OCCASIONAL:** Diarrhea, abdominal pain, esophagitis, stomatitis (redness/burning of oral mucous membranes, inflammation of gums/tongue), transverse pigmentation of fingernails/toenails. **RARE:** Transient fever, chills.

ADVERSE REACTIONS/TOXIC EFFECTS

Bone marrow depression mani-

fested as hematologic toxicity (generally severe leukopenia, anemia, thrombocytopenia). Decrease in platelet count, WBC occurs in 10–14 days, returns to normal level by third week.

Cardiotoxicity noted as either acute, transient, abnormal EKG findings and/or cardiomyopathy manifested as CHF (risk increases when cumulative dose exceeds 550 mg/m^2 in adults and 300 mg/m^2 in children >2 yrs, or total dosage more than 10 mg/kg in children <2 yrs).

NURSING IMPLICATIONS
BASELINE ASSESSMENT

Obtain WBC, platelet, erythrocyte counts prior to and at frequent intervals during therapy. EKG should be obtained prior to therapy. Antiemetics may be effective in preventing, treating nausea.

INTERVENTION/EVALUATION:

Monitor for stomatitis (burning, erythema of oral mucosa). May lead to ulceration within 2–3 days. Assess skin, nailbeds for hyperpigmentation. Monitor hematologic status, renal/hepatic function studies, serum uric acid level. Assess pattern of daily bowel activity and stool consistency. Monitor for hematologic toxicity (fever, sore throat, signs of local infection, easy bruising, or unusual bleeding from any site), symptoms of anemia (excessive tiredness, weakness).

PATIENT/FAMILY TEACHING:

Urine may turn reddish color for 1–2 days after beginning therapy. Alopecia is reversible, but new hair growth may have different color or texture. New hair growth resumes about 5 wks after last therapy dose. Maintain fastidious oral hygiene. Do not have immunizations w/o physician's approval (drug lowers body's resistance). Avoid contact w/those who have recently received live virus vaccine. Promptly report fever, sore throat, signs of local infection, easy bruising, or unusual bleeding from any site. Increase fluid intake (may protect against hyperuricemia). Contact physician if nausea/vomiting continues at home.

deferoxamine

deaf-er-**ox**-ah-meen
(Desferal Mesylate)

CANADIAN AVAILABILITY:
Desferal

CLASSIFICATION

Antidote

AVAILABILITY (Rx)

Injection: 500 mg

PHARMACOKINETICS

Well absorbed after IM, SubQ administration. Widely distributed. Rapidly metabolized in tissues, plasma. Excreted in urine, eliminated in feces via biliary excretion. Removed by hemodialysis. Half-life: 6 hrs.

ACTION / *THERAPEUTIC EFFECT*

Binds w/iron to form complex, *promoting urine excretion of acute iron poisoning.*

USES / *UNLABELED*

Treatment of acute iron toxicity, chronic iron toxicity secondary to multiple transfusions associated w/some chronic anemia (e.g., thalassemia). *Treatment/diagnosis of aluminum toxicity.*

STORAGE / HANDLING

Store parenteral powder at room temperature.

IM / SUBQ / IV ADMINISTRATION

Note: Reconstitute each 500 mg vial w/2 ml sterile water to provide a concentration of 250 mg/ml.

Sub Q:
Administer SubQ very slowly; may give undiluted.

IM:
1. Inject deeply into upper outer quadrant of buttock.
2. May give undiluted.

IV:
1. For IV infusion, further dilute w/0.9% NaCl, 5% dextrose, and administer at maximum rate of 15 mg/kg/hr.
2. A too-rapid IV administration may produce skin flushing, urticaria, hypotension, shock.

INDICATIONS / DOSAGE / ROUTES

Acute iron intoxication:
IM: Adults: Initially, 90 mg/kg, then 45 mg/kg up to 1 g q4–12h. **Maximum:** 6 g/day.
IV: Adults: 15 mg/kg/hr up to 90 mg/kg q8hrs. **Maximum:** 6 g/day. **Children:** 15 mg/kg/hr.

Chronic iron overload:
SubQ: Adults: 1–2 g/day (20–40 mg/kg) over 8–24 hrs. **Children:** 10 mg/kg/day.
IM: Adults: 0.5–1 g/day. **IV:** In addition to IM, 2 g infused at rate not to exceed 15 mg/kg/hr.

PRECAUTIONS

CONTRAINDICATIONS: Severe renal disease, anuria, primary hemochromatosis. **CAUTIONS:** None significant. **PREGNANCY/LACTATION:** Unknown if drug crosses placenta or is distributed in breast milk. Use only when absolutely necessary. Skeletal anomalies may present in neonate. **Pregnancy Category C**.

INTERACTIONS

DRUG INTERACTIONS: Vitamin C may increase effect. **ALTERED LAB VALUES:** May cause a falsely high total iron-binding capacity (TIBC).

SIDE EFFECTS

FREQUENT: Pain, induration at injection site, urine color change (to orange-rose). **OCCASIONAL:** Abdominal discomfort, diarrhea, leg cramps, impaired vision.

ADVERSE REACTIONS/TOXIC EFFECTS

Neurotoxicity, including high-frequency hearing loss, has been noted.

NURSING IMPLICATIONS
BASELINE ASSESSMENT:

Inform pt injection may produce discomfort at IM or SubQ injection site. Assess serum iron levels, iron binding capacity before and during therapy.

INTERVENTION/EVALUATION:

Question pt for evidence of hearing loss (neurotoxicity). Periodic slit-lamp ophthalmic exams should be obtained in those treated for chronic iron overload. If using SubQ technique, monitor for pruritus, erythema, skin irritation, and swelling.

PATIENT/FAMILY TEACHING:

Urine will appear reddish. Discomfort may occur at site of injection.

delavirdine
(Rescriptor)
See Supplement

demecarium
(Humorsol)
See Classification section under: Antiglaucoma agents

demeclocycline hydrochloride
deh-meh-clo-**sigh**-clean
(Declomycin)

CANADIAN AVAILABILITY: Declomycin

CLASSIFICATION

Antibiotic: Tetracycline

AVAILABILITY (Rx)

Capsules: 150 mg. **Tablets:** 150 mg, 300 mg.

PHARMACOKINETICS

Readily absorbed from GI tract (food decreases absorption). Widely distributed. Primarily excreted unchanged in urine. Half-life: 10–17 hrs (increased in decreased renal function).

ACTION/THERAPEUTIC EFFECT

Bacteriostatic due to binding to ribosomes, *inhibiting protein synthesis*. Inhibits ADH-induced water reabsorption, *producing water diuresis.*

USES

Treatment of respiratory and urinary tract infections, uncomplicated gonorrhea, brucellosis, rheumatic fever prophylaxis, trachoma, Rocky Mountain spotted fever, typhus, Q fever, rickettsialpox, psittacosis, ornithosis, granuloma inguinale, lymphogranuloma venereum. Treatment of syndrome of inappropriate ADH secretion (SIADH).

PO ADMINISTRATION

Give w/full glass of water 1 hr before or 2 hrs after meals/milk.

INDICATIONS/DOSAGE/ROUTES

Note: Space doses evenly around the clock.

Mild to moderate infections:
PO: Adults, elderly: 600 mg/day in 2–4 divided doses. **Children >8 yrs:** 6–12 mg/kg/day in 2–4 divided doses.

Uncomplicated gonorrhea:
PO: Adults: Initially, 600 mg, then 300 mg q12h for 4 days for total of 3 g.

Chronic form of SIADH:
PO: Adults, elderly: 600 mg–1.2 g/day in 3–4 divided doses, or 3.25–3.75 mg/kg q6h.

PRECAUTIONS

CONTRAINDICATIONS: Hypersensitivity to tetracyclines, last half of pregnancy, infants–8 yrs. **CAUTIONS:** Renal impairment, sun or ultraviolet exposure (severe photosensitivity reaction). **PREGNANCY/LACTATION:** Readily crosses placenta, distributed in breast milk. Avoid use during last half of pregnancy. May produce permanent teeth discoloration, enamel hypoplasia, inhibit fetal skeletal growth in children <8 yrs. **Pregnancy Category D.**

INTERACTIONS

DRUG INTERACTIONS: Antacids containing aluminum/calcium/magnesium, laxatives containing magnesium, oral iron preparations, dairy products impair absorption of tetracyclines (give 1–2 hrs before or after tetracyclines). Cholestyramine, colestipol may decrease absorption. May decrease effect of oral contraceptives. **ALTERED LAB VALUES:** May increase BUN, SGOT (AST), SGPT (ALT), alkaline phosphatase, amylase, bilirubin concentrations.

SIDE EFFECTS

FREQUENT: Anorexia, nausea, vomiting, diarrhea, dysphagia, exaggerated sunburn reaction w/moderate to high dosage. **OCCASIONAL:** Urticaria, rash. Long-term therapy may result in diabetes insipidus syndrome: polydipsia, polyuria, weakness.

ADVERSE REACTIONS/TOXIC EFFECTS

Superinfection (especially fungal) anaphylaxis, increased intracranial pressure occur rarely. Bulging fontanelles occur rarely in infants.

NURSING IMPLICATIONS

BASELINE ASSESSMENT:

Question for history of allergies, especially to tetracyclines. Obtain culture, sensitivity test before giving first dose (therapy may begin before results are known).

INTERVENTION/EVALUATION:

Determine pattern of bowel activity and stool consistency. Check food intake, tolerance. Monitor I&O, renal function test results. Assess for rash. Be alert to superinfection: diarrhea, ulceration or changes of oral mucosa, tongue, anal/genital pruritus. Monitor B/P and LOC because of potential for increased intracranial pressure.

PATIENT/FAMILY TEACHING:

Continue antibiotic for full length of treatment. Space doses evenly. Take oral doses on empty stomach w/full glass of water. Avoid bedtime doses. Notify physician in event of diarrhea, rash, other new symptom. Avoid sun/ultraviolet light exposure. Consult physician before taking any other medication.

---

denileukin
(Ontak)
See Supplement

---

desipramine hydrochloride

deh-**sip**-rah-meen
(Norpramin)

CANADIAN AVAILABILITY:
Norpramin

CLASSIFICATION

Antidepressant: Tricyclic

AVAILABILITY (Rx)

Tablets: 10 mg, 25 mg, 50 mg, 75 mg, 100 mg, 150 mg. **Capsules:** 25 mg, 50 mg.

PHARMACOKINETICS

Rapid, well absorbed from GI tract. Metabolized in liver. Primarily excreted in urine. Half-life: 12–27 hrs.

ACTION/*THERAPEUTIC EFFECT*

Increases synaptic concentration of norepinephrine and/or serotonin (inhibits reuptake by presynaptic membrane), *producing antidepressant effect.* Strong anticholinergic activity.

USES/*UNLABELED*

Treatment of various forms of depression, often in conjunction w/ psychotherapy. *Treatment of panic disorder, neurogenic pain, attention deficit hyperactivity disorder, narcolepsy/cataplexy, bulimia nervosa, cocaine withdrawal.*

PO ADMINISTRATION

Give w/food or milk if GI distress occurs.

INDICATIONS/DOSAGE/ROUTES

Depression:
PO: Adults: Initially, 75–150 mg daily as single daily dose, or in divided doses. Gradually increase to lowest effective therapeutic level. Do not exceed 300 mg daily.

Usual elderly dosage:
PO: 25–100 mg/day. **Maximum:** 150 mg/day.

PRECAUTIONS

CONTRAINDICATIONS: Acute recovery period following MI, within 14 days of MAO inhibitor ingestion. **CAUTIONS:** Prostatic hypertrophy, history of urinary retention or obstruction, glaucoma, diabetes mellitus, history of seizures, hyperthyroidism, cardiac/hepatic/ renal disease, schizophrenia, increased intraocular pressure, hiatal hernia. **PREGNANCY/LACTATION:** Crosses placenta; minimally distributed in breast milk. **Pregnancy Category C**.

INTERACTIONS

DRUG INTERACTIONS: Alcohol,

CNS depressants may increase CNS, respiratory depression, hypotensive effects. Antithyroid agents may increase risk of agranulocytosis. Phenothiazines may increase sedative, anticholinergic effects. Cimetidine may increase concentration, toxicity. May decrease effects of clonidine, guanadrel. May increase cardiac effects w/sympathomimetics. May increase risk of hypertensive crisis, hyperpyrexia, convulsions w/MAO inhibitors. Phenytoin may decrease desipramine concentration. **ALTERED LAB VALUES:** May alter EKG readings, glucose serum level.

SIDE EFFECTS

FREQUENT: Drowsiness, fatigue, dry mouth, blurred vision, constipation, delayed micturition, postural hypotension, excessive sweating, disturbed concentration, increased appetite, urinary retention. **OCCASIONAL:** GI disturbances (nausea, GI distress, metallic taste sensation). **RARE:** Paradoxical reaction (agitation, restlessness, nightmares, insomnia), extrapyramidal symptoms (particularly fine hand tremor).

ADVERSE REACTIONS/TOXIC EFFECTS

High dosage may produce confusion, seizures, severe drowsiness, fast/slow/irregular heartbeat, fever, hallucinations, agitation, shortness of breath, vomiting, unusual tiredness/weakness. Abrupt withdrawal from prolonged therapy may produce severe headache, malaise, nausea, vomiting, vivid dreams.

NURSING IMPLICATIONS
BASELINE ASSESSMENT:

For those on long-term therapy, liver/renal function tests, blood counts should be performed periodically.

INTERVENTION/EVALUATION:

Supervise suicidal risk pt closely during early therapy (as depression lessens, energy level improves, increasing suicide potential). Assess appearance, behavior, speech pattern, level of interest, mood. Monitor pattern of daily bowel activity and stool consistency. Monitor B/P, pulse for hypotension, arrhythmias. Assess for urinary retention by monitoring I&O and by bladder palpation.

PATIENT/FAMILY TEACHING:

Change positions slowly to avoid hypotensive effect. Tolerance to postural hypotension, sedative, and anticholinergic effects usually develops during early therapy. Maximum therapeutic effect may be noted in 2–4 wks. Photosensitivity to sun may occur. Dry mouth may be relieved by sugarless gum or sips of tepid water. Do not abruptly discontinue medication. Report visual disturbances. Avoid tasks that require alertness, motor skills until response to drug is established. Avoid alcohol.

desmopressin
des-moe-**press**-in
(DDAVP, Stimate)

CANADIAN AVAILABILITY:
DDAVP, Octostim

CLASSIFICATION
Antidiuretic

AVAILABILITY (Rx)
Tablets: 0.1 mg, 0.2 mg. **Nasal**

Solution: 0.1 mg/ml, 1.5 mg/ml. **Nasal spray. Injection:** 4 mcg/ml.

PHARMACOKINETICS

	ONSET	PEAK	DURATION
PO	1 hr	4–7 hrs	—
Intranasal			
	15 min–1 hr	1–5 hrs	5–21 hrs
IV	15–30 min	1.5–3 hrs	—

Absorption 10–20% from nasal administration. Metabolized renally. Half-life: 75 min.

ACTION/ *THERAPEUTIC EFFECT*

Increases reabsorption of water by increasing permeability of collecting ducts of the kidneys, *decreasing urinary output. Increases plasma factor VIII (antihemophilic factor),* plasminogen activator.

USES

DDAVP *Intranasal:* Primary nocturnal enuresis, central cranial diabetes insipidus. *Parenteral:* Central cranial diabetes insipidus, hemophilia A, von Willebrand's disease (type I).

Stimate *Intranasal:* Hemophilia A, von Willebrand's disease (type I) .

Oral: Central cranial diabetes insipidus.

STORAGE/HANDLING

Refrigerate nasal solution, injection. Nasal solution stable for up to 3 wks at room temperature. Nasal spray stored at room temperature.

SUBQ/IV/INTRANASAL ADMINISTRATION

SubQ

1. Evening dosage should consider satisfactory sleep response.

2. Morning and evening doses should be adjusted separately.

IV:

1. For preop use, administer 30 min before procedure.

2. Monitor B/P and pulse during IV infusion.

3. IV dose = 1/10 intranasal dose.

4. IV infusion: dilute in 10–50 ml 0.9% NaCl; infuse over 15–30 min.

INTRANASAL:

1. A calibrated catheter (rhinyle) is used to draw up a measured quantity of desmopressin; w/one end inserted in the nose, the patient blows on the other end to deposit the solution deep in the nasal cavity.

2. For infants, young children, obtunded pts, an air-filled syringe may be attached to the catheter to deposit the solution.

INDICATIONS/DOSAGE/ROUTES

Primary nocturnal enuresis:
Intranasal: Children ≥6 yrs: Initially, 20 mcg (0.2 ml) at bedtime ($^{1}/_{2}$ dose each nostril). Adjust up to 40 mcg.

Central cranial diabetes insipidus:
PO: Adults, elderly: Initially, 0.05 mg 2 times/day. **Range:** 0.1–1.2 mg/day in 2–3 divided doses. **Children:** 0.05 mg initially.
Intranasal: Adults, elderly: 0.1–0.4 ml/day as single or 2–3 divided doses. **Children (3 mos–12 yrs):** 0.05–0.3 ml/day as single or 2 divided doses.
SubQ/IV: Adults, elderly: 0.5–1 ml/day in 2 divided doses.

Hemophilia A, von Willebrand's disease (type I):
IV Infusion: Adults, elderly, children >10 kg: 0.3 mcg/kg diluted in 50 ml 0.9% NaCl. **Children <10 kg:** 0.3 mcg/kg diluted in 10 ml 0.9% nacl.
Intranasal: Adults, elderly >50 kg: 300 mcg (1 spray each nos-

tril). **Adults, elderly <50 kg:** 150 mcg as single spray.

PRECAUTIONS

CONTRAINDICATIONS: Hypersensitivity to desmopressin; type IIB or platelet-type von Willebrand's disease; nasal scarring, blockage, or other impairment w/intranasal administration. Intranasal administration with impaired level of consciousness. **CAUTIONS:** Coronary artery insufficiency, hypertensive cardiovascular disease, infants, and children < 6 yrs. **PREGNANCY/LACTATION:** Pregnancy Category B.

INTERACTIONS

DRUG INTERACTIONS: Carbamazepine, chlorpropamide, clofibrate may increase effect. Demeclocycline, lithium, norepinephrine may decrease effect. **ALTERED LAB VALUES:** None significant.

SIDE EFFECTS

OCCASIONAL: *IV:* Pain/redness/swelling at injection site, headache, abdominal cramps, vulval pain, flushed skin; mild elevation of B/P; nausea w/high doses. *Nasal:* Runny/stuffy nose; slight elevation of B/P.

ADVERSE REACTIONS/TOXIC EFFECTS

Water intoxication or hyponatremia (coma, confusion, drowsiness, headache, decreased urination, seizures, rapid weight gain) may occur in overhydration. Elderly, infants, children are esp. at risk.

NURSING IMPLICATIONS
BASELINE ASSESSMENT:

Question for hypersensitivity to desmopressin. Establish baselines for B/P, pulse, weight, electrolytes, urine specific gravity.

Check lab values for factor VIII coagulant concentration for hemophilia A and von Willebrand's disease; bleeding times, ristocetin colactor, and Willebrand factor for von Willebrand's disease.

INTERVENTION/EVALUATION:

Monitor I&O closely, restrict intake as necessary to prevent water intoxication. Weigh daily if indicated. Check B/P and pulse q15min during IV administration, 2 times/day for other routes. Monitor electrolytes, urine specific gravity, and other lab results (see Baseline Assessment). Evaluate parenteral injection site for erythema, pain. Report side effects to physician for dose reduction. Assess bleeding as appropriate. Check for nasal mucosa changes w/intranasal route. Be alert for early signs of water intoxication: drowsiness, listlessness, headache.

PATIENT/FAMILY TEACHING:

Teach pt/family proper technique for intranasal administration. Report headache, nausea, shortness of breath, or other symptoms promptly. Stress importance of I&O. Notify physician if bleeding is not controlled.

desonide
(Otic Tridesilon, Tridesilon)
See Classification section under: Corticosteroids: topical

desoximetasone
(Topicort)
See Classification section under: Corticosteroids: topical

dexamethasone
dex-a-**meth**-a-sone
(Decadron, Hexadrol)

dexamethasone acetate
(Dalalone L.A., Decadron L.A., Dexone L.A.)

dexamethasone sodium phosphate
(Decadron, Respihaler)

FIXED-COMBINATION(S):
Dexamethasone phosphate w/ neomycin sulfate, an anti-infective (**NeoDecadron**); dexamethasone sodium phosphate w/lidocaine, a local anesthetic

CANADIAN AVAILABILITY:
Decadron, Dexasone, Maxidex

CLASSIFICATION
Corticosteroid

AVAILABILITY (Rx)
Tablets: 0.25 mg, 0.5 mg, 0.75 mg, 1 mg, 1.5 mg, 2 mg, 4 mg, 6 mg. **Elixir:** 0.5 mg/5 ml. **Oral Solution:** 0.5 mg/5 ml, 0.5 mg/0.5 ml. **Injection:** 4 mg/ml, 8 mg/ml (suspension), 10 mg/ml, 16 mg/ml (suspension), 20 mg/ml, 24 mg/ml. **Inhalant, Intranasal, Ophthalmic:** Solution, suspension, ointment. **Topical:** Aerosol, cream.

PHARMACOKINETICS
Rapid, complete absorption from GI tract, after IM administration. Widely distributed. Metabolized in liver. Primarily excreted in urine. Half-life: 3–4.5 hrs.

ACTION/*THERAPEUTIC EFFECT*
Inhibits accumulation of inflammatory cells at inflammation sites, phagocytosis, lysosomal enzyme release and synthesis and/or release of mediators of inflammation. *Prevents/suppresses cell and tissue immune reactions, inflammatory process.*

USES
Substitution therapy in deficiency states: acute/chronic adrenal insufficiency, congenital adrenal hyperplasia, adrenal insufficiency secondary to pituitary insufficiency.
Nonendocrine disorders: arthritis, rheumatic carditis, allergic, collagen, intestinal tract, liver, ocular, renal, and skin diseases, bronchial asthma, cerebral edema, malignancies.
Ophthalmic: Treatment of responsive inflammatory conditions of palpebral and bulbar conjunctiva, cornea, and anterior segment of globe. *Nasal:* Maintenance treatment of asthma. Allergic/inflammatory nasal conditions and nasal polyps. *Topical:* Relief of inflammatory/pruritic conditions of steroid-responsive dermatoses. *Respiratory:* Control of bronchial asthma in pts requiring chronic steroid therapy.

PO/IM/IV/TOPICAL/ OPHTHALMIC ADMINISTRATION
PO:
Give w/milk or food.
IM:
Give deep IM, preferably in gluteus maximus.

IV:

Note: Dexamethasone sodium phosphate may be given by direct IV injection or IV infusion.

1. For IV infusion, mix w/0.9% NaCl or 5% dextrose.

2. For neonate, solution must be preservative free.

3. IV solution must be used within 24 hrs.

OPHTHALMIC:

1. Place finger on lower eyelid and pull out until a pocket is formed between eye and lower lid. Hold dropper above pocket and place correct number of drops ($1/4$–$1/2$ inch ointment) into pocket. Close eye gently. *Solution:* Apply digital pressure to lacrimal sac for 1–2 min (minimizes drainage into nose and throat, reducing risk of systemic effects). *Ointment:* Close eye for 1–2 min, rolling eyeball (increases contact area of drug to eye). Remove excess solution or ointment around eye w/tissue.

2. Ointment may be used at night to reduce frequency of solution administration.

3. As w/other corticosteroids, taper dosage slowly when discontinuing.

TOPICAL:

1. Gently cleanse area prior to application.

2. Use occlusive dressings only as ordered.

3. Apply sparingly and rub into area thoroughly.

INDICATIONS/DOSAGE/ROUTES

Dexamethasone, oral:
PO: Adults, elderly: 0.75–9 mg/day.

Dexamethasone acetate:
IM: Adults, elderly: 8–16 mg, may repeat in 1–3 wks. **Intralesional: Adults, elderly:** 0.8–1.6 mg.
Intra-Articular and Soft Tissues:

Adults, elderly: 4–16 mg; may repeat ql–3 wks.

Dexamethasone sodium phosphate:
IM/IV: Adults, elderly: Initially, 0.5–9 mg/day.
Intra-Articular, Intralesional, or Soft Tissue: 0.4–6 mg.

Usual topical dosage:
Topical: Adults, elderly: 2–4 times/day.

Respiratory inhalant:
Respiratory Inhalation: Adults, elderly: 3 inhalations 3–4 times/day; **Maximum:** 12/day. **Children:** 2 inhalations 3–4 times/day. **Maximum:** 8/day.

Usual intranasal dosage:
Adults, elderly: 2 sprays each nostril 2–3 times/day. **Maximum:** 12/day. **Children:** 1–2 sprays 2 times/day; **Maximum:** 8/day.

PRECAUTIONS

CONTRAINDICATIONS: Hypersensitivity to any corticosteroid or components, systemic fungal infection, peptic ulcers (except life-threatening situations). Avoid live virus vaccine such as smallpox. *Topical:* Marked circulation impairment. Do not instill ocular solutions when topical corticosteroids are being used on eyelids or surrounding skin. **CAUTIONS:** Thromboembolic disorders, history of tuberculosis (may reactivate disease), hypothyroidism, cirrhosis, nonspecific ulcerative colitis, CHF, hypertension, psychosis, renal insufficiency, seizure disorders. Prolonged therapy should be discontinued slowly. *Topical:* Do not apply to extensive areas. **PREGNANCY/LACTATION:** Crosses placenta, distributed in breast milk. **Pregnancy Category C.**

INTERACTIONS

DRUG INTERACTIONS: Amphotericin may increase hypokalemia. May decrease effect of oral hypoglycemics, insulin, diuretics, potassium supplements. May increase digoxin toxicity (due to hypokalemia). Hepatic enzyme inducers may decrease effect. Live virus vaccines may potentiate virus replication, increase vaccine side effects, decrease pt's antibody response to vaccine. **ALTERED LAB VALUES:** May decrease calcium, potassium, thyroxine. Increases cholesterol, glucose, lipids, sodium, amylase serum levels.

SIDE EFFECTS

FREQUENT: *Inhalation:* Cough, dry mouth, hoarseness, throat irritation. *Intranasal:* Burning, dryness inside nose. *Ophthalmic:* Blurred vision. *Systemic:* Insomnia, facial swelling ("moon face"), moderate abdominal distention, indigestion, increased appetite, nervousness, facial flushing, increased sweating. **OCCASIONAL:** *Inhalation:* Localized fungal infection (thrush). *Intranasal:* Crusting inside nose, nosebleed, sore throat, ulceration of nasal mucosa. *Ophthalmic:* Decreased vision, watering of eyes, eye pain, nausea, vomiting, burning, stinging, redness of eyes. *Systemic:* Dizziness, decreased/blurred vision. *Topical:* Allergic contact dermatitis, purpura (blood-containing blisters), thinning of skin w/easy bruising, telangiectasis (raised dark red spots on skin). **RARE:** *Inhalation:* Increased bronchospasm, esophageal candidiasis. *Intranasal:* Nasal/pharyngeal candidiasis, eye pain. *Systemic:* General allergic reaction (rash, hives), pain, redness, swelling at injection site, psychic changes, false sense of well-being, hallucinations, depression.

ADVERSE REACTIONS/TOXIC EFFECTS

Long-term therapy: Muscle wasting (esp. arms, legs), osteoporosis, spontaneous fractures, amenorrhea, cataracts, glaucoma, peptic ulcer, CHF. *Abrupt withdrawal following long-term therapy:* Severe joint pain, severe headache, anorexia, nausea, fever, rebound inflammation, fatigue, weakness, lethargy, dizziness, orthostatic hypotension. *Ophthalmic:* Glaucoma, ocular hypertension, cataracts.

NURSING IMPLICATIONS

BASELINE ASSESSMENT:

Question for hypersensitivity to any of the corticosteroids, components. Obtain baselines for height, weight, B/P, glucose, electrolytes. Check results of initial tests (e.g., TB skin test, X-rays, EKG).

INTERVENTION/EVALUATION:

Monitor I&O, daily weight: Assess for edema. Check lab results for blood coagulability and clinical evidence of thromboembolism. Evaluate food tolerance and bowel activity; report hyperacidity promptly. Check B/P, temperature, respirations, pulse at least 2 times/day. Be alert to infection: sore throat, fever, or vague symptoms. Monitor electrolytes. Watch for hypercalcemia (muscle twitching, cramps, positive Trousseau's or Chvostek's signs), hypokalemia (weakness and muscle cramps, numbness/tingling esp. lower extremities, nausea and vomiting, irritability, EKG changes). Assess emotional status, ability to sleep. Provide assistance w/ambulation.

PATIENT/FAMILY TEACHING:

Take w/food or milk. Carry identification of drug and dose, physician's name and phone number. Do not change dose/schedule or stop taking drug. *Must taper off gradually under medical supervision* Notify physician of fever, sore throat, muscle aches, sudden weight gain/swelling. W/dietician give instructions for prescribed diet (usually sodium-restricted w/high vitamin D, protein, and potassium). Maintain careful personal hygiene, avoid exposure to disease or trauma. Severe stress (serious infection, surgery, or trauma) may require increased dosage. Do not take any other medication w/o consulting physician. Follow-up visits, lab tests are necessary; children must be assessed for growth retardation. Inform dentist or other physicians of dexamethasone therapy now or within past 12 mos. Caution against overuse of joints injected for symptomatic relief. *Topical:* Apply after shower or bath for best absorption. Do not cover unless physician orders; do not use tight diapers, plastic pants, or coverings. Avoid contact w/eyes. Do not expose treated area to sunlight.

dexfenfluramine

dex-fen-**flur**-ah-mean
(Redux)

CLASSIFICATION

Appetite suppressant

AVAILABILITY (Rx)

Capsules:15 mg

PHARMACOKINETICS

Completely absorbed, widely distributed. Undergoes significant first-pass metabolism in liver to active metabolite. Primarily eliminated via renal excretion. Half-life: 17–20 hrs; metabolite: 32 hrs. Steady state plasma concentration: 8 days.

ACTION/ *THERAPEUTIC EFFECT*

Stimulates release and inhibits serotonin reuptake, *suppressing appetite for carbohydrates.*

USES

Management of obesity including weight loss and maintenance of weight loss in those on reduced calorie diet.

INDICATIONS/DOSAGE/ROUTES

Appetite suppression:
PO: Adults, elderly: 15 mg twice daily w/meals.

PRECAUTIONS

CONTRAINDICATIONS: Concurrent MAO inhibitors, diagnosed primary pulmonary hypertension, hypersensitivity to dexfenfluramine, fenfluramine, or related compounds. CAUTIONS: Glaucoma, elderly, renal or hepatic impairment, cardiac arrhythmias. PREGNANCY/LACTATION: May significantly reduce body weight and weight gain during pregnancy. Not recommended during pregnancy or in nursing mothers. Pregnancy Category C.

INTERACTIONS

DRUG INTERACTIONS: MAO inhibitors, serotoninergic agents (fluoxetine, fluvoxamine, paroxetine, sertraline, venlafaxine), concurrent migraine therapy. May potentiate sedative effects of alcohol, CNS depressants. ALTERED LAB VAL-

UES: May produce false-positive urine drug test for amphetamines up to 24 hrs after 30 mg dose.

SIDE EFFECTS

Generally mild and transient effects. **FREQUENT:** Insomnia (20%), diarrhea (17.5%), asthenia (loss of strength), headache (16%), dry mouth (12.5%). **OCCASIONAL:** Mild to moderate drowsiness, abdominal pain (7%), pharyngitis (6%), dizziness (5.5%), depression (5%). **RARE:** Cough, bronchitis, vertigo, emotional lability, thirst, urinary frequency, rash.

ADVERSE REACTIONS/TOXIC EFFECTS

Overdosage results in severe drowsiness, agitation, sweating, mydriasis (large pupils), shivering, nausea and vomiting. Primary pulmonary hypertension (dyspnea, angina, lower extremity edema) occurs rarely.

NURSING IMPLICATIONS
INTERVENTION/EVALUATION:

Question sleep pattern. Determine pattern of bowel activity and stool consistency.

PATIENT/FAMILY TEACHING:

Due to potential of mild to moderate drowsiness, assess ability to perform tasks that require alertness, coordination, or physical dexterity. Contact physician if any decrease in exercise tolerance, chest pain, difficulty breathing, or swelling of feet or lower legs occur (signs of pulmonary hypertension [see CONTRAINDICATIONS]) or if nausea or vomiting occurs (symptoms of intolerance to drugs). Dry mouth may be relieved by sips of tepid water, sugarless gum. A false-positive urine drug test for amphetamines may occur for up to 24 hrs following dose. Take w/food. Avoid alcohol.

dexrazoxane
dex-rah-**zox**-ann
(Zinecard)

CANADIAN AVAILABILITY: Zinecard

CLASSIFICATION

Antineoplastic adjunct, cardioprotective agent

AVAILABILITY (Rx)

Powder for Injection: 250 mg (10 mg/ml reconstituted in 25 ml single-use vial), 500 mg (10 mg/ml reconstituted in 50 ml single-use vial)

PHARMACOKINETICS

Rapidly distributed following IV administration. Primarily excreted in urine. Elimination half-life: 2.1–2.5 hrs.

ACTION/THERAPEUTIC EFFECT

Readily penetrates cell membranes converting intracellularly to a chelating agent, *binding iron and preventing free radical formation by anthracycline, protecting against anthracycline-induced cardiomyopathy.*

USES

Reduction of incidence and severity of cardiomyopathy associated w/doxorubicin therapy in women w/metastatic breast cancer. Not recommended w/initiation of doxorubicin therapy.

STORAGE/HANDLING

Store vials at room temperature. Reconstituted solution stable for 6 hrs at room temperature or refrigeration. Discard unused solution.

IV ADMINISTRATION

Note: Do not mix w/other drugs. Use caution in handling and preparation of reconstituted solution (glove use recommended).

1. Reconstitute w/0.167 molar (M/6) sodium lactate injection to give concentration of 10 mg dexrazoxane for each ml of sodium lactate.

2. Give reconstituted solution by slow IV push or rapid drip IV infusion from a bag.

3. After infusion is completed, and before a total elapsed time of 30 min from beginning of dexrazoxane infusion, give IV injection of doxorubicin.

INDICATIONS/DOSAGE/ROUTES

Note: Dexrazoxane should only be used in those who have received a cumulative doxorubicin dose of 300 mg/m^2 and are continuing w/doxorubicin therapy. The reconstituted dexrazoxane solution may be diluted w/0.9% NaCl injection or 5% dextrose injection to a concentration range of 1.3 to 5 mg/ml in IV infusion bags.

Cardioprotective:
IV: Adults: Recommended dosage ratio of dexrazoxane:doxorubicin is 10:1 (e.g., 500 mg/m^2 dexrazoxane: 50 mg/m^2 doxorubicin).

PRECAUTIONS

CONTRAINDICATIONS: Chemotherapy regimens that do not contain an anthracycline. **CAUTIONS:** Chemotherapeutic agents that are additive to myelosuppression, concurrent FAC therapy (fluorouracil, doxorubicin, cyclophosphamide). **PREGNANCY/LACTATION:** May be embryotoxic, tetragenic. Unknown if distributed in breast milk. Recommended not to breast-feed during therapy. **Pregnancy Category C**.

INTERACTIONS

DRUG INTERACTIONS: Concurrent FAC therapy (fluorouracil, doxorubicin, cyclophosphamide) may produce severe blood dyscrasias. **ALTERED LAB VALUES:** Concurrent FAC (fluorouracil, doxorubicin, cyclophosphamide) therapy may produce abnormal hepatic or renal function tests.

SIDE EFFECTS

FREQUENT: Alopecia, nausea, vomiting, fatigue, malaise, anorexia, stomatitis, fever, infection, diarrhea. **OCCASIONAL:** Pain w/injection, neurotoxicity, phlebitis, dysphagia, streaking/erythema. **RARE:** Urticaria, skin reaction.

ADVERSE REACTIONS/TOXIC EFFECTS

FAC therapy w/dexrazoxane may produce more severe leukopenia, granulocytopenia, and thrombocytopenia than those receiving FAC w/o dexrazoxane. Overdosage can be removed w/peritoneal or hemodialysis.

NURSING IMPLICATIONS
BASELINE ASSESSMENT:

Use gloves when preparing solution. If powder or solution comes in contact w/skin, wash immediately w/soap and water. Antiemetics may be effective in preventing, treating nausea.

INTERVENTION/EVALUATION:

Frequently monitor blood

counts for evidence of blood dyscrasias. Monitor for stomatitis (burning/erythema of oral mucosa at inner margin of lips, sore throat, difficulty swallowing). Monitor hematologic status, renal/hepatic function studies, cardiac function. Assess pattern of daily bowel activity, stool consistency. Monitor for hematologic toxicity (fever, signs of local infection, easy bruising, unusual bleeding from any site).

PATIENT/FAMILY TEACHING:

Alopecia is reversible, but new hair growth may have different color or texture. New hair growth resumes 2–3 mos after last therapy dose. Maintain fastidious oral hygiene. Do not have immunizations w/o physician approval (drug lowers body's resistance). Avoid those who have recently taken live virus vaccine. Promptly report fever, sore throat, signs of local infection. Contact physician if nausea/vomiting continues at home.

dextran, low molecular weight (dextran 40)

dex-tran
(Gentran, Rheomacrodex)

dextran, high molecular weight (dextran 75)

(Macrodex)

CANADIAN AVAILABILITY:
Hyskon, Rheomacrodex

CLASSIFICATION

Plasma volume expander

AVAILABILITY (Rx)

Injection: 10% dextran 40 in NaCl or D5W, 6% dextran 75 in NaCl or D5W

PHARMACOKINETICS

Evenly distributed in vascular circulation. Enzymatically degraded to glucose. Excreted in urine, feces.

ACTION/ *THERAPEUTIC EFFECT*

Draws fluid from interstitial to intravascular space (colloidal osmotic effect) *resulting in increased central venous pressure, cardiac output, stroke volume, B/P, urine output, capillary perfusion, pulse pressure, and decreased heart rate, peripheral resistance, blood viscosity.* Reduces aggregation of erythrocytes. Enhances blood flow *(corrects hypovolemia, improves circulation)*.

USES

Adjunctive treatment of shock or impending shock (due to burns, surgery, hemorrhage); primary fluid in pump oxygenation during extracorporeal circulation. Prophylaxis against deep vein thrombosis, pulmonary embolism in those having procedures associated w/high risk of thromboembolic complications.

STORAGE/HANDLING

Store at room temperature. Use only clear solutions. Discard partially used containers.

IV ADMINISTRATION

1. Give by IV infusion only.
2. Monitor pt closely during first minutes of infusion for anaphylactoid reaction. Monitor vital signs q5min.

3. Monitor urine flow rates during administration (if oliguria or anuria occurs, dextran 40 should be discontinued and osmotic diuretic given—minimizes vascular overloading).

4. Monitor central venous pressure (CVP) when given by rapid infusion. If there is a precipitous rise in CVP, immediately discontinue drug (overexpansion of blood volume).

5. Monitor B/P diligently during infusion; if marked hypotension occurs, stop infusion immediately (imminent anaphylactoid reaction).

6. If evidence of blood volume overexpansion occurs, discontinue IV until blood volume adjusts via urine output.

INDICATIONS/DOSAGE/ROUTES

USUAL LOW MOLECULAR WEIGHT DEXTRAN DOSAGES

Adjunct to shock therapy:
IV: Adults, elderly: Total dose for first 24 hrs not to exceed 20 ml/kg. Infuse first 10 ml/kg rapidly. Therapy beyond 24 hrs not to exceed 10 ml/kg/day or 5 days duration.

Hemodilution in extracorporeal solutions:
IV: Adults, elderly: 10–20 ml/kg added to perfusion circuit. Do not exceed 20 ml/kg.

Prophylactic use in deep vein thrombosis and pulmonary embolism:
IV: Adults, elderly: 500–1,000 ml (10 ml/kg) on day of surgery; continue 500 ml/day for 2–3 additional days. Thereafter, continue therapy at 500 ml q2–3days up to 2 wks (based on risk of complications).

USUAL HIGH MOLECULAR WEIGHT DEXTRAN DOSAGES

IV: Adults, elderly: 500–1,000 ml given up to 20–40 ml/min. **Maxi-**mum dose: 20 ml/kg in first 24 hrs, then 10 ml/kg/24 hrs thereafter. **Children:** 20 ml/kg in first 24 hrs, then 10 ml/kg/24 hrs.

PRECAUTIONS

CONTRAINDICATIONS: Marked hemostatic defects, including drug-induced, marked cardiac decompensation, renal disease with severe oliguria or anuria, hypervolemic conditions, severe bleeding disorders, when use of sodium or chloride could be detrimental. **CAUTIONS:** Those w/thrombocytopenia, CHF, pulmonary edema, severe renal insufficiency, those on corticosteroids or corticotropin, presence of edema w/sodium retention, impaired renal clearance, chronic liver disease, pathologic abdominal conditions, those undergoing bowel surgery. **PREGNANCY/LACTATION:** Unknown if drug crosses placenta or is distributed in breast milk. **Pregnancy Category C.**

INTERACTIONS

DRUG INTERACTIONS: None significant. **ALTERED LAB VALUES:** Prolongs bleeding time, increases bleeding tendency, depresses platelet count. Decreases factor VIII, factor V, factor IX.

SIDE EFFECTS

OCCASIONAL: Mild hypersensitivity reaction (urticaria, nasal congestion, wheezing).

ADVERSE REACTIONS/TOXIC EFFECTS

Severe or fatal anaphylaxis (marked hypotension, cardiac/respiratory arrest) may occur, noted early during IV infusion, generally in those not previously exposed to IV dextran.

NURSING IMPLICATIONS

INTERVENTION/EVALUATION:

Monitor urine output closely (increase in output generally occurs in oliguric pts after dextran administration). If no increase is observed after 500 ml dextran is infused, discontinue drug until diuresis occurs. Monitor for fluid overload (peripheral and/or pulmonary edema, impending CHF symptoms). Assess lung sounds for rales. Monitor central venous pressure (detects overexpansion of blood volume). Observe closely for allergic reaction. Assess for bleeding esp. following surgery or those on anticoagulant therapy (overt bleeding esp. at surgical site and bruising, petechiae development).

dextroamphetamine sulfate

dex-tro-am-**fet**-ah-meen
(Dexedrine)

CANADIAN AVAILABILITY:
Dexedrine

CLASSIFICATION

CNS stimulant

AVAILABILITY (Rx)

Tablets: 5 mg, 10 mg. **Capsules (sustained-release):** 5 mg, 10 mg, 15 mg. **Elixir:** 5 mg/5 ml.

PHARMACOKINETICS

	ONSET	PEAK	DURATION
PO	1–2 hrs	—	2–10 hrs

Well absorbed from GI tract. Widely distributed. Primarily excreted in urine. Half-life: 10–12 hrs (children 6–8 hrs).

ACTION/*THERAPEUTIC EFFECT*

Enhances release, action of catecholamine (dopamine, norepinephrine) by blocking reuptake, inhibiting MAO. *Increases motor activity, mental alertness, decreases drowsiness, fatigue.*

USES

Treatment of narcolepsy; treatment of attention deficit disorder in hyperactive children; short-term treatment to assist caloric restriction in exogenous obesity.

STORAGE/HANDLING

Store elixir form at room temperature.

PO ADMINISTRATION

1. Give single daily dose, initial daily dose upon awakening.
2. When given in 2–3 divided doses/day, give at 4–6 hr intervals.
3. Give last dose at least 6 hrs before retiring (prevents insomnia).
4. Give sustained-release form (one capsule daily), 10–14 hrs before bedtime.
5. If used as anorexic, give dose 30–60 min before meals.
6. Do not break capsule or tablet form.

INDICATIONS/DOSAGE/ROUTES

Narcolepsy:
PO: **Adults, children >12 yrs:** Initially, 10 mg/day. Increase by 10 mg at weekly intervals until therapeutic response achieved. **Usual dose:** 5–60 mg/day. **Children 6–12 yrs:** Initially, 5 mg/day. Increase by 5 mg/day at weekly intervals until therapeutic response achieved.

Attention deficit disorder:
PO: **Children >6 yrs:** Initially, 5 mg 1–2 times/day. Increase by 5 mg/day

at weekly intervals until therapeutic response achieved. **Maximum daily dose:** 40 mg. **Children 3–5 yrs:** Initially, 2.5 mg/day. Increase by 2.5 mg/day at weekly intervals until therapeutic response achieved.

Appetite suppressant:
PO: Adults: 5–30 mg daily in divided doses of 5–10 mg each dose, given 30–60 min before meals. **Extended-Release:** 1 capsule in morning.

PRECAUTIONS

CONTRAINDICATIONS: Hyperthyroidism, advanced arteriosclerosis, agitated states, moderate to severe hypertension, symptomatic cardiovascular disease, history of drug abuse, glaucoma, history of hypersensitivity to sympathomimetic amines, within 14 days of MAO inhibitor ingestion. **CAUTIONS:** Elderly, debilitated, tartrazine-sensitive pts. **PREGNANCY/LACTATION:** Distributed in breast milk. Significant agitation in neonates of mothers dependent on amphetamines. **Pregnancy Category C.**

INTERACTIONS

DRUG INTERACTIONS: Tricyclic antidepressants may increase cardiovascular effects. Beta blockers may increase risk of hypertension, bradycardia, heart block. CNS stimulants may increase effects. May increase risk of arrhythmias w/digoxin. Meperidine may increase risk of hypotension, respiratory depression, convulsions, vascular collapse. MAO inhibitors may prolong, intensify effects. May increase effects of thyroid hormone. Thyroid hormones may increase effects. **ALTERED LAB VALUES:** May increase plasma corticosteroid concentrations.

SIDE EFFECTS

FREQUENT: Irregular heartbeat, CNS stimulation, false sense of well-being, nervousness, insomnia. Increased motor activity, talkativeness, nervousness, mild euphoria, insomnia. **OCCASIONAL:** Headache, chilliness, dry mouth, GI distress, increased depression in depressed pts, tachycardia, palpitations, chest pain.

ADVERSE REACTIONS/TOXIC EFFECTS

Overdose may produce pallor or flushing, cardiac irregularities, psychotic syndrome. Abrupt withdrawal following prolonged administration of high dosage may produce lethargy (may last for weeks). Prolonged administration to children w/ADD may produce a temporary suppression of weight and/or height patterns.

NURSING IMPLICATIONS
PATIENT/FAMILY TEACHING:

Normal dosage levels may produce tolerance to drug's anorexic mood-elevating effects within a few weeks. Avoid tasks that require alertness, motor skills until response to drug is established. Dry mouth may be relieved by sugarless gum, sips of tepid water. Take early in day. May mask extreme fatigue. Report pronounced nervousness, dizziness, decreased appetite, dry mouth.

dezocine
dez-oh-seen
(Dalgan)

CLASSIFICATION

Opioid analgesic (**Schedule V**)

AVAILABILITY (Rx)

Injection: 5 mg/ml, 10 mg/ml, 15 mg/ml

PHARMACOKINETICS

	ONSET	PEAK	DURATION
IM	<30 min	30–45 min	2–4 hrs
IV	<15 min	30 min	2–4 hrs

Rapid, complete absorption after IM administration. Metabolized in liver. Primarily excreted in urine. Half-life: IM 2.2 hrs; IV 2.4–2.6 hrs.

ACTION / *THERAPEUTIC EFFECT*

Binds w/opiate receptors in CNS (probably in limbic system), *producing impaired pain perception.*

USES

Relief of moderate to severe pain.

STORAGE / HANDLING

Store parenteral form at room temperature. Discard if solution contains a precipitate.

INDICATIONS / DOSAGE / ROUTES

Analgesia:
IM: Adults, >18 yrs, elderly: 5–20 mg q3–6h as needed. **Maximum:** 120 mg/day.
IV: Adults, >18 yrs, elderly: 2.5–10 mg q2–4h as needed.

PRECAUTIONS

CONTRAINDICATIONS: None significant. **CAUTIONS:** Impaired hepatic/renal function, elderly, debilitated, head injury, respiratory disease, hypertension, hypothyroidism, acute alcoholism, urethral stricture. **PREGNANCY/LACTATION:** Unknown if drug crosses placenta or is distributed in breast milk (breast-feeding not recommended). Prolonged use during pregnancy may produce withdrawal symptoms (irritability, excessive crying, tremors, hyperactive reflexes, fever, vomiting, diarrhea, yawning, sneezing, seizures) in neonate. **Pregnancy Category C.**

INTERACTIONS

DRUG INTERACTIONS: CNS depressants, MAO inhibitors may increase CNS or respiratory depression, hypotensive effects. May decrease effects of other opioid analgesics, may also precipitate withdrawal symptoms. **ALTERED LAB VALUES:** May increase SGOT (AST), alkaline phosphatase.

SIDE EFFECTS

FREQUENT (3–9%): Drowsiness, nausea, vomiting. **OCCASIONAL (1–3%):** Anxiety, confusion, dizziness, slurred speech, flushed skin, abdominal pain, diarrhea, constipation, altered vision. **RARE (<1%):** Coughing, difficulty breathing, chest pain, delirium, skin rash, thrombophlebitis.

ADVERSE REACTIONS / TOXIC EFFECTS

Overdosage results in acute respiratory depression, skeletal muscle flaccidity, cyanosis, extreme somnolence progressing to convulsions, stupor, coma. Naloxone given as antidote.

NURSING IMPLICATIONS
BASELINE ASSESSMENT:

Raise bed rails. Obtain vital signs before giving medication. If respirations are 12/min or lower (20/min or lower in children), withhold medication, contact physician. Assess onset, type, location, and duration of pain. Effect of medication is reduced if full pain recurs before next dose.

D

INTERVENTION/EVALUATION:

Increase fluid intake and environmental humidity to improve viscosity of lung secretions. Monitor for change in respirations, B/P, change in rate or quality of pulse. Monitor daily bowel activity and prevent constipation. Initiate deep breathing and coughing exercises, particularly in those w/impaired pulmonary function. Change pt's position q2–4h and ambulate w/assistance. Assess for clinical improvement and record onset of relief of pain.

PATIENT/FAMILY TEACHING:

Change positions slowly to avoid dizziness. Avoid tasks that require alertness, motor skills until response to drug is established. Avoid alcohol.

---

diazepam

dye-**az**-eh-pam
(Diastat, Dizac, Valium, Valrelease)

CANADIAN AVAILABILITY:
Apo-Diazepam, Diazemuls, Valium, Vivol

CLASSIFICATION

Antianxiety: Benzodiazepine (Schedule IV)

AVAILABILITY (Rx)

Tablets: 2 mg, 5 mg, 10 mg. **Capsules (sustained-release):** 15 mg. **Oral Solution:** 5 mg/5 ml, 5 mg/ml. **Injection:** 5 mg/ml. **Injectable Emulsion:** 5 mg/ml. **Rectal Gel:** 2.5 mg, 10 mg, 15 mg, 20 mg.

PHARMACOKINETICS

	ONSET	PEAK	DURATION
IV	1–5 min	—	15–60 min

Well absorbed from GI tract. Widely distributed. Metabolized in liver to active metabolite. Excreted in urine. Half-life: 20–70 hrs (increased in elderly, liver dysfunction).

ACTION/*THERAPEUTIC EFFECT*

Enhances action of neurotransmitter gamma-aminobutyric acid (GABA) neurotransmission at CNS, *producing anxiolytic effect.* Enhances presynaptic inhibition, *elevating seizure threshold* in response to electrical/chemical stimulation. Inhibits spinal afferent pathways, *producing skeletal muscle relaxation.*

USES/*UNLABELED*

Short-term relief of anxiety symptoms, preanesthetic medication, relief of acute alcohol withdrawal. Adjunct for relief of acute musculoskeletal conditions, treatment of seizures (IV route used for termination of status epilepticus). Gel: Control of increased seizure activity in refractory epilepsy in those on stable regimens. *Treatment of panic disorders, tension headache, tremors.*

STORAGE/HANDLING

Store tablets, extended-release capsules, oral/parenteral solutions at room temperature.

PO/IM/IV ADMINISTRATION

PO:

1. Give w/o regard to meals.
2. Dilute oral concentrate w/ water, juice, carbonated beverages; may also be mixed in semi-solid food (applesauce, pudding).
3. Tablets may be crushed.
4. Do not crush or break capsule.

Parenteral form:

Do not mix w/other injections (produces precipitate).

IM:

Injection may be painful. Inject deeply into deltoid muscle.

IV:

1. Give by direct IV injection.

2. Administer directly into a large vein (reduces risk of thrombosis/phlebitis). If not possible, administer into tubing of a flowing IV solution as close to the vein insertion point as possible. Do not use small veins (e.g., wrist/dorsum of hand).

3. Administer IV rate not exceeding 5 mg/min. For children, give over a 3 min period (a too rapid IV may result in hypotension, respiratory depression).

4. Monitor respirations q5–15 min for 2h. May produce arrhythmias when used prior to cardioversion.

INDICATIONS/DOSAGE/ROUTES

Note: Use smallest effective dose in those w/liver disease, low serum albumin.

Anxiety:
PO/IM/IV: Adults: 2–10 mg 2–4 times/day. **Elderly/debilitated:** 2.5 mg 2 times/day. **Children >6 mos:** 1–2.5 mg 3–4 times/day.

Preanesthesia:
IV: Adults, elderly: 5–15 mg 5–10 min prior to procedure.

Alcohol withdrawal:
PO: Adults, elderly: 10 mg 3–4 times during first 24 hrs, then reduce to 5–10 mg 3–4 times/day as needed.
IM/IV: Adults, elderly: Initially, 10 mg, followed by 5–10 mg q3–4h.

Musculoskeletal spasm:
PO: Adults: 2–10 mg 2–4 times/day.
Elderly: 2–5 mg 2–4 times/day.
IM/IV: Adults: 5–10 mg q3–4h.

Seizures:
PO: Adults: 2–10 mg 2–4 times/day. **Elderly, debilitated:** 2.5 mg 2 times/day.
IM/IV: Adults: 5–10 mg, repeated at 10–15 min intervals to total of 30 mg. **Elderly, debilitated:** 2–5 mg, increase gradually as needed.
Gel: Adults, elderly, children: 0.2–0.5 mg/kg depending on age. May repeat in 4–12 hrs.

PRECAUTIONS

CONTRAINDICATIONS: Acute narrow-angle glaucoma, acute alcohol intoxication. **CAUTIONS:** Impaired kidney/liver function. **PREGNANCY/LACTATION:** Crosses placenta; distributed in breast milk. May increase risk of fetal abnormalities if administered during first trimester of pregnancy. Chronic ingestion during pregnancy may produce withdrawal symptoms, CNS depression in neonates. **Pregnancy Category D.**

INTERACTIONS

DRUG INTERACTIONS: Alcohol, CNS depressants may increase CNS depressant effect. **ALTERED LAB VALUES:** May produce abnormal renal function tests, elevate SGOT (AST), SGPT (ALT), LDH, alkaline phosphatase, serum bilirubin.

SIDE EFFECTS

FREQUENT: Pain w/IM injection, drowsiness, fatigue, ataxia (muscular incoordination). **OCCASIONAL:** Slurred speech, orthostatic hypotension, headache, hypoactivity, constipation, nausea, blurred vision. **RARE:** Paradoxical CNS hyperactivity/nervousness in children, excitement/restlessness in elderly/debilitated (generally noted during first 2 wks of therapy, particularly noted in presence of uncontrolled pain).

ADVERSE REACTIONS/TOXIC EFFECTS

IV route may produce pain, swelling, thrombophlebitis, carpal tunnel syndrome. Abrupt or too rapid withdrawal may result in pronounced restlessness, irritability, insomnia, hand tremors, abdominal/muscle cramps, sweating, vomiting, seizures. Abrupt withdrawal in pts w/epilepsy may produce increase in frequency and/or severity of seizures. Overdosage results in somnolence, confusion, diminished reflexes, coma.

NURSING IMPLICATIONS

BASELINE ASSESSMENT:

Assess B/P, pulse, respirations immediately before administration. Pt must remain recumbent for up to 3 hrs (individualized) after parenteral administration to reduce hypotensive effect. *Anxiety:* Assess autonomic response (cold, clammy hands, sweating) and motor response (agitation, trembling, tension). Offer emotional support to anxious pt. *Musculoskeletal spasm:* Record onset, type, location, duration of pain. Check for immobility, stiffness, swelling. *Seizures:* Review history of seizure disorder (length, intensity, frequency, duration, LOC). Observe frequently for recurrence of seizure activity. Initiate seizure precautions.

INTERVENTION/EVALUATION:

Monitor IV site for swelling, phlebitis (heat, pain, red streaking of skin over vein, hardness to vein). Assess children, elderly for paradoxical reaction, particularly during early therapy. Assist w/ambulation if drowsiness, ataxia occur. For those on long-term therapy, liver/renal function tests, blood counts should be performed periodically. Evaluate for therapeutic response: a decrease in intensity/frequency of seizures; a calm, facial expression, decreased restlessness; decreased intensity of skeletal muscle pain.

PATIENT/FAMILY TEACHING:

Discomfort may occur w/IM injection. Drowsiness usually diminishes w/continued therapy. Avoid tasks that require alertness, motor skills until response to drug is established. Smoking reduces drug effectiveness. Do not abruptly withdraw medication after long-term therapy. Strict maintenance of drug therapy is essential for seizure control. Avoid alcohol.

diazoxide
dye-ah-**zocks**-eyd
(Hyperstat, Proglycem)

CANADIAN AVAILABILITY:
Hyperstat, Proglycem

CLASSIFICATION

Antihypertensive, antihypoglycemic

AVAILABILITY (Rx)

Capsules: 50 mg. **Oral Suspension:** 50 mg/ml. **Injection:** 15 mg/ml.

PHARMACOKINETICS

	ONSET	PEAK	DURATION
PO: hypoglycemia	1 hr	—	Up to 8 hrs
IV: hypotensive	1 min	2–5 min	3–12 hrs

Readily absorbed from GI tract. Metabolized in liver. Excreted in urine. Removed by hemodialysis. Half-life: 21–36 hrs (increased in decreased renal function).

ACTION/*THERAPEUTIC EFFECT*

Directly relaxes smooth muscle in peripheral arterioles, *reducing peripheral vascular resistance, B/P.* Inhibits insulin release from pancreas, *increasing blood glucose.*

USES

Emergency lowering of B/P in adults w/severe, nonmalignant and malignant hypertension; children w/acute severe hypertension. Management of hypoglycemia caused by hyperinsulinism associated w/islet cell adenoma, carcinoma, or extrapancreatic malignancy.

STORAGE/HANDLING

Store capsules, oral suspension at room temperature. Parenteral forms should appear clear, colorless. Discard darkened solution (may be subpotent), or if precipitate is present.

PO/IV ADMINISTRATION

PO:

1. Shake well before using oral suspension.
2. May give w/o regard to food.

IV:

Note: IV form frequently produces a feeling of warmth along injection vein. Extravasation produces severe burning, cellulitis, phlebitis.

1. Place pt in supine position during and for 1 hr after IV dosing, monitor B/P diligently, follow by standing B/P in ambulatory pts.
2. Administer only in peripheral vein.
3. Give over 30 secs or less.
4. Do not use longer than 10 days.

INDICATIONS/DOSAGE/ROUTES

Severe hypertension:
IV: **Adults, elderly, children:** 1–3 mg/kg (up to max of 150 mg). Repeat q5–15min until adequate decrease in B/P occurs. Thereafter, give at intervals of 4–24 hrs.

Hypoglycemia:
PO: Adults, elderly, children: Initially, 3 mg/kg/day in 3 divided doses q8h. **Maintenance:** 3–8 mg/kg/day in 2–3 divided doses at 12 or 8 hr intervals. **Maximum:** Up to 15 mg/kg/day. **Infants, neonates:** Initially, 10 mg/kg/day in 3 divided doses q8h. **Maintenance:** 8–15 mg/kg/day in 2–3 divided doses at 12 or 8 hr intervals.

PRECAUTIONS

CONTRAINDICATIONS: History of hypersensitivity to thiazide derivatives. *IV:* Hypertension associated w/aortic coarctation, arteriovenous shunt. *Oral:* Management of functional hypoglycemia. **CAUTIONS:** Impaired renal function, cardiac reserve; caution when reducing severely elevated B/P. **PREGNANCY/LACTATION:** Crosses placenta; unknown if distributed in breast milk. May produce fetal or neonatal hyperbilirubinemia, thrombocytopenia, altered carbohydrate metabolism, alopecia, hypertrichosis. May produce cessation of uterine contractions if given during labor via IV. **Pregnancy Category C**.

INTERACTIONS

DRUG INTERACTIONS: Beta blockers, vasodilators, hypotension-producing medications may increase hypotensive effect. *Oral:* May decrease effect of phenytoin. **ALTERED LAB VALUES:** May increase SCOT (AST), alkaline phosphatase, free fatty acids, sodium, uric acid, glucose, BUN. May decrease hemoglobin, hematocrit, creatinine clearance.

SIDE EFFECTS

FREQUENT: Edema (increased weight, swelling of feet). **OCCASIONAL:** Tachycardia, altered taste, constipation, anorexia, nausea, vomiting, abdominal pain. *Parenteral:* Back pain, tinnitus, facial flushing, headache, pain/warmth along injection site. **RARE:** *IV/oral:* Sensitivity reaction (rash, fever), confusion, paresthesia, orthostatic hypotension.

ADVERSE REACTIONS/TOXIC EFFECTS

Overdose may cause hyperglycemia/ketoacidosis (increased urination, thirst, fruitlike breath). Angina, myocardial infarction, thrombocytopenia occur rarely.

NURSING IMPLICATIONS

BASELINE ASSESSMENT:

Establish baseline B/P, blood glucose. When administering IV, achieve desired B/P over as long a period of time as possible.

INTERVENTION/EVALUATION:

If excessive reduction in B/P occurs, place pt in supine position w/legs elevated. If parenteral form leaks in SubQ tissue, apply warm compresses to decrease pain sensation. Monitor for development of hyperglycemia, particularly in those w/renal or liver disease, diabetes mellitus, concurrent therapy that may increase blood glucose concentrations. Monitor blood glucose concentrations daily in those receiving IV therapy. Monitor serum uric acid in those w/history of gout, hyperuricemia.

PATIENT/FAMILY TEACHING:

Blood glucose or daily urine testing should be attained in those on chronic oral therapy. Report increases in urinary frequency, thirst, or fruity breath odor. Inform physician if pregnant.

---

dibucaine
(Nupercainal)
See Classification section under:
Anesthetics: local

---

diclofenac sodium
dye-**klo**-feh-nak
(Voltaren, Voltaren XR)
diclofenac potassium
(Cataflam)

FIXED-COMBINATION(S)
w/misoprostil, an antisecretory gastric protectant (Arthrotec)

CANADIAN AVAILABILITY:
Diclotek, Novo-Difenac, Voltaren

CLASSIFICATION

Nonsteroidal anti-inflammatory

AVAILABILITY (Rx)

Tablets: 50 mg (Cataflam). **Tablets (delayed-release):** 25 mg, 50 mg, 75 mg. **Tablets (extended-release):** 100 mg. **Ophthalmic Solution:** 0.1%.

PHARMACOKINETICS

	ONSET	PEAK	DURATION
PO	—	2–3 hrs	—

Completely absorbed from GI tract, penetrates cornea after ophthalmic administration (may be systemically absorbed). Widely distributed. Metabolized in liver. Primarily excreted in urine. Half-life: 1.2–2 hrs.

ACTION/THERAPEUTIC EFFECT

Inhibits prostaglandin synthesis,

reducing inflammatory response and intensity of pain stimulus reaching sensory nerve endings, *producing analgesic and anti-inflammatory effect.* Constricts iris sphincter, *preventing miosis during cataract surgery.*

USES / *UNLABELED*

Symptomatic treatment of acute and/or chronic rheumatoid arthritis, osteoarthritis, ankylosing spondylitis; postop inflammation of cataract extraction; analgesic, primary dysmenorrhea. Treatment of photophobia, relief of pain in incisional refractive surgery. *Ophthalmic: Reduces occurrence/severity of cystoid macular edema post cataract surgery. Oral: Treatment of vascular headaches.*

PO / OPHTHALMIC ADMINISTRATION

PO:

1. Do not crush or break enteric-coated form.

2. May give w/food, milk, or antacids if GI distress occurs.

OPHTHALMIC:

1. Place finger on lower eyelid and pull out until pocket is formed between eye and lower lid. Hold dropper above pocket and place prescribed number of drops in pocket.

2. Close eye gently. Apply digital pressure to lacrimal sac for 1–2 min (minimized drainage into nose and throat, reducing risk of systemic effects).

3. Remove excess solution w/ tissue.

INDICATIONS / DOSAGE / ROUTES

Osteoarthritis:
PO: Adults, elderly: 100–150 mg/day in 2–3 divided doses. *Extended release:* 100 mg/day as single dose.

Rheumatoid arthritis:
PO: Adults, elderly: 150–200 mg/day in 2–4 divided doses. *Extended-release:* 100 mg/day.

Ankylosing spondylitis:
PO: Adults, elderly: 100–125 mg/day in 4–5 divided doses.

Analgesic, primary dysmenorrhea:
PO: Adults: 150 mg/day in 3 divided doses.

Usual ophthalmic dosage:
Adults, elderly: Apply 1 drop to eye 4 times/day commencing 24 hrs after cataract surgery. Continue for 2 wks after surgery.

Photophobia:
Adults, elderly: 1 drop to affected eye 1 hr preop, within 15 min postop, then 4 times/day for 3 days.

PRECAUTIONS

CONTRAINDICATIONS: History of severe reaction induced by aspirin, other NSAIDs, nasal polyps associated w/bronchospasm, bone marrow depression, blood dyscrasias. **CAUTIONS:** History of inflammatory or ulcerative disease of GI tract (e.g., peptic ulcer, Crohn's disease), hemophilia or other bleeding problem. Impaired renal or liver function. Stomatitis. **PREGNANCY/LACTATION:** Crosses placenta, unknown if distributed in breast milk. Avoid use during last trimester (may adversely affect fetal cardiovascular system: premature closure of ductus arteriosus). **Pregnancy Category B.** (Category D if used in 3rd trimester or near delivery.)

INTERACTIONS

DRUG INTERACTIONS: May increase effects of oral anticoagulants, heparin, thrombolytics. May decrease effect of antihypertensives, diuretics. Salicylates, aspirin may increase risk of GI side effects, bleeding. Bone marrow depressants may increase risk of hematologic reactions. May increase concentration, toxicity of lithium. May increase methotrexate toxicity. Probenecid may increase concentration. *Ophthalmic:* May decrease effect of acetylcholine, carbachol. May decrease antiglaucoma effect of epinephrine, other antiglaucoma medications. **ALTERED LAB VALUES:** May increase alkaline phosphatase, LDH, serum transaminase, potassium urine protein, BUN, serum creatinine. May decrease uric acid.

SIDE EFFECTS

FREQUENT (3–9%): *Oral:* Headache, abdominal cramping, constipation, diarrhea, nausea, dyspepsia. *Ophthalmic:* Burning, stinging on instillation, ocular discomfort. **OCCASIONAL (1–3%):** *Oral:* Flatulence, dizziness, epigastric pain. *Ophthalmic:* Itching, tearing. **RARE (<1%):** *Oral:* Rash, peripheral edema/fluid retention, visual disturbances, vomiting, drowsiness.

ADVERSE REACTIONS/TOXIC EFFECTS

Overdosage may result in acute renal failure. In those treated chronically, peptic ulcer, GI bleeding, gastritis, severe hepatic reaction (jaundice), nephrotoxicity (hematuria, dysuria, proteinuria), severe hypersensitivity reaction (bronchospasm, angiofacial edema) occur rarely.

NURSING IMPLICATIONS
BASELINE ASSESSMENT:

Anti-inflammatory: **Assess onset, type, location, and duration of pain or inflammation. Inspect appearance of affected joints for immobility, deformities, and skin condition.**

INTERVENTION/EVALUATION:

Monitor for headache, dys- pepsia. Monitor pattern of daily bowel activity and stool consistency. Evaluate for therapeutic response: relief of pain, stiffness, swelling, increase in joint mobility, reduced joint tenderness, improved grip strength.

PATIENT/FAMILY TEACHING:

Swallow tablet whole; do not crush or chew. Avoid aspirin, alcohol during therapy (increases risk of GI bleeding). If GI upset occurs, take w/food, milk. Report GI distress, visual disturbances, rash, edema, headache. Report skin rash, itching, weight gain, changes in vision, black stools, persistent headache. Avoid tasks requiring alertness, motor skills until response to drug is established.

dicloxacillin sodium

dye-**clocks**-ah-sill-in
(Dynapen, Dycill, Pathocil)

CLASSIFICATION

Antibiotic: Penicillin

AVAILABILITY (Rx)

Capsules: 250 mg, 500 mg.
Oral Solution: 125 mg/5 ml.

PHARMACOKINETICS

Moderately absorbed from GI tract (food decreases absorption). Metabolized in liver. Primarily excreted in urine. Not removed by hemodialysis. Half-life: 0.5–1.1 hrs (increase in decreased renal function).

ACTION/*THERAPEUTIC EFFECT*

Inhibits cell wall synthesis by binding to bacterial membranes, *producing bactericidal effect.*

USES

Treatment of mild to moderate infections of respiratory tract and skin/skin structure, chronic osteomyelitis, urinary tract infection; follow-up to parenteral therapy for acute, severe infections. Predominantly treatment of infections caused by penicillinase-producing *Staphylococcus*.

STORAGE/HANDLING

Store capsules at room temperature. Oral solution, after reconstitution, is stable for 7 days at room temperature, 14 days if refrigerated.

PO ADMINISTRATION

1. Give 1 hr before or 2 hrs after meals.

2. Space doses evenly around the clock.

INDICATIONS/DOSAGE/ROUTES

Mild to moderate upper respiratory, localized skin/skin structure infections:
PO: Adults, elderly, children >40 kg: 125 mg q6h. Children <40 kg: 12.5 mg/kg/day in divided doses q6h.

Severe infections, lower respiratory tract, disseminated infections:
PO: Adults, elderly, children >40 kg: 250 mg q6h. Maximum: 4 g/day. Children <40 kg: 25 mg/kg/day in divided doses q6h.

PRECAUTIONS

CONTRAINDICATIONS: Hypersensitivity to any penicillin. CAUTIONS: History of allergies, particularly cephalosporins. PREGNANCY/LACTATION: Readily crosses placenta, appears in cord blood, amniotic fluid. Distributed in breast milk in low concentrations. May lead to allergic sensitization, diarrhea, candidiasis, skin rash in infant. Pregnancy Category B.

INTERACTIONS

DRUG INTERACTIONS: Probenecid may increase concentration, toxicity risk. ALTERED LAB VALUES: May increase SGOT (AST), SGPT (ALT), alkaline phosphatase, LDH. May cause positive Coombs' test.

SIDE EFFECTS

FREQUENT: Mild hypersensitivity reaction (fever, rash, pruritus), nausea, vomiting, diarrhea, flatulence.

ADVERSE REACTIONS/TOXIC EFFECTS

Superinfections, potentially fatal antibiotic-associated colitis may result from altered bacterial balance. Hematologic effects, severe hypersensitivity reactions, anaphylaxis occur rarely.

NURSING IMPLICATIONS

BASELINE ASSESSMENT:

Question for history of allergies, esp. penicillins, cephalosporins. Obtain specimen for culture and sensitivity before giving first dose (therapy may begin before results are known).

INTERVENTION/EVALUATION:

Hold medication and promptly report rash (may indicate hypersensitivity) or diarrhea (w/fever, abdominal pain, mucus and blood in stool may indicate antibiotic-associated colitis). Assess food tolerance. Check hematology reports (esp. WBCs), periodic renal or hepatic reports in prolonged therapy. Be alert for superinfection: increased fever, sore throat, diarrhea, ulceration or changes of oral mucosa, vaginal discharge, anal/genital pruritus.

Patient/Family Teaching:

Continue antibiotic for full length of treatment. Space doses evenly. Notify physician in event of diarrhea, rash, other new symptom.

dicyclomine hydrochloride

dye-**sigh**-clo-meen
(Antispaz, Bentyl, Dibent, Di-Spaz, Neoquess, OrTyl, Spasmoject)

CANADIAN AVAILABILITY: Bentylol, Formulex, Lomine

CLASSIFICATION

Antispasmodic, anticholinergic

AVAILABILITY (Rx)

Capsule: 10 mg, 20 mg. **Tablet:** 20 mg. **Syrup:** 10 mg/5 ml. **Injection:** 10 mg/ml.

PHARMACOKINETICS

Readily absorbed from GI tract. Widely distributed. Metabolized in liver. Half-life: 9–10 hrs.

ACTION/ *THERAPEUTIC EFFECT*

Direct relaxant action on smooth muscle, *reducing tone, motility of GI tract.*

USES

Treatment of functional disturbances of GI motility (i.e., irritable bowel syndrome).

STORAGE/HANDLING

Store capsules, tablets, syrup, parenteral form at room temperature. Injection should appear colorless.

PO/IM ADMINISTRATION

PO:

1. Dilute oral solution w/equal volume of water just before administration.

2. May give w/o regard to meals (food may slightly decrease absorption).

IM:

1. Do not administer IV or SubQ.

2. Inject deep into large muscle mass.

3. Do not give longer than 2 days.

INDICATIONS/DOSAGE/ROUTES

Functional disturbances of GI motility:
PO: Adults: 10–20 mg 3–4 times/day up to 40 mg 4 times/day. **Children 6 mos–2 yrs:** 5–10 mg 3–4 times/day. **Children >2 yrs:** 10 mg 3–4 times/day.
IM: Adults: 20 mg q4–6h.

Usual elderly dosage:
PO: 10–20 mg 4 times/day. May increase up to 160 mg/day.

PRECAUTIONS

CONTRAINDICATIONS: Narrow-angle glaucoma, severe ulcerative colitis, toxic megacolon, obstructive disease of GI tract, paralytic ileus, intestinal atony, bladder neck obstruction due to prostatic hypertrophy, myasthenia gravis in those not treated w/neostigmine, tachycardia secondary to cardiac insufficiency or thyrotoxicosis, cardiospasm, unstable cardiovascular status in acute hemorrhage. **EXTREME CAUTION:** Autonomic neuropathy, known or suspected GI infections, diarrhea, mild to moderate ulcerative colitis. **CAUTIONS:** Hyperthyroidism, hepatic or renal disease, hypertension, tachyarrhythmias, CHF, coronary artery disease, gastric ulcer, esophageal reflux or hiatal hernia associated w/reflux esophagitis, infants, elderly, those w/COPD. **PREGNANCY/LACTATION:** Unknown if drug crosses placenta or is distributed in breast milk. **Pregnancy Category B**.

INTERACTIONS

DRUG INTERACTIONS: Antacids, antidiarrheals may decrease absorption. Anticholinergics may increase effects. May decrease absorption of ketoconazole. May increase severity of GI lesions with KCl (wax matrix). **ALTERED LAB VALUES:** None significant.

SIDE EFFECTS

FREQUENT: Dry mouth (sometimes severe), constipation, decreased sweating. **OCCASIONAL:** Blurred vision, intolerance to light, urinary hesitancy, drowsiness (with high dosage), agitation/excitement/drowsiness noted in elderly (even with low doses). IM may produce transient lightheadedness, irritation at injection site. **RARE:** Confusion, hypersensitivity reaction, increased intraocular pressure, nausea, vomiting, unusual tiredness.

ADVERSE REACTIONS/TOXIC EFFECTS

Overdosage may produce temporary paralysis of ciliary muscle, pupillary dilation, tachycardia, palpitation, hot/dry/flushed skin, absence of bowel sounds, hyperthermia, increased respiratory rate, EKG abnormalities, nausea, vomiting, rash over face/upper trunk, CNS stimulation, psychosis (agitation, restlessness, rambling speech, visual hallucination, paranoid behavior, delusions), followed by depression.

NURSING IMPLICATIONS

BASELINE ASSESSMENT:

Before giving medication, instruct pt to void (reduces risk of urinary retention).

INTERVENTION/EVALUATION:

Monitor daily bowel activity and stool consistency. Assess for urinary retention. Monitor changes in B/P, temperature. Assess skin turgor, mucous membranes to evaluate hydration status (encourage adequate fluid intake), bowel sounds for peristalsis. Be alert for fever (increased risk of hyperthermia).

PATIENT/FAMILY TEACHING:

Do not become overheated during exercise in hot weather (may result in heat stroke). Avoid hot baths, saunas. Avoid tasks that require alertness, motor skills until response to drug is established. Sugarless gum, sips of tepid water may relieve dry mouth. Do not take antacids or medicine for diarrhea within 1 hr of taking this medication (decreased effectiveness).

didanosine

dye-**dan**-oh-sin
(Videx)

CANADIAN AVAILABILITY:
Videx

CLASSIFICATION

Antiviral

AVAILABILITY (Rx)

Tablets: 25 mg, 50 mg, 100 mg, 150 mg, 200 mg. **Powder for Oral Solution (packets):** 100 mg, 167 mg, 250 mg, 375 mg. **Powder for Oral Solution (bottles):** 2 g, 4 g.

PHARMACOKINETICS

Variably absorbed from GI tract. Rapidly metabolized intracellularly to active form. Primarily excreted in urine. Half-life: 1.5 hrs; metabolite: 8–24 hrs.

ACTION / *THERAPEUTIC EFFECT*

Intracellularly converted into a triphosphate, interfering w/RNA-directed DNA polymerase (reverse transcriptase). *Virustatic,* inhibiting replication of retroviruses, including human immunodeficiency virus (HIV).

USES

Management (not cure) of advanced HIV disease in pts who cannot tolerate zidovudine or who have had clinically or immunologically significant deterioration during zidovudine therapy. Initial therapy in AIDS.

STORAGE / HANDLING

Store at room temperature. If tablets dispersed in water, stable for 1 hr at room temperature; after reconstitution of buffered powder, oral solution stable for 4 hrs at room temperature. Pediatric powder for oral solution after reconstitution as directed, stable for 30 days refrigerated.

PO ADMINISTRATION

1. Give 1 hr before or 2 hrs after meals (food decreases rate and extent of absorption).

2. Chewable tablets: thoroughly crushed and dispersed in at least 30 ml water before swallowing. Mixture should be stirred well (2–3 min) and swallowed immediately.

3. Buffered powder for oral solution: reconstitute prior to administration by pouring contents of packet into about 4 oz water; stir until completely dissolved (up to 2–3 min). Do not mix w/fruit juice or other acidic liquid because didanosine is unstable at acidic pH.

4. Unbuffered pediatric powder: add 100–200 ml water to 2 or 4 g, respectively, to provide concentration of 20 mg/ml. Immediately mix w/equal amount of antacid to provide concentration of 10 mg/ml. Shake thoroughly prior to removing each dose.

INDICATIONS / DOSAGE / ROUTES

Note: Each dose consists of 2 tablets (prevents degradation of drug). Children <1 yr need only 1 tablet/dose.

HIV infections (adults):
Note: May give tablets 400 mg/day once daily in HIV-infected adults. Powder only in renal impairment.
PO (Tablets): Adults >60 kg: 200 mg q12h. **<60 kg:** 125 mg q12h. **(Buffered oral solution): Adults >60 kg:** 250 mg q12h. **<60 kg:** 167 mg q12h.

HIV infections (children):
PO (Tablets): Children BSA 1.1–1.4 m²: 100 mg q12h; **BSA 0.8–1.0 m²:** 75 mg q12h; **BSA 0.5–0.7 m²:** 50 mg q12h; **BSA <0.4 m²:** 25 mg q12h. **(Pediatric oral solution): Children BSA 1.1–1.4 m²:** 125 mg q12h; **BSA 0.8–1.0 m²:** 94 mg q12h; **BSA 0.5–0.7 m²:** 62 mg q12h; **BSA <0.4 m²:** 31 mg q12h.

PRECAUTIONS

CONTRAINDICATIONS: Hypersensitivity to drug or any component of preparation. **CAUTIONS:** Renal or hepatic dysfunction, alcoholism, elevated triglycerides, T cell counts less than 100 cells/mm^3; extreme caution w/history of pancreatitis. Phenylketonuria and sodium-restricted diets due to phenylalanine and sodium content of preparations. **PREGNANCY/LACTATION:** Use during pregnancy only if clearly needed. Discontinue nursing during didanosine therapy. Pregnancy Category B.

INTERACTIONS

DRUG INTERACTIONS: May increase risk of pancreatitis, peripheral neuropathy w/medications producing pancreatitis, peripheral neuropathy, respectively. May decrease absorption of dapsone, itraconazole, ketoconazole, tetracyclines, fluoroquinolones. **ALTERED LAB VALUES:** May increase alkaline phosphatase, SGOT (AST), SGPT (ALT), bilirubin, amylase, lipase, triglycerides, uric acid. May decrease potassium.

SIDE EFFECTS

FREQUENT: *Adults (>10%):* Diarrhea, neuropathy, chills/fever. *Children (>25%):* Chills, fever, decreased appetite, pain, malaise, nausea, diarrhea, vomiting, abdominal pain, headache, nervousness, cough, rhinitis, dyspnea, asthenia, rash, itching. **OCCASIONAL:** *Adults (2–9%):* Rash, itching, headache, abdominal pain, nausea, vomiting, pneumonia, myopathy, decreased appetite, dry mouth, dyspnea. *Children (10–25%):* Failure to thrive, decreased weight, stomatitis, oral thrush, ecchymosis, arthritis, myalgia, insomnia, epistaxis, pharyngitis.

ADVERSE REACTIONS/TOXIC EFFECTS

Pneumonia, opportunistic infection occur occasionally. Peripheral neuropathy, potentially fatal pancreatitis are the major toxicities.

NURSING IMPLICATIONS
BASELINE ASSESSMENT:

Obtain baseline values for CBC, renal and hepatic function tests, vital signs, weight. Question for hypersensitivity to didanosine or components of preparation.

INTERVENTION/EVALUATION:

In event of abdominal pain and nausea, vomiting, or elevated serum amylase, triglycerides, contact physician before administering medication (potential pancreatitis). Be alert to burning feet, "restless leg syndrome" (unable to find comfortable position for legs and feet), lack of coordination and other signs of peripheral neuropathy. Check food intake and assure availability of desired foods. Monitor consistency and frequency of stools. Check skin for rash, eruptions. Assess temperature, respiration, pulse, B/P at least b.i.d. Assess for opportunistic infections: onset of fever, oral mucosa changes, cough, or other respiratory symptoms. Monitor lab values carefully. Assess children for epistaxis or other bleeding, petechiae. Evaluate for dehydration (esp. children): decreased skin turgor, dry skin and mucous membranes, decreased urinary output. Check weight at least twice a week. Assess for visual or hearing difficulty; provide protection from light if photophobia develops. Auscultate lungs and assess for difficult breathing. If dizziness occurs, provide assistance w/ambulation.

PATIENT/FAMILY TEACHING:

Explain correct administration of medication. Small, frequent meals of favorite foods to offset anorexia, vomiting. Accurate I&O record. Report development of fever or any new symptom promptly.

dienestrol

dye-en-**ess**-troll
(Ortho Dienestrol)

CANADIAN AVAILABILITY:
Ortho Dienestrol

CLASSIFICATION

Estrogen

AVAILABILITY (Rx)

Vaginal cream: 0.01%

PHARMACOKINETICS

Extensively absorbed into systemic circulation. Widely distributed. Metabolized in liver. Primarily excreted in urine.

ACTION/THERAPEUTIC EFFECT

Increases synthesis of DNA, RNA, and various proteins in responsive tissues, *alleviating signs and symptoms of vulvovaginal epithelial atrophy (atrophic vaginitis), kraurosis vulvae associated w/ menopause.*

USES

Treatment of atrophic vaginitis, kraurosis vulvae.

VAGINAL ADMINISTRATION

1. Apply at bedtime for best absorption.
2. Assemble and fill applicator per manufacturer's directions.
3. Insert end of applicator into vagina, direct slightly toward sacrum; push plunger down completely.
4. Avoid skin contact w/cream due to absorption.

INDICATIONS/DOSAGE/ROUTES

Atrophic vaginitis, kraurosis vulvae:
Intravaginal: Adults, elderly: Initially, 1–2 applicatorsful/day for 7–14 days. Reduce dose by $1/2$ for additional 1–2 wks. **Maintenance:** 1 applicatorful 1–3 times/wk.

PRECAUTIONS

CONTRAINDICATIONS: Known or suspected breast cancer, estrogen-dependent neoplasia; undiagnosed abnormal genital bleeding; active thrombophlebitis or thromboembolic disorders; history of thrombophlebitis, thrombosis, or thromboembolic disorders w/previous estrogen use, hypersensitivity to estrogen or ingredients of cream. **CAUTIONS:** Conditions that may be aggravated by fluid retention: cardiac, renal, or hepatic dysfunction, epilepsy, migraine. Mental depression, hypercalcemia, history of jaundice during pregnancy, or strong family history of breast cancer, fibrocystic disease, or breast nodules. **PREGNANCY/LACTATION:** Possibly excreted in breast milk. May be harmful to fetus. **Pregnancy Category X.**

INTERACTIONS

DRUG INTERACTIONS: May interfere w/effects of bromocriptine. May increase concentration cyclosporine, increase hepatic, nephrotoxicity. Hepatotoxic medications may increase hepatotoxicity. **ALTERED LAB VALUES:** May affect metapyrone, thyroid function tests. May decrease cholesterol, LDH. May increase calcium, glucose, HDL, triglycerides.

SIDE EFFECTS

FREQUENT: Breast pain/tenderness, enlarged breasts, edema (swelling of feet, increased weight), decreased appetite, abdominal cramping. **OCCASIONAL:** Diarrhea, dizziness, headache, increased libido, abnormal vaginal bleeding, (amenorrhea, breakthrough bleeding, spotting, menorrhagia), breast tumors, gallbladder obstructions. Local irritation (itching, redness, swelling).

ADVERSE REACTIONS/TOXIC EFFECTS

Prolonged administration increases risk of gallbladder, thromboembolic disease, and breast, cervical, vaginal, endometrial, and liver carcinoma.

NURSING IMPLICATIONS

BASELINE ASSESSMENT:

Question hypersensitivity to estrogen or ingredients of cream, previous jaundice or thromboembolic disorders associated w/pregnancy or estrogen therapy. Establish baseline B/P, blood glucose.

INTERVENTION/EVALUATION:

Initially assess B/P, weight daily. Monitor blood glucose 4 times/day for pts w/diabetes. Check for swelling. Assess for vaginal discharge, local irritation. Promptly report signs and symptoms of thromboembolic or thrombotic disorders: weakness, pain or numbness of an extremity, chest pain, shortness of breath. Note estrogen therapy on specimens.

PATIENT/FAMILY TEACHING:

Importance of medical supervision. W/systemic absorption, smoking may increase risk of heart attack or blood clots. Notify physician of abnormal vaginal bleeding pain or numbness of an extremity, other symptoms. Teach breast self-exam. Use protection from sun or ultraviolet light. Check weight weekly; report weekly gain of 5 lbs or more. Remain recumbent at least 30 min after application and do not use tampons. Stop using dienestrol, contact physician at once if suspect pregnancy. Give labeling from drug package.

---

diethylstilbestrol

dye-eth-ill-still-**bess**-trole
(DES, Stilphostrol)

diethylstilbestrol diphosphate

(Stilphostrol)

CANADIAN AVAILABILITY:
Honvol

CLASSIFICATION

Antineoplastic, estrogen

AVAILABILITY (Rx)

Tablets: 1 mg, 5 mg. **Tablets (as diphosphate):** 50 mg. **Injection (as diphosphate):** 250 mg.

PHARMACOKINETICS

Well absorbed from GI tract. Widely distributed. Metabolized in liver. Primarily excreted in urine.

ACTION / *THERAPEUTIC EFFECT*

Increases synthesis of DNA, RNA, and various proteins in responsive tissues. Reduces release of gonadotopin-releasing hormone, *reducing follicle-stimulating hormone (FSH) and luteinizing hormone (LH); decreases serum concentration of testosterone.*

USES / *UNLABELED*

Palliative therapy for inoperable cancer of the prostate and advanced metastatic cancer of the breast in men and postmenopausal women. *Prophylaxis of postmenopausal osteoporosis, estrogen deficiency–induced premenopausal osteoporosis.*

STORAGE / HANDLING

Injection is colorless to light yellow solution. Discard if solution is cloudy or precipitate forms.

PO / IV ADMINISTRATION

PO:

1. Enteric tablets should not be crushed.
2. Give w/food to reduce nausea.

IV:

1. Dilute in 300 ml normal saline or 5% dextrose for injection.
2. Administer slowly (12 ml/min) the first 10–15 min, then increase rate to infuse over 1 hr.

INDICATIONS / DOSAGE / ROUTES

Breast carcinoma:
PO: Adults, elderly: 15 mg/day.

Prostatic carcinoma:
PO: Adults, elderly: Initially, 1–3 mg/day. **Maintenance:** 1 mg/day.

Usual dosage for diethylstilbestrol diphosphate:
PO: Adults, elderly: Initially, 50 mg 3 times/day; increase to 200 mg 3 times/day.
IV: Adults, elderly: Initially, 500 mg, then 1 g/day for 5 or more days. **Maintenance:** 250–500 mg 1–2 times/wk.

PRECAUTIONS

CONTRAINDICATIONS: Known or suspected breast cancer (except select cases), estrogen-dependent neoplasia; undiagnosed abnormal genital bleeding; active thrombophlebitis or thromboembolic disorders; history of thrombophlebitis, thrombosis, or thromboembolic disorders w/previous estrogen use, hypersensitivity to estrogen. Stilphostrol (diethylstilbestrol diphosphate) is not for use in women. **CAUTIONS:** Conditions that may be aggravated by fluid retention: cardiac, renal, or hepatic dysfunction, epilepsy, migraine. Metabolic bone disease w/potential hypercalcemia, mental depression, history of jaundice during pregnancy, or strong family history of breast cancer, fibrocystic disease, or breast nodules, young pts in whom bone growth is not complete. **PREGNANCY/LACTATION:** Not for use during lactation. May cause serious fetal toxicity (increased risk of congenital anomalies). **Pregnancy Category X.**

INTERACTIONS

DRUG INTERACTIONS: May interfere w/effects of bromocriptine. May increase concentration of cyclosporine, increase hepatic, nephrotoxicity. Hepatotoxic medications may increase hepatotoxicity. **ALTERED LAB VALUES:** May affect metapyrone, thyroid function tests. May decrease cholesterol, LDH. May increase calcium, glucose, HDL, triglycerides.

SIDE EFFECTS

FREQUENT: Change in vaginal bleeding (spotting, breakthrough, heavy, or prolonged bleeding), breast tenderness, gynecomastia, peripheral edema. *High-dose therapy:* Anorexia, nausea. **OCCASIONAL:** Headache, intolerance to contact lenses. **RARE:** Hirsutism, loss of scalp hair, depression.

ADVERSE REACTIONS/TOXIC EFFECTS

Prolonged administration may have possibility of increased risk of gallbladder, thromboembolic disease, and cervical, vaginal, endometrial, and liver carcinoma.

NURSING IMPLICATIONS

BASELINE ASSESSMENT:

Question for possibility of pregnancy before initiating therapy. Question hypersensitivity to estrogen, previous jaundice, or thromboembolic disorders associated w/pregnancy or estrogen therapy. Establish baseline B/P, blood glucose.

INTERVENTION/EVALUATION:

Assess B/P at least daily. Monitor blood glucose 4 times/day in diabetic pts. Check for swelling, weigh daily. Promptly report signs and symptoms of thromboembolic or thrombotic disorders: sudden severe headache, shortness of breath, vision or speech disturbance, weakness or numbness of an extremity, loss of coordination, pain in chest, groin, or leg. Estrogen therapy should be noted on specimens.

PATIENT/FAMILY TEACHING:

Importance of medical supervision. Avoid smoking due to increased risk of heart attack or blood clots. Do not take other medications w/o physician approval. Teach how to perform Homan's test, signs and symptoms of blood clots (report these to physician immediately). Notify physician of vaginal discharge or bleeding, difficulty or discomfort w/urination, other symptoms. Teach female patients to perform breast self-exam. Cyclic treatment of atrophic vaginitis may take several years. Avoid exposure to sun or ultraviolet light. Check weight daily; report weekly gain of 5 lbs or more. Use nonhormonal contraceptive or inform physician if suspect pregnancy. Libido improves, gynecomastia is reduced when medication stopped.

diflunisal

dye-**flew**-neh-sol
(Dolobid)

CANADIAN AVAILABILITY:
Apo-Diflunisal, Dolobid, Novo-Diflunisal

CLASSIFICATION

Nonsteroidal anti-inflammatory

AVAILABILITY (Rx)

Tablets: 250 mg, 500 mg

PHARMACOKINETICS

	ONSET	PEAK	DURATION
PO	1 hr	2–3 hrs	—

Completely absorbed from GI tract. Widely distributed. Metabolized in liver. Primarily excreted in urine. Half-life: 8–12 hrs.

ACTION/THERAPEUTIC EFFECT

Inhibits prostaglandin synthesis, reducing inflammatory response and intensity of pain stimulus reaching sensory nerve endings, *producing analgesic and anti-inflammatory effect.*

USES/UNLABELED

Treatment of acute or long-term mild to moderate pain associated w/acute and/or chronic rheumatoid arthritis, osteoarthritis. *Treatment of psoriatic arthritis, vascular headache.*

PO ADMINISTRATION

1. May give w/water, milk, or meals.
2. Do not crush or break film-coated tablets.

INDICATIONS/DOSAGE/ROUTES

Mild to moderate pain:
PO: Adults, elderly: Initially, 0.5–1 g, then 250–500 mg q8–12h.

Rheumatoid arthritis, osteoarthritis:
PO: Adults, elderly: 0.5–1 g/day in 2 divided doses.

PRECAUTIONS

CONTRAINDICATIONS: History of severe allergic reaction induced by aspirin, other NSAIDs, nasal polyps associated w/bronchospasm, bone marrow depression, blood dyscrasias. **CAUTIONS:** History of inflammatory or ulcerative disease of GI tract (e.g., peptic ulcer, Crohn's disease), hemophilia or other bleeding problem. Impaired renal or liver function. Stomatitis. **PREGNANCY/LACTATION:** Crosses placenta; distributed in breast milk. Avoid use during last trimester (may adversely affect fetal cardiovascular system: premature closure of ductus arteriosus). **Pregnancy Category C**. (Category D if used in 3rd trimester or near delivery.)

INTERACTIONS

DRUG INTERACTIONS: May increase effects of oral anticoagulants, heparin, thrombolytics. May decrease effect of antihypertensives, diuretics. Salicylates, aspirin may increase risk of GI side effects, bleeding. Bone marrow depressants may increase risk of hematologic reactions. May increase concentration, toxicity of lithium. May increase methotrexate toxicity. Probenecid may increase concentration. **ALTERED LAB VALUES:** May increase serum transaminase activity. May decrease uric acid.

SIDE EFFECTS

Side effects appear less frequently with short-term treatment. **OCCASIONAL (3–9%):** Nausea, dyspepsia (heartburn, indigestion, epigastric pain), diarrhea, headache, rash. **RARE (1–3%):** Vomiting, constipation, flatulence, dizziness, insomnolence, insomnia, fatigue, tinnitus.

ADVERSE REACTIONS/TOXIC EFFECTS

Overdosage may produce drowsiness, vomiting, nausea, diarrhea, hyperventilation, tachycardia, sweating, stupor, coma. Peptic ulcer, GI bleeding, gastritis, severe hepatic reaction (cholestasis, jaundice) occur rarely. Nephrotoxicity (dysuria, hematuria, proteinuria, nephrotic syndrome) and severe hypersensitivity reaction (bronchospasm, angiofacial edema) occur rarely.

NURSING IMPLICATIONS
BASELINE ASSESSMENT:

Assess onset, type, location, and duration of pain or inflammation. Inspect appearance of affected joints for immobility, deformities, and skin condition.

INTERVENTION/EVALUATION:

Monitor for nausea, dyspepsia. Assess skin for evidence of rash. Monitor pattern of daily bowel activity and stool consistency. Evaluate for therapeutic response: relief of pain, stiffness, swelling, increase in joint mobility, reduced joint tenderness, improved grip strength.

PATIENT/FAMILY TEACHING:

Swallow tablet whole; do not crush or chew. If GI upset occurs, take w/food, milk. Avoid aspirin, alcohol during therapy (increases risk of GI bleeding). Report GI distress, headache, rash.

digoxin
di-**jox**-in
(Lanoxin, Lanoxicaps)

CANADIAN AVAILABILITY:
Lanoxin

CLASSIFICATION

Antiarrhythmic, cardiotonic

AVAILABILITY (Rx)

Tablets: 0.125 mg, 0.25 mg, 0.5 mg. **Capsules:** 0.05 mg, 0.1 mg, 0.2 mg. **Elixir:** 0.05 mg/ml. **Injection:** 0.25 mg/ml, 0.1 mg/ml.

PHARMACOKINETICS

Readily absorbed from GI tract. Widely distributed. Partially metabolized in liver. Primarily excreted in urine. Half-life: 36–48 hrs (increased in decreased renal function, elderly).

ACTION/THERAPEUTIC EFFECT

Direct action on cardiac muscle, conduction system. Decreases conduction rate through SA, AV node. *Increases force, velocity of myocardial contraction.*

USES

Prophylactic management and treatment of CHF, control of ventricular rate in pts w/atrial fibrillation. Treatment and prevention of recurrent paroxysmal atrial tachycardia.

PO/IV ADMINISTRATION

Note: IM rarely used (produces severe local irritation, erratic absorption). If no other route possible, give deep into muscle followed by massage. Give no more than 2 ml at any one site.

PO:

1. May be given w/o regard to meals.
2. Tablets may be crushed.

IV:

1. May give undiluted or dilute w/at least a 4-fold volume of sterile water for injection, or 5% dextrose (less than this may cause a precipitate). Use immediately.
2. Give IV slowly over at least 5 min.

INDICATIONS/DOSAGE/ROUTES

Note: Adjust dose in elderly, pts w/renal dysfunction. Larger doses often required for adequate control of ventricular rate in pts w/atrial fibrillation or flutter. Administer loading dosage in several doses at 4–8 hr intervals.

USUAL DOSAGE FOR ADULTS

Rapid loading dosage:
IV: Adults, elderly: 0.6–1 mg.
PO: Adults, elderly: Initially, 0.5–0.75 mg, additional doses of 0.125–0.375 mg at 6–8 hr intervals. **Range:** 0.75–1.25 mg..

Maintenance dosage:
PO/IV: Adults, elderly: 0.125–0.375 mg/day.

USUAL DOSAGE FOR CHILDREN

Rapid loading dosage:
IV: Children (>10 yrs): 8–12 mcg/kg; **(5–10 yrs):** 15–30 mcg/kg; **(2–5 yrs):** 25–35 mcg/kg; **(1–24 mos):** 30–50 mcg/kg; **(Full term):** 20–30 mcg/kg; **(Premature):** 15–25 mcg/kg.
PO: Children (>10 yrs): 10–15 mcg/kg; **(5–10 yrs):** 20–35 mcg/kg; **(2–5 yrs):** 30–40 mcg/kg; **(1–24 mos):** 35–60 mcg/kg; **(Full term):** 25–35 mcg/kg; **(Premature):** 20–30 mcg/kg.

Maintenance dosage:
PO/IV: Children: 25–35% loading dose (20–30% for premature).

PRECAUTIONS

CONTRAINDICATIONS: Ventricular fibrillation, ventricular tachycardia unrelated to CHF. **CAUTIONS:** Impaired renal function, impaired hepatic function, hypokalemia, advanced cardiac disease, acute myocardial infarction, incomplete AV block, cor pulmonale, hypothyroidism, pulmonary disease. **PREGNANCY/ LACTATION:** Crosses placenta; distributed in breast milk. **Pregnancy Category C.**

INTERACTIONS

DRUG INTERACTIONS: Glucocorticoids, amphotericin, potassium-depleting diuretics may increase toxicity (due to hypokalemia). Amiodarone may increase concentration, toxicity; additive effect on SA, AV nodes. Antiarrhythmics, parenteral calcium, sympathomimetics may increase risk of arrhythmias. Antidiarrheals, cholestyramine, colestipol, sucralfate may decrease absorption. Diltiazem, verapamil, fluoxetine, quinidine may increase concentration. Parenteral magnesium may cause conduction changes, heart block. **ALTERED LAB VALUES:** None significant.

SIDE EFFECTS

None significant; however, there is a very narrow margin of safety between a therapeutic and toxic result. See Adverse Reactions/ Toxic Effects.

ADVERSE REACTIONS/TOXIC EFFECTS

The most common early manifestations of toxicity are GI disturbances (anorexia, nausea, vomiting) and neurologic abnormalities (fatigue, headache, depression, weakness, drowsiness, confusion, nightmares). Facial pain, personality change, ocular disturbances (photophobia, light flashes, halos around bright objects, yellow or green color perception) may be noted.

NURSING IMPLICATIONS
BASELINE ASSESSMENT:

Assess apical radial pulse for 60 secs (30 secs if on maintenance therapy). If pulse is 60/min or below (70/min or below for children), withhold drug and contact physician. Blood samples are best taken 6–8 hrs after dose or just prior to next dose.

INTERVENTION/EVALUATION:

Monitor pulse for bradycardia, EKG for arrhythmias for 1–2 hrs after administration (excessive slowing of pulse may be a first clinical sign of toxicity). Assess for GI disturbances, neurologic abnormalities (signs of toxicity) q2–4h during digitalization (daily during maintenance). Monitor serum potassium, magnesium levels. Monitor for therapeutic plasma level (0.5–2.0 ng/ml).

PATIENT/FAMILY TEACHING:

Importance of follow-up visits, tests. Teach pt to take pulse correctly and to report pulse below 60/min (or as indicated by physician). Assure pt understands signs of toxicity and need to notify physician if any occur. Wear/carry identification of digoxin therapy and inform dentist or other physician of taking digoxin. Take medication as directed; do not increase or skip doses. Do not take OTC medications w/o consulting physician. Chronic therapy may produce mammary gland enlargement in women but is reversible when drug is withdrawn. Report nausea, vomiting, extremely slow pulse.

digoxin immune FAB
(Digibind)

CANADIAN AVAILABILITY: Digibind

CLASSIFICATION

Antidote

AVAILABILITY (Rx)

Powder for Injection: 38 mg vial

PHARMACOKINETICS

	ONSET	PEAK	DURATION
IV	30 min	—	3–4 days

Widely distributed into extracellular space. Excreted in urine. Half-life: 15–20 hrs.

ACTION/ THERAPEUTIC EFFECT

Acts in extracellular space. Binds molecules of digoxin, *making digoxin unavailable for binding at its site of action on cells in the body.*

USES

Treatment of potentially life-threatening digoxin intoxication.

STORAGE/HANDLING

Refrigerate vials. After reconstitution, stable for 4 hrs if refrigerated. Use immediately after reconstitution.

IV ADMINISTRATION

1. Reconstitute each 38 mg vial w/4 ml sterile water for injection to provide a concentration of 9.5 mg/ml.
2. Further dilute w/50 ml 0.9% NaCl and infuse over 30 min (recommended that solution be infused through a 0.22 micron filter).
3. If cardiac arrest imminent, may give IV push.

INDICATIONS/DOSAGE/ROUTES

Dosage varies according to amount of digoxin to be neutralized. Refer to manufacturer's dosing guidelines.

PRECAUTIONS

CONTRAINDICATIONS: None significant. **CAUTIONS:** Impaired cardiac, renal function. **PREGNANCY/LACTATION:** Unknown if drug crosses placenta or is distributed in breast milk. **Pregnancy Category C.**

INTERACTIONS

DRUG INTERACTIONS: None significant. **ALTERED LAB VALUES:** May alter potassium concentration. Serum digoxin concentration may increase precipitously and persist for up to 1 wk (until FAB/digoxin complex is eliminated from body).

SIDE EFFECTS

None significant.

ADVERSE REACTIONS/TOXIC EFFECTS

As result of digitalis intoxication, hyperkalemia may present (diarrhea, paresthesia of extremities, heaviness of legs, decreased B/P, cold skin, grayish pallor, hypotension, mental confusion, irritability, flaccid paralysis, tented T waves, widening QRS, ST depression). When effect of digitalis is reversed, hypokalemia may develop rapidly (muscle cramping, nausea, vomiting, hypoactive bowel sounds, abdominal distension, difficulty breathing, postural hypotension). Rarely, low cardiac output, CHF may occur.

NURSING IMPLICATIONS

BASELINE ASSESSMENT:

Obtain serum digoxin level before administering drug. If drawn <6 hrs before last digoxin dose, serum digoxin level may be unreliable. Those w/impaired renal function may require >1 wk before serum digoxin assay is reliable. Assess baseline electrolytes, particularly potassium levels. Assess muscle strength, mental status. Note skin temperature, moisture. Obtain baseline weight. Initiate I&O.

INTERVENTION/EVALUATION:

Closely monitor temperature, B/P, EKG, and potassium serum level during and after drug is administered. Watch for changes from initial assessment (hypokalemia may result in muscle strength changes, tremor, muscle cramps, change in mental status, cardiac arrhythmias; hyponatremia may result in confusion, thirst, cold/clammy skin).

---

diltiazem hydrochloride

dill-**tie**-ah-zem
(Cardizem, Cardizem CD, Dilacor XR, Tiazac)

FIXED-COMBINATION(S)
W/enalapril, an ACE inhibitor **(Teczem)**

CANADIAN AVAILABILITY:
Apo-Diltiaz, Cardizem, Novo-Diltiazem, Tiazac

CLASSIFICATION

Calcium channel blocker

AVAILABILITY (Rx)

Tablets: 30 mg, 60 mg, 90 mg, 120 mg. **Capsules (sustained-release):** 60 mg, 90 mg, 120 mg, 180 mg, 240 mg, 300 mg, 360 mg. **Injection:** 5 mg/ml vials, 100 mg Monovial..

PHARMACOKINETICS

	ONSET	PEAK	DURATION
PO	30–60 min	—	—

Well absorbed from GI tract. Undergoes first-pass metabolism in liver. Metabolized in liver to active metabolite. Primarily excreted in urine. Not removed by hemodialysis. Half-life: 3–8 hrs.

ACTION/*THERAPEUTIC EFFECT*

Inhibits calcium movement across cell membranes of cardiac and vascular smooth muscle (dilates coronary arteries, peripheral arteries/arterioles); *decreases heart rate, myocardial contractility, slows SA and AV conduction. Decreases total peripheral vascular resistance by vasodilation.*

USES

Oral: Treatment of angina due to coronary artery spasm (Prinzmetal's variant angina), chronic stable angina (effort-associated angina). *Extended-release:* Treatment of essential hypertension, angina. *Parenteral:* Temporary control of rapid ventricular rate in atrial fibrillation/flutter. Rapid conversion of PSVT to normal sinus rhythm.

PO/IV ADMINISTRATION

PO:

1. Give before meals and at bedtime.

2. Tablets may be crushed.

3. Do not crush sustained-release capsules.

IV:

1. Add 125 mg to 100 ml 5% dextrose, 0.9% NaCl, or 5% dextrose/0.45% NaCl to provide a concentration of 1 mg/ml. Add 250 mg to 250 or 500 ml diluent to provide a concentration of 0.83 mg/ml or 0.45 mg/ml, respectively.

2. After dilution, stable for 24 hrs.

3. Infuse per dilution/rate chart provided by manufacturer.

4. Do not mix directly w/ furosemide.

INDICATIONS/DOSAGE/ROUTES

Angina:
PO: Adults, elderly: Initially, 30 mg 4 times/day. Increase up to 180–360 mg/day in 3–4 divided doses at 1–2 day intervals.
(CD capsules): Adults, elderly: Initially, 120–180 mg/day; titrate over 7–14 days. **Range:** Up to 480 mg/day.

Essential hypertension:
PO (Extended-release): Adults, elderly: Initially, 60–120 mg 2 times/day.
(CD capsules): Adults, elderly: Initially, 180–240 mg/day. **Range:** 240–360 mg in 2 divided doses.
(Dilacor XR): Adults, elderly: Initially, 180–240 mg/day. **Range:** 180–480 mg/day.

Usual parenteral dosage:
IV Push: Adults, elderly: Initially, 0.25 mg/kg actual body weight over 2 min. May repeat in 15 min at dose of 0.35 mg/kg actual body weight. Subsequent doses individualized.
IV Infusion: Adults, elderly: After initial bolus injection, 5–10 mg/ hr, may increase at 5 mg/hr up to 15 mg/hr. Maintain over 24 hrs. **Note:** Refer to manufacturer's information for dose concentration/infusion rates.

PRECAUTIONS

CONTRAINDICATIONS: Sick sinus syndrome/second- or third-degree AV block (except in presence of pacemaker), severe hypotension (<90 mm Hg, systolic), acute MI, pulmonary congestion. **CAUTIONS:** Impaired renal/hepatic function, CHF. **PREGNANCY/LACTATION:** Distributed in breast milk. **Pregnancy Category C.**

INTERACTIONS

DRUG INTERACTIONS: Beta blockers may have additive effect.

May increase digoxin concentration. Procainamide, quinidine may increase risk of QT interval prolongation. Carbamazepine, quinidine, theophylline may increase concentration, toxicity. **ALTERED LAB VALUES:** PR interval may be increased.

SIDE EFFECTS

FREQUENT (5–10%): Peripheral edema, dizziness, lightheadedness, headache, bradycardia, asthenia (loss of strength, weakness). **OCCASIONAL (2–5%):** Nausea, constipation, flushing, altered EKG. **RARE (<2%):** Rash, micturation disorder (polyuria, nocturia, dysuria, frequency of urination), abdominal discomfort, somnolence.

ADVERSE REACTIONS/TOXIC EFFECTS

Abrupt withdrawal may increase frequency/duration of angina. CHF, second- and third-degree AV block occur rarely. Overdosage produces nausea, drowsiness, confusion, slurred speech, profound bradycardia.

NURSING IMPLICATIONS
Baseline Assessment:

Concurrent therapy of sublingual nitroglycerin may be used for relief of anginal pain. Record onset, type (sharp, dull, squeezing), radiation, location, intensity, and duration of anginal pain, and precipitating factors (exertion, emotional stress). Assess baseline renal/liver function tests. Assess B/P, apical pulse immediately before drug is administered.

Intervention/Evaluation:

Assist w/ambulation if dizziness occurs. Assess for peripheral edema behind medial malleolus (sacral area in bedridden patients).

Monitor pulse rate for bradycardia. Question for asthenia, headache.

Patient/Family Teaching:

Do not abruptly discontinue medication. Compliance w/therapy regimen is essential to control anginal pain. To avoid hypotensive effect rise slowly from lying to sitting position, wait momentarily before standing. Avoid tasks that require alertness, motor skills until response to drug is established. Contact physician/nurse if irregular heartbeat, shortness of breath, pronounced dizziness, nausea, or constipation occurs.

---

dimenhydrinate
(Dramamine)
See Classification section under: Antihistamines

---

dinoprostone
dye-noe-**pros**-tone
(Cervidil, Prepidil Gel, Prostaglandin E$_2$, Prostin E$_2$)

CANADIAN AVAILABILITY:
Cervidil, Prepidil Gel, Prostin E$_2$

CLASSIFICATION
Prostaglandin

AVAILABILITY (Rx)
Vaginal Suppository: 20 mg.
Vaginal Gel: 0.5 mg (Prepidil).
Vaginal Inserts: 10 mg (Cervidil).

PHARMACOKINETICS
Undergoes rapid enzymatic deactivation primarily in maternal lungs. Primarily excreted in urine.

ACTION/*THERAPEUTIC EFFECT*

Direct action on myometrium. Direct softening, dilation effect on cervix. *Stimulates myometrial contractions in gravid uterus.*

USES/*UNLABELED*

Suppository: To induce abortion from the 12th wk of pregnancy through the second trimester; to evacuate uterine contents in missed abortion or intrauterine fetal death up to 28 wks gestational age (as calculated from the first day of the last normal menstrual period), benign hydatidiform mole. *Gel:* Ripening unfavorable cervix in pregnant women at or near term w/medical or obstetrical need for labor induction. *Suppository: Treatment of postpartum/postabortion hemorrhage, induction labor at or near term. Gel: Induction labor at or near term.*

STORAGE/HANDLING

Suppository: Keep frozen (<4°F); bring to room temperature just prior to use. *Gel:* Refrigerate.

INTRAVAGINAL ADMINISTRATION (SUPPOSITORY)

1. Administer only in hospital setting w/emergency equipment available.
2. Warm suppository to room temperature before removing foil wrapper.
3. Avoid skin contact because of risk of absorption.
4. Insert high in vagina.
5. Pt should remain supine for 10 min after administration.

INTRACERVICAL ADMINISTRATION (GEL)

1. Use caution in handling, prevent skin contact. Wash hands thoroughly w/soap and water after administration.
2. Bring to room temperature just before use (avoid forcing the warming process).
3. Assemble dosing apparatus as described in manufacturer insert.
4. Have pt in dorsal position w/cervix visualized using a speculum.
5. Introduce gel into cervical canal just below level of internal os.
6. Have pt remain in supine position at least 15–30 min (minimizes leakage from cervical canal).

INDICATIONS/DOSAGE/ROUTES

Abortifacient:
Intravaginally: Adults: 20 mg (one suppository) high into vagina. May repeat at 3–5 hr intervals until abortion occurs. Do not administer >2 days.

Ripening unfavorable cervix:
Intracervical: (*Prepidil*): **Adults:** Initially, 0.5 mg (2.5 ml); if no cervical/uterine response, may repeat 0.5 mg dose in 6 hrs. **Maximum:** 1.5 mg (7.5 ml) for a 24 hr period. (*Cervidil*): **Adults:** 10 mg over 12 hr period. Remove upon onset of active labor or 12 hrs after insertion.

PRECAUTIONS

CONTRAINDICATIONS: Hypersensitivity to dinoprostone or other prostaglandins; acute pelvic inflammatory disease; active cardiac, renal, hepatic, or pulmonary disease; fetal malpresentation or significant cephalopelvic disproportion. **CAUTIONS:** Cervicitis, infected endocervical lesions or acute vaginitis, history of asthma, hypo/hypertension, anemia, jaundice, diabetes, epilepsy, uterine fibroids, compromised (scarred) uterus, cardiovascular, renal, or hepatic disease. **PREGNANCY/LACTATION:** *Suppository:* Teratogenic; therefore abortion must be complete. *Gel:* Sustained uterine hyperstimulation may affect fetus (e.g., abnormal heart rate). **Pregnancy Category C.**

INTERACTIONS

DRUG INTERACTIONS: Oxytocics may cause uterine hypertonus, possibly causing uterine rupture or cervical laceration. **ALTERED LAB VALUES:** None significant.

SIDE EFFECTS

FREQUENT: Abdominal/stomach cramps, diarrhea, fever, nausea, vomiting. **OCCASIONAL:** Headache, chills/shivering, hives, shortness of breath, wheezing, bradycardia, bronchoconstriction, increased uterine pain accompanying abortion, peripheral vasoconstriction. **RARE:** Flushing, ileus, vulvae edema.

ADVERSE REACTIONS/TOXIC EFFECTS

Excessive dosage may cause uterine hypertonicity w/spasm and tetanic contraction, leading to cervical laceration/perforation, uterine rupture or hemorrhage.

NURSING IMPLICATIONS

BASELINE ASSESSMENT:

Suppository: Question for hypersensitivity to dinoprostone or other prostaglandins. Establish baseline B/P, temperature, respirations, pulse. Obtain orders for antiemetics and antidiarrheals, meperidine or other pain medication for abdominal cramps. Assess any uterine activity or vaginal bleeding. *Gel:* Question pt regarding conditions where prolonged uterine contractions are inappropriate. Assess Bishop score. Assess degree of effacement (determines size of shielded endocervical catheter).

INTERVENTION/EVALUATION:

Suppository: Check strength, duration, and frequency of contractions and monitor vital signs q15min until stable, then hourly until abortion complete. Check resting uterine tone. Administer medications for relief of GI effects if indicated, abdominal cramps. Provide emotional support as necessary. *Gel:* Monitor uterine activity (onset of uterine contractions), fetal status (heart rate), character of cervix (dilation, effacement). Have pt remain recumbent 12 hrs after application w/continuous electronic monitoring of fetal heart rate and uterine activity. Record maternal vital signs at least hourly in presence of uterine activity. Reassess Bishop score.

PATIENT/FAMILY TEACHING:

Suppository: Report fever, chills, foul smelling/increased vaginal discharge, uterine cramps, or pain promptly.

diphenhydramine hydrochloride

dye-phen-**high**-dra-meen **(Benadryl)**

FIXED-COMBINATION(S): W/calamine, an astringent, and camphor, a counter-irritant **(Caladryl)**

CLASSIFICATION

Antihistamine

AVAILABILITY (OTC)

Capsules: 25 mg, 50 mg.
Tablets: 25 mg, 50 mg. **Elixir:** 12.5
mg/5 ml. **Injection (Rx):** 10 mg/ml,
50 mg/ml.

PHARMACOKINETICS

	ONSET	PEAK	DURATION
PO	15–30 min	1–4 hrs	4–6 hrs
IM/IV	<15 min	1–4 hrs	4–6 hrs

Well absorbed following oral,
parenteral administration. Widely
distributed. Metabolized in liver.
Primarily excreted in urine. Half-
life: 1–4 hrs.

ACTION / THERAPEUTIC EFFECT

Competes w/histamine at histaminic receptor sites, *resulting in
anticholinergic, antipruritic, antitussive, antiemetic effects.* Inhibits
central acetylcholine, *producing
antidyskinetic, sedative effect.*

USES

Treatment of allergic reactions,
parkinsonism, prevention and
treatment of nausea, vomiting, vertigo due to motion sickness; antitussive, short-term management
of insomnia. Topical form used for
relief of pruritus, insect bites, skin
irritations.

STORAGE/HANDLING

Store oral, elixir, topical, parenteral forms at room temperature. Powder slowly darkens on
exposure to light (does not alter
effectiveness).

PO/IM/IV ADMINISTRATION

PO:
1. Give w/o regard to meals.
2. Scored tablets may be crushed.
3. Do not crush capsules or film-
coated tablets.

IM:
Give deep IM into large muscle
mass.

IV:

Note: Compatible w/most IV infusion solutions.
1. May be given undiluted.
2. Give IV injection over at
least 1 min.

INDICATIONS/DOSAGE/ROUTES

*Allergic reaction, parkinsonism,
treatment of motion sickness:*
PO: Adults: 25–50 mg 3–4 times/
day q4–6h. **Elderly:** Initially, 25 mg
2–3 times/day. May increase as
needed. **Children >20 lbs:** 5 mg/
kg/24 hrs in divided doses 4
times/day.
IM/IV: Adults: 10–50 mg. **Maximum daily dose:** 400 mg. **Children >20 lbs:** 5 mg/kg/24 hrs 4
times/day.

Prevention of motion sickness:
PO: Adults: 25–50 mg 30 min before exposure to motion. Give subsequent doses q4–6h.

Nighttime sleep aid:
PO: Adults: 50 mg 20 min before
bedtime.

Cough:
PO: Adults: 25 mg q4h.
Syrup: Children: 6.25–12.5 mg q4h.

Pruritus relief:
Topical: Adults: Apply to affected
area 3–4 times/day.

PRECAUTIONS

CONTRAINDICATIONS: Acute

asthmatic attack, those receiving MAO inhibitors. **CAUTIONS:** Narrow-angle glaucoma, peptic ulcer, prostatic hypertrophy, pyloro-duodenal or bladder neck obstruction, asthma, COPD, increased intraocular pressure, cardiovascular disease, hyperthyroidism, hypertension, seizure disorders. **PREGNANCY/LACTATION:** Crosses placenta; detected in breast milk (may produce irritability in nursing infants). Increased risk of seizures in neonates, premature infants if used during third trimester of pregnancy. May prohibit lactation. **Pregnancy Category B**.

INTERACTIONS

DRUG INTERACTIONS: Alcohol, CNS depressants may increase CNS depressant effects. MAO inhibitors may increase anticholinergic, CNS depressant effects. Anticholinergics may increase anticholinergic effects. **ALTERED LAB VALUES:** May suppress wheal and flare reactions to antigen skin testing unless antihistamines are discontinued 4 days prior to testing.

SIDE EFFECTS

FREQUENT: Drowsiness, dizziness, muscular weakness, hypotension, dry mouth/nose/throat/lips, urinary retention, thickening of bronchial secretions. Sedation, dizziness, hypotension more likely noted in elderly. **OCCASIONAL:** Epigastric distress, flushing, visual disturbances, hearing disturbances, paresthesia, sweating, chills.

ADVERSE REACTIONS/TOXIC EFFECTS

Children may experience domi-

nant paradoxical reactions (restlessness, insomnia, euphoria, nervousness, tremors). Overdosage in children may result in hallucinations, convulsions, death. Hypersensitivity reaction (eczema, pruritus, rash, cardiac disturbances, photosensitivity) may occur. Overdosage may vary from CNS depression (sedation, apnea, cardiovascular collapse, death) to severe paradoxical reaction (hallucinations, tremor, seizures).

NURSING IMPLICATIONS
BASELINE ASSESSMENT:

If pt is undergoing allergic reaction, obtain history of recently ingested foods, drugs, environmental exposure, recent emotional stress. Monitor rate, depth, rhythm, type of respiration, and quality and rate of pulse. Assess lung sounds for rhonchi, wheezing, rales.

INTERVENTION/EVALUATION:

Monitor B/P, esp. in elderly (increased risk of hypotension). Monitor children closely for paradoxical reaction.

PATIENT/FAMILY TEACHING:

Tolerance to antihistaminic effect generally does not occur; tolerance to sedative effect may occur. Avoid tasks that require alertness, motor skills until response to drug is established. Dry mouth, drowsiness, dizziness may be an expected response of drug. Avoid alcoholic beverages during antihistamine therapy. Sugarless gum, sips of tepid water may relieve dry mouth. Coffee or tea may help reduce drowsiness.

diphenoxylate hydrochloride w/ atropine sulfate

dye-pen-**ox**-e-late
(Lofene, Logen, Lomanate, Lomotil)

CANADIAN AVAILABILITY:
Lomotil

CLASSIFICATION

Antidiarrheal

AVAILABILITY (Rx)

Tablets: 2.5 mg. **Liquid:** 2.5 mg/5 ml.

PHARMACOKINETICS

Well absorbed from GI tract. Metabolized in liver to active metabolite. Primarily eliminated in feces. Half-life: 2.5 hrs; metabolite: 12–24 hrs.

ACTION / THERAPEUTIC EFFECT

Acts locally, centrally *to reduce intestinal motility.*

USES

Adjunctive treatment of acute, chronic diarrhea.

PO ADMINISTRATION

1. Give w/o regard to meals. If GI irritation occurs, give w/food or meals.

2. Use liquid for children under 12 yrs (use dropper for administration of liquids).

INDICATIONS/DOSAGE/ROUTES

Antidiarrheal:
PO: Adults, elderly: Initially, 2.5 mg 4 times/day. **Maintenance:** 2.5 mg 2–3 times/day. **Children:** Initially, 0.3–0.4 mg/kg/day in 4 divided doses. **Maintenance:** As low as $\frac{1}{4}$ initial dose (0.075–0.1 mg/kg/day in divided doses).

PRECAUTIONS

CONTRAINDICATIONS: Obstructive jaundice, diarrhea associated w/pseudomembranous enterocolitis due to broad-spectrum antibiotics or w/organisms that invade intestinal mucosa (*E. coli, Shigella, Salmonella*), acute ulcerative colitis (may produce toxic megacolon). **CAUTIONS:** Advanced hepatorenal disease, abnormal liver function. **PREGNANCY/LACTATION:** Unknown if drug crosses placenta or is distributed in breast milk. **Pregnancy Category C.**

INTERACTIONS

DRUG INTERACTIONS: Alcohol, CNS depressants may increase effect. Anticholinergics may increase effect of atropine. MAO inhibitors may precipitate hypertensive crisis. **ALTERED LAB VALUES:** May increase amylase.

SIDE EFFECTS

FREQUENT: Drowsiness, lightheadedness, dizziness, nausea. **OCCASIONAL:** Headache, dry mouth. **RARE:** Flushing, tachycardia, urinary retention, constipation, paradoxical reaction (restlessness, agitation), blurred vision.

ADVERSE REACTIONS/TOXIC EFFECTS

Dehydration may predispose to toxicity. Paralytic ileus, toxic megacolon (constipation, decreased appetite, stomach pain w/nausea/vomiting) occurs rarely. Severe anticholinergic effects (severe drowsiness, hypotonic reflexes, hyperthermia) may result in severe respiratory depression, coma.

NURSING IMPLICATIONS

BASELINE ASSESSMENT:

Check baseline hydration status: skin turgor, mucous membranes for dryness, urinary status.

INTERVENTION/EVALUATION:

Encourage adequate fluid intake. Assess bowel sounds for peristalsis. Monitor daily bowel activity, stool consistency (watery loose, soft, semisolid, solid) and record time of evacuation. Assess for abdominal disturbances. Discontinue medication if abdominal distention occurs. Check I&O. Monitor for paradoxical reaction.

PATIENT/FAMILY TEACHING:

Avoid tasks that require alertness, motor skills until response to drug is established. Do not ingest alcohol or barbiturates. Contact physician if fever, palpitations occur or diarrhea persists. Cola, unsalted crackers, dry toast may relieve nausea. Dry mouth may be relieved by sugarless gum, sips of tepid water. Report abdominal distention.

---

dipivefrin
(Propine)
See Classification section under: Antiglaucoma agents

---

dipyridamole
die-pie-**rid**-ah-mole
(Persantine)

FIXED-COMBINATION(S):
W/aspirin, an antiplatelet (**Aggrenox**).

CANADIAN AVAILABILITY:
Apo-Dipyridamole, Novodipiradol, Persantine

CLASSIFICATION
Antiplatelet, antianginal

AVAILABILITY (Rx)
Tablets: 25 mg, 50 mg, 75 mg.
Injection: 10 mg

PHARMACOKINETICS
Slow, variably absorbed from GI tract. Widely distributed. Metabolized in liver. Primarily eliminated via biliary excretion. Half-life: 10–15 hrs.

ACTION/*THERAPEUTIC EFFECT*
Direct action on small vessels of coronary vascular bed, *increasing coronary blood flow, coronary sinus oxygen saturation.*

USES/*UNLABELED*
Adjunct to coumarin anticoagulant in prevention of postop thromboembolic complications of cardiac valve replacement. IV use: alternative to exercise in thallium myocardial perfusion imaging for evaluation of coronary artery disease. *Prophylaxis of myocardial reinfarction, treatment of transient ischemic attacks (TIAs).*

PO/IV ADMINISTRATION
PO:
Best taken on empty stomach w/full glass of water.

IV:
1. Dilute to at least 1:2 ratio w/0.9% NaCl or 5% dextrose in water for total volume of 20–50 ml (undiluted may cause irritation).
2. Infuse over 4 min.
3. Inject thallium within 5 min after dipyridamole infusion.

INDICATIONS/DOSAGE/ROUTES
Prevention of thromboembolic disorders:
PO: **Adults, elderly:** 75–100 mg 4 times/day in combination w/other medications.

Diagnostic:
IV: Adults, elderly (based on weight): 0.142 mg/kg/min infused over 4 min; doses >60 mg not needed for any pt.

PRECAUTIONS

CONTRAINDICATIONS: None significant. **CAUTIONS:** Those w/hypotension. **PREGNANCY/LACTATION:** Distributed in breast milk. **Pregnancy Category C**.

INTERACTIONS

DRUG INTERACTIONS: May increase risk of bleeding w/ anticoagulants, heparin, thrombolytics, aspirin, salicylates. **ALTERED LAB VALUES:** None significant.

SIDE EFFECTS

FREQUENT (14%): Dizziness. **OCCASIONAL (2–6%):** Abdominal distress, headache, rash. **RARE (<2%):** Diarrhea, vomiting, flushing, pruritis.

ADVERSE REACTIONS/TOXIC EFFECTS

Overdosage produces peripheral vasodilation, resulting in hypotension.

NURSING IMPLICATIONS
BASELINE ASSESSMENT:

Assess chest pain, B/P, pulse. When used as antiplatelet, check hematologic levels.

INTERVENTION/EVALUATION:

Assist w/ambulation if dizziness occurs. Monitor heart sounds by auscultation. Assess B/P for hypotension. Assess skin for flushing, rash.

PATIENT/FAMILY TEACHING:

If nausea occurs, cola, unsalted crackers, or dry toast may relieve effect. Therapeutic response may not be achieved before 2–3 mos of continuous therapy. Use caution when getting up suddenly from lying or sitting position.

dirithromycin

dih-**rith**-row-my-sin
(Dynabac)

CLASSIFICATION

Antibiotic: Macrolide

AVAILABILITY (Rx)

Tablets, enteric coated: 250 mg

PHARMACOKINETICS

Rapidly absorbed from GI tract. Widely distributed into tissues and within cells. Eliminated primarily unchanged via biliary excretion. Half-life: 30–44 hrs.

ACTION/*THERAPEUTIC EFFECT*

Binds to ribosomal receptor sites of susceptible organisms, *inhibiting protein synthesis.*

USES

Treatment of mild to moderate infections of upper respiratory tract (pharyngitis, tonsillitis), acute bronchitis, chronic bronchitis, uncomplicated skin/skin structure infections, community-acquired pneumonia.

PO ADMINISTRATION

1. Administer w/food or within an hour of having eaten (food increases absorption).
2. Swallow whole (tablets not to be cut, crushed, or chewed).

INDICATIONS/DOSAGE/ROUTES

Pharyngitis/tonsillitis:
    PO: Adults, elderly, children

≥12 yrs: 500 mg once daily for 10 days.

Acute bronchitis, chronic bronchitis:
PO: Adults, elderly, children ≥12 yrs: 500 mg once daily for 7 days.

Community-acquired pneumonia:
PO: Adults, elderly, children ≥12 yrs: 500 mg once daily for 14 days.

Skin, skin structure infections:
PO: Adults, elderly, children ≥12 yrs: 500 mg once daily for 7 days.

PRECAUTIONS

CONTRAINDICATIONS: Hypersensitivity to dirithromycin, erythromycins, any macrolide antibiotic, concurrent terfenadine therapy, electrolyte disturbances (may cause cardiac dysrhythmias), bacteremia. CAUTIONS: Hepatic/renal dysfunction. PREGNANCY/LACTATION: Unknown if distributed in breast milk. Pregnancy Category C.

INTERACTIONS

DRUG INTERACTIONS: H_2 antagonists increase dirithromycin absorption. Aluminum/magnesium containing antacids may decrease concentration (give 1 hr before or 2 hrs after antacid). ALTERED LAB VALUES: May increase platelet count, potassium CPK, eosinophils, neutrophils. Decreases bicarbonate level.

SIDE EFFECTS

FREQUENT: Abdominal pain (10%), headache (9%), nausea, diarrhea (8%). OCCASIONAL: Vomiting, dyspepsia (3%), dizziness, nonspecific pain, asthenia (2%). RARE: Increased cough, flatulence, rash, dyspnea, pruritus/urticaria, insomnia.

ADVERSE REACTIONS/TOXIC EFFECTS

Superinfections, esp. antibiotic-associated colitis (abdominal cramps, watery severe diarrhea, fever) may result from altered bacterial balance.

NURSING IMPLICATIONS
BASELINE ASSESSMENT:

Question pt for history of allergies to dirithromycin, erythromycins. Obtain specimens for culture, sensitivity before giving first dose (therapy may begin before results are known).

INTERVENTION/EVALUATION:

Check for GI discomfort, nausea, headache, diarrhea. Determine pattern of bowel activity and stool consistency. Evaluate for superinfection: genital/anal pruritus, sore mouth or tongue, moderate to severe diarrhea.

PATIENT/FAMILY TEACHING:

Continue therapy for full length of treatment. Doses should be evenly spaced. Take medication w/food or within an hour of having eaten.

disopyramide phosphate

dye-so-**peer**-ah-myd
(Norpace)

CANADIAN AVAILABILITY:
Rythmodan

CLASSIFICATION

Antiarrhythmic

AVAILABILITY (Rx)

Capsules: 100 mg, 150 mg. **Capsules (extended-release):** 100 mg, 150 mg.

PHARMACOKINETICS

	ONSET	PEAK	DURATION
PO	0.5–3.5 hrs	—	1.5–8.5 hrs

Rapidly, completely absorbed from GI tract. Metabolized in liver. Primarily excreted in urine. Removed by hemodialysis. Half-life: 7 hrs (increased in reduced renal function).

ACTION / THERAPEUTIC EFFECT

Prolongs refractory period by direct effect, decreasing myocardial excitability and conduction velocity. *Depresses myocardial contractility. Has anticholinergic, negative inotropic effects.*

USES / UNLABELED

Suppression and prevention of unifocal/multifocal premature ventricular contractions (ectopic), paired ventricular contractions (couplets), episodes of ventricular tachycardia. *Prophylaxis/treatment of supraventricular tachycardia.*

PO ADMINISTRATION

1. May be given w/o regard to meals but best absorbed 1 hr before or 2 hrs after meals.
2. Do not crush or break extended-release capsules.

INDICATIONS / DOSAGE / ROUTES

Usual dosage:
PO: **Adults, elderly >50 kg:** 150 mg q6h (300 mg q12h w/extended-release). **Adults, elderly <50 kg:** 100 mg q6h (200 mg q12h w/extended-release). **Children 12–18 yrs:** 6–15 mg/kg/day in divided doses q6h. **Children 4–12 yrs:** 10–15 mg/kg/day in divided doses q6h. **Children 1–4 yrs:** 10–20 mg/kg/day in divided doses q6h. **Children <1 yr:** 10–30 mg/kg/day in divided doses q6h.

Rapid control of arrhythmias:
Note: Do not use extended-release capsules.
PO: **Adults, elderly >50 kg:** Initially, 300 mg, then 150 mg q6h. **Adults, elderly <50 kg:** Initially, 200 mg, then 100 mg q6h.

Severe refractory arrhythmias:
PO: **Adults, elderly:** Up to 400 mg q6h.

Dosage in renal impairment:
With or without loading dose of 150 mg:

CREATININE CLEARANCE	DOSAGE
>40 ml/min	100 mg q6h (extended-release 200 mg q12h)
30–40 ml/min	100 mg q8h
15–30 ml/min	100 mg q12h
<15 ml/min	100 mg q24h

Dosage in hepatic impairment:
100 mg q6h (200 mg q12h w/extended-release).

Dosage in cardiomyopathy, decompensated myocardium:
No loading dose; 100 mg q6–8h w/gradual dosage adjustments.

PRECAUTIONS

CONTRAINDICATIONS: Preexisting urinary retention, preexisting second- or third-degree AV block, cardiogenic shock, narrow-angle glaucoma, unless pt is undergoing cholinergic therapy. **CAUTIONS:** CHF, myasthenia gravis, narrow-angle glaucoma, prostatic hypertrophy, sick-sinus syndrome (bradycardia/tachycardia), Wolff-Parkinson-White syndrome, bundle-branch block, impaired renal/hepatic function. **PREGNANCY/LACTATION:** Crosses placenta; distributed in breast milk. May stimulate contractions of pregnant uterus. **Pregnancy Category C.**

INTERACTIONS

DRUG INTERACTIONS: Other antia rrhythmics (e.g., propranolol, diltiazem, verapamil) may prolong conduction, decrease cardiac output. Pimozide may increase cardiac arrhythmias. **ALTERED LAB VALUES:** May decrease glucose. May cause ECG changes.

SIDE EFFECTS

FREQUENT (>9%): Dry mouth (32%), urinary hesitancy, constipation. **OCCASIONAL (3–9%):** Blurred vision, dry eyes, nose, or throat, urinary retention, headache, dizziness, fatigue, nausea. **RARE (<1%):** Impotence, hypotension, edema, weight gain, shortness of breath, syncope, chest pain, nervousness, diarrhea, vomiting, decreased appetite, rash, itching.

ADVERSE REACTIONS/TOXIC EFFECTS

May produce or aggravate CHF. May produce severe hypotension, compounded w/shortness of breath, chest pain, syncope (esp. in those w/primary cardiomyopathy or in inadequately compensated CHF). Hepatic toxicity occurs rarely.

NURSING IMPLICATIONS

BASELINE ASSESSMENT:

Assess baseline hepatic, renal function studies. Before giving medication, instruct pt to void (reduces risk of urinary retention).

INTERVENTION/EVALUATION:

Monitor EKG for cardiac changes, particularly widening of QRS complex, prolongation of PR and QT intervals. Notify physician of any significant interval changes. Assess pattern of daily bowel activity, stool consistency. Monitor I&O (be alert to urinary retention). Assess for evidence of CHF (cough, dyspnea [particularly on exertion], rales at base of lungs, fatigue). Assess for edema directly behind medial malleolus in ambulatory pts, sacral area in bedridden pts (usually first areas showing impending edema). Assist w/ambulation if dizziness occurs. Monitor for therapeutic serum level (2–8 mcg/ml).

PATIENT/FAMILY TEACHING:

Report shortness of breath, productive cough. Compliance w/therapy regimen is essential to control cardiac dysrhythmias. Do not use nasal decongestants, OTC cold preparations (stimulants) w/o physician approval. Restrict salt, alcohol intake. Sugarless gum, sips of tepid water may relieve dry mouth. Report visual disturbances, headache, dizziness.

disulfiram

dye-**sul**-fi-ram
(Antabuse)

CANADIAN AVAILABILITY: Antabuse

CLASSIFICATION

Alcohol deterrent

AVAILABILITY (Rx)

Tablets: 250 mg, 500 mg

PHARMACOKINETICS

Slowly absorbed from GI tract. Metabolized in liver. Primarily excreted in urine. Up to 20% of dose remains in body for at least 1 wk.

ACTION/*THERAPEUTIC EFFECT*

Inhibits enzyme aldehyde dehydrogenase, responsible for breakdown of ethanol metabolite acetaldehyde. Increased acetaldehyde responsible for *disulfiram reaction after alcohol ingestion.*

USES

Adjunct in management of selected chronic alcoholic pts who want to remain in state of enforced sobriety.

PO ADMINISTRATION

1. Scored tablets may be crushed.

2. Give w/o regard to meals.

INDICATIONS/DOSAGE/ROUTES

Note: Pts must abstain from alcohol for at least 12 hrs before initial dose is administered.

PO: Adults, elderly: Initially, administer maximum of 500 mg daily given as a single dose for 1–2 wks. **Maintenance:** 250 mg daily (normal range: 125–500 mg). Do not exceed maximum daily dose of 500 mg.

PRECAUTIONS

CONTRAINDICATIONS: Severe heart disease, psychosis. **CAUTIONS:** Alcoholic disease. **PREGNANCY/LACTATION: Category C.** Safety during pregnancy not established.

INTERACTIONS

DRUG INTERACTIONS: Alcohol within 14 days results in disulfiram/alcohol reaction. Oral anticoagulant effect may be increased. May increase concentration, toxicity of phenytoin. Isoniazid may increase CNS effects. Metronidazole may increase toxicity. **ALTERED LAB VALUES:** May increase cholesterol concentrations. May decrease VMA concentrations.

SIDE EFFECTS

FREQUENT: Drowsiness. **OCCASIONAL:** Neurotoxicity, optic neuritis (eye pain, altered vision), peripheral neuritis (numbness of hands or feet), mental changes, headache, impotence, metallic or garlic taste, skin rash, unusual tiredness. **RARE:** Liver toxicity.

ADVERSE REACTIONS/TOXIC EFFECTS

Disulfiram-alcohol reaction to ingestion of alcohol in any form: flushing/throbbing in head and neck, throbbing headache, nausea, copious vomiting, diaphoresis, dyspnea, hyperventilation, tachycardia, hypotension, marked uneasiness, vertigo, blurred vision, confusion. Can produce death.

NURSING IMPLICATIONS

INTERVENTION/EVALUATION:

Do not give w/o pt's knowledge. Fully inform pt of consequences of alcohol ingestion. Therapy cannot be started until a minimum of 12 hrs has elapsed since pt's last ingestion of alcohol.

PATIENT/FAMILY TEACHING:

Avoid cough syrups, vinegars, fluid extracts, elixirs because of their alcohol content. Even external application of liniments, shaving or body lotion may precipitate a crisis. Effects of medication may occur several days after discontinuance. Avoid alcohol in all forms, including beverages, vinegar, liquid medications, colognes, etc. Use caution driving, performing tasks requiring alertness.

dobutamine hydrochloride

do-**byew**-ta-meen
(Dobutrex)

CANADIAN AVAILABILITY:
Dobutrex

CLASSIFICATION

Sympathomimetic

AVAILABILITY (Rx)

Injection: 250 mg vial. **Infusion:** 500 mg/250 ml solution.

PHARMACOKINETICS

	ONSET	PEAK	DURATION
IV	1–2 min	10 min	Length of infusion

Metabolized in liver. Primarily excreted in urine. Half-life: 2 min.

ACTION/*THERAPEUTIC EFFECT*

Direct acting inotropic agent acting primarily on beta$_1$-adrenergic receptors, *enhancing myocardial contractility, stroke volume, cardiac output.* Decreases preload, afterload. Excessive doses *increase heart rate. Improves renal blood flow, urine output.*

USES

Prophylaxis/treatment of acute hypotension, shock (associated w/myocardial infarction, trauma, renal failure, cardiac decompensation, open heart surgery), treatment of low cardiac output, CHF.

STORAGE/HANDLING

Store at room temperature. Freezing produces crystallization. Pink discoloration of solution (due to oxidation) does not indicate loss of potency if used within recommended time period. Reconstituted, concentrated solution maintains potency for 6 hrs at room temperature, 48 hrs if refrigerated. Further diluted solutions for infusion must be used within 24 hrs.

IV ADMINISTRATION

Note: Correct hypovolemia w/volume expanders before dobutamine infusion. Those w/atrial fibrillation should be digitalized prior to infusion. Administer by IV infusion only.

IV:

1. Dilute 250 mg ampule w/10 ml sterile water for injection or 5% dextrose for injection. Resulting solution: 25 mg/ml. Add additional 10 ml of diluent if not completely dissolved (resulting solution: 12.5 mg/ml).
2. Dilute further to at least 50 ml w/5% dextrose, 0.9% NaCl, or sodium lactate injection before administration.
3. Use infusion pump to control flow rate.
4. Titrate dosage to individual response.

INDICATIONS/DOSAGE/ROUTES

Note: Dosage determined by pt response.
IV Infusion: Adults, elderly: 2.5–10 mcg/kg/min. Rarely, infusion rate up to 40 mcg/kg/min to increase cardiac output.

PRECAUTIONS

CONTRAINDICATIONS: Idiopathic hypertrophic subaortic stenosis, hypovolemic pts, sulfite sensitivity. **CAUTIONS:** Atrial fibrillation, hypertension. Safety in children not established. **PREGNANCY/LACTATION:** Unknown if drug crosses placenta or is distributed in breast milk. Has not been administered to pregnant women. **Pregnancy Category C**.

INTERACTIONS

DRUG INTERACTIONS: Tricyclic antidepressants, MAO inhibitors, oxytocics may increase effect (arrhythmias, hypertension), beta blockers may antagonize effects, digoxin may increase risk of arrhythmias, additional inotropic effect. **ALTERED LAB VALUES:** Decreases potassium serum levels.

SIDE EFFECTS

FREQUENT (5%): Increased heart rate, blood pressure. **OCCASIONAL (3–5%):** Pain at injection site. **RARE (1–3%):** Nausea, headache, anginal pain, shortness of breath, fever.

ADVERSE REACTIONS/TOXIC EFFECTS

Overdosage may produce marked increase in heart rate (30 beats/min or greater), marked increase in systolic B/P (50 mm Hg or greater), anginal pain, premature ventricular beats.

NURSING IMPLICATIONS

BASELINE ASSESSMENT:

Pt must be on continuous cardiac monitoring. Determine weight (for dosage calculation). Obtain initial B/P, heart rate, and respirations.

INTERVENTION/EVALUATION:

Continuously monitor for cardiac rate, arrhythmias. W/physician, establish parameters for adjusting rate or stopping infusion. Maintain accurate I&O; measure urine output frequently. Assess potassium levels and dobutamine plasma level (therapeutic range = 40–190 ng/ml). Check cardiac output. Monitor B/P continuously (hypertension greater risk in pts w/preexisting hypertension) and pulmonary wedge pressure or central venous pressure frequently. Immediately notify physician of decreased urine output, cardiac arrhythmias, significant increase in B/P or heart rate, and less commonly hypotension.

PATIENT/FAMILY TEACHING:

Explain rationale for therapy. Report chest pain, discomfort at IV site.

---

docetaxel

dox-eh-**tax**-el
(Taxotere)

CANADIAN AVAILABILITY:
Taxotere

CLASSIFICATION

Antineoplastic

AVAILABILITY (Rx)

Injection: 20 mg in 0.5 ml w/diluent, 80 mg in 2 ml w/diluent

PHARMACOKINETICS

Distributed into peripheral compartments. Extensively metabolized. Excreted primarily in feces w/lesser amount in urine.

ACTION/*THERAPEUTIC EFFECT*

Disrupts the microtubular cell network, essential for cellular function, *inhibiting cell mitosis.*

USES/*UNLABELED USES*

Treatment of locally advanced or metastatic breast carcinoma after the failure of any prior chemotherapy.

STORAGE/HANDLING

Refrigerate vial. Protect from light. Stand vial at room temperature for 5 min before administering (do not store in PVC bags). Premixed solution stable for 8 hrs either at room temperature or if refrigerated.

IV ADMINISTRATION

Note: Dilution is required before administration. Pt should be premedicated w/oral corticosteroids (dexamethasone 16 mg/day for 5 days beginning day 1 before docetaxel therapy; reduces severity of fluid retention, hypersensitivity reaction).

1. Dilute with 0.9% NaCl injection or 5% dextrose injection.

2. Those dosed initially at 100 mg/m^2 who experience febrile neutropenia, neutrophils <500 cells/mm^3 for >1 wk, severe or cumulative cutaneous reactions, or severe peripheral neuropathy during therapy should have dose adjusted from 100 to 75 mg/m^2. If reaction continues, lower dose from 75 to 55 mg/m^2 or stop therapy. Those dosed at 60 mg/m^2 and do not experience above symptoms may tolerate increased dose.

3. Monitor closely for hypersensitivity reaction, i.e., flushing, localized skin reaction, bronchospasm (may occur within a few minutes after infusion).

INDICATIONS/DOSAGE/ROUTES

Breast carcinoma:
IV Infusion: Adults: 60–100 mg/m^2 given over 1 hr q3 wks.

PRECAUTIONS

CONTRAINDICATIONS: Neutrophil count <1,500 cells/mm^3, history of severe hypersensitivity to docetaxel or other drugs formulated w/polysorbate 80. **EXTREME CAUTION:** Abnormal liver function, those receiving higher doses than normal (increased risk of mortality). **PREGNANCY/LACTATION:** May cause fetal harm. Unknown if distributed in breast milk; do not breast-feed. **Pregnancy Category D.**

INTERACTIONS

DRUG INTERACTIONS: Cyclosporine, terfenadine, ketoconazole, erythromycin, troleandomycin may significantly modify docetaxel metabolism. **ALTERED LAB VALUES:** May significantly increase bilirubin, BUN, serum creatinine, transaminase, alkaline phosphatase. Reduces neutrophils, thrombocytes, WBC count.

SIDE EFFECTS

FREQUENT: Alopecia (80%), asthenia, i.e., loss of strength (62%), hypersensitivity reaction, i.e., dermatitis (59%). Hypersensitivity reaction decreases to 16% in those treated w/premedicated oral corticosteroids. Fluid retention (49%), stomatitis (redness/burning of oral mucous membranes, gum/tongue inflammation—43%), nausea, diarrhea (40%), fever (30%), nail changes (28%), vomiting (24%), myalgia (19%). **OCCASIONAL:** Hypotension, erythema, rash, edema, anorexia, headache, weight gain, infection (urinary tract, injection site, catheter tip), dizziness. **RARE:** Dry skin, sensory disorders (vision, speech, taste), dermatitis, arthralgia, myalgia, weight loss, conjunctivitis, hematuria, proteinuria.

ADVERSE REACTIONS/TOXIC EFFECTS

In those w/normal liver function tests, neutropenia (<2,000 cells/

mm³) and leukopenia (<4000 cells/mm³) occurs in 96% of pts. Anemia (<11 g/dl) occurs in 90%. Thrombocytopenia (<100,000 cells/mm³) occurs in 8%. Infection occurs in 28%. Neurosensory, neuromotor (distal extremity weakness) occur in 54% and 13%, respectively.

NURSING IMPLICATIONS
BASELINE ASSESSMENT:

CBC, differential and platelet counts, blood chemistries including electrolytes, renal and hepatic function tests, chest x-ray should be performed before therapy begins and routinely thereafter. Obtain baseline B/P, temperature, pulse, weight. Offer emotional support to pt and family. Antiemetics may be effective in preventing, treating nausea, vomiting.

INTERVENTION/EVALUATION:

Frequent monitoring of blood counts is essential, particularly neutrophil count (<1,500 cells/mm³ requires discontinuation of therapy), renal, hepatic function studies, serum uric acid levels. Assess pattern of daily bowel activity, stool consistency. Assess weight gain or loss. Assess skin, nailbeds for cutaneous reaction, hyperpigmentation of nails. Monitor for cutaneous reactions characterized by rash w/eruptions, mainly on hands or feet. Assess for extravascular fluid accumulation: rales in lungs, edema in dependent areas, dyspnea at rest, pronounced abdominal distension (due to ascites).

PATIENT/FAMILY TEACHING:

Alopecia is reversible, but new hair growth may have different color or texture. New hair growth resumes 2–3 mos after last therapy dose. Maintain fastidious oral hygiene. Do not have immunizations w/o physician approval (drug lowers body's resistance). Avoid those who have recently taken live virus vaccine. Promptly report fever, sore throat, signs of local infection.

docusate calcium
dock-cue-sate
(Pro-Cal-Sof, Surfak)

docusate potassium
(Dialose, Diocto-K, Kasof)

docusate sodium
(Colace, Doxinate, Modane Soft)

FIXED-COMBINATION(S):
W/casanthranol, a stimulant laxative (**Peri-colace**); w/phenolphthalein, a laxative (**Correctol, Doxidan**)

CANADIAN AVAILABILITY:
Colace, Surfak

CLASSIFICATION
Laxative: Stool softener

AVAILABILITY (OTC)
Calcium: Capsules: 50 mg, 240 mg
Potassium: Capsules: 100 mg, 240 mg
Sodium: Tablets: 100 mg. **Capsules:** 50 mg, 100 mg, 240 mg, 250 mg. **Syrup:** 60 mg/15 ml, 50 mg/15 ml. **Liquid:** 150 mg/15 ml. **Solution:** 50 mg/ml.

PHARMACOKINETICS
Minimal absorption from GI tract. Acts in small/large intestine. Results occur 1–2 days after first dose (may take 3–5 days).

ACTION/ *THERAPEUTIC EFFECT*

Decreases surface film tension by mixing liquid and bowel contents, *increasing infiltration of liquid to form a softer stool.*

USES

Prophylaxis/treatment of constipation.

PO ADMINISTRATION

Drink 6–8 glasses of water/day (aids stool softening). Give each dose w/glass of water or fruit juice.

INDICATIONS/DOSAGE/ROUTES

STOOL SOFTENER:

Calcium docusate:
PO: **Adults, elderly:** 240 mg/day until evacuation. **Children >6 yrs:** 50–150 mg/day.

Potassium docusate:
PO: **Adults, elderly:** 100–300 mg/day until evacuation. **Children >6 yrs:** 100 mg at bedtime.

Sodium docusate:
PO: **Adults, elderly:** 50–500 mg/day. **Children 6–12 yrs:** 40–120 mg/day. **Children 3–6 yrs:** 20–60 mg/day. **Children <3 yrs:** 10–40 mg/day.

PRECAUTIONS

CONTRAINDICATIONS: Abdominal pain, nausea, vomiting, appendicitis. **CAUTIONS:** None significant. **PREGNANCY/LACTATION:** Unknown if drug is distributed in breast milk. **Pregnancy Category C.**

INTERACTIONS

DRUG INTERACTIONS: May increase absorption of mineral oil, danthron, phenolphthalein. **ALTERED LAB VALUES:** None significant.

SIDE EFFECTS

OCCASIONAL: Mild GI cramping, throat irritation (liquid preparation). **RARE:** Rash.

ADVERSE REACTIONS/TOXIC EFFECTS

None significant.

NURSING IMPLICATIONS

INTERVENTION/EVALUATION:

Encourage adequate fluid intake. Assess bowel sounds for peristalsis. Monitor daily bowel activity and stool consistency (watery, loose, soft, semisolid, solid) and record time of evacuation.

PATIENT/FAMILY TEACHING:

Institute measures to promote defecation: increase fluid intake, exercise, high-fiber diet.

---

dofetilide
(Tikosyn)
See Supplement
See Classification section under:
Antiarrhythmics

---

dolesetron
(Anzemet)
See Supplement

---

donepezil
(Aricept)
See Supplement

---

dopamine hydrochloride
dope-a-meen
(Intropin, Dopastat)

CANADIAN AVAILABILITY:
Intropin

CLASSIFICATION

Cardiac stimulant, vasopressor

AVAILABILITY (Rx)

Injection: 40 mg/ml, 80 mg/ml,

160 mg/ml. **Injection w/Dextrose:** 80 mg/100 ml, 160 mg/100 ml, 320 mg/100 ml.

PHARMACOKINETICS

	ONSET	PEAK	DURATION
IV	1–2 min	<5 min	<10 min

Widely distributed. Does not cross blood-brain barrier. Metabolized in liver, kidney, plasma. Primarily excreted in urine. Half-life: 2 min.

ACTION/*THERAPEUTIC EFFECT*

Stimulates adrenergic receptors; effects are dose dependent. *Low doses:* Stimulates dopaminergic receptors causing renal vasodilation *(increases renal blood flow, urine flow, sodium excretion). Low to moderate doses:* Positive inotropic effect by direct action, release of norepinephrine *(increases myocardial contractility, stroke volume, cardiac output). High doses:* Stimulates alpha receptors *(increased peripheral resistance, renal vasoconstriction, increases systolic and diastolic B/P).*

USES

Prophylaxis/treatment of acute hypotension, shock (associated w/myocardial infarction, trauma, renal failure, cardiac decompensation, open heart surgery), treatment of low cardiac output, CHF.

STORAGE/HANDLING

Do not use solutions darker than slightly yellow or discolored to yellow, brown, or pink to purple (indicates decomposition of drug).

IV ADMINISTRATION

Note: Blood volume depletion must be corrected before administering dopamine (may be used concurrently with fluid replacement).

IV:

1. Dilute each 5 ml (200 mg) ampule in 250–500 ml of compatible solution (concentration is dependent on dosage and fluid requirement of pt); 250 ml solution yields 800 mcg/ml; 500 ml solution yields 400 mcg/ml.
2. Administer into large vein (antecubital fossa) to prevent extravasation.
3. Use infusion pump to control rate of flow.
4. Titrate each pt to the desired hemodynamic or renal response.

INDICATIONS/DOSAGE/ROUTES

IV: Adults, elderly: Begin with rate of 1–5 mcg/kg/min in those likely to respond to minimal treatment. May be gradually increased in 1–4 mcg/kg/min increments at 10–30 min intervals until optimum response achieved. Most pts are maintained on dose of 20 mcq/kg/ min or less.

Seriously ill:
IV: Adults, elderly: Begin with 5 mcg/kg/min rate; gradually increase in 5–10 mcg/kg/min increments up to rate of 20–50 mcg/ kg/min. Those who do not respond may require further increments.

Pts with occlusive vascular disease:
IV: Adults, elderly: Begin with rate of 1 mcg/kg/min.

Pts on MAO inhibitors:
IV: Adults, elderly: Reduce dose to one-tenth the calculated amount.

PRECAUTIONS

CONTRAINDICATIONS: Pheochromocytoma, uncorrected tachyarrhythmias, ventricular fibrillation, sulfite sensitivity. **CAUTIONS:** Ischemic heart disease, occlusive vascular disease. Safety and efficacy for use in children has not been established. **PREGNANCY/LACTATION:** Unknown if drug crosses placenta or is distributed in breast milk. **Pregnancy Category C.**

INTERACTIONS

DRUG INTERACTIONS: Tricyclic antidepressants, may increase cardiovascular effects. Beta blockers may decrease effects. May increase risk of arrhythmias w/ digoxin. Ergot alkaloids may increase vasoconstriction. MAO inhibitors may increase cardiac stimulation, vasopressor effects. **ALTERED LAB VALUES:** Increases urea nitrogen in blood.

SIDE EFFECTS

FREQUENT: Headache, ectopic beats, tachycardia, anginal pain, palpitations, vasoconstriction, hypotension, nausea, vomiting, dyspnea. **OCCASIONAL:** Piloerection (goose bumps), bradycardia, widening of QRS complex. **RARE:** Increased urination.

ADVERSE REACTIONS/TOXIC EFFECTS

High doses may produce ventricular arrhythmias. Pts with occlusive vascular disease are high-risk candidates for further compromise of circulation to extremities, which may result in gangrene. Extravasation resulting in tissue necrosis with sloughing may occur w/IV administration.

NURSING IMPLICATIONS

BASELINE ASSESSMENT:

Check for MAO inhibitor therapy within last 2–3 wks

(dosage reduction). Pt must be on continuous cardiac monitoring. Determine weight (for dosage calculation). Obtain initial B/P, heart rate, and respirations.

INTERVENTION/EVALUATION:

Continuously monitor for cardiac arrhythmias. W/physician, establish parameters for adjusting rate or stopping infusion. Maintain accurate I&O: Measure urine output frequently. Assure proper placement of IV catheter: If extravasation occurs, immediately infiltrate the affected tissue w/10–15 ml 0.9% NaCl solution containing 5–10 mg phentolamine mesylate. Monitor B/P, heart rate, and respirations every 15 min during administration (or more often if indicated). Assess cardiac output, pulmonary wedge pressure or central venous pressure frequently. Assess peripheral circulation (palpate pulses, note color and temperature of extremities). Immediately notify physician of decreased urine output, cardiac arrhythmias, significant changes in B/P or heart rate (or failure to respond to increase/decrease in infusion rate), decreased peripheral circulation (cold, pale, or mottled extremities). Taper dosage before discontinuing because abrupt cessation of therapy may result in marked hypotension. Be alert to excessive vasoconstriction (as evidenced by decreased urine output, increased heart rate or arrhythmias, and a disproportionate increase in diastolic B/P and decrease in pulse pressure); slow or temporarily stop the infusion and notify physician at once.

PATIENT/FAMILY TEACHING:

Explain rationale for therapy. Report cold extremities, chest pain, difficulty breathing, or discomfort at IV site.

dornase alfa

door-naze **al**-fah
(Pulmozyme)

CANADIAN AVAILABILITY:
Pulmozyme

CLASSIFICATION

Enzyme

AVAILABILITY (Rx)

Solution for Inhalation: 1 mg/ml

PHARMACOKINETICS

	ONSET	PEAK	DURATION
Inhalant			
	15 min	3 days	—

Minimal systemic absorption after inhalation.

ACTION/*THERAPEUTIC EFFECT*

Selectively splits, hydrolyzes DNA in sputum, *reducing sputum viscid elasticity.*

USES

Management (w/standard therapy) of cystic fibrosis pts (including pts w/advanced disease) to reduce frequency of respiratory infections, improve pulmonary function.

STORAGE/HANDLING

Refrigerate. Ampules are clear, colorless (discard if cloudy, discolored, or left at room temperature for a total time >24 hrs).

NEBULIZATION ADMINISTRATION

Note: Administer only w/compressed-air-driven nebulizers and compressors. Do not mix/dilute w/other drugs.

1. Wash hands thoroughly w/soap and water before preparation.

2. Pour entire contents of one single-use ampule into nebulizer.

3. Hold tab at base of ampule firmly, twist off top, and squeeze contents into nebulizer cup (use full dose of drug).

4. Attach nebulizer cup, connect plastic T to nebulizer cup.

5. Connect open end to port at bottom of nebulizer cup.

6. Instruct pt to breathe normally by inhaling and exhaling through mouth only.

INDICATIONS/DOSAGE/ROUTES

Management of pulmonary function:
Nebulization: Adults, children >5 yrs: 2.5 mg (1 ampule) once daily via recommended nebulizer. (Twice daily dosing may be beneficial for some pts.)

PRECAUTIONS

CONTRAINDICATIONS: None significant. **CAUTIONS:** None significant. **PREGNANCY/LACTATION:** Unknown whether drug crosses placenta or is distributed in breast milk. **Pregnancy Category B**.

INTERACTIONS

DRUG INTERACTIONS: None significant. **ALTERED LAB VALUES:** None significant.

SIDE EFFECTS

FREQUENT: Pharyngitis (36%), chest pain or discomfort (18%), sore throat, changes in voice (12%).

OCCASIONAL (3–10%): Conjunctivitis, hoarseness, skin rash.

ADVERSE REACTIONS/TOXIC EFFECTS

None significant.

NURSING IMPLICATIONS
BASELINE ASSESSMENT:

Assess ABGs, lung sounds, dyspnea and fatigue, pulmonary secretions (amount, color, viscosity).

INTERVENTION/EVALUATION:

Provide emotional support to pt, family, parents. Encourage activity within limits of physical ability. Assess for relief of dyspnea, fatigue. Monitor ABGs, lung sounds, and observe for decreased viscosity of pulmonary secretions. Encourage fluid intake.

PATIENT/FAMILY TEACHING:

Refrigerate. Do not dilute/mix w/other medications. Treatment lasts 10–15 min. Inhale full-treatment dose. May have hoarseness or other upper airway irritation. Not a replacement for other components of therapy (e.g., antibiotics, bronchodilators, and daily physical exercise) or a cure.

dorzolamide
(Trusopt)
See Supplement
See Classification section under:
Antiglaucoma agents

doxacurium chloride
(Nuromax)
See Classification section under:
Neuromuscular blockers

doxazosin mesylate

docks-ah-**zoe**-sin
(Cardura)

CANADIAN AVAILABILITY:
Cardura

CLASSIFICATION

Antihypertensive

AVAILABILITY (Rx)

Tablets: 1 mg, 2 mg, 4 mg, 8 mg

PHARMACOKINETICS

	ONSET	PEAK	DURATION
PO	—	2–6 hrs	—

Well absorbed from GI tract. Metabolized in liver. Primarily eliminated in feces. Half-life: 19–22 hrs.

ACTION/*THERAPEUTIC EFFECT*

Selectively blocks alpha$_1$-adrenergic receptors, decreasing peripheral vascular resistance. Resulting peripheral vasodilation *lowers B/P, relaxes smooth muscle of bladder/prostate.*

USES

Treatment of mild to moderate hypertension. Used alone or in combination w/other antihypertensives. Treatment of benign prostatic hyperplasia.

PO ADMINISTRATION

May give w/o regard to food.

INDICATIONS/DOSAGE/ROUTES

Hypertension:
PO: **Adults:** Initially, 1 mg/day. May increase to 2, 4, 8, and 16 mg if necessary. **Elderly:** Initially, 0.5 mg/day. **Note:** Doses >4 mg increase potential postural effects.

Benign prostatic hyperplasia:
PO: **Adults, elderly:** 2–16 mg/day.

PRECAUTIONS

CONTRAINDICATIONS: None significant. CAUTIONS: Chronic renal failure, impaired hepatic function. PREGNANCY/LACTATION: Unknown if drug crosses placenta or is distributed in breast milk. Pregnancy Category B.

INTERACTIONS

DRUG INTERACTIONS: NSAIDs, estrogen may decrease effect. Hypotension-producing medications may increase effect. ALTERED LAB VALUES: None significant.

SIDE EFFECTS

FREQUENT (10–20%): Dizziness, asthenia, headache, edema. OCCASIONAL (3–9%): Nausea, pharyngitis, rhinitis, pain in extremities, somnolence. RARE (1–3%): Palpitations, diarrhea, constipation, dyspnea, muscle pain, altered vision, dizziness, nervousness.

ADVERSE REACTIONS/TOXIC EFFECTS

First-dose syncope (hypotension w/sudden loss of consciousness) generally occurs 30–90 min after giving initial dose of 2 mg or greater, a too rapid increase in dose, or addition of another hypotensive agent to therapy. May be preceded by tachycardia (120–160 beats/min).

NURSING IMPLICATIONS

BASELINE ASSESSMENT:

Give first dose at bedtime. If initial dose is given during daytime, pt must remain recumbent for 3–4 hrs. Assess B/P, pulse immediately before each dose, and q15–30min until stabilized (be alert to B/P fluctuations).

INTERVENTION/EVALUATION:

Monitor pulse diligently (first-dose syncope may be preceded by tachycardia). Monitor pattern of daily bowel activity and stool consistency. Assist w/ambulation if dizziness, lightheadedness occurs.

PATIENT/FAMILY TEACHING:

Dry mouth may be relieved by sugarless gum, sips of tepid water. Cola, unsalted crackers, dry toast may relieve nausea. Nasal congestion may occur. Full therapeutic effect may not occur for 3–4 wks. May cause syncope (fainting). Avoid driving for 12–24 hrs after first dose or increase in dosage. Use caution driving or operating machinery, or when rising from sitting or lying position. Report dizziness or palpitations if bothersome.

doxepin hydrochloride

dox-eh-pin
(Adapin, Sinequan, Zonalon)

CANADIAN AVAILABILITY:
Novo-Doxepin, Sinequan, Zonalon

CLASSIFICATION

Antidepressant: Tricyclic

AVAILABILITY (Rx)

Capsules: 10 mg, 25 mg, 50 mg, 75 mg, 100 mg, 150 mg. Oral Concentrate: 10 mg/ml. Cream: 5%.

PHARMACOKINETICS

Rapid, well absorbed from GI tract. Metabolized in liver to active metabolite. Primarily excreted in urine. Half-life: 11–23 hrs. *Topical:* Absorbed through skin, distributed to body tissues, metabolized to active metabolite, eliminated renally.

ACTION/*THERAPEUTIC EFFECT*

Increases synaptic concentration of norepinephrine and/or serotonin (inhibits reuptake by presynaptic membrane), *producing antidepressant, anxiolytic effect.* Strong anticholinergic activity. Topical may produce antihistamine/sedative effect.

USES/*UNLABELED*

Treatment of various forms of depression, often in conjunction w/psychotherapy. Treatment of anxiety. *Topical:* Treatment of pruritus associated w/eczema. *Treatment of panic disorder, neurogenic pain, prophylaxis vascular headache, pruritus in idiopathic cold urticaria.*

PO ADMINISTRATION

1. Give w/food or milk if GI distress occurs.

2. Dilute concentrate in 8 oz glass of water, milk, orange, grapefruit, tomato, prune, pineapple juice. Incompatible w/carbonated drinks.

INDICATIONS/DOSAGE/ROUTES

Mild to moderate depression/anxiety:
PO: Adults: 25 mg 3 times/day (75 mg/day). **Usual therapeutic range:** 75–150 mg/day. Alternately, 150 mg/day as single dose at bedtime.

Severe depression/anxiety:
PO: Adults: 50 mg 3 times/day. Gradually increase to 300 mg/day, if needed.

Emotional symptoms accompanying organic brain disease:
PO: Adults: 25–50 mg/day.

Usual elderly dosage:
PO: Initially, 10–25 mg at bedtime. May increase by 10–25 mg/day every 3–7 days. **Maximum:** 75 mg/day.

Usual topical dosage:
Topical: Adults, elderly: Apply thin film 4 times/day.

PRECAUTIONS

CONTRAINDICATIONS: Acute recovery period following MI, within 14 days of MAO inhibitor ingestion. **CAUTIONS:** Prostatic hypertrophy, history of urinary retention/obstruction, glaucoma, diabetes mellitus, history of seizures, hyperthyroidism, cardiac/hepatic/renal disease, schizophrenia, increased intraocular pressure, hiatal hernia. **PREGNANCY/LACTATION:** Crosses placenta; distributed in breast milk. **Pregnancy Category C**. *Topical:* **Pregnancy Category B**.

INTERACTIONS

DRUG INTERACTIONS: Alcohol, CNS depressants may increase CNS, respiratory depression, hypotensive effects. Antithyroid agents may increase risk of agranulocytosis. Phenothiazines may increase sedative, anticholinergic effects. Cimetidine may increase concentration, toxicity. May decrease effects of clonidine, guanadrel. May increase cardiac effects w/sympathomimetics. May increase risk of hypertensive crisis, hyperpyretic, convulsions w/MAO inhibitors. **ALTERED LAB VALUES:** May alter ECG readings, glucose.

SIDE EFFECTS

FREQUENT: *Oral:* Orthostatic hypotension, drowsiness, dry mouth, headache, increased appetite/weight, nausea, unusual tiredness, unpleasant taste. *Topical:* Edema at application site, increased itching/eczema, burning, stinging of skin, altered taste, dizziness, drowsiness, dry skin, dry mouth, fatigue, headache, thirst. **OCCASIONAL:** *Oral:* Blurred vision, confusion, constipation, hallucinations, difficult urination, eye pain, irregular heartbeat, fine muscle tremors, Parkinson syndrome, nervousness, impaired sexual function, diarrhea, increased sweating, heartburn, insomnia. *Topical:* Anxiety, skin irritation/cracking, nausea. **RARE:** Allergic reaction, alopecia, tinnitus, breast enlargement. *Topical:* Fever.

ADVERSE REACTIONS/TOXIC EFFECTS

High dosage may produce confusion, seizures, severe drowsiness, fast/slow/irregular heartbeat, fever, hallucinations, agitation, shortness of breath, vomiting, unusual tiredness/weakness. Abrupt withdrawal from prolonged therapy may produce headache, malaise, nausea, vomiting, vivid dreams.

NURSING IMPLICATIONS
BASELINE ASSESSMENT:

For those on long-term therapy, liver/renal function tests, blood counts should be performed periodically.

INTERVENTION/EVALUATION:

Supervise suicidal risk pt closely during early therapy (as depression lessens, energy level improves, increasing suicide potential). Assess appearance, behavior, speech pattern, level of interest, mood. Monitor pattern of daily bowel activity, stool consistency. Monitor B/P, pulse for hypotension, arrhythmias. Assess for urinary retention by bladder palpation. Avoid alcohol.

PATIENT/FAMILY TEACHING:

Change positions slowly to avoid hypotensive effect. Tolerance to postural hypotension, sedative and anticholinergic effects usually develops during early therapy. Therapeutic effect may be noted within 2–5 days, maximum effect within 2–3 wks. Photosensitivity to sun may occur. Dry mouth may be relieved by sugarless gum, sips of tepid water. Report visual disturbances. Do not abruptly discontinue medication. Avoid tasks that require alertness, motor skills until response to drug is established.

---

doxercalciferol
(Hectorol)
See Supplement

---

doxorubicin
dox-o-**roo**-bi-sin
(Adriamycin, Doxil, Rubex)

CANADIAN AVAILABILITY:
Adriamycin

CLASSIFICATION

Antineoplastic

AVAILABILITY (Rx)

Powder for Injection: 10 mg, 20 mg, 50 mg, 100 mg, 150 mg. **Lipid Complex (Doxil):** 20 mg.

PHARMACOKINETICS

Widely distributed. Does not cross blood-brain barrier. Metabolized rapidly in liver to active metabolite. Primarily eliminated via biliary system. Half-life: 16 hrs; metabolite: 32 hrs.

ACTION/ *THERAPEUTIC EFFECT*

Inhibits DNA, DNA-dependent RNA synthesis by binding w/DNA strands, *preventing cellular divi-*

sion. Cell cycle-specific for S phase of cell division.

USES / *UNLABELED*

Produces regression in breast, ovarian, thyroid, transitional cell bladder, bronchogenic, gastric carcinoma; soft tissue and bone sarcomas, neuroblastoma, Wilms' tumor, lymphomas of Hodgkin's and non-Hodgkin's type, acute lymphoblastic and myeloblastic leukemia. *Doxil:* Treatment of AIDS-related Kaposi's sarcoma, metastatic ovarian cancer. *Treatment of head/neck, cervical, liver, pancreatic, prostatic, testicular, endometrial carcinoma; treatment of germ cell tumors, multiple myeloma.*

STORAGE / HANDLING

Note: May be carcinogenic, mutagenic, or teratogenic. Handle w/extreme care during preparation/administration.

Reconstituted solution stable for 24 hrs at room temperature or 48 hrs if refrigerated. Protect from prolonged exposure to sunlight; discard unused solution.

IV ADMINISTRATION

Note: Give by IV injection. Wear gloves. If powder or solution comes in contact w/skin, wash thoroughly. Avoid small veins, swollen or edematous extremities, and areas overlying joints, tendons. *Doxil:* Do not use w/in-line filter or mix w/any diluent except D₅W.

1. Reconstitute each 10 mg vial w/5 ml preservative-free 0.9% NaCl injection (10 ml for 20 mg; 25 ml for 50 mg) to provide concentration of 2 mg/ml.

2. Shake vial; allow contents to dissolve.

3. Withdraw appropriate volume of air from vial during reconstitution (avoids excessive pressure buildup).

4. For IV injection, administer into tubing of freely running IV infusion of 5% dextrose or 0.9% NaCl, preferably via butterfly needle, at rate no faster than 3–5 min (avoids local erythematous streaking along vein and facial flushing).

5. Extravasation produces immediate pain, severe local tissue damage. Terminate immediately; flood site w/normal saline.

INDICATIONS / DOSAGE / ROUTES

Note: Dosage individualized based on clinical response, tolerance to adverse effects. When used in combination therapy, consult specific protocols for optimum dosage, sequence of drug administration.

Usual dose:
IV: Adults: 60–75 mg/m² single dose every 21 days, 20 mg/m² once weekly, or 25–30 mg/m² daily on 2–3 successive days q4 wks. Due to cardiotoxicity, do not exceed cumulative dose of 550 mg/m² (400–450 mg/m² for those whose previous therapy included related compounds or irradiation of cardiac region). **Children** 25–40 mg/m² or per individual protocol.

Kaposi's sarcoma: (Doxil)
IV Infusion: Adults: 20 mg/m² q3wks (infuse over 30 min).

Ovarian cancer: (Doxil)
IV Infusion: Adults: 50 mg/m² q4wks.

Dosage in hepatic impairment:

SERUM BILIRUBIN CONCENTRATION	DOSAGE
1.2–3 mg/dl	50% usual dose
>3 mg/dl	25% usual dose

PRECAUTIONS

CONTRAINDICATIONS: Preexisting myelosuppression, impaired cardiac function, previous treatment w/complete cumulative doses of doxorubicin and/or daunorubicin. **CAUTIONS:** Impaired hepatic, renal function. Children at increased risk of cardiotoxicity. **PREGNANCY/LACTATION:** If possible, avoid use during pregnancy, esp. first trimester. Breast-feeding not recommended. **Pregnancy Category D**.

INTERACTIONS

DRUG INTERACTIONS: May decrease effect of antigout medication. Bone marrow depressants may increase bone marrow depression. May increase cardiotoxicity w/daunorubicin. Live virus vaccines may potentiate virus replication, increase vaccine side effects, decrease pt's antibody response to vaccine. **ALTERED LAB VALUES:** May cause EKG changes. May increase uric acid. *Doxil:* Reduces neutrophil, RBC count.

SIDE EFFECTS

FREQUENT: Complete alopecia (scalp, axillary, pubic hair), nausea, vomiting, stomatitis, esophagitis (esp. if drug given daily on several successive days), reddish urine. *Doxil:* Nausea. **OCCASIONAL:** Anorexia, diarrhea, hyperpigmentation of nailbeds, phalangeal and dermal creases. **RARE:** Fever, chills, conjunctivitis, lacrimation.

ADVERSE REACTIONS/TOXIC EFFECTS

Bone marrow depression manifested as hematologic toxicity (principally leukopenia, and to lesser extent anemia, thrombocytopenia). Generally occurs within 10–15 days, returns to normal levels by third week. Cardiotoxicity noted as either acute, transient ab-

normal EKG findings and for cardiomyopathy manifested as CHF.

NURSING IMPLICATIONS

BASELINE ASSESSMENT:

Obtain WBC, platelet, erythrocyte counts before and at frequent intervals during therapy. Obtain EKG prior to therapy, liver function studies prior to each dose. Antiemetics may be effective in preventing, treating nausea.

INTERVENTION/EVALUATION:

Monitor for stomatitis (burning/erythema of oral mucosa at inner margin of lips, sore throat, difficulty swallowing). May lead to ulceration within 2–3 days. Assess skin, nailbeds for hyperpigmentation. Monitor hematologic status, renal/hepatic function studies, serum uric acid levels. Assess pattern of daily bowel activity, stool consistency. Monitor for hematologic toxicity (fever, sore throat, signs of local infection, easy bruising, unusual bleeding from any site), symptoms of anemia (excessive tiredness, weakness).

PATIENT/FAMILY TEACHING:

Alopecia is reversible, but new hair growth may have different color or texture. New hair growth resumes 2–3 mos after last therapy dose. Maintain fastidious oral hygiene. Do not have immunizations w/o physician's approval (drug lowers body's resistance). Avoid contact w/those who have recently received live virus vaccine. Promptly report fever, sore throat, signs of local infection, easy bruising, or unusual bleeding from any site. Contact physician if nausea/vomiting continues at home. Avoid alcohol.

doxycycline calcium

dock-see-**sigh**-clean
(Vibramycin Calcium syrup)

doxycycline hyclate, monohydrate

(Doryx, Periostat, Vibra-Tabs, Vibramycin)

CANADIAN AVAILABILITY:
Apo-Doxy, Doxycin, Vibra-Tabs

CLASSIFICATION

Antibiotic: Tetracycline

AVAILABILITY (Rx)

Capsules: 20 mg, 50 mg, 100 mg. **Tablets:** 50 mg, 100 mg. **Powder for Oral Suspension:** 25 mg/5 ml, 50 mg/5 ml. **Syrup:** 50 mg/5 ml. **Powder for Injection:** 100 mg, 200 mg.

PHARMACOKINETICS

Well absorbed from GI tract (may give w/food). Widely distributed. Partially inactivated in intestine. Excreted in urine, eliminated in feces via biliary secretion. Not removed by hemodialysis. Half-life: 12–22 hrs.

ACTION/ *THERAPEUTIC EFFECT*

Bacteriostatic due to binding to ribosomes, *inhibiting protein synthesis.*

USES/ *UNLABELED*

Treatment of periodontis, respiratory, skin/ soft tissue, urinary tract infections, syphilis, uncomplicated gonorrhea, pelvic inflammatory disease, rheumatic fever prophylaxis, brucellosis, trachoma, Rocky Mountain spotted fever, typhus, Q fever, rickettsia, smallpox, psittacosis, ornithosis, granuloma inguinale, lymphogranuloma venereum, adjunctive treatment of intestinal amebiasis. *Treatment of gonorrhea, malaria, atypical mycobacterial infections, prophylaxis/treatment of traveler's diarrhea, rheumatoid arthritis.*

STORAGE/HANDLING

Store capsules, tablets at room temperature. Oral suspension stable for 2 wks at room temperature. After reconstitution, IV infusion (piggyback) is stable for 12 hrs at room temperature, 72 hrs if refrigerated. Protect from direct sunlight. Discard if precipitate forms.

PO/IV ADMINISTRATION

Note: Do not administer IM or SubQ. Space doses evenly around clock.

PO:
Give w/full glass of fluid. May take w/food or milk.

IV:

Note: Give by intermittent IV infusion (piggyback).
   1. Reconstitute each 100 mg vial w/10 ml sterile water for injection for concentration of 10 mg/ml.
   2. Further dilute each 100 mg w/at least 100 ml 5% dextrose, 0.9% NaCl, or other compatible IV fluid. Infuse >1–4 hrs.

INDICATIONS/DOSAGE/ROUTES

Usual dosage:
PO: Adults, elderly: Initially, 200 mg (100 mg q12h), then 100 mg/day as single dose or in 2 divided doses (100 mg q12h in severe infections). **Children >8 yrs, >45 kg:** Initially, 4.4 mg/kg divided in 2 doses, then 2.2 mg/kg as single dose or in 2 divided doses (4.4 mg/kg in severe infections).

IV: Adults, elderly: Initially, 200 mg as 1–2 infusions; then 100–200 mg/day (200 mg as 12 infusions). **Children:** Initially, 4.4 mg/kg on first day as 1–2 infusions; then 2.2–4.4 mg/kg as 12 infusions.

Acute gonococcal infections:
PO: Adults: Initially, 200 mg, then 100 mg at bedtime on first day; then 100 mg 2 times/day for 3 days.

Syphilis:
PO/IV: Adults: 300 mg/day in divided doses for 10 days.

Traveler's diarrhea:
PO: Adults, elderly: 100 mg daily during a period of risk (up to 14 days) and for 2 days after returning home.

Periodonitis:
PO: Adults: 20 mg 2 times/day.

PRECAUTIONS

CONTRAINDICATIONS: Hypersensitivity to tetracyclines, sulfite, last half of pregnancy, children <8 yrs. **CAUTIONS:** Sun/ultraviolet light exposure (severe photosensitivity reaction). **PREGNANCY/ LACTATION:** Readily crosses placenta; distributed in breast milk. Avoid use in women during last half of pregnancy. May produce permanent teeth discoloration, enamel hypoplasia, inhibits skeletal growth in children <8 yrs. **Pregnancy Category D.**

INTERACTIONS

DRUG INTERACTIONS: Antacids containing aluminum/calcium/ magnesium, laxatives containing magnesium. Oral iron preparations impair absorption of tetracyclines (give 1–2 hrs before or after tetracyclines). Barbiturates, phenytoin, carbamazepine may decrease doxycycline concentrations. Cholestyramine, colestipol may decrease absorption. May decrease effect of oral contraceptives. Carbamazepine, phenytoin may decrease concentrations. **ALTERED LAB VALUES:** May increase SCOT (AST), SGPT (ALT), alkaline phosphatase, amylase, bilirubin concentrations; alter CBC.

SIDE EFFECTS

FREQUENT: Anorexia, nausea, vomiting, diarrhea, dysphagia, photosensitivity. **OCCASIONAL:** Rash, urticaria.

ADVERSE REACTIONS/TOXIC EFFECTS

Superinfection (esp. fungal), benign intracranial hypertension (headache, visual changes). Liver toxicity, fatty degeneration of liver, pancreatitis occur rarely.

NURSING IMPLICATIONS

BASELINE ASSESSMENT:

Question for history of allergies esp. to tetracyclines, sulfite. Obtain culture and sensitivity test before giving first dose (therapy may begin before results are known).

INTERVENTION/EVALUATION:

Check IV site for phlebitis (heat, pain, red streaking over vein). Determine pattern of bowel activity, stool consistency. Monitor food intake, tolerance. Assess skin for rash. Monitor B/P and LOC because of potential for increased intracranial pressure. Be alert for superinfection: diarrhea, ulceration or changes of oral mucosa, anal/genital pruritus.

PATIENT/FAMILY TEACHING:

Continue antibiotic for full length of treatment. Space doses evenly. Drink full glass of water w/capsules or tablets. May take w/food or milk. Notify physician in event of diarrhea, rash, or other new symptoms. Protect skin from sun/ultraviolet light exposure. Consult physician before taking any other medication.

dronabinol

drow-**nab**-in-all
(Marinol)

CANADIAN AVAILABILITY:
Marinol

CLASSIFICATION

Antinausea, antiemetic (**Schedule III**)

AVAILABILITY (Rx)

Capsules: 2.5 mg, 5 mg, 10 mg

PHARMACOKINETICS

Poorly absorbed from GI tract. Metabolized in liver. Primarily eliminated via biliary excretion. Half-life: 15–18 hrs (metabolite).

ACTION

May inhibit vomiting control mechanisms in medulla oblongata.

USES

Prevention, treatment of nausea, vomiting due to cancer chemotherapy; appetite stimulant in AIDS pts.

INDICATIONS/DOSAGE/ROUTES

Nausea, vomiting:
PO: Adults: Initially, 5 mg/m², 1–3 hrs before chemotherapy, then q2–4h after chemotherapy for total of 4–6 doses/day. May increase by 2.5 mg/m² up to 15 mg/m²/dose.

Appetite stimulant:
PO: Adults: Initially, 2.5 mg 2 times/day (before lunch, dinner). **Range:** 2.5–20 mg/day.

PRECAUTIONS

CONTRAINDICATIONS: Nausea, vomiting other than due to chemotherapy. **CAUTIONS:** Hypertension, heart disease; manic, depressive, or schizophrenic pts. Not recommended in children. **PREGNANCY/LACTATION:** Unknown if drug crosses placenta. Distributed in breast milk. **Pregnancy Category B**.

INTERACTIONS

DRUG INTERACTIONS: CNS depressants may enhance sedative effects. **ALTERED LAB VALUES:** None significant.

SIDE EFFECTS

FREQUENT (3–10%): Nausea, vomiting, euphoria, dizziness, somnolence. **OCCASIONAL (1–3%):** Asthenia, ataxia, confusion, abnormal thinking, altered vision. **RARE (<1%):** Diarrhea, depression, nightmares, speech difficulties, headache, anxiety, ringing in ears, flushed skin.

ADVERSE REACTIONS/TOXIC EFFECTS

Overdosage may produce increased sensory awareness (e.g., taste, smell, sound), altered time perception, reddened conjunctiva, memory impairment, urinary retention, constipation, slurred speech.

NURSING IMPLICATIONS
BASELINE ASSESSMENT:

Assess for dehydration if excessive vomiting occurs (poor

skin turgor, dry mucous membranes, decreased urine output).

INTERVENTION/EVALUATION:

Provide emotional support. Supervise closely for serious mood and behavior responses. Do not continue drug after a psychotic episode until pt and situation have been fully evaluated.

PATIENT/FAMILY TEACHING:

Potentially abusable drug— take only as directed. Report visual disturbances. Dry mouth is expected response to medication. Relief from nausea/vomiting generally occurs within 15 min of drug administration. Avoid alcohol, barbiturates. Avoid tasks that require alertness, motor skills until response to drug is established. Remain under supervision of a responsible adult because mood alterations and adverse behavioral effects can occur. For appetite stimulation take before lunch and dinner.

droperidol

droe-**pear**-ih-dall
(Inapsine)

FIXED-COMBINATION(S):
W/fentanyl, a narcotic (**Innovar**)

CLASSIFICATION

Antiemetic

AVAILABILITY (Rx)

Injection: 2.5 mg/ml

PHARMACOKINETICS

	ONSET	PEAK	DURATION
IM	3–10 min	30 min	2–4 hrs
IV	3–10 min	30 min	2–4 hrs

Well absorbed after IM administration. Crosses blood-brain barrier. Metabolized in liver. Primarily excreted in urine.

ACTION/ *THERAPEUTIC EFFECT*

Antagonizes dopamine neurotransmission at synapses by blocking postsynaptic dopamine receptor sites; partially blocks adrenergic receptor binding sites, *producing tranquilization, antiemetic effect.*

USES

Tranquilization, control of nausea/vomiting during surgical, diagnostic procedures. Used preoperatively w/opiate analgesics during general anesthesia as anxiolytic, to increase analgesic effect of opiate.

STORAGE/HANDLING

Store parenteral form at room temperature. Precipitate occurs if mixed w/barbiturate.

IM/IV ADMINISTRATION

Note: Pt must remain recumbent for 30–60 min in head-low position w/legs raised, to minimize hypotensive effect.
IM: Inject slow, deep IM into upper outer quadrant of gluteus maximus.
IV: Dose for high-risk pts should be added to 5% dextrose or lactated Ringer's injection to a concentration of 1 mg/50 ml; give by slow IV infusion.

INDICATIONS/DOSAGE/ROUTES

Preop:
IM/IV: Adults, elderly: 2.5–10 mg 30–60 min before induction of

general anesthesia. **Children 2–12 yrs:** 0.088–0.165 mg/kg.

Adjunct for induction of general anesthesia:
IV: **Adults, elderly:** 0.22–0.275 mg/kg. **Children 2–12 yrs:** 0.088–0.165 mg/kg.

Adjunct for maintenance of general anesthesia:
IV: **Adults, elderly:** 1.25–2.5 mg.

Diagnostic procedures w/o general anesthesia:
IM: **Adults, elderly:** 2.5–10 mg 30–60 min before procedure. If needed, may give additional doses of 1.25–2.5 mg (usually by IV injection).

Adjunct to regional anesthesia:
IM/IV: **Adults, elderly:** 2.5–5 mg.

PRECAUTIONS

CONTRAINDICATIONS: Known intolerance to drug. **CAUTIONS:** Impaired hepatic/renal/cardiac function. **PREGNANCY/LACTATION:** Crosses placenta; unknown if drug is distributed in breast milk. **Pregnancy Category C**.

INTERACTIONS

DRUG INTERACTIONS: CNS depressants may increase CNS depressant effect. Hypotensives may increase hypotension. **ALTERED LAB VALUES:** None significant.

SIDE EFFECTS

FREQUENT: Mild to moderate hypotension. **OCCASIONAL:** Tachycardia, postop drowsiness, dizziness, chills, shivering. **RARE:** Postop nightmares, facial sweating, bronchospasm.

ADVERSE REACTIONS/TOXIC EFFECTS

Extrapyramidal symptoms may appear as akathisia (motor restlessness) and dystonias: torticollis (neck muscle spasm), opisthotonos (rigidity of back muscles), and oculogyric crisis (rolling back of eyes).

NURSING IMPLICATIONS
BASELINE ASSESSMENT:

Assess vital signs. Have pt void. Prepare for surgery. Raise side rails. Instruct to remain recumbent.

INTERVENTION/EVALUATION:

Monitor B/P and pulse diligently for hypotensive reaction during and after procedure. Assess pulse for tachycardia. Monitor for extrapyramidal symptoms. Evaluate for therapeutic response from anxiety: a calm facial expression, decreased restlessness.

---

echothiophate
(Phospholine Iodide)
See Classification section under:
Antiglaucoma agents

---

edetate calcium disodium (calcium EDTA)
ed-eh-tate
(Calcium Disodium Versehate)

CLASSIFICATION

Antidote

AVAILABILITY (Rx)

Injection: 200 mg/ml

PHARMACOKINETICS

	ONSET	PEAK	DURATION
IV	1 hr	24–48 hrs	—

Well absorbed after parenteral administration. Primarily distributed in extracellular fluid. Excreted unchanged in urine. Half-life: 20–90 min.

ACTION/*THERAPEUTIC EFFECT*

Reduces blood concentration of heavy metals, esp. lead, forming stable complexes, *allowing heavy metal excretion in urine.*

USES

Acute and chronic lead poisoning, lead encephalopathy.

STORAGE/HANDLING

Store parenteral form at room temperature.

IM/IV ADMINISTRATION

IM:
Add 1 ml 1% procaine to each ml calcium EDTA prior to administration.

IV:
1. Dilute each calcium EDTA ampule (1 g) w/5% dextrose or 0.9% NaCl to provide a concentration of 2–4 mg/ml.
2. For intermittent IV administration, solution containing $1/2$ daily dose infused over 1–2 hrs; second dose infused at least 6 hrs after first infusion.
3. For IV infusion, give over 12–24 hrs. **Note:** Interrupt infusion for 1 hr before blood lead concentration measured (avoids falsely elevated reading).

INDICATIONS/DOSAGE/ROUTES

Note: When administered IV, calcium EDTA may be given in 2 divided doses at 12 hr intervals or 12–24 hr infusions; when administered IM and

used alone, may be given in divided doses at 8–12 hr intervals; when given IM w/dimercaprol in divided doses, administer at 4 hr intervals.

Diagnosis of lead poisoning:
IM/IV Infusion: Adults, elderly: 500 mg/m². **Maximum:** 1 g.
IV Infusion: Children: 500 mg/ m².
IM: Children: 500 mg/m² as single dose or 500 mg/m² each at 12 hr intervals.

Lead poisoning (w/o encephalopathy):
Note: Total dose dependent on severity of lead poisoning, pt response/tolerance to medication. Consult specific protocols.
IM/IV: Adults, elderly, children: 1–1.5 g/m² daily for 3–5 days. (If blood lead concentration >100 mcg/dl, calcium edetate usually given w/dimercaprol.) Allow at least 2–4 days, up to 2–3 wks between courses of therapy. Adults should not be given more than 2 courses of therapy.

Lead poisoning (w/encephalopathy):
IM: Adults, elderly, children: Initially, dimercaprol 4 mg/kg; then give dimercaprol 4 mg/kg and calcium EDTA 250 mg/m²; then 4 hrs later and q4h for 5 days .

PRECAUTIONS

CONTRAINDICATIONS: Anuria. **CAUTIONS:** None significant. **PREGNANCY/LACTATION:** Unknown if drug crosses placenta or is distributed in breast milk. Do not use in pregnancy unless benefits outweigh potential risk to fetus. **Pregnancy Category C.**

INTERACTIONS

DRUG INTERACTIONS: May decrease effects of zinc. **ALTERED LAB VALUES:** None significant.

SIDE EFFECTS

FREQUENT: Chills, fever, anorexia, headache, histaminelike reaction (sneezing, stuffy nose, watery eyes), decreased B/P, nausea, vomiting, thrombophlebitis. **OCCASIONAL:** Transient anemia/bone marrow depression, hypercalcemia (constipation, drowsiness, dry mouth, metallic taste). **RARE:** Frequent urination, secondary gout (severe pain in feet, knees, elbows).

ADVERSE REACTIONS/TOXIC EFFECTS

Renal tubular necrosis.

NURSING IMPLICATIONS

BASELINE ASSESSMENT:

Assure urine flow before start of therapy. Determine serum and urine, lead levels, BUN. Assess family members for lead poisoning.

INTERVENTION/EVALUATION:

Monitor EKG during therapy. Assess vital signs, neurologic status. Maintain careful I&O. Avoid rapid IV infusion (may be lethal due to increased ICP). Periodically check serum and urine lead levels, BUN; obtain daily urinalysis. Stop drug immediately and notify physician of anuria or urinalysis report of increased proteinuria, increased erythrocytes, or presence of large renal epithelial cells.

PATIENT/FAMILY TEACHING:

Necessity of follow-up visits for tests and possible further therapy. Evaluation of home to prevent future poisoning.

emedastine
(Emadine)
See Supplement

efavirenz
(Sustiva)
See Supplement
See Classification section inder:
Antivirals, Human immunodeficiency virus (HIV) infection

E

enalapril maleate

en-**al**-ah-prill
(Vasotec)

FIXED-COMBINATION(S):
W/hydrochlorothiazide, a diuretic (**Vaseretic**); w/diltrazem., a calcium channel blocker (**Teczem**); w/felodipine, a calcium channel blocker (**Lexxel**)

CANADIAN AVAILABILITY:
Vasotec

CLASSIFICATION

Angiotensin-converting enzyme (ACE) inhibitor, antihypertensive

AVAILABILITY (Rx)

Tablets: 2.5 mg, 5 mg, 10 mg, 20 mg. **Injection:** 1.25 mg/ml.

PHARMACOKINETICS

	ONSET	PEAK	DURATION
PO	1 hr	4–6 hrs	24 hrs
IV	15 min	1–4 hrs	6 hrs

Readily absorbed from GI tract (not affected by food). Converted to active metabolite enalapril. Primarily excreted in urine. Removed by hemodialysis. Half-life: 11 hrs (increased in reduced renal function).

ACTION/THERAPEUTIC EFFECT

Suppresses renin-angiotensin-aldosterone system (prevents conversion of angiotensin I to angiotensin II, a potent vasoconstrictor; may inhibit angiotensin II at local vascular, renal sites). Decreases plasma angiotensin II, increases plasma renin activity, decreases aldosterone secretion. *In hypertension, reduces peripheral arterial resistance. In CHF, increases cardiac output, decreases peripheral vascular resistance, B/P, pulmonary capillary wedge pressure, heart size.*

USES / *UNLABELED*

Treatment of hypertension alone or in combination w/other antihypertensives. Adjunctive therapy for CHF (in combination w/cardiac glycosides, diuretics). *Treatment of diabetic nephropathy, hypertension, or renal crisis in scleroderma.*

STORAGE / HANDLING

Store tablets, parenteral form at room temperature. For parenteral form, use only clear, colorless solution. Diluted IV solution is stable for 24 hrs at room temperature.

PO / IV ADMINISTRATION

PO:

1. May give w/o regard to food.

2. Tablets may be crushed.

IV:

1. For direct IV, give undiluted over 5 min.

2. May dilute w/5% dextrose or 0.9% NaCl. Infuse over 10–15 min.

INDICATIONS / DOSAGE / ROUTES

Hypertension (used alone):
PO: Adults, elderly: Initially, 5 mg/day. **Maintenance:** 10–40 mg/day as single or in 2 divided doses. **IV: Adults, elderly:** 1.25 mg q6h.

Hypertension (w/diuretics):
Note: Discontinue diuretic 2–3 days before initiating enalapril therapy; if unable, initiate w/2.5 mg enalapril (0.625 mg IV).

Dose in renal impairment:
(Based on creatinine clearance.)
PO: Adults, elderly: Initially, 2.5–5 mg/day titrate up to maximum of 40 mg/day.
IV: Adults, elderly (Ccr <30 ml/min): Initially, 0.625 mg. May repeat in 1 hr if no response, then 1.25 mg q6h.

CHF:
PO: Adults, elderly: Initially, 2.5–5 mg/day. **Maintenance:** 5–20 mg/day in 2 divided doses. **Maximum:** 40 mg/day in 2 divided doses.

Dosage in renal impairment, hyponatremia (Na <130, Creat >1.6):
Initially, 2.5 mg/day, increase to 2.5 mg 2 times/day, then 5 mg 2 times/day at 4 day intervals (minimum) up to 40 mg/day.

PRECAUTIONS

CONTRAINDICATIONS: History of angioedema w/previous treatment w/ACE inhibitors. **CAUTIONS:** Renal impairment, those w/sodium depletion or on diuretic therapy, dialysis, hypovolemia, coronary/cerebrovascular insufficiency. **PREGNANCY/LACTATION:** Crosses placenta; distributed in breast milk. May cause fetal/neonatal mortality/morbidity. **Pregnancy Category D**.

INTERACTIONS

DRUG INTERACTIONS: Alcohol, diuretics, hypotensive agents may increase effects. NSAIDs may decrease effect. Potassium-sparing diuretics, potassium supplements may cause hyperkalemia. May increase lithium concentration, toxicity. **ALTERED LAB VALUES:** May increase potassium, SGOT (AST), SGPT (ALT), alkaline phosphatase, bilirubin, BUN, creatinine. May decrease sodium. May cause positive ANA titer.

SIDE EFFECTS

FREQUENT (5–7%): Postural hypotension, headache, dizziness. **OCCASIONAL (2–3%):** Orthostatic hypotension, fatigue, diarrhea, cough, syncope. **RARE (<2%):** Angina, abdominal pain, vomiting, nausea, rash, asthenia (loss of strength/energy), fainting.

ADVERSE REACTIONS/TOXIC EFFECTS

Excessive hypotension ("first-dose syncope") may occur in those w/CHF, severely salt/volume depleted. Angioedema (swelling of face, lips), hyperkalemia occur rarely. Agranulocytosis, neutropenia may be noted in those w/impaired renal function or collagen vascular disease (systemic lupus erythematosus, scleroderma). Nephrotic syndrome may be noted in those w/history of renal disease.

NURSING IMPLICATIONS

BASELINE ASSESSMENT:

Obtain B/P immediately before each dose in addition to regular monitoring (be alert to fluctuations). Renal function tests should be performed before therapy begins. In those w/renal impairment, autoimmune disease, or taking drugs that affect leukocytes or immune response, CBC and differential count should be performed before therapy begins and q2wks for 3 mos, then periodically thereafter.

INTERVENTION/EVALUATION:

Assist w/ambulation if dizziness occurs. Assess skin for development of rash. Monitor serum potassium, BUN, serum creatinine levels. Monitor pattern of daily bowel activity, stool consistency. Assess for anorexia due to decreased taste sensa-

tion. If excessive reduction in B/P occurs, place pt in supine position w/legs elevated.

PATIENT/FAMILY TEACHING:

To reduce hypotensive effect, rise slowly from lying to sitting position and permit legs to dangle from bed momentarily before standing. If nausea occurs, noncaffeinated carbonated beverages, unsalted crackers, or dry toast may relieve effect. Report any sign of infection (sore throat, fever). Several weeks may be needed for full therapeutic effect of B/P reduction. Skipping doses or voluntarily discontinuing drug may produce severe, rebound hypertension.

---

enoxacin

en-**ox**-ah-sin
(Penetrex)

CLASSIFICATION

Anti-infective: quinolone

AVAILABILITY (Rx)

Tablets: 200 mg, 400 mg

PHARMACOKINETICS

Well absorbed from GI tract. Partially metabolized in liver. Primarily excreted in urine. Half-life: 3–6 hrs.

ACTION/ *THERAPEUTIC EFFECT*

Inhibits DNA-gyrase in susceptible microorganisms, *interfering w/bacterial DNA replication and repair.*

USES/ *UNLABELED*

Treatment of uncomplicated urethral or cervical gonorrhea, uncomplicated (cystitis) or complicated urinary tract infections. *Treatment of chancroid.*

PO ADMINISTRATION.

Give 1 hr before or 2 hrs after meals.

INDICATIONS/DOSAGE/ROUTES

Uncomplicated (cystitis) urinary tract infection:
PO: Adults >18 yrs, elderly: 200 mg q12h for 7 days.

Complicated urinary tract infection:
PO: Adults >18 yrs, elderly: 400 mg q12h for 14 days.

Uncomplicated gonorrhea:
PO: Adults >18 hrs: 400 mg given as single dose.

Dosage in renal impairment:
The dose and/or frequency is modified based on degree of renal impairment.

CREATININE CLEARANCE	DOSAGE
<30 ml/min	Normal initial dose, then $1/2$ regular dose q12h

PRECAUTIONS

CONTRAINDICATIONS: Do not use in children <18 years of age. **CAUTIONS:** Impaired renal function, any predisposition to seizures. **PREGNANCY/LACTATION:** May produce maternal toxicity (weight loss, venous irritation), fetal toxicity. Unknown whether distributed in breast milk. Should not be used in pregnant women. **Pregnancy Category C.**

INTERACTIONS

DRUG INTERACTIONS: Antacids, bismuth subsalicylate, sucralfate may decrease absorption (give at least 4 hrs before or 2 hrs after enoxacin). Decreases clearance, may increase concentration, toxicity of theophylline. May increase effects of oral anticoagulants. **ALTERED LAB VALUES:** May increase SGOT (AST), SGPT (ALT), alkaline phosphatase, LDH, bilirubin, BUN, creatinine.

SIDE EFFECTS

FREQUENT (5–10%): Nausea, vomiting. **OCCASIONAL (1–5%):** Abdominal pain, diarrhea, headache, dizziness. **RARE (<1%):** Dry mouth, heartburn, constipation, flatulence, fatigue, drowsiness, insomnia, seizures, confusion, photosensitivity.

ADVERSE REACTIONS/TOXIC EFFECTS

Superinfection (particularly enterococcal, fungal). Hypersensitivity reactions, serious and occasionally fatal, have occurred in pts receiving quinolone therapy. Arthropathy may occur if given to children <18 yrs.

NURSING IMPLICATIONS

BASELINE ASSESSMENT:

Question for history of hypersensitivity to fluoroquinolones, quinolone group of antibacterials (cinoxacin, nalidixic acid).

INTERVENTION/EVALUATION:

Monitor stool frequency and consistency. Be alert for superinfection, e.g., genital pruritus, vaginitis, fever, sores, and discomfort in mouth.

PATIENT/FAMILY TEACHING:

Drink fluids liberally. Complete full course of therapy. Instruct pt regarding meals/medications (see PO Administration). Do not drive or perform activities requiring alertness or dexterity if dizziness occurs. Avoid sunlight/ultraviolet exposure; wear sunscreen and protective clothing.

enoxaparin sodium

en-**ox**-ah-pear-in
(**Lovenox**)

CANADIAN AVAILABILITY:
Lovenox

CLASSIFICATION

Anticoagulant

AVAILABILITY (Rx)

Injection: 30 mg/0.3 ml, 40 mg/0.4 ml, 60 mg/0.6 ml, 80 mg/0.8 ml, 100 mg/1 ml, prefilled syringes

PHARMACOKINETICS

	ONSET	PEAK	DURATION
SubQ	—	3–5 hrs	12 hrs

Well absorbed after SubQ administration. Eliminated primarily in urine. Half-life: 4.5 hrs.

ACTION / *THERAPEUTIC EFFECT*

Antithrombin; in presence of low molecular weight heparin, *produces anticoagulation* by inhibition of factor Xa. Enoxaparin causes less inactivation of thrombin, inhibition of platelets, and bleeding than standard heparin. Does not significantly influence bleeding time, prothrombin time (PT), activated partial thromboplastin time (APTT).

USES / *UNLABELED*

Prevention of postop deep vein thrombosis (DVT) following hip or knee replacement surgery, abdominal surgery. Long-term DVT prevention following hip replacement surgery. Treatment of unstable angina, non-Q-wave myocardial infarction, acute DVT (w/warfarin). *Prevents DVT following general surgical procedures.*

STORAGE / HANDLING

Parenteral form appears clear and colorless to pale yellow. Store at room temperature.

SUBQ ADMINISTRATION

Note: Do not mix w/other injections or infusions. Do not give IM.

SubQ:

1. Instruct pt to lie down before administering by deep SubQ injection.

2. Inject between left and right anterolateral and left and right posterolateral abdominal wall.

3. Introduce entire length of needle ($1/2$ inch) into skin fold held between thumb and forefinger, holding skin fold during injection.

INDICATIONS / DOSAGE / ROUTES

Note: Give initial dose as soon as possible after surgery but not more than 24 hrs after surgery.

Prevent deep vein thrombosis (hip, knee surgery):
SubQ: Adults, elderly: 30 mg twice daily, generally for 7–10 days.

Prevent DVT abdominal surgery:
SubQ: Adults, elderly: 40 mg daily for 7–10 days.

Prevent long-term DVT:
SubQ: Adults, elderly: 40 mg once daily for 3 wks.

Angina, myocardial infarction:
SubQ: Adults, elderly: 1 mg/kg q12 hrs.

Acute DVT:
SubQ: Adults, elderly: 1 mg/kg q12h or 1.5 mg/kg once daily.

PRECAUTIONS

CONTRAINDICATIONS: Active major bleeding, concurrent heparin therapy, thrombocytopenia associated w/positive in vitro test for antiplatelet antibody, hypersensitivity to heparin or pork products. **CAUTIONS:** Conditions w/increased risk of hemorrhage, history of heparin-induced thrombocytopenia, impaired renal function, elderly, uncontrolled arterial hypertension, history of recent GI ulceration and hemorrhage. **PREGNANCY/LACTATION:** Use w/caution, particularly during last trimester, immediate postpartum period (increased risk of maternal hemorrhage). Unknown whether it is excreted in breast milk. **Pregnancy Category B**.

INTERACTIONS

DRUG INTERACTIONS: Anticoagulants, platelet inhibitors may increase bleeding (use w/care). **ALTERED LAB VALUES:** Reversible increases in SGOT (AST), SGPT (ALT), alkaline phosphatase, lactic dehydrogenase (LDH).

SIDE EFFECTS

OCCASIONAL (1–4%): Bleeding, pain, or irritation at injection site, nausea, asthenia (unusual tiredness or weakness), confusion, peripheral edema.

ADVERSE REACTIONS/TOXIC EFFECTS

Accidental overdosage may lead to bleeding complications ranging from local ecchymoses to major hemorrhage. *Antidote:* Dose of protamine sulfate (1% solution) should be equal to the dose of enoxaparin injected. One mg protamine sulfate neutralizes 1 mg enoxaparin. A second dose of 0.5 mg/mg protamine sulfate may be given if APTT tested 2–4 hrs after the first infusion remains prolonged.

NURSING IMPLICATIONS
BASELINE ASSESSMENT:

Assess complete blood count, including platelet count. Determine initial B/P.

INTERVENTION/EVALUATION:

Periodically monitor CBC, platelet count, stool for occult blood (no need for daily monitoring in pts w/normal presurgical coagulation parameters). Assess for any sign of bleeding: bleeding at surgical site, hematuria, blood in stool, bleeding from gums, petechiae, bruising, bleeding from injection sites; monitor B/P for hypotension.

PATIENT/FAMILY TEACHING:

Usual length of therapy is 7–10 days. Report any sign of bleeding (as above). Do not take any OTC medication (esp. aspirin) w/o consulting physician.

---

entacapone
(Comtan)
See Supplement

---

epinephrine

eh-pih-**nef**-rin
(Adrenalin, Sus-Phrine, Primatene, Bronkaid, AsthmaHaler, Bronitin, MedihalerEpi, EpiPen)

CANADIAN AVAILABILITY:
Adrenalin, Bronkaid, Epi-Pen, Vaponefrin

CLASSIFICATION

Sympathomimetic

AVAILABILITY (Rx)

Solution for Inhalation: 2%, 2.25%. **Aerosol:** 0.2 mg/spray, 0.25 mg/spray, 0.3 mg/spray. **Injection:** 1 mg/ml, 0.1 mg/ml, 0.01 mg/ml. **Injection (suspension):** 5 mg/ml. **Ophthalmic Solution:** 0.1%, 0.5%, 1%, 2%.

PHARMACOKINETICS

	ONSET	PEAK	DURATION
SubQ	5–10 min	20 min	1–4 hrs
IM	5–10 min	20 min	1–4 hrs
Inhalation	3–5 min	20 min	1–3 hrs
Ophthalmic	1 hr	4–8 hrs	12–24 hrs

Minimal absorption after inhalation, well absorbed after parenteral administration. Metabolized in liver, other tissues, sympathetic nerve endings. Excreted in urine. *Ophthalmic:* May have systemic absorption from drainage into nasal pharyngeal passages. Mydriasis occurs within several minutes, persists several hours; vasoconstriction occurs within 5 min, lasts <1 hr.

ACTION/*THERAPEUTIC EFFECT*

Stimulates alpha-adrenergic receptors (vasoconstriction, pressor effects), beta$_1$-adrenergic receptors (cardiac stimulation), and beta$_2$-adrenergic receptors (bronchial dilation, vasodilation), *resulting in relaxation of smooth muscle of bronchial tree, peripheral vasculature. Ophthalmic:* Increases outflow of aqueous humor from anterior eye chamber, *dilates pupils (constricts conjunctival blood vessels).*

USES/*UNLABELED*

Treatment of acute bronchial asthma attacks, reversible bronchospasm in pts w/chronic bronchitis, emphysema, hypersensitivity reactions. Restores cardiac rhythm in cardiac arrest. *Ophthalmic:* Management of chronic open-angle glaucoma alone or in combination w/other agents. *Systemic: Treatment of gingival/pulpal hemorrhage; priapism. Ophthalmic: Treatment of conjunctival congestion during surgery; secondary glaucoma.*

STORAGE/HANDLING

Store parenteral forms at room temperature. Do not use if solution appears discolored or contains a precipitate.

INHALATION/OPHTHALMIC/ SUBQ/IV ADMINISTRATION

INHALATION:

1. Shake container well, exhale completely then holding mouthpiece 1 inch away from lips,

inhale and hold breath as long as possible before exhaling.

2. Wait 1–10 min before inhaling second dose (allows for deeper bronchial penetration).

3. Rinse mouth w/water immediately after inhalation (prevents mouth/throat dryness).

OPHTHALMIC:

1. For topical ophthalmic use only.

2. Instruct pt to tilt head backward and look up.

3. Gently pull lower lid down to form pouch and instill medication.

4. Do not touch tip of applicator to lids or any surface.

5. When lower lid is released, have pt keep eye open w/o blinking for at least 30 secs.

6. Apply gentle finger pressure to lacrimal sac (bridge of the nose, inside corner of the eye) for 1–2 min.

7. Remove excess solution around eye w/a tissue. Wash hands immediately to remove medication on hands.

SubQ:

1. Shake ampule thoroughly.

2. Use tuberculin syringe for SubQ into lateral deltoid region.

3. Massage rejection site (minimizes vasoconstriction effect).

IV:

1. For injection, dilute each 1 mg of 1:1,000 solution w/10 ml normal saline to provide 1:10,000 solution.

2. For infusion, further dilute w/5% dextrose in water.

INDICATIONS/DOSAGE/ROUTES

Cardiac arrest:
IV: Adults, elderly: 0.1–1 mg (1–10 ml of 1:10,000 concentration). May repeat q5min (or may be followed by 0.3 mg SubQ or IV infusion initially at 1 mcg/min up to 4 mcg/min).

Children: 0.01 mg/kg (0.1 ml/kg of 1:10,000 concentration). May repeat q5min (or may give IV infusion initially at 0.1 mcg/kg/min increased at 0.1 mcg/kg/min increments up to maximum of 1 mcg/kg/min). **Neonates:** 0.01–0.03 mg/kg (0.1–0.3 ml/kg of 1:10,000 concentration). May repeat q5min.
Intracardiac: Adults, elderly: 0.1–1 mg (1–10 ml of 1:10,000 concentration). **Children:** 0.005–0.01 mg/kg (0.05–0.1 ml/kg of 1:10,000 concentration).

Severe anaphylaxis or asthma:
SubQ/IM: Adults, elderly: 0.1–0.5 mg (0.1–0.5 ml of 1:1,000 concentration). May repeat at 10–15 min intervals for anaphylaxis; 20 min–4 hrs for asthma.
SubQ: Children: 0.01 mg/kg (0.01 ml/kg of 1:1,000 concentration). **Maximum single dose:** 0.5 mg. May repeat at 20 min–4 hr intervals.

Asthma (prolonged effect):
SubQ: Adults, elderly: Initially, 0.5 mg (0.1 ml of 1:200 concentration). May repeat w/0.5–1.5 mg no sooner than 6 hrs from previous dose. **Children:** 0.02–0.025 mg/kg (0.004–0.005 ml/kg of 1:200 concentration). **Maximum single dose:** 0.75 mg. May repeat no sooner than 6 hrs from previous dose.

Severe anaphylactic shock:
IV: Adults, elderly: 0.1–0.25 mg (1–2.5 ml of 1:10,000 concentration) over 5–10 min. May repeat q5–15 min, or continuous IV infusion initially at 1 mcg/min up to 4 mcg/min. **Children:** 0.1 mg (10 ml of 1: 100,000 concentration) over 5–10 min followed w/IV infusion of 0.1 mcg/kg/ min up to 1.5 mcg/kg/min.

Usual inhalation dosage:
Inhalation: Adults, elderly, children >4 yrs: 1 inhalation, may repeat in at least 1 min; subsequent doses no sooner than 3 hrs.

Nebulizer: Adults, elderly, children >4 yrs: 1–3 deep inhalations; subsequent doses no sooner than 3 hrs.

Glaucoma:
Ophthalmic: Adults, elderly: 1–2 drops 1–2 times/day.

PRECAUTIONS

CONTRAINDICATIONS: Hypertension, hyperthyroidism, ischemic heart disease, cardiac arrhythmias, cerebrovascular insufficiency, narrow-angle glaucoma, shock. **CAUTIONS:** Elderly, diabetes mellitus, angina pectoris, tachycardia, MI, severe renal/hepatic impairment, psychoneurotic disorders, hypoxia. **PREGNANCY/LACTATION:** Crosses placenta; distributed in breast milk. **Pregnancy Category C**.

INTERACTIONS

DRUG INTERACTIONS: Tricyclic antidepressants may increase cardiovascular effects. May decrease effects of beta blockers. Ergonovine, methergine, oxytocin may increase vasoconstriction. Digoxin, sympathomimetics may increase risk of arrhythmias. **ALTERED LAB VALUES:** May decrease serum potassium levels.

SIDE EFFECTS

FREQUENT: *Systemic:* Fast/pounding heartbeat, nervousness. *Ophthalmic:* Headache/brow ache, stinging, burning, other eye irritation, watering of eyes. **OCCASIONAL:** *Systemic:* Dizziness, lightheadedness, facial flushing, headache, diaphoresis, increased B/P, nausea, trembling, insomnia, vomiting, weakness. *Ophthalmic:* Blurred/decreased vision, eye pain. **RARE:** *Systemic:* Chest discomfort/pain, irregular heartbeats, bronchospasm, dry mouth/throat.

ADVERSE REACTIONS/TOXIC EFFECTS

Excessive doses may cause acute

hypertension, arrhythmias. Prolonged or excessive use may result in metabolic acidosis (due to increased serum lactic acid concentrations). Observe for disorientation, weakness, hyperventilation, headache, nausea, vomiting, diarrhea.

NURSING IMPLICATIONS
BASELINE ASSESSMENT:

Offer emotional support (high incidence of anxiety due to difficulty in breathing and sympathomimetic response to drug).

INTERVENTION/EVALUATION:

Monitor B/P: rate, depth, rhythm, type of respiration; quality and rate of pulse. Assess lung sounds for rhonchi, wheezing, rales. Monitor arterial blood gases. Observe lips, fingernails for blue or dusky color in light-skinned patients; gray in dark-skinned patients. In cardiac arrest, monitor EKG, B/P, pulse. Evaluate for clinical improvement (quieter, slower respirations, relaxed facial expression, cessation of clavicular retractions).

PATIENT/FAMILY TEACHING:

Increase fluid intake (decreases lung secretion viscosity). Avoid excessive use of caffeine derivatives (chocolate, coffee, tea, cola, cocoa). *Ophthalmic:* Teach proper administration. Slight burning, stinging may occur on initial instillation. Report any new symptoms (rapid pulse, shortness of breath, or dizziness immediately: may be systemic effects).

epirubicin
(Ellene)
See Supplement
See Classification section under: Antineoplastics

epoetin alfa
eh-po-**ee**-tin
(Epogen, Procrit)

CANADIAN AVAILABILITY
Eprex

CLASSIFICATION
Erythropoietin

AVAILABILITY (Rx)
Injection: 2,000 units, 3,000 units, 4,000 units, 10,000 units

PHARMACOKINETICS
Well absorbed after SubQ administration. After administration, an increase in reticulocyte count seen within 10 days; increases in Hgb, Hct, and RBC count within 2–6 wks. Half-life: 4–13 hrs.

ACTION/ *THERAPEUTIC EFFECT*
Stimulates division, differentiation of erythroid progenitor cells in bone marrow, *induces erythropoiesis, release of reticulocytes from marrow.*

USES/ *UNLABELED*
Treatment of anemia associated w/chronic renal failure or related to zidovudine (AZT) therapy in HIV-infected pts or to chemotherapy in cancer pts, those scheduled for elective nonvascular surgery, reducing need for allogenic blood transfusions. *Prevents anemia in patients donating blood prior to elective surgery, autologous transfusion; treatment of anemia associated w/neoplastic diseases.*

STORAGE/HANDLING
Refrigerate; stable for up to 14 days at room temperature. Use 1 dose/vial; do not reenter vial. Discard unused portion.

INDICATIONS/DOSAGE/ROUTES

Note: May give IV or SubQ.

Chronic renal failure:
IV/SubQ: Adults, elderly: Initially 50–100 units/kg 3 times/wk. Target Hct range: 30–36%. Dosage adjustments not earlier than 1 mo intervals unless clinically indicated. *Decrease dose:* Hct increasing and approaching 36% (temporarily hold doses if Hct continues to rise, reinstate lower dose when Hct begins to decrease); Hct increases by >4 points in 2 wk period (monitor Hct 2 times/wk for 2–6 wks). *Increase dose:* Hct does not increase 5–6 points after 8 wks (w/iron stores adequate) and Hct below target range. **Maintenance:** *(Dialysis):* 75 units/kg 3 times/wk. **Range:** 12.5–525 units/kg. *(Nondialysis):* 75–150 units/kg/wk.

AZT-treated, HIV-infected patients:
Note: Pt receiving AZT w/serum erythropoietin levels >500 milliunits likely not to respond to therapy. **IV/SubQ: Adults:** Initially, 100 units/kg 3 times/wk for 8 wks; may increase by 50–100 units/kg 3 times/wk. Evaluate response q4–8 wks thereafter; adjust dose by 50–100 units/kg 3 times/wk. If doses >300 units/kg 3 times/wk are not eliciting response, unlikely pt will respond. **Maintenance:** Titrate to maintain desired Hct.

Chemotherapy patients:
SubQ: Adults, elderly: Initially, 150 units/kg 3 times/wk up to 300 units/kg 3 times/wk.

Reduce allogenic blood transfusions:
SubQ: Adults, elderly: 300 units/kg/day 10 days prior to, on day of, and 4 days after surgery.

PRECAUTIONS

CONTRAINDICATIONS: Uncontrolled hypertension, history of sensitivity to mammalian cell–derived products or human albumin. **CAUTIONS:** Pts w/known porphyria (impairment of erythrocyte formation in bone marrow or responsible for liver impairment). **PREGNANCY/LACTATION:** Unknown if drug crosses placenta or is distributed in breast milk. **Pregnancy Category C**.

INTERACTIONS

DRUG INTERACTIONS: May need to increase heparin (increase in RBC volume may enhance blood clotting). **ALTERED LAB VALUES:** May decrease bleeding time, iron concentration, serum ferritin. May increase BUN, creatinine, phosphorus, potassium, sodium, uric acid.

SIDE EFFECTS

Chronic renal failure: **FREQUENT (11–24%):** Hypertension, headache, nausea, arthralgia. **OCCASIONAL (7–9%):** Fatigue, edema, diarrhea, vomiting, chest pain, reactions at administration site, asthenia, dizziness. *AZT-treated HIV-infected:* **FREQUENT (15–38%):** Fever, fatigue, headache, cough, diarrhea, rash, nausea. **OCCASIONAL (9–14%):** Shortness of breath, asthenia (loss of strength, weakness), skin reaction at injection site, dizziness.

ADVERSE REACTIONS/TOXIC EFFECTS

Hypertensive encephalopathy, thrombosis, cerebrovascular accident, MI, seizures have occurred rarely. Hyperkalemia occurs occasionally, usually in those who do not conform to medication compliance, dietary guidelines, frequency of dialysis.

NURSING IMPLICATIONS

BASELINE ASSESSMENT:

Assess B/P before drug initiation (80% of those w/CRF have history of hypertension). B/P often rises during early therapy in those w/history of hypertension. Consider that all pts will eventually need supplemental iron therapy. Assess serum iron (transferrin saturation: should be >20%) and serum ferritin (>100 ng/ml) prior to and during therapy. Establish baseline CBC, differential and platelet counts (esp. note hematocrit). Monitor B/P aggressively for increased B/P (25% of those on medication require antihypertension therapy, dietary restrictions).

INTERVENTION/EVALUATION:

Monitor Hct level diligently (if level increases >4 points in 2 wk period, dosage should be reduced); assess CBC, differential, platelet counts routinely. Monitor temperature, esp. in cancer pts on chemotherapy and zidovudine-treated HIV pts, and BUN, uric acid, creatinine, phosphorus, potassium, esp. in CRF pts. Evaluate food tolerance and stool frequency, consistency. Provide assistance for dizziness, fatigue, and safety for possible seizures.

PATIENT/FAMILY TEACHING:

Compliance w/dietary guidelines and frequency of dialysis is essential (improved sense of well-being may be misleading in CRF pts). Evidence of response to epoetin alfa may be seen in increased reticulocyte count within 10 days; however, Hct changes take 2–6 wks. Does not substitute for emergency transfusions. Avoid tasks that require alertness, motor skills until response to drug is established.

---

eprosartan
(Teveten)
See Supplement

---

epoprostenol sodium, PG$_2$, PGX, prostacyclin

ep-oh-**pros**-ten-awl
(Flolan)

CANADIAN AVAILABILITY:
Flolan

CLASSIFICATION

Antihypertensive

AVAILABILITY (Rx)

Powder for Injection: 0.5 mg, 1.5 mg

PHARMACOKINETICS

After IV administration, rapidly hydrolyzed, subject to enzymatic degradation. Metabolized to active metabolite. Half-life: 6 min.

ACTION/*THERAPEUTIC EFFECT*

Directly vasodilates pulmonary and systemic arterial vascular beds and inhibits platelet aggregation. *Reduces right and left ventricular afterload, increases cardiac output, stroke volume.*

USES/*UNLABELED*

Long-term treatment of primary pulmonary hypertension in class III and class IV pts (New York Heart Association). *Pulmonary hypertension associated w/adult respiratory syndrome, systemic lupus erythematosus, or congenital heart disease; neonatal pulmonary hypertension, cardiopulmonary bypass surgery, hemodialysis, refractory CHF, severe community-acquired pneumonia.*

STORAGE/HANDLING

Store unopened vials at room temperature. Protect both unopened vial and reconstituted solution from light. After reconstitution, refrigerate, protect from light. Do not freeze (discard any frozen solution). Discard any solution refrigerated >48 hrs.

IV ADMINISTRATION

Note: Refer to manufacturer for concentration and proper dilutions. Give reconstituted solution at room temperature for duration of 8 hrs or may be used w/cold pouch and given ≤24 hrs w/2 frozen 6 oz gel packs. Insulate from temp >77°F or <32°F. Do not expose to direct sunlight.

IV:

1. Administer through central venous catheter using ambulatory infusion pump. During dose ranging, may administer peripherally.
2. Do not give w/other solutions or medications.

INDICATIONS/DOSAGE/ROUTES

Pulmonary hypertension:
Note: Infused continuously through permanent indwelling central venous catheter using an ambulatory infusion pump. May give through peripheral vein on temporary basis.
IV Infusion: Adults, elderly: *(Acute dose-ranging procedure):* Initially, 2 ng/kg/min increased in increments of 2 ng/kg/min every 15 min until dose-limiting adverse effects occur. *(Chronic infusion):* Start at 4 ng/kg/min less than the maximum dose rate tolerated during acute dose ranging (or $1/2$ maximum rate if rate was below 5 ng/kg/min).

PRECAUTIONS

CONTRAINDICATIONS: Chronic use in those w/CHF (severe ventricular systolic dysfunction), hypersensitivity to drug or structurally related compounds. **CAUTIONS:** Elderly. **PREGNANCY/LACTATION:** Unknown if distributed in breast milk. **Pregnancy Category B.**

INTERACTIONS

DRUG INTERACTIONS: Hypotensive effects may be increased by other vasodilators or using acetate in dialysis fluids. Anticoagulants, antiplatelets may increase risk of bleeding. Vasoconstrictors may decrease effect. **ALTERED LAB VALUES:** None significant.

SIDE EFFECTS

FREQUENT: *Acute phase:* Flushing (**58%**), headache (**49%**), nausea (**32%**), vomiting (**32%**), hypotension (**16%**), anxiety (**11%**), chest pain (**11%**), dizziness (**8%**). **OCCASIONAL (2–5%):** Bradycardia, abdominal pain, muscle pain, dyspnea, back pain. **RARE (<2%):** Diaphoresis, dyspepsia, paresthesia, tachycardia. *Chronic phase:* **FREQUENT (>20%):** Dyspnea, asthenia, dizziness, headache, chest pain, nausea, vomiting, palpitations, edema, jaw pain, tachycardia, flushing, myalgia, nonspecific muscle pain, paresthesia, diarrhea, anxiety, chills/fever/flulike symptoms. **OCCASIONAL (10–20%):** Rash, depression, hypotension, pallor, syncope, bradycardia, ascites.

ADVERSE REACTIONS/TOXIC EFFECTS

Overdose may cause hyperglycemia/ketoacidosis (increased urination, thirst, fruitlike breath). Angina, myocardial infarction, thrombocytopenia occur rarely. Abrupt withdrawal (including large reduction in dosage, interruption in drug delivery) may produce rebound pulmonary hypertension (dyspnea, dizziness, asthenia).

NURSING IMPLICATIONS

INTERVENTION/EVALUATION:

Monitor functioning of pump devices/catheters. Monitor standing/supine B/P w/any dosage adjustment for several hours after adjustment. Assess for therapeutic response: improvement in pulmonary function, decreased dyspnea on exertion (DOE), fatigue, syncope, chest pain, pulmonary vascular resistance, pulmonary arterial pressure.

PATIENT/FAMILY TEACHING:

Instruct pt on drug reconstitution, drug administration, care of the permanent central venous catheter. Brief interruptions in drug delivery may result in rapid, deteriorating symptoms. Drug therapy will be necessary for a prolonged period, possibly years.

---

eptifibate
(Intergrillin)
See Supplement

---

ergoloid mesylates

ur-go-loyd mess-**ah**-lates
(Gerimal, Hydergine)

CANADIAN AVAILABILITY:
Hydergine

CLASSIFICATION

Psychotherapeutic

AVAILABILITY (Rx)

Tablets (sublingual): 0.5 mg, 1 mg. **Tablets:** 0.5 mg, 1 mg. **Capsules:** 1 mg. **Liquid:** 1 mg/ml.

PHARMACOKINETICS

Rapidly, incompletely absorbed from GI tract. Metabolized in liver. Eliminated primarily in feces. Half-life: 2–5 hrs.

ACTION/*THERAPEUTIC EFFECT*

Central action decreases vascular tone, slows heart rate. Peripheral action blocks alpha adrenergic receptors. *Improves O_2 uptake and improves cerebral metabolism.*

USES

Treatment of age-related (those >60 yrs) mental capacity decline (cognitive and interpersonal skills, mood, self-care, apparent motivation).

PO ADMINISTRATION

1. Instruct pt to allow sublingual tablets to completely dissolve under tongue; do not crush or chew.
2. Do not break capsule or tablet form.

INDICATIONS/DOSAGE/ROUTES

Age-related decline in mental capacity:
PO: Adults, elderly: Initially, 1 mg 3 times/day. **Range:** 1.5–12 mg/day.

PRECAUTIONS

CONTRAINDICATIONS: Acute or chronic psychosis, regardless of etiology. **CAUTIONS:** None significant.

INTERACTIONS

DRUG INTERACTIONS: None significant. **ALTERED LAB VALUES:** None significant.

SIDE EFFECTS

OCCASIONAL: GI distress, transient nausea, sublingual irritation.

ADVERSE REACTIONS/TOXIC EFFECTS

Overdose may produce blurred vision, dizziness, syncope, headache, flushed face, nausea, vomiting, decreased appetite, stomach cramps, stuffy nose.

NURSING IMPLICATIONS

BASELINE ASSESSMENT:

Exclude possibility that pt's signs and symptoms arise from a possibly reversible and treatable condition secondary to systemic disease, neurologic disease, or primary disturbance of mood before administering medication.

INTERVENTION/EVALUATION:

Periodically reassess benefit of current therapy.

PATIENT/FAMILY TEACHING:

Elimination of symptoms appears gradual: Results may not be noted for 3–4 wks. May cause nausea, GI upset. Allow sublingual tablets to dissolve completely under tongue.

ergonovine maleate

er-goe-**noe**-veen
(Ergotrate)

CLASSIFICATION

Uterine stimulant

AVAILABILITY (Rx)

Injection: 0.2 mg/ml

PHARMACOKINETICS

	ONSET	PEAK	DURATION
IM	3–5 min	—	>3 hrs
IV	40 secs	—	>45 min

Rapidly absorbed after IM administration. Distributed to plasma, extracellular fluid. Metabolized in liver. Excreted in urine.

ACTION/*THERAPEUTIC EFFECT*

Directly stimulates uterine muscle *(increases force, frequency of contractions). Induces cervical contractions.* Stimulates alpha adrenergic, serotonin receptors *producing arterial vasoconstriction.* Causes vasospasm of coronary arteries.

USES/*UNLABELED*

To prevent and treat postpartum, postabortal hemorrhage due to atony or involution (not for induction or augmentation of labor). *Treatment of incomplete abortion, diagnosis of angina pectoris.*

STORAGE/HANDLING

Refrigerate; protect from light.

IM/IV ADMINISTRATION

IV use in life-threatening emergencies only; may dilute to volume of 5 ml w/0.9% NaCl injection; give over at least 1 min, carefully monitoring B/P.

INDICATIONS/DOSAGE/ROUTES

Oxytocic:
IM/IV: Adults: Initially, 0.2 mg. May repeat no more often than q2–4h for no more than 5 doses total.

PRECAUTIONS

CONTRAINDICATIONS: Hypersensitivity to ergot, induction of labor, threatened spontaneous abortions. **CAUTIONS:** Renal/hepatic impairment, coronary artery disease, occlusive peripheral vascular disease, sepsis. **PREGNANCY/LACTATION:** Contraindicated during pregnancy. Small amounts in breast milk.

INTERACTIONS

DRUG INTERACTIONS: Vasoconstrictors, vasopressors may increase effect. **ALTERED LAB VALUES:** May decrease prolactin concentration.

SIDE EFFECTS

FREQUENT: Nausea, vomiting, uterine cramping. **OCCASIONAL:** Diarrhea, headache, dizziness, nasal congestion, sweating, ringing in ears, unpleasant taste. **RARE:** Allergic reaction, pain in arms, legs, or lower back.

ADVERSE REACTIONS/TOXIC EFFECTS

Severe hypertensive episodes may result in cerebrovascular accident, serious arrhythmias, seizures; hypertensive effects more frequent w/pt susceptibility, rapid IV administration, concurrent regional anesthesia or vasoconstrictors. Peripheral ischemia may lead to gangrene. *Overdose:* Angina, bradycardia, confusion, drowsiness, fast, weak pulse; miosis, severe peripheral vasoconstriction (numbness in arms or legs, blue skin color), seizures, tachycardia, thirst, severe uterine cramping.

NURSING IMPLICATIONS

BASELINE ASSESSMENT:

Question for hypersensitivity to any ergot derivatives. Determine calcium, B/P, and pulse baselines. Assess bleeding prior to administration.

INTERVENTION/EVALUATION:

Monitor uterine contractions (frequency, strength, duration), bleeding, B/P, and pulse every 15 min until stable (about 1–2 hrs). Assess extremities for color, warmth, movement, pain. Report chest pain promptly. Provide support w/ambulation if dizziness occurs.

PATIENT/FAMILY TEACHING:

Avoid smoking because of added vasoconstriction. Report increased cramping, bleeding, or foul-smelling lochia. Pale, cold hands/feet should be reported because may mean decreased circulation.

E

ergotamine tartrate

er-**got**-a-meen
(Ergostar Medihaler Ergotamine)

dihydroergotamine

(D.H.E., Migranal)

FIXED-COMBINATION(S):
W/caffeine, a stimulant (**Cafergot, Wigraine**). W/belladonna, an anticholinergic, and phenobarbital, a sedative-hypnotic (**Bellergal-S**)

CANADIAN AVAILABILITY:
Ergomar, Migranal

CLASSIFICATION

Antimigraine

AVAILABILITY (Rx)

Tablets (sublingual): 2 mg. **Injection:** 1 mg/ml. **Aerosol:** 9 mg/ml (0.36 mg/dose). **Nasal Spray.**

PHARMACOKINETICS

Slow, incomplete absorption from GI tract, rapid, extensive absorption rectally. Undergoes extensive first-pass metabolism in liver. Metabolized to active metabolite. Eliminated in feces via biliary system. Half-life: 21 hrs.

ACTION/*THERAPEUTIC EFFECT*

May have agonist/antagonist actions w/alpha adrenergic, serotonergic, dopaminergic receptors. Directly stimulates vascular smooth muscle, *constricting arteries and veins.* May inhibit reuptake of norepinephrine.

USES

Prevents or aborts vascular headaches (e.g., migraine, cluster headaches).

SUBLINGUAL/INHALATION ADMINISTRATION

SUBLINGUAL:

Place under tongue; do not swallow.

INHALATION:

1. Shake container well; exhale completely; then holding mouthpiece 1 inch away from lips, inhale and hold breath as long as possible before exhaling.

2. Wait at least 5 min before inhaling second dose, if needed.

3. Rinse mouth w/water immediately after inhalation (prevents mouth/throat dryness).

INDICATIONS/DOSAGE/ROUTES

Note: Initiate therapy as soon as possible after first signs of attack.

Vascular headaches:
Sublingual: Adults, elderly: Initially, 2 mg (1 tablet). May repeat at 30 min intervals. **Maximum:** 3 tablets/24 hrs or 5 tablets/wk.
Aerosol: Adults, elderly: Initially, 1 inhalation. May repeat in 5 min. **Maximum:** 6 inhalations/24 hrs or 15 inhalations/wk.
Intranasal: Adults, elderly: 1 spray (0.5 mg) in each nostril; follow in 15 min w/1 additional spray in each nostril.
IM: Adults, elderly: 1 mg at first sign of headache; repeat at 1 hr intervals. **Maximum:** 3 mg.
IV: Adults, elderly: As above. **Maximum:** 2 mg. Do not exceed 6 mg/wk.

PRECAUTIONS

CONTRAINDICATIONS: Hypersensitivity to ergot alkaloids, peripheral vascular disease (thromboangiitis obliterans, syphilitic arteritis, severe arteriosclerosis, thrombophlebitis, Raynaud's disease), impaired renal/hepatic function, severe pruritus, coronary artery disease, hypertension, sepsis, malnutrition. **CAUTIONS:** None significant. **PREGNANCY/LACTATION:** Contraindicated in pregnancy (produces uterine stimulant action, resulting in possible fetal death or retarded fetal growth); increases vasoconstriction of placental vascular bed. Drug distributed in breast milk. May produce diarrhea, vomiting in neonate. May prohibit lactation. **Pregnancy Category D**.

INTERACTIONS

DRUG INTERACTIONS: Beta blockers, erythromycin may increase risk of vasospasm. May decrease effect of nitroglycerin. Ergot alkaloids, systemic vasoconstrictors may increase pressor effect. **ALTERED LAB VALUES:** None significant.

SIDE EFFECTS

OCCASIONAL (2–5%): Cough, dizziness. **RARE (<2%):** Muscle pain, fatigue, diarrhea, upper respiratory infection, dyspepsia.

ADVERSE REACTIONS/TOXIC EFFECTS

Prolonged administration or excessive dosage may produce ergotamine poisoning: nausea, vomiting, weakness of legs, pain in limb muscles, numbness and tingling of fingers/toes, precordial pain, tachycardia or bradycardia, hyper/hypotension. Localized edema, itching due to vasoconstriction of peripheral arteries and arterioles. Feet, hands will become cold, pale, numb. Muscle pain occurs when walking and later, even at rest. Gangrene may occur. Occasionally confusion, depression, drowsiness, convulsions appear.

NURSING IMPLICATIONS
BASELINE ASSESSMENT:

Question pt regarding history of peripheral vascular disease, renal/hepatic impairment, or possibility of pregnancy. Contact physician w/findings before administering drug. Question pt regarding onset, location, and duration of migraine and possible precipitating symptoms.

INTERVENTION/EVALUATION:

Monitor closely for evidence of ergotamine overdosage as result of prolonged administration or excessive dosage (see Adverse Reactions/Toxic Effects). Notify physician of any signs and symptoms of ergotamine poisoning.

PATIENT/FAMILY TEACHING:

Initiate therapy at first sign of migraine attack. Report if there is need to progressively increase dose to relieve vascular headaches or if irregular heartbeat, nausea, vomiting, numbness/tingling of fingers/toes, or pain or weakness of extremities is noted. Discuss contraception w/physician; report suspected pregnancy immediately.

---

erythrityl
(Cardilate)
See Classification section under: Nitrates

---

erythromycin base

eh-rith-row-**my**-sin
(E-Mycin, Eryc, Ery-tab, PCE Dispertab, Ilotycin)

erythromycin estolate
(Ilosone)
erythromycin ethylsuccinate
(EES, Pediamycin, EryPed)
erythromycin lactobionate
(Erythrocin)
erythromycin stearate
(Erythrocin, Wyamycin)
erythromycin topical
(Akne-mycin, Eryderm, Erymax)

FIXED-COMBINATION(S):
Erythromycin ethylsuccinate combined w/sulfisoxazole, a sulfonamide (Pediazole)

CANADIAN AVAILABILITY:
Erybid, EES, Eryc, Erythrocin, Erythromid, Novoryihro, PCE

CLASSIFICATION
Antibiotic: Macrolide

AVAILABILITY (Rx)

Powder for Injection: 500 mg, 1 g.
Base: Tablets: 250 mg, 333 mg, 500 mg. **Tablets (delayed-release):** 333 mg. **Capsules (delayed-release):** 250 mg.
Estolate: Tablets: 500 mg. **Capsules:** 250 mg. **Oral Suspension:** 125 mg/5 ml, 250 mg/5 ml.
Ethylsuccinate: Tablets (chewable): 200 mg. **Tablets:** 400 mg. **Oral Suspension:** 200 mg/5 ml, 400 mg/5 ml. **Oral Drops:** 100 mg/2.5 ml.
Stearate: Tablets: 250 mg, 500 mg.

Ophthalmic Ointment: 5 mg/g. **Topical Solution:** 1.5%, 2%. **Topical Gel:** 2%. **Topical Ointment:** 2%.

PHARMACOKINETICS

Variably absorbed from GI tract (affected by dosage form used). Widely distributed. Metabolized in liver. Primarily eliminated in feces via bile. Not removed by hemodialysis. Half-life: 1.4–2 hrs (increased in reduced renal function).

ACTION/ *THERAPEUTIC EFFECT*

Bacteriostatic. Penetrates bacterial cell membrane and reversibly binds to bacterial ribosomes, *inhibiting protein synthesis.*

USES/ *UNLABELED*

Respiratory infections, otitis media, pertussis, inflammatory acne vulgaris, diphtheria (adjunctive therapy), Legionnaires' disease, intestinal amebiasis, preop intestinal antisepsis. Prophylaxis for rheumatic fever, bacterial endocarditis, respiratory tract surgery/invasive procedures, gonococcal ophthalmia neonatorum; if penicillin, tetracycline is contraindicated: gonorrheal pelvic inflammatory disease, coexisting chlamydial infections, uncomplicated urogenital infections, Lyme disease (younger than 9 yrs). *Topical:* Treatment of acne vulgaris. *Ophthalmic:* Treatment of ocular infections, prophylaxis of neonatal conjunctivitis, ophthalmia neonatorium. *Systemic: Treatment of acne vulgaris, chancroid, Campylobacter enteritis, gastroparesis, Lyme disease. Topical: Treatment of minor skin bacterial infections. Ophthalmic: Treatment of blepharitis, conjunctivitis, chlamydia, keratitis, trachoma.*

STORAGE/HANDLING

Store capsules, tablets at room temperature. Oral suspension stable for 14 days at room temperature. Diluted IV solutions stable for 8 hrs at room temperature, 24 hrs if refrigerated. Discard if precipitate forms.

PO/IV/OPHTHALMIC ADMINISTRATION

PO:

1. Administer erythromycin base, stearate 1 hr before or 2 hrs after food. Erythromycin estolate, ethylsuccinate may be given w/o regard to meals, but optimal absorption occurs when given on empty stomach.

2. Give w/8 oz water.

3. If swallowing difficulties exist, sprinkle capsule contents on teaspoon of applesauce, follow w/water.

4. Do not swallow chewable tablets whole.

IV:

1. For intermittent IV infusion, infuse over 20–60 min.

2. Alternating IV sites, use large veins to reduce risk of phlebitis.

OPHTHALMIC:

1. Place finger on lower eyelid and pull out until a pocket is formed between eye and lower lid. Place 1/4–1/2 inch ointment into pocket.

2. Have pt close eye gently for 1–2 min, rolling eyeball (increases contact area of drug to eye).

3. Remove excess ointment around eye w/tissue.

INDICATIONS/DOSAGE/ROUTES

Note: Space doses evenly around the clock. 400 mg erythromycin ethylsuccinate = 250 mg erythromycin base, stearate, or estolate.

Usual parenteral dosage:
IV: Adults, elderly, children: 15–20 mg/kg/day in divided doses. **Maximum:** 4 g/day.

Usual oral dosage:
PO: Adults, elderly: 250 mg q6h; 500 mg q12h; or 333 mg q8h. Increase up to 4 g/day. **Children:** 30–50 mg/kg/day in divided doses up to 60–100 mg/kg/day for severe infections.

Preop intestinal antisepsis:
PO: Adults, elderly: Give 1 g at 1, 2, and 11 PM on day prior to surgery (w/neomycin).

Acne vulgaris:
Topical: Adults: Apply to skin 2 times/day.

Gonococcal ophthalmia neonatorum:
Ophthalmic: Neonates: 0.5–2 cm no later than 1 hr after delivery.

PRECAUTIONS

CONTRAINDICATIONS: Hypersensitivity to erythromycins, preexisting liver disease, history of hepatitis due to erythromycins. Do not administer Pediazole to infants <2 mos. **CAUTIONS:** Hepatic dysfunction. If combination used (Pediazole), consider precautions of sulfonamides. IV may cause increased HR, prolonged QT interval. **PREGNANCY/LACTATION:** Crosses placenta, distributed in breast milk. Erythromycin estolate may increase liver function test results in pregnant women. **Pregnancy Category B.**

INTERACTIONS

DRUG INTERACTIONS: May inhibit metabolism of carbamazepine. May decrease effects of chloramphenicol, clindamycin. May increase concentration, toxicity of buspirone, cyclosporine, felodipine, lovastatin, simvastatin. Hepatotoxic medications may increase hepatotoxicity. May increase risk of cardiotoxicity w/cisapride. May increase risk of toxicity w/theophylline. May increase effect of warfarin. **ALTERED LAB VALUES:** May increase SGOT (AST), SGPT (ALT), alkaline, phosphatase, bilirubin.

SIDE EFFECTS

FREQUENT: Abdominal discomfort/cramping, phlebitis/thrombophlebitis w/IV administration. *Topical:* Dry skin (50%). **OCCASIONAL:** Nausea, vomiting, diarrhea, rash, urticaria. **RARE:** *Ophthalmic:* Sensitivity reaction w/ increased irritation, burning, itching, inflammation. *Topical:* Urticaria.

ADVERSE REACTIONS/TOXIC EFFECTS

Superinfections, esp. antibiotic-associated colitis, reversible cholestatic hepatitis may occur. High dosage in renal impairment may lead to reversible hearing loss. Anaphylaxis occurs rarely.

NURSING IMPLICATIONS
BASELINE ASSESSMENT:

Question pt for history of allergies (particularly erythromycins), hepatitis. Obtain specimens for culture and sensitivity before giving first dose (therapy may begin before results are known).

INTERVENTION/EVALUATION:

Check for GI discomfort, nausea, vomiting. Determine pattern of bowel activity, stool consistency. Assess skin for rash. Monitor hepatic function tests, assess for hepatotoxicity: malaise, fever, abdominal pain, GI disturbances.

Evaluate for superinfection: genital/anal pruritus, sore mouth or tongue, moderate to severe diarrhea. Check for phlebitis (heat, pain, red streaking over vein).

PATIENT/FAMILY TEACHING:

Continue therapy for full length of treatment. Doses should be evenly spaced. Do *not* swallow chewable tablets whole. Take medication w/8 oz water 1 hr before or 2 hrs after food/beverage. Notify physician in event of GI upset, rash, diarrhea, or other new symptom. *Ophthalmic:* Report burning, itching, or inflammation: Inquire about use of eye makeup. *Topical:* Report excessive dryness, itching, burning. Improvement of acne may not occur for 1–2 mos; maximum benefit may take 3 mos; therapy may last months or years. Use caution in use of other topical acne preparations containing peeling or abrasive agents, medicated or abrasive soaps, cosmetics containing alcohol (e.g., astringents, aftershave lotion).

esmolol hydrochloride

ez-moe-lol
(Brevibloc)

CANADIAN AVAILABILITY:
Brevibloc

CLASSIFICATION

Beta$_1$-adrenergic blocker

AVAILABILITY (Rx)

Injection: 10 mg/ml, 250 mg/ml

PHARMACOKINETICS

Widely distributed. Rapidly hydrolyzed by esterases in RBCs. Primarily excreted in urine. Half-life: 9 min.

ACTION/THERAPEUTIC EFFECT

Selectively blocks beta$_1$-adrenergic receptors, *slowing sinus heart rate, decreasing cardiac output, decreasing B/P* (exact mechanism unknown but may block peripheral adrenergic receptors, decrease sympathetic outflow from CNS or decrease renin release from kidney). Antiarrhythmic activity due to blocking stimulation of cardiac pacemaker potentials.

USES

Rapid, short-term control of ventricular rate in those w/supraventricular arrhythmias, sinus tachycardia. Intra/postop control of tachycardia/hypertension.

STORAGE/HANDLING

Use only clear and colorless to light yellow solution. Alter dilution, solution is stable for 24 hrs. Discard solution if it is discolored or if precipitate forms.

IV ADMINISTRATION

Note: Give by IV infusion. Avoid butterfly needles, very small veins.

1. Must be diluted to concentration of 10 mg/ml (prevents vein irritation).

2. For IV infusion, remove 20 ml from 500 ml container of 5% dextrose, 0.9% NaCl, or other compatible IV fluid and dilute 5 g vial esmolol hydrochloride w/remaining 480 ml to provide concentration of 10 mg/ml.

3. Administer by controlled infusion device set at rate judged by tolerance and response. Hypoten-

sion (systolic B/P below 90 mm Hg) is greatest during first 30 min of IV infusion.

INDICATIONS/DOSAGE/ROUTES

IV: Adults, elderly: Initially, loading dose of 500 mcg/kg/min for 1 min, followed by 50 mcg/kg/min for 4 min. If optimum response is not attained in 5 min, give second loading dose of 500 mcg/kg/min for 1 min, followed by infusion of 100 mcg/kg/min for 4 min. Additional loading doses can be given and infusion increased by 50 mcg/kg/min (up to 200 mcg/kg/min) for 4 min. Once desired response is attained, cease loading dose and increase infusion by no more than 25 mcg/kg/min. Interval between doses may be increased to 10 min. Infusion usually administered over 24–48 hrs in most pts.

PRECAUTIONS

CONTRAINDICATIONS: Overt cardiac failure, cardiogenic shock, heart block greater than first degree, sinus bradycardia. **CAUTIONS:** History of allergy, bronchial asthma, emphysema, bronchitis, CHF, diabetes, impaired renal function. **PREGNANCY/LACTATION:** Unknown if drug crosses placenta or is distributed in breast milk. Pregnancy Category C.

INTERACTIONS

DRUG INTERACTIONS: Sympathomimetics, xanthines may mutually inhibit effects. May mask symptoms of hypoglycemia, prolong hypoglycemic effect of insulin, oral hypoglycemics. MAO inhibitors may cause significant hypertension. **ALTERED LAB VALUES:** None significant.

SIDE EFFECTS

Generally well tolerated, w/transient and mild side effects. **FREQUENT:** Hypotension (systolic B/P below 90 mm Hg) manifested as dizziness, nausea, diaphoresis, headache, cold extremities, fatigue. **OCCASIONAL:** Anxiety, drowsiness, flushed skin, headache, nausea, vomiting, confusion, cold hands or feet, redness, inflammation at injection site, fever.

ADVERSE REACTIONS/TOXIC EFFECTS

Excessive dosage may produce profound hypotension, bradycardia, dizziness, syncope, drowsiness, breathing difficulty, bluish fingernails/palms of hands, seizures. May potentiate insulin-reduced hypoglycemia in diabetic pts.

NURSING IMPLICATIONS

BASELINE ASSESSMENT:

Assess B/P, apical pulse immediately before drug is administered (if pulse is 60/min or below, or systolic B/P is below 90 mm Hg, withhold medication, contact physician).

INTERVENTION/EVALUATION:

Monitor B/P for hypotension, development of diaphoresis or dizziness (usually first sign of impending hypotension). Assess pulse for strength/weakness, irregular rate, bradycardia. Monitor EKG for cardiac changes, particularly shortening of QT interval, prolongation of PR interval. Assess extremities for coldness. Assist w/ambulation if dizziness occurs. Assess for nausea, diaphoresis, headache, fatigue.

estazolam

es-**tay**-zoe-lam
(ProSom)

CLASSIFICATION

Sedative-hypnotic

AVAILABILITY (Rx)

Tablets: 1 mg, 2 mg

PHARMACOKINETICS

Well absorbed from GI tract. Crosses blood-brain barrier. Metabolized in liver. Primarily excreted in urine. Half-life: 10–24 hrs.

ACTION / *THERAPEUTIC EFFECT*

Enhances action of inhibitory neurotransmitter gamma-amino-butyric acid (GABA). *Depressant effects occur at all levels of CNS.*

USES

Short-term treatment of insomnia (up to 6 wks). Reduces sleep induction time, number of nocturnal awakenings; increases length of sleep.

PO ADMINISTRATION

1. Give w/o regard to meals.
2. Tablet may be crushed.

INDICATIONS / DOSAGE / ROUTES

Note: Use smallest effective dose in those w/liver disease, low serum albumin.

Insomnia:
PO: Adults >18 yrs: 1–2 mg at bedtime. **Elderly/debilitated:** 0.5–1 mg at bedtime.

PRECAUTIONS

CONTRAINDICATIONS: Sensitivity to other benzodiazepines. Pregnancy. **CAUTIONS:** Impaired renal/hepatic function. **PREGNANCY/LACTATION:** Crosses placenta; may be distributed in breast milk. Chronic ingestion during pregnancy may produce withdrawal symptoms, CNS depression in neonates. **Pregnancy Category X.**

INTERACTIONS

DRUG INTERACTIONS: Alcohol, CNS depressants may increase CNS depressant effect. **ALTERED LAB VALUES:** None significant.

SIDE EFFECTS

FREQUENT: Drowsiness, sedation, rebound insomnia (may occur for 1–2 nights after drug is discontinued), dizziness, confusion, euphoria. **OCCASIONAL:** Weakness, anorexia, diarrhea. **RARE:** Paradoxical CNS excitement, restlessness (particularly noted in elderly/debilitated).

ADVERSE REACTIONS / TOXIC EFFECTS

Abrupt or too rapid withdrawal may result in pronounced restlessness, irritability, insomnia, hand tremors, abdominal/muscle cramps, sweating, vomiting, seizures. Overdosage results in somnolence, confusion, diminished reflexes, coma.

NURSING IMPLICATIONS

BASELINE ASSESSMENT:

Assess B/P, pulse, respirations immediately before administration. Raise bed rails. Provide environment conductive to sleep (backrub, quiet environment, low lighting).

INTERVENTION / EVALUATION:

Assess sleep pattern of pt. Assess elderly/debilitated for paradoxical reaction, particularly during early therapy. Evaluate for therapeutic response: decrease in number of nocturnal awakenings, increase in length of sleep.

PATIENT/FAMILY TEACHING:

Smoking reduces drug effectiveness. Do not abruptly withdraw medication following long-term use. Rebound insomnia may occur when drug is discontinued after short-term therapy. Do not use during pregnancy. Avoid alcohol. Use caution while driving or operating machinery.

estradiol
ess-tra-**dye**-ole
(Alora, Climara, Esclim, Estrace, Estring, Estraderm, FemPatch, Vivelle, Vivelle Dot)

estradiol cypionate
(Depo-Estradiol, Depogen)

estradiol valerate
(Delestrogen, Dioval, Valergen 10)

ethinyl estradiol
(Estinyl)

FIXED-COMBINATION(S):
W/medroxyprogesterone, a progestin **(Lunelle)**; w/norethindrone, a progestogen **(Femhrt 1/5) (Combi-Patch)**; w/norgestimate, a progestogen **(Ortho-Prefest)**; estradiol cypionate w/testosterone cypionate, an androgen **(DepoTestadiol)**; estradiol valerate w/testosterone enanthate, an androgen **(Deladumone, Estra-Testrin)**; ethinyl estradiol w/fluoxymesterone, an androgen **(Halodrin)**; esterified estrogens w/methyltestosterone, an androgen **(Estratest)**

CANADIAN AVAILABILITY:
Climara, Estrace, Estraderm, Estring, Delestrogen, Vivelle

CLASSIFICATION
Antineoplastic, estrogen

AVAILABILITY (Rx)
Injection: (Valerate): 10 mg/ml, 20 mg/ml, 40 mg/ml. (Cypionate): 5 mg/ml. Tablet (ethinyl estradiol): 0.02 mg, 0.05 mg, 0.5 mg. Extended-Release Insert (Estring), Vaginal Cream: 0.1 mg/g. Topical (transdermal patch): 0.025 mg, 0.0375 mg, 0.05 mg, 0.075 mg, 0.1 mg.

PHARMACOKINETICS
Well absorbed from GI tract. Widely distributed. Metabolized in liver. Primarily excreted in urine. Half-life: 50–60 min.

ACTION/ *THERAPEUTIC EFFECT*
Increases synthesis of DNA, RNA, and various proteins in responsive tissues. Reduces release of gonadotropin-releasing hormone, reducing follicle-stimulating hormone (FSH) and leuteinizing hormone (LH). *Promotes normal growth, development of female sex organs, maintaining GU function, vasomotor stability. Prevents accelerated bone loss by inhibiting bone resorption, restoring balance of bone resorption and formation.* Inhibits LH, decreases serum concentration of testosterone.

USES/ *UNLABELED*
Management of moderate to severe vasomotor symptoms associated w/menopause, female hypogonadism. Palliative treatment of advanced, inoperable metastatic carcinoma of the breast in postmenopausal women (estradiol, ethinyl estradiol), prostate in men (estradiol, estradiol valerate, ethinyl estradiol). Prevention of postpartum breast engorgement (estradiol valerate). Treatment of

atrophic vaginitis, kraurosis vulvae (estradiol, estradiol valerate). Treatment of postmenopausal osteoporosis (estradiol transdermal system). Prevention of osteoporosis. *Treatment of Turner's syndrome.*

PO/IM/VAGINAL/TRANSDERMAL ADMINISTRATION

PO:

1. Administer at the same time each day.
2. Give w/milk or food if nausea occurs.

IM:

1. Rotate vial to disperse drug in solution.
2. Inject deep IM in gluteus maximus.

VAGINAL:

1. Apply at bedtime for best absorption.
2. Assemble and fill applicator per manufacturer's directions.
3. Insert end of applicator into vagina, directed slightly toward sacrum; push plunger down completely.
4. Avoid skin contact w/cream (prevents skin absorption).

TRANSDERMAL:

1. Remove old patch; select new site (buttocks an alternative application site).
2. Peel off protective strip to expose adhesive surface.
3. Apply immediately to clean, dry, intact skin on the trunk of the body (area w/as little hair as possible).
4. Press in place for at least 10 secs.
5. Do not apply to the breasts or waistline.

INDICATIONS/DOSAGE/ROUTES
ESTRADIOL ORAL, INTRAVAGINAL, TRANSDERMAL

Vasomotor symptoms, atrophic vaginitis, kraurosis vulvae, female hypogonadism, castration, primary ovarian failure:
PO: Adults, elderly: Initially, 1–2 mg/day cyclically.
Intravaginally: Adults, elderly: Initially, 2–4 g/day for 12 wks; reduce dose by $^1/_2$ over 1–2 wks. **Maintenance:** 1 g 1–3 times/wk cyclically.
Topical: Adults, elderly: Initially, 0.05 mg/24 hrs 2 times/wk cyclically; maintenance dose adjusted to pt's needs. *Climara:* Initially, 12.5 cm^2 patch once weekly. *FemPatch:* 0.025 mg once weekly.

Breast cancer:
PO: Adults, elderly: 10 mg 3 times/day.

Prostate cancer:
PO: Adults, elderly: 1–2 mg 3 times/day.

Osteoporosis prevention:
PO: Adults, elderly: 0.5 mg/day (3 wks on, 1 wk off). **Topical (Climara):** 0.025–0.1 mg/wk.

ESTRADIOL CYPIONATE

Vasomotor symptoms:
IM: Adults, elderly: 1–5 mg q3–4 wks.

Female hypogonadism:
IM: Adults, elderly: 1.5–2 mg every month.

ESTRADIOL VALERATE

Vasomotor symptoms, atrophic vaginitis, kraurosis vulvae, female hypogonadism, castration, primary ovarian failure:
IM: Adults, elderly: 10–20 mg q4wks.

Prevention of postpartum breast engorgement:

IM: **Adults, elderly:** 10–25 mg as single dose at end of first stage of labor.

Prostate cancer:
IM: **Adults, elderly:** 30 mg or more q1–2wks.

ETHINYL ESTRADIOL

Vasomotor symptoms:
PO: **Adults, elderly:** 0.02–0.15 mg/day cyclically.

Female hypogonadism:
PO: **Adults, elderly:** 0.05 mg 1–3 times/day during first 2 wks menstrual cycle.

Breast cancer:
PO: **Adults, elderly:** 1 mg 3 times/day.

Prostate cancer:
PO: **Adults, elderly:** 0.15–0.2 mg/day.

Urogenital atrophy:
Vaginally: (Extended-release insert): Once q3mos.

PRECAUTIONS

CONTRAINDICATIONS: Known or suspected breast cancer (except select pts w/metastasis), estrogen-dependent neoplasia; undiagnosed abnormal genital bleeding; active thrombophlebitis or thromboembolic disorders; history of thrombophlebitis, thrombosis or thromboembolic disorders w/previous estrogen use, hypersensitivity to estrogen. **CAUTIONS:** Conditions that may be aggravated by fluid retention: cardiac, renal/hepatic dysfunction, epilepsy, migraine. Mental depression, metabolic bone disease w/potential hypercalcemia, history of jaundice during pregnancy or strong family history of breast cancer, fibrocystic disease, or breast nodules, children in whom bone growth is not complete. **PREGNANCY/LACTATION:** Distributed in breast milk. May be harmful to offspring. Not for use during lactation. **Pregnancy Category X.**

INTERACTIONS

DRUG INTERACTIONS: May interfere w/effects of bromocriptine. May increase concentration of cyclosporine, increase hepatic, nephrotoxicity. Hepatotoxic medications may increase hepatotoxicity. **ALTERED LAB VALUES:** May affect metapyrone, thyroid function tests. May decrease cholesterol, LDH. May increase calcium, glucose, HDL, triglycerides.

SIDE EFFECTS

FREQUENT: Anorexia, nausea, swelling of breasts, peripheral edema evidenced by swollen ankles, feet. *Transdermal route:* Skin irritation, redness. **OCCASIONAL:** Vomiting (esp. w/high dosages), headache (may be severe), intolerance to contact lenses, increased B/P, glucose intolerance, brown spots on exposed skin. *Vaginal route:* Local irritation, vaginal discharge, changes in vaginal bleeding (spotting, breakthrough or prolonged bleeding). **RARE:** Chorea, cholestatic jaundice, hirsutism, loss of scalp hair, depression.

ADVERSE REACTIONS/TOXIC EFFECTS

Prolonged administration increases risk of gallbladder, thromboembolic disease, and breast, cervical, vaginal, endometrial, and liver carcinoma.

NURSING IMPLICATIONS
BASELINE ASSESSMENT:

Question hypersensitivity to estrogen, previous jaundice or

thromboembolic disorders associated w/pregnancy or estrogen therapy. Establish baseline B/P, blood glucose.

INTERVENTION/EVALUATION:

Assess B/P at least daily. Check for swelling. Weigh daily. Monitor blood glucose 4 times/day for pts w/diabetes. Promptly report signs and symptoms of thromboembolic or thrombotic disorders: sudden severe headache, shortness of breath, vision or speech disturbance, weakness or numbness of an extremity, loss of coordination, pain in chest, groin, or leg. Assess skin for irritation due to transdermal application or brown blotches. Note estrogen therapy on specimens.

PATIENT/FAMILY TEACHING:

Importance of medical supervision. Avoid smoking due to increased risk of heart attack or blood clots. Do not take other medications w/o physician approval. Teach how to perform Homan's test, signs and symptoms of blood clots (report these to physician immediately). Notify physician of abnormal vaginal bleeding, depression, other symptoms. Teach female pts to perform breast self-exam. Avoid exposure to sun/ultraviolet light. Check weight daily; report weekly gain of 5 lbs or more. W/vaginal application: Remain recumbent at least 30 min after application and do not use tampons. Stop taking the medication and contact physician at once if pregnancy is suspected. Give labeling from drug package.

estramustine phosphate sodium

es-trah-**mew**-steen
(Emcyt)

CANADIAN AVAILABILITY:
Emcyt

CLASSIFICATION

Antineoplastic

AVAILABILITY (Rx)

Capsule: 140 mg

PHARMACOKINETICS

Well absorbed from GI tract. Highly localized in prostatic tissue. Rapidly dephosphorylated during absorption into peripheral circulation. Metabolized in liver. Primarily eliminated in feces via biliary system. Half-life: 20 hrs.

ACTION/*THERAPEUTIC EFFECT*

Action may be due to direct effect of estrogen component or antimitotic activity. *Reduces serum testosterone concentration.*

USES

Treatment of metastatic or progressive carcinoma of prostate gland.

STORAGE/HANDLING

Note: May be carcinogenic, mutagenic, or teratogenic. Handle w/extreme care during administration.

Refrigerate capsules (may remain at room temperature for 24–48 hrs w/o loss of potency).

PO ADMINISTRATION

Give w/water 1 hr before or 2 hrs after meals.

INDICATIONS/DOSAGE/ROUTES

Prostatic carcinoma:
PO: Adults, elderly: 10–16 mg/kg/day (140 mg for each 10 kg weight) in 3–4 doses/day.

PRECAUTIONS

CONTRAINDICATIONS: Hypersensitivity to estradiol or nitrogen mustard, active thrombophlebitis or thrombolic disorders unless tumor is cause for thrombolic disorders and benefits outweigh risk. **CAUTIONS:** History of thrombophlebitis, thrombosis, or thromboembolic disorders, cerebrovascular or coronary artery disease, impaired hepatic function, metabolic bone disease in those w/hypercalcemia or renal insufficiency.

INTERACTIONS

DRUG INTERACTIONS: Hepatotoxic drugs may increase risk of hepatotoxicity. **ALTERED LAB VALUES:** May increase SGOT (AST), LDH, bilirubin, cortisol, glucose, phospholipids, prolactin, prothrombin, sodium, triglycerides. May decrease antithrombin 3, folate, pregnanediol excretion, phosphate. May alter thyroid function tests.

SIDE EFFECTS

FREQUENT: Peripheral edema of lower extremities, breast tenderness or enlargement, diarrhea, flatulence, nausea. **OCCASIONAL:** Increase in B/P, thirst, dry skin, easy bruising, flushing, thinning hair, night sweats. **RARE:** Headache, rash, fatigue, insomnia, vomiting.

ADVERSE REACTIONS/TOXIC EFFECTS

May exacerbate CHF, pulmonary emboli, thrombophlebitis, cerebrovascular accident.

NURSING IMPLICATIONS

INTERVENTION/EVALUATION:

Monitor B/P periodically.

PATIENT/FAMILY TEACHING:

Do not take w/milk, milk products or calcium-rich food, calcium-containing antacids. Use contraceptive measures during therapy. If headache (migraine or severe), vomiting, disturbed speech or vision, dizziness, numbness, shortness of breath, calf pain, heaviness in chest, unexplained cough occurs, contact physician. Do not have immunizations w/o physician's approval (drug lowers body's resistance). Avoid contact w/those who have recently received live virus vaccine. Contact physician if nausea/vomiting continues at home.

estropipate

ess-troe-**pie**-pate
(Ogen)

CANADIAN AVAILABILITY:
Ogen

CLASSIFICATION

Estrogen

AVAILABILITY (Rx)

Tablets: 0.625 mg, 1.25 mg, 2.5 mg. **Vaginal Cream:** 1.5 mg/g.

PHARMACOKINETICS

Well absorbed from GI tract. Widely distributed. Metabolized in liver. Primarily excreted in urine.

ACTION/THERAPEUTIC EFFECT

Increases synthesis of DNA, RNA, and various proteins in responsive tissues. Reduces release of gonadotropin-releasing hormone, reducing follicle-stimulating hormone (FSH) and leuteinizing hormone (LH). *Promotes normal growth, development of female sex organs, maintaining GU function, vasomotor stability. Prevents accelerated bone loss by inhibiting bone resorption, restoring balance of bone resorption and formation.*

USES

Management of moderate to severe vasomotor symptoms associated w/menopause. Treatment of atrophic vaginitis, kraurosis vulvae, female hypogonadism and castration, primary ovarian failure. Prevention of osteoporosis.

PO/VAGINAL ADMINISTRATION

PO:
Administer at the same time each day.

VAGINAL:
1. Apply at bedtime for best absorption.
2. Assemble and fill applicator per manufacturer's directions.
3. Insert end of applicator into vagina, directed slightly toward sacrum; push plunger down completely.
4. Avoid skin contact w/cream (prevents skin absorption).

INDICATIONS/DOSAGE/ROUTES

Vasomotor symptoms, atrophic vaginitis, kraurosis vulvae:
PO: Adults, elderly: 0.625–5 mg/day cyclically.

Atrophic vaginitis, kraurosis vulvae:
Intravaginally: Adults, elderly: 2–4 g/day cyclically.

Female hypogonadism, castration, primary ovarian failure:
PO: Adults, elderly: 1.25–7.5 mg/day × 21 days; off 8–10 days. Repeat if bleeding does not occur by end of rest period.

Osteoporosis prevention:
PO: Adults, elderly: 0.625 mg/day (25 days of 31 day cycle/month).

PRECAUTIONS

CONTRAINDICATIONS: Known or suspected breast cancer, estrogen-dependent neoplasia; undiagnosed abnormal genital bleeding; active thrombophlebitis or thromboembolic disorders; history of thrombophlebitis, thrombosis, or thromboembolic disorders w/previous estrogen use, hypersensitivity to estrogen. **CAUTIONS:** Conditions that may be aggravated by fluid retention: cardiac, renal, or hepatic dysfunction, epilepsy, migraine. Mental depression, hypercalcemia, history of jaundice during pregnancy or strong family history of breast cancer, fibrocystic disease, or breast nodules, children in whom bone growth is not complete. **PREGNANCY/LACTATION:** Distributed in breast milk. May be harmful to fetus. Not for use during lactation. **Pregnancy Category X**.

INTERACTIONS

DRUG INTERACTIONS: May interfere w/effects of bromocriptine. May increase concentration of cyclosporine, increase hepatic/nephrotoxicity. Hepatotoxic medications may increase hepatotoxicity. **ALTERED LAB VALUES:** May affect metapyrone, thyroid function tests. May decrease cholesterol, LDH. May increase calcium, glucose, HDL, triglycerides.

SIDE EFFECTS

FREQUENT: Anorexia, nausea, swelling of breasts, peripheral edema evidenced by swollen ankles, feet. **OCCASIONAL:** Vomiting (esp. w/high dosages), headache (may be severe), intolerance to contact lenses, increased B/P, glucose intolerance, brown spots on exposed skin. *Vaginal route:* Local irritation, vaginal discharge, changes in vaginal bleeding (spotting, breakthrough or prolonged bleeding). **RARE:** Chorea, cholestatic jaundice, hirsutism, loss of scalp hair, depression.

ADVERSE REACTIONS/TOXIC EFFECTS

Prolonged administration increases risk of gallbladder, thromboembolic disease, and breast, cervical, vaginal, endometrial, and liver carcinoma.

NURSING IMPLICATIONS
BASELINE ASSESSMENT:

Question for hypersensitivity to estrogen, previous jaundice, or thromboembolic disorders associated w/pregnancy or estrogen therapy. Establish baseline B/P, blood glucose.

INTERVENTION/EVALUATION:

Assess B/P at least daily. Check for swelling, weigh daily. Check blood glucose 4 times/day for pts w/diabetes. Promptly report signs and symptoms of thromboembolic or thrombotic disorders: sudden severe headache, shortness of breath, vision or speech disturbance, weakness or numbness of an extremity, loss of coordination, pain in chest, groin, or leg. Note estrogen therapy on specimens.

PATIENT/FAMILY TEACHING:

Importance of medical supervision. Avoid smoking because of increased risk of heart attack or blood clots. Do not take other medications w/o physician approval. Teach how to perform Homan's test, signs and symptoms of blood clots (report these to physician immediately). Also notify physician of abnormal vaginal discharge or bleeding, depression. Teach breast self-exam. Avoid exposure to sun/ultraviolet light. Check weight daily; report weekly gain of 5 lbs or more. W/vaginal application: Remain recumbent at least 30 min after application and do not use tampons. Stop taking estropipate and contact physician if pregnancy suspected. Give labeling from drug package.

---

etanercept
(Enbrel)
See Supplement

---

ethacrynic acid
eth-ah-**krin**-ick
(Edecrin)

ethacrynate sodium
eth-ah-**krin**-ate
(Edecrin Sodium)

CANADIAN AVAILABILITY:
Edecrin

CLASSIFICATION

Diuretic: Loop

AVAILABILITY (Rx)

Tablets: 25 mg, 50 mg. **Powder for Injection:** 50 mg.

PHARMACOKINETICS

	ONSET	PEAK	DURATION
PO	<30 min	2 hrs	6–8 hrs
IV	<5 min	15–30 min	2 hrs

Rapidly absorbed from GI tract. Metabolized in liver to active metabolite. Primarily excreted in urine.

ACTION/ *THERAPEUTIC EFFECT*

Enhances excretion of sodium, chloride, potassium at ascending limb of loop of Henle and distal renal tubule *producing diuretic effect.*

USES/ *UNLABELED*

Treatment of edema associated w/CHF, severe renal impairment, nephrotic syndrome, hepatic cirrhosis; short-term management of ascites, children w/congenital heart disease. *Treatment of hypertension, hypercalcemia.*

STORAGE/HANDLING

Store oral, parenteral form at room temperature. Discard if parenteral form appears hazy or opalescent. Discard unused reconstituted solution after 24 hrs.

PO/IV ADMINISTRATION

PO:

Give w/food to avoid GI upset, preferably w/breakfast (may prevent nocturia).

IV:

1. For direct IV, administer slowly over several minutes.

2. For IV infusion, reconstitute each 50 mg ethacrynate sodium w/50 ml 5% dextrose injection or NaCl injection.

3. Infuse slowly, over 20–30 min, through tubing of running IV infusion.

INDICATIONS/DOSAGE/ROUTE

Edema:

PO: Adults: 50–100 mg daily. Dosage may be increased in 25–50 mg increments until therapeutic response is achieved. **Elderly:** Initially, 25–50 mg/day; increase as needed. **Children:** Initially, 25 mg. Dosage may be increased in increments of 25 mg until therapeutic response is achieved. Alternate day scheduling may be used for maintenance therapy.

IV: Adults >18 yrs, elderly: 0.5–1.0 mg/kg or 50 mg for average-sized adult. Single IV dose should not exceed 100 mg.

PRECAUTIONS

CONTRAINDICATIONS: Anuria, severe renal impairment. **CAUTIONS:** Hepatic cirrhosis, ascites, history of gout, pancreatitis, systemic lupus erythematosus, diabetes mellitus, elderly, debilitated. **PREGNANCY/LACTATION:** Unknown if drug crosses placenta or is distributed in breast milk. **Pregnancy Category D**.

INTERACTIONS

DRUG INTERACTIONS: Amphotericin, ototoxic and nephrotoxic agents may increase toxicity. May decrease effect of anticoagulants, heparin. Hypokalemia-causing agents may increase risk hypokalemia. May increase risk of lithium toxicity. **ALTERED LAB VALUES:** May increase glucose, BUN, uric acid, urinary phosphate. May decrease calcium, chloride, magnesium, potassium, sodium.

SIDE EFFECTS

FREQUENT: Expected: Increase in urine frequency/volume. **OCCASIONAL:** Nausea, gastric upset w/cramping, diarrhea, headache, fatigue, apprehension. **RARE:** Severe, watery diarrhea.

ADVERSE REACTIONS/TOXIC EFFECTS

Vigorous diuresis may lead to profound water loss and electrolyte depletion, resulting in hypokalemia, hyponatremia, dehydration, coma, circulatory collapse. Acute hypotensive episodes may also occur, sometimes several days after beginning of therapy. Ototoxicity manifested as deafness, vertigo, tinnitus (ringing/roaring in ears) may occur, especially in those w/severe renal impairment. Can exacerbate diabetes mellitus, systemic lupus erythematosus, gout, pancreatitis. Blood dyscrasias have been reported.

NURSING IMPLICATIONS
BASELINE ASSESSMENT:

Check vital signs, esp. B/P for hypotension prior to administration. Obtain baseline electrolytes. Particularly check for low potassium. Check edema, skin turgor, mucous membranes for hydration status. Assess muscle strength, mental status. Note skin temperature, moisture. Obtain baseline weight. Initiate I&O.

INTERVENTION/EVALUATION:

Monitor B/P, vital signs, electrolytes, I&O, weight. Note extent of diuresis. Watch for changes from initial assessment (hypokalemia may result in muscle strength changes, tremor, muscle cramps, change in mental status, cardiac arrhythmias; hyponatremia may result in confusion, thirst, cold/clammy skin).

PATIENT/FAMILY TEACHING:

Expect increased frequency and volume of urination. Report irregular heartbeat, signs of electrolyte imbalances (noted above), hearing abnormalities (such as sense of fullness in ears, ringing/roaring in ears). Eat foods high in potassium such as whole grains (cereals), legumes, meat, bananas, apricots, orange juice, potatoes (white, sweet), raisins.

E

ethambutol
eth-**am**-byoo-toll
(Myambutol)

CANADIAN AVAILABILITY:
Etibi, Myambutol

CLASSIFICATION

Antitubercular

AVAILABILITY (Rx)

Tablets: 100 mg, 400 mg

PHARMACOKINETICS

Rapidly, well absorbed from GI tract. Widely distributed. Metabolized in liver. Primarily excreted in urine. Removed by hemodialysis. Half-life: 3–4 hrs (increased in reduced renal function).

ACTION/ *THERAPEUTIC EFFECT*

Interferes w/cell metabolism and multiplication by inhibiting one or more metabolites in susceptible bacteria. Active only during cell division. *Bacteriostatic.*

USES/ *UNLABELED*

In conjunction w/at least one other antitubercular agent for initial treatment and retreatment of clinical tuberculosis. *Treatment of atypical mycobacterial infections.*

PO ADMINISTRATION

1. Give w/food (decreases GI upset).
2. Give once q24h.

INDICATIONS/DOSAGE/ROUTES

Tuberculosis:
PO: Adults, elderly: Initially (no prior anti-TB medication): 15 mg/kg q24h. (Prior anti-TB medication): 25 mg/kg/day q24h for 60 days then decrease to 15 mg/kg/day. **Note:** When used in combination therapy and given 2 times/wk, dose is 50 mg/kg. Decrease dose in those w/renal impairment.

PRECAUTIONS

CONTRAINDICATIONS: Hypersensitivity to ethambutol, optic neuritis. **CAUTIONS:** Renal dysfunction, gout, ocular defects: diabetic retinopathy, cataracts, recurrent ocular inflammatory conditions. Not recommended for children under 13 yrs of age. **PREGNANCY/LACTATION:** Crosses placenta; excreted in breast milk. **Pregnancy Category B**.

INTERACTIONS

DRUG INTERACTIONS: Neurotoxic medications may increase risk of neurotoxicity. **ALTERED LAB VALUES:** May increase uric acid.

SIDE EFFECTS

OCCASIONAL: Acute gouty arthritis (chills, pain, swelling of joints w/hot skin), confusion, abdominal pain, nausea, vomiting, loss of appetite, headache. **RARE:** Rash, fever, blurred vision, eye pain, red-green color blindness, any vision loss.

ADVERSE REACTIONS/TOXIC EFFECTS

Optic neuritis (occurs more often w/high dosage, long-term therapy), peripheral neuritis, thrombocytopenia, anaphylactoid reaction occur rarely.

NURSING IMPLICATIONS
BASELINE ASSESSMENT:

Question for hypersensitivity to ethambutol. Assure collection of specimens for culture, sensitivity. Evaluate initial CBC, renal and hepatic test results.

INTERVENTION/EVALUATION:

Assess for vision changes (altered color perception, decreased visual acuity may be first signs): Discontinue drug and notify physician immediately. Give w/food if GI distress occurs. Monitor uric acid concentrations and assess for hot/painful/swollen joints, esp. big toe, ankle, or knee (gout). Check CBC, culture and sensitivity tests, renal and hepatic function results. Monitor I&O in event of renal dysfunction. Report numbness, tingling, burning of extremities (peripheral neuritis). Assess for dizziness and assure assistance w/ambulation. Check mental status. Evaluate skin for rash.

PATIENT/FAMILY TEACHING:

Do not skip doses; take for full length of therapy (may take months, years). Not affected by food. Office visits, vision and lab tests are essential part of treatment. Do not take any other medication w/o consulting physician. Notify physician immediately of any visual problem (visual effects generally reversible w/discontinuation of ethambutol, but in rare cases may take up to a year to disappear or may be permanent); promptly report rash, swelling and pain of joints, numbness/tingling/burning of hands or feet. Do not drive or use machinery if visual problems or dizziness occurs.

ethosuximide
(Zarontin)
See Classification section under:
Anticonvulsants

etidronate disodium
eh-**tye**-droe-nate
(Didronel)

CANADIAN AVAILABILITY:
Didronel

CLASSIFICATION

Calcium regulator

AVAILABILITY (Rx)

Tablets: 200 mg, 400 mg. **Injection:** 50 mg/ml.

PHARMACOKINETICS

Minimally absorbed from GI tract (1–6%). Chemically adsorbed to bone in areas of elevated osteogenesis. Absorbed dose excreted in urine; unabsorbed dose eliminated in feces. Half-life: 5–7 hrs.

ACTION/*THERAPEUTIC EFFECT*

Binds to calcium phosphate surface of calcium crystals, retarding *bone resorption, bone formation. May also retard accelerated rate of bone turnover in Paget's disease.*

USES

Oral: Treatment of symptomatic Paget's disease of the bone, prevention and treatment of heterotopic ossification following hip replacement or due to spinal injury. *Parenteral (IV):* Treatment of hypercalcemia associated w/malignant neoplasms inadequately managed by dietary modification or oral hydration; treatment of hypercalcemia of malignancy persisting after adequate hydration has been restored.

STORAGE/HANDLING

Store tablets at room temperature. After dilution, IV stable for at least 48 hrs.

PO/IV ADMINISTRATION

PO:

1. Give on empty stomach, 2 hrs before meals.
2. Do not give within 2 hrs of vitamins w/mineral supplements, antacids, or medications high in calcium, magnesium, iron, or aluminum.

IV INFUSION:

1. Dilute in at least 250 ml 0.9% NaCl.
2. Infuse slowly, over a minimum of 2 hrs regardless of volume of solution.

INDICATIONS/DOSAGE/ROUTES

Paget's disease:
PO: Adults, elderly: Initially, 5–10 mg/kg/day not to exceed 6 mos or 11–20 mg/kg/day not to exceed 3 mos. Repeat only after drug-free period of at least 90 days.

Heterotopic ossification (due to spinal cord injury):
PO: Adults, elderly: 20 mg/kg/day for 2 wks; then 10 mg/kg/day for 10 wks.

Heterotopic ossification (complicating total hip replacement):
PO: Adults, elderly: 20 mg/kg/day for 1 mo preop; follow w/20 mg/kg/day for 3 mos postop.

Usual parenteral dosage:
IV: Adults, elderly: 7.5 mg/kg/day

× 3 days; retreatment no sooner than 7 day intervals between courses. Follow w/oral therapy on day after last infusion (20 mg/kg/day for 30 days; may extend up to 90 days).

PRECAUTIONS

CONTRAINDICATIONS: Children, severe renal function. **CAUTIONS:** Enterocolitis, renal impairment, pts unable to maintain adequate intake of vitamin D or calcium. **PREGNANCY/LACTATION:** Unknown if drug crosses placenta or is distributed in breast milk. **Pregnancy Category B** (oral). **Pregnancy Category C** (parenteral).

INTERACTIONS

DRUG INTERACTIONS: Antacids w/calcium, magnesium, aluminum, foods w/calcium, mineral supplements may decrease absorption. **ALTERED LAB VALUES:** None significant.

SIDE EFFECTS

FREQUENT: Nausea, diarrhea increased, continuing or more frequent bone pain in those with Paget's disease. **OCCASIONAL:** Bone fractures (esp. femur). *Parenteral:* Metallic, altered, or loss of taste. **RARE:** Hypersensitivity reaction (rash, pruritus, urticaria, angioedema).

ADVERSE REACTIONS/TOXIC EFFECTS

Nephrotoxicity (hematuria, dysuria, proteinuria) noted w/parenteral route.

NURSING IMPLICATIONS
BASELINE ASSESSMENT:

Obtain lab baselines, esp. electrolytes, renal function.

INTERVENTION/EVALUATION:

Assess food tolerance. Check for diarrhea. Monitor electrolytes. Check I&O, BUN, creatinine in pts w/impaired renal function. Evaluate pain in pts w/Paget's disease. Assess skin for eruptions.

PATIENT/FAMILY TEACHING:

May take up to 3 mos for therapeutic response; do not stop taking medication, discuss w/physician. Taste may be altered, usually disappears w/continuation of therapy. Assure milk, dairy products in diet for calcium, vitamin D. Do not take any other medications w/o physician approval. Take medication on empty stomach, 2 hrs from food, vitamins, antacids. Report nausea, diarrhea, rash, or other symptoms. Follow-up office visits are necessary even when therapy is discontinued.

etodolac
eh-**toe**-doe-lack
(Lodine, Lodine XL)

CANADIAN AVAILABILITY:
Apo-Etodolac, Ultradol

CLASSIFICATION

Nonsteroidal anti-inflammatory

AVAILABILITY (Rx)

Capsules: 200 mg, 300 mg, 400 mg, 500 mg. **Capsules (extended-release):** 400 mg, 500 mg, 600 mg, 1,200 mg.

PHARMACOKINETICS

	ONSET	PEAK	DURATION
PO analgesic			
	30 min	—	4–12 hrs

E

Completely absorbed from GI tract. Widely distributed. Metabolized in liver. Primarily excreted in urine. Half-life: 6–7 hrs.

ACTION/*THERAPEUTIC EFFECT*

Produces analgesic and anti-inflammatory effect by inhibiting prostaglandin synthesis, *reducing inflammatory response and intensity of pain stimulus reaching sensory nerve endings.*

USES/*UNLABELED*

Acute and long-term treatment of osteoarthritis, management of pain, treatment of rheumatoid arthritis. *Treatment of acute gouty arthritis, vascular headache.*

PO ADMINISTRATION

1. Do not crush or break capsules, extended-release capsules.
2. May give w/food, milk, or antacids if GI distress occurs.

INDICATIONS/DOSAGE/ROUTES

Note: Reduce dosage in elderly; maximum dose for pts weighing <60 kg: 20 mg/kg.

Osteoarthritis:
PO: Adults, elderly: Initially, 800–1,200 mg/day in 2–4 divided doses. **Maintenance:** 600–1,200 mg/day.

Rheumatoid arthritis:
PO: Adults, elderly: Initially, 300 mg 2–3 times/day or 400–500 mg 2 times/day. **Maintenance:** 600–1,200 mg/day.

Analgesia:
PO: Adults, elderly: 200–400 mg q6–8h as needed. **Maximum:** 1,200 mg/day.

PRECAUTIONS

CONTRAINDICATIONS: Active peptic ulcer, GI ulceration, chronic inflammation of GI tract, GI bleeding disorders, history of hypersensitivity to aspirin or NSAIDs. **CAUTIONS:** Impaired renal/hepatic function, history of GI tract disease, predisposition to fluid retention. **PREGNANCY/LACTATION:** Unknown if drug crosses placenta or is distributed in breast milk. Avoid use during last trimester (may adversely affect fetal cardiovascular system: premature closure of ductus arteriosus). **Pregnancy Category C.**

INTERACTIONS

DRUG INTERACTIONS: May increase effects of oral anticoagulants, heparin, thrombolytics. May decrease effect of antihypertensives, diuretics. Salicylates, aspirin may increase risk of GI side effects, bleeding. Bone marrow depressants may increase risk of hematologic reactions. May increase concentration, toxicity of lithium. May increase methotrexate toxicity. Probenecid may increase concentration. **ALTERED LAB VALUES:** May increase bleeding time, creatinine, liver function tests. May decrease uric acid.

SIDE EFFECTS

FREQUENT (3–9%): Dizziness, headache, abdominal pain or cramps, bloated feeling, diarrhea, nausea, indigestion. **OCCASIONAL (1–3%):** Constipation, rash, itching, visual changes, ringing in ears.

ADVERSE REACTIONS/TOXIC EFFECTS

Overdosage may result in acute renal failure. In those treated chronically, peptic ulcer, GI bleeding, gastritis, severe hepatic reaction (jaundice), nephrotoxicity (hematuria, dysuria, proteinuria), severe hypersensitivity reaction (bronchospasm, angiofacial edema) occur rarely.

NURSING IMPLICATIONS
BASELINE ASSESSMENT:

Assess onset, type, location, duration of pain or inflammation. Inspect appearance of affected joints for immobility, deformities, skin condition.

INTERVENTION/EVALUATION:

Monitor for headache, dyspepsia. Monitor pattern of daily bowel activity, stool consistency. Evaluate for therapeutic response: relief of pain, stiffness, swelling, increase in joint mobility, reduced joint tenderness, improved grip strength.

PATIENT/FAMILY TEACHING:

Swallow capsule whole; do not crush or chew. Avoid aspirin, alcohol during therapy (increases risk of GI bleeding). If GI upset occurs, take w/food, milk. Report GI distress, visual disturbances, rash, edema, headache.

etoposide, VP-16

eh-**toe**-poe-side
(Etopophos, VePesid)

CANADIAN AVAILABILITY:
VePesid

CLASSIFICATION

Antineoplastic

AVAILABILITY (Rx)

Capsules: 50 mg. **Injection:** 20 mg/ml. **Injection (water soluble)** Etopophos: 20 mg/ml.

PHARMACOKINETICS

Variably absorbed from GI tract. Rapidly distributed. Low concentrations in CSF. Metabolized in liver. Primarily excreted in urine. Half-life: 3–12 hrs.

ACTION/THERAPEUTIC EFFECT

Induces single- and double-stranded breaks in DNA, *inhibiting or altering DNA synthesis.* Cell cycle-dependent and phase specific w/maximum effect on S, G_2 phase of cell division.

USES/UNLABELED

Treatment of refractory testicular tumors, small cell lung carcinoma. *Treatment of bladder carcinoma, Hodgkin's, non-Hodgkin's lymphoma, acute myelocytic leukemia, Ewing's sarcoma, AIDS-associated Kaposi's sarcoma.*

STORAGE/HANDLING

Note: May be carcinogenic, mutagenic, or teratogenic. Handle w/extreme care during preparation/administration.

Refrigerate gelatin capsules. Concentrate for injection is clear, yellow. Diluted solutions are stable at room temperature for 96 hrs at 0.2 mg/ml, 48 hrs at 0.4 mg/ml. Discard if crystallization occurs.

IV ADMINISTRATION

Note: Administer by slow IV infusion. Wear gloves when preparing solution. If powder or solution comes in contact w/skin, wash immediately and thoroughly w/soap, water.

1. Syringes w/Luer-Lock fittings should be used for handling concentrate (prevents displacement of needle from syringe).

2. Dilute concentrate (20 mg/ml) w/50 ml 5% dextrose or 0.9% NaCl to provide concentration of 0.4 mg/ml (100 ml for concentration of 0.2 mg/ml). Avoid concentrations above 0.4 mg/ml (solutions may precipitate).

3. Infuse slowly, over 30–60 min (rapid IV may produce transient hypotension, local pain).

4. Monitor for anaphylactic reaction during infusion (chills, fever, dyspnea, sweating, lacrimation, sneezing, throat/back/chest pain).

INDICATIONS/DOSAGE/ROUTES

Note: Dosage individualized based on clinical response, tolerance to adverse effects. When used in combination therapy, consult specific protocols for optimum dosage, sequence of drug administration. Treatment repeated at 3–4 wk intervals.

Refractory testicular tumors:
IV: Adults: Combination therapy: 50–100 mg/m^2/day on days 1 to 5 to 100 mg/m^2/day on days 1, 3, 5.

Small cell lung carcinoma:
PO: Adults: 2 times IV dose rounded to nearest 50 mg.
IV: Adults: *Combination therapy:* 35 mg/m^2 daily for 4 consecutive days up to 50 mg/m^2 daily for 5 consecutive days.

PRECAUTIONS

CONTRAINDICATIONS: None significant. **CAUTIONS:** Impaired hepatic function. **PREGNANCY/ LACTATION:** If possible, avoid use during pregnancy, esp. first trimester. May cause fetal harm. Breast-feeding not recommended. **Pregnancy Category D**.

INTERACTIONS

DRUG INTERACTIONS: Bone marrow depressants may increase bone marrow depression. Live virus vaccines may potentiate virus replication, increase vaccine side effects, decrease pt's antibody response to vaccine. **ALTERED LAB VALUES:** None significant.

SIDE EFFECTS

FREQUENT (43–66%): Mild to moderate nausea and vomiting, alopecia. **OCCASIONAL (6–13%):** Diarrhea, anorexia, stomatitis. **RARE (≤2%):** Hypotension, peripheral neuropathy.

ADVERSE REACTIONS/TOXIC EFFECTS

Bone marrow depression manifested as hematologic toxicity (principally leukopenia, thrombocytopenia, anemia, and to lesser extent, pancytopenia). Leukopenia occurs within 7–14 days after drug administration, thrombocytopenia occurs within 9–16 days after administration. Bone marrow recovery occurs by day 20. Hepatotoxicity occurs occasionally.

NURSING IMPLICATIONS

BASELINE ASSESSMENT:

Obtain hematology tests prior to and at frequent intervals during therapy. Antiemetics readily control nausea, vomiting.

INTERVENTION/EVALUATION:

Monitor Hgb, Hct, WBC, differential, platelet count. Assess pattern of daily bowel activity and stool consistency. Monitor for hematologic toxicity (fever, sore throat, signs of local infection, easy bruising, unusual bleeding from any site), symptoms of anemia (excessive tiredness, weakness). Assess for paresthesias (peripheral neuropathy).

PATIENT/FAMILY TEACHING:

Alopecia is reversible, but new

hair growth may have different color or texture. Do not have immunizations w/o physician's approval (drug lowers body's resistance). Avoid contact w/those who have recently received live virus vaccine. Promptly report fever, sore throat, signs of local infection, easy bruising, or unusual bleeding from any site. Contact physician if nausea/vomiting continues at home. Teach signs of peripheral neuropathy.

exemestane
(Aromasin)
See Supplement
See Classification section under: Antineoplastics

factor IX complex (human)
(Benefix, Konyne, Profilnine, Heat-treated Propex T)

CANADIAN AVAILABILITY:
Immunine VH

AVAILABILITY (Rx)

Injection: Number of units indicated on each vial

CLASSIFICATION

Antihemophilic

ACTION/*THERAPEUTIC EFFECT*

Raises plasma levels of factor IX, restores hemostasis in pts w/factor IX deficiency. *Increases blood clotting factors II, VII, IX, and X.*

USES

Note: Only Propex T controls bleeding in pts w/factor VII deficiency.
Treatment of bleeding caused by hemophilia B (deficiency of factor IX is demonstrated). Treatment of bleeding in pts w/hemophilia A who have factor VIII inhibitors. Reversal of anticoagulant effect of coumarin anticoagulants.

STORAGE/HANDLING

Store in refrigerator. Do not freeze. Reconstituted solutions stable for 12 hrs at room temperature. Begin administration within 3 hrs. Do not refrigerate reconstituted solutions.

IV ADMINISTRATION

1. Administer by slow IV injection or IV infusion.
2. Filter before administration.
3. Before reconstitution, warm diluent to room temperature.
4. Gently agitate vial until powder is completely dissolved (prevents removal of active components during administration through filter).
5. Infuse slowly, not to exceed 3 ml/min. A too rapid IV may produce headache, flushing, change in B/P and pulse rate, tingling sensation. Discontinuing infusion will eliminate effects immediately. Resume IV at slower rate.
6. If evidence of disseminated intravascular coagulation (DIC) occurs (change in B/P and pulse rate, respiratory distress, chest pain, cough), stop infusion immediately.

INDICATIONS/DOSAGE/ROUTES

Note: Amount of factor IX required is individualized.
Dosage depends on degree of deficiency, level of each factor desired, weight of pt, severity of bleeding. Give sufficient drug to achieve/maintain plasma level at least 20% of normal until hemostasis achieved.

PRECAUTIONS

CONTRAINDICATIONS: Sensitivity

to mouse protein. **CAUTIONS:** Sensitivity to factor IX, liver impairment, recent surgery. **PREGNANCY/LACTATION:** Unknown if drug crosses placenta or is distributed in breast milk. **Pregnancy Category C.**

INTERACTIONS

DRUG INTERACTIONS: Aminocaproic acid may increase risk of thrombosis. **ALTERED LAB VALUES:** None significant.

SIDE EFFECTS

RARE: Mild hypersensitivity reaction (fever, chills, change in B/P and pulse rate, rash, tingling urticaria [hives]).

ADVERSE REACTIONS/TOXIC EFFECTS

High risk of venous thrombosis during postop period. Acute hypersensitivity reaction, anaphylactoid reaction may occur. *Antidote:* Epinephrine 1:1,000. High dosage may produce DIC, MI, thrombosis, pulmonary embolism. There is a risk of transmitting viral hepatitis, other viral diseases.

NURSING IMPLICATIONS
BASELINE ASSESSMENT:

When monitoring B/P, avoid overinflation of cuff. Remove adhesive tape from any pressure dressing very carefully and slowly. Assess results of coagulation studies and extent of existing bleeding (overt bleeding, bruising, joint pain, and swelling).

INTERVENTION/EVALUATION:

Monitor vital signs, I&O. Assess for hypersensitivity reaction (slow infusion and notify physician). Monitor results of coagulation studies closely. Avoid IM or SubQ injections or rectal temperatures. After IV administration, apply direct pressure to venipuncture site for a full 5 min or longer to assure bleeding has stopped. Monitor IV site for oozing q5–15min for 1–2 hrs after administration. Report any evidence of hematuria or change in vital signs immediately. Assess for decrease in B/P, increase in pulse rate, complaint of abdominal/back pain, severe headache (may be evidence of hemorrhage). Question for increase in amount of discharge during menses. Assess peripheral pulses; skin for bruises, petechiae. Check for excessive bleeding from minor cuts, scratches. Assess gums for erythema, gingival bleeding. Evaluate for therapeutic relief of pain, reduction of swelling, and restricted joint movement.

PATIENT/FAMILY TEACHING:

Use electric razor, soft toothbrush to prevent bleeding. Report any sign of red/dark urine, black/red stool, coffee-ground vomitus, red-speckled mucus from cough. Do not use OTC medication w/o physician approval (may interfere w/platelet aggregation). Carry identification that indicates disease.

famciclovir
fam-**sigh**-klo-vir
(Famvir)

CANADIAN AVAILABILITY:
Famvir

CLASSIFICATION
Antiviral

AVAILABILITY (Rx)
Tablets: 125 mg, 250 mg, 500 mg

PHARMACOKINETICS

Rapidly, extensively absorbed following oral administration. Rapidly metabolized to penciclovir by enzymes in gut wall, plasma, and liver. Penciclovir eliminated unchanged in urine. Half-life: 2 hrs.

ACTION / THERAPEUTIC EFFECT

Suppresses herpes simplex virus and varicella zoster virus replication by inhibition of viral DNA synthesis.

USES

Treatment of herpes simplex virus (HSV), acute herpes zoster in immunocompromised pts, recurrent genital herpes, prevention of genital herpes, recurrent herpes simplex.

PO ADMINISTRATION

May be given w/o regard to meals.

INDICATIONS/DOSAGE/ROUTES

Herpes zoster:
PO: Adults: 500 mg q8h for 7 days.

Genital herpes:
PO: Adults: 125 mg twice daily for 7 days.

Prevention of genital herpes:
PO: Adults: 500 mg twice daily for 7 days.

Recurrent herpes simplex:
PO: Adults: 500 mg twice daily for 7 days.

Dosage in renal impairment:
Dosage based upon creatinine clearance (ml/min):

CREATININE CLEARANCE	HERPES ZOSTER	GENITAL HERPES
40–59	500 mg q12h	125 mg q12h
20–39	500 mg q24h	125 mg q24h
<20	250 mg q48h	125 mg q48h

Hemodialysis pts:
PO: Adults: 250 mg (herpes zoster) or 125 mg (genital herpes) following each dialysis treatment.

PRECAUTIONS

CONTRAINDICATIONS: Hypersensitivity to famciclovir. **CAUTIONS:** Renal function impairment. **PREGNANCY/LACTATION:** Increase in mammary adenocarcinoma in animals. Unknown if excreted in breast milk. **Pregnancy Category B.**

INTERACTIONS

DRUG INTERACTIONS: None significant. **ALTERED LAB VALUES:** None significant.

SIDE EFFECTS

FREQUENT: Headache (23%), nausea (12%). **OCCASIONAL (2–10%):** Dizziness, somnolence, numbness of feet, diarrhea, vomiting, constipation, decreased appetite, fatigue, fever, pharyngitis, sinusitis, pruritus. **RARE (<2%):** Inability to sleep, abdominal pain, dyspepsia, flatulence, back pain, arthralgia.

ADVERSE REACTIONS/TOXIC EFFECTS

None significant.

NURSING IMPLICATIONS

BASELINE ASSESSMENT:

Tissue cultures for herpes simplex virus and varicella zoster virus should be done before giving first dose (therapy may proceed before results are known).

INTERVENTION/EVALUATION:

Evaluate cutaneous lesions. Be alert to neurologic effects: headache, dizziness. Provide analgesics and comfort measures; esp. exhausting to elderly. Encourage fluids. Keep pt's fingernails short, hands clean.

PATIENT/FAMILY TEACHING:

Drink adequate fluids. Notify physician if side effects develop. Do not touch lesions with fingers to avoid spreading infection to new site. *Genital herpes:* Continue therapy for full length of treatment. Space doses evenly. Use finger cot or rubber glove to apply topical ointment. Avoid sexual intercourse during duration of lesions to prevent infecting partner. Notify physician if lesions do not improve or recur. Avoid driving or operating machinery if dizziness is present. Pap smears should be done at least annually.

famotidine

fah-**mow**-tih-deen
(Mylanta AR, Pepcid, Pepcid AC, Pepcid RPD)

CANADIAN AVAILABILITY:
Maalox H_2 Acid Controller, Novo-Famotidine, Pepcid, Ulcidine

CLASSIFICATION

H-2 receptor antagonist

AVAILABILITY (Rx)

Tablets: 10 mg (OTC), 20 mg, 40 mg. **Chewable Tablets:** 10 mg. **Powder for Oral Suspension:** 40 mg/5 ml. **Injection:** 10 mg/ml, 20 mg/50 ml NaCl infusion.

PHARMACOKINETICS

Rapid, incompletely absorbed from GI tract. Partially metabolized in liver. Primarily excreted in urine. Half-life: 2.5–3.5 hrs (increased in reduced renal function).

ACTION/*THERAPEUTIC EFFECT*

Inhibits histamine action at H-2 receptors of parietal cells, *inhibiting gastric acid secretion (fasting, nocturnal, or when stimulated by food, caffeine, insulin).*

USES/*UNLABELED*

Short-term treatment of active duodenal ulcer. Prevention of duodenal ulcer recurrence. Treatment of active benign gastric ulcer, pathologic GI hypersecretory conditions. Short-term treatment of gastroesophageal reflux disease including erosive esophagitis. *Prophylaxis vs. aspiration pneumonitis. Autism.*

STORAGE/HANDLING

Store tablets, suspension at room temperature. After reconstitution, suspension is stable for 30 days at room temperature. Refrigerate unreconstituted vials. IV solution appears clear, colorless. After dilution, IV solution is stable for 48 hrs at room temperature.

PO/IV ADMINISTRATION

PO:

1. Give w/o regard to meals or antacids. Best given after meals or at bedtime.
2. Shake suspension well before use.
3. Pepcid RPD dissolves under tongue; does not require water for dosing.

IV:

1. For direct IV injection, dilute 20 mg vial w/5–10 ml 0.9% NaCl or other compatible IV solution. Inject over not less than 2 min.
2. For intermittent IV infusion (piggyback), dilute w/100 ml 5% dextrose or other compatible IV fluid. Infuse over 15–30 min.

INDICATIONS/DOSAGE/ROUTES

Acute therapy—duodenal ulcer:
PO: **Adults, elderly:** 40 mg at bedtime or 20 mg q12h. **Maintenance:** 20 mg at bedtime. **Children 1–6 yrs:** 0.5 mg/kg/day. **Maximum:** 40 mg.

Acute therapy—benign gastric ulcer:
PO: **Adults, elderly:** 40 mg at bedtime.

Gastroesophageal reflux disease:
PO: Adults, elderly: 20 mg 2 times/day up to 6 wks; 20–40 mg 2 times/day up to 12 wks in pts w/esophagitis (including erosions, ulcerations). **Children 1–16 yrs:** 1 mg/kg/day in 2 divided doses. **Maximum:** 80 mg/day.

Pathologic hypersecretory conditions:
PO: Adults, elderly: Initially, 20 mg q6h up to 160 mg q6h.

Usual parenteral dosage:
IV: Adults, elderly: 20 mg q12h. **Children:** 0.25 mg/kg q12h. **Maximum:** 40 mg/day.

Dosage in renal impairment:
Creatinine clearance equal to or less than 10 ml/min: Decrease dose to 20 mg at bedtime or increase dosage interval to 36–48 hrs.

PRECAUTIONS

CONTRAINDICATIONS: None significant. **CAUTIONS:** Impaired renal/hepatic function. **PREGNANCY/LACTATION:** Unknown if drug crosses placenta or is distributed in breast milk. **Pregnancy Category B.**

INTERACTIONS

DRUG INTERACTIONS: Antacids may decrease absorption (do not give within $1/2$–1 hr). May decrease absorption of ketoconazole (give at least 2 hrs after). **ALTERED LAB VALUES:** Interferes w/skin tests using allergen extracts. May increase liver function tests.

SIDE EFFECTS

FREQUENT (4–6%): Headache. **OCCASIONAL (1–3%):** Constipation, diarrhea, dizziness, decreased appetite, joint pain, nausea, vomiting, ringing in ears, skin rash.

ADVERSE REACTIONS/TOXIC EFFECTS

None significant.

NURSING IMPLICATIONS
INTERVENTION/EVALUATION:

Monitor daily bowel activity and stool consistency. Assess for abdominal pain, GI bleeding signs. Monitor for diarrhea/constipation.

PATIENT/FAMILY TEACHING:

IV may produce transient discomfort at injection site. May take w/o regard to meals or antacids. Report headache. Avoid tasks that require alertness, motor skills until drug response is established. Avoid smoking (decreases effectiveness). Do not use OTC medications/alcohol w/o consulting physician.

---

felodipine

feh-**low**-dih-peen
(Plendil)

FIXED-COMBINATION(S):
W/enalapril, an ACE inhibitor
(Lexxel)

CANADIAN AVAILABILITY:
Plendil, Renedil

CLASSIFICATION

Calcium channel blocker

AVAILABILITY (Rx)

Tablets (extended-release): 2.5 mg, 5 mg, 10 mg

PHARMACOKINETICS

	ONSET	PEAK	DURATION
PO	2–5 hrs	—	—

Rapidly, completely absorbed from GI tract. Undergoes first-pass metabolism in liver. Metabolized in liver. Primarily excreted in urine. Half-life: 11–16 hrs.

ACTION/*THERAPEUTIC EFFECT*

Inhibits calcium movement across cardiac, vascular smooth muscle. Potent peripheral vasodilator (does not depress SA, AV nodes). *Increases myocardial contractility, heart rate, cardiac output; decreases peripheral vascular resistance.*

USES/*UNLABELED*

Management of hypertension. May be used alone or w/other antihypertensives. *Treatment of chronic angina pectoris, Raynaud's phenomena.*

PO ADMINISTRATION

1. May take w/o regard to food.
2. Do not crush or break tablets.

INDICATIONS/DOSAGE/ROUTES

Hypertension:
PO: Adults: Initially, 5 mg/day as single dose. **Elderly, pts w/impaired liver function:** Initially, 2.5 mg/day. Adjust dosage at no less than 2 wk intervals. **Maintenance:** 2.5–10 mg/day.

PRECAUTIONS

CONTRAINDICATIONS: Sick-sinus syndrome/second- or third-degree AV block (except in presence of pacemaker). Severe hypotension, extreme bradycardia, CHF. **CAUTIONS:** Impaired renal/hepatic function, CHF. Grapefruit jiuce may increase concentration of felodipine. **PREGNANCY/LACTATION:** Unknown if drug crosses placenta or is distributed in breast milk. **Pregnancy Category C**.

INTERACTIONS

DRUG INTERACTIONS: Beta blockers may have additive effect. May increase digoxin concentration. Procainamide, quinidine may increase risk of QT interval prolongation. Erythromycin may increase concentration/toxicity. Hypokalemia-producing agents may increase risk of arrhythmias. **ALTERED LAB VALUES:** None significant.

SIDE EFFECTS

FREQUENT (18–22%): Headache, peripheral edema. **OCCASIONAL (4–6%):** Flushing, respiratory infection, dizziness, lightheadedness, asthenia (loss of strength, weakness). **RARE (<3%):** Paresthesia, abdominal discomfort, nervousness, muscle cramping, cough, diarrhea, constipation.

ADVERSE REACTIONS/TOXIC EFFECTS

Overdosage produces nausea, drowsiness, confusion, slurred speech.

NURSING IMPLICATIONS

BASELINE ASSESSMENT:

Assess baseline renal/liver function tests. Assess B/P, apical pulse immediately before drug is administered (if pulse is 60/min or below, or systolic B/P is below 90 mm Hg, withhold medication, contact physician).

INTERVENTION/EVALUATION:

Assist w/ambulation if lightheadedness, dizziness occur. Assess for peripheral edema behind media/malleolus (sacral area in bedridden pts). Monitor pulse rate for bradycardia. Assess skin for flushing. Monitor liver enzyme tests. Question for headache, asthenia.

PATIENT/FAMILY TEACHING:

Do not abruptly discontinue medication. Compliance w/therapy regimen is essential to control hypertension. To avoid hypotensive effect, rise slowly from lying to sitting position. Wait momentarily before standing. Avoid tasks that require alertness, motor skills until response to drug is established. Contact physician/nurse if

F

irregular heartbeat, shortness of breath, pronounced dizziness, or nausea occurs. Swallow whole; do not crush or chew. Avoid grapefruit juice.

fenofibrate

(Tricor)
See Supplement
See Classification section under:
Antihyperlipedemics

fenoldopam

(Corlopam)
See Supplement

fenoprofen calcium

fen-oh-**pro**-fen
(Nalfon)

CANADIAN AVAILABILITY:
Nalfon

CLASSIFICATION

Nonsteroidal anti-inflammatory

AVAILABILITY (Rx)

Capsules: 200 mg, 300 mg.
Tablets: 600 mg.

PHARMACOKINETICS

ONSET	PEAK	DURATION
PO (antirheumatic)		
2 days	—	2–3 wks

Rapidly absorbed from GI tract. Widely distributed. Metabolized in liver. Primarily excreted in urine. Half-life: 3 hrs.

ACTION / *THERAPEUTIC EFFECT*

Produces analgesic and anti-inflammatory effect by inhibiting prostaglandin synthesis, *reducing inflammatory response and intensi-ty of pain stimulus reaching sensory nerve endings.*

USES / *UNLABELED*

Treatment of acute or long-term mild to moderate pain, symptomatic treatment of acute and/or chronic rheumatoid arthritis, osteoarthritis. *Treatment of vascular headaches, ankylosing spondylitis, psoriatic arthritis.*

PO ADMINISTRATION

May give w/food, milk, or antacids if GI distress occurs.

INDICATIONS / DOSAGE / ROUTES

Note: Do not exceed 3.2 g/day.

Mild to moderate pain:
PO: Adults, elderly: 200 mg q4–6h as needed.

Rheumatoid arthritis, osteoarthritis:
PO: Adults, elderly: 300–600 mg 3–4 times/day.

PRECAUTIONS

CONTRAINDICATIONS: Active peptic ulcer, GI ulceration, chronic inflammation of GI tract, GI bleeding disorders, history of hypersensitivity to aspirin/NSAIDs, history of significantly impaired renal function. **CAUTIONS:** Impaired renal/hepatic function, history of GI tract diseases, predisposition to fluid retention. **PREGNANCY/LACTATION:** Distributed in low concentration in breast milk. Avoid use during last trimester (may adversely affect fetal cardiovascular system: premature closure of ductus arteriosus). **Pregnancy Category B**. (Category D if used in 3rd trimester or near delivery.)

INTERACTIONS

DRUG INTERACTIONS: May increase effects of oral anticoagulants, heparin, thrombolytics. May decrease effect of antihypertensives, diuretics. Salicylates, aspirin may increase risk of GI side effects, bleeding. Bone marrow depressants may increase risk of hematologic reactions. May increase concentration, toxicity of lithium. May increase methotrexate toxicity. Probenecid may increase concentrations. **ALTERED LAB VALUES:** May increase serum transaminase, LDH, alkaline phosphatase, BUN, creatinine, potassium, glucose, protein, bleeding time.

SIDE EFFECTS

FREQUENT (3–9%): Headache, somnolence/drowsiness, dyspepsia (heartburn, indigestion, epigastric pain), nausea, vomiting, constipation. **OCCASIONAL (1–3%):** Dizziness, pruritus, nervousness, asthenia (loss of strength), diarrhea, abdominal cramps, flatulence, tinnitus, blurred vision, peripheral edema/fluid retention.

ADVERSE REACTIONS/TOXIC EFFECTS

Overdosage may result in acute hypotension, tachycardia. Peptic ulcer, GI bleeding, nephrotoxicity (dysuria, cystitis, hematuria, proteinuria, nephrotic syndrome), gastritis, severe hepatic reaction (cholestasis, jaundice), severe hypersensitivity reaction (bronchospasm, angiofacial edema) occur rarely.

NURSING IMPLICATIONS

BASELINE ASSESSMENT:

Assess onset, type, location, duration of pain or inflammation. Inspect appearance of affected joints for immobility, deformities, skin condition.

INTERVENTION/EVALUATION:

Assist w/ambulation if somnolence/drowsiness/dizziness occurs. Monitor for evidence of dyspepsia. Monitor pattern of daily bowel activity, stool consistency. Check behind medial malleolus for fluid retention (usually first area noted). Evaluate for therapeutic response: relief of pain, stiffness, swelling, increase in joint mobility, reduced joint tenderness, improved grip strength.

PATIENT/FAMILY TEACHING:

Swallow capsule whole; do not crush or chew. Avoid tasks that require alertness, motor skills until response to drug is established. If GI upset occurs, take w/food, milk. Avoid aspirin, alcohol during therapy (increases risk of GI bleeding). Report headache, GI distress, visual disturbances, edema, itching, black stools.

fentanyl

fen-**tah**-nil

(Actiq, Duragesic)

fentanyl citrate

(Fentanyl Oralet, Sublimaze)

FIXED-COMBINATION(S): W/droperidol, an antianxiety, antiemetic **(Innovar)**

CANADIAN AVAILABILITY: Duragesic

CLASSIFICATION

Opioid: Analgesic **(Schedule II)**

AVAILABILITY (Rx)

Injection: 0.05 mg/ml. **Transdermal Patch:** 25 mcg/hr, 50 mcg/hr, 75 mcg/hr, 100 mcg/hr. **Lozenges:** 200 mcg, 300 mcg, 400 mcg.

PHARMACOKINETICS

	ONSET	PEAK	DURATION
IM	7–15 min	20–30 min	1–2 hrs
IV	1–2 min	3–5 min	0.5–1 hr

Well absorbed after topical, IM administration. Transmucosal absorbed through mucosal tissue of mouth, GI tract. Metabolized in liver. Primarily eliminated via biliary system. Half-life: 3.6 hrs (increased in elderly).

ACTION/*THERAPEUTIC EFFECT*

Binds at opiate receptor sites within CNS, reducing stimuli from sensory nerve endings, *affecting pain perception, emotional response to pain.*

USES

Analgesic action for short duration surgery, outpatient minor surgery, diagnostic procedures requiring pt to be awake or lightly anesthetized; during surgery, immediately after surgery to prevent/relieve tachypnea, postop delirium, adjunct to general/regional anesthesia. Transdermal for management of chronic pain. Transmucosal for anesthetic premedication. *Actiq:* treatment breakthrough for pain in chronic cancer or AIDS-related pain.

STORAGE/HANDLING

Store parenteral form at room temperature.

IM/IV/TRANSDERMAL/ TRANSMUCOSAL ADMINISTRATION

IV/IM:

Note: Incompatible w/methohexital, pentobarbital, thiopental.

1. For initial anesthesia induction dosage, give small amount, via tuberculin syringe.

2. Give by slow IV injection (over 1–2 min).

3. Too rapid IV increases risk of severe adverse reactions (skeletal and thoracic muscle rigidity resulting in apnea, laryngospasm, bronchospasm, peripheral circulatory collapse, anaphylactoid effects, cardiac arrest).

4. Opiate antagonist (naloxone) should be readily available.

TRANSDERMAL:

1. Apply to nonhairy area of intact skin of upper torso.

2. Use flat, nonirritated site.

3. Firmly press evenly for 10–20 secs assuring adhesion is in full contact w/skin and edges are completely sealed.

4. Use only water to cleanse site prior to application (soaps, oils, etc., may irritate skin).

5. Rotate sites of application.

6. Used patches are carefully folded so system adheres to itself; discard in toilet.

TRANSMUCOSAL:

Suck lozenge vigorously.

INDICATIONS/DOSAGE/ROUTES

Note: Reduce initial dose by 25–33% in those receiving CNS depressants. Reduce dose in elderly, debilitated. Obese (>20% ideal body weight): Adjust dosage based on lean body weight.

PREOP:

IM: Adults, elderly: 50–100 mcg (0.05–0.1 mg) 30–60 min before surgery.

PRIMARY AGENT ANESTHESIA:

IV: Adults, elderly: 50–100 mcg/kg, administered w/oxygen and skeletal muscle relaxant. **Children 2–12 yrs:** 1.7–3.3 mcg/kg.

ADJUNCT TO LOCAL ANESTHESIA:

IM/IV: Adults, elderly: 50–100 mcg.

ADJUNCT TO GENERAL ANESTHESIA:

Total low dose:
IV: **Adults, elderly:** 2 mcg/kg one time.

Total moderate dose:
IV/IM: **Adults, elderly:** Initially, 2–20 mcg/kg IV, then 25–100 mcg IM/IV as necessary.

Total high dose:
IV: **Adults, elderly:** Initially, 20–50 mcg/kg. May give additional doses ranging from 25 mcg up to one-half initial dose.

POSTOP (RECOVERY ROOM):

IM: **Adults, elderly:** 50–100 mcg q1–2h, as needed.

USUAL TRANSDERMAL DOSAGE:

Transdermal: **Adults, elderly:** Individualized. Use lowest effective dose based on previous analgesics given, opioid tolerance, pt condition, medical status.

USUAL TRANSMUCOSAL DOSAGE:

Transmucosal: **Adults, children:** 200–400 mcg.

PRECAUTIONS

CONTRAINDICATIONS: *Transdermal:* Diarrhea, acute respiratory depression. **EXTREME CAUTION:** Bradyarrhythmias, severe CNS depression, anoxia, hypercapnia, respiratory depression, seizures, acute alcoholism, shock, untreated myxedema, respiratory dysfunction. **CAUTIONS:** *Transdermal:* Acute asthma attack, chronic respiratory disease, severe inflammatory bowel disease, impaired liver/renal function, increased intracranial pressure, head injury. **PREGNANCY/LACTATION:** Readily crosses placenta; unknown if distributed in breast milk. May prolong labor if administered in latent phase of first stage of labor, or before cervical dilation of 4–5 cm has occurred. Respiratory depression may occur in neonate if mother received opiates during labor. **Pregnancy Category B**. (Category D if used for prolonged periods or in high doses at term.)

INTERACTIONS

DRUG INTERACTIONS: Benzodiazepines may increase risk of hypotension, respiratory depression. Buprenorphine may decrease effect. CNS depressants may increase CNS, respiratory depression, hypotension. **ALTERED LAB VALUES:** May increase amylase, lipase plasma concentrations.

SIDE EFFECTS

FREQUENT: *Transdermal (3–10%):* Headache, itching skin, nausea, vomiting, sweating, difficulty breathing, confusion, dizziness, drowsiness, diarrhea, constipation, decreased appetite. *IV:* Post-op drowsiness, nausea, vomiting. **OCCASIONAL:** *Transdermal (1–3%):* Chest pain, irregular heartbeat, redness, itching, swelling of skin, fainting, agitation, tingling/burning of skin. *IV:* Post-op confusion, blurred vision, chills, orthostatic hypotension, constipation, difficulty urinating.

ADVERSE REACTIONS/TOXIC EFFECTS

Overdosage or too rapid IV results in severe respiratory depression, skeletal and thoracic muscle rigidity resulting in apnea, laryngospasm, bronchospasm, cold and clammy skin, cyanosis, coma. Tolerance to analgesic effect may occur w/repeated use.

NURSING IMPLICATIONS
BASELINE ASSESSMENT:

Resuscitative equipment and opiate antagonist (naloxone, 0.5 mcg/kg) must be available. Establish baseline B/P and respirations. Assess type, location, intensity, and duration of pain.

INTERVENTION/EVALUATION:

Monitor B/P and respirations closely. Assist w/ambulation. Encourage pt to turn, cough, and deep breathe q2h. Check for constipation; increase fluids, bulk, and exercise as appropriate. Assess for relief of pain.

PATIENT/FAMILY TEACHING:

Avoid alcohol; do not take other medications w/o consulting physician. Do not drive or perform other activities requiring alertness, coordination. Teach pt proper application of transdermal. Use as directed to avoid overdosage; potential for physical dependence w/prolonged use. After long-term use, must be discontinued slowly.

ferrous fumarate

fair-us **fume**-ah-rate
(Feostat)

ferrous gluconate

fair-us **glue**-kuh-nate
(Fergon, Ferralet, Simron)

ferrous sulfate

fair-us **sul**-fate
(Feosol, Slow-Fe)

FIXED-COMBINATION(S):

W/docusate sodium, a stool softener **(Ferro-Sequels)**; w/aluminum and magnesium hydroxide, antacids **(Fermalox)**

CANADIAN AVAILABILITY:

Apo-Ferrous Gluconate, Apo-Ferrous Sulfate, Fer-In-Sol, Palafer, Slow Fe

CLASSIFICATION

Iron preparation

AVAILABILITY (OTC)

Ferrous Fumarate: **Tablets:** 63 mg, 195 mg, 200 mg, 324 mg, 350 mg. **Tablets (chewable):** 100 mg. **Capsules (controlled-release):** 325 mg. **Suspension:** 100 mg/5 ml. **Oral Drops:** 45 mg/0.6 ml.

Ferrous Gluconate: **Tablets:** 300 mg, 320 mg. **Tablets (sustained-release):** 320 mg.

Ferrous Sulfate: **Tablets:** 195 mg, 300 mg, 324 mg. **Capsules:** 250 mg. **Tablets (timed-release):** 525 mg. **Syrup:** 90 mg/5 ml. **Elixir:** 220 mg/5 ml. **Oral Drops:** 125 mg/ml.

Ferrous Sulfate (exsiccated): **Tablets:** 200 mg. **Capsules:** 190 mg. **Capsules (timed-release):** 159 mg, 250 mg. **Tablets (slow-release):** 160 mg.

PHARMACOKINETICS

Absorption increased when iron stores depleted. Primarily absorbed in duodenum, proximal jejunum and stored in hepatocytes and reticuloendothelial system. No physiologic system of elimination (small amounts lost daily in shedding skin, hair, nails). Half-life: 6 hrs.

ACTION/*THERAPEUTIC EFFECT*

Essential component in formation of hemoglobin, myoglobin, and enzymes, *necessary for effective erythropoiesis and for transport and utilization of oxygen.*

USES

Prevention and treatment of iron deficiency anemia due to inadequate diet, malabsorption, pregnancy, and/or blood loss.

STORAGE/HANDLING

Store all forms (tablets, capsules, suspension, drops) at room temperature.

PO ADMINISTRATION

1. Ideally, give between meals w/water but may give w/meals if GI discomfort occurs.

2. Transient staining of mucous membranes and teeth will occur w/liquid iron preparation. Place liquid on back of tongue w/dropper or straw.

3. Avoid simultaneous administration of antacids or tetracycline.

4. Do not crush sustained-release preparations.

INDICATIONS/DOSAGE/ROUTES

Note: Dosage expressed in terms of elemental iron. Elemental iron content: ferrous fumarate: 33% (99 mg iron/300 mg tablet); ferrous gluconate: 11.6% (35 mg iron/300 mg tablet); ferrous sulfate: 20% (60 mg iron/300 mg tablet).

Deficiency:
PO: Adults, elderly: 2–3 mg/kg/day in 3 divided doses. **Children 2–12 yrs:** 3 mg/kg/day in 3–4 divided doses. **Children 6 mos–2 yrs:** Up to 6 mg/kg/day in 3–4 divided doses. **Infants:** 10–25 mg/day in 3–4 divided doses.

PRECAUTIONS

CONTRAINDICATIONS: Hemochromatosis, hemosiderosis, hemolytic anemias, those w/peptic ulcer, regional enteritis, or ulcerative colitis. **CAUTIONS:** Those w/bronchial asthma, iron hypersensitivity. **PREGNANCY/LACTATION:** Crosses placenta; excreted in breast milk. **Pregnancy Category A.**

INTERACTIONS

DRUG INTERACTIONS: Antacids, calcium supplements, pancreatin, pancrelipase may decrease absorption. May decrease absorption of quinolones, etidronate, tetracyclines. **ALTERED LAB VALUES:** May increase bilirubin. May decrease calcium. May obscure occult blood in stools.

SIDE EFFECTS

OCCASIONAL: Mild, transient nausea. **RARE:** Heartburn, anorexia, constipation, or diarrhea.

ADVERSE REACTIONS/TOXIC EFFECTS

Large doses may aggravate existing GI tract disease (peptic ulcer, regional enteritis, ulcerative colitis). Severe iron poisoning occurs mostly in children and is manifested as vomiting, severe abdominal pain, diarrhea, dehydration, followed by hyperventilation, pallor or cyanosis, cardiovascular collapse.

NURSING IMPLICATIONS

BASELINE ASSESSMENT:

To prevent mucous membrane and teeth staining w/liquid preparation, use dropper or straw and allow solution to drop on back of tongue. Eggs, milk inhibit absorption. Obtain Hgb, Hct results.

INTERVENTION/EVALUATION:

Those w/normal iron balance should not take iron preparation routinely. Monitor daily pattern of bowel activity and stool consistency. Assess for clinical improvement and record relief of iron deficiency symptoms (fatigue, irritability, pallor, paresthesia of extremities, headache). Monitor Hgb, Hct results.

PATIENT/FAMILY TEACHING:

Expect stools to darken in color. Take on empty stomach. If GI discomfort occurs, take after meals or w/food. Do not take within 2 hrs of antacids (prevents absorption).

fexofenadine

fecks-**oh**-fen-ah-deen
(Allegra)

FIXED-COMBINATION(S):
W/pseudoephedrine, a sympathomimetic **(Allegra-D).**

CANADIAN AVAILABILITY:
Allegra

CLASSIFICATION

Antihistamine

AVAILABILITY (Rx)

Capsules: 60 mg

PHARMACOKINETICS

Rapidly absorbed following oral
administration. Does not cross
blood-brain barrier. Minimally
metabolized. Eliminated in feces,
excreted in urine. Half-life: 14.4
hrs (increased in those w/reduced
renal function).

ACTION/*THERAPEUTIC EFFECT*

Prevents, antagonizes most histamine effects (e.g., urticaria, pruritus). *Relieves allergic rhinitis
symptoms.*

USES

Relief of symptoms associated
w/seasonal allergic rhinitis (sneezing, rhinorrhea, itching of throat/
eyes) in adults, children >12 yrs.

PO ADMINISTRATION

May take w/o regard to food.

INDICATIONS/DOSAGE/ROUTES

Allergic rhinitis:
PO: Adults, elderly, children >12
yrs: 60 mg 2 times/day.

Dosage in renal impairment:
PO: Adults, elderly, children >12
yrs: 60 mg once daily.

PRECAUTIONS

CONTRAINDICATIONS: Hyper-
sensitivitiy to fexofenadine or its ingredients. **CAUTIONS:** Severe renal
impairment. **PREGNANCY/LAC-
TATION:** Unknown if drug crosses
placenta or is distributed in breast
milk. **Pregnancy Category C.**

INTERACTIONS

DRUG INTERACTIONS: None significant. **ALTERED LAB VALUES:**
May suppress wheal and flare reactions to antigen skin testing. Discontinue at least 4 days before testing.

SIDE EFFECTS

RARE (<2%): Drowsiness, headache, fatigue, nausea, vomiting, abdominal distress, dysmenorrhea.

ADVERSE REACTIONS/TOXIC EFFECTS

None significant.

NURSING IMPLICATIONS
BASELINE ASSESSMENT:

If patient is undergoing allergic
reaction, obtain history of recently
ingested foods, drugs, environmental exposure, recent emotional
stress. Monitor rate, depth, rhythm,
type of respiration; quality and
rate of pulse. Assess lung sounds
for rhonchi, wheezing, rales.

INTERVENTION/EVALUATION:

Assess for therapeutic response from allergy: itching, red,
watery eyes, relief from rhinorrhea, sneezing.

PATIENT/FAMILY TEACHING:

Avoid tasks that require alertness, motor skills until response
to drug is established. Avoid alcoholic beverages during antihistamine therapy. Coffee or tea
may help reduce drowsiness.

filgrastim

fill-**grass**-tim
(Neupogen)

CANADIAN AVAILABILITY:
Neupogen

CLASSIFICATION

Colony stimulating factor

AVAILABILITY (Rx)

Injection: 300 mcg/ml

PHARMACOKINETICS

Readily absorbed after SubQ administration. Half-life: 3.5 hrs.

ACTION/*THERAPEUTIC EFFECT*

Regulates production of neutrophils within bone marrow. Primarily affects neutrophil progenitor proliferation, differentiation, and selected end-cell functional activation (*e.g., increased phagocytic ability, antibody-dependent killing*).

USES/*UNLABELED*

Decrease infection incidence in pt w/nonmyeloid malignancies receiving myelosuppressive therapy associated w/severe neutropenia, fever. Reduce neutropenia duration (and sequelae) in pt w/nonmyeloid malignancies having myeloablative therapy followed by bone marrow transplant (BMT). Mobilization of hematopoietic progenitor cells into peripheral blood for collection by leukapheresis. Improve neutrophil recovery, reduce fever duration following chemotherapy for acute myeloid leukemia (AML). *Treatment of AIDS-related neutropenia; chronic, severe neutropenia, drug-induced neutropenia; myelodysplastic syndrome.*

STORAGE/HANDLING

Refrigerate. Do not shake vial. Use 1 dose/vial, do not reenter vial. Stable for up to 24 hrs at room temperature (provided vial contents are clear, contain no particulate matter). Remains stable if accidentally exposed to freezing temperature.

SUBQ/IV ADMINISTRATION

May be given by SubQ bolus injection or short IV infusion (15–30 min) or by continuous SubQ or IV infusion.

INDICATIONS/DOSAGE/ROUTES

Note: Begin at least 24 hrs after last dose of chemotherapy, discontinue at least 24 hrs prior to next dose of chemotherapy.

Myelosuppressive:
SubQ/IV or SubQ Infusion: Adults, elderly: Initially, 5 mcg/kg/day. May increase by 5 mcg/kg for each chemotherapy cycle based on duration/severity of absolute neutrophil count (ANC) nadir.
Note: Begin at least 24 hrs after last dose of chemotherapy and at least 24 hrs after bone marrow infusion.

BMT:
IV or SubQ Infusion: Adults, elderly: 10 mcg/kg/day. Adjust dose daily during period of neutrophil recovery based on neutrophil response.

Mobilize progenitor cells:
IV/SubQ: Adults: 10 mcg/kg/day beginning at least 4 days before first leukapheresis and continuing until last leukapheresis.

PRECAUTIONS

CONTRAINDICATIONS: Hypersensitivity to *Escherichia coli*–derived proteins, 24 hrs before or after cytotoxic chemotherapy, use w/other drugs that may result in lowered platelet count. **CAUTIONS:** Concurrent use w/my-

coloid properties. **PREGNAN-CY/LACTATION:** Unknown if drug crosses placenta or is distributed in breast milk. **Pregnancy Category C.**

INTERACTIONS

DRUG INTERACTIONS: None significant. **ALTERED LAB VALUES:** May increase alkaline phosphatase, LDH, uric acid, leukocyte (LAP) scores.

SIDE EFFECTS

FREQUENT (>10%): Bone pain, mild to severe (occurs more frequently in those receiving high dose via IV form, less frequently in low dose, SubQ form), nausea, vomiting, alopecia, diarrhea, fever, fatigue. **OCCASIONAL (5–10%):** Anorexia, dyspnea, headache, cough, skin rash. **RARE (<5%):** Psoriasis, hematuria/proteinuria, osteoporosis.

ADVERSE REACTIONS/TOXIC EFFECTS

Chronic administration occasionally produces chronic neutropenia, splenomegaly. Thrombocytopenia, MI arrhythmias occur rarely. Adult respiratory distress syndrome may occur in septic pts.

NURSING IMPLICATIONS
Baseline Assessment:

A CBC, platelet count (differential) should be obtained before initiation of therapy and twice weekly thereafter.

Intervention/Evaluation:

In septic pts, be alert to adult respiratory distress syndrome. Closely monitor those w/preexisting cardiac conditions. Monitor B/P (transient decrease in B/P may occur).

finasteride
fin-**ah**-stir-eyd
(Propecia, Proscar)

CANADIAN AVAILABILITY: Propecia, Proscar

CLASSIFICATION
5-alpha reductase inhibitor

AVAILABILITY (Rx)
Tablets: 1 mg, 5 mg

PHARMACOKINETICS

	ONSET	PEAK	DURATION
PO	24 hrs	1–2 days	5–7 days

Rapidly absorbed from GI tract. Widely distributed. Metabolized in liver. Half-life: 6–8 hrs.

ACTION/*THERAPEUTIC EFFECT*

Inhibits steroid 5-alpha reductase, an intracellular enzyme that converts testosterone into dihydrotestosterone (DHT) in the prostate gland, providing a reduction in serum DHT, *regressing the enlarged prostate gland.*

USES

Reduce risk of acute urinary retention, need for surgery in symptomatic benign prostatic hypertrophy (BPH). Most improvement noted in hesitancy, feeling of incomplete bladder emptying, interruption of urinary stream, difficulty initiating flow, dysuria, impaired size and force of urinary stream. Treatment for hair loss.

PO ADMINISTRATION

1. Do not break or crush film-coated tablets.
2. May take w/o regard to meals.

INDICATIONS/DOSAGE/ROUTES

Benign prostatic hypertrophy:
PO: **Adults, elderly:** 5 mg once daily (minimum 6 mos).

Hair loss:
PO: **Adults:** 1 mg daily.

PRECAUTIONS

CONTRAINDICATIONS: Physical handling of tablet in those who may become, or are, pregnant, exposure to semen in those who may become pregnant. **CAUTIONS:** Liver function abnormalities. **PREGNANCY/LACTATION:** Physical handling of tablet in those who may become, or are, pregnant. Exposure to semen in those who may become pregnant may harm male fetus. **Pregnancy Category X.**

INTERACTIONS

DRUG INTERACTIONS: None significant. **ALTERED LAB VALUES:** Produces decrease in serum prostate-specific antigen (PSA) levels (even in presence of prostate cancer).

SIDE EFFECTS

OCCASIONAL (2–4%): Impotence, decreased libido, gynecomastia, decreased volume of ejaculate.

ADVERSE REACTIONS/TOXIC EFFECTS

None significant.

NURSING IMPLICATIONS

BASELINE ASSESSMENT:

Digital rectal exam, serum PSA determination should be performed in those w/benign prostatic hypertrophy before initiating therapy and periodically thereafter.

INTERVENTION/EVALUATION:

Diligent monitoring of I&O, esp. in those w/large residual urinary volume or severely diminished urinary flow for obstructive uropathy.

PATIENT/FAMILY TEACHING:

Pt should be aware of potential impotence. May not notice improved urinary flow even if prostate gland shrinks, need to take medication >6 mos, and it is not known if medication decreases need for surgery. Regular visits to physician and monitoring tests are necessary. Because of potential risk to male fetus, a woman who is or may become pregnant should not handle tablets or be exposed to pt's semen. Volume of ejaculate may be decreased during treatment (decrease does not interfere w/sexual function).

flavoxate

flay-**vocks**-ate
(Urispas)

CANADIAN AVAILABILITY:
Urispas

CLASSIFICATION

Antispasmodic

AVAILABILITY (Rx)

Tablets: 100 mg

PHARMACOKINETICS

Well absorbed from GI tract. Primarily excreted in urine.

ACTION/ *THERAPEUTIC EFFECT*

Relaxes detrusor and other smooth muscle by cholinergic blockade, counteracting muscle spasm of urinary tract. *Produces anticholinergic, local anesthetic, analgesic effects.*

USES

Symptomatic relief of dysuria, urgency, nocturia, frequency, incontinence associated w/cystitis, prostatitis, urethritis, urethrocystitis, or urethrotrigonitis.

PO ADMINISTRATION

May be given w/o regard to food.

INDICATIONS/DOSAGE/ROUTES

Urinary antispasmodic:
PO: Adults, elderly, adolescent: 100–200 mg 3–4 times/day.

PRECAUTIONS

CONTRAINDICATIONS: GI tract obstructive disease, GI hemorrhage, paralytic ileus, obstructive uropathy. **CAUTIONS:** None significant. **PREGNANCY/LACTATION:** Pregnancy Category B.

INTERACTIONS

DRUG INTERACTIONS: None significant. **ALTERED LAB VALUES:** None significant.

SIDE EFFECTS

Generally well tolerated. Side effects usually mild and transient. **FREQUENT:** Drowsiness, dry mouth, throat. **OCCASIONAL:** Constipation, difficult urination, blurred vision, dizziness, headache, increased light sensitivity, nausea, vomiting, stomach pain. **RARE:** Confusion (primarily in elderly), hypersensitivity, increase intraocular pressure, leukopenia.

ADVERSE REACTIONS/TOXIC EFFECTS

Anticholinergic effect w/overdose (unsteadiness, severe dizziness, drowsiness, fever, flushed face, shortness of breath, nervousness, irritability).

NURSING IMPLICATIONS

BASELINE ASSESSMENT:

Assess dysuria, urgency, frequency, incontinence, or suprapubic pain.

INTERVENTION/EVALUATION:

Monitor for symptomatic relief. Observe elderly esp. for mental confusion.

PATIENT/FAMILY TEACHING:

Avoid driving or other tasks requiring alertness, coordination, or manual dexterity (blurred vision, drowsiness). Dry mouth may be relieved by sips of water, sugarless gum, or hard candy.

---

flecainide acetate

fleh-kun-eyed
(Tambocor)

CANADIAN AVAILABILITY:
Tambocor

CLASSIFICATION

Antiarrhythmic

AVAILABILITY (Rx)

Tablets: 50 mg, 100 mg, 150 mg

PHARMACOKINETICS

Completely absorbed from GI tract. Widely distributed. Metabolized in liver. Primarily excreted in urine. Minimal removal by hemodialysis. Half-life: 12–27 hrs (increased in decreased renal, liver function, CHF).

ACTION/THERAPEUTIC EFFECT

Slows atrial, AV, His-Purkinje, intraventricular conduction *(decreases excitability, conduction velocity, automaticity)*. Greatest effect on His-Purkinje system.

USES

Prevention of documented life-threatening ventricular arrhythmias, paroxysmal supraventricular tachycardias (PSVT) without structural heart disease, and paroxysmal atrial fibrillation (PAF).

PO ADMINISTRATION

1. Scored tablets may be crushed.
2. Monitor EKG for cardiac changes, particularly widening of QRS, prolongation of PR interval. Notify physician of any significant interval changes.

INDICATIONS/DOSAGE/ROUTES

Life-threatening ventricular arrhythmias, sustained ventricular tachycardia:
PO: Adults, elderly: Initially, 100 mg q12h, increased by 100 mg (50 mg 2 times/day) every 4 days until effective dose or maximum of 400 mg/day attained.

PSVT, PAF:
PO: Adults, elderly: Initially, 50 mg q12h, increased by 100 mg (50 mg 2 times/day) every 4 days until effective dose or maximum of 300 mg/day attained. **Dose in pts w/CHF or myocardial dysfunction:** Initially, 50–100 mg q12h. Increase by 50 mg 2 times/day every 4 days up to 200 mg q12h (400 mg/day). **Dose in pts w/renal or hepatic impairment:** Initially, 100 mg q12h increased at intervals greater than 4 days. Creatinine clearance <35 ml/min/m² dose is reduced by 25–50%.

PRECAUTIONS

CONTRAINDICATIONS: Cardiogenic shock, preexisting second- or third-degree AV block, right bundle branch block (w/o presence of pacemaker). **CAUTIONS:** Impaired myocardial function, second- or third-degree AV block (w/pacemaker), CHF, sick-sinus syndrome. **PREGNANCY/LACTATION:** Unknown if drug crosses placenta. May be distributed in breast milk. **Pregnancy Category C**.

INTERACTIONS

DRUG INTERACTIONS: Urinary acidifiers may increase excretion; urinary alkalizers may decrease excretion. Other antiarrhythmics may have additive effects. Beta blockers may increase negative inotropic effects. May increase digoxin concentrations. **ALTERED LAB VALUES:** None significant.

SIDE EFFECTS

Note: Most effects appear mild, transient. **FREQUENT (>10%):** Dizziness, dyspnea, visual disturbances. **OCCASIONAL (3–10%):** Headache, nausea, fatigue, palpitations, chest pain, asthenia (loss of strength), tremor, constipation, abdominal pain. **RARE (1–3%):** Vomiting, diarrhea, decreased appetite, dry mouth, insomnia, eye pain, fever.

ADVERSE REACTIONS/TOXIC EFFECTS

Has ability to worsen existing arrhythmias or produce new ones. May also produce or worsen CHF. Overdosage may increase QRS duration, QT interval and conduction disturbances, reduce myocardial contractility, conduction disturbances, hypotension.

NURSING IMPLICATIONS
BASELINE ASSESSMENT:

Obtain medication history (esp other antiarrhythmics), cardiovascular history. Assess liver function studies.

INTERVENTION/EVALUATION:

Assess pulse for strength/weakness, irregular rate. Monitor EKG for cardiac changes, particularly widening of QRS, prolongation of PR interval. Notify physician of any significant interval changes. Question for visual disturbances, headache, GI upset. Monitor fluid and electrolyte serum levels. Assess for evidence of CHF: dyspnea (particularly on exertion or lying down), night cough, peripheral edema, distended neck veins. Monitor I&O (increase in weight, decrease in urine output may indicate CHF). Assess hand movement for sign of tremor. Monitor for therapeutic serum level (0.2–1 mcg/ml).

PATIENT/FAMILY TEACHING:

Side effects generally disappear w/continued use or decreased dosage. Do not abruptly discontinue medication. Compliance w/therapy regimen is essential to control arrhythmias. Do not use nasal decongestants, OTC cold preparations (stimulants) w/o physician approval. Restrict salt, alcohol intake. Use caution driving and in tasks requiring mental alertness (may cause dizziness).

floxuridine
flocks-**your**-ih-deen
(FUDR)

CLASSIFICATION
Antineoplastic

AVAILABILITY (Rx)
Injection (preservative free): 100 mg/ml. **Powder for Injection:** 500 mg.

PHARMACOKINETICS
Metabolized in liver, tissues to active metabolites. After continuous intra-arterial infusion primarily converted to FUDR-MP; converted to 5-fluorouracil after IV or intra-arterial injection. Partially crosses blood-brain barrier. Active metabolites localized intracellularly. Excreted via lungs, urine.

ACTION/*THERAPEUTIC EFFECT*
Inhibits action of thymidylate synthetase, an essential component of DNA, RNA synthesis, *inducing cell death.* Cell cycle-specific for S phase cell division.

USES/*UNLABELED*
Palliative management of GI adenocarcinoma metastatic to liver. *Treatment of breast, cervical, ovarian, bladder, renal, prostate carcinoma.*

STORAGE/HANDLING
Note: May be carcinogenic, mutagenic, or teratogenic. Handle w/extreme care during preparation/administration.

Reconstituted solutions stable for 2 wks, if refrigerated.

INTRA-ARTERIAL ADMINISTRATION
Note: Give by continuous intra-arterial infusion via catheter inserted into arterial blood supply of tumor.

1. Reconstitute each 500 mg vial w/5 ml sterile water for injection to provide concentration of 100 mg/ml.
2. Further dilute w/5% dex-

trose or 0.9% NaCl to volume appropriate for specific infusion apparatus used.

INDICATIONS/DOSAGE/ROUTES

Note: Dosage individualized based on clinical response, tolerance to adverse effects. When used in combination therapy, consult specific protocols for optimum dosage, sequence of drug administration.

Intra-arterial Infusion: Adults: 0.1–0.6 mg/kg/day (0.4–0.6 mg/kg/day for hepatic artery infusion). Continue therapy until toxicity or as long as response continues.

PRECAUTIONS

CONTRAINDICATIONS: Poor nutritional state, depressed bone marrow function (WBC less than 5,000/mm³ and/or platelet count less than 100,000/mm³), serious infection. **EXTREME CAUTION:** Previous high-dose pelvic irradiation therapy or alkylating agents, impaired liver, kidney function. **PREGNANCY/LACTATION:** If possible, avoid use during pregnancy, esp. first trimester. Breastfeeding not recommended. **Pregnancy Category D.**

INTERACTIONS

DRUG INTERACTIONS: Bone marrow depressants may increase bone marrow depression. Live virus vaccines may potentiate virus replication, increase vaccine side effects, decrease pt's antibody response to vaccine. **ALTERED LAB VALUES:** May increase SGOT (AST), SGPT (ALT), alkaline phosphatase, LDH, bilirubin. Interferes w/bromosulfophthalein (BSP) test, prothrombin, sedimentation rate assays.

SIDE EFFECTS

FREQUENT: Nausea, vomiting, diarrhea, leukopenia, anemia, localized erythema, anorexia, abdominal cramping, thrombocytopenia, alopecia, rash, pruritus. **OCCASIONAL:** Duodenal ulcer, gastritis, glossitis, pharyngitis, ataxia, blurred vision, vertigo, weakness, mental depression, lethargy.

ADVERSE REACTIONS/TOXIC EFFECTS

Toxicity manifested as stomatitis, enteritis. Hepatic arterial infusion associated w/sclerosis of bile ducts, cirrhosis of liver.

NURSING IMPLICATIONS

BASELINE ASSESSMENT:

Notify physician if WBC falls below 3,500 mm³ or rapidly decreases, platelet count falls below 100,000/mm³, intractable vomiting, diarrhea, stomatitis, GI bleeding occurs (drug may need to be discontinued).

INTERVENTION/EVALUATION:

Monitor leukocyte, platelet counts diligently. Check for stomatitis (burning/erythema of oral mucosa at inner margin of lips, sore throat, difficulty swallowing). May lead to ulceration within 2–3 days. Avoid IM and SubQ injections or rectal temperatures; other trauma. Apply direct pressure to venipuncture sites for full 5 min. Assess intra-arterial site for signs of bleeding, infection, or catheter displacement. Monitor I&O, food tolerance, and stool frequency/consistency. Assess vital signs. Use infusion pump to overcome pressure and provide consistent rate of infusion.

PATIENT/FAMILY TEACHING:

Maintain fastidious but gentle oral hygiene. Do not have immunizations w/o physician's approval (drug lowers body's resistance). Avoid contact w/those who have recently received live virus vaccine. Promptly report fever, sore throat, signs of local infection, easy bruising, unusual bleeding from any site. Increase fluids. Do not take medications or alcohol w/o consulting physician. Contact physician if nausea/vomiting continue at home.

fluconazole

flu-**con**-ah-zole
(Diflucan)

CANADIAN AVAILABILITY:
Diflucan

CLASSIFICATION

Antifungal

AVAILABILITY (Rx)

Tablets: 50 mg, 100 mg, 150 mg, 200 mg. **Powder for Oral Suspension:** 10 mg/ml, 40 mg/ml. **Injection:** 2 mg/ml (in 100 or 200 ml containers).

PHARMACOKINETICS

Well absorbed from GI tract. Widely distributed (including CSF). Partially metabolized in liver. Primarily excreted unchanged in urine. Partially removed by hemodialysis. Half-life: 20–50 hrs (increased in reduced renal function).

ACTION/ *THERAPEUTIC EFFECT*

Directly damages fungal membrane, altering membrane function. Interferes w/cytochrome (necessary for ergosterol formation). *Fungistatic.*

USES/ *UNLABELED*

Treatment of oropharyngeal, esophageal, vaginal candidiasis, serious systemic candidal infections (e.g., urinary tract infections, peritonitis, pneumonia), *Cryptococcus neoformans* meningitis. Prevent candidiasis in bone marrow transplants. *Treatment of coccidiomycosis, cryptococcosis, onychomycosis, fungal pneumonia/septicemia, ringworm of the hand.*

STORAGE/HANDLING

Store at room temperature. Do not use parenteral form if solution is cloudy, precipitate forms, seal is not intact, or it is discolored.

PO/IV ADMINISTRATION

PO:

1. Give w/o regard to meals.
2. Not affected by gastric pH.
3. Oral and IV therapy equally effective; IV therapy for pt intolerant of the drug or unable to take orally.

IV:

1. Do not remove from outer wrap until ready to use.
2. Squeeze inner bag to check for minute leaks.
3. Discard if solution is cloudy or precipitate is noted.
4. Do not add supplementary medication.
5. Plastic containers are not to be used in series connections (could cause air embolism).
6. Maximum flow rate is 200 mg/hr.

INDICATIONS/DOSAGE/ROUTES

Oropharyngeal candidiasis:
PO/IV: Adults, elderly: Initially, 200 mg once, then 100 mg/day for at least 14 days. **Children:** Initially,

6 mg/kg/day once, then 3 mg/kg/day.

Esophageal candidiasis:
PO/IV: Adults, elderly: 200 mg once, then 100 mg/day (up to 400 mg/day) for 21 days and at least 14 days following resolution of symptoms. **Children:** 6 mg/kg/day once, then 3 mg/kg/day (up to 12 mg/kg/day).

Vaginal candidiasis:
PO: Adults: 150 mg once.

Candidiasis prevention:
PO: Adults: 400 mg/day.

Systemic candidiasis:
PO/IV: Adults, elderly: Initially, 400 mg once, then 200 mg/day (up to 400 mg/day) for at least 28 days and at least 14 days following resolution of symptoms. **Children:** 6–12 mg/kg/day.

Cryptococcal meningitis:
PO/IV: Adults, elderly: Initially, 400 mg once, then 200 mg/day (up to 400 mg/day). Continue for 10–12 wks after CSF becomes negative (200 mg/day for suppression of relapse in pts w/AIDS). **Children:** 12 mg/kg/day once, then 6–12 mg/kg/day; 6 mg/kg/day for suppression.

Onychomycosis:
PO: Adults: 150 mg weekly.

Dosage in renal impairment:
After loading dose of 400 mg, daily dose based on creatinine clearance:

CREATININE CLEARANCE	% OF RECOMMENDED DOSE
>50	100
21–50	50
11–20	25
Dialysis	Dose after dialysis

PRECAUTIONS

CONTRAINDICATIONS: Hypersensitivity to fluconazole or any component of preparation. **CAUTIONS:** Hepatic impairment. Hypersensitivity to other triazoles (e.g., itraconazole, terconazole) or imidazoles (butoconazole, ketoconazole, etc.). **PREGNANCY/LACTATION:** Unknown if excreted in breast milk. **Pregnancy Category C.**

INTERACTIONS

DRUG INTERACTIONS: May increase concentration, effects of oral hypoglycemics. High doses increase cyclosporine concentration. May decrease metabolism of phenytoin, warfarin. Rifampin may increase metabolism. May decrease metabolism; increase cisapride concentration, risk of cardiotoxicity. **ALTERED LAB VALUES:** May increase SGOT (AST), SGPT (ALT), alkaline phosphatase, bilirubin.

SIDE EFFECTS

OCCASIONAL (1–4%): Hypersensitivity reaction (fever, chills, rash, itching), dizziness, drowsiness, headache, constipation, diarrhea, nausea, vomiting, abdominal pain.

ADVERSE REACTIONS/TOXIC EFFECTS

Exfoliative skin disorders, serious hepatic effects, blood dyscrasias (eosinophilia, thrombocytopenia, anemia, leukopenia) have been reported rarely.

NURSING IMPLICATIONS
Baseline Assessment:

Question for hypersensitivity to fluconazole or components of preparation. Confirm that a culture or histologic test was done for accurate diagnosis; therapy may begin before results are known. Establish baselines for CBC, potassium.

INTERVENTION/EVALUATION:

Monitor hepatic function tests; be alert for hepatotoxicity: dark urine, pale stools, anorexia/nausea/vomiting, yellow skin or sclera. Report rash, itching promptly. Check CBC and potassium lab results. Evaluate food tolerance. Monitor temperature at least daily. Determine pattern of bowel activity, stool consistency. Assess for dizziness and provide assistance as needed.

PATIENT/FAMILY TEACHING:

Do not drive car, machinery if dizziness, drowsiness occur. Notify physician of dark urine, pale stool, yellow skin/eyes or rash w/or w/o itching. Pts w/oropharyngeal infections should be taught good oral hygiene. Consult physician before taking any other medication.

fludarabine phosphate

flew-**dare**-ah-bean
(Fludara)

CANADIAN AVAILABILITY:
Fludara

CLASSIFICATION

Antineoplastic

AVAILABILITY (Rx)

Injection: 50 mg

PHARMACOKINETICS

Rapidly dephosphorylated in serum, then phosphorylated intracellularly to active triphosphate. Primarily excreted in urine. Half-life: 10 hrs.

ACTION/THERAPEUTIC EFFECT

Interferes w/DNA polymerase alpha, ribonucleotide reductase, and DNA primase, *inhibiting DNA synthesis, inducing cell death.*

USES

Treatment of chronic lymphocytic leukemia in pt who has not responded to or has progressed w/another standard alkylating agent.

STORAGE/HANDLING

Store in refrigerator. Handle w/extreme care during preparation and administration. If contact w/skin or mucous membranes, wash thoroughly w/soap and water; rinse eyes profusely w/plain water. After reconstitution, use within 8 hrs; discard unused portion.

IV ADMINISTRATION

Note: Give by IV infusion. Do not add to other IV infusions. Avoid small veins, swollen or edematous extremities, areas overlying joints, tendons.

1. Reconstitute 50 mg vial w/2 ml sterile water for injection to provide a concentration of 25 mg/ml.

2. Further dilute w/100–125 ml 0.9% NaCl or 5% dextrose and infuse over 30 min.

INDICATIONS/DOSAGE/ROUTES

Note: Dosage is individualized on basis of clinical response and tolerance to adverse effects. When used in combination therapy, consult specific protocols for optimum dosage, sequence of drug administration. Dosage based on pt's actual weight. Use ideal body weight in obese or edematous pts.

Chronic lymphocytic leukemia:
IV: Adults: 25 mg/m² daily for 5

consecutive days. Continue up to 3 additional cycles. Begin each course of treatment every 28 days.

PRECAUTIONS

CONTRAINDICATIONS: None significant. **CAUTIONS:** Impaired renal function. **PREGNANCY/LACTATION:** If possible, avoid use during pregnancy, esp. first trimester. May cause fetal harm. Not known whether distributed in breast milk. Breast-feeding not recommended. **Pregnancy Category D**.

INTERACTIONS

DRUG INTERACTIONS: May decrease effect of antigout medications. Bone marrow depressants may increase risk of bone marrow depression. Live virus vaccines may potentiate virus replication, increase vaccine side effects, decrease pt's antibody response to vaccine. **ALTERED LAB VALUES:** May increase uric acid, alkaline phosphatase, SGOT (AST).

SIDE EFFECTS

OCCASIONAL: Anorexia, nausea, diarrhea, peripheral edema, dry skin, rash, erythema, aches/pains, confusion, chilliness, fatigue, weakness, sinusitis. **RARE:** Paresthesia, headaches, hearing loss, visual disturbances, urinary difficulties, GI bleeding.

ADVERSE REACTIONS/TOXIC EFFECTS

Pneumonia occurs frequently. Severe bone marrow toxicity (anemia, thrombocytopenia, neutropenia) may occur, evidenced by fever, chills, infection, nausea, vomiting, fatigue, anorexia, weakness. High dosage may produce acute leukemia, blindness, coma.

NURSING IMPLICATIONS

BASELINE ASSESSMENT:

Drug should be discontinued if intractable vomiting, diarrhea, stomatitis, GI bleeding occurs.

INTERVENTION/EVALUATION:

Monitor CBC, platelet, differential count, serum creatinine routinely. Assess for weakness, agitation, confusion, visual disturbances, peripheral neuropathy. Assess lung sounds for evidence of pneumonia. Monitor for dyspnea, cough, rapidly falling WBC and/or intractable diarrhea, GI bleeding (bright red or tarry stool). Avoid IM, SubQ injections; protect from trauma; do not take rectal temperatures. Apply direct pressure to IV sites for full 5 min. Assess oral mucosa for mucosal erythema, ulceration at inner margin of lips, sore throat, difficulty swallowing (stomatitis). Assess skin for rash. Monitor for and report diarrhea. Check food tolerance, provide antiemetics as needed. Be alert to possible tumor lysis syndrome (onset w/flank pain and hematuria). This syndrome may include hypercalcemia, hyperphosphatemia, hyperuricemia and result in renal failure.

PATIENT/FAMILY TEACHING:

Avoid crowds and exposure to infection. Do not take alcohol or other medications w/o consulting physician. Maintain fastidious oral hygiene. Do not have immunizations w/o physician's approval (drug lowers body's resistance). Promptly report fever, sore throat, signs of local infection, easy bruising, unusual bleeding from any site. Contact physician if nausea/vomiting continues at home.

fludrocortisone

floo-droe-**kor**-tih-sone
(Florinef)

CANADIAN AVAILABILITY:
Florinef

CLASSIFICATION

Mineralocorticoid

AVAILABILITY (Rx)

Tablets: 0.1 mg

PHARMACOKINETICS

Well absorbed from GI tract. Widely distributed. Metabolized in liver, kidney. Primarily excreted in urine. Half-life: 3.5 hrs.

ACTION/ THERAPEUTIC EFFECT

High mineralocorticoid, moderate glucocorticoid activity. Acts at distal tubules to *increase potassium, hydrogen ion excretion, sodium reabsorption, and water retention.*

USES/ UNLABELED

Partial replacement therapy for primary and secondary adrenocortical insufficiency in Addison's disease. Adjunctive treatment of salt-losing forms of congenital adrenogenital syndrome. *Treatment of idiopathic orthostatic hypotension, acidosis in renal tubular disorders.*

PO ADMINISTRATION

1. Give w/food or milk.
2. Administer w/glucocorticoid.

INDICATIONS/DOSAGE/ROUTES

Addison's disease:
PO: Adults, elderly: 0.05–0.1 mg/day. **Range:** 0.1 mg 3 times/wk–0.2 mg/day. Administration w/cortisone/hydrocortisone preferred.

Salt-losing adrenogenital syndrome:
PO: Adults, elderly: 0.1–0.2 mg/day.

PRECAUTIONS

CONTRAINDICATIONS: Hypersensitivity to fludrocortisone, any condition except those requiring high mineralocorticoid activity. **CAUTIONS:** CHF, hypertension, renal insufficiency. Prolonged therapy should be discontinued slowly. **PREGNANCY/LACTATION:** Not known whether drug crosses placenta or is distributed in breast milk. **Pregnancy Category C.**

INTERACTIONS

DRUG INTERACTIONS: May increase digoxin toxicity (hypokalemia). Hepatic enzyme inducers (e.g., phenytoin) may increase metabolism. Hypokalemia-causing medications may increase effect. Sodium-containing medication may increase sodium, edema, B/P. **ALTERED LAB VALUES:** May increase sodium. May decrease potassium, hematocrit.

SIDE EFFECTS

FREQUENT: Increased appetite, exaggerated sense of well-being, abdominal distention, weight gain, insomnia, mood swings. *High dose, prolonged therapy, too rapid withdrawal:* Increased susceptibility to infection (signs/symptoms masked); delayed wound healing, hypokalemia, hypocalcemia, GI distress, diarrhea or constipation, hypertension. **OCCASIONAL:** Headache (frontal or occipital), dizziness, menstrual difficulty or amenorrhea, ulcer development. **RARE:** Hypersensitivity reaction.

ADVERSE REACTIONS/TOXIC EFFECTS

Long-term therapy: muscle wasting (esp. arms, legs), osteoporosis, spontaneous fractures, amenorrhea, cataracts, glaucoma, peptic ulcer, CHF. *Abrupt withdrawal following long-term therapy:* anorexia, nausea, fever, headache, joint pain, rebound inflammation, fatigue, weakness, lethargy, dizziness, orthostatic hypotension.

NURSING IMPLICATIONS

BASELINE ASSESSMENT:

Question for hypersensitivity to any corticosteroids. Obtain baselines for weight, B/P, blood glucose, electrolytes, chest x-ray, EKG.

INTERVENTION/EVALUATION:

Monitor I&O, daily weight. Check B/P, pulse at least 2 times/day. Assess for signs of edema. Monitor blood glucose and electrolytes. Provide assistance w/ambulation, notify physician of dizziness. Be alert to signs/symptoms of hypokalemia (weakness and muscle cramps, numbness/tingling, esp. lower extremities, nausea and vomiting, irritability, EKG changes). Evaluate food tolerance and bowel activity; report hyperacidity promptly. Assess emotional status, ability to sleep. Assess for infection: fever, sore throat, vague symptoms.

PATIENT/FAMILY TEACHING:

Take w/food or milk. Usually given in conjunction w/glucocorticoids, electrolytes. Carry identification of drug and dose, physician name and phone number. Do not change dose/schedule or stop taking drug; must taper off gradually under medical supervision. Notify physician of fever, sore throat, muscle aches, sudden weight gain/swelling, continuing headaches. W/dietician give instructions for prescribed diet (usually high potassium). Maintain careful personal hygiene, avoid exposure to disease or trauma. Severe stress (serious infection, surgery, or trauma) may require increased dosage. Do not take aspirin or any other medication w/o consulting physician. Follow-up visits, lab tests are necessary; children must be assessed for growth retardation. Inform dentist or other physicians of fludrocortisone therapy now or within past 12 mos.

flumazenil

flew-**maz**-ah-nil
(Romazicon)

CANADIAN AVAILABILITY:
Anexate

CLASSIFICATION

Benzodiazepine receptor antagonist

AVAILABILITY (Rx)

Injection: 0.1 mg/ml

PHARMACOKINETICS

	ONSET	PEAK	DURATION
IV	1–2 min	6–10 min	—

Duration, degree of benzodiazepine reversal related to dosage, plasma concentration. Metabolized by liver; excreted in urine.

ACTION/THERAPEUTIC EFFECT

Antagonizes sedation, impairment of recall and psychomotor impairment due to benzodiazepine activity on CNS.

USES

Complete or partial reversal of sedative effects of benzodiazepines when general anesthesia has been induced and/or maintained w/benzodiazepines, when sedation has been produced w/benzodiazepines for diagnostic and therapeutic procedures, management of benzodiazepine overdosage.

STORAGE/HANDLING

Store parenteral form at room temperature. Discard after 24 hrs once medication is drawn into syringe, is mixed w/any solutions, or if particulate or discoloration is noted.

IV ADMINISTRATION

Note: Compatible w/5% dextrose in water, lactated Ringer's, 0.9% NaCl solutions.

1. Rinse spilled medication from skin w/cool water.

2. Administer through freely running IV infusion into large vein (local injection produces pain, inflammation at injection site).

INDICATIONS/DOSAGE/ROUTES

Reversal of conscious sedation, in general anesthesia:
IV: Adults, elderly: Initially, 0.2 mg (2 ml) over 15 secs; may repeat 0.2 mg dose in 45 secs; then at 60 sec intervals. **Maximum:** 1 mg (10 ml total dose).
Note: If resedation occurs, repeat dose at 20 min intervals. **Maximum:** 1 mg (given as 0.2 mg/min) at any one time, 3 mg in any 1 hr.

Benzodiazepine overdose:
IV: Adults, elderly: Initially, 0.2 mg (2 ml) over 30 secs; may repeat after 30 secs w/0.3 mg (3 ml) over 30 secs if desired level of consciousness not achieved. Further doses of 0.5 mg (5 ml) over 30 secs may be administered at 60 sec intervals. **Maximum:** 3 mg (30 ml) total dose.
Note: If resedation occurs, repeat dose at 20 min intervals. **Maximum:** 1 mg (given as 0.5 mg/min) at any one time, 3 mg in any 1 hr.

PRECAUTIONS

CONTRAINDICATIONS: History of hypersensitivity to benzodiazepines, in those who have been given a benzodiazepine for control of a potentially life-threatening condition (control of intracranial pressure, status epilepticus), those showing signs of serious cyclic antidepressant overdose manifested by motor abnormalities, dysrhythmias, anticholinergic signs, cardiovascular collapse. **CAUTIONS:** Head injury, impaired hepatic function, alcoholism, drug dependency. **PREGNANCY/LACTATION:** Not known whether drug crosses placenta or is distributed in breast milk. Not recommended during labor, delivery. **Pregnancy Category C**.

INTERACTIONS

DRUG INTERACTIONS: Seizure-induced medications may increase risk of seizures. **ALTERED LAB VALUES:** None significant.

SIDE EFFECTS

FREQUENT (3–11%): Agitation, anxiety, dry mouth, dyspnea, insomnia, palpitations, tremors, headache, blurred vision, dizziness, ataxia, nausea, vomiting, pain at injection site, increased sweating. **OCCASIONAL (1–3%):** Fatigue, flushing, hearing disturbances, thrombophlebitis, skin rash. **RARE (<1%):** Hives, itching, hallucinations.

ADVERSE REACTIONS/TOXIC EFFECTS

May produce onset of seizures (particularly those on long-term benzodiazepine use), overdosage, concurrent sedative-hypnotic drug withdrawal, recent therapy w/repeated doses of parenteral benzodiazepine, myoclonic jerking, concurrent cyclic antidepressant poisoning. May provoke panic attack in those w/history of panic disorder.

NURSING IMPLICATIONS

BASELINE ASSESSMENT:

Arterial blood gases should be obtained before and at 30 min intervals during IV administration. Prepare to intervene in reestablishing airway, assisting ventilation (drug may not fully reverse ventilatory insufficiency induced by benzodiazepines). Note that effects of flumazenil may wear off before effects of benzodiazepines.

INTERVENTION/EVALUATION:

Properly manage airway, assisted breathing, circulatory access and support, internal decontamination by lavage and charcoal, adequate clinical evaluation. Monitor for reversal of benzodiazepine effect. Assess for possible resedation, respiratory depression, hypoventilation. Assess closely for return of unconsciousness (narcosis) for at least 1 hr after pt is fully alert.

PATIENT/FAMILY TEACHING:

Avoid tasks that require alertness, motor skills, ingestion of alcohol, or taking nonprescription drugs until at least 18–24 hrs after discharge.

flunisolide
flew-**nis**-oh-lide
(AeroBid, Nasalide, Nasarel)

CANADIAN AVAILABILITY:
Bronalide aerosol, Rhinalar

CLASSIFICATION

Corticosteroid

AVAILABILITY (Rx)

Aerosol: 250 mcg/activation. **Nasal Spray:** 25 mcg/activation.

PHARMACOKINETICS

Minimally absorbed from pulmonary, nasal, and GI tissue. Primarily metabolized in liver, lung. Primarily excreted in urine. Half-life: 1–1.5 hrs (nasal: 1–2 hrs).

ACTION/*THERAPEUTIC EFFECT*

Decreases number, activity of anti-inflammatory cells. *Inhibits bronchoconstriction, produces smooth muscle relaxation. Decreases immediate and late-phase allergic reactions.*

USES/*UNLABELED*

Inhalation: Control of bronchial asthma in those requiring chronic steroid therapy. *Intranasal:* Relief of symptoms of seasonal/perennial rhinitis. *Prevent recurrence of postsurgical nasal polyps.*

INHALATION/INTRANASAL ADMINISTRATION

INHALATION:

1. Shake container well; exhale completely; holding mouth-

piece 1 inch away from lips, inhale and hold breath as long as possible before exhaling; then exhale slowly.

2. Wait 1 min between inhalations when multiple inhalations ordered (allows for deeper bronchial penetration).

3. Rinse mouth w/water immediately after inhalation (prevents mouth/throat dryness).

INTRANASAL:

1. Clear nasal passages before use (topical nasal decongestants may be needed 5–15 min before use).

2. Tilt head slightly forward.

3. Insert spray tip up in 1 nostril, pointing toward inflamed nasal turbinates, away from nasal septum.

4. Pump medication into 1 nostril while holding other nostril closed and concurrently inspire through nose.

5. Discard used nasal solution after 3 mos.

INDICATIONS/DOSAGE/ROUTES

Usual inhalation dosage:
Inhalation: Adults, elderly: 2 inhalations 2 times/day, morning and evening. **Maximum:** 4 inhalations 2 times/day. **Children (6–15 yrs):** 2 inhalations 2 times/day.

Usual intranasal dosage:
Note: Improvement seen within few days; may take 3 wks. Do not continue beyond 3 wks if no significant improvement occurs.
Intranasal: Adults, elderly: Initially, 2 sprays each nostril 2 times/day, may increase to 2 sprays 3 times/day. **Maximum:** 8 sprays each nostril/day. **Children (6–14 yrs):** Initially, 1 spray 3 times/day or 2 sprays 2 times/day. **Maximum:** 4 sprays each nostril/day.

Maintenance: Smallest amount to control symptoms.

PRECAUTIONS

CONTRAINDICATIONS: Hypersensitivity to any corticosteroid or components, primary treatment of status asthmaticus, systemic fungal infections, persistently positive sputum cultures for *Candida albicans.* **CAUTIONS:** Adrenal insufficiency. **PREGNANCY/LACTATION:** Not known whether drug crosses placenta or is distributed in breast milk. **Pregnancy Category C.**

INTERACTIONS

DRUG INTERACTIONS: None significant. **ALTERED LAB VALUES:** None significant.

SIDE EFFECTS

FREQUENT: *Inhalation* (10–25%): Unpleasant taste, nausea, vomiting, sore throat, diarrhea, upset stomach, cold symptoms, nasal congestion. **OCCASIONAL:** *Inhalation* (3–9%): Dizziness, irritability, nervousness, shakiness, abdominal pain, heartburn, fungal infection in mouth, pharynx, larynx, edema. *Intranasal:* Mild nasopharyngeal irritation, dryness, rebound congestion, bronchial asthma, rhinorrhea, loss of sense of taste.

ADVERSE REACTIONS/TOXIC EFFECTS

Acute hypersensitivity reaction (urticaria, angioedema, severe bronchospasm) occurs rarely. Transfer from systemic to local steroid therapy may unmask previously suppressed bronchial asthma condition.

NURSING IMPLICATIONS
BASELINE ASSESSMENT:

Question for hypersensitivity

to any corticosteroids, components. Offer emotional support (high incidence of anxiety due to difficulty in breathing and sympathomimetic response to drug).

INTERVENTION/EVALUATION:

In those receiving bronchodilators by inhalation concomitantly w/steroid inhalation therapy, advise pts to use bronchodilator several minutes before corticosteroid aerosol (enhances penetration of steroid into bronchial tree). Monitor rate, depth, rhythm, type of respiration; quality and rate of pulse. Assess lung sounds for rhonchi, wheezing, rales. Monitor arterial blood gases. Observe lips, fingernails for blue or dusky color in light-skinned pts; gray in dark-skinned pts. Observe for clavicular retractions, hand tremor. Evaluate for clinical improvement (quieter, slower respirations, relaxed facial expression, cessation of clavicular retractions).

PATIENT/FAMILY TEACHING:

Do not change dose schedule or stop taking drug; must taper off gradually under medical supervision. Maintain careful mouth hygiene. Rinse mouth w/water immediately after inhalation (prevents mouth/throat dryness, fungal infection of mouth). Contact physician/nurse if sore throat/mouth occurs. Increase fluid intake (decreases lung secretion viscosity). Do not take more than 2 inhalations at any one time (excessive use may produce paradoxical bronchoconstriction or a decreased bronchodilating effect). Avoid excessive use of caffeine derivatives (chocolate, coffee, tea, cola).

fluocinolone acetonide
(Flurosyn, Synalar, Synemol)

fluocinonide
(Lidex, Vasoderm)
See Classification section under: Corticosteroids: topical.

fluoride
flur-eyd
(Fluoritab, Luride)

CANADIAN AVAILABILITY:
Fluor-A-Day, Fluotic

CLASSIFICATION
Dietary supplement

AVAILABILITY (OTC)
Tablets (Chewable): 0.5 mg, 1 mg. **Oral Drops:** 0.125 mg/drop, 0.25 mg/drop.

PHARMACOKINETICS
Rapid, completely absorbed from GI tract. Concentrated primarily in bone, developing teeth. Primarily excreted in urine.

ACTION/*THERAPEUTIC EFFECT*
Increases tooth resistance to acid dissolution by *promoting remineralization of decalcified enamel, inhibiting dental plaque bacteria, increasing resistance to development of caries.* Maintains bone strength.

USES
Dietary supplement for prevention of dental caries in children. Treatment of osteoporosis.

PO ADMINISTRATION

1. May take w/o regard to food.
2. May crush chewable tablets. Liquid: Avoid glass (causes etching of glass), may mix w/cereal, juice, food.

INDICATIONS/DOSAGE/ROUTES

Dietary supplement:
WATER

FLUORIDE	AGE	MG/DAY
<0.3 ppm	<2 yrs	0.25 mg/day
	2–3 yrs	0.5 mg/day
	3–13 yrs	1 mg/day
0.3–0.7 ppm	<2 yrs	None
	2–3 yrs	0.25 mg/day
	3–13 yrs	0.5 mg/day
>0.7 ppm	None	None

Osteoporosis:
PO: **Adults, elderly:** 50–75 mg/day in divided doses.

PRECAUTIONS

CONTRAINDICATIONS: Arthralgia, GI ulceration, severe renal insufficiency. **CAUTIONS:** None significant. **PREGNANCY/LACTATION:** Readily crosses placenta; minimal amount distributed in breast milk.

INTERACTIONS

DRUG INTERACTIONS: Aluminum hydroxide, calcium may decrease absorption. **ALTERED LAB VALUES:** May increase SGOT (AST), alkaline phosphatase.

SIDE EFFECTS

Generally well tolerated. Side effects usually mild and transient. **RARE:** Oral mucous membrane ulceration.

ADVERSE REACTIONS/TOXIC EFFECTS

Hypocalcemia, tetany, bone pain (esp. ankles, feet), electrolyte disturbances, arrhythmias, may cause cardiac failure, respiratory arrest. May cause skeletal fluorosis, osteomalacia, osteosclerosis.

NURSING IMPLICATIONS
PATIENT/FAMILY TEACHING:

Use only as directed and keep out of reach of children to avoid overdosage. Do not take w/milk or other dairy products (decreases absorption). Rinses and gels should be used at bedtime after brushing or flossing. Expectorate excess—do not swallow. Do not eat, drink, or rinse mouth after application.

fluorouracil

phlur-oh-**your**-ah-sill
(Adrucil, Efudex, Fluoroplex)

CANADIAN AVAILABILITY:
Adrucil, Efudex, Fluoroplex

CLASSIFICATION

Antineoplastic

AVAILABILITY (Rx)

Injection: 50 mg/ml. **Cream:** 1%, 5%. **Topical Solution:** 1%, 2%, 5%.

PHARMACOKINETICS

Crosses blood-brain barrier. Widely distributed. Rapidly metabolized in tissues to active metabolite, which is localized intracellularly. Primarily excreted via lungs as carbon dioxide. Half-life: 20 hrs.

ACTION/ *THERAPEUTIC EFFECT*

Blocks formation of thymidylic acid, *inhibiting DNA, RNA synthesis. Topical:* Destroys rapidly proliferating cells. Cell cycle-specific for S phase of cell division.

USES / *UNLABELED*

Parenteral: Treatment of carcinoma of colon, rectum, breast, stomach, pancreas. Used in combination w/levamisole after surgical resection in patients w/Duke's stage C colon cancer. *Topical:* Treatment of multiple actinic or solar keratoses, superficial basal cell carcinomas. *Systemic: Treatment of bladder, prostate, ovarian, cervical, endometrial, lung, liver, head/neck carcinomas; treatment of pericardial, peritoneal, pleural effusions. Topical: Treatment of actinic cheilitis, radiodermatitis.*

STORAGE / HANDLING

Note: May be carcinogenic, mutagenic, or teratogenic. Handle w/extreme care during preparation/administration.

Solution appears colorless to faint yellow. Slight discoloration does not adversely affect potency or safety. If precipitate forms, redissolve by heating, shaking vigorously; allow to cool to body temperature.

IV ADMINISTRATION

Note: Give by IV injection or IV infusion. Do not add to other IV infusions. Avoid small veins, swollen or edematous extremities, areas overlying joints, tendons.

1. IV injection does not need to be diluted or reconstituted.

2. Give IV injection slowly over 1–2 min.

3. Apply prolonged pressure to IV injection site if thrombocytopenia is demonstrated by platelet count.

4. For IV infusion, further dilute with 5% dextrose or 0.9% NaCl and infuse over 30 min–24 hrs.

5. Extravasation produces immediate pain, severe local tissue damage. Notify physician and apply ice packs to area.

INDICATIONS / DOSAGE / ROUTES

Note: Dosage is individualized on basis of clinical response and tolerance to adverse effects. When used in combination therapy, consult specific protocols for optimum dosage, sequence of drug administration. Dosage based on pt's actual weight. Use ideal body weight in obese or edematous pts.

Initial course:
IV: Adults: 12 mg/kg daily for 4 consecutive days; if no toxicity, then 6 mg/kg on days 6, 8, 10, and 12. Do not exceed 800 mg/day. **Adults, poor risk:** 6 mg/kg daily for 3 consecutive days; if no toxicity, then 3 mg/kg on days 5, 7, and 9. Do not exceed 400 mg/day. Repeat at 30 day intervals after last dose of previous schedule.

Maintenance:
IV: Adults: 10–15 mg/kg 1 time/ week not to exceed 1 g/week. Reduce dosage in poor-risk pts.

Usual topical dosage:
Topical: Adults: Apply 2 times/ day to cover lesions.

PRECAUTIONS

CONTRAINDICATIONS: Poor nutritional status, depressed bone marrow function, potentially serious infections, major surgery within previous month. **CAUTIONS:** History of high-dose pelvic irradiation, metastatic cell infiltration of bone marrow, impaired hepatic, renal function. **PREGNANCY/ LACTATION:** If possible, avoid use during pregnancy, esp. first trimester. May cause fetal harm. Not known whether distributed in breast milk. Breast-feeding not recommended. **Pregnancy Category D**.

INTERACTIONS

DRUG INTERACTIONS: Bone marrow depressant may increase risk of bone marrow depression. Live virus vaccines may potentiate virus replication, increase vaccine side effects, decrease pt's antibody response to vaccine. **ALTERED LAB VALUES:** May decrease albumin. May increase excretion of 5-HIAA in urine. *Topical:* May cause eosinophilia, leukocytosis, thrombocytopenia, toxic granulation.

SIDE EFFECTS

OCCASIONAL: Anorexia, diarrhea, minimal alopecia, fever, dry skin, fissuring, scaling, erythema. *Topical:* pain, pruritus, hyperpigmentation, irritation, inflammation, burning at application site. **RARE:** Nausea, vomiting, anemia, esophagitis, proctitis, GI ulcer, confusion, headache, lacrimation, visual disturbances, angina, allergic reactions.

ADVERSE REACTIONS/TOXIC EFFECTS

Earliest sign of toxicity (4–8 days after beginning of therapy) is stomatitis (dry mouth, burning sensation, mucosal erythema, ulceration at inner margin of lips). Most common dermatologic toxicity is pruritic rash (generally appears on extremities, less frequently on trunk). Leukopenia generally occurs within 9–14 days after drug administration (may occur as late as 25th day). Thrombocytopenia occasionally occurs within 7–17 days after administration. Hematologic toxicity may also manifest itself as pancytopenia, agranulocytosis.

NURSING IMPLICATIONS

BASELINE ASSESSMENT:

Monitor hematology test results. Drug should be discontinued if intractable vomiting, diarrhea, stomatitis, GI bleeding occurs.

INTERVENTION/EVALUATION:

Monitor for rapidly falling WBC and/or intractable diarrhea, GI bleeding (bright red or tarry stool). Assess oral mucosa for mucosal erythema, ulceration of inner margin of lips, sore throat, difficulty swallowing (stomatitis). Assess skin for rash, check for diarrhea.

PATIENT/FAMILY TEACHING:

Transient alopecia may occur. Contraceptive measures should be used during therapy. Drink plenty of fluids. Maintain fastidious oral hygiene. Do not have immunizations w/o physician's approval (drug lowers body's resistance). Avoid contact w/those who have recently taken oral polio vaccine. Promptly report fever, sore throat, signs of local infection, easy bruising, unusual bleeding from any site. Contact physician if diarrhea, nausea/vomiting continue at home. Avoid ultraviolet rays w/topical or parenteral therapy. *Topical:* Apply only to affected area. Do not use occlusive coverings. Be careful near eyes, nose, and mouth. Wash hands thoroughly after application. Treated areas may be unsightly for several weeks after therapy.

fluoxetine hydrochloride

flew-**ox**-eh-teen
(Prozac)

CANADIAN AVAILABILITY:
Novo-Fluoxetine, Prozac

CLASSIFICATION

Antidepressant

AVAILABILITY (Rx)

Capsules: 10 mg, 20 mg. **Liquid:** 20 mg/5 ml. **Tablets:** 10 mg.

PHARMACOKINETICS

Well absorbed from GI tract. Crosses blood-brain barrier. Metabolized in liver to active metabolite. Primarily excreted in urine. Half-life: 2–3 days; metabolite: 7–9 days.

ACTION/*THERAPEUTIC EFFECT*

Selectively inhibits serotonin uptake in CNS, enhancing serotonergic function. *Resulting enhancement of synaptic activity produces antidepressant effect.*

USES

Outpatient treatment of major depression exhibited as persistent, prominent dysphoria (occurring nearly every day for at least 2 wks) manifested by 4 of 8 symptoms: change in appetite, change in sleep pattern, increased fatigue, impaired concentration, feelings of guilt or worthlessness, loss of interest in usual activities, psychomotor agitation or retardation, or suicidal tendencies. Treatment of obsessive-compulsive disorder (OCD). Treatment of panic disorder, premenstrual disorder, bulimia.

PO ADMINISTRATION

Give w/food or milk if GI distress occurs.

INDICATIONS/DOSAGE/ROUTES

Note: Use lower or less frequent doses in those w/renal, hepatic impairment, elderly, those w/concurrent disease or on multiple medications.

Depression, OCD:
PO: Adults: Initially, 20 mg each morning. If therapeutic improvement does not occur after 2 wks, gradually increase dose to maximum 80 mg/day in 2 equally divided doses in morning, noon. **Elderly:** Initially, 10 mg/day. May increase by 10–20 mg q2wks. Avoid administration at night.

Bulimia:
PO: Adults: 60 mg once daily in morning.

PRECAUTIONS

CONTRAINDICATIONS: Within 14 days of MAO inhibitor ingestion. **CAUTIONS:** Impaired renal or hepatic function. **PREGNANCY/LACTATION:** Not known whether drug crosses placenta or is distributed in breast milk. **Pregnancy Category B**.

INTERACTIONS

DRUG INTERACTIONS: Alcohol, CNS depressants antagonize CNS depressant effect. May displace highly protein-bound medications from protein-binding sites (e.g., oral anticoagulants). MAO inhibitors may produce serotonin syndrome. May increase phenytoin concentration, toxicity. **ALTERED LAB VALUES:** None significant.

SIDE EFFECTS

FREQUENT (>10%): Headache, asthenia (loss of strength), inability to sleep, anxiety, nervousness, drowsiness, nausea, diarrhea, decreased appetite. **OCCASIONAL (2–9%):** Dizziness, tremor, fatigue, vomiting, constipation, dry mouth, abdominal pain, nasal congestion, increased sweating. **RARE (<2%):** Flushed skin, lightheadedness, decreased ability to concentrate.

ADVERSE REACTIONS/TOXIC EFFECTS

Overdosage may produce seizures, nausea, vomiting, excessive agitation, restlessness.

NURSING IMPLICATIONS

BASELINE ASSESSMENT:

For those on long-term therapy, liver/renal function tests, blood counts should be performed periodically.

INTERVENTION/EVALUATION:

Supervise suicidal risk pt closely during early therapy (as energy level improves, suicide potential increases). Assess appearance, behavior, speech pattern, level of interest, mood. Assist w/ambulation if dizziness occurs. Monitor stool frequency and consistency. Assess skin for appearance of rash.

PATIENT/FAMILY TEACHING:

Maximum therapeutic response may require 4 or more wks of therapy. Dry mouth may be relieved by sugarless gum, sips of tepid water. Report visual disturbances. Do not abruptly discontinue medication. Avoid tasks that require alertness, motor skills until response to drug is established. Avoid alcohol.

fluoxymesterone

floo-ox-ih-**mes**-teh-rone
(**Android-F, Halotestin**)

FIXED-COMBINATION(S):
W/ethinyl estradiol, an estrogen
(**Halodrin**)

CANADIAN AVAILABILITY:
Halotestin

CLASSIFICATION

Androgen

AVAILABILITY (Rx)

Tablets: 2 mg, 5 mg, 10 mg

PHARMACOKINETICS

Metabolized in liver. Primarily excreted in urine. Half-life: 9.2 hrs.

ACTION/ *THERAPEUTIC EFFECT*

Suppresses gonadotropin-releasing hormone, LH, and FSH. *Stimulates spermatogenesis, development of male secondary sex characteristics, sexual maturation at puberty.* Stimulates production of RBCs.

USES/ *UNLABELED*

Treatment of delayed puberty; testicular failure due to cryptorchidism, bilateral orchism, orchitis, vanishing testis syndrome, or orchidectomy; hypogonadotropic hypogonadism due to pituitary/hypothalamic injury (tumors, trauma, or radiation), idiopathic gonadotropin or LHRH deficiency. Palliative therapy in women 1–5 years past menopause w/advancing, inoperable metastatic breast cancer or premenopausal women who have benefited from oophorectomy and have a hormone-responsive tumor. Prevention of postpartum breast pain and engorgement. In combination w/estrogens for management of moderate to severe vasomotor symptoms associated w/menopause when estrogens alone are not effective. *Treatment of anemia.*

PO ADMINISTRATION

Take w/food if GI upset occurs.

INDICATIONS/DOSAGE/ROUTES

Males (hypogonadism):
PO: Adults: 5–20 mg/day.

Males (delayed puberty):
PO: Adults: 2.5–20 mg/day for 4–6 mos.

Females (inoperable breast cancer):
PO: Adults: 10–40 mg/day in divided doses for 1–3 mos.

Females (prevent postpartum breast pain/engorgement):
PO: Adults: Initially, 2.5 mg shortly after delivery, then 5–10 mg/day in divided doses for 4–5 days.

PRECAUTIONS

CONTRAINDICATIONS: Hypersensitivity to drug or components of preparation, serious cardiac, renal, or hepatic dysfunction. Do not use for men w/carcinomas of the breast or prostate. **CAUTIONS:** Decreased renal or liver function, benign prostate hypertrophy, hypercalcemia (may be aggravated in pts w/metastatic breast cancer), history of myocardial infarction, diabetes mellitus. **PREGNANCY/ LACTATION:** Contraindicated during lactation. **Pregnancy Category X.**

INTERACTIONS

DRUG INTERACTIONS: May increase effect of oral anticoagulants. Hepatotoxic medications may increase hepatotoxicity. **ALTERED LAB VALUES:** May increase alkaline phosphatase, SGOT (AST), bilirubin, calcium, potassium, sodium, Hgb, Hct, LDL. May decrease HDL.

SIDE EFFECTS

FREQUENT: *Females:* Amenorrhea, virilism (e.g., acne, decreased breast size, enlarged clitoris, male pattern baldness), deepening voice. *Males:* UTI, breast soreness, gynecomastia, priapism, virilism (e.g., acne, early pubic hair growth). **OCCASIONAL:** Edema, nausea, vomiting, mild acne, diarrhea, stomach pain. *Males:* Impotence, testicular atrophy. **RARE:** Hepatic necrosis, leukopenia.

ADVERSE REACTIONS/TOXIC EFFECTS

Peliosis hepatitis (liver, spleen replaced w/blood-filled cysts), hepatic neoplasms, and hepatocellular carcinoma have been associated w/prolonged high dosage.

NURSING IMPLICATIONS

BASELINE ASSESSMENT:

Question for hypersensitivity to drug or components (sensitivity to aspirin may indicate tartrazine sensitivity). Establish baseline weight, B/P, Hgb, Hct. Check liver function test results, electrolytes, and cholesterol if ordered. Wrist x-rays may be ordered to determine bone maturation in children.

INTERVENTION/EVALUATION:

Weigh daily and report weekly gain of more than 5 lbs; evaluate for edema. Monitor I&O. Check B/P at least 2 times/day. Assess electrolytes, cholesterol, Hgb, Hct (periodically for high dosage), liver function test results. W/ breast cancer or immobility, check for hypercalcemia (lethargy, muscle weakness, confusion, irritability). Assure adequate intake of protein, calories. Be alert to signs of virilization. Monitor sleep patterns. Assess for hepatitis: nausea, yellowing of eyes and skin, dark urine, light stools.

PATIENT/FAMILY TEACHING:

Regular visits to physician and monitoring tests are necessary. Do not take any other medications w/o consulting physician. Teach diet high in protein, calories. Food may be tolerated better in small, frequent feedings. Weigh daily, report weekly gain of 5 lbs or more. Teach signs of jaundice; notify physician if these, nausea, vomiting, acne, ankle swelling occur. *Female:* Promptly report menstrual irregularities, hoarseness, deepening of voice. *Male:* Report frequent erections, difficulty urinating, gynecomastia.

fluphenazine decanoate

flew-**phen**-ah-zeen
(Prolixin)

fluphenazine enanthate

(Prolixin)

fluphenazine hydrochloride

(Prolixin, Permitil)

CANADIAN AVAILABILITY:
Apo-Fluphenazine, Moditen

CLASSIFICATION

Antipsychotic

AVAILABILITY (Rx)

Tablets: 1 mg, 2.5 mg, 5 mg, 10 mg. **Elixir:** 2.5 mg/5 ml. **Oral Concentrate:** 5 mg/ml. **Injection:** 2.5 mg/ml.

PHARMACOKINETICS

Variably absorbed after oral administration; well absorbed after IM administration. Metabolized in liver to active metabolites. Primarily excreted in urine. Half-life: 33 hrs.

ACTION/*THERAPEUTIC EFFECT*

Antagonizes dopamine neurotransmission at synapses by blocking postsynaptic dopaminergic receptors in brain, *decreasing psychotic behavior.* Produces weak anticholinergic, sedative, antiemetic effects, strong extrapyramidal activity.

USES/*UNLABELED*

Management of psychotic disturbances (schizophrenia, delusions, hallucinations). *Treatment of neurogenic pain (adjunct to tricyclic antidepressants).*

STORAGE/HANDLING

Store oral and parenteral form at room temperature. Yellow discoloration of solution does not affect potency, but discard if markedly discolored or if precipitate forms.

PO/IM ADMINISTRATION

PO:

1. Mix oral concentrate w/ water, carbonated orange or lemon-lime drink, milk, vegetable, pineapple, apricot, prune, orange, tomato, grapefruit juice.

2. Do not mix oral concentrate w/caffeine (coffee, cola), tea, apple

juice because of physical incompatibility.

IM:

Note: Pt must remain recumbent for 30–60 min in head-low position w/legs raised, to minimize hypotensive effect.

    1. Use a dry 21 gauge needle, syringe for administering fluphenazine decanoate or enanthate (wet needle and syringe turn solution cloudy).

    2. Inject slow, deep IM into upper outer quadrant of gluteus maximus. If irritation occurs, further injections may be diluted w/0.9% NaCl or 2% procaine hydrochloride.

    3. Massage IM injection site to reduce discomfort.

INDICATIONS/DOSAGE/ROUTES

Psychotic disorders:
PO: Adults: Initially, 0.5–10 mg/day fluphenazine HCl in divided doses q6–8h. Increase gradually until therapeutic response is achieved (usually under 20 mg daily); decrease gradually to maintenance level (1–5 mg/day).
Elderly: Initially, 1–2.5 mg/day.
IM: Adults: Initially, 1.25 mg, followed by 2.5–10 mg/day in divided doses q6–8h.

Chronic schizophrenic disorder:
IM: Adults: Initially, 12.5–25 mg of fluphenazine decanoate q1–6 wks, or 25 mg fluphenazine enanthate q2wks.

Usual elderly dosage (nonpsychotic):
PO: Initially, 1–2.5 mg/day. May increase by 1–2.5 mg/day q4–7 days. **Maximum:** 20 mg/day.

PRECAUTIONS

CONTRAINDICATIONS: Severe CNS depression, comatose states, severe cardiovascular disease, bone marrow depression, subcortical brain damage. **CAUTIONS:** Impaired respiratory/hepatic/renal/cardiac function, alcohol withdrawal, history of seizures, urinary retention, glaucoma, prostatic hypertrophy, hypocalcemia (increased susceptibility to dystonias). **PREGNANCY/LACTATION:** Crosses placenta; distributed in breast milk. **Pregnancy Category C.**

INTERACTIONS

DRUG INTERACTIONS: Alcohol, CNS depressants may increase CNS, respiratory depression, hypotensive effects. Tricyclic antidepressants, MAO inhibitors may increase sedative, anticholinergic effects. Antithyroid agents may increase risk of agranulocytosis. Extrapyramidal symptoms (EPS) may increase w/EPS-producing medications. Hypotensives may increase hypotension. May decrease levodopa effects. Lithium may decrease absorption, produce adverse neurologic effects. **ALTERED LAB VALUES:** May produce false-positive pregnancy test, PKU. EKG changes may occur, including Q and T wave disturbances.

SIDE EFFECTS

FREQUENT: Hypotension, dizziness, and fainting occur frequently after first injection, occasionally after subsequent injections, and rarely w/oral dosage. **OCCASIONAL:** Drowsiness during early therapy, dry mouth, blurred vision, lethargy, constipation or diarrhea, nasal congestion, peripheral edema, urinary retention. **RARE:** Ocular changes, skin pigmentation (those on high doses for prolonged periods).

ADVERSE REACTIONS/TOXIC EFFECTS

Extrapyramidal symptoms appear dose related (particularly high dosage), divided into 3 categories: akathisia (inability to sit still, tapping of feet, urge to move around); parkinsonian symptoms (mask-like face, tremors, shuffling gait, hypersalivation); and acute dystonias: torticollis (neck muscle spasm), opisthotonos (rigidity of back muscles), and oculogyric crisis (rolling back of eyes). Dystonic reaction may also produce profuse sweating, pallor. Tardive dyskinesia (protrusion of tongue, puffing of cheeks, chewing/puckering of the mouth) occurs rarely (may be irreversible). Abrupt withdrawal after long-term therapy may precipitate nausea, vomiting, gastritis, dizziness, tremors. Blood dyscrasias, particularly agranulocytosis, mild leukopenia (sore mouth/gums/throat) may occur. May lower seizure threshold.

NURSING IMPLICATIONS
BASELINE ASSESSMENT:

Avoid skin contact w/solution (contact dermatitis). Assess behavior, appearance, emotional status, response to environment, speech pattern, thought content.

INTERVENTION/EVALUATION:

Monitor B/P for hypotension. Assess for extrapyramidal symptoms. Monitor WBC, differential count for blood dyscrasias. Monitor for fine tongue movement (may be early sign of tardive dyskinesia). Supervise suicidal risk pt closely during early therapy (as depression

lessens, energy level improves, increasing suicide potential). Assess for therapeutic response (interest in surroundings, improvement in self-care, increased ability to concentrate, relaxed facial expression).

PATIENT/FAMILY TEACHING:

Full therapeutic effect may take up to 6 wks. Urine may darken. Do not abruptly withdraw from long-term drug therapy. Report visual disturbances. Sugarless gum, sips of tepid water may relieve dry mouth. Drowsiness generally subsides during continued therapy. Avoid tasks that require alertness, motor skills until response to drug is established. Avoid alcohol.

---

flurandrenolide
(Cordran)
See Classification section under: Corticosteroids: topical

---

flurazepam hydrochloride
flur-**aye**-zah-pam
(Dalmane)

CANADIAN AVAILABILITY:
Apo-Flurazepam, Dalmane

CLASSIFICATION

Sedative-hypnotic (**Schedule IV**)

AVAILABILITY (Rx)

Capsules: 15 mg, 30 mg

PHARMACOKINETICS

	ONSET	PEAK	DURATION
PO	15–45 min	—	7–8 hrs

Well absorbed from GI tract. Crosses blood-brain barrier. Widely distributed. Metabolized in liver to active metabolite. Primarily excreted in urine. Half-life: 2.3 hrs; metabolite: 40–114 hrs.

ACTION/ *THERAPEUTIC EFFECT*

Enhances action of inhibitory neurotransmitter gamma-aminobutyric acid (GABA), *producing hypnotic effect due to CNS depression.*

USES

Short-term treatment of insomnia (up to 4 wks). Reduces sleep-induction time, number of nocturnal awakenings; increases length of sleep.

PO ADMINISTRATION

1. Give w/o regard to meals.
2. Capsules may be emptied and mixed w/food.

INDICATIONS/DOSAGE/ROUTES

Insomnia:
PO: Adults: 15–30 mg at bedtime. **Elderly/debilitated/liver disease/low serum albumin:** 15 mg at bedtime.

PRECAUTIONS

CONTRAINDICATIONS: Acute narrow-angle glaucoma, acute alcohol intoxication. **CAUTIONS:** Impaired renal/hepatic function. **PREGNANCY/LACTATION:** Crosses placenta; may be distributed in breast milk. Chronic ingestion during pregnancy may produce withdrawal symptoms, CNS depression in neonates. **Pregnancy Category X.**

INTERACTIONS

DRUG INTERACTIONS: Alcohol, CNS depressants may increase CNS depressant effect. **ALTERED LAB VALUES:** None significant.

SIDE EFFECTS

FREQUENT: Drowsiness, dizziness, ataxia, sedation. Morning drowsiness may occur initially. **OCCASIONAL:** Dizziness, GI disturbances, nervousness, blurred vision, dry mouth, headache, confusion, skin rash, irritability, slurred speech. **RARE:** Paradoxical CNS excitement/restlessness (particularly noted in elderly/debilitated).

ADVERSE REACTIONS/TOXIC EFFECTS

Abrupt or too rapid withdrawal may result in pronounced restlessness and irritability, insomnia, hand tremors, abdominal/muscle cramps, sweating, vomiting, seizures. Overdosage results in somnolence, confusion, diminished reflexes, coma.

NURSING IMPLICATIONS

BASELINE ASSESSMENT:

Assess B/P, pulse, respirations immediately before administration. Raise bed rails. Provide environment conducive to sleep (back rub, quiet environment, low lighting).

INTERVENTION/EVALUATION:

Assist w/ambulation. Assess for paradoxical reaction, particularly during early therapy. Evaluate for therapeutic response: decrease in number of nocturnal awakenings, increase in length of sleep duration.

PATIENT/FAMILY TEACHING:

Smoking reduces drug effectiveness. Do not abruptly withdraw medication after long-term use. Avoid alcohol. May have disturbed sleep 1–2 nights after discontinuing. Use caution driving, performing other tasks requiring alertness. Notify physician if pregnant or planning to become pregnant.

flurbiprofen

fleur-bih-pro-fen
(Ansaid)

flurbiprofen sodium

(Ocufen)

CANADIAN AVAILABILITY:
Ansaid, Froben, Ocufen

CLASSIFICATION

Nonsteroidal anti-inflammatory

AVAILABILITY (Rx)

Tablets: 50 mg, 100 mg. **Ophthalmic Solution:** 0.03%.

PHARMACOKINETICS

Well absorbed from GI tract, penetrates cornea after ophthalmic administration (may be systemically absorbed). Widely distributed. Metabolized in liver. Primarily excreted in urine. Half-life: 3–4 hrs.

ACTION / THERAPEUTIC EFFECT

Produces analgesic and anti-inflammatory effect by inhibiting prostaglandin synthesis, *reducing inflammatory response and intensity of pain stimulus reaching sensory nerve endings.* Prevents, reduces miosis by relaxing iris sphincter.

USES

Symptomatic treatment of acute and/or chronic rheumatoid arthritis, osteoarthritis; inhibits intraoperative miosis.

PO/OPHTHALMIC ADMINISTRATION

PO:

1. Do not crush or break enteric-coated form.
2. May give w/food, milk, or antacids if GI distress occurs.

OPHTHALMIC:

Place finger on lower eyelid and pull out until pocket is formed between eye and lower lid. Hold dropper above pocket and place prescribed number of drops into pocket. Close eye gently. Apply digital pressure to lacrimal sac for 1–2 min (minimizes drainage into nose and throat, reducing risk of systemic effects). Remove excess solution w/tissue.

INDICATIONS/DOSAGE/ROUTES

Rheumatoid arthritis, osteoarthritis:
PO: Adults, elderly: 200–300 mg/day in 2–4 divided doses. Do not give >100 mg/dose or 300 mg/day.

Usual ophthalmic dosage:
Ophthalmic: Adults, elderly: Apply 2 drops into conjunctival sac 3, 2, and 1 hr before surgery or 2 drops q4h while pt is awake day before surgery.

PRECAUTIONS

CONTRAINDICATIONS: Active peptic ulcer, GI ulceration, chronic inflammation of GI tract, GI bleeding disorders, history of hypersensitivity to aspirin or NSAIDs. **CAUTIONS:** Impaired renal/hepatic function, history of GI tract disease, predisposition to fluid retention, those wearing soft contact lenses, surgical pts w/bleeding tendencies. **PREGNANCY/LACTATION:** Crosses placenta; not known whether distributed in breast milk. Avoid use during last trimester (may adversely affect fetal cardiovascular system: premature closure of ductus arteriosus). **Pregnancy Category B.** (Category D if used in 3rd trimester or near delivery.) *Ophthalmic:* **Pregnancy Category C**.

INTERACTIONS

DRUG INTERACTIONS: May increase effects of oral anticoagulants, heparin, thrombolytics. May decrease effect of antihypertensives, diuretics. Salicylates, aspirin may increase risk of GI side effects, bleeding. Bone marrow depressants may increase risk of hematologic reactions. May increase concentration, toxicity of lithium. May increase methotrexate toxicity. Probenecid may increase concentration. *Ophthalmic:* May decrease effect of acetylcholine, carbachol. May decrease antiglaucoma effect of epinephrine, other antiglaucoma medications. **ALTERED LAB VALUES:** May increase serum transaminase, alkaline phosphatase, LDH, bleeding time.

SIDE EFFECTS

OCCASIONAL: *Oral (3–9%):* Headache, abdominal pain, diarrhea, indigestion, nausea, fluid retention. *Ophthalmic:* Burning, stinging on instillation, keratitis, elevated intraocular pressure. **RARE (<3%):** Blurred vision, flushed skin, dizziness, drowsiness, nervousness, insomnia, unusual weakness, constipation, decreased appetite, vomiting, confusion.

ADVERSE REACTIONS/TOXIC EFFECTS

Overdosage may result in acute renal failure. In those treated chronically, peptic ulcer, GI bleeding, gastritis, severe hepatic reaction (jaundice), nephrotoxicity (hematuria, dysuria, proteinuria), severe hypersensitivity reaction (bronchospasm, angiofacial edema), cardiac arrhythmias occur rarely.

NURSING IMPLICATIONS

BASELINE ASSESSMENT:

Anti-inflammatory: Assess onset, type, location, and duration of pain or inflammation. Inspect appearance of affected joints for immobility, deformities, and skin condition.

INTERVENTION/EVALUATION:

Monitor for headache, dyspepsia, dizziness. Monitor pattern of daily bowel activity and stool consistency. Evaluate for therapeutic response: relief of pain, stiffness, swelling, increase in joint mobility, reduced joint tenderness, improved grip strength.

PATIENT/FAMILY TEACHING:

Swallow tablet whole; do not crush or chew. Avoid aspirin, alcohol during therapy (increases risk of GI bleeding). If GI upset occurs, take w/food, milk. Report GI distress, visual disturbances, rash, edema, headache. *Ophthalmic:* Eye burning may occur w/instillation.

flutamide
flew-tah-myd
(Eulexin)

CANADIAN AVAILABILITY:
Euflex, Novo-Flutamide

CLASSIFICATION

Antineoplastic

AVAILABILITY (Rx)

Capsules: 125 mg

PHARMACOKINETICS

Completely absorbed from GI tract. Metabolized in liver to active metabolite. Primarily excreted in urine. Half-life: 6 hrs (increase in elderly).

ACTION/THERAPEUTIC EFFECT

Inhibits androgen uptake and/or binding of androgen in tissues. Interferes w/testosterone at cellular level (complements leuprolide, *suppressing testicular androgen production* by inhibiting LH secretion).

USES

Treatment of metastatic carcinoma of prostate (in combination w/ LHRH analogues—i.e., leuprolide). Management of locally confined stage B_2–C and stage D_2.

INDICATIONS/DOSAGE/ROUTES

Prostatic carcinoma:
PO: Adults, elderly: 250 mg q8h.

PRECAUTIONS

CONTRAINDICATIONS: None significant. **CAUTIONS:** None significant.

INTERACTIONS

DRUG INTERACTIONS: None significant. **ALTERED LAB VALUES:** May increase estradiol, testosterone, SGOT (AST), SGPT (ALT), bilirubin, creatinine.

SIDE EFFECTS

FREQUENT: Hot flashes, loss of libido, impotence, diarrhea, nausea/vomiting, gynecomastia. **OCCASIONAL:** Rash, anorexia. **RARE:** Photosensitivity.

ADVERSE REACTIONS/TOXIC EFFECTS

Hepatitis, hypertension may be noted.

NURSING IMPLICATIONS
INTERVENTION/EVALUATION:

Monitor B/P periodically and hepatic function tests in long-term therapy. Check for diarrhea, nausea, and vomiting.

PATIENT/FAMILY TEACHING:

Do not stop taking medication (both drugs must be continued). Explain side effects and action on carcinoma. Contact physician if nausea/vomiting continues at home.

fluticasone propionate

flew-**tih**-cah-sewn
(Flonase, Cutivate, Flovent)

CANADIAN AVAILABILITY:
Flonase, Flovent

CLASSIFICATION

Corticosteroid

AVAILABILITY (Rx)

Cream: 0.05%. **Ointment:** 0.005%. **Intranasal:** 0.05%. **Inhalation:** 44 mcg/actuation, 110 mcg/actuation, 220 mcg/actuation. **Powder for Inhalation:** 50 mcg, 100 mcg, 250 mcg.

PHARMACOKINETICS

Inhalation/intranasal: Undergoes extensive first-pass metabolism in liver. Excreted in urine. Half-life: 3–7.8 hrs. *Topical:* Amount absorbed dependent on drug, area, skin condition (absorption increased w/elevated skin temperature, hydration, inflamed/denuded skin).

ACTION/*THERAPEUTIC EFFECT*

Nasal: Inhibits early activation of inflammatory cells, release of inflammatory mediators, generally on late-phase allergic reactions, *decreasing response to seasonal and perennial rhinitis. Topical:* Stimulates protein synthesis of inhibitory enzymes responsible for anti-inflammatory effects. *Inhalation:* Inhibits inflammatory cascade reducing airway hyper-responsiveness. *Decreases bronchial reactivity inhibiting early/late bronchoconstriction* occurring when exposed to inhaled allergens.

USES

Nasal: Relief of seasonal/perennial allergic rhinitis. *Topical:* Relief of inflammation/pruritus associated w/steroid-responsive disorders (e.g., contact dermatitis, eczema). *Inhalation:* Maintenance treatment of asthma for those requiring oral corticosteroid therapy for asthma. *Powder:* Maintenance of asthma treatment in children 4 yrs and older.

INHALATION/INTRANASAL ADMINISTRATION

INHALATION:

1. Shake container well; exhale completely; holding mouthpiece 1 inch away from lips, inhale and hold breath as long as possible before exhaling; then exhale slowly.

2. Wait 1 min between inhalations when multiple inhalations ordered (allows for deeper bronchial penetration).

3. Rinse mouth w/water immediately after inhalation (prevents mouth/throat dryness).

INTRANASAL:

1. Clear nasal passages before use (topical nasal decongestants may be needed 5–15 min before use).

2. Tilt head slightly forward.

3. Insert spray tip up in 1 nostril, pointing toward inflamed nasal turbinates, away from nasal septum.

4. Pump medication into 1 nostril while holding other nostril closed and concurrently inspire through nose.

5. Discard used nasal solution after 3 mos.

INDICATIONS/DOSAGE/ROUTES

Allergic rhinitis:
Intranasal: Adults, elderly: Initially, 200 mcg (2 sprays each nostril once daily or 1 spray each nostril q12h). **Maintenance:** 1 spray each nostril once daily. **Maximum:** 200 mcg/day. **Children >4 yrs:** Initially, 100 mcg (1 spray each nostril once daily). **Maximum:** 200 mcg/day.

Usual topical dosage:
Topical: Adults, elderly, children > 3 mos: Apply sparingly to affected area 1–2 times/day.

Usual inhalation dosage (dry powder formulation):
Inhalation: Children (4–11 yrs): 50–100 mcg twice daily.

Previous treatment: bronchodilators:
Inhalation: Adults, elderly, children >12 yrs: Initially 88 mcg q12h. **Maximum:** 440 mcg/day.

Previous treatment: inhaled steroids:
Inhalation: Adults, elderly, children >12 yrs: Initially 88–220 mcg q12h. **Maximum:** 440 mcg q12h.

Previous treatment: oral steroids:
Inhalation: Adults, elderly, children >12 yrs: Initially, 880 mcg q12h.

PRECAUTIONS

CONTRAINDICATIONS: Untreated localized infection of nasal mucosa, hypersensitivity of drug or component. *Inhalation:* Primary treatment of status asthmaticus or other acute asthma episodes. **CAUTIONS:** Active or quiescent tuberculosis, untreated fungal, bacterial, or systemic viral infection of ocular herpes simplex. **PREGNANCY/LACTATION:** Unknown if drug crosses placenta or is distributed in breast milk. **Pregnancy Category C**.

INTERACTIONS

DRUG INTERACTIONS: None significant. **ALTERED LAB VALUES:** None significant.

SIDE EFFECTS

FREQUENT: *Inhalation:* Throat irritation, hoarseness, dry mouth, coughing, temporary wheezing, localized fungal infection in mouth, pharynx, larynx (particularly if mouth is not rinsed w/water after each administration). *Intranasal:* Mild nasopharyngeal irritation; nasal irritation, burning, stinging, dryness, rebound congestion, rhinorrhea, loss of sense of taste. **OCCASIONAL:** *Intranasal:* Nasal/pharyngeal candidiasis, headache. *Inhalation:* Oral candidiasis. *Topical:* Burning/itching of skin.

ADVERSE REACTIONS/TOXIC EFFECTS

None significant.

NURSING IMPLICATIONS
BASELINE ASSESSMENT:

Question for hypersensitivity to any fluticasone. Establish baseline assessment of skin disorder, asthma, or rhinitis.

INTERVENTION/EVALUATION:

In those receiving bronchodilators by inhalation concomitantly with inhalation of steroid therapy, advise pt to use bronchodilator several minutes before corticosteroid aerosol (enhances penetration of steroid into bronchial tree). Monitor rate, depth, rhythm, type of respiration; quality and rate of pulse. Assess lung sounds for rhonchi, wheezing, rales. Monitor arterial blood gases. Observe lips, fingernails for blue or dusky color in light-skinned pts; gray in dark-skinned pts. Observe for clavicular retractions, hand tremor. Evaluate for clinical improvement (quieter, slower respirations, relaxed facial expression, cessation of clavicular retractions). *Topical:* Assess involved area for therapeutic response to irritation.

PATIENT/FAMILY TEACHING:

Do not change dose schedule or stop taking drug; must taper off gradually under medical supervision. *Inhalation:* Teach proper use of inhaler. Maintain careful mouth hygiene. Rinse mouth w/water immediately after inhalation (prevents mouth/throat dryness, fungal infection of mouth). Increase fluid intake (decreases lung secretion viscosity). Contact physician/nurse if sore throat or mouth occurs. *Intranasal:* Teach proper use of nasal spray. Clear nasal passages prior to use. Contact physician if no improvement in symptoms, sneezing or nasal irritation occur. Improvement seen in several days. *Topical:* Rub thin film gently into affected area. Use only for prescribed area and no longer than ordered. Report adverse local reaction. Avoid contact w/eyes.

---

fluvastatin

flu-vah-**stah**-tin
(Lescol)

CANADIAN AVAILABILITY:
Lescol

CLASSIFICATION

Antihyperlipoproteinemic

AVAILABILITY (Rx)

Capsules: 20 mg, 40 mg

PHARMACOKINETICS

Well absorbed from GI tract (unaffected by food). Does not cross blood-brain barrier. Primarily eliminated in feces.

ACTION / *THERAPEUTIC EFFECT*

Inhibits HMG-CoA reductase, the enzyme that catalyzes the early step in cholesterol synthesis. *Decreases LDL cholesterol, VLDL, plasma triglycerides.* Increases HDL cholesterol concentration slightly.

USES

Adjunct to diet therapy to decrease elevated total and LDL cholesterol concentrations in those w/primary hypercholesterolemia (types IIa and IIb) and in those w/combined hypercholesterolemia, hypertriglyceridemia. Treatment of elevated triglycerides and apolipoprotein.

PO ADMINISTRATION

May give w/o regard to food.

INDICATIONS / DOSAGE / ROUTES

Hyperlipoproteinemia:
PO: Adults, elderly: Initially, 20 mg/day in the evening. May increase up to 40 mg/day. **Maintenance:** 20–40 mg/day in single or divided doses.

PRECAUTIONS

CONTRAINDICATIONS: Hypersensitivity to fluvastatin, active liver disease, unexplained increased serum transaminase. **CAUTIONS:** Anticoagulant therapy, history of liver disease, substantial alcohol consumption. Withholding/discontinuing fluvastatin may be necessary when pt at risk for renal failure (secondary to rhabdomyolysis); major surgery, severe acute infection, trauma, hypotension, severe metabolic, endocrine, or electrolyte disorders, or uncontrolled seizures. **PREGNANCY/LACTATION:** Contraindicated in pregnancy (suppression of cholesterol biosynthesis may cause fetal toxicity) and lactation. Unknown whether drug is distributed in breast milk. **Pregnancy Category X.**

INTERACTIONS

DRUG INTERACTIONS: Increased risk of rhabdomyolysis, acute renal failure w/cyclosporine, erythromycin, gemfibrozil, niacin, other immunosuppressants. **ALTERED LAB VALUES:** May increase creatinine kinase (CK), serum transaminase concentrations.

SIDE EFFECTS

FREQUENT (5–8%): Headache, dyspepsia, back pain, myalgia, arthralgia, diarrhea, abdominal cramping, rhinitis. **OCCASIONAL (2–4%):** Nausea, vomiting, insomnia, constipation, flatulence, rash, fatigue, cough, dizziness.

ADVERSE REACTIONS / TOXIC EFFECTS

Myositis (inflammation of voluntary muscle), w/ or w/o increased

CK, muscle weakness, occurs rarely. May progress to frank rhabdomyolysis and renal impairment.

NURSING IMPLICATIONS
BASELINE ASSESSMENT:

Question for possibility of pregnancy before initiating therapy **(Pregnancy Category X).** Question history of hypersensitivity to fluvastatin. Assess baseline lab results: cholesterol, triglycerides, liver function tests.

INTERVENTION/EVALUATION:

Evaluate food tolerance. Determine pattern of bowel activity. Check for headache, dizziness, blurred vision. Assess for rash, pruritus. Monitor cholesterol and triglyceride lab results for therapeutic response. Be alert for malaise, muscle cramping or weakness. Monitor temperature at least twice a day.

PATIENT/FAMILY TEACHING:

Follow special diet (important part of treatment). Periodic lab tests are essential part of therapy. Do not take other medications w/o physician knowledge. Do not stop medication w/o consulting physician. Report promptly any muscle pain or weakness, esp. if accompanied by fever or malaise. Do not drive or perform activities that require alert response if dizziness occurs.

fluvoxamine maleate

flew-**vox**-ah-meen
(Luvox)

CANADIAN AVAILABILITY:
Luvox

CLASSIFICATION
Antidepressant

AVAILABILITY (Rx)
Tablets: 50 mg, 100 mg

PHARMACOKINETICS
Well absorbed following oral administration. Metabolized in liver (none of metabolites possess actions of parent drug). Primarily excreted in urine. Half-life: 13–15 hrs.

ACTION/THERAPEUTIC EFFECT
Selectively inhibits serotonin neuronal uptake in CNS, *producing antidepressant effect.*

USES/UNLABELED
Treatment of obsessive-compulsive disorder (OCD). *Treatment of depression.*

PO ADMINISTRATION
May give w/o regard to food.

INDICATIONS/DOSAGE/ROUTES
Note: Use lower or less frequent dosing in impaired hepatic function, elderly.

Obsessive-compulsive disorder:
PO: Adults: 50 mg at bedtime, increased by 50 mg q4–7days. Doses >100 mg/day in 2 divided doses. **Maximum:** 300 mg/day. **Children 8–17 yrs:** 25 mg at bedtime, increased by 25 mg q4–7 days. Doses >50 mg/day in 2 divided doses. **Maximum:** 200 mg/day. .

PRECAUTIONS
CONTRAINDICATIONS: Within 14 days of MAO inhibitor ingestion, concurrent astemizole or terfenadine therapy. **CAUTIONS:** Impaired renal or hepatic function, elderly. **PREGNANCY/LACTATION:** Not known whether drug crosses placenta or is distributed in breast milk. **Pregnancy Category C.**

INTERACTIONS

DRUG INTERACTIONS: MAO inhibitors may produce serious reactions (hyperthermia, rigidity, myoclonus). Tryptophan, lithium may enhance serotonergic effects. Tricyclic antidepressants may increase concentration. Fluvoxamine may increase concentration/toxicity of astemizole, benzodiazepines, carbamazepine, clozapine, terfenadine, theophylline. May increase effects of warfarin. **ALTERED LAB VALUES:** None significant.

SIDE EFFECTS

FREQUENT (40%): Nausea **(21–22%):** Headache, somnolence, insomnia. **OCCASIONAL (8–14%):** Nervousness, dizziness, diarrhea/loose stools, dry mouth, asthenia (loss of strength, weakness), dyspepsia, constipation, abnormal ejaculation. **RARE (3–6%):** Anorexia, anxiety, tremor, vomiting, flatulence, urinary frequency, sexual dysfunction, taste change.

ADVERSE REACTIONS/TOXIC EFFECTS

Overdosage may produce seizures, nausea, vomiting, excessive agitation, restlessness.

NURSING IMPLICATIONS

BASELINE ASSESSMENT:

For those on long-term therapy, liver/renal function tests, blood counts should be performed periodically.

INTERVENTION/EVALUATION:

Supervise suicidal risk pt closely during early therapy (as energy level improves, suicide potential increases). Assess appearance, behavior, speech pattern, level of interest, mood. Assist w/ambulation if dizziness occurs. Monitor stool frequency and consistency. Assess skin for appearance of rash.

PATIENT/FAMILY TEACHING:

Change positions slowly to avoid hypotensive effect. Maximum therapeutic response may require 4 or more wks of therapy. Photosensitivity to sun may occur. Dry mouth may be relieved by sugarless gum, sips of tepid water. Report visual disturbances. Do not abruptly discontinue medication. Avoid tasks that require alertness, motor skills until response to drug is established. Avoid alcohol.

folic acid (vitamin B₉)

foe-lick
(Folvite)

sodium folate

(Folvite—parenteral)

CANADIAN AVAILABILITY: Apo-Folic

CLASSIFICATION

Coenzyme

AVAILABILITY (Rx)

Tablets: 0.4 mg, 0.8 mg **(OTC),** 1 mg **(Rx). Injection (Rx):** 5 mg/ml.

PHARMACOKINETICS

Almost completely absorbed from GI tract (upper duodenum). Metabolized in liver, plasma to active form. Excreted in urine. Removed by hemodialysis.

ACTION/*THERAPEUTIC EFFECT*

Stimulates production of red and white blood cells and platelets, *essen-*

tial for nucleoprotein synthesis, maintenance of normal erythropoiesis.

USES/ UNLABELED

Treatment of megaloblastic, macrocytic anemia associated w/pregnancy, infancy, childhood, inadequate dietary intake. *Decreases risk of colon cancer.*

PO/SUBQ/IM/IV ADMINISTRATION

Note: Parenteral form used in acutely ill, parenteral or enteral alimentation, those unresponsive to oral route in GI malabsorption syndrome. Dosage >0.1 mg daily may conceal pernicious anemia.

INDICATIONS/DOSAGE/ROUTES

Deficiency:
PO/IM/IV: **Adults, children:** Up to 1 mg/day.

Supplement:
PO/IM/IV: **Adults, elderly, children >4 yrs:** 0.4 mg/day. **Children <4 yrs:** 0.3 mg/day. **Children <1 yr:** 0.1 mg/day. **Pregnancy:** 0.8 mg/day.

PRECAUTIONS

CONTRAINDICATIONS: Anemias (pernicious, aplastic, normocytic, refractory). **CAUTIONS:** None significant. **PREGNANCY/LACTATION:** Distributed in breast milk. **Pregnancy Category A**. If more than RDA: **Pregnancy Category C**.

INTERACTIONS

DRUG INTERACTIONS: May decrease effects of hydantoin anticonvulsants. Analgesics, anticonvulsants, carbamazepine, estrogens may increase folic acid requirements. Antacids, cholestyramine may decrease absorption. Methotrexate, triamterene, trimethoprim may antagonize effects. **ALTERED LAB VALUES:** May decrease vitamin B$_{12}$ concentration.

SIDE EFFECTS

None significant.

ADVERSE REACTIONS/TOXIC EFFECTS

Allergic hypersensitivity occurs rarely w/parenteral form. Oral folic acid is nontoxic.

NURSING IMPLICATIONS
BASELINE ASSESSMENT:

Pernicious anemia should be ruled out by Schilling test and vitamin B$_{12}$ blood level before therapy is initiated (may produce irreversible neurologic damage). Resistance to treatment may occur if decreased hematopoiesis, alcoholism, antimetabolic drugs or deficiency of vitamin B$_6$, B$_{12}$, C, or E is evident.

INTERVENTION/EVALUATION:

Assess for therapeutic improvement: improved sense of wellbeing, relief from iron deficiency symptoms (fatigue, shortness of breath, sore tongue, headache, pallor).

PATIENT/FAMILY TEACHING:

Take only under medical supervision. Follow diet as ordered. Eat foods rich in folic acid including fruits, vegetables, and organ meats. Report rash or hives promptly.

follitropin alpha
(Gonal-F)
See Supplement

fomivirsen
(Vitravene)
See Supplement
See Classification section under:
Antivirals

foscarnet sodium

fos-**car**-net

(Foscavir)

CLASSIFICATION

Antiviral

AVAILABILITY (Rx)

Injection: 24 mg/ml

PHARMACOKINETICS

Sequestered into bone, cartilage. Primarily excreted unchanged in urine. Removed by hemodialysis. Half-life: 3.3–6.8 hrs (increased in decreased renal function).

ACTION / THERAPEUTIC EFFECT

Provides selective inhibition at binding site on virus-specific DNA polymerases and reverse transcriptases, *inhibiting replication of herpes virus.*

USES / UNLABELED

Treatment of CMV retinitis in pts w/AIDS; in combination w/ganciclovir for relapsed AIDS-related CMV retinitis;acyclovir-resistant herpes simplex virus (HSV) in immunocompromised pts. *Treatment of CMV disease, herpes simplex, varicella zoster.*

STORAGE / HANDLING

Store parenteral vials at room temperature. After dilution, stable for 24 hrs at room temperature.

IV ADMINISTRATION

1. Do not give IV injection or rapid infusion (increases toxicity).

2. Administer only by IV infusion over a minimum of 1 hr (no more than 1 mg/kg/min).

3. To minimize toxicity and phlebitis, use central venous lines or veins w/adequate blood to permit rapid dilution and dissemination of foscarnet.

4. Use IV infusion pump to prevent accidental overdose.

5. The standard 24 mg/ml solution may be used w/o dilution when central venous catheter is used for infusion; 24 mg/ml solution *must* be diluted to 12 mg/ml when peripheral vein catheter is being used. Only 5% dextrose in water or normal saline solution for injection should be used for dilution.

6. Since dosage is calculated on body weight, unneeded quantity may be removed before start of infusion to avoid overdosage. Aseptic technique must be used and solution administered within 24 hrs of first entry into sealed bottle.

7. Do not use if solution is discolored or contains particulate material.

INDICATIONS / DOSAGE / ROUTES

CMV retinitis:

IV: Adults: Initially, 60 mg/kg q8h for 2–3 wks. **Maintenance:** 90 mg/kg/day; may increase up to 120 mg/kg/day if retinitis progresses.

Herpes simplex:

IV: Adults: 40 mg/kg q8–12h for 2–3 wks or until healed.

Dosage in renal impairment:

Dosage individualized according to pt's creatinine clearance. Refer to dosing guide provided by manufacturer.

PRECAUTIONS

CONTRAINDICATIONS: Hypersensitivity to foscarnet sodium. **CAUTIONS:** Neurologic or cardiac abnormalities, history of renal impairment, altered calcium or other electrolyte levels. **PREG-NANCY/LACTATION:** Unknown if excreted in breast milk. **Pregnancy Category C**.

INTERACTIONS

DRUG INTERACTIONS: Nephrotoxic medications may increase risk of renal toxicity. Pentamidine (IV) may cause reversible hypocalcemia, hypomagnesemia, nephrotoxicity. Zidovudine may increase anemia. **ALTERED LAB VALUES:** May increase SGOT (AST), SGPT (ALT), alkaline phosphatase, bilirubin, creatinine. May decrease magnesium, potassium. May alter calcium, phosphate concentrations.

SIDE EFFECTS

FREQUENT: Fever **(65%)**, nausea **(47%)**, vomiting, diarrhea **(30%)**. **OCCASIONAL** (≥5%): Anorexia, pain and inflammation at injection site, fever, rigors, malaise, hyper/hypotension, headache, paresthesia, dizziness, rash, increased sweating, nausea, vomiting, abdominal pain. **RARE (1–5%):** Back/chest pain, edema, hyper/hypotension, flushing, pruritus, constipation, dry mouth.

ADVERSE REACTIONS/TOXIC EFFECTS

Renal impairment is a major toxicity that occurs to some extent in most pts. Seizures and mineral/electrolyte imbalances may be life threatening.

NURSING IMPLICATIONS

BASELINE ASSESSMENT:

Question for hypersensitivity to foscarnet. Obtain baseline mineral and electrolyte levels, vital signs, CBC values, renal functioning.

INTERVENTION/EVALUATION:

Monitor electrolyte results closely; assess for signs of electrolyte imbalance, esp. hypocalcemia (perioral tingling, numbness/paresthesia of extremities) or hypokalemia (weakness, muscle cramps, numbness/tingling of extremities, irritability). Maintain accurate I&O, provide adequate hydration to assure diuresis before and during dosing, and monitor renal function tests to avoid or identify promptly renal impairment. Assess for tremors; provide safety measures for potential seizures. Evaluate vital signs at least 2 times/day. Provide small, attractive meals; avoid unattractive sights, smells, esp. at mealtimes, and administer ordered antiemetics to support nutrition. Monitor number, consistency of stools. Assess for bleeding, anemia, or developing superinfections.

PATIENT/FAMILY TEACHING:

Foscarnet is not a cure for CMV retinitis; regular ophthalmologic examinations are part of therapy. Dose modifications may be necessary, esp. w/regard to controlling side effects; close medical supervision is essential. Infusion rate must be controlled to prevent overdosage (no more than 1 mg/kg/min). Important to report perioral tingling, numbness in the extremities, or paresthesias during or after infusion (may indicate electrolyte abnormalities). Risk of renal impairment can be reduced by sufficient fluid intake to assure diuresis before and during dosing. Tremors should be reported promptly because of potential for seizures.

fosfomycin
(Monural)
See Supplement

fosinopril
foh-**sin**-oh-prill
(Monopril)

CANADIAN AVAILABILITY:
Monopril

CLASSIFICATION

Angiotensin-converting enzyme (ACE) inhibitor

AVAILABILITY (Rx)

Tablets: 10 mg, 20 mg

PHARMACOKINETICS

	ONSET	PEAK	DURATION
PO	1 hr	2–6 hrs	24 hrs

Slowly absorbed from GI tract. Metabolized in liver, GI mucosa to active metabolite. Primarily excreted in urine. Minimal removal by hemodialysis. Half-life: 11.5 hrs.

ACTION/ *THERAPEUTIC EFFECT*

Suppresses renin-angiotensin-aldosterone system (prevents conversion of angiotensin I to angiotensin II, a potent vasoconstrictor; may also inhibit angiotensin II at local vascular and renal sites). Decreases plasma angiotensin II, increases plasma renin activity, decreases aldosterone secretion. *Reduces peripheral arterial resistance, pulmonary capillary wedge pressure, improves cardiac output, exercise tolerance.*

USES/ *UNLABELED*

Treatment of hypertension. Used alone or in combination w/other antihypertensives. Treatment of heart failure. *Treatment of renal crisis in scleroderma.*

PO ADMINISTRATION

1. May give w/o regard to food.
2. Tablets may be crushed.

INDICATIONS/DOSAGE/ROUTES

Hypertension (used alone):
PO: Adults, elderly: Initially, 10 mg/day. **Maintenance:** 20–40 mg/day. **Maximum:** 80 mg/day.

Hypertension (w/diuretic):
Note: Discontinue diuretic 2–3 days before initiation of fosinopril therapy.
PO: Adults, elderly: Initially, 10 mg/day titrated to pt's needs.

Heart failure:
PO: Adults, elderly: Initially, 5–10 mg. **Maintenance:** 20–40 mg/day.

PRECAUTIONS

CONTRAINDICATIONS: History of angioedema w/previous treatment w/ACE inhibitors. **CAUTIONS:** Renal impairment, those w/sodium depletion or on diuretic therapy, dialysis, hypovolemia, coronary or cerebrovascular insufficiency. **PREGNANCY/LACTATION:** Crosses placenta; distributed in breast milk. May cause fetal/neonatal mortality/morbidity. **Pregnancy Category D**.

INTERACTIONS

DRUG INTERACTIONS: Alcohol, diuretics, hypotensive agents may increase effects. NSAIDs may decrease effect. Potassium-sparing diuretics, potassium supplements may cause hyperkalemia. May increase lithium concentration, toxicity. **ALTERED LAB VALUES:** May increase potassium, SGOT (AST), SGPT (ALT), alkaline phosphatase, bilirubin, BUN, creatinine. May decrease sodium. May cause positive ANA titer.

SIDE EFFECTS

FREQUENT (9–12%): Dizziness, cough. **OCCASIONAL (2–4%):** Hypotension, nausea, vomiting, upper respiratory infection.

ADVERSE REACTIONS/TOXIC EFFECTS

Excessive hypotension ("first-dose syncope") may occur in pts w/CHF, severely salt/volume depleted. Angioedema (swelling of face/lips), hyperkalemia occur rarely. Agranulocytosis, neutropenia may be noted in those w/impaired renal function or collagen vascular disease (systemic lupus erythematosus, scleroderma). Nephrotic syndrome may be noted in those w/history of renal disease.

NURSING IMPLICATIONS
BASELINE ASSESSMENT:

Obtain B/P immediately before each dose, in addition to regular monitoring (be alert to fluctuations). Renal function tests should be performed before therapy begins. In pts w/renal impairment, autoimmune disease, or taking drugs that affect leukocytes or immune response, CBC and differential count should be performed before therapy begins and q2wks for 3 mos, then periodically thereafter.

INTERVENTION/EVALUATION:

If excessive reduction in B/P occurs, place pt in supine position w/legs elevated. Assist w/ambulation if dizziness occurs. Assess

for urinary frequency. Auscultate lung sounds for rales, wheezing in those w/CHF. Monitor urinalysis for proteinuria. Monitor serum potassium levels in those on concurrent diuretic therapy. Monitor pattern of daily bowel activity and stool consistency.

PATIENT/FAMILY TEACHING:

Report any sign of infection (sore throat, fever). Several weeks may be needed for full therapeutic effect of B/P reduction. Skipping doses or voluntarily discontinuing drug may produce severe, rebound hypertension. To reduce hypotensive effect, rise slowly from lying to sitting position and permit legs to dangle from bed momentarily before standing.

fosphenytoin
fos-**phen**-ih-twon
(Cerebyx)

CANADIAN AVAILABILITY:
Cerebyx

CLASSIFICATION
Anticonvulsant

AVAILABILITY (Rx)
Injection: 75 mg/ml (50 mg phenytoin sodium)

PHARMACOKINETICS
Completely absorbed following IM administration. After IM or IV administration, rapidly/completely hydrolyzed to phenytoin. Half-life for conversion to phenytoin: 8–15 min.

ACTION/THERAPEUTIC EFFECT
Stabilizes neuronal membranes,

limits spread of seizure activity. *Decreases sodium, calcium, ion influx in neurons. Decreases post-tetanic potentiation and repetitive afterdischarge. Decreases seizure activity.*

USES

Acute treatment, control of generalized convulsive status epilepticus, prevention, treatment of seizures occurring during neurosurgery, short-term substitution of oral phenytoin.

STORAGE/HANDLING

Refrigerate. Do not store at room temperature >48 hrs. After dilution, solution stable for 8 hrs at room temperature or 24 hrs if refrigerated.

IM/IV ADMINISTRATION

1. Dilute in 5% dextrose or 0.9% NaCl to a concentration ranging from 1.5 to 25 mg PE/ml (PE: phenytoin equivalent).

2. Administer at rate of ≤150 mg PE/min (decreases risk of hypotension).

INDICATIONS/DOSAGE/ROUTES

Note: 150 mg fosphenytoin yields 100 mg phenytoin. Dose, concentration solution, infusion rate of fosphenytoin expressed in terms of phenytoin equivalents (PE). Lower, less frequent dosing in elderly may be required. Not approved for pediatric use.

Status epilepticus:
IV: Adults: Loading dose: 15–20 mg PE/kg infused at rate of 100–150 mg PE/min.

Nonemergent seizures:
IV: Adults: Loading dose: 10–20 mg PE/kg. **Maintenance:** 4–6 mg PE/kg/day.

PRECAUTIONS

CONTRAINDICATIONS: Hypersensitivity to fosphenytoin, phenytoin, or any of its ingredients, severe bradycardia, SA block, second- or third-degree AV block, Adams-Stokes syndrome. **CAUTIONS:** Porphyria, hypotension, severe myocardial insufficiency, renal/hepatic disease, hypoalbuminemia. **PREGNANCY/LACTATION:** May increase frequency of seizures during pregnancy. Increased risk of congenital malformations. Unknown if excreted in breast milk. **Pregnancy Category D.**

INTERACTIONS

DRUG INTERACTIONS: May decrease effect of glucocorticoids. Alcohol, CNS depressants may increase CNS depression. Antacids may decrease absorption. Amiodarone, anticoagulants, cimetidine, disulfiram, fluoxetine, isoniazid, sulfonamides may increase fosphenytoin concentration, effects, toxicity. Fluconazole, ketoconazole, miconazole may increase concentration. Lidocaine, propranolol may increase cardiac depressant effects. Valproic acid may increase concentration, decrease metabolism. May increase xanthine metabolism. **ALTERED LAB VALUES:** May increase alkaline phosphatase, GGT, glucose.

SIDE EFFECTS

FREQUENT: Dizziness, paresthesia, tinnitus, pruritus, headache, somnolence. **OCCASIONAL:** Morbilliform rash.

ADVERSE REACTIONS/TOXIC EFFECTS

A too high fosphenytoin blood concentration may produce ataxia (muscular incoordination), nystagmus (rhythmic oscillation of eyes), double vision, lethargy, slurred speech, nausea, vomiting, hypotension. As level increases, extreme lethargy to comatose states occur.

NURSING IMPLICATIONS
BASELINE ASSESSMENT:

Review history of seizure disorder (intensity, frequency, duration, level of consciousness). Initiate seizure precautions. Obtain vital signs, medication history (esp. use of phenytoin or other anticonvulsants). Observe clinically.

INTERVENTION/EVALUATION:

Measure cardiac function, EKG, determination of respiratory function, B/P during and immediately after infusion (10–20 min). Discontinue if skin rash appears. Interrupt or decrease rate if hypotension or arrhythmias are detected. Assess pt postinfusion (may feel dizzy, ataxic, or drowsy). Assess blood levels of fosphenytoin (2 hrs post IV infusion or 4 hrs post IM injection).

PATIENT/FAMILY TEACHING:

Teach pts about their seizure condition and role in its management. If noncompliance is an issue in causing acute seizures, discuss reasons for noncompliance and address them.

furosemide
feur-**oh**-sah-mide
(Lasix)

CANADIAN AVAILABILITY:
Apo-Furosemide, Lasix

CLASSIFICATION
Diuretic: Loop

AVAILABILITY (Rx)
Tablets: 20 mg, 40 mg, 80 mg.
Oral Solution: 10 mg/ml, 40 mg/5 ml. **Injection:** 10 mg/ml.

PHARMACOKINETICS

	ONSET	PEAK	DURATION
PO	30–60 min	1–2 hrs	6–8 hrs
IM	—	30 min	—
IV	5 min	20–60 min	2 hrs

Well absorbed from GI tract. Partially metabolized in liver. Primarily excreted in urine (in severe renal impairment, nonrenal clearance increases). Half-life: 30–90 min (increased in decreased renal, liver function and in neonates).

ACTION/THERAPEUTIC EFFECT

Enhances excretion of sodium, chloride, potassium by direct action at ascending limb of loop of Henle, producing diuretic effect.

USES/UNLABELED

Treatment of edema associated w/CHF, chronic renal failure including nephrotic syndrome, hepatic cirrhosis, acute pulmonary edema. Treats hypertension, either alone or in combination w/other antihypertensives. Treatment of hypercalcemia.

STORAGE/HANDLING

Solution appears clear, colorless. Discard yellow injections or discolored tablet.

PO/IM/IV ADMINISTRATION
PO:
Give w/food to avoid GI upset, preferably w/breakfast (may prevent nocturia).

IM:

Temporary pain at injection site may be noted.

IV:

1. May give undiluted but is compatible w/5% dextrose in water, 0.9% NS, or lactated Ringer's solutions.
2. Administer direct IV over 1–2 min, preferably through Y tube or 3-way stopcock.
3. Do not exceed administration rate of 4 mg/min in those w/renal impairment.

INDICATIONS/DOSAGE/ROUTE

Edema:
PO: Adults: 20–80 mg daily given as single dose in morning. May increase in 20–40 mg increments q6–8h. Give effective dose 1–2 times/day. **Maximum:** 600 mg.
IM/IV: Adults: 20–40 mg given as single injection. May increase in 20 mg increments no sooner than 2 hrs after previous dose. May give effective dose 1–2 times/day.

Acute pulmonary edema:
IV: Adults: 40 mg slow IV, given over 1–2 min. If satisfactory response is not reached in 1 hr, may increase to 80 mg slow IV, given over 1–2 min.

Hypertension:
PO: Adults: Initially 40 mg 2 times/day based on pt response.

Usual elderly dosage:
IM/IV/PO: Initially, 20 mg/day. May increase slowly to desired response.

Usual dosage for children:
PO: 2 mg/kg given as single dose. May be increased in 1–2 mg/kg increments q6–8h. **Maximum:** 6 mg/kg/day.
IV/IM: 1 mg/kg given as single dose. May increase by 1 mg/kg no sooner than 2 hrs after previous dose. **Maximum:** 6 mg/kg/day.

PRECAUTIONS

CONTRAINDICATIONS: Anuria, hepatic coma, severe electrolyte depletion. **CAUTIONS:** Acute MI, oliguria, hepatic cirrhosis, history of gout, diabetes, systemic lupus erythematosus, pancreatitis. **PREGNANCY/LACTATION:** Crosses placenta; distributed in breast milk. **Pregnancy Category C**.

INTERACTIONS

DRUG INTERACTIONS: Amphotericin, ototoxic, nephrotoxic agents may increase toxicity. May decrease effect of anticoagulants, heparin. Hypokalemia-causing agents may increase risk of hypokalemia. May increase risk of lithium toxicity. Probenecid may increase concentrations. **ALTERED LAB VALUES:** May increase glucose, BUN, uric acid. May decrease calcium, chloride, magnesium, potassium, sodium.

SIDE EFFECTS

EXPECTED: Increase in urinary frequency/volume. **FREQUENT:** Nausea, gastric upset w/cramping, diarrhea, or constipation, electrolyte disturbances. **OCCASIONAL:** Dizziness, lightheadedness, headache, blurred vision, paresthesia, photosensitivity, rash, weakness, urinary frequency/bladder spasm, restlessness, diaphoresis. **RARE:** Flank pain, loin pain.

ADVERSE REACTIONS/TOXIC EFFECTS

Vigorous diuresis may lead to profound water loss and electrolyte depletion, resulting in hypokalemia, hyponatremia, dehydration. Sudden volume depletion may result in increased risk of thrombosis, circulatory collapse, sudden death. Acute hypotensive episodes may also occur, sometimes several days after beginning of therapy. Ototoxicity manifested as deafness, vertigo, tinnitus (ringing/roaring in ears) may occur, especially in those w/severe renal impairment. Can exacerbate diabetes mellitus, systemic lupus erythematosus, gout, pancreatitis. Blood dyscrasias have been reported.

NURSING IMPLICATIONS
BASELINE ASSESSMENT:

Check vital signs, esp. B/P for hypotension before administration. Assess baseline electrolytes, particularly check for low potassium. Assess edema, skin turgor, mucous membranes for hydration status. Assess muscle strength, mental status. Note skin temperature, moisture. Obtain baseline weight. Initiate I&O monitoring.

INTERVENTION/EVALUATION:

Monitor B/P, vital signs, electrolytes, I&O, weight. Note extent of diuresis. Watch for changes from initial assessment (hypokalemia may result in changes in muscle strength, tremor, muscle cramps, change in mental status, cardiac arrhythmias). Hyponatremia may result in confusion, thirst, cold/clammy skin.

PATIENT/FAMILY TEACHING:

Expect increased frequency and volume of urination. Report irregular heartbeat, signs of electrolyte imbalances (noted above), hearing abnormalities (such as sense of fullness in ears, ringing/roaring in ears). Eat foods high in potassium such as whole grains (cereals), legumes, meat, bananas, apricots, orange juice, potatoes (white, sweet), raisins. Avoid sun/sunlamps.

---

gabapentin
gah-bah-**pen**-tin
(**Neurontin**)

CANADIAN AVAILABILITY:
Neurontin

CLASSIFICATION

Anticonvulsant

AVAILABILITY (Rx)

Capsules: 100 mg, 300 mg, 400 mg. **Tablets.**

PHARMACOKINETICS

Well absorbed from GI tract (not affected by food). Widely distributed. Crosses blood-brain barrier. Primarily excreted unchanged in urine. Removed by hemodialysis. Half-life: 5–7 hrs (increased in decreased renal function, elderly).

ACTION/*THERAPEUTIC EFFECT*

Exact mechanism unknown. May be due to increased gamma-aminobutyric acid (GABA) synthesis rate, increased GABA accumulation, or binding to as yet undefined receptor sites in brain tissue *to produce anticonvulsant activity.*

USES/*UNLABELED*

Adjunctive therapy in treatment of partial seizures and partial seizures w/secondary generalization in adults. *Neuropathic pain. Psychiatric disorders.*

PO ADMINISTRATION

1. May be given w/o regard to meals; may give w/food to avoid or reduce GI upset.

2. If treatment is discontinued or anticonvulsant therapy is added, do so gradually over at least 1 wk (reduces risk of loss of seizure control).

INDICATIONS/DOSAGE/ROUTES

Seizure control:
Note: Maximum time between doses should not exceed 12 hrs.
PO: Adults, elderly: 900–1,800 mg/day given in divided doses q8h. May titrate to effective dose rapidly: *Day 1:* 300 mg (give at bedtime). *Day 2:* 300 mg q12h. *Day 3:* 300 mg q8h.

Renal function impairment:
Based on creatinine clearance:

CREATININE CLEARANCE	DOSAGE
>60 ml/min	400 mg q8h
30–60 ml/min	300 mg q12h
15–30 ml/min	300 mg daily
<15 ml/min	300 mg every other day
Hemodialysis	200–300 mg after each 4 hr hemodialysis

PRECAUTIONS

CONTRAINDICATIONS: None significant. **CAUTIONS:** Renal impairment. Discontinue/add anticonvulsant therapy gradually (reduces loss of seizure control). Children <18 yrs of age. **PREGNANCY/LACTATION:** Unknown whether it is distributed in breast milk. **Pregnancy Category C**.

INTERACTIONS

DRUG INTERACTIONS: None significant. **ALTERED LAB VALUES:** May decrease WBCs.

SIDE EFFECTS

FREQUENT (>10%): Fatigue, somnolence, dizziness, ataxia. **OCCASIONAL (2–10%):** Weight gain, dyspepsia, muscle pain, rhinitis, tremor, nystagmus (rolling eye movements), loss of memory. **RARE (<2%):** Back pain, peripheral edema, dry mouth, constipation, increased appetite, cough, altered thinking/coordination, itching, impotence.

ADVERSE REACTIONS/TOXIC EFFECTS

Abrupt withdrawal may increase seizure frequency. Overdosage may result in double vision, slurred speech, drowsiness, lethargy, diarrhea.

NURSING IMPLICATIONS
BASELINE ASSESSMENT:

Review history of seizure disorder (type, onset, intensity, frequency, duration, level of consciousness). Routine laboratory monitoring of blood serum levels unnecessary for safe use. Obtain vital signs, medication history.

INTERVENTION/EVALUATION:

Provide safety measures as needed. Assess for seizure activity.

PATIENT/FAMILY TEACHING:

Take gabapentin only as prescribed; do not abruptly stop taking drug because seizure frequency may be increased. Do not drive, operate machinery, or perform activities requiring mental acuity due to potential dizziness, somnolence. Avoid alcohol. Carry identification card/bracelet to note anticonvulsant therapy. Teach pt about his/her seizure condition and role in its management. If noncompliance is an issue in causing acute seizures, discuss reasons for noncompliance and address them.

gallium nitrate

gal-lee-um
(Ganite)

CLASSIFICATION

Antihypercalcemic

AVAILABILITY (Rx)

Injection: 25 mg/ml

PHARMACOKINETICS

Primarily excreted in urine. Half-life: 24 hrs.

ACTION/ *THERAPEUTIC EFFECT*

Inhibits abnormal bone resorption, reduces flow of calcium from resorbing bone into blood, *decreasing calcium serum levels.*

USES

Treatment of hypercalcemia or malignancy that is inadequately managed by oral hydration alone. Use concomitantly w/saline (increases urine output) and diuretics (increases rate of calcium excretion).

STORAGE/HANDLING

Store undiluted vials at room temperature. After dilution, stable for 48 hrs at room temperature or up to 7 days refrigerated.

IV ADMINISTRATION

Must dilute daily dose in 1,000 ml 0.9% NaCl or 5% dextrose.

INDICATIONS/DOSAGE/ROUTES

Hypercalcemia:
IV Infusion: Adults, elderly: 100–200 mg/m^2/day over 24 hrs for 5 days. May repeat after waiting 3–4 wks.

PRECAUTIONS

CONTRAINDICATIONS: Decreases renal function when serum creatinine >2.5 mg/dl. **CAUTIONS:** Renal function when serum creatinine 2–2.5 mg/dl. **PREGNANCY/LACTATION:** Unknown whether excreted in breast milk. **Pregnancy Category C.**

INTERACTIONS

DRUG INTERACTIONS: Calcium-containing medications, products, vitamin D may decrease effect. Nephrotoxic medications may increase nephrotoxicity. **ALTERED LAB VALUES:** None significant.

SIDE EFFECTS

FREQUENT: Hypophosphatemia (e.g., bone pain, muscle weakness, anorexia), nephrotoxicity (blood in urine, nausea, vomiting), diarrhea, metallic taste. **OCCASIONAL:** Hypocalcemia (abnormal cramps, confusion, muscle spasms). **RARE:** Anemia.

ADVERSE REACTIONS/TOXIC EFFECTS

None significant.

NURSING IMPLICATIONS

BASELINE ASSESSMENT:

Assure no other nephrotoxic drugs are being given concurrently. Determine initial serum calcium and creatinine levels. Establish adequate hydration w/oral or IV fluids, preferably saline, to counteract dehydration (caused by hypercalcemia) and increase excretion of calcium. Assure satisfactory urine output (2 L/day recommended) before starting gallium therapy.

INTERVENTION/EVALUATION:

Throughout therapy maintain adequate hydration w/o overhydrating pt w/compromised cardiovascular status. Monitor urinary output. Assess serum calcium, phosphorus, creatinine, and BUN frequently (therapy should be discontinued if serum creatinine level exceeds 2.5 mg/dl).

PATIENT/FAMILY TEACHING:

Explain rationale of therapy and importance of fluids, I&O.

ganciclovir sodium

gan-**sye**-klo-vir
(Cytovene, Vitrasert)

CANADIAN AVAILABILITY:
Cytovene

CLASSIFICATION

Antiviral

AVAILABILITY (Rx)

Capsules: 250 mg, 500 mg. **Powder for Injection:** 500 mg. **Implant.**

PHARMACOKINETICS

Widely distributed. Undergoes minimal metabolism. Primarily excreted unchanged in urine. Removed by hemodialysis. Half-life: 2.5–3.6 hrs (increased in decreased renal function).

ACTION/*THERAPEUTIC EFFECT*

Converted intracellularly, competes w/viral DNA polymerases and direct incorporation into growing viral DNA chains, *interfering w/DNA synthesis and viral replication.* Congener of acyclovir.

USES/*UNLABELED*

Treatment of cytomegalovirus (CMV) retinitis in immunocompromised pts (e.g., AIDS, bone marrow recipients); in combination w/foscarnet for relapsed AIDS-related CMV retinitis; prevention of CMV in transplant pts. *Oral:* Maintenance treatment of CMV. *Vitrasert: intraocular implant:* Treatment of CMV in pts w/AIDS. *Intravenous: Treatment of other CMV infections (e.g., pneumonitis, gastroenteritis, hepatitis).*

STORAGE/HANDLING

Store vials at room temperature. Reconstituted solution in vial stable for 12 hrs at room temperature. Do not refrigerate. After dilution, refrigerate, use within 24 hrs. Discard if precipitate forms, discoloration occurs. Avoid exposure to skin, eyes, mucous membranes. Wear latex gloves.

PO/IV ADMINISTRATION

PO:
Take w/food.

IV:

1. Latex gloves and safety glasses should be used during preparation and handling of solution. Avoid inhalation. (If solution contacts skin, mucous membrane wash carefully w/soap and water; rinse eyes thoroughly w/plain water.)

2. Reconstitute 500 mg vial w/10 ml sterile water for injection to provide a concentration of 50 mg/ml; do *not* use bacteriostatic water (contains parabens, which is incompatible w/ganciclovir).

3. Further dilute w/100 ml D_5W, 0.9% NaCl, or other compatible fluid to provide a concentration of 5 mg/ml.

4. Administer only by IV infusion over 1 hr.

5. Do not give IV injection or rapid infusion (increases toxicity).

6. Do not give IM or SubQ; protect from infiltration (high pH causes severe tissue irritation).

7. Use veins w/adequate blood to permit rapid dilution and dissemination of ganciclovir (minimize phlebitis); central venous catheters tunneled under subcutaneous tissue may reduce catheter-associated infection.

INDICATIONS/DOSAGE/ROUTES

Note: Do not give if neutrophil count <500 cells/mm^3 or platelets <25,000/mm^3.

CMV retinitis treatment:
IV: Adults: Initially, 5 mg/kg q12h for 14–21 days.

CMV disease prevention:
IV: Adults: Initially, 5 mg/kg q12h for 7–14 days.

Maintenance:
IV: Adults: 5 mg/kg/day for 7 days or 6 mg/kg for 5 days.
PO: Adults: 1,000 mg 3 times/day or 500 mg 6 times/day q3h given w/food.

Dosage in renal impairment:

CREATININE CLEARANCE	DOSAGE	DOSING INTERVAL
≥80 ml/min	5 mg/kg	12 hrs
50–79 ml/min	2.5 mg/kg	12 hrs
25–49 ml/min	2.5 mg/kg	24 hrs
<25 ml/min	1.25 mg/kg	24 hrs

PRECAUTIONS

CONTRAINDICATIONS: Hypersensitivity to ganciclovir or acyclovir. Not for use in immunocompetent persons or those w/congenital or neonatal CMV disease. **CAUTIONS:** Extreme caution in children because of long-term carcinogenicity, reproductive toxicity. Renal impairment, preexisting cytopenias or history of cytopenic reactions to other drugs, elderly (at greater risk of renal impairment). **PREGNANCY/LACTATION:** Effective contraception should be used during therapy; ganciclovir should not be used during pregnancy. Nursing should be discontinued. May be resumed no sooner than 72 hrs after the last dose of ganciclovir. **Pregnancy Category C**.

INTERACTIONS

DRUG INTERACTIONS: Bone marrow depressants may increase bone marrow depression. May increase risk of seizures w/imipenem-cilastatin. May increase hematologic toxicity w/zidovudine. **ALTERED LAB VALUES:** May increase SGOT (AST), SGPT (ALT), alkaline phosphatase, bilirubin.

SIDE EFFECTS

FREQUENT (>10%): Fever (40%), diarrhea (41%), nausea (25%), abdominal pain, vomiting, decreased appetite, anemia, leukopenia. *Intraocular insert:* Visual acuity loss, vitreous hemorrhage, retinal detachment. **OCCASIONAL (1–10%):** Infection, chills, flatulence, numbness in hands/feet, itching, pneumonia, neutropenia. **RARE (<1%):** Headache, dizziness, thought disorders, behavioral changes, psychosis, coma, seizures, abnormal dreams, intention tremor, chills, malaise, cardiac arrhythmias, hyper/hypotension, pruritus, hematuria, diarrhea, paresthesia, ataxia, edema, alopecia.

ADVERSE REACTIONS/TOXIC EFFECTS

Hematologic toxicity, GI hemorrhage occur rarely.

NURSING IMPLICATIONS
BASELINE ASSESSMENT:

Question for hypersensitivity to ganciclovir or acyclovir. Evaluate hematologic baseline. Obtain specimens for support of differential diagnosis (urine, feces, blood, throat) because usually retinal infection due to hematogenous dissemination.

INTERVENTION/EVALUATION:

Monitor I&O and assure adequate hydration (minimum 1,500 ml/24 hrs). Check IV site, rate of infusion every 15 min during dosage administration. Diligently evaluate hematology reports for potentially life-threatening neutropenia, thrombocytopenia, decreased platelets (hold ganciclovir and notify physician immediately of neutrophil count less than 500/mm³, platelet count less than 25,000/mm³). Monitor B/P at least 2 times/day for hyper/hypotension. Check temperature at least 2 times/day for onset or increase in fever. Assess pt carefully for change (i.e., increased bleeding tendency, signs of infection). Question pt regarding vision, therapeutic improvement, or complications. Be alert for behavior changes, thought disorders, confusion, or other nervous system effects and report promptly. Assess for rash, pruritus.

PATIENT/FAMILY TEACHING:

Ganciclovir provides suppression, not cure of CMV retinitis. Frequent blood tests and eye exams are necessary during therapy because of toxic nature of drug. It is essential to report any new symptom promptly. May temporarily or permanently inhibit sperm production in men, suppress fertility in women. Barrier contraception should be used during and for 90 days after therapy because of mutagenic potential.

---

ganirelix
(Antagon)
See Supplement

---

gatifloxacin
(Tequin)
See Supplement
See Classification section under:
Antibiotic: fluoroquinolones

---

gemcitabine hydrochloride
gem-**cih**-tah-bean
(Gemzar)

G

CANADIAN AVAILABILTY:
Gemzar

CLASSIFICATION

Antineoplastic

AVAILABILITY (Rx)

Powder for Reconstitution: 200 mg, 1 g vials

PHARMACOKINETICS

Following IV infusion, not extensively distributed (increased w/length of infusion). Excreted primarily in urine as metabolite. Half-life: 42–94 min (influenced by gender/duration of infusion).

ACTION/*THERAPEUTIC EFFECT*

Inhibits ribonucleotide reductase, the enzyme necessary for catalyzing DNA synthesis, thereby *producing cell death in those cells undergoing DNA synthesis.*

USES

Treatment of locally advanced (stage II or stage III) or metastatic (stage IV) adenocarcinoma of pancreas. Indicated for pts previously treated w/5-fluorouracil. Monotherapy or in combination w/cisplatin for treatment for locally advanced/metastatic non-small cell lung cancer.

STORAGE/HANDLING

Store at room temperature (refrigeration may cause crystallization). Reconstituted solution stable for 24 hrs at room temperature.

IV ADMINISTRATION

1. Use gloves when handling/preparing gemcitabine.

2. Reconstitute 200 mg or 1 g vial w/0.9% NaCl injection w/o preservative (5 ml or 25 ml, respectively) to provide a concentration of 40 mg/ml.

3. Shake to dissolve.

4. Infuse over 30 min.

INDICATIONS/DOSAGE/ROUTES

Note: Dosage is individualized on basis of clinical response and tolerance to adverse effects. When used in combination therapy, consult specific protocols for optimum dosage, sequence of drug administration.

Pancreatic cancer:
IV Infusion: Adults: 1,000 mg/m^2 once weekly for up to 7 wks (or until toxicity necessitates decreasing/holding the dose), followed by 1 wk of rest. Subsequent cycles should consist of once weekly for 3 consecutive weeks out of every 4 wks.

Pts completing cycles at 1,000 mg/m^2 may increase dose to 1,250 mg/m^2 as tolerated. Dose for next cycle may be increased to 1,500 mg/m^2. **Note:** May increase dose provided the absolute granulocyte count (AGC) and platelet nadirs exceed 1,500 × 10^6/L and 100,000 × 10^6/L, respectively.

DOSE REDUCTION GUIDELINES

AGC (10^6/L)		PLATELETS (10^6/L)	% FULL DOSE
1,000	and	100,000	100
500–999	or	50,000–99,000	75
<500	or	<50,000	Hold

PRECAUTIONS

CONTRAINDICATIONS: History of hypersensitivity to gemcitabine. **CAUTIONS:** Impaired renal function, hepatic insufficiency. **PREGNANCY/LACTATION:** If possible, avoid use during pregnancy, esp. first trimester. May cause fetal harm. Not known whether distributed in breast milk. Breast-feeding not recommended. **Pregnancy Category D**.

INTERACTIONS

DRUG INTERACTIONS: Bone marrow depressants may increase risk of bone marrow depression. Live virus vaccines may potentiate virus replication, increase vaccine side effects, decrease pt's antibody response to vaccine. **ALTERED LAB VALUES:** May increase SGOT (AST), SGPT (ALT), alkaline phosphatase, bilirubin, creatinine, BUN.

SIDE EFFECTS

FREQUENT: Nausea, vomiting, fever, mild to moderate pruritic rash, dyspnea, constipation/diarrhea, proteinuria, hematuria, mild dyspnea, peripheral edema. **OCCASIONAL:** "Flu syndrome," alopecia, stomatitis (mucosal erythema, gingivitis, glossitis), somnolence, paresthesia, petechiae. **RARE:** Sweating, rhinitis, insomnia, malaise.

ADVERSE REACTIONS/TOXIC EFFECTS

Severe bone marrow suppression evidenced by anemia, thrombocytopenia, leukopenia.

NURSING IMPLICATIONS

BASELINE ASSESSMENT:

CBC, including differential and platelet count, renal and hepatic function lab tests should be performed prior to initiation of therapy and periodically thereafter. Drug should be suspended or dose modified if bone marrow suppression is detected.

INTERVENTION/EVALUATION:

Assess all lab results before each dose is given. Monitor for dyspnea, fever, pruritic rash. Assess oral mucosa for mucosal erythema, ulceration at inner margin of lips, sore throat, difficulty swallowing (stomatitis). Assess skin for rash. Monitor for and report diarrhea. Check food tolerance, provide antiemetics as needed.

PATIENT/FAMILY TEACHING:

Avoid crowds and exposure to infection. Do not take alcohol or other medications w/o consulting physician. Maintain fastidious oral hygiene. Do not have immunizations w/o physician's approval (drug lowers body's resistance). Promptly report fever, sore throat, signs of local infection, easy bruising, unusual bleeding from any site. Contact physician if nausea/vomiting continues at home.

gemfibrozil

gem-**fie**-bro-zill
(Lopid)

CANADIAN AVAILABILITY:
Lopid

CLASSIFICATION

Antihyperlipoproteinemic

AVAILABILITY (Rx)

Tablets: 600 mg

PHARMACOKINETICS

Well absorbed from GI tract. Metabolized in liver. Primarily excreted in urine. Half-life: 1.5 hrs.

ACTION/THERAPEUTIC EFFECT

Inhibits lipolysis of fat in adipose tissue; decreases liver uptake of free fatty acids (reduces hepatic triglyceride production). Inhibits synthesis of VLDL carrier apolipoprotein B. *Lowers serum cholesterol and triglycerides (decreases VLDL, LDL, increases HDL).*

USES

Treatment of hyperlipidemia, decreases risk of coronary heart disease in pts w/type IIB hyperlipidemia. Treatment of severe primary hyperlipidemia (types IV, V).

PO ADMINISTRATION

Give 30 min before morning and evening meals.

INDICATIONS/DOSAGE/ROUTES

Hyperlipidemia:
PO: Adults, elderly: 900 mg to 1.5 g/day in 2 divided doses.

PRECAUTIONS

CONTRAINDICATIONS: Hypersensitivity to gemfibrozil, hepatic dysfunction (including primary biliary cirrhosis), severe renal dysfunction, preexisting gallbladder disease. **CAUTIONS:** Hypothroidism, diabetes mellitus, estrogen or anticoagulant therapy. **PREGNANCY/LACTATION:** Not known whether drug crosses placenta or is distributed in breast milk. Decision to discontinue nursing or drug should be based on potential for serious adverse effects. **Pregnancy Category C.**

INTERACTIONS

DRUG INTERACTIONS: May increase effect of warfarin. May cause rhabdomyolysis, leading to acute renal failure w/lovastatin.

ALTERED LAB VALUES: May increase SGOT (AST), SGPT (ALT), alkaline phosphatase, bilirubin, creatinine kinase, LDH. May decrease Hgb, Hct, potassium, leukocyte counts.

SIDE EFFECTS

FREQUENT (20%): Dyspepsia. **OCCASIONAL (2–10%):** Abdominal pain, diarrhea, nausea, vomiting, fatigue. **RARE (<2%):** Constipation, acute appendicitis, vertigo, headache, rash, altered taste.

ADVERSE REACTIONS/TOXIC EFFECTS

Cholelithiasis, cholecystitis, acute appendicitis, pancreatitis, malignancy occur rarely.

NURSING IMPLICATIONS
BASELINE ASSESSMENT:

Question for history of hypersensitivity to gemfibrozil. Assess baseline lab results: serum glucose, triglyceride, cholesterol levels, liver function tests, CBC.

INTERVENTION/EVALUATION:

Evaluate food tolerance. Determine pattern of bowel activity. Monitor LDL, VLDL, serum triglyceride, and cholesterol lab results for therapeutic response. Assess for rash, pruritus. Check for headache and dizziness, blurred vision. Monitor liver function and hematology tests. Assess for pain, esp. right upper quadrant/epigastric pain suggestive of adverse gallbladder effects. Monitor serum glucose for those receiving insulin or oral antihyperglycemics.

PATIENT/FAMILY TEACHING:

Follow special diet (important part of treatment). Do not take other medication w/o checking w/physician. Do not stop medication w/o physician's knowledge. Periodic lab tests are essential part of therapy. Notify physician in event of new symptoms, particularly abdominal/epigastric pain. Do not drive or perform other activities that require alert response if dizziness occurs.

gentamicin sulfate
jen-tah-**my**-sin
(Garamycin, Genoptic, Gentacidin, Jenamicin)

CANADIAN AVAILABILITY: Alcomicin, Cidomycin, Garamycin

CLASSIFICATION

Antibiotic: Aminoglycoside

AVAILABILITY (Rx)

Injection: 10 mg/ml, 40 mg/ml, 2 mg/ml (Intrathecal). **Ophthalmic Solution:** 3 mg/ml. **Ophthalmic Ointment:** 3 mg/g. **Cream:** 0.5%. **Ointment:** 0.1%.

PHARMACOKINETICS

Rapid, complete absorption after IM administration. Widely distributed (does not cross blood-brain barrier, low concentrations in CSF). Excreted unchanged in urine. Removed by hemodialysis. Half-life: 2–4 hrs (increased in decreased renal function, neonates; decreased in cystic fibrosis, burn or febrile pts).

ACTION/THERAPEUTIC EFFECT

Bactericidal. Irreversibly binds to protein of bacterial ribosomes, *interfering in protein synthesis of susceptible microorganisms.*

USES/*UNLABELED*

Parenteral: Treatment of skin/skin structure, bone, joint, respiratory tract, intra-abdominal, complicated urinary tract, and acute pelvic infections; postop, burns, septicemia, meningitis. *Ophthalmic:* Ointment/solution for superficial eye infections. *Topical:* Cream/ointment for superficial skin infections. Ophthalmic or topical applications may be combined w/systemic administration for serious, extensive infections. *Topical: Prophylaxis of minor bacterial skin infections, treatment of dermal ulcer.*

STORAGE/HANDLING

Store vials, ophthalmic, topical preparations at room temperature. Solutions appear clear or slightly yellow. Intermittent IV infusion (piggyback) stable for 24 hrs at room temperature. Discard if precipitate forms. Use intrathecal forms immediately after preparation. Discard unused portion.

IM/IV/INTRATHECAL/OPHTHALMIC ADMINISTRATION

Note: Coordinate peak and trough lab draws w/administration times.

IM:

To minimize discomfort, give deep IM slowly. Less painful if injected into gluteus maximus rather than lateral aspect of thigh.

IV:

1. Dilute w/50–200 ml 5% dextrose, 0.9% NaCl, or other compatible fluid. Amount of diluent for infants, children depends on individual needs.

2. Infuse over 30–60 min for adults, older children, and over 60–120 min for infants, young children.

3. Alternating IV sites, use large veins to reduce risk of phlebitis.

INTRATHECAL:

1. Use only 2 mg/ml intrathecal preparation w/o preservative.

2. Mix w/10% estimated CSF volume or sodium chloride.

3. Give over 3–5 min.

OPHTHALMIC:

1. Place finger on lower eyelid and pull out until a pocket is formed between eye and lower lid.

2. Hold dropper above pocket and place correct number of drops ($1/4$–$1/2$ inch ointment) into pocket. Close eye gently.

3. *Solution:* Apply digital pressure to lacrimal sac for 1–2 min (minimizes drainage into nose and throat, reducing risk of systemic effects). *Ointment:* Close eye for 1–2 min, rolling eyeball (increases contact area of drug to eye).

4. Remove excess solution or ointment around eye w/tissue.

INDICATIONS/DOSAGE/ROUTES

Note: Space parenteral doses evenly around the clock. Dosage based on ideal body weight. Peak, trough level determined periodically to maintain desired serum concentrations (minimizes risk of toxicity). *Recommended peak level:* 4–10 mcg/ml; *trough level:* 1–2 mcg/ml.

Moderate to severe infections:

IM/IV: Adults, elderly: 3 mg/kg/day in divided doses q8h. **Children:** 6–7.5 mg/kg/day in divided doses q8h. **Infants, neonates:** 7.5 mg/kg/day in divided doses q8h. **Premature or full-term neonates <7 days:** 5/mg/kg/day in divided doses q12h.

Life-threatening infections:
IM/IV: Adults, elderly: Up to 5 mg/kg/day in divided doses 3–4 times/day.
Intrathecal: Adults, elderly: 4–8 mg as single daily dose (w/IM/IV doses). **Children >3 mos:** 1–2 mg as single daily dose (w/IM/IV doses).

Dosage in renal impairment:
Dose and/or frequency is modified according to degree of renal impairment, serum concentration of drug. After loading dose of 1–2 mg/kg, maintenance dose/frequency based on serum creatinine or creatinine clearance.

Usual ophthalmic dosage:
Adults, elderly: *Ointment:* Thin strip to conjunctiva q6–12h. *Solution:* 1 drop q4–8h to conjunctiva.

Usual topical dosage:
Adults, elderly: Apply 3–4 times/day.

PRECAUTIONS

CONTRAINDICATIONS: Hypersensitivity to gentamicin, other aminoglycosides (cross sensitivity). Sulfite sensitivity may result in anaphylaxis, especially in asthmatics. **CAUTIONS:** Elderly, neonates because of renal insufficiency or immaturity; neuromuscular disorders (potential for respiratory depression), prior hearing loss, vertigo, renal impairment. Cumulative effects may occur w/concurrent systemic administration and topical application to large areas. **PREGNANCY/LACTATION:** Readily crosses placenta, not known whether distributed in breast milk. May produce fetal nephrotoxicity. **Pregnancy Category C**.

INTERACTIONS

DRUG INTERACTIONS: Other aminoglycosides, nephrotoxic, ototoxic-producing medications may increase toxicity. May increase effects of neuromuscular blocking agents. **ALTERED LAB VALUES:** May increase BUN, SGPT (ALT), SGOT (AST), bilirubin, creatinine, LDH concentrations; may decrease serum calcium, magnesium, potassium, sodium concentrations.

SIDE EFFECTS

OCCASIONAL: Pain, induration at IM injection site; phlebitis, thrombophlebitis w/IV administration; hypersensitivity reactions: rash, fever, urticaria, pruritus. *Ophthalmic:* Burning, tearing, itching, blurred vision. *Topical:* Redness, itching. **RARE:** Alopecia, hypertension, weakness.

ADVERSE REACTIONS/TOXIC EFFECTS

Nephrotoxicity (evidenced by increased BUN and serum creatinine, decreased creatinine clearance) may be reversible if drug stopped at first sign of symptoms; irreversible ototoxicity (tinnitus, dizziness, ringing/roaring in ears, reduced hearing) and neurotoxicity (headache, dizziness, lethargy, tremors, visual disturbances) occur occasionally. Risk is greater w/higher dosages, prolonged therapy, or if solution is applied directly to mucosa. Superinfections, particularly w/fungi, may result from bacterial imbalance via any route of administration. Ophthalmic application may cause paresthesia of conjunctiva, mydriasis.

NURSING IMPLICATIONS
BASELINE ASSESSMENT:

Dehydration must be treated before parenteral therapy is begun. Establish baseline hearing acuity. Question for history of allergies, especially to aminoglycosides and sulfite (and parabens for topical/ophthalmic routes). Obtain specimens for culture, sensitivity before giving first dose (therapy may begin before results are known).

INTERVENTION/EVALUATION:

Monitor I&O (maintain hydration), urinalysis (casts, RBCs, WBCs, decrease in specific gravity). Monitor results of peak/trough blood tests. Be alert to ototoxic and neurotoxic symptoms (see Adverse Reactions/Toxic Effects). Check IM injection site for pain, induration. Evaluate IV site for phlebitis (heat, pain, red streaking over vein). Assess for rash (*ophthalmic:* assess for redness, burning, itching, tearing; *topical:* assess for redness, itching). Be alert for superinfection, particularly genital/anal pruritus, changes in oral mucosa, diarrhea. When treating those w/neuromuscular disorders, assess respiratory response carefully.

PATIENT/FAMILY TEACHING:

Continue antibiotic for full length of treatment. Space doses evenly. Discomfort may occur w/IM injection. Blurred vision or tearing may occur briefly after each ophthalmic dose. Notify physician in event of any hearing, visual, balance, urinary problems, even after therapy is completed. *Ophthalmic:* Contact physician if tearing, redness, or irritation continues. *Topical:* Cleanse area gently before applying; notify physician if redness, itching occurs. Do not take other medication w/o consulting physician. Lab tests are an essential part of therapy.

glatiramer
(Copaxone)
See Supplement

glimepiride
glim-**eh**-purr-eyd
(Amaryl)

CLASSIFICATION
Hypoglycemic: Oral

AVAILABILITY (Rx)
Tablets: 1 mg, 2 mg, 4 mg

PHARMACOKINETICS

	ONSET	PEAK	DURATION
PO	—	2–3 hrs	24 hrs

Completely absorbed from GI tract. Metabolized in liver. Excreted in urine and eliminated in feces. Half-life: 5–9.2 hrs.

ACTION/*THERAPEUTIC EFFECT*
Promotes release of insulin from beta cells of pancreas, increases insulin sensitivity at peripheral sites, *lowering blood glucose concentration.*

USES
Adjunct to diet/exercise in management of noninsulin-dependent diabetes mellitus (type II, NIDDM). Use in combination w/insulin or metformin in pts not controlled by diet/exercise in conjunction w/oral hypoglycemic agent.

PO ADMINISTRATION

Take w/breakfast or first main meal.

INDICATIONS/DOSAGE/ROUTES

Diabetes mellitus:
PO: Adults: Initially, 1–2 mg once daily, w/breakfast or first main meal. **Maintenance:** 1–4 mg once daily. After dose of 2 mg is reached, dosage should be increased in increments of up to 2 mg every 1–2 wks, based on blood glucose response. **Maximum:** 8 mg/day.

Combination therapy w/insulin:
PO: Adults: 8 mg once daily w/breakfast or first main meal w/low-dose insulin.

Renal function impairment:
PO: Adults: 1 mg once/day.

PRECAUTIONS

CONTRAINDICATIONS: Sole therapy for type I diabetes mellitus, diabetic complications (ketosis, acidosis, diabetic coma), stress situations (severe infection, trauma, surgery), hypersensitivity to drug, severe renal or hepatic impairment. **CAUTIONS:** Severe diarrhea, intestinal obstruction, prolonged vomiting, liver disease, hyperthyroidism (not controlled), impaired renal function, adrenal insufficiency, debilitation, malnutrition, pituitary insufficiency. **PREGNANCY/LACTATION:** Not recommended for use during pregnancy. Unknown if distributed in breast milk. **Pregnancy Category C**.

INTERACTIONS

DRUG INTERACTIONS: May increase effect of oral anticoagulants. Fluconazole, cimetidine, ranitidine, ciprofloxacin, MAO inhibitors, quinidine, salicylates (large doses) may increase effect. Beta blockers may increase hypoglycemic effect, mask signs of hypoglycemia. Corticosteroids, thiazide diuretics, lithium may decrease effect. **ALTERED LAB VALUES:** May increase alkaline phosphatase, SGOT (AST), LDH, creatinine, BUN.

SIDE EFFECTS

FREQUENT: Altered taste sensation, dizziness, drowsiness, weight gain, constipation, diarrhea, heartburn, nausea, vomiting, stomach fullness, headache. **OCCASIONAL:** Increased sensitivity of skin to sunlight, peeling of skin, itching, rash.

ADVERSE REACTIONS/TOXIC EFFECTS

Hypoglycemia may occur due to overdosage, insufficient food intake esp. w/increased glucose demands. GI hemorrhage, cholestatic hepatic jaundice, leukopenia, thrombocytopenia, pancytopenia, agranulocytosis, aplastic or hemolytic anemia occurs rarely.

NURSING IMPLICATIONS
BASELINE ASSESSMENT:

Question for hypersensitivity to glimepiride. Check blood glucose level. Discuss lifestyle to determine extent of learning, emotional needs. Assure follow-up instruction if pt/family do not thoroughly understand diabetes management or glucose-testing technique.

INTERVENTION/EVALUATION:

Monitor blood glucose and food intake. Assess for hypoglycemia (cool wet skin, tremors, dizziness, anxiety, headache, tachycardia, numbness in mouth, hunger, diplopia) or hyperglycemia (polyuria, polyphagia, polydipsia, nausea, vomiting, dim vision, fatigue, deep rapid breathing). Check for adverse skin reactions, jaundice. Monitor hematology reports. Assess for bleeding or bruising. Be alert to conditions that alter glucose requirements: fever, increased activity or stress, surgical procedure.

PATIENT/FAMILY TEACHING:

Prescribed diet is principal part of treatment; do not skip or delay meals. Diabetes mellitus requires lifelong control. Check blood glucose/urine as ordered. Carry candy, sugar packets, or other sugar supplements for immediate response to hypoglycemia. Wear medical alert identification. Check w/physician when glucose demands are altered (e.g., fever, infection, trauma, stress, heavy physical activity). Avoid alcoholic beverages. Do not take other medication w/o consulting physician. Weight control, exercise, hygiene (including foot care), and nonsmoking are essential part of therapy. Notify physician promptly of skin eruptions, itching, bleeding, yellow skin, dark urine. Inform dentist, physician, or surgeon of this medication before any treatment.

glipizide

glip-ih-zide
(Glucotrol, Glucotrol XL)

CLASSIFICATION

Hypoglycemic: Oral

AVAILABILITY (Rx)

Tablets: 5 mg, 10 mg. **Tablets (extended-release):** 5 mg, 10 mg.

PHARMACOKINETICS

	ONSET	PEAK	DURATION
PO	10–30 min	0.5–2 hrs	24 hrs

Well absorbed from GI tract. Metabolized in liver. Excreted in urine. Half-life: 2–4 hrs.

ACTION/*THERAPEUTIC EFFECT*

Promotes release of insulin from beta cells of pancreas, increases insulin sensitivity at peripheral sites, *lowering blood glucose concentration.*

USES

Adjunct to diet/exercise in management of stable, mild to moderately severe noninsulin-dependent diabetes mellitus (type II, NIDDM). May be used to supplement insulin in those w/type I diabetes mellitus.

PO ADMINISTRATION

1. May take w/food (response better if taken 15–30 min before meals).
2. Do not crush extended-release tablets.

INDICATIONS/DOSAGE/ROUTES

Diabetes mellitus:
PO: Adults: Initially, 5 mg/day (2.5 mg in geriatric or those w/liver disease). Adjust dosage in 2.5–5 mg increments at intervals of several days. **Maximum single dose:** 15 mg. **Maximum dose/day:** 40 mg. **Maintenance:** 10 mg/day.

Usual elderly dosage:
PO: Initially, 2.5–5 mg/day. May increase by 2.5–5 mg/day q1–2 wks.

PRECAUTIONS

CONTRAINDICATIONS: Sole therapy for type I diabetes mellitus, diabetic complications (ketosis, acidosis, diabetic coma), stress situations (severe infection, trauma, surgery), hypersensitivity to drug, severe renal or hepatic impairment. **CAUTIONS:** Severe diarrhea, intestinal obstruction, prolonged vomiting, liver disease, hyperthyroidism (not controlled), impaired renal function, adrenal insufficiency, debilitation, malnourishment, pituitary insufficiency. **PREGNANCY/LACTATION:** Insulin is drug of choice during pregnancy; glipizide given within 1 mo of delivery may produce neonatal hypoglycemia. Drug crosses placenta; distributed in breast milk. **Pregnancy Category C**.

INTERACTIONS

DRUG INTERACTIONS: May increase effect of oral anticoagulants. Fluconazole, cimetidine, ranitidine, ciprofloxacin, MAO inhibitors, quinidine, salicylates (large doses) may increase effect. Beta blockers may increase hypoglycemic effect, mask signs of hypoglycemia. Corticosteroids, thiazide diuretics, lithium may decrease effect. **ALTERED LAB VALUES:** May increase alkaline phosphatase, SGOT (AST), LDH, creatinine, BUN.

SIDE EFFECTS

FREQUENT: Altered taste sensation, dizziness, drowsiness, weight gain, constipation, diarrhea, heartburn, nausea, vomiting, stomach fullness, headache. **OCCASIONAL:** Increased sensitivity of skin to sunlight, peeling of skin, itching, rash.

ADVERSE REACTIONS/TOXIC EFFECTS

Hypoglycemia may occur because of overdosage, insufficient food intake esp. w/increased glucose demands. GI hemorrhage, cholestatic hepatic jaundice, leukopenia, thrombocytopenia, pancytopenia, agranulocytosis, aplastic or hemolytic anemia occurs rarely.

NURSING IMPLICATIONS

BASELINE ASSESSMENT:

Question for hypersensitivity to glipizide. Check blood glucose level. Discuss lifestyle to determine extent of learning, emotional needs. Assure follow-up instruction if pt/family do not thoroughly understand diabetes management or glucose-testing technique.

INTERVENTION/EVALUATION:

Monitor blood glucose and food intake. Assess for hypoglycemia (cool wet skin, tremors, dizziness, anxiety, headache, tachycardia, numbness in mouth, hunger, diplopia) or hyperglycemia (polyuria, polyphagia, polydipsia, nausea, vomiting, dim vision, fatigue, deep rapid breathing). Check for adverse skin reactions, jaundice. Monitor hematology reports. Assess for bleeding or bruising. Be alert to conditions that alter glucose requirements: fever, increased activity or stress, surgical procedure.

PATIENT/FAMILY TEACHING:

Prescribed diet is principal part of treatment; do not skip or delay meals. Diabetes mellitus requires lifelong control. Check blood glucose/urine as ordered. Carry candy, sugar packets, or other sugar supplements for immediate response to hypoglycemia. Wear medical alert identification. Check w/physician when glucose demands are altered (e.g., fever, infection, trauma, stress, heavy physical activity). Avoid alcoholic beverages. Do not take other medication w/o consulting physician. Weight control, exercise, hygiene (including foot care), and nonsmoking are essential part of therapy. Inform dentist, physician, or surgeon of this medication before any treatment.

glucagon hydrochloride

glue-ka-gon
(Glucagon Emergency Kit)

CANADIAN AVAILABILITY:
Glucagon Emergency Kit

CLASSIFICATION

Antihypoglycemic

AVAILABILITY (Rx)

Powder for Injection: 1 mg, 10 mg

PHARMACOKINETICS

Well absorbed after IM, SubQ administration. Undergoes enzymatic proteolysis in liver/kidney. Half-life: 10 min. Peak hyperglycemia occurs within 30 min, lasting 1–2 hrs. Return to consciousness in 5–20 min.

ACTION/ *THERAPEUTIC EFFECT*

Promotes hepatic glycogenolysis, gluconeogenesis. Stimulates enzyme to increase production of cAMP, *resulting in increased plasma glucose concentration, relaxant effect on smooth muscle, and inotropic myocardial effect.*

USES/ *UNLABELED*

Treatment of severe hypoglycemia in diabetic pts. Not for use in chronic hypoglycemia or hypoglycemia due to starvation, adrenal insufficiency, since liver glycogen unavailable. Diagnostic aid in radiographic examination of GI tract. *Treatment of toxicity associated w/beta blockers, calcium channel blockers; esophageal obstruction due to foreign bodies.*

STORAGE/HANDLING

Store vial at room temperature. After reconstitution, stable for 48 hrs if refrigerated. If reconstituted w/sterile water for injection, use immediately. Do not use glucagon solution unless clear.

SUBQ/IM/IV ADMINISTRATION

Note: Place pt on side to avoid potential aspiration (glucagon, as well as hypoglycemia, may produce nausea and vomiting).
   1. Reconstitute powder w/manufacturer's diluent when preparing 2 mg doses or less. For doses exceeding 2 mg, dilute w/sterile water for injection.
   2. To provide 1 mg glucagon/ml, use 1 ml diluent. For 1 mg vial of glucagon, use 10 ml diluent for 10 mg vial.
   3. Pt will usually awaken in 5–20 min. Although 1–2 additional doses may be administered, the concern for effects of continuing cerebral hypoglycemia requires consideration of parenteral glucose.
   4. When pt awakens, give supplemental carbohydrate to restore liver glycogen and prevent secondary hypoglycemia. If pt fails to respond to glucagon, IV glucose is necessary.

INDICATIONS/DOSAGE/ROUTES

Note: Administer IV dextrose if pt fails to respond to glucagon.

Hypoglycemia:
SubQ/IM/IV: Adults, elderly: 0.5–1 mg (0.5–1 unit). May repeat 1–2 additional doses if response is delayed.

Diagnostic aid:
IM: Adults, elderly: 1–2 mg (1–2 units).
IV: Adults, elderly: 0.25–2 mg (0.25–2 units).

PRECAUTIONS

CONTRAINDICATIONS: Pheochromocytoma, hypersensitivity to glucagon (protein). CAUTIONS: History of insulinoma or pheochromocytoma. PREGNANCY/LACTATION: Not known whether drug crosses placenta or is distributed in breast milk. Pregnancy Category B.

INTERACTIONS

DRUG INTERACTIONS: May increase anticoagulant effect. ALTERED LAB VALUES: May decrease potassium.

SIDE EFFECTS

OCCASIONAL: Nausea, vomiting. RARE: Allergic reaction (urticaria, respiratory distress, hypotension).

ADVERSE REACTIONS/TOXIC EFFECTS

Overdose may produce continuing nausea, vomiting, hypokalemia (severe weakness, decreased appetite, irregular heartbeat, muscle cramps).

NURSING IMPLICATIONS
BASELINE ASSESSMENT:

Obtain immediate assessment, including history, clinical signs, and symptoms. If hypoglycemic coma is established, give glucagon promptly as described above.

INTERVENTION/EVALUATION:

Monitor response time carefully. Have IV dextrose readily available in event pt does not awaken within 5–20 min. Assess for possible allergic reaction (urticaria, respiratory difficulty, hypotension). When pt is conscious, give carbohydrate and review insulin/diet needs w/physician.

PATIENT/FAMILY TEACHING:

Recognize significance of recognizing symptoms of hypoglycemia: pale cool skin, anxiety, difficulty concentrating, headache, hunger, nausea, nervousness, shakiness, sweating, unusual tiredness, weakness, unconsciousness. Instruct pt, family, or friend to give sugar form first (orange juice, honey, hard candy, sugar cubes, or table sugar dissolved in water or juice) if symptoms of hypoglycemia develop, followed by cheese and crackers or half a sandwich or glass of milk. Inform physician of hypoglycemic episode and use of glucagon so that regimen can be regulated appropriately. Replace glucagon as soon as possible.

glyburide
glye-byoo-ride
(Diabeta, Micronase)

CANADIAN AVAILABILITY:
Diabeta, Euglucon

CLASSIFICATION
Hypoglycemic: Oral

AVAILABILITY (Rx)
Tablets: 1.25 mg, 2.5 mg, 5 mg

PHARMACOKINETICS

	ONSET	PEAK	DURATION
PO	0.25–1 hr	1–2 hrs	24 hrs

Well absorbed from GI tract. Metabolized in liver to weakly active metabolite. Primarily excreted in urine. Half-life: 10 hrs.

ACTION/ *THERAPEUTIC EFFECT*

Promotes release of insulin from beta cells of pancreas, increases insulin sensitivity at peripheral sites, *lowering blood glucose concentration.*

USES

Adjunct to diet/exercise in management of stable, mild to moderately severe noninsulin-dependent diabetes mellitus (type II, NIDDM). May be used to supplement insulin in those w/type I diabetes mellitus.

PO ADMINISTRATION

May take w/food (response better if taken 15–30 min before meals).

INDICATIONS/DOSAGE/ROUTES

Diabetes mellitus:
PO: Adults: Initially, 2.5 mg up to 20 mg/day. **Range:** 1.25–20 mg/day as a single or in divided doses. **Maintenance:** 7.5 mg/day.

Usual elderly dosage:
PO: Initially, 1.25–2.5 mg/day. May increase by 1.25–2.5 mg/day q1–3 wks.

PRECAUTIONS

CONTRAINDICATIONS: Sole therapy for type I diabetes mellitus, diabetic complications (ketosis, acidosis, diabetic coma), stress situations (severe infection, trauma, surgery), hypersensitivity to drug, severe renal or hepatic impairment. **CAUTIONS:** Severe diarrhea, intestinal obstruction, prolonged vomiting, liver disease, hyperthyroidism (not controlled), impaired renal function, adrenal insufficiency, debilitation, malnourishment, pituitary insufficiency. **PREGNANCY/LACTATION:** Crosses placenta, distributed in breast milk. May produce neonatal hypoglycemia if given within 2 wks of delivery. **Pregnancy Category C**.

INTERACTIONS

DRUG INTERACTIONS: May increase effect of oral anticoagulants. Fluconazole, cimetidine, ranitidine, ciprofloxacin, MAO inhibitors, quinidine, salicylates (large doses) may increase effect. Beta blockers may increase hypoglycemic effect, mask signs of hypoglycemia. Corticosteroids, thiazide diuretics, lithium may decrease effect. **ALTERED LAB VALUES:** May increase alkaline phosphatase, SGOT (AST), LDH, creatinine, BUN.

SIDE EFFECTS

FREQUENT: Altered taste sensation, dizziness, drowsiness, weight gain, constipation, diarrhea, heartburn, nausea, vomiting, stomach fullness, headache. **OCCASIONAL:** Increased sensitivity of skin to sunlight, peeling of skin, itching, rash.

ADVERSE REACTIONS/TOXIC EFFECTS

Overdosage, insufficient food intake may produce hypoglycemia, esp. w/increased glucose demands. Cholestatic jaundice, leukopenia, thrombocytopenia, pancytopenia, agranulocytosis, aplastic or hemolytic anemia occurs rarely.

NURSING IMPLICATIONS

BASELINE ASSESSMENT:

Question for hypersensitivity to glyburide. Check blood glucose level. Discuss lifestyle to determine extent of learning,

emotional needs. Assure follow-up instruction if pt/family does not thoroughly understand diabetes management or glucose-testing techniques.

INTERVENTION/EVALUATION:

Monitor blood glucose and food intake. Assess for hypoglycemia (cool wet skin, tremors, dizziness, anxiety, headache, tachycardia, numbness in mouth, hunger, diplopia) or hyperglycemia (polyuria, polyphagia, polydipsia, nausea and vomiting, dim vision, fatigue, deep rapid breathing). Be alert to conditions altering glucose requirements: fever, increased activity or stress, surgical procedure. Check for adverse skin reactions, jaundice. Monitor hematology reports. Assess for bleeding or bruising.

PATIENT/FAMILY TEACHING:

Prescribed diet is principal part of treatment; do not skip or delay meals. Diabetes mellitus requires lifelong control. Check blood glucose/urine as ordered. Signs and symptoms, treatment of hypo/hyperglycemia. Carry candy, sugar packets, or other sugar supplements for immediate response to hypoglycemia; wear medical alert identification. Check w/physician when glucose demands change (e.g., fever, infection, trauma, stress, heavy physical activity). Avoid alcoholic beverages. Do not take other medication w/o consulting physician. Weight control, exercise, hygiene (including foot care), and nonsmoking are essential part of therapy. Inform dentist, physician, or surgeon of this medication before any treatment.

glycopyrrolate

gly-ko-**pie**-roll-ate
(Robinul)

CANADIAN AVAILABILITY: Robinul

CLASSIFICATION

Anticholinergic

AVAILABILITY (Rx)

Tablets: 1 mg, 2 mg. **Injection:** 0.2 mg/ml.

PHARMACOKINETICS

Incompletely absorbed from GI tract. Well absorbed after IM administration. Metabolized in liver. Primarily excreted in urine. Half-life: 1.7 hrs.

ACTION/*THERAPEUTIC EFFECT*

Inhibits action of acetylcholine on structures innervated by postganglionic sites: smooth, cardiac muscle, SA, AV nodes, exocrine glands. Larger doses may decrease motility, secretory activity of GI system, tone of ureter, urinary bladder. *Reduces salivation and excessive secretions of respiratory tract; reduces gastric secretions, acidity.*

USES

Treatment of peptic ulcer disease. Preop medication to prevent cholinergic effect during surgery (i.e., arrhythmias; reduces salivation, secretions). Given concurrently w/anticholinesterase agents to block adverse muscarinic effects. Blocks vagal inhibitory reflexes during anesthesia induction and intubation. Used intraoperatively to counter vagal reflexes w/arrhythmias. Protects against peripheral muscarinic effects (bradycardia, secretions) of cholinergic agents.

PO/IM/IV ADMINISTRATION

PO:

Administer before meals (food decreases absorption) and bedtime.

IM:

For preop, may be given in same syringe w/other compatible preop medication.

IV:

1. Give by direct IV injection.

2. May be given via tubing or running IV infusion of compatible solution.

3. When used concurrently w/neostigmine or physostigmine, may be administered via same syringe.

INDICATIONS/DOSAGE/ROUTES

Peptic ulcer disease:
PO: Adults, elderly: Initially, 1 mg 3 times/day. **Maintenance:** 1 mg 2 times/day. **Maximum:** 8 mg/day.
IM/IV: Adults, elderly: 0.1–0.2 mg q4h (3–4 times/day). **Maximum:** 4 doses/day.

Preop:
IM: Adults, elderly, children >2 yrs: 0.004 mg/kg 30–60 min before anesthesia. **Children <2 yrs:** Up to 0.004 mg/lb.

Intraoperative (prevent cholinergic effects):
IV: Adults, elderly, children: 0.1 mg (0.5 ml). May repeat at 2–3 min intervals.

Block effects of anticholinesterase agents:
IV: Adults, elderly: 0.2 mg for each 1 mg neostigmine or 5 mg pyridostigmine.

PRECAUTIONS

CONTRAINDICATIONS: Narrow-angle glaucoma, severe ulcerative colitis, toxic megacolon, obstructive disease of GI tract, paralytic ileus, intestinal atony, bladder neck obstruction due to prostatic hypertrophy, myasthenia gravis in those not treated w/neostigmine, tachycardia secondary to cardiac insufficiency or thyrotoxicosis, cardiospasm, unstable cardiovascular status in acute hemorrhage. **EXTREME CAUTION:** Autonomic neuropathy, known or suspected GI infections, diarrhea, mild to moderate ulcerative colitis. **CAUTIONS:** Hyperthyroidism, hepatic or renal disease, hypertension, tachyarrhythmias, CHF, coronary artery disease, gastric ulcer, esophageal reflux or hiatal hernia associated w/reflux esophagitis, infants, elderly, those w/COPD. **PREGNANCY/LACTATION:** Not known whether drug crosses placenta or is distributed in breast milk. **Pregnancy Category B.**

INTERACTIONS

DRUG INTERACTIONS: Antacids, antidiarrheals may decrease absorption. Anticholinergics may increase effects. May decrease absorption of ketoconazole. May increase severity of GI lesions with potassium chloride (wax matrix). **ALTERED LAB VALUES:** May decrease uric acid.

SIDE EFFECTS

FREQUENT: Dry mouth (sometimes severe), decreased sweating, constipation. **OCCASIONAL:** Blurred vision, bloated feeling, urinary hesitancy, drowsiness (w/high dosage), headache, intolerance to light, loss of taste, nervousness, flushing, insomnia, impotence, mental confusion/excitement (particularly in elderly, children). Parenteral form may produce temporary lightheadedness, local irritation. **RARE:** Dizziness, faintness.

ADVERSE REACTIONS/TOXIC EFFECTS

Overdosage may produce temporary paralysis of ciliary muscle, pupillary dilation, tachycardia, palpitation, hot/dry/flushed skin, absence of bowel sounds, hyperthermia, increased respiratory rate, EKG abnormalities, nausea, vomiting, rash over face/upper trunk, CNS stimulation, psychosis (agitation, restlessness, rambling speech, visual hallucination, paranoid behavior, delusions), followed by depression.

NURSING IMPLICATIONS
Baseline Assessment:

Before giving medication, instruct pt to void (reduces risk of urinary retention).

Intervention/Evaluation:

Monitor daily bowel activity and stool consistency. Palpate bladder for urinary retention. Monitor changes in B/P, temperature. Assess skin turgor, mucous membranes to evaluate hydration status (encourage adequate fluid intake), bowel sounds for peristalsis. Be alert for fever (increased risk of hyperthermia).

Patient/Family Teaching:

Take 30 min before meals (food decreases absorption of medication). Use care not to become overheated during exercise in hot weather (may result in heat stroke). Avoid hot baths, saunas. Avoid tasks that require alertness, motor skills until response to drug is established. Sugarless gum, sips of tepid water may relieve dry mouth. Do not take antacids or medicine for diarrhea within 1 hr of taking this medication (decreased effectiveness).

gold sodium thiomalate

gold sodium thigh-oh-**mal**-ate **(Myochrysine)**

CANADIAN AVAILABILITY: Myochrysine

CLASSIFICATION

Antirheumatic, anti-inflammatory

AVAILABILITY (Rx)

Injection: 25 mg/ml, 50 mg/ml

PHARMACOKINETICS

Rapidly absorbed after IM administration. Widely distributed. Metabolic fate unknown. Primarily excreted in urine. Half-life: 3–27 days after single dose up to 168 days w/multiple doses. Contains approximately 50% gold.

ACTION/ *THERAPEUTIC EFFECT*

Inhibits phagocytosis, lysomal enzyme activity, decreasing concentration of rheumatoid factor, immunoglobulins. *Decreases synovial inflammation, retards cartilage and bone destruction (suppresses or prevents, but does not cure, arthritis, synovitis).*

USES/ *UNLABELED*

Management of rheumatoid arthritis in those w/insufficient therapeutic response to non-steroidal anti-inflammatory agents. *Treatment of psoriatic arthritis.*

IM ADMINISTRATION

1. Give in upper outer quadrant of gluteus maximus.

2. Pt to be lying down when administered.

INDICATIONS/DOSAGE/ROUTES

Rheumatoid arthritis:
Note: Give as weekly injections.
IM: Adults, elderly: Initially, 10 mg, then 25 mg for second dose. Follow w/25 mg/wk until improvement noted or total of 1 g administered. **Maintenance:** 25–50 mg q2 wks for 2–20 wks; if stable, may increase to q3–4 wk intervals. **Children:** Initially, 10 mg, then 1 mg/kg/wk. **Maximum single dose:** 50 mg.

PRECAUTIONS

CONTRAINDICATIONS: History of gold-induced pathoses (necrotizing enterocolitis, exfoliative dermatitis, pulmonary fibrosis, blood dyscrasias), hepatic dysfunction or history of hepatitis, uncontrolled diabetes or CHF, urticaria, eczema, colitis, hemorrhagic conditions, systemic lupus erythematosus, recent radiation therapy. **CAUTIONS:** Renal/hepatic disease, inflammatory bowel disease. **PREGNANCY/LACTATION:** Crosses placenta, distributed in breast milk. Use only when benefits outweigh hazard to fetus. **Pregnancy Category C.**

INTERACTIONS

DRUG INTERACTIONS: Bone marrow depressants, hepatotoxic, nephrotoxic medications may increase toxicity. Penicillamine may increase risk of hematologic or renal adverse effects. **ALTERED LAB VALUES:** May decrease Hgb, Hct, platelets, WBCs. May alter liver function tests. May increase urine protein.

SIDE EFFECTS

FREQUENT: Diarrhea/loose stools, rash, pruritus, abdominal pain, nausea. **OCCASIONAL:** Vomiting, anorexia, flatulence, dyspepsia, conjunctivitis, photosensitivity. **RARE:** Constipation, urticaria, rash.

ADVERSE REACTIONS/TOXIC EFFECTS

Signs of gold toxicity: decreased hemoglobin, leukopenia (WBC below 4,000 mm^3), reduced granulocyte counts (below 150,000/mm^3), proteinuria, hematuria, stomatitis, blood dyscrasias (anemia, leukopenia, thrombocytopenia, eosinophilia), glomerulonephritis, nephrotic syndrome, cholestatic jaundice.

NURSING IMPLICATIONS

BASELINE ASSESSMENT:

Rule out pregnancy before beginning treatment; CBC, urinalysis, platelet and differential, renal and liver function tests should be performed before therapy begins.

INTERVENTION/EVALUATION:

Monitor daily bowel activity and stool consistency. Assess urine tests for proteinuria or hematuria. Monitor WBC, hemoglobin, differential, platelet count, renal and hepatic function studies. Question for skin pruritus (may be first sign of impending rash). Assess skin daily for rash, purpura, or ecchymoses. Assess oral mucous membranes, borders of tongue, palate, pharynx for ulceration, complaint of metallic taste sensation (signs of stomatitis). Evaluate for therapeutic response: relief of pain, stiffness, swelling, increase in

G

joint mobility, reduced joint tenderness, improved grip strength.

PATIENT/FAMILY TEACHING:

Therapeutic response may take 6 mos or longer. Avoid exposure to sunlight (gray to blue pigment may appear). Contact physician/nurse if pruritus, rash, sore mouth, indigestion, or metallic taste occurs. Maintain diligent oral hygiene.

---

gonadorelin acetate

go-nad-oh-**rell**-in
(Lutrepulse)

gonadorelin hydrochloride

(Factrel)

CANADIAN AVAILABILITY:
Factrel, Lutrepulse

CLASSIFICATION

Gonadotropin-releasing hormone

AVAILABILITY (Rx)

Powder for Injection: (acetate): 0.8 mg, 3.2 mg; **(hydrochloride):** 100 mcg, 500 mcg

PHARMACOKINETICS

Rapidly metabolized. Primarily excreted in urine. Half-life: 10–40 min.

ACTION/THERAPEUTIC EFFECT

Diagnostic aid. *Stimulates synthesis, release of luteinizing hormone (LH), follicle-stimulating hormone (FSH)* from anterior pituitary. *Stimulates release of gonadotropin-releasing hormone* from hypothalamus.

USES/UNLABELED

As a single dose, to evaluate the functional capacity and response of gonadotropes of anterior pituitary in suspected gonadotropic deficiency (does not differentiate between hypothalamus or pituitary disorders). Multiple injection testing is used to evaluate residual gonadotropic function of pituitary after removal of a pituitary tumor by surgery and/or irradiation. Induction of ovulation in women w/primary hypothalamic amenorrhea. *Acetate: Treatment of delayed puberty, infertility.*

STORAGE/HANDLING

Solution should appear clear, colorless, free of particulate matter. Do not use if discolored/precipitate formed. Discard unused portion.

SUBQ/IV ADMINISTRATION

GONADORELIN ACETATE:

1. Reconstitute vial w/8 ml diluent immediately before use. Inject diluent onto dry product cake.
2. Shake a few seconds.
3. Transfer solution to plastic reservoir.
4. Set Lutrepulse pump to deliver appropriate volume/pulse over 1 min q90 min.
5. Solution will supply doses for approximately 7 days.

GONADORELIN HYDROCHLORIDE:

1. Reconstitute 100 mcg w/1.0 ml of sterile diluent supplied.
2. Reconstitute 500 mcg w/2.0 ml of sterile diluent supplied.
3. Prepare solution immediately before use.

INDICATIONS/DOSAGE/ROUTES

Note: Test should be conducted in

the absence of other drugs that affect pituitary secretion of gonadotropins.

GONADORELIN ACETATE:

Primary hypothalamic amenorrhea:
IV Pump: Adults: 5 mcg q90min (range 1–20 mcg); treatment interval 21 days. Refer to manufacturer's manual for proper dilutions/settings on pump. Response usually occurs 2–3 wks after initiation. Continue additional 2 wks after ovulation occurs (maintains corpus luteum).

GONADORELIN HYDROCHLORIDE:

Diagnostic agent:
IV/SubQ: Adults: 100 mcg. In females, perform test in early follicular phase of menstrual cycle.

PRECAUTIONS

CONTRAINDICATIONS: Hypersensitivity to gonadorelin, components. *Gonadorelin acetate:* Women w/any condition exacerbated by pregnancy, ovarian cysts, or causes of anovulation other than hypothalamic in origin. CAUTIONS: None significant. PREGNANCY/LACTATION: Pregnancy Category B.

INTERACTIONS

DRUG INTERACTIONS: None significant. ALTERED LAB VALUES: None significant.

SIDE EFFECTS

OCCASIONAL: *Gonadorelin acetate:* Multiple pregnancy, inflammation, infection, mild phlebitis, hematoma at catheter site. *Gonadorelin hydrochloride:* Swelling, pain, or itching at injection site w/SubQ administration. Local or generalized skin rash w/chronic SubQ administration. RARE: *Gonadorelin acetate:* Ovarian hyperstimulation. *Gonadorelin hydrochloride:* Headache, nausea, lightheadedness, abdominal discomfort, hypersensitivity reactions (bronchospasm, tachycardia, flushing, urticaria), induration at injection site.

ADVERSE REACTIONS/TOXIC EFFECTS

Anaphylactic reaction occurs rarely.

NURSING IMPLICATIONS

BASELINE ASSESSMENT:

Before test is started, assure that pt understands procedure. Question for hypersensitivity to gonadorelin or components. *Gonadorelin acetate:* Pt instructions included w/kit from manufacturer. *Gonadorelin hydrochloride:* Venous blood sample (for LH) to be drawn immediately before gonadorelin hydrochloride administration.

INTERVENTION/EVALUATION:

Gonadorelin acetate: W/baseline pelvic ultrasound, follow-up studies. *Gonadorelin hydrochloride:* At 7 and 14 days of therapy. Change cannula and IV site at 48 hr intervals. Assure protocol for test is maintained: usually venous blood samples (for LH) drawn after administration at intervals of 15, 30, 45, 60, and 120 min.

goserelin acetate

gos-**er**-ah-lin
(Zoladex)

CANADIAN AVAILABILITY: Zoladex

CLASSIFICATION

Antineoplastic

AVAILABILITY (Rx)

Implant: 3.6 mg, 10.8 mg

PHARMACOKINETICS

Well absorbed (slower first 8 days after injection than remainder of 28 day cycle). Half-life: 4.2 hrs.

ACTION / THERAPEUTIC EFFECT

Synthetic luteinizing hormone-releasing hormone analogue. Stimulates release of luteinizing hormone (LH), follicle-stimulating hormone (FSH) from anterior pituitary *(increases testosterone concentrations). After initial increase, decreases release of LH, FSH, testosterone.*

USES

Treatment of advanced carcinoma of prostate as alternative when orchiectomy or estrogen therapy is either not indicated or unacceptable to pt. In combination w/flutamide prior to and during radiation therapy for early stages of prostate cancer. Management of endometriosis. Treatment of advanced breast cancer in premenopausal and perimenopausal women. Endometrial thinning before ablation for dysfunctional uterine bleeding.

STORAGE / HANDLING

Store at room temperature.

SUBQ ADMINISTRATION

Administer into upper abdominal wall (local anesthesia acceptable).

INDICATIONS / DOSAGE / ROUTES

Prostatic carcinoma, endometriosis:
SubQ Implant: Adults >18 yrs, elderly: 3.6 mg q28days or 10.8 mg q12wks into upper abdominal wall.

Endometrial thinning:
SubQ: Adults: 3.6 mg once or 4 wks apart times 2 doses.

PRECAUTIONS

CONTRAINDICATIONS: Pregnancy. **CAUTIONS:** None significant. **PREGNANCY/LACTATION:** Produces atrophic secondary sex organs, implantation loss; suppresses ovarian function, ovarian weight and size. Not known whether drug is distributed in breast milk. Do not use during pregnancy or in those who may become pregnant. **Pregnancy Category X** (endometriosis), **Category D** (breast cancer).

INTERACTIONS

DRUG INTERACTIONS: None significant. **ALTERED LAB VALUES:** May increase serum acid phosphatase, testosterone concentrations.

SIDE EFFECTS

FREQUENT (>10%): Headache (60%), depression (54%), hot flashes (55%), sweating, sexual dysfunction, decreased erection, lower urinary tract symptoms, nausea. **OCCASIONAL (5–10%):** Pain, lethargy, dizziness, insomnia, decreased appetite, nausea, rash, CHF, upper respiratory infections, hair growth, abdominal pain. **RARE:** Itching.

ADVERSE REACTIONS / TOXIC EFFECTS

Arrhythmias, CHF, hypertension occur rarely. Ureteral obstruction, spinal cord compression observed (immediate orchiectomy may be necessary).

NURSING IMPLICATIONS

INTERVENTION / EVALUATION:

Monitor pt closely for worsening signs and symptoms of prostatic cancer, esp. during first month of therapy.

PATIENT/FAMILY TEACHING:

Use contraceptive measures during therapy. Do not have immunizations w/o doctor's approval (drug lowers body's resistance). Avoid contact w/those who have recently received live virus vaccine. Inform physician if regular menstruation persists, become pregnant. Breakthrough menstrual bleeding may occur if dose is missed. Use nonhormonal methods of contraception.

granisetron

gran-**is**-eh-tron
(Kytril)

CANADIAN AVAILABILITY:
Kytril

CLASSIFICATION

Antiemetic

AVAILABILITY (Rx)

Tablets: 1 mg, 2 mg. **Injection:** 1 mg/ml.

PHARMACOKINETICS

Rapid, widely distributed to tissues. Metabolized in liver to active metabolite. Excreted in urine, eliminated in feces. Half-life: 10–12 hrs (increased in elderly).

ACTION/ *THERAPEUTIC EFFECT*

Selectively blocks serotonin stimulation at receptor sites on abdominal vagal afferent nerve and chemoreceptor trigger zone, *preventing nausea, vomiting.*

USES/ *UNLABELED*

Prevents nausea, vomiting associated w/emetogenic cancer therapy (includes high-dose cisplatin).

Prophylaxis of nausea/vomiting associated w/cancer radiotherapy. Oral: prevention of nausea/vomiting associated w/radiation therapy.

STORAGE/HANDLING

Clear, colorless solution. Store at room temperature. After dilution, stable for at least 24 hrs at room temperature. Inspect for particulates, discoloration.

IV ADMINISTRATION

1. Dilute calculated dose w/20–50 ml 0.9% NaCl or 5% dextrose. Do not mix w/other medications.

2. Infuse IV over 5 min.

3. May give undiluted over 30 sec.

INDICATIONS/DOSAGE/ROUTES

Antiemetic:
IV: Adults, elderly, children >2 yrs: 10 mcg/kg beginning within 30 min before initiating chemotherapy. **PO: Adults, elderly:** 1 mg up to 1 hr before chemotherapy and 12 hrs after first dose or 2 mg once 1 hr prior to chemotherapy.

Give only on days that chemotherapy is administered.

PRECAUTIONS

CONTRAINDICATIONS: None significant. **CAUTIONS:** Safety in children <2 yrs of age not established. **PREGNANCY/LACTATION:** Not known whether drug is distributed in breast milk. **Pregnancy Category B**.

INTERACTIONS

DRUG INTERACTIONS: Hepatic enzyme inducers may decrease effect. **ALTERED LAB VALUES:** May increase SGOT (AST), SGPT (ALT).

SIDE EFFECTS

FREQUENT (10–20%): Headache, constipation, asthenia (loss of strength), nausea, leukopenia. **OCCASIONAL (2–10%):** Abdominal pain, diarrhea, vomiting, decreased appetite, chills, hair loss. **RARE (<2%):** Chest pain, angina, hypertension, altered taste, hypersensitivity reaction.

ADVERSE REACTIONS/TOXIC EFFECTS

None significant.

NURSING IMPLICATIONS
BASELINE ASSESSMENT:

Assure granisetron is given within 30 min before start of chemotherapy.

INTERVENTION/EVALUATION:

Monitor for therapeutic effect. Assess for headache. Monitor frequency and consistency of stools.

PATIENT/FAMILY TEACHING:

Granisetron is effective shortly after administration; prevents nausea, vomiting. Explain that transitory taste disorder may occur.

---

griseofulvin

griz-ee-oh-**full**-vin
(Fulvicin, Grisactin, GrisPEG)

CANADIAN AVAILABILITY:
Fulvicin, Grisovin-FP

CLASSIFICATION

Antifungal

AVAILABILITY (Rx)

Microsize: **Tablets:** 250 mg, 500 mg. **Capsules:** 125 mg, 250 mg. **Oral Suspension:** 125 mg/5 ml.
Ultra Microsize: **Tablets:** 125 mg, 165 mg, 250 mg, 330 mg.

PHARMACOKINETICS

Microsize: Variably absorbed from GI tract. *Ultra microsize:* Completely absorbed from GI tract. Primarily deposited in keratin layer of skin, hair, nails. Metabolized in liver. Primarily excreted in urine. Half-life: 24 hrs.

ACTION/*THERAPEUTIC EFFECT*

Inhibits fungal cell mitosis by disrupting mitotic spindle structure. *Fungistatic.*

USES

Treatment of tineas (ringworm): t. capitis, t. corporis, t. cruris, t. pedis, t. unguium.

PO ADMINISTRATION

1. Take w/or after meals (decreases GI irritation, increases absorption).
2. Shake suspension well before administration.
3. Distinguish carefully between microsize and ultra microsize doses.

INDICATIONS/DOSAGE/ROUTES

Note: Give orally as a single dose or in 2–4 divided doses. Dosage is individualized.

Tinea corporis, tinea cruris, tinea capitis:
PO: Adults, elderly: Ultra microsize: 330–375 mg/day. Microsize: 500 mg/day.

Tinea pedis, tinea unguium:
PO: Adults, elderly: Ultra microsize: 660–750 mg/day. Microsize: 750 mg to 1 g/day. **Children >2**

yrs: Ultra microsize: 7.3 mg/kg/day. **Microsize:** 10–11 mg/kg/day.

PRECAUTIONS

CONTRAINDICATIONS: Hypersensitivity to griseofulvin, porphyria, hepatocellular failure. **CAUTIONS:** Exposure to sun or ultraviolet light (photosensitivity), hypersensitivity to penicillins. **PREGNANCY/LACTATION:** Not known whether drug crosses placenta or is distributed in breast milk. **Pregnancy Category C**.

INTERACTIONS

DRUG INTERACTIONS: May decrease effects of warfarin, oral contraceptives. **ALTERED LAB VALUES:** None significant.

SIDE EFFECTS

OCCASIONAL: Hypersensitivity reaction (rash, pruritus, urticaria), headache, nausea, diarrhea, excessive thirst, flatulence, oral thrush, dizziness, insomnia. **RARE:** Paresthesia of hands/feet, proteinuria.

ADVERSE REACTIONS/TOXIC EFFECTS

Granulocytopenia should cause discontinuation of drug.

NURSING IMPLICATIONS

BASELINE ASSESSMENT:

Question for history of allergies, esp. to griseofulvin, penicillins. Confirm that a culture/histologic test was done for accurate diagnosis.

INTERVENTION/EVALUATION:

Assess skin for rash and response to therapy. Evaluate food intake, tolerance. Determine pattern of bowel activity and stool consistency. Question presence of headache: onset, location, type of discomfort. Assess mental status for dizziness and provide ambulation assistance when necessary.

PATIENT/FAMILY TEACHING:

Prolonged therapy (weeks or months) is usually necessary. Do not miss a dose; continue therapy as long as ordered. Avoid alcohol (may produce tachycardia, flushing). Maintain good hygiene (prevents superinfection). Separate personal items in direct contact w/affected areas. Do not apply other preparations or take other medications w/o consulting physician. Avoid exposure to sunlight. Keep areas dry; wear light clothing for ventilation. Take w/foods high in fat such as milk, ice cream (reduces GI upset and assists absorption).

---

guaifenesin (glyceryl guaiacolate)

guay-**fen**-ah-sin
(Glycotuss, Humibid, Robitussin)

FIXED-COMBINATION(S):
W/phenylephrine and phenylpropanolamine, sympathomimetics **(Entex)**.

CANADIAN AVAILABILITY:
Balminil, Benylin E, Robitussin

CLASSIFICATION

Expectorant

AVAILABILITY (OTC)

Tablets: 100 mg, 200 mg. **Tablets (sustained-release):** 600 mg. **Capsules:** 200 mg. **Capsules (sustained-release):** 300 mg. **Syrup:** 100 mg/5 ml. **Liquid:** 200 mg/5 ml.

PHARMACOKINETICS

Well absorbed from GI tract. Metabolized in liver. Excreted in urine.

ACTION/*THERAPEUTIC EFFECT*

Enhances fluid output of respiratory tract by decreasing adhesiveness and surface tension, *promoting removal of viscous mucus*.

USES

Symptomatic relief of cough in presence of mucus in respiratory tract. Not for use w/persistent cough due to smoking, asthma, emphysema or cough accompanied by excessive secretions.

STORAGE/HANDLING

Store syrup, liquid, capsules at room temperature.

PO ADMINISTRATION

1. Give w/o regard to meals.
2. Do not crush or break sustained-release capsule. May sprinkle contents on soft food, then swallow w/o crushing/chewing.

INDICATIONS/DOSAGE/ROUTES

Note: Give extended-release at 12 hr intervals.

Expectorant:
PO: Adults, elderly, children >12 yrs: 200–400 mg q4h. **Maximum:** 2.4 g/day. **Children 6–12 yrs:** 100–200 mg q4h. **Maximum:** 1.2 g/day. **Children 2–6 yrs:** 50–100 mg q4h. **Maximum:** 600 mg/day.

PRECAUTIONS

CONTRAINDICATIONS: None significant. **CAUTIONS:** None significant. **PREGNANCY/LACTATION:** Not known whether drug crosses placenta or is distributed in breast milk. **Pregnancy Category C.**

INTERACTIONS

DRUG INTERACTIONS: None significant. **ALTERED LAB VALUES:** None significant.

SIDE EFFECTS

RARE: Dizziness, headache, rash, diarrhea, nausea, vomiting, stomach pain.

ADVERSE REACTIONS/TOXIC EFFECTS

Excessive dosage may produce nausea, vomiting.

NURSING IMPLICATIONS

BASELINE ASSESSMENT:

Assess type, severity, frequency of cough and productions. Increase fluid intake and environmental humidity to lower viscosity of lung secretions.

INTERVENTION/EVALUATION:

Initiate deep breathing and coughing exercises, particularly in those w/impaired pulmonary function. Assess for clinical improvement and record onset of relief of cough.

PATIENT/FAMILY TEACHING:

Avoid tasks that require alertness, motor skills until response to drug is established. Do not take for chronic cough. Inform physician if cough persists or if fever, rash, headache, or sore throat is present w/cough. Maintain adequate hydration.

guanabenz acetate

gwan-ah-benz
(Wytensin)

CLASSIFICATION

Antihypertensive

AVAILABILITY (Rx)

Tablets: 4 mg, 8 mg

guanabenz acetate / 483

PHARMACOKINETICS

	ONSET	PEAK	DURATION
PO	1 hr	2–4 hrs	6–8 hrs

Well absorbed from GI tract. Widely distributed. Metabolized in liver. Primarily excreted in urine. Half-life: 7–10 hrs.

ACTION/*THERAPEUTIC EFFECT*

Stimulates alpha$_2$-adrenergic receptors. Inhibits sympathetic cardioaccelerator and vasoconstrictor center to heart, kidneys, peripheral vasculature. *Decreases systolic, diastolic B/P.* Chronic use *decreases peripheral vascular resistance.*

USES

Treatment of hypertension. Used alone or in combination w/thiazide-type diuretics.

PO ADMINISTRATION

1. May give w/food if GI distress occurs.
2. Tablets may be crushed.
3. Give last dose at bedtime (ensures control of B/P at night, minimizing daytime drowsiness).

INDICATIONS/DOSAGE/ROUTES

Hypertension:
PO: **Adults:** Initially, 4 mg 2 times/day. Increase by 4–8 mg at 1–2 wk intervals. **Elderly:** Initially, 4 mg/day. May increase q1–2 wks. **Maintenance:** 8–16 mg/day. **Maximum:** 32 mg/day.

PRECAUTIONS

CONTRAINDICATIONS: None significant. **CAUTIONS:** Severe coronary insufficiency, recent MI, cerebrovascular disease, severe hepatic, renal failure. **PREGNANCY/LACTATION:** Not known whether drug crosses placenta or is distributed in breast milk. May cause fetal harm. Pregnancy Category C.

INTERACTIONS

DRUG INTERACTIONS: Beta-adrenergic blockers, hypotension-producing medications may increase antihypertensive effect. **ALTERED LAB VALUES:** May decrease cholesterol, total triglyceride concentrations.

SIDE EFFECTS

FREQUENT (>10%): Dizziness, drowsiness (20–39%), dry mouth (28–38%), weakness. **OCCASIONAL (3–10%):** Headache, nausea, decreased sexual ability. **RARE (<3%):** Ataxia, sleep disturbances, rash, itching, diarrhea, constipation, altered taste, muscle aches.

ADVERSE REACTIONS/TOXIC EFFECTS

Abrupt withdrawal may result in rebound hypertension manifested as nervousness, agitation, anxiety, insomnia, hand tingling, tremor, flushing, sweating. Overdosage produces hypotension, somnolence, lethargy, irritability, bradycardia, miosis (pupillary constriction).

NURSING IMPLICATIONS

BASELINE ASSESSMENT:

Obtain B/P immediately before each dose administration, in addition to regular monitoring (be alert to B/P fluctuations).

INTERVENTION/EVALUATION:

Sedative effect, drowsiness may require assistance w/ambulation, esp. during early therapy. Assess for peripheral edema of hands, feet (usually, first area of low extremity swelling is behind medial malleolus). Assess skin for development of rash. If excessive reduction in B/P occurs, place pt in supine position w/legs elevated. Assess for anorexia secondary to decreased taste perception. Monitor pattern of daily bowel activity and stool consistency.

PATIENT/FAMILY TEACHING:

Side effects may occur during first 2 wks of therapy but generally diminish or disappear during continued therapy. Sugarless gum, sips of tepid water may relieve dry mouth. Skipping doses or voluntarily discontinuing drug may produce severe, rebound hypertension. Avoid alcohol; use caution driving or operating machinery until tolerance to medication is established.

guanadrel sulfate

gwan-ah-drel
(Hylorel)

CLASSIFICATION

Antihypertensive

AVAILABILITY (Rx)

Tablets: 10 mg, 25 mg

PHARMACOKINETICS

	ONSET	PEAK	DURATION
PO	2 hrs	4–6 hrs	—

Rapidly, completely absorbed from GI tract. Widely distributed. Metabolized in liver. Primarily excreted in urine. Half-life: 10 hrs.

ACTION/THERAPEUTIC EFFECT

Depletes norepinephrine from adrenergic nerve endings, *reducing B/P.* Prevents release of norepinephrine normally produced by nerve stimulation.

USES

Treatment of hypertension in those not controlled w/thiazide-type diuretic. Combine w/diuretic therapy for optimum control of B/P.

PO ADMINISTRATION

1. May give w/o regard to food.
2. Tablets may be crushed.

INDICATIONS/DOSAGE/ROUTES

Hypertension:
PO: Adults: Initially, 5 mg 2 times/day. Increase at 1–4 wk intervals. **Elderly:** Initially, 5 mg/day. May gradually increase at 1–4 wk intervals. **Maintenance:** 20–75 mg/day in 2 divided doses.

PRECAUTIONS

CONTRAINDICATIONS: Frank CHF, pheochromocytoma. **EXTREME CAUTION:** CHF, regional vascular disease. **CAUTIONS:** Elderly, bronchial asthma, peptic ulcer. **PREGNANCY/LACTATION:** Not known whether drug crosses placenta or is distributed in breast milk. **Pregnancy Category B.**

INTERACTIONS

DRUG INTERACTIONS: Tricyclic antidepressants, MAO inhibitors, phenothiazines, sympathomimetics may decrease antihypertensive effect. **ALTERED LAB VALUES:** None significant.

SIDE EFFECTS

FREQUENT (30–65%): Fatigue, headache, faintness, drowsiness, nocturia, urinary frequency, change in weight, aching limbs. **OCCASIONAL (10–30%):** Cough, shortness of breath (resting), change in vision, confusion, constipation, decreased appetite, peripheral edema, leg cramps. **RARE (<10%):** Depression, altered sleep, nausea, vomiting, dry

mouth, throat, impotence, backache, joint pain.

ADVERSE REACTIONS/TOXIC EFFECTS

Overdose may produce blurred
vision, severe dizziness/faintness.

NURSING IMPLICATIONS
BASELINE ASSESSMENT:

Obtain B/P immediately before each dose, in addition to
regular monitoring (be alert to
B/P fluctuations). Therapy should
be discontinued 2–3 days before
elective surgery. Advise anesthe-
siologist of drug therapy if emergency surgery is necessary.

INTERVENTION/EVALUATION:

Monitor pattern of daily bowel
activity and stool consistency. If
excessive reduction in B/P occurs, place pt in supine position
w/legs elevated. Assess for peripheral edema of hands, feet
(usually, first area of low extremity swelling is behind medial
malleolus in ambulatory, sacral
area in bedridden). Monitor
both erect and supine B/P.

PATIENT/FAMILY TEACHING:

To reduce hypotensive effect,
rise slowly from lying to sitting
position and permit legs to dangle from bed momentarily before standing. Avoid sudden or
prolonged standing, exercise,
hot environment or hot shower,
alcohol ingestion, particularly in
morning (may aggravate orthostatic hypotension). If dizziness
or weakness occurs, sit or lie
down immediately. If nausea occurs, cola, unsalted crackers, or
dry toast may relieve effect. Sugarless gum, sips of tepid water
may relieve dry mouth.

guanfacine
gwan-fah-seen
(Tenex)

CLASSIFICATION

Antihypertensive

AVAILABILITY (Rx)

Tablets: 1 mg, 2 mg

PHARMACOKINETICS

	ONSET	PEAK	DURATION
PO	—	1–4 hrs	—

Rapidly, completely absorbed
from GI tract. Widely distributed.
Metabolized in liver. Primarily excreted in urine. Half-life: 10–30 hrs.

ACTION/*THERAPEUTIC EFFECT*

Stimulates alpha$_2$-adrenergic receptors. Inhibits sympathetic cardioaccelerator and vasoconstrictor
center to heart, kidneys, peripheral vasculature. *Decreases systolic,
diastolic B/P. Chronic use decreases peripheral vascular resistance.*

USES/*UNLABELED*

Management of hypertension
alone or in combination w/other
antihypertensives, especially thi-
azide-type diuretics. *Attention
deficit hyperactivity disorder
(ADHD), tic disorders.*

PO ADMINISTRATION

1. Give w/o regard to food.
2. Tablets may be crushed.
3. Administer at bedtime (minimizes daytime drowsiness).

INDICATIONS/DOSAGE/ROUTES

Hypertension:
PO: Adults, elderly: Initially, 1
mg/day. Increase by 1 mg/day at
intervals of 3–4 wks up to 3 mg/
day in single or divided doses.

PRECAUTIONS

CONTRAINDICATIONS: None significant. **CAUTIONS:** Impaired renal function. **PREGNANCY/LACTATION:** Not known whether drug crosses placenta or is distributed in breast milk. Not recommended in treatment of acute hypertension associated w/preeclampsia. **Pregnancy Category B**.

INTERACTIONS

DRUG INTERACTIONS: Beta-adrenergic blockers, hypotension-producing medications may increase antihypertensive effect. **ALTERED LAB VALUES:** May increase growth hormone concentration. May decrease urinary catecholamine, VMA excretion.

SIDE EFFECTS

FREQUENT (>10%): Constipation, dizziness, drowsiness, dry mouth. **OCCASIONAL (2–10%):** Confusion, depression, conjunctivitis (dry, itching, burning eyes), decreased sexual ability, headache, nausea, vomiting, inability to sleep, unusual tiredness.

ADVERSE REACTIONS/TOXIC EFFECTS

Overdosage may produce difficult breathing, dizziness, faintness, severe drowsiness, bradycardia.

NURSING IMPLICATIONS
BASELINE ASSESSMENT:

Obtain B/P and pulse immediately before each dose. Withhold medication and notify physician if systolic B/P <90 mm Hg and/or pulse rate <60/min.

INTERVENTION/EVALUATION:

Monitor B/P, pulse. Sedative effect, drowsiness may require assistance w/ambulation, esp. during early therapy. If excessive B/P reduction occurs, place pt in supine position w/legs elevated.

PATIENT/FAMILY TEACHING:

Sugarless gum or sips of tepid water may help relieve dry mouth. Avoid tasks that require alertness, motor skills until drug response is established. Side effects usually diminish w/continued therapy. Tolerance to alcohol or other CNS depressants may be reduced. Do not abruptly withdraw medication after long-term use. Therapeutic effect may take 1 wk; peak effect noted in 1–3 mos. Best taken at bedtime.

halcinonide
(Halog)
See Classification section under: Corticosteroids: topical

halobetasol
(Ultravate)
See Classification section under: Corticosteroids: topical

haloperidol

hal-oh-**pear**-ih-dawl
(Haldol)

CANADIAN AVAILABILITY:
Apo-Haloperidol, Haldol, Novo-peridol, Peridol

CLASSIFICATION

Antiemetic, antipsychotic

AVAILABILITY (Rx)

Tablets: 0.5 mg, 1 mg, 2 mg, 5 mg, 10 mg, 20 mg. **Oral Concen-**

trate: 2 mg/ml. **Injection:** 5 mg/ml. **Injection (Decanoate):** 50 mg/ml, 100 mg/ml.

PHARMACOKINETICS

Readily absorbed from GI tract. Extensively metabolized in liver. Primarily excreted in urine. Half-life: *oral:* 12–37 hrs; *IM:* 17–25 hrs, *IV:* 10–19 hrs.

ACTION / *THERAPEUTIC EFFECT*

Competitively blocks postsynaptic dopamine receptors, increases turnover of brain dopamine, *producing tranquilizing effect.* Has anticholinergic, alpha-adrenergic blocking activity.

USES / *UNLABELED*

Management of psychotic disorders, control of tics, vocal utterances in Tourette's syndrome. Used in management of severe behavioral problems in children, short-term treatment of hyperactivity in children. *Treatment of infantile autism, Huntington's chorea, nausea/vomiting associated w/cancer chemotherapy.*

STORAGE / HANDLING

Store all preparations at room temperature. Discard if precipitate forms, discoloration occurs.

PO / IM ADMINISTRATION

PO:

1. Give w/o regard to meals.
2. Scored tablets may be crushed.

IM:

Parenteral administration: Pt must remain recumbent for 30–60 min in head-low position w/legs raised to minimize hypotensive effect.

1. Prepare Decanoate IM injection using 21 gauge needle.

2. Do not exceed maximum volume of 3 ml per IM injection site.

3. Inject slow, deep IM into upper outer quadrant of gluteus maximus.

INDICATIONS / DOSAGE / ROUTES

Note: Increase dosage gradually to optimum response, then decrease to lowest effective level for maintenance. Replace parenteral therapy w/oral therapy as soon as possible.

Moderate symptoms:
PO: Adults, elderly: Initially, 0.5–2 mg 2–3 times/day; may titrate up to 100 mg/day. **Maintenance:** Lowest effective dose.

Severe symptoms:
PO: Adults, elderly: Initially, 3–5 mg 2–3 times/day; may titrate up to 100 mg/day. **Maintenance:** Lowest effective dose.

Usual parenteral dosage:
IM: Adults, elderly: 2–5 mg; may repeat at 1–8 hr intervals. Give oral dose 12–24 hrs after last parenteral dose administered.

Usual elderly dosage (nonpsychotic):
PO: Initially, 0.25–0.5 mg 1–2 times/day. May increase by 0.25–0.5 mg q4–7 days. **Maximum:** 50 mg/day.

Usual pediatric dosage:
PO: Children (3–12 yrs): Initially, 0.5 mg/day. May increase by 0.5 mg q5–7 days. Total daily dose given in 2–3 doses/day. **Psychotic disorders:** 0.05–0.15 mg/kg/day. **Nonpsychiatric disorders, Tourette's disorder:** 0.05–0.075 mg/kg/day.

PRECAUTIONS

CONTRAINDICATIONS: Coma, alcohol ingestion, Parkinson's disease, thyrotoxicosis. **CAUTIONS:** Impaired respiratory/hepatic/cardiovascular function, alcohol withdrawal, history of seizures, urinary retention, glaucoma, prostatic hypertrophy, elderly. **PREGNANCY/LACTATION:** Crosses placenta; distributed in breast milk. **Pregnancy Category C.**

INTERACTIONS

DRUG INTERACTIONS: Alcohol, CNS depressants may increase CNS depression. Epinephrine may block alpha-adrenergic effects. Extrapyramidal symptom (EPS)–producing medications may increase EPS. Lithium may increase neurologic toxicity. **ALTERED LAB VALUES:** None significant.

SIDE EFFECTS

FREQUENT: Blurred vision, constipation, dry mouth, swelling or soreness of female breasts, weight gain. **OCCASIONAL:** Allergic reaction, difficulty urinating, decreased thirst, dizziness, lightheadedness, decreased sexual ability, drowsiness, nausea, vomiting, increased sensitivity of skin to sunlight, lethargy, transient leukopenia.

ADVERSE REACTIONS/TOXIC EFFECTS

Extrapyramidal symptoms appear to be dose related and may be noted in first few days of therapy. Marked drowsiness and lethargy, excessive salivation, fixed stare may be mild to severe in intensity. Less frequently seen are severe akathisia (motor restlessness) and acute dystonias: torticollis (neck muscle spasm), opisthotonos (rigidity of back muscles), and oculogyric crisis (rolling back of eyes). Tardive dyskinesia (protrusion of tongue, puffing of cheeks, chewing/puckering of the mouth) may occur during long-term administration or following drug discontinuance, and may be irreversible. Risk is greater in female geriatric pts. Abrupt withdrawal following long-term therapy may provoke transient dyskinesia signs.

NURSING IMPLICATIONS

BASELINE ASSESSMENT:

Assess behavior, appearance, emotional status, response to environment, speech pattern, thought content.

INTERVENTION/EVALUATION:

Supervise suicidal risk pt closely during early therapy (as depression lessens, energy level improves, causing increased suicide potential). Monitor B/P for hypotension. Assess for peripheral edema behind medial malleolus (sacral area in bedridden pts). Assess stool consistency and frequency. Monitor for rigidity, tremor, masklike facial expression, fine tongue movement. Assess for therapeutic response (interest in surroundings, improvement in self-care, increased ability to concentrate, relaxed facial expression).

PATIENT/FAMILY TEACHING:

Full therapeutic effect may take up to 6 wks. Do not abruptly withdraw from long-term drug therapy. Report visual disturbances. Sugarless gum, sips of tepid water may relieve dry mouth. Drowsiness generally subsides during continued therapy. Avoid tasks that require alertness, motor skills until response to drug is established. Avoid alcohol. Report muscle stiffness. Avoid exposure to sunlight, overheating, and dehydration (increased risk of heat stroke).

haloprogin
(Halotex)
*See Classification section under:
Antifungals: topical*

heparin sodium
hep-ah-rin
(Liquaemin)

CANADIAN AVAILABILITY:
Hepalean

CLASSIFICATION
Anticoagulant

AVAILABILITY (Rx)
Injection: 10 units/ml, 100 units/ml, 1,000 units/ml, 2,500 units/ml, 5,000 units/ml, 7,500 units/ml, 10,000 units/ml, 20,000 units/ml, 40,000 units/ml, 25,000 units/500 ml infusion

PHARMACOKINETICS
Well absorbed after SubQ administration. Metabolized in liver, removed from circulation by uptake by reticuloendothelial system. Primarily excreted in urine. Half-life: 1–6 hrs.

ACTION/ *THERAPEUTIC EFFECT*
Blocks conversion of prothrombin to thrombin and fibrinogen to fibrin. *Prevents further extension of existing thrombi or new clot formation.* No effect on existing clots.

USES
Prophylaxis, treatment of venous thrombosis, pulmonary embolism, peripheral arterial embolism, atrial fibrillation w/embolism. Prevention of thromboembolus in cardiac and vascular surgery, dialysis procedures, blood transfusions, and blood sampling for laboratory purposes. Adjunct in treatment of coronary occlusion w/acute MI. Maintains patency of indwelling intravascular devices. Diagnoses and treatment of acute/chronic consumptive coagulation pathology (e.g., DIC). Prevents cerebral thrombosis in progressive strokes.

STORAGE/HANDLING
Store parenteral form at room temperature.

SUBQ/IV ADMINISTRATION
Note: Do *not* give by IM injection (pain, hematoma, ulceration, erythema).
SubQ: Note: Used in low-dose therapy.
　1. After withdrawal of heparin from vial, change needle before injection (prevents leakage along needle track).
　2. Inject above iliac crest or in abdominal fat layer. Do not inject within 2 inches of umbilicus, or any scar tissue.
　3. Withdraw needle rapidly, apply prolonged pressure at injection site. Do not massage.
　4. Rotate injection sites.
IV: Note: Used in full-dose therapy. Intermittent IV produces higher incidence of bleeding abnormalities. Continuous IV preferred.
　1. Dilute IV infusion in isotonic sterile saline, 5% dextrose in water, or lactated Ringer's.
　2. Invert container at least 6 times (ensures mixing, prevents pooling of medication).
　3. Use constant-rate IV infusion pump or microdrip.

INDICATIONS/DOSAGE/ROUTES
Note: Dosage expressed in USP

units. Dosage requirements highly individualized.

SubQ: Adults, elderly: 5,000 units IV injection and 10,000–20,000 units SubQ, followed by 8,000–10,000 units q8h or 15,000–20,000 units q12h.

Prophylaxis of postoperative thrombosis:
SubQ: Adults, elderly: 5,000 units given 2 hrs before surgery, then q8–12h after surgery for 5–7 days or when pt is ambulatory.

Full-dose therapy:
Continuous IV: Adults, elderly: 5,000 units IV injection to start, followed by 20,000–40,000 units IV infusion given over 24 hrs. **Children:** 50 units/kg IV to start, followed by 20,000 units/m² continuous IV infusion per 24 hrs.
Intermittent IV: Adults, elderly: 10,000 units to start, followed by 5,000–10,000 units q4–6h. **Children:** 100 units/kg to start, followed by 50–100 units/kg q4h.

Maintaining patency of indwelling intravascular devices:
IV: Adults, elderly: 10–100 units injected into diaphragm of device after each use, designated interval, or as necessary.

PRECAUTIONS

CONTRAINDICATIONS: Bleeding abnormalities, vitamin K insufficiency, chronic alcoholism, severe hepatic/renal disease, salicylate therapy, severe hypertension, pregnancy, hypersensitivity to heparin, ergot alkaloids, lidocaine; peripheral artery disease, coronary insufficiency, angina, sepsis, thrombocytopenia, brain/spinal cord surgery, spinal anesthesia, eye surgery, oral anticoagulants. **CAUTIONS:** Severe hypertension, peripheral vascular disease, indwelling catheters, those >60 yrs, factors increasing risk of hemorrhage, diabetes, mild hepatic/renal disease. **PREGNANCY/LACTATION:** Use w/caution, particularly during last trimester, immediate postpartum period (increased risk of maternal hemorrhage). Does not cross placenta; not distributed in breast milk. **Pregnancy Category B.**

INTERACTIONS

DRUG INTERACTIONS: Anticoagulants, platelet aggregation inhibitors, thrombolytics may increase risk of bleeding. Antithyroid medications, cefoperazone, cefotetan, valproic acid may cause hypoprothrombinemia. Probenecid may increase effect. **ALTERED LAB VALUES:** May increase free fatty acids, SGOT (AST), SGPT (ALT). May decrease triglycerides, cholesterol.

SIDE EFFECTS

OCCASIONAL: Itching, burning, particularly on soles of feet (due to vasospastic reaction). **RARE:** Pain, cyanosis of extremity 6–10 days after initial therapy, lasts 4–6 hrs; hypersensitivity reaction (chills, fever, pruritus, urticaria, asthma, rhinitis, lacrimation, headache).

ADVERSE REACTIONS/TOXIC EFFECTS

Bleeding complications ranging from local ecchymoses to major hemorrhage occur more frequently in high-dose therapy, intermittent IV infusion, and in women >60 yrs. *Antidote:* Protamine sulfate 1–1.5 mg for q 100 units heparin SubQ if overdosage occurred before 30 min, 0.5–0.75 mg for q 100 units heparin SubQ if overdosage occurred within 30–60 min, 0.25–0.375 mg for q 100 units heparin SubQ if 2 hrs have elapsed since overdosage, 25–50 mg if heparin given by IV infusion.

NURSING IMPLICATIONS
BASELINE ASSESSMENT:

Cross-check dose w/co-worker. Determine activated partial thromboplastin time (APTT) before administration and 24 hrs after initiation of therapy, then 24–48 hrs for first week of therapy or until maintenance dose is established. Follow with APTT determinations 1–2 times weekly for 3–4 wks. Long-term therapy: 1–2 times/month.

INTERVENTION/EVALUATION:

Monitor APTT (therapeutic dosage at 1.5–2.5 times normal) diligently. Assess hematocrit, platelet count, urine/stool culture for occult blood, SGOT (AST), SGPT (ALT), regardless of route of administration. Assess for decrease in B/P, increase in pulse rate, complaint of abdominal or back pain, severe headache (may be evidence of hemorrhage). Question for increase in amount of discharge during menses. Check peripheral pulses; skin for bruises, petechiae. Check for excessive bleeding from minor cuts, scratches. Assess gums for erythema, gingival bleeding. Assess urine output for hematuria. Avoid IM injections of other medications because of potential for hematomas. When converting to coumadin therapy, monitor PT results (will be 10–20% higher while heparin is given concurrently).

PATIENT/FAMILY TEACHING:

Use electric razor, soft toothbrush to prevent bleeding. Report any sign of red or dark urine, black or red stool, coffee-ground vomitus, red-speckled mucus from cough. Do not use any OTC medication w/o physician approval (may interfere w/platelet aggregation). Wear/carry identification that notes anticoagulant therapy. Inform dentist, other physicians of heparin therapy.

hepatitis A
(Havrix, Vaqta)
See Supplement

hepatitis B immune globulin
(Nabi-HB)
See Supplement

hetastarch
het-ah-starch
(Hespan, Hextend)

CLASSIFICATION

Plasma volume expander

AVAILABILITY (Rx)

Injection: 6 g/100 ml 0.9% NaCl (500 ml infusion container)

PHARMACOKINETICS

Smaller molecules (<50,000 molecular weight) rapidly excreted by kidneys; larger molecules (>50,000 molecular weight) slowly degraded to smaller sized molecules, then excreted. Half-life: 17 days.

ACTION/*THERAPEUTIC EFFECT*

Exerts osmotic pull on tissue fluids; *reducing hemoconcentration and blood viscosity, increasing circulating blood volume.*

USES

Fluid replacement and plasma volume expansion in treatment of shock due to hemorrhage, burns, surgery, sepsis, trauma, leukapheresis.

STORAGE/HANDLING

Store solutions at room temperature. Solution should appear clear, pale yellow to amber. Do not use if discolored (deep turbid brown) or if precipitate forms.

IV ADMINISTRATION

1. Administer only by IV infusion.

2. Do not add drugs or mix w/other IV fluids.

3. In acute hemorrhagic shock, administer at rate approaching 1.2 g/kg (20 ml/kg) per hour. Use slower rates for burns, septic shock.

4. Monitor central venous pressure (CVP) when given by rapid infusion. If there is a precipitous rise in CVP, immediately discontinue drug (overexpansion of blood volume).

INDICATIONS/DOSAGE/ROUTES

Plasma volume expansion:
IV: Adults, elderly: 500–1,000 ml/day up to 1,500 ml/day (20 mg/kg) at a rate up to 20 ml/kg/hr in hemorrhagic shock (slower rates for burns or septic shock).

Leukapheresis:
IV: Adults, elderly: 250–700 ml infused at constant rate, usually 1:8 to venous whole blood.

PRECAUTIONS

CONTRAINDICATIONS: Severe bleeding disorders, severe CHF, oliguria, anuria. **CAUTIONS:** Thrombocytopenia, elderly or very young, pulmonary edema, CHF, impaired renal function, hepatic disease, those on sodium restriction. **PREGNANCY/LACTATION:** Do not use in pregnancy unless benefits outweigh risk to fetus. **Pregnancy Category C**.

INTERACTIONS

DRUG INTERACTIONS: None significant. **ALTERED LAB VALUES:** May prolong prothrombin time (PT), partial thromboplastin time (PTT), bleeding, and clotting times; decrease hematocrit.

SIDE EFFECTS

RARE: Allergic reaction resulting in vomiting, mild temperature elevation, chills, itching; submaxillary and parotid gland enlargement, peripheral edema of lower extremities, mild flulike symptoms: headache, muscle aches.

ADVERSE REACTIONS/TOXIC EFFECTS

Fluid overload (headache, weakness, blurred vision, behavioral changes, incoordination, isolated muscle twitching) and pulmonary edema (rapid breathing, rales, wheezing, coughing, increased B/P, distended neck veins) may occur. Anaphylactoid reaction may be observed as periorbital edema, urticaria, wheezing.

NURSING IMPLICATIONS

INTERVENTION/EVALUATION:

Monitor for fluid overload (peripheral and/or pulmonary edema, impending CHF symptoms). Assess lung sounds for wheezing, rales. During leukapheresis, monitor CBC, leukocyte and platelet counts, differential, hemoglobin, hematocrit, PT, PTT, I&O. Monitor central venous B/P (detects overexpansion of blood volume). Monitor urine output closely (increase in output generally occurs in oliguric pts after administration). Assess for periorbital edema, itching, wheezing, urticaria (allergic reaction). Monitor for oliguria, anuria, any change in output ratio. Monitor for bleeding from surgical or trauma sites.

hyaluronate sodium
(Hyalgan, Synvisc)
See Supplement

hydralazine hydrochloride
hy-**dral**-ah-zeen
(Apresoline)

FIXED-COMBINATION(S):
W/hydrochlorothiazide, a diuretic **(Apresodex, Apresoline-Esidrex, Apresazide, Hydralazine PLUS, Hydrazide)**; w/reserpine, an antihypertensive **(Serpasil-Apresoline)**; w/hydrochlorothiazide and reserpine **(Cherapas, Ser-Ap-Es, Serathide).**

CANADIAN AVAILABILITY:
Apresoline, Novohylazin

CLASSIFICATION
Antihypertensive

AVAILABILITY (Rx)
Tablets: 10 mg, 25 mg, 50 mg, 100 mg. **Injection:** 20 mg/ml.

PHARMACOKINETICS

	ONSET	PEAK	DURATION
PO	10–20 min	0.5–2 hrs	2–4 hrs

Well absorbed from GI tract. Widely distributed. Metabolized in liver to active metabolite. Primarily excreted in urine. Half-life: 3–7 hrs (increased in decreased renal function).

ACTION / *THERAPEUTIC EFFECT*
Directly relaxes vascular smooth muscle (greater effect on arterioles), *reducing B/P*. Produces decreased peripheral vascular resistance, increased heart rate, cardiac output. Decreases afterload (increases CO, decreases systemic resistance).

USES / *UNLABELED*
Management of moderate/severe hypertension. *Treatment of congestive heart failure.*

STORAGE / HANDLING
Store oral form at room temperature.

PO ADMINISTRATION
1. Best given w/food or regularly spaced meals.
2. Tablets may be crushed.

INDICATIONS / DOSAGE / ROUTES
Hypertension:
PO: Adults: Initially, 10 mg 4 times/day for 2–4 days. Increase to 25 mg 4 times/day for remainder of first week. Increase second week and subsequent weeks to 50 mg 4 times/day. **Elderly:** Initially, 10 mg 2–3 times/day. May increase by 10–25 mg/day q2–5 days. **Children:** Initially, 0.75 mg/kg in 4 divided doses (maximum 25 mg). May be increased over 1–4 wks up to 7.5 mg/kg/day or 200 mg/day. **IM/IV: Adults, elderly:** 20–40 mg. **Children:** 0.1–0.2 mg/kg/dose.

PRECAUTIONS
CONTRAINDICATIONS: Coronary artery disease, rheumatic heart disease, lupus erythematosus. **CAUTIONS:** Impaired renal function, cerebrovascular disease. **PREGNANCY/LACTATION:** Drug crosses placenta; unknown if drug is distributed in breast milk. Thrombocytopenia, leukopenia, petechial bleeding, hematomas have occurred in newborns (re-

solved within 1–3 wks). **Pregnancy Category C**.

INTERACTIONS

DRUG INTERACTIONS: Diuretics, other hypotensives may increase hypotensive effect. **ALTERED LAB VALUES:** May produce positive direct Coombs' test.

SIDE EFFECTS

FREQUENT: Headache, palpitations, tachycardia (generally disappears in 7–10 days). **OCCASIONAL:** GI disturbance (nausea, vomiting, diarrhea), paresthesia, fluid retention, peripheral edema, dizziness, flushed face, nasal congestion.

ADVERSE REACTIONS/TOXIC EFFECTS

High dosage may produce lupus erythematosis-like reaction (fever, facial rash, muscle and joint aches, splenomegaly). Severe orthostatic hypotension, skin flushing, severe headache, myocardial ischemia, cardiac arrhythmias may develop. Profound shock may occur in cases of severe overdosage.

NURSING IMPLICATIONS

BASELINE ASSESSMENT:

Obtain B/P, pulse immediately before each dose administration, in addition to regular monitoring (be alert to fluctuations). Keep tissues readily available at pt's bedside for lacrimation, nasal congestion.

INTERVENTION/EVALUATION:

Assess for peripheral edema of hands, feet (usually, first area of low extremity swelling is behind medial malleolus in ambulatory, sacral area in bedridden). Monitor temperature for fever (lupus-like reaction). Monitor pattern of daily bowel activity and stool consistency.

PATIENT/FAMILY TEACHING:

To reduce hypotensive effect, rise slowly from lying to sitting position and permit legs to dangle from bed momentarily before standing. Unsalted crackers, dry toast may relieve nausea. Report muscle and joint aches, fever (lupus-like reaction).

---

hydrochlorothiazide

high-drow-chlor-oh-**thigh**-ah-zide
(**HydroDIURIL, Esidrix, Microzide, Oretic**)

FIXED-COMBINATION(S):
W/methyldopa, an antihypertensive (**Aldoril**); w/propranolol, a beta blocker (**Inderide**); w/hydralazine, a vasodilator (**Apresazide**); w/captopril, an ACE inhibitor (**Capozide**); w/enalapril, an ACE inhibitor (**Vaseretic**); w/irbesartan, an angiotensin II inhibitor (**Avalide**); w/losartan, an angiotensin II inhibitor (**Hyzaar**); w/metoprolol, a beta blocker (**Lopressor HCT**); w/moexipril, an ACE inhibitor (**Uniretic**); w/timolol, a beta blocker (**Timolide**); w/labetolol, an alpha-beta blocker (**Normozide**); w/potassium-sparing diuretics (amiloride) [**Moduretic**]; (spironolactone) [**Aldactazide**] (triamterene) [**Dyazide, Maxzide**]; w/valsartan, an angiotensin II inhibitor (**Diovan HCT**).

CANADIAN AVAILABILITY:
Apo-Hydro, Hydrodiuril,

CLASSIFICATION

Diuretic: Thiazide

AVAILABILITY (Rx)

Capsules: 12.5 mg, **Tablets:** 25

mg, 50 mg, 100 mg. **Oral Solution:** 50 mg/5 ml, 100 mg/ml.

PHARMACOKINETICS

	ONSET	PEAK	DURATION
PO **(diuretic)**	2 hrs	4–6 hrs	6–12 hrs

Variably absorbed from GI tract. Primarily excreted unchanged in liver. Half-life: 5.6–14.8 hrs.

ACTION/THERAPEUTIC EFFECT

Diuretic: Blocks reabsorption of water, electrolytes (sodium, potassium) at cortical diluting segment of distal tubule, *promoting renal excretion. Antihypertensive:* Reduces plasma, extracellular fluid volume, decreases peripheral vascular resistance (PVR) by direct effect on blood vessels, *reducing B/P.*

USES/UNLABELED

Adjunctive therapy in edema associated w/CHF, hepatic cirrhosis, corticoid or estrogen therapy, renal impairment. In treatment of hypertension, may be used alone or w/other antihypertensive agents. *Treatment of diabetes insipidus; prevents calcium-containing renal stones.*

PO ADMINISTRATION

May give w/food or milk if GI upset occurs, preferably w/breakfast (may prevent nocturia).

INDICATIONS/DOSAGE/ROUTES

Edema:
PO: Adults: Initially, 25–200 mg in 1–3 divided doses. **Maintenance:** 25–100 mg/day. **Maximum:** 200 mg/day.

Hypertension:
PO: Adults: Initially, 12.5–25 mg/day. Gradually increase up to 50 mg/day. **Maintenance:** 25–50 mg/day.

Usual elderly dosage:
PO: 12.5–25 mg/day.

Usual dosage for children:
PO: Children 2–12 yrs: 37.5–100 mg/day. **Children <2 yrs:** 12.5–37.5 mg/day.

PRECAUTIONS

CONTRAINDICATIONS: History of hypersensitivity to sulfonamides or thiazide diuretics, renal decompensation, anuria. **CAUTIONS:** Severe renal disease, impaired hepatic function, diabetes mellitus, elderly/debilitated, thyroid disorders. **PREGNANCY/LACTATION:** Crosses placenta; small amount distributed in breast milk—nursing not advised. **Pregnancy Category D**.

INTERACTIONS

DRUG INTERACTIONS: Cholestyramine, colestipol may decrease absorption, effects. May increase digoxin toxicity (due to hypokalemia). May increase lithium toxicity. **ALTERED LAB VALUES:** May increase bilirubin, serum calcium, LDL, cholesterol, triglycerides, creatinine, glucose, uric acid. May decrease urinary calcium, magnesium, potassium, sodium.

SIDE EFFECTS

EXPECTED: Increase in urine frequency/volume. **FREQUENT:** Potassium depletion. **OCCASIONAL:** Postural hypotension, headache, GI disturbances, photosensitivity reaction.

ADVERSE REACTIONS/TOXIC EFFECTS

Vigorous diuresis may lead to profound water loss and electrolyte depletion, resulting in hypokalemia, hyponatremia, dehydration. Acute hypotensive episodes may occur. Hyperglycemia may be noted during prolonged therapy. GI upset, pancreatitis, dizziness, paresthesias, headache, blood dyscrasias, pulmonary edema, allergic pneumonitis, dermatologic reactions occur rarely. Overdosage can lead to lethargy, coma w/o changes in electrolytes or hydration.

NURSING IMPLICATIONS
BASELINE ASSESSMENT:

Check vital signs, esp. B/P for hypotension prior to administration. Assess baseline electrolytes; particularly check for low potassium. Evaluate edema, skin turgor, mucous membranes for hydration status. Assess muscle strength, mental status. Note skin temperature, moisture. Obtain baseline weight. Initiate I&O.

INTERVENTION/EVALUATION:

Continue to monitor B/P, vital signs, electrolytes, I&O, weight. Note extent of diuresis. Watch for changes from initial assessment (hypokalemia may result in weakness, tremor, muscle cramps, nausea, vomiting, change in mental status, tachycardia; hyponatremia may result in confusion, thirst, cold/clammy skin). Be esp. alert for potassium depletion in pts taking digoxin (cardiac arrhythmias). Potassium supplements are frequently ordered. Check for constipation (may occur w/exercise diuresis).

PATIENT/FAMILY TEACHING:

Expect increased frequency and volume of urination. To reduce hypotensive effect, rise slowly from lying to sitting position and permit legs to dangle momentarily before standing. Eat foods high in potassium such as whole grains (cereals), legumes, meat, bananas, apricots, orange juice, potatoes (white, sweet), raisins. Protect skin from sun/ultraviolet rays (photosensitivity may occur).

hydrocodone bitartrate

high-drough-**koe**-doan

FIXED-COMBINATION(S):
W/acetaminophen (**Anexsia, Lortab, Vicodin, Vicodin HP, Zydone**); w/aspirin (**Lortab ASA**); w/chlorpheniramine, an antihistamine (**Tussionex**); w/ibuprofen, a NSAD (**Vicoprofen**); w/phenypropanolamine, a sympathomimetic (**Hycomine**).

CANADIAN AVAILABILITY:
Hycodan, Robidone

CLASSIFICATION

Opioid: Analgesic (**Schedule III**)

PHARMACOKINETICS

	ONSET	PEAK	DURATION
PO	—	—	4–6 hrs

Well absorbed from GI tract. Metabolized in liver. Primarily excreted in urine. Half-life: 3.8 hrs (increased in elderly).

ACTION/THERAPEUTIC EFFECT

Binds at opiate receptor sites in CNS. *Reduces intensity of pain stimuli incoming from sensory nerve endings, altering pain perception and emotional response to pain; suppresses cough reflex.*

USES

Relief of moderate to moderately severe pain, nonproductive cough.

PO ADMINISTRATION

1. Give w/o regard to meals.
2. Tablets may be crushed.

INDICATIONS/DOSAGE/ROUTES

Analgesia:
PO: Adults, children >12 yrs: 5–10 mg q4–6h. **Elderly:** 2.5–5 mg q4–6h.

Antitussive:
PO: Adults: 5–10 mg q4–6h as needed. **Maximum:** 15 mg/dose. **Children:** 0.6 mg/kg/day in 3–4 divided doses at intervals of no less than 4 hrs. **Maximum single dose in children 2–12 yrs:** 5 mg. **Maximum single dose in children <2 yrs:** 1.25 mg.

Extended-release:
PO: Adults: 10 mg q12h. **Children 6–12 yrs:** 5 mg q12h.

PRECAUTIONS

CONTRAINDICATIONS: None significant. **EXTREME CAUTION:** CNS depression, anoxia, hypercapnia, respiratory depression, seizures, acute alcoholism, shock, untreated myxedema, respiratory dysfunction. **CAUTIONS:** Increased intracranial pressure, impaired hepatic function, acute abdominal conditions, hypothyroidism, prostatic hypertrophy, Addison's disease, urethral stricture, COPD. **PREGNANCY/LACTATION:** Readily crosses placenta; distributed in breast milk. May prolong labor if administered in latent phase of first stage of labor, or before cervical dilation of 4–5 cm has occurred. Respiratory depression may occur in neonate if mother received opiates during labor. Regular use of opiates during pregnancy may produce withdrawal symptoms (irritability, excessive crying, tremors, hyperactive reflexes, fever, vomiting, diarrhea, yawning, sneezing, seizures) in the neonate. **Pregnancy Category C.** (Category D if used for prolonged periods or high doses at term.)

INTERACTIONS

DRUG INTERACTIONS: Alcohol, CNS depressants may increase CNS or respiratory depression, hypotension. MAO inhibitors may produce severe, fatal reaction (reduce dose to $1/4$ usual dose). **ALTERED LAB VALUES:** May increase amylase, lipase plasma concentrations.

SIDE EFFECTS

Note: Effects are dependent on dosage amount but occur infrequently w/oral antitussives. Ambulatory pts and those not in severe pain may experience dizziness, nausea, vomiting, hypotension more frequently than those who are in supine position or having severe pain. **FREQUENT:** Sedation, decreased B/P, increased sweating, flushed face, dizziness, drowsiness, hypotension. **OCCASIONAL:** Decreased urination, blurred vision, constipation, dry mouth, headache, nausea, vomiting, difficult/painful urination, euphoria, dysphoria.

ADVERSE REACTIONS/TOXIC EFFECTS

Overdosage results in respiratory depression, skeletal muscle flaccidity, cold clammy skin, cyanosis, extreme somnolence progressing to convulsions, stupor, coma. Tolerance to analgesic effect, physical dependence may occur w/repeated use. Prolonged duration of action, cumulative effect may occur in those w/impaired hepatic, renal function.

NURSING IMPLICATIONS
BASELINE ASSESSMENT:

Obtain vital signs before giving medication. If respirations are 12/min or lower (20/min or lower in children), w/hold medication, contact physician. *Analgesic:* Assess onset, type, location, and duration of pain. Effect of medication is reduced if full pain recurs before next dose. *Antitussive:* Assess type, severity, frequency of cough, and productions.

INTERVENTION/EVALUATION:

Increase fluid intake and environmental humidity to improve viscosity of lung secretions. Palpate bladder for urinary retention. Monitor pattern of daily bowel activity and stool consistency. Initiate deep breathing and coughing exercises, particularly in those w/impaired pulmonary function. Assess for clinical improvement and record onset of relief of pain or cough.

PATIENT/FAMILY TEACHING:

Change positions slowly to avoid orthostatic hypotension. Avoid tasks that require alertness, motor skills until response to drug is established. Tolerance/dependence may occur w/prolonged use of high doses. Avoid alcohol. Report nausea, vomiting, constipation, shortness of breath, difficulty breathing. May take w/food.

hydrocortisone

high-droe-**core**-tah-sewn
(Cortef, Cort-Dome, Cortenema, Hydrocortone, Hytone, Locoid, Pandel)

hydrocortisone acetate
(Cortaid, Corticaine, Proctocort)

hydrocortisone cypionate
(Cortef Suspension)

hydrocortisone sodium phosphate
(Hydrocortone Phosphate)

hydrocortisone sodium succinate
(A-hydroCort, Solu-Cortef)

hydrocortisone valerate
(WestCort)

FIXED-COMBINATION(S):
W/Neomycin, an antibiotic (**Neo-Cort-Dome**); w/Bacitracin, Neomycin, Polymyxin B, anti-infectives (**Cortisporin**); hydrocortisone acetate w/Neomycin, an antibiotic (**Neo-Cortef**); w/ciprofloxacin, an antibiotic (**Cipro HC Otic**).

CANADIAN AVAILABILITY:
Cortamed, Cortef, Cortenema, SoluCortef, Westcort

CLASSIFICATION

Corticosteroid

AVAILABILITY (Rx)

Hydrocortisone: Tablets: 5 mg, 10 mg, 20 mg. **Gel:** 0.5%, 1% (OTC). **Lotion:** 0.25%, 0.5%, 1%, 2%, 2.5%. **Cream:** 0.5%, 1% (OTC), 2.5%. **Ointment:** 0.5%, 1% (OTC), 2.5%. **Topical Solution:** 1%

Cypionate: Oral Suspension: 10 mg/5 ml

Sodium phosphate: Injection: 50 mg/ml

Sodium succinate: Injection: 100 mg, 250 mg, 500 mg, 1,000 mg

Acetate: Injection: 25 mg/ml, 50 mg/ml. **Suppository:** 10 mg, 25 mg, 30 mg. **Cream:** 0.5%, 1%. Ointment: 0.5%, 1%.

Valerate: Cream: 0.2%. **Cream:** 0.2%

PHARMACOKINETICS

Well absorbed from GI tract, after IM administration. Widely distributed. Metabolized in liver. Half-life: *plasma:* 1.5–2 hrs; *biologic:* 8–12 hrs.

ACTION/*THERAPEUTIC EFFECT*

Inhibits accumulation of inflammatory cells at inflammation sites, phagocytosis, lysosomal enzyme release and synthesis and/or release of mediators of inflammation. *Prevents/suppresses cell-mediated immune reactions. Decreases/prevents tissue response to inflammatory process.*

USES

Substitution therapy in deficiency states (acute/chronic adrenal insufficiency, congenital adrenal hyperplasia, adrenal insufficiency secondary to pituitary insufficiency); nonendocrine disorders (arthritis, rheumatic carditis, allergic, collagen, intestinal tract, liver, ocular, renal, skin diseases, bronchial asthma, cerebral edema, malignancies). *Rectal:* Adjunctive therapy in treatment of ulcerative colitis.

STORAGE/HANDLING

Store parenteral forms at room temperature. *Hydrocortisone sodium succinate:* After reconstitution, use solution within 72 hrs. Use immediately if further diluted w/5% dextrose, 0.9% NaCl, or other compatible diluent.

PO/IM/IV/TOPICAL/ RECTAL ADMINISTRATION

PO:

1. Give w/milk or food (decreases GI upset).
2. Give single dose before 9 AM; give multiple doses at evenly spaced intervals.

IM/IV:

1. Once reconstituted, solution stable for 72 hrs at room temperature.
2. May further dilute w/5% dextrose or 0.9% NaCl.

TOPICAL:

1. Gently cleanse area prior to application.
2. Use occlusive dressings only as ordered.
3. Apply sparingly and rub into area thoroughly.

RECTAL:

1. Shake homogeneous suspension well.
2. Instruct pt to lie on left side w/left leg extended, right leg flexed.
3. Gently insert applicator tip into rectum, pointed slightly toward navel (umbilicus).
4. Aim nozzle to back, then slowly instill medication.

INDICATIONS/DOSAGE/ROUTES

Hydrocortisone:
PO: Adults, elderly: 20–240 mg/day.
IM: Adults, elderly: $^1/_3$–$^1/_2$ oral dose q12h.

Hydrocortisone sodium phosphate:
IM/IV/SubQ: Adults, elderly: 15–

240 mg/day, usually $^1/_3$–$^1/_2$ oral dose q12h.

Hydrocortisone sodium succinate:
IM/IV: Adults, elderly: Initially, 100–500 mg/day.

Hydrocortisone acetate:
Intra-articular, intralesional, soft tissue: Adults, elderly: 5–50 mg.

Usual rectal dosage:
Rectal: Adults, elderly: 100 mg at bedtime for 21 nights or until clinical and proctologic remission occurs (may require 2–3 mos therapy).
Cortifoam: Adults, elderly: 1 applicator 1–2 times/day for 2–3 wks, then every second day thereafter.

Usual topical dosage:
Adults, elderly: Apply sparingly 2–4 times/day.

PRECAUTIONS

CONTRAINDICATIONS: Hypersensitivity to any corticosteroid or sulfite, systemic fungal infection, peptic ulcers (except life-threatening situations). Avoid live virus vaccine such as smallpox. *Topical:* Marked circulation impairment. Do not instill ocular solution when topical corticosteroids are being used on eyelids or surrounding skin. **CAUTIONS:** Thromboembolic disorders, history of tuberculosis (may reactivate disease), hypothyroidism, cirrhosis, nonspecific ulcerative colitis, CHF, hypertension, psychosis, renal insufficiency, seizure disorders. Prolonged therapy should be discontinued slowly. *Topical:* Do not apply to extensive areas. **PREGNANCY/LACTATION:** Crosses placenta, distributed in breast milk. May produce cleft palate if used chronically during first trimester. Nursing contraindicated. **Pregnancy Category D.**

INTERACTIONS

DRUG INTERACTIONS: Amphotericin may increase hypokalemia. May decrease effect of oral hypoglycemics, insulin, diuretics, potassium supplements. May increase digoxin toxicity (due to hypokalemia). Hepatic enzyme inducers may decrease effect. Live virus vaccines may potentiate virus replication, increase vaccine side effects, decrease pt's antibody response to vaccine. **ALTERED LAB VALUES:** May decrease calcium, potassium, thyroxine. May increase cholesterol, lipids, glucose, sodium, amylase.

SIDE EFFECTS

FREQUENT: Insomnia, heartburn, nervousness, abdominal distension, increased sweating, acne, mood swings, increased appetite, facial flushing, delayed wound healing, increased susceptibility to infection, diarrhea/constipation. **OCCASIONAL:** Headache, edema, change in skin color, frequent urination. *Topical:* Itching, redness, irritation. **RARE:** Tachycardia, allergic reaction (rash, hives), psychic changes, hallucinations, depression. *Topical:* Allergic contact dermatitis, purpura. Systemic absorption more likely w/occlusive dressings or extensive application in young children.

ADVERSE REACTIONS/TOXIC EFFECTS

Long-term therapy: Hypocalcemia, hypokalemia, muscle wasting (esp. arms, legs), osteoporosis, spontaneous fractures, amenorrhea, cataracts, glaucoma, peptic ulcer, CHF. *Abrupt withdrawal following long-term therapy:* Anorexia, nausea, fever, headache, sudden severe joint pain, rebound inflammation, fatigue, weakness, lethargy, dizziness, orthostatic hypertension.

NURSING IMPLICATIONS
BASELINE ASSESSMENT:

Question for hypersensitivity to any of the corticosteroids. Obtain baseline values for weight, B/P, glucose, cholesterol, electrolytes. Check results of initial tests, e.g., TB skin test, x-rays, EKG.

INTERVENTION/EVALUATION:

Monitor I&O, daily weight; assess for edema. Check B/P, vital signs at least 2 times/day. Be alert to infection (reduced immune response): sore throat, fever, or vague symptoms. Evaluate bowel activity. Monitor electrolytes. Watch for hypocalcemia (muscle twitching, cramps, positive Trousseau's or Chvostek's signs) or hypokalemia (weakness and muscle cramps, numbness/tingling esp. lower extremities, nausea and vomiting, irritability, EKG changes). Assess emotional status, ability to sleep.

PATIENT/FAMILY TEACHING:

Take oral dose w/food or milk. Carry identification of drug and dose, physician's name and phone number. Do not change dose/schedule or stop taking drug; *must* taper off under medical supervision. Notify physician of fever, sore throat, muscle aches, sudden weight gain/swelling. W/dietician, give instructions for prescribed diet (usually sodium restricted w/high vitamin D, protein, and potassium). Maintain fastidious oral hygiene. Severe stress (serious infection, surgery, or trauma) may require increased dosage. Do not take aspirin or any other medication w/o consulting physician. Follow-up visits, lab tests are necessary; children must be assessed for growth retardation. Inform dentist or other physicians of cortisone therapy now or within past 12 mos. Caution against overuse of joints injected for symptomatic relief. *Topical:* Apply after shower or bath for best absorption. Do not cover unless physician orders; do not use tight diapers, plastic pants, or coverings. Avoid contact w/eyes.

hydromorphone hydrochloride

high-dro-**more**-phone
(Dilaudid, Dilaudid HP)

FIXED-COMBINATION(S):
W/guaifenesin, an expectorant **(Dilaudid Cough Syrup).**

CANADIAN AVAILABILITY:
Dilaudid, Hydromorph Contin

CLASSIFICATION

Opioid: Analgesic **(Schedule II)**

AVAILABILITY (Rx)

Tablets: 1 mg, 2 mg, 3 mg, 4 mg. **Injection:** 1 mg/ml, 2 mg/ml, 3 mg/ml, 4 mg/ml, 10 mg/ml. **Suppository:** 3 mg.

PHARMACOKINETICS

	ONSET	PEAK	DURATION
PO	30 min	90–120 min	4 hrs
SubQ	15 min	30–90 min	4 hrs
IM	15 min	30–60 min	4–5 hrs
IV	10–15 min	15–30 min	2–3 hrs
Rectal			
	15–30 min	—	—

Well absorbed from GI tract, after IM administration. Widely distributed. Metabolized in liver. Excreted in urine. Half-life: 1–3 hrs.

ACTION/ *THERAPEUTIC EFFECT*

Binds at opiate receptor sites in CNS. *Reduces intensity of pain stimuli incoming from sensory nerve endings, altering pain perception and emotional response to pain; suppresses cough reflex.*

USES

Relief of moderate to severe pain, persistent nonproductive cough.

STORAGE/HANDLING

Store oral/parenteral form at room temperature. Slight yellow discoloration of parenteral form does not indicate loss of potency. Refrigerate suppositories.

PO/SUBQ/IM/IV/RECTAL ADMINISTRATION

PO:

1. Give w/o regard to meals.
2. Tablets may be crushed.

SubQ/IM:

1. Use short 30 gauge needle for SubQ injection.
2. Administer slowly, rotating injection sites.
3. Pts w/circulatory impairment experience higher risk of overdosage because of delayed absorption of repeated administration.

IV:

Note: High concentration injection (10 mg/ml) should only be used in those tolerant to opiate agonists, currently receiving high doses of another opiate agonist for severe, chronic pain due to cancer.

1. Administer very slowly (over 2–3 min).
2. Rapid IV increases risk of severe adverse reactions (chest wall rigidity, apnea, peripheral circulatory collapse, anaphylactoid effects, cardiac arrest).

RECTAL:

Moisten suppository w/cold water before inserting well up into rectum.

INDICATIONS/DOSAGE/ROUTES

Analgesia:
PO/SubQ/IM/IV: Adults, elderly: 2 mg q4–6h, as needed. Severe pain may require up to 4 mg q4–6h. **Rectal: Adults, elderly:** 3 mg q6–8h.

Antitussive:
PO: Adults, children >12 yrs, elderly: 1 mg q3–4h. Children 6–12 yrs: 0.5 mg q3–4h.

PRECAUTIONS

CONTRAINDICATIONS: None significant. **EXTREME CAUTION:** CNS depression, anoxia, hypercapnia, respiratory depression, seizures, acute alcoholism, shock, untreated myxedema, respiratory dysfunction. **CAUTIONS:** Increased intracranial pressure, impaired hepatic function, acute abdominal conditions, hypothyroidism, prostatic hypertrophy, Addison's disease, urethral stricture, COPD. **PREGNANCY/LACTATION:** Readily crosses placenta; unknown if distributed in breast milk. May prolong labor if administered in latent phase of first stage of labor or before cervical dilation of 4–5 cm has occurred. Respiratory depression may occur in neonate if mother receives opiates during labor. Regular use of opiates during pregnancy may produce withdrawal symptoms in the neonate (irritability, excessive crying, tremors, hyperactive reflexes, fever, vomiting, diarrhea, yawning, sneezing, seizures). **Pregnancy Category B.** (Category D if used for prolong periods or high doses at term.)

INTERACTIONS

DRUG INTERACTIONS: Alcohol, CNS depressants may increase CNS or respiratory depression, hypotension. MAO inhibitors may produce severe, fatal reaction (reduce dose to $1/4$ usual dose). **ALTERED LAB VALUES:** May increase amylase, lipase plasma concentrations.

SIDE EFFECTS

Note: Effects are dependent on dosage amount, route of administration but occur infrequently w/oral antitussives. Ambulatory pts and those not in severe pain may experience dizziness, nausea, vomiting, hypotension more frequently than those in supine position or having severe pain. **FREQUENT:** Drowsiness, dizziness, hypotension, decreased appetite. **OCCASIONAL:** Confusion, diaphoresis, facial flushing, urinary retention, constipation, dry mouth, nausea, vomiting, headache, pain at injection site. **RARE:** Allergic reaction, depression.

ADVERSE REACTIONS/TOXIC EFFECTS

Overdosage results in respiratory depression, skeletal muscle flaccidity, cold clammy skin, cyanosis, extreme somnolence progressing to convulsions, stupor, coma. Tolerance to analgesic effect, physical dependence may occur w/repeated use. Prolonged duration of action, cumulative effect may occur in those w/impaired hepatic, renal function.

NURSING IMPLICATIONS
BASELINE ASSESSMENT:

Obtain vital signs before giving medication. If respirations are 12/min or lower (20/min or lower in children), withhold medication, contact physician. *Analgesic:* Assess onset, type, location, and duration of pain. Effect of medication is reduced if full pain recurs before next dose. *Antitussive:* Assess type, severity, frequency of cough and productions.

INTERVENTION/EVALUATION:

Monitor B/P, pulse, respirations. Assess cough, lung sounds. Increase fluid intake and environmental humidity to improve viscosity of lung secretions. To prevent pain cycles, instruct pt to request pain medication as soon as discomfort begins. Check for constipation (esp. in long-term use) and increase fiber, fluids, and exercise as appropriate. Initiate deep breathing and coughing exercises, particularly in those w/impaired pulmonary function. Assess for clinical improvement and record onset of relief of pain or cough.

PATIENT/FAMILY TEACHING:

Discomfort may occur w/injection. Change positions slowly to avoid orthostatic hypotension. Avoid tasks that require alertness, motor skills until response to drug is established. Tolerance/dependence may occur w/prolonged use of high doses. Avoid alcohol. Report difficulty breathing.

H

hydroxychloroquine sulfate

hi-drocks-ee-**klor**-oh-kwin
(Plaquenil Sulfate)

CANADIAN AVAILABILITY:
Plaquenil

CLASSIFICATION

Antimalarial, antirheumatic

AVAILABILITY (Rx)

Tablets: 200 mg

PHARMACOKINETICS

Variably absorbed from GI tract. Widely distributed. Slowly excreted in urine. Minimal removal by hemodialysis. Half-life: 1.9–5.5 hrs.

ACTION/THERAPEUTIC EFFECT

Concentrates in parasite acid vesicles, interfering w/parasite protein synthesis, increasing pH *(inhibits parasite growth)*. Antirheumatic action unknown, but may involve suppressing formation of antigens responsible for hypersensitivity reactions.

USES/UNLABELED

Treatment of falciparum malaria (terminates acute attacks and cures nonresistant strains), suppression of acute attacks and prolongation of interval between treatment/relapse in vivax, ovale, malariae malaria. Treatment of discoid or systematic lupus erythematosus, acute and chronic rheumatoid arthritis. *Treatment of juvenile arthritis, sarcoid-associated hypercalcemia.*

ADMINISTRATION

Administer w/meals to reduce GI upset.

INDICATIONS/DOSAGE/ROUTES

Note: 200 mg hydroxychloroquine = 155 mg base.

Suppression of malaria:
PO: Adults: 310 mg base weekly on same day each week. **Children:** 5 mg base/kg/wk. Begin 2 wks prior to exposure; continue 6–8 wks after leaving endemic area or if therapy is not begun prior to exposure.
PO: Adults: 620 mg base. **Children:** 10 mg base/kg given in 2 divided doses 6 hrs apart.

Treatment of malaria (acute attack): Dose (mg base)

DOSE	TIMES	ADULTS	CHILDREN
Initial	Day 1	620 mg	10 mg/kg
2nd	6 hrs later	310 mg	5 mg/kg
3rd	Day 2	310 mg	5 mg/kg
4th	Day 3	310 mg	5 mg/kg

Rheumatoid arthritis:
PO: Adults: Initially, 400–600 mg (310–465 mg base) daily for 5–10 days; gradually increase dose to optimum response level. **Maintenance (usually within 4–12 wks):** Decrease dose by 50%, continue at level of 200–400 mg/day. Maximum effect may not be seen for several months.

Lupus erythematosus:
PO: Adults: Initially, 400 mg 1–2 times/day for several weeks or months. **Maintenance:** 200–400 mg/day.

PRECAUTIONS

CONTRAINDICATIONS: Hypersensitivity to 4-aminoquinolones, retinal or visual field changes, long-term therapy for children, psoriasis, porphyria. After weighing risk/benefit ratio, physician may still elect to use drug, esp. w/plasmodial forms. **CAUTIONS:** Alcoholism, hepatic disease, G-6-

PD deficiency. Children are esp. susceptible to hydroxychloroquine fatalities. **PREGNANCY/LACTATION:** Unknown if drug crosses placenta; small amount excreted in breast milk. If possible, avoid use in pregnancy. **Pregnancy Category C**.

INTERACTIONS

DRUG INTERACTIONS: May increase concentration of penicillamine, increase risk of hematologic/renal or severe skin reaction. **ALTERED LAB VALUES:** None significant.

SIDE EFFECTS

FREQUENT: Mild transient headache, anorexia, nausea, vomiting. **OCCASIONAL:** Visual disturbances (blurring and difficulty focusing); nervousness; fatigue; pruritus (esp. of palms, soles, scalp); bleaching of hair; irritability, personality changes, diarrhea, skin eruptions. **RARE:** Stomatitis, exfoliative dermatitis, reduced hearing (nerve deafness).

ADVERSE REACTIONS/TOXIC EFFECTS

Ocular toxicity (esp. retinopathy, which may progress even after drug is discontinued). *Prolonged therapy:* peripheral neuritis, neuromyopathy, hypotension, EKG changes, agranulocytosis, aplastic anemia, thrombocytopenia, convulsions, psychosis. *Overdosage:* headache, vomiting, visual disturbance, drowsiness, convulsions, hypokalemia followed by cardiovascular collapse, death.

NURSING IMPLICATIONS
BASELINE ASSESSMENT:

Question for hypersensitivity to hydroxychloroquine sulfate or chloroquine. Evaluate CBC, hepatic function results.

INTERVENTION/EVALUATION:

Monitor and report any visual disturbances promptly. Evaluate for GI distress: Give dose w/food (for malaria); discuss w/physician dividing the dose into separate days during week. Monitor hepatic function tests and check for fatigue, jaundice, other signs of hepatic effects. Assess skin and buccal mucosa; inquire about pruritus. Check vital signs. Be alert to signs/symptoms of overdosage (esp. w/children). Monitor CBC results for adverse hematologic effects. Report reduced hearing immediately. W/prolonged therapy, test for muscle weakness.

PATIENT/FAMILY TEACHING:

Continue drug for full length of treatment. In long-term therapy therapeutic response may not be evident for up to 6 mos. Immediately notify physician of *any* new symptom of visual difficulties, muscular weakness, decreased hearing, tinnitus. Do not take any other medication w/o consulting physician. Periodic lab and visual tests are important part of therapy. Keep out of reach of children (small amount can cause serious effects, death).

hydroxyurea

high-**drocks**-ee-your-e-ah
(Droxia, Hydrea)

CANADIAN AVAILABILITY:
Hydrea

CLASSIFICATION

Antineoplastic

AVAILABILITY (Rx)

Capsules: 500 mg

PHARMACOKINETICS

Well absorbed from GI tract. Crosses blood-brain barrier. Metabolized in liver. Primarily excreted in urine; partially removed in lungs as CO_2. Half-life: 3–4 hrs.

ACTION/*THERAPEUTIC EFFECT*

Cell cycle-specific for S phase. Inhibits DNA synthesis w/o interfering w/RNA synthesis or protein, *interfering with the normal repair process of cells damaged by irradiation.*

USES/*UNLABELED*

Treatment of melanoma, resistant chronic myelocytic leukemia, recurrent, metastatic, or inoperable ovarian carcinoma. Also used in combination w/radiation therapy for local control of primary squamous cell carcinoma of head and neck, excluding lip. Treatment of sickle-cell anemia. *Treatment of cervical carcinoma, polycythemia vera. Long-term suppression of HIV.*

PO ADMINISTRATION

Note: May be carcinogenic, mutagenic, or teratogenic. Handle w/extreme care during administration. If pt is unable to swallow, dissolve contents of capsule in water immediately before administration.

INDICATIONS/DOSAGE/ROUTES

Note: Dosage individualized based on clinical response, tolerance to adverse effects. When used in combination therapy, consult specific protocols for optimum dosage, sequence of drug administration. Dosage based on actual or ideal body weight, whichever is less. Therapy interrupted when platelets fall below 100,000/mm³ or leukocytes fall below 2,500/mm³. Resume when counts rise toward normal.

Solid tumors, carcinoma of head and neck (with irradiation):
PO: Adults: 60–80 mg/kg (2–3 g/m²) as single dose every third day, or 20–30 mg/kg as single daily dose begun at least 7 days prior to start of irradiation.

Resistant chronic myelocytic leukemia:
PO: Adults: 20–30 mg/kg as single daily dose or 2 divided doses.

PRECAUTIONS

CONTRAINDICATIONS: WBC less than 2,500/mm³ or platelet count <100,000/mm³. **CAUTIONS:** Previous irradiation therapy, other cytoxic drugs, impaired renal, hepatic function. **PREGNANCY/LACTATION:** If possible, avoid use during pregnancy, esp. first trimester. Breast-feeding not recommended. **Pregnancy Category D.**

INTERACTIONS

DRUG INTERACTIONS: May decrease effect of antigout medications. Bone marrow depressants may increase bone marrow depression. Live virus vaccines may potentiate virus replication, increase vaccine side effects, decrease pt's antibody response to vaccine. **ALTERED LAB VALUES:** May increase BUN, creatinine, uric acid.

SIDE EFFECTS

FREQUENT: Nausea, vomiting, anorexia, constipation/diarrhea. **OCCASIONAL:** Mild reversible rash, facial flushing, pruritus, fever, chills, malaise. **RARE:** Alopecia, headache, drowsiness, dizziness, disorientation.

ADVERSE REACTIONS/TOXIC EFFECTS

Bone marrow depression manifested as hematologic toxicity (leukopenia, and to lesser extent, thrombocytopenia, anemia).

NURSING IMPLICATIONS
BASELINE ASSESSMENT:

Obtain bone marrow studies, liver, kidney function tests before therapy begins, periodically thereafter. Obtain Hgb, WBC, platelet count weekly during therapy. Those w/marked renal impairment may develop visual, auditory hallucinations, marked hematologic toxicity.

INTERVENTION/EVALUATION:

Assess pattern of daily bowel activity and stool consistency. Monitor for hematologic toxicity (fever, sore throat, signs of local infection, easy bruising, or unusual bleeding from any site), symptoms of anemia (excessive tiredness, weakness). Assess skin for rash, erythema.

PATIENT/FAMILY TEACHING:

Alopecia is reversible, but new hair growth may have different color or texture. Do not have immunizations w/o physician's approval (drug lowers body's resistance). Avoid contact w/those who have recently received live virus vaccine. Promptly report fever, sore throat, signs of local infection, easy bruising, or unusual bleeding from any site. Contact physician if nausea/vomiting continues at home.

hydroxyzine hydrochloride
high-**drox**-ih-zeen
(Atarax, Vistaril)
hydroxyzine pamoate
(Vistaril)

CANADIAN AVAILABILITY:
Apo-Hydroxyzine, Atarax, Novohydroxyzin

CLASSIFICATION

Antihistamine

AVAILABILITY (Rx)

Tablets: 10 mg, 25 mg, 50 mg, 100 mg. **Capsules:** 25 mg, 50 mg, 100 mg. **Syrup:** 10 mg/5 ml. **Oral Suspension:** 25 mg/5 ml. **Injection:** 25 mg/ml, 50 mg/ml.

PHARMACOKINETICS

	ONSET	PEAK	DURATION
PO	15–30 min	—	—

Well absorbed from GI tract, parenteral administration. Metabolized in liver. Primarily excreted in urine. Half-life: 20–25 hrs (increased in elderly).

ACTION/ *THERAPEUTIC EFFECT*

Suppresses activity at subcortical levels of CNS, *producing anticholinergic, antihistaminic, analgesic effects, skeletal muscle relaxation.* Diminishes vestibular stimulation and depresses labyrinthine function, *controlling nausea, vomiting.*

USES

Relief of anxiety, tension; pruritus caused by allergic conditions, preop and postop sedation, control of muscle spasm, nausea, and vomiting.

STORAGE/HANDLING

Store oral solution/suspension, parenteral form at room temperature.

PO/IM ADMINISTRATION

PO:

1. Shake oral suspension well.
2. Scored tablets may be crushed.
3. Do not crush or break capsule.

IM:

Note: Significant tissue damage, thrombosis, gangrene may occur if injection is given SubQ, intra-arterial, or IV injection.

1. IM may be given undiluted.
2. Use Z-track technique of injection to prevent SubQ infiltration.
3. Inject deep IM into gluteus maximus or midlateral thigh in adults, midlateral thigh in children.

INDICATIONS/DOSAGE/ROUTES

Anxiety, tension:
PO: Adults, elderly: 25–100 mg 3–4 times/day. **Children >6 yrs:** 50–100 mg/day in divided doses. **Children <6 yrs:** 50 mg/day in divided doses.
IM: Adults, elderly: 25–100 mg q4–6h, as needed. **Children:** 0.5 mg/kg.

Nausea, vomiting:
IM: Adults, elderly: 25–100 mg. **Children:** 1.1 mg/kg.

Pruritus:
PO: Adults, elderly: 25 mg 3–4 times/day. **Children >6 yrs:** 50–100/day in divided doses. **Children <6 yrs:** 50 mg/day in divided doses.

Agitation due to alcohol withdrawal:
IM: Adults, elderly: 50–100 mg. May be repeated q4–6h, as needed.

PRECAUTIONS

CONTRAINDICATIONS: None significant. **CAUTIONS:** None significant. **PREGNANCY/LACTATION:** Unknown if hydroxyzine crosses placenta or is distributed in breast milk. **Pregnancy Category C**.

INTERACTIONS

DRUG INTERACTIONS: Alcohol, CNS depressants may increase CNS depressant effects. MAO inhibitors may increase anticholinergic, CNS depressant effects. **ALTERED LAB VALUES:** May cause false positives w/17-hydroxy corticosteroid determinations.

SIDE EFFECTS

Side effects are generally mild and transient. **FREQUENT:** Drowsiness, dry mouth, marked discomfort w/IM injection. **OCCASIONAL:** Dizziness, ataxia (muscular incoordination), weakness, slurred speech, headache, agitation, increased anxiety. **RARE:** Paradoxical CNS hyperactivity/nervousness in children, excitement/restlessness in elderly/debilitated pts (generally noted during first 2 wks of therapy, particularly noted in presence of uncontrolled pain).

ADVERSE REACTIONS/TOXIC EFFECTS

Hypersensitivity reaction (wheezing, dyspnea, tightness of chest).

NURSING IMPLICATIONS
BASELINE ASSESSMENT:

Anxiety: **Offer** emotional support to anxious pt. Assess motor responses (agitation, trembling, tension) and autonomic responses (cold, clammy hands, sweating). *Antiemetic:* Assess for dehydration (poor skin turgor, dry mucous membranes, longitudinal furrows in tongue).

INTERVENTION/EVALUATION:

For those on long-term therapy, liver/renal function tests, blood counts should be performed periodically. Monitor lung sounds for signs of hypersensitivity reaction. Monitor serum electrolytes in those w/severe vomiting. Assess for paradoxical reaction, particularly during early therapy. Assist w/ambulation if drowsiness, lightheadedness occurs.

PATIENT/FAMILY TEACHING:

Marked discomfort may occur w/IM injection. Sugarless gum, sips of tepid water may relieve dry mouth. Drowsiness usually diminishes w/continued therapy. Avoid tasks that require alertness, motor skills until response to drug is established.

hyoscyamine hydrobromide

high-oh-**sigh**-ah-meen

hyoscyamine sulfate

(Anaspaz, Levsin, Levsinex, Neoquess, Cystospaz)

FIXED-COMBINATION(S): W/phenobarbital, a sedative-hypnotic (**Levsinex w/PB, Anaspaz PB**).

CANADIAN AVAILABILITY: Buscopan, Levsin

CLASSIFICATION

Anticholinergic

AVAILABILITY (Rx)

Tablets: 0.125 mg, 0.15 mg. **Capsules (timed-release):** 0.375 mg. **Oral Solution:** 0.125 mg/ml. **Elixir:** 0.125 mg/5 ml. **Injection:** 0.5 mg/ml. **Ophthalmic Solution:** 0.25%.

PHARMACOKINETICS

Well absorbed from GI tract. Widely distributed. Protein binding: 50%. Metabolized in liver. Primarily excreted in urine. Half-life: 3.5 hrs.

ACTION/*THERAPEUTIC EFFECT*

Inhibits action of acetylcholine at postganglionic (muscarinic) receptor sites, *decreasing secretions (bronchial, salivary, sweat glands, gastric juices). Reduces motility of GI and urinary tract.*

USES

Adjunct in treatment of peptic ulcer disease; GI hypermotility (i.e., irritable bowel syndrome). Treatment of neurogenic bowel syndrome. Drying agent in acute rhinitis. Aid in controlling gastric secretion, visceral spasm, hypermotility in spastic colitis, spastic bladder, pylorospasm, associated abdominal cramps. Reduces duodenal motility to facilitate diagnostic radiologic procedure. Preop to reduce salivary, tracheobronchial, pharyngeal secretions. Reduces volume, acidity of gastric secretions.

PO/SUBQ/IM/IV ADMINISTRATION

PO:

1. May give w/o regard to meals.

H

2. Tablets may be crushed, chewed.

3. Extended-release capsule should be swallowed whole.

INDICATIONS/DOSAGE/ROUTES

Usual oral dose:
PO: Adults, elderly: 0.125–0.25 mg 3–4 times/day. **(Extended-release):** 0.375–0.750 mg q12h. **Children:** Based on weight q4h as needed.

Usual parenteral dosage:
IM/IV/SubQ: Adults, elderly: 0.25–0.5 mg 2–4 times/day.

Duodenography:
IV: Adults, elderly: 0.25–0.5 mg 10 min prior to procedure.

Preop:
IM: Adults, elderly: 0.5 mg (0.005 mg/kg) 30–60 min prior to induction of anesthesia or administration of preop medications.

PRECAUTIONS

CONTRAINDICATIONS: Narrow-angle glaucoma, severe ulcerative colitis, toxic megacolon, obstructive disease of GI tract, paralytic ileus, intestinal atony, bladder neck obstruction due to prostatic hypertrophy, myasthenia gravis in those not treated w/neostigmine, tachycardia secondary to cardiac insufficiency or thyrotoxicosis, cardiospasm, unstable cardiovascular status in acute hemorrhage. **EXTREME CAUTION:** Autonomic neuropathy, known or suspected GI infections, diarrhea, mild to moderate ulcerative colitis, bronchial asthma. **CAUTIONS:** Hyperthyroidism, hepatic or renal disease, hypertension, tachyarrhythmias, CHF, coronary artery disease, gastric ulcer, esophageal reflux or hiatal hernia associated w/reflux esophagitis, infants, elderly, those w/COPD. **PREGNANCY/LACTATION:** Crosses placenta; distributed in breast milk. Parenteral form near term may produce tachycardia in fetus. **Pregnancy Category C.**

INTERACTIONS

DRUG INTERACTIONS: Antacids, antidiarrheals may decrease absorption. Anticholinergics may increase effects. May decrease absorption of ketoconazole. May increase severity of GI lesions with potassium chloride (wax matrix). **ALTERED LAB VALUES:** None significant.

SIDE EFFECTS

FREQUENT: Dry mouth (sometimes severe), decreased sweating, constipation. **OCCASIONAL:** Blurred vision, bloated feeling, urinary hesitancy, drowsiness (w/ high dosage), headache, intolerance to light, loss of taste, nervousness, flushing, insomnia, impotence, mental confusion/excitement (particularly in elderly, children). Parenteral form may produce temporary lightheadedness, local irritation. **RARE:** Dizziness, faintness.

ADVERSE REACTIONS/TOXIC EFFECTS

Overdosage may produce temporary paralysis of ciliary muscle, pupillary dilation, tachycardia, palpitation, hot/dry/flushed skin, absence of bowel sounds, hyperthermia, increased respiratory rate, EKG abnormalities, nausea, vomiting, rash over face/upper trunk, CNS stimulation, psychosis (agitation, restlessness, rambling speech, visual hallucination, paranoid behavior, delusions), followed by depression.

NURSING IMPLICATIONS
BASELINE ASSESSMENT:

Before giving medication, instruct pt to void (reduces risk of urinary retention).

INTERVENTION/EVALUATION:

Monitor daily bowel activity and stool consistency. Palpate bladder for urinary retention. Monitor changes in B/P, temperature. Assess skin turgor, mucous membranes to evaluate hydration status (encourage adequate fluid intake), bowel sounds for peristalsis. Be alert for fever (increased risk of hyperthermia).

PATIENT/FAMILY TEACHING:

Do not become overheated during exercise in hot weather (may result in heat stroke). Avoid hot baths, saunas. Avoid tasks that require alertness, motor skills until response to drug is established. Sugarless gum, sips of tepid water may relieve dry mouth. Do not take antacids or medicine for diarrhea within 1 hr of taking this medication (decreased effectiveness).

ibuprofen

eye-byew-**pro**-fen
(Advil, Motrin, Nuprin, Rufen, Trendar)

FIXED COMBINATION(S)
W/hydrocodone, an opioid analgesic (Vicoprofen)

CANADIAN AVAILABILITY:
Advil, Motrin, Novoprofen

CLASSIFICATION

Nonsteroidal anti-inflammatory

AVAILABILITY (Rx)

Tablets: 100 mg, 200 mg (OTC), 400 mg, 600 mg, 800 mg. **Tablets (chewable):** 50 mg, 100 mg. **Oral Suspension:** 100 mg/5 ml (OTC). **Oral Drops:** 40 mg/ml.

PHARMACOKINETICS

	ONSET	PEAK	DURATION
PO (analgesic)	0.5 hrs	—	4–6 hrs
PO (antirheumatic)	2 days	1–2 wks	—

Rapidly absorbed from GI tract. Metabolized in liver. Primarily excreted in urine. Half-life: 2–4 hrs.

ACTION/*THERAPEUTIC EFFECT*

Produces analgesic and anti-inflammatory effect by inhibiting prostaglandin synthesis, *reducing inflammatory response and intensity of pain stimulus reaching sensory nerve endings.* Antipyresis produced by effect on hypothalamus, producing vasodilation, *thereby decreasing elevated body temperature.*

USES/*UNLABELED*

Symptomatic treatment of acute/chronic rheumatoid arthritis and osteoarthritis; reduces fever. Relief of mild to moderate pain, primary dysmenorrhea. Temporary relief of minor aches/pain associated w/common cold, headache, toothache, muscular aches, backaches, menstrual cramps. *Treatment of psoriatic arthritis, vascular headaches.*

PO ADMINISTRATION

1. Do not crush or break enteric-coated form.
2. May give w/food, milk, or antacids if GI distress occurs.

INDICATIONS/DOSAGE/ROUTES

Note: Do not exceed 3.2 g/day.

Acute/chronic rheumatoid arthritis, osteoarthritis:
PO: **Adults, elderly:** 300–800 mg 3–4 times/day.

Mild to moderate pain, primary dysmenorrhea:
PO: **Adults, elderly:** 400 mg q4–6h.

Fever, minor aches/pain:
PO: **Adults, elderly:** 200–400 mg q4–6h. **Maximum:** 1.2 g/day. **Children:** 5–10 mg/kg/dose. **Maximum:** 40 mg/kg/day.

Juvenile arthritis:
PO: **Children:** 30–70 mg/kg/day in 3–4 divided doses.

PRECAUTIONS

CONTRAINDICATIONS: Active peptic ulcer, GI ulceration, chronic inflammation of GI tract, GI bleeding disorders, history of hypersensitivity to aspirin or NSAIDs. **CAUTIONS:** Impaired renal/hepatic function, history of GI tract disease, predisposition to fluid retention. **PREGNANCY/LACTATION:** Unknown if drug crosses placenta or is distributed in breast milk. Avoid use during third trimester (may adversely affect fetal cardiovascular system: premature closure of ductus arteriosus). **Pregnancy Category B**. (Category D if used in 3rd trimester or near delivery.)

INTERACTIONS

DRUG INTERACTIONS: May increase effects of oral anticoagulants, heparin, thrombolytics. May decrease effect of antihypertensives, diuretics. Salicylates, aspirin may increase risk of GI side effects, bleeding. Bone marrow depressants may increase risk of hematologic reactions. May increase concentration, toxicity of lithium. May increase methotrex-

ate toxicity. Probenecid may increase concentration. **ALTERED LAB VALUES:** May prolong bleeding time. May alter blood glucose. May increase BUN, creatinine, potassium, liver function tests. May decrease Hgb, Hct.

SIDE EFFECTS

FREQUENT (3–9%): Nausea (with or without vomiting), dyspepsia, dizziness, rash. **OCCASIONAL (<3%):** Diarrhea/constipation, flatulence, abdominal cramping/pain, itching. **RARE:** Confusion, increased B/P, blurred vision.

ADVERSE REACTIONS/TOXIC EFFECTS

Acute overdosage may result in metabolic acidosis. Peptic ulcer, GI bleeding, gastritis, severe hepatic reaction (cholestasis, jaundice) occur rarely. Nephrotoxicity (dysuria, hematuria, proteinuria, nephrotic syndrome) and severe hypersensitivity reaction (particularly those w/systemic lupus erythematosus, other collagen diseases) occur rarely.

NURSING IMPLICATIONS
BASELINE ASSESSMENT:

Assess onset, type, location, and duration of pain or inflammation. Inspect appearance of affected joints for immobility, deformities, and skin condition.

INTERVENTION/EVALUATION:

Monitor for evidence of nausea, dyspepsia. Monitor pattern of daily bowel activity and stool consistency. Check behind medial malleolus for fluid retention (usually first area noted). Assess skin for evidence of rash. Assist w/ambulation if dizziness occurs. Evaluate for therapeutic response: relief of pain, stiffness, swelling, increase in joint mobility, reduced joint tenderness, improved grip strength.

PATIENT/FAMILY TEACHING:

Avoid aspirin, alcohol during therapy (increases risk of GI bleeding). If GI upset occurs, take w/food, milk, or antacids. Report blurred vision, ringing/roaring in ears. Avoid tasks that require alertness until response to drug is established. Do not crush or chew enteric-coated tablet.

ibutilide fumarate

eye-**byew**t-ih-lied
(Corvert)

CLASSIFICATION

Antiarrhythmic

AVAILABILITY (Rx)

Injection: 0.1 mg/ml solution

PHARMACOKINETICS

After IV administration, highly distributed, rapidly cleared. Primarily excreted in urine as metabolite. Half-life: 2–12 hrs (avg: 6 hrs).

ACTION/THERAPEUTIC EFFECT

Prolongs both atrial and ventricular action potential duration and increases atrial and ventricular refractory period. Activates slow, inward current (sodium), produces mild slowing of sinus rate and AV conduction, dose-related prolongation of QT interval. Converts arrhythmias to sinus rhythm.

USES/UNLABELED

Rapid conversion of atrial fibril-lation or flutter of recent onset to sinus rhythm (arrhythmias of longer duration less likely to respond to therapy).

STORAGE/HANDLING

Admixtures w/diluent stable at room temperature for 24 hrs, 48 hrs if refrigerated.

IV ADMINISTRATION

Note: Compatible w/5% dextrose injection, 0.9% NaCl diluents. Compatible w/polyvinyl chloride plastic and polyolefin bag admixtures.

1. Give undiluted or diluted in 50 ml diluent.
2. Give infusion over 10 min.
3. Monitor pt w/continuous EKG reading for at least 4 hrs following infusion or until QT interval has returned to baseline.

INDICATIONS/DOSAGE/ROUTES

Atrial arrhythmias:
IV Infusion: Adults, elderly ≥60 kg (132 lbs): One vial (1 mg) given over 10 min. If arrhythmia does not stop within 10 min after end of initial infusion, a second 10 min infusion may be given 10 min after completion of first infusion. **Adults, elderly <60 kg (132 lbs):** 0.1 ml/kg (0.01 mg/kg) given over 10 min. If arrhythmia does not stop within 10 min after end of initial infusion, a second 10 min infusion may be given 10 min after completion of first infusion.

PRECAUTIONS

CONTRAINDICATIONS: Hypersensitivity to ibutilide. **CAUTIONS:** Abnormal liver function, heart block. **PREGNANCY/LACTATION:** Teratogenic, embryocidal in animals. Discourage breast-feeding during therapy. **Pregnancy Category C**.

INTERACTIONS

DRUG INTERACTIONS: Do not give concurrently w/class Ia (disopyramide, quinidine, procainamide, moricizine) or class III (amiodarone, sotalol, bretylium) antiarrhythmics or within 4 hrs postinfusion of ibutilide. Phenothiazines, tricyclic and tetracyclic antidepressants, H_1 receptor antagonists may prolong QT interval. **ALTERED LAB VALUES:** None significant.

SIDE EFFECTS

Generally well tolerated. **OCCASIONAL:** Ventricular extrasystoles (5.1%), ventricular tachycardia (4.9%), headache (3.6%), hypotension, postural hypotension (2%). **RARE:** Bundle-branch block, AV block, bradycardia, hypertension.

ADVERSE REACTIONS/TOXIC EFFECTS

Sustained polymorphic ventricular tachycardia, occasionally w/QT prolongation (torsades de pointes) occurs rarely. Overdosage results in CNS toxicity (CNS depression, rapid gasping breathing, seizures). May exaggerate expected prolongation of repolarization. May worsen existing arrhythmias or produce new arrhythmias.

NURSING IMPLICATIONS

BASELINE ASSESSMENT:

Those w/atrial fibrillation of >2–3 days duration must be treated w/anticoagulants generally for at least 2 wks prior to ibutilide therapy. Cardiac monitoring equipment, intracardiac pacing facility, cardioverter/defibrillator, medications for treatment of sustained ventricular tachycardia (VT), including polymorphic VT, must be available during and after administration. Anticipate proarrhythmic events.

INTERVENTION/EVALUATION:

Observe pt w/continuous EKG monitoring for at least 4 hrs following infusion or until QT interval has returned to baseline. If any arrhythmic activity is noted, continue EKG monitoring. Monitor for symptoms of electrolyte abnormalities, esp. magnesium and potassium, and overdrive cardiac pacing, electrical cardioversion, or defibrillation.

idarubicin hydrochloride

eye-dah-**roo**-bi-sin
(Idamycin, Idamycin PFS)

CANADIAN AVAILABILITY:
Idamycin

CLASSIFICATION

Antineoplastic

AVAILABILITY (Rx)

Injection: 5 mg, 10 mg, 20 mg

PHARMACOKINETICS

Widely distributed. Rapidly metabolized in liver to active metabolite. Primarily eliminated via biliary excretion. Not removed by hemodialysis. Half-life: 4–46 hrs; metabolite: 8–92 hrs.

ACTION/*THERAPEUTIC EFFECT*

Inhibits nucleic acid synthesis by interacting with the enzyme topoisomerase II (an enzyme promoting DNA strand supercoiling), *producing death of rapidly dividing cells.*

USES

Treatment of acute myeloid leukemia (AML) in adults.

STORAGE/HANDLING

Reconstituted solution stable for 72 hrs (3 days) at room temperature or 168 hrs (7 days) if refrigerated. Discard unused solution.
Note: Idamycin PFS does not require reconstitution and is stored refrigerated.

IV ADMINISTRATION

Note: Give by free-flowing IV infusion (*never* SubQ or IM). Gloves, gowns, eye goggles recommended during preparation and administration of medication. If powder or solution comes in contact with skin, wash thoroughly. Avoid small veins, swollen or edematous extremities, and areas overlying joints, tendons.

1. Reconstitute each 10 mg vial with 10 ml 0.9% NaCl injection (5 ml/5 mg vial) to provide a concentration of 1 mg/ml.

2. Administer into tubing of freely running IV infusion of 5% dextrose or 0.9% NaCl, preferably via butterfly needle, *slowly* (>10–15 min).

3. Extravasation produces immediate pain, severe local tissue damage. Terminate infusion immediately. Apply cold compresses for $1/2$ hr immediately, then $1/2$ hr 4 times/day for 3 days. Keep extremity elevated.

INDICATIONS/DOSAGE/ROUTES

Note: Dosage individualized based on clinical response, tolerance to adverse effects. When used in combination therapy, consult specific protocols for optimum dosage, sequence of drug administration.

Usual dose:
IV: Adults: 12 mg/m²/day for 3 days (combined with Ara-C).

Dosage in hepatic/renal impairment:
Dosage may be decreased in pts with liver/renal dysfunction.

PRECAUTIONS

CONTRAINDICATIONS: None significant. **EXTREME CAUTION:** Preexisting myelosuppression, cardiac disease, impaired hepatic/renal function. **PREGNANCY/LACTATION:** If possible, avoid use during pregnancy (may be embryotoxic). Unknown if drug is distributed in breast milk (advise to discontinue nursing before drug initiation). **Pregnancy Category D.**

INTERACTIONS

DRUG INTERACTIONS: May decrease effect of antigout medications. Bone marrow depressants may increase bone marrow depression. Live virus vaccines may potentiate virus replication, increase vaccine side effects, decrease pt's antibody response to vaccine. **ALTERED LAB VALUES:** May increase uric acid, SGOT (AST), SGPT (ALT), alkaline phosphatase, bilirubin. May cause EKG changes.

SIDE EFFECTS

FREQUENT: Complete alopecia (scalp, axillary, pubic hair), nausea, vomiting, abdominal pain (suggestive of stomatitis), diarrhea, esophagitis (esp. if drug given daily on several successive days). **OCCASIONAL:** Anorexia, hyperpigmentation of nailbeds, phalangeal and dermal creases. **RARE:** Fever, chills, conjunctivitis, lacrimation.

ADVERSE REACTIONS/TOXIC EFFECTS

Bone marrow depression manifested as hematologic toxicity (principally leukopenia and, to lesser extent, anemia, thrombocytopenia). Generally occurs within 10–15 days, returns to normal levels by third week. Cardiotoxicity noted as either acute, transient abnormal EKG findings and/or cardiomyopathy manifested as CHF.

NURSING IMPLICATIONS

BASELINE ASSESSMENT:

Determine baseline renal and hepatic function, CBC results. Obtain EKG before therapy. Antiemetic before and during therapy may prevent, relieve nausea.

INTERVENTION/EVALUATION:

Severe myelosuppression of idarubicin requires frequent CBC assessment and close observation of pt: thrombocytopenia (easy bruising, unusual bleeding to frank hemorrhage), leukemia (fever, sore throat, signs of infection), and anemia (excessive fatigue, weakness, dyspnea). Avoid IM injections, rectal temperatures, and other trauma that may precipitate bleeding. Check infusion site frequently for extravasation (causes severe local necrosis). Assess for potentially fatal CHF dyspnea, rales, edema, and life-threatening arrhythmias.

PATIENT/FAMILY TEACHING:

Total body alopecia is frequent but reversible. Assist w/ways to cope w/hair loss. New hair growth resumes 2–3 mos after last therapy dose and may have different color, texture. Maintain fastidious oral hygiene. Do not have immunizations without physician's approval (drug lowers body's resistance). Avoid crowds, those w/infections. Teach pt and family the early signs of bleeding and infection.

ifosfamide

eye-**fos**-fah-mid
(Ifex)

CANADIAN AVAILABILITY:
Ifex

CLASSIFICATION

Antineoplastic

AVAILABILITY (Rx)

Powder for Injection: 1 g, 3 g

PHARMACOKINETICS

Metabolized in liver to active metabolite. Crosses blood-brain barrier (limited). Primarily excreted in urine. Half-life: 15 hrs.

ACTION/*THERAPEUTIC EFFECT*

Converted to active metabolite, binds with intracellular structures. Action primarily due to cross-linking strands of DNA, RNA, *inhibiting protein synthesis.*

USES/*UNLABELED*

Third-line chemotherapy of germ cell testicular carcinoma (used in combination w/agents that protect against hemorrhagic cystitis). *Treatment of soft tissue sarcoma, Ewing's sarcoma, non-Hodgkin's lymphomas, lung, pancreatic carcinoma.*

STORAGE/HANDLING

Note: May be carcinogenic, mutagenic, or teratogenic. Handle w/extreme care during preparation/administration. Store vial at room temperature. After reconstitution w/bacteriostatic water for injection, solution stable for 1 wk at room temperature; stable for 3 wks if refrigerated (further diluted solution stable for 6 wks, refrigerated). Solutions prepared w/other diluents should be used within 6 hrs.

IV ADMINISTRATION

1. Reconstitute 1 g vial w/20 ml sterile water for injection or bacteriostatic water for injection to provide concentration of 50 mg/ml. Shake to dissolve.
2. Further dilute w/5% dextrose or 0.9% NaCl to provide concentration of 0.6–20 mg/ml.
3. Infuse over 30 min minimum.
4. Give w/at least 2,000 ml oral or IV fluid (prevents bladder toxicity).
5. Give w/protector against hemorrhagic cystitis (e.g., mesna).

INDICATIONS/DOSAGE/ROUTES

Note: Dosage individualized based on clinical response, tolerance to adverse effects. When used in combination therapy, consult specific protocols for optimum dosage, sequence of drug administration.

Germ cell testicular carcinoma:
IV: Adults: 1.2 g/m^2/day for 5 consecutive days. Repeat q3 wks or after recovery from hematologic toxicity. Administer w/mesna.

PRECAUTIONS

CONTRAINDICATIONS: Severely depressed bone marrow function. **CAUTIONS:** Impaired renal, liver function, compromised bone marrow function. **PREGNANCY/LACTATION:** If possible, avoid use during pregnancy, esp. first trimester. May cause fetal damage. Drug is distributed in breast milk. Breast-feeding not recommended. **Pregnancy Category D.**

INTERACTIONS

DRUG INTERACTIONS: Bone marrow depressants may increase bone marrow depression. Live virus vaccines may potentiate virus replication, increase vaccine side effects, decrease pt's antibody response to vaccine. **ALTERED LAB VALUES:** May increase BUN, creatinine, uric acid, SGOT (AST), SGPT (ALT), LDH, bilirubin.

SIDE EFFECTS

FREQUENT (>30%): Nausea, vomiting (58%), hematuria (92%), alopecia (83%), hemorrhagic cystitis, dysuria, increased urinary frequency. **OCCASIONAL (5–15%):** Confusion, somnolence, psychosis, hallucinations, infection. **RARE (<5%):** Dizziness, seizures, disorientation, fever, malaise, stomatitis (mucosal irritation, glossitis, gingivitis).

ADVERSE REACTIONS/TOXIC EFFECTS

Hemorrhagic cystitis (occurs frequently), severe myelosuppression, pulmonary toxicity (cough, SOB), hepatotoxicity, nephrotoxicity, cardiotoxicity, CNS toxicity (confusion, hallucinations, somnolence, coma) may require discontinuation of therapy.

NURSING IMPLICATIONS

BASELINE ASSESSMENT:

Obtain urinalysis before each dose. If hematuria occurs (>10 RBCs per field), withhold therapy until resolution occurs. Obtain WBC, platelet count, Hgb before each dose.

INTERVENTION/EVALUATION:

Monitor hematologic studies, urinalysis diligently. Assess for fever, sore throat, signs of local infection, easy bruising, unusual bleeding from any site, symptoms of anemia (excessive tiredness, weakness).

PATIENT/FAMILY TEACHING:

Maintain copious daily fluid intake (protects against cystitis). Therapy may interfere w/wound healing. Do not have immunizations w/o physician's approval (drug lowers body's resistance). Avoid contact w/those who have recently received live virus vaccine. Contact physician if nausea/vomiting continues at home. Report unusual bleeding/bruising, fever, chills, sore throat, cough, SOB, seizures, joint pain, sores in mouth or on lips, yellowing skin/eyes.

---

imiglucerase
(Cerezyme)
See Supplement

---

imipenem/ cilastatin sodium

im-ih-**peh**-nem/sill-as-**tah**-tin
(Primaxin)

CANADIAN AVAILABILITY:
Primaxin

CLASSIFICATION

Antibiotic

AVAILABILITY (Rx)

Injection for IM: 500 mg, 750 mg.
Injection for IV: 250 mg, 500 mg.

PHARMACOKINETICS

Readily absorbed after IM administration. Widely distributed. Metabolized in kidney. Primarily excreted in urine. Removed by hemodialysis. Half-life: 1 hr (increased in decreased renal function).

ACTION/ *THERAPEUTIC EFFECT*

Imipenem: Bactericidal. Binds to bacterial membranes, *inhibiting bacterial cell wall synthesis. Cilastatin:* Prevents renal metabolism of imipenem.

USES

Treatment of respiratory tract, skin/skin structure, gynecologic, bone/joint, intra-abdominal, complicated/uncomplicated urinary tract infections, endocarditis, polymicrobic infections, septicemia; serious nosocomial infections.

STORAGE/HANDLING

Solution appears colorless to yellow; discard if solution turns brown. IV infusion (piggyback) stable for 4 hrs at room temperature, 24 hrs if refrigerated. Discard if precipitate forms.

IM/IV ADMINISTRATION
IM:

1. Prepare w/1% lidocaine w/o epinephrine; 500 mg vial w/2 ml, 750 mg vial w/3 ml lidocaine HCl.
2. Administer suspension within 1 hr of preparation.
3. Do not mix w/any other medications.
4. Inject deep in large muscle; aspirate to decrease risk of injection into a blood vessel.

IV:

1. Give by intermittent IV infusion (piggyback). Do not give IV push.

2. Dilute each 250 mg or 500 mg vial w/100 ml 5% dextrose; 0.9% NaCl, or other compatible IV fluid. Infuse >20–30 min (1 g dose >40–60 min).

3. Use large veins to reduce risk of phlebitis; alternate sites.

4. Observe pt during first 30 min of infusion to observe for possible hypersensitivity reaction.

INDICATIONS/DOSAGE/ROUTES

Note: Space doses evenly around the clock.

Uncomplicated urinary tract infections:
IV: Adults, elderly: 250 mg q6h.

Complicated urinary tract infections:
IV: Adults, elderly: 500 mg q6h.

Mild infections:
IV: Adults, elderly: 250–500 mg q6h.

Moderate infections:
IV: Adults, elderly: 500 mg q6–8h.

Severe, life-threatening infections:
IV: Adults, elderly: 500 mg q6h.

Usual pediatric dosage:
IV: Children (≥3 mos): 10–25 mg/kg/dose q6h.

Dosage in renal impairment:
Dose and/or frequency is modified based on creatinine clearance and/or severity of infection.

CREATININE CLEARANCE	DOSAGE
31–70 ml/min	500 mg q8h
21–30 ml/min	500 mg q12h
0–20 ml/min	250 mg q12h

USUAL INTRAMUSCULAR DOSAGE:

Note: Do not use for severe or life-threatening infections.

Mild to moderate lower respiratory tract, skin/skin structure, gynecologic infections:
IM: Adults, elderly: 500–750 mg q12h.

Mild to moderate intra-abdominal infections:
IM: Adults, elderly: 750 mg q12h.

PRECAUTIONS

CONTRAINDICATIONS: Hypersensitivity to imipenem/cilastatin sodium, other beta lactams. *IM:* Hypersensitivity to any local anesthetics of amide type; pts w/severe shock or heart block (due to use of lidocaine diluent). **CAUTIONS:** Hypersensitivity to penicillins, cephalosporins, other allergens; renal dysfunction, CNS disorders, particularly w/history of seizures. **PREGNANCY/LACTATION:** Crosses placenta; distributed in cord blood, amniotic fluid, breast milk. **Pregnancy Category C**.

INTERACTIONS

DRUG INTERACTIONS: None significant. **ALTERED LAB VALUES:** May increase SGOT (AST), SGPT (ALT), alkaline phosphatase, LDH, bilirubin, BUN, creatinine. May decrease Hgb, Hct.

SIDE EFFECTS

OCCASIONAL (2–3%): Diarrhea, nausea, vomiting. **RARE (1–2%):** Rash.

ADVERSE REACTIONS/TOXIC EFFECTS

Antibiotic-associated colitis, other superinfections may occur. Anaphylactic reactions in those receiving beta lactams have occurred.

NURSING IMPLICATIONS

BASELINE ASSESSMENT:

Question pt for history of allergies, particularly to imipenem/cilastatin sodium, other beta lactams, penicillins, cephalosporins. Inquire about history of seizures. Obtain culture and sensitivity tests before giving first dose (therapy may begin before results are known).

INTERVENTION/EVALUATION:

Evaluate for phlebitis (heat, pain, red streaking over vein), pain at IV injection site. Assess for GI discomfort, nausea, vomiting. Determine pattern of bowel activity and stool consistency. Assess skin for rash. Monitor I&O, renal function tests. Check mental status, be alert to tremors and possible seizures. Assess temperature, B/P twice daily, more often if necessary. Assess for hearing loss, tinnitus. Monitor electrolytes, esp. potassium.

PATIENT/FAMILY TEACHING:

Continue therapy for full length of treatment. Doses should be evenly spaced. Do not take any other medication unless approved by physician. Notify physician in event of tremors, seizures, rash, diarrhea, or other new symptom.

imipramine hydrochloride

ih-**mih**-prah-meen
(Janimine, Tofranil)

imipramine pamoate

(Tofranil-PM)

CANADIAN AVAILABILITY:
Api-Imipramine, Tofranil

CLASSIFICATION

Antidepressant: Tricyclic

AVAILABILITY (Rx)

Hydrochloride: **Tablets:** 10 mg, 25 mg, 50 mg. **Injection:** 25 mg/ml.
Pamoate: **Capsules:** 75 mg, 100 mg, 125 mg, 150 mg.

PHARMACOKINETICS

Rapidly, well absorbed from GI tract. Widely distributed. Metabolized in liver, undergoing first-pass effect. Primarily excreted in urine. Half-life: 11–25 hrs.

ACTION/*THERAPEUTIC EFFECT*

Blocks reuptake of neurotransmitters (norepinephrine, serotonin) at presynaptic membranes, increasing concentration at postsynaptic receptor sites, *resulting in antidepressant effect*. Anticholinergic effect *controls nocturnal enuresis.*

USES/*UNLABELED*

Treatment of various forms of depression, often in conjunction w/psychotherapy. Treatment of nocturnal enuresis in children >6 yrs. *Treatment of panic disorder, neurogenic pain, attention deficit hyperactivity disorder (ADHD), cataplexy associated w/narcolepsy.*

STORAGE/HANDLING

Parenteral form takes on yellow or reddish hue when exposed to light. Slight discoloration does not affect potency but marked discoloration is associated w/potency loss.

PO/IM ADMINISTRATION

PO:

1. Give w/food or milk if GI distress occurs.
2. Do not crush or break film-coated tablets.

IM:

1. Give by IM only if oral administration is not feasible.

2. Crystals may form in injection. Redissolve by immersing ampule in hot water for 1 min.

3. Give deep IM slowly.

INDICATIONS/DOSAGE/ROUTES

Depression:

PO: Adults: Initially, 75–100 mg daily. Dosage may be gradually increased to 300 mg daily for hospitalized pts, 200 mg for outpatients, then reduce dosage to effective maintenance level (50–150 mg daily). **Elderly:** Initially, 10–25 mg/day at bedtime. May increase by 10–25 mg q3–7 days. **Range:** 50–150 mg. **Adolescents:** 30–40 mg daily in divided doses to maximum of 100 mg/day.

IM: Adults: Do not exceed 100 mg/day, administered in divided doses.

Childhood enuresis:

PO: Children >6 yrs: 25 mg 1 hr before bedtime.

PRECAUTIONS

CONTRAINDICATIONS: Acute recovery period following MI, within 14 days of MAO inhibitor ingestion. **CAUTIONS:** Prostatic hypertrophy, history of urinary retention or obstruction, glaucoma, diabetes mellitus, history of seizures, hyperthyroidism, cardiac/hepatic/renal disease, schizophrenia, increased intraocular pressure, hiatal hernia. **PREGNANCY/LACTATION:** Crosses placenta; distributed in breast milk. **Pregnancy Category D.**

INTERACTIONS

DRUG INTERACTIONS: Alcohol, CNS depressants may increase CNS, respiratory depression, hypotensive effects. Antithyroid agents may increase risk of agranulocytosis. Phenothiazines may increase sedative, anticholinergic effects. Cimetidine may increase concentration, toxicity. May decrease effects of clonidine, guanadrel. May increase cardiac effects w/sympathomimetics. May increase risk of hypertensive crisis, hyperpyretic, convulsions w/MAO inhibitors. Phenytoin may decrease concentrations. **ALTERED LAB VALUES:** May alter EKG readings, glucose.

SIDE EFFECTS

FREQUENT: Drowsiness, fatigue, dry mouth, blurred vision, constipation, delayed micturition, postural hypotension, excessive sweating, disturbed concentration, increased appetite, urinary retention. **OCCASIONAL:** GI disturbances (nausea, metallic taste sensation). **RARE:** Paradoxical reaction (agitation, restlessness, nightmares, insomnia), extrapyramidal symptoms (particularly fine hand tremor).

ADVERSE REACTIONS/TOXIC EFFECTS

High dosage may produce cardiovascular effects (severe postural hypotension, dizziness, tachycardia, palpitations, arrhythmias) and seizures. May also result in altered temperature regulation (hyperpyrexia or hypothermia). Abrupt withdrawal from prolonged therapy may produce headache, malaise, nausea, vomiting, vivid dreams.

NURSING IMPLICATIONS
BASELINE ASSESSMENT:

For those on long-term therapy, liver/renal function tests, blood counts should be performed periodically.

INTERVENTION/EVALUATION:

Supervise suicidal risk pt closely during early therapy (as depression lessens, energy level improves, causing increased suicide potential). Assess appearance, behavior, speech pattern, level of interest, mood. Monitor pattern of daily bowel activity and stool consistency. Monitor B/P, pulse for hypotension, arrhythmias. Assess for urinary retention by bladder palpation.

PATIENT/FAMILY TEACHING:

Change positions slowly to avoid hypotensive effect. Tolerance to postural hypotension, sedative, and anticholinergic effects usually develops during early therapy. Therapeutic effect may be noted within 2–5 days, maximum effect within 2–3 wks. Photosensitivity to sun may occur. Dry mouth may be relieved by sugarless gum, sips of tepid water. Report visual disturbances. Do not abruptly discontinue medication. Avoid tasks that require alertness, motor skills until response to drug is established. Avoid alcohol.

---

imiquimod
(Aldara)
See Supplement

---

immune globulin IM (IGIM, gamma globulin, ISG)
(Gamastan, Gammar)

immune globulin IV (IGIV)
(Gamimune N, Gammagard, Gammar-IV, Iveegam, Sandoglobulin, Venoglobulin-I)

CANADIAN AVAILABILITY:
Gamimune N, Iveegam

CLASSIFICATION

Immune serum

AVAILABILITY (Rx)

Injection: 5%, 10%. **Powder for Injection:** 50 mg/ml, 1 g, 3 g, 6 g, 12 g.

PHARMACOKINETICS

Evenly distributed between intravascular and extravascular space. Half-life: 21–23 days.

ACTION/*THERAPEUTIC EFFECT*

Increases antibody titer and antigen-antibody reaction, *providing passive immunity against infection.* Induces rapid increase in platelet counts. Produces anti-inflammatory effect.

USES/*UNLABELED*

IGIM: Provides passive immunity to those exposed to hepatitis A virus, hepatitis B virus, or hepatitis B surface antigen (HBsAg); prevents or modifies symptoms of measles (rubeola) in susceptible individuals exposed <6 days previously; provides replacement therapy in prophylactic management of infections with those with IgG or other antibody deficiency diseases. *IGIV:* Maintenance treatment in those unable to produce sufficient amounts of IgG antibodies; treatment of idiopathic thrombocytopenic purpura (ITP); prevents bacterial infections in those with hypogammaglobulinemia and/or recurrent bacterial infections associated with B-cell chronic lymphocytic leukemia (CLL). Treatment of Kawasaki disease. *Prevents acute infections in immunosuppressed pts, controls/prevents infections in infants/children immunosuppressed in association w/AIDs or ARC. Prophylaxis/treatment of infections in high-risk, preterm, low birth weight neonates, treatment of chronic inflammatory demyelinating polyneuropathies.*

STORAGE/HANDLING

Refrigerate IM vials; refer to individual IV preparations for storage requirements, stability after reconstitution. Reconstitute only with diluent provided by manufacturer. Discard partially used or turbid preparations.

IM/IV ADMINISTRATION

Note: Do not mix with other medications. Do not perform skin testing prior to administration.

IM:

1. Inject into deltoid muscle or anterolateral aspect of thigh.
2. Use upper outer quadrant of gluteal muscle only for large volumes or multiple injections (when dose >10 ml).

IV:

1. Give by infusion only.
2. After reconstituted, administer via separate tubing.
3. Avoid mixing with other medication/IV infusion fluids.
4. Rate of infusion varies with product used.
5. Monitor vital signs and B/P diligently during and immediately following IV administration (precipitous fall in B/P may produce picture of anaphylactic reaction). Stop infusion immediately. Epinephrine should be readily available.

INDICATIONS/DOSAGE/ROUTES

Hepatitis A infection:
IM: Adults, elderly, children: (after exposure): 0.02 ml/kg as single dose as soon as possible after exposure; (before exposure): 0.02 ml/kg as single dose; 0.06 ml/kg if exposure >3 mos, repeat every 4–6 mos.

Non-A, non-B hepatitis:
IM: Adults, elderly, children: 0.06 ml/kg as single dose as soon as possible after exposure.

Measles (after exposure):
IM: Adults, children: 0.25 ml/kg as single dose within 6 days of exposure; 0.5 ml/kg if pt suspected of having leukemia, lymphoma, generalized malignancy, or immunodeficiency disorder, receiving steroids, or other immunosuppression therapy.

Immunodeficiency diseases:
IM: Adults, elderly, children: Initially, 1.2 ml/kg. **Maintenance:** 0.6 ml/kg (at least 100 mg/kg) q2–4 wks. **Maximum single dose:** 30–50 ml (adults); 20–30 ml (infants, small children).

Primary immunodeficiency diseases:
IV Infusion: Adults, elderly, children: *(Gamimune N):* 100–200 mg/kg or 2–4 ml/kg once monthly; may increase to 400 mg/kg or 8 ml/kg once monthly or more frequently. *(Gammagard):* 200–400 mg/kg once monthly. **Minimum:** 100 mg/kg once monthly. *(Gammar-IV):* 100–200 mg/kg q3–4 wks. Loading dose 200 mg/kg may be given at more frequent intervals until therapeutic concentration attained.

(Iveegam): 200 mg/kg once monthly. *(Sandoglobulin):* 200 mg/kg once monthly, may increase to 300 mg/kg once monthly or at more frequent intervals. *(Venoglobulin-I):* 200 mg/kg once monthly, may increase to 300–400 mg/kg once monthly or at more frequent intervals.

Idiopathic thrombocytopenic purpura (ITP):
IV Infusion: Adults, elderly, children: *(Gamimune-N, Sandoglobulin):* Initially, 400 mg/kg/day for 2–5 days depending on platelet count/clinical response. *(Gammagard):* 1 g/kg as single dose; may give up to 3 doses on alternate days. *(Venoglobulin-I):* Initially, 500 mg/kg/day for 2–7 days; then, if necessary, 500–2,000 mg/kg q2 wks or less to maintain platelets >30,000/m^3 in children or >20,000/m^3 in adults.

Kawasaki disease:
IV: Adults: 2 g/kg as single dose (w/aspirin 80–100 mg/kg/day).

Hypogammaglobulinemia and/or recurrent bacterial infections in B-cell CLL:
IV Infusion: Adults, elderly, children: *(Gammagard):* 400 mg/kg q3–4 wks.

PRECAUTIONS

CONTRAINDICATIONS: History of allergic response to gamma globulin or anti-immunoglobulin A (IgA) antibodies, allergic response to thimerosal, those with isolated immunoglobulin A (IgA) deficiency. IM also contraindicated in those who have severe thrombocytopenia and any coagulation disorder. **CAUTIONS:** Prior systemic allergic reactions following administration of human immunoglobulin preparations. Pre-existing renal dysfunction, diabetes; those >65

are at increased risk of acute renal failure. **PREGNANCY/LACTATION:** Unknown if drug crosses placenta or is distributed in breast milk. **Pregnancy Category C**.

INTERACTIONS

DRUG INTERACTIONS: Live virus vaccines may potentiate virus replication, increase vaccine side effects, decrease pt's antibody response to vaccine. **ALTERED LAB VALUES:** None significant.

SIDE EFFECTS

FREQUENT: Tachycardia, backache or pain, headache, joint or muscle pain. **OCCASIONAL:** Fatigue, wheezing, rash or pain at injection site, leg cramps, hives, bluish color of lips/ nailbeds, lightheadedness.

ADVERSE REACTIONS/TOXIC EFFECTS

Anaphylactic reactions occur rarely but increased incidence when given large IM doses or in those receiving repeated injections of immune globulin. Epinephrine should be readily available. Overdose may produce chest tightness, chills, diaphoresis, dizziness, flushed face, nausea, vomiting, fever, hypotension.

NURSING IMPLICATIONS
BASELINE ASSESSMENT:

Inquire about history of exposure to disease for both pt and family as appropriate. Have epinephrine readily available. Well hydrate pt prior to use.

INTERVENTION/EVALUATION:

Control rate of IV infusion carefully; too rapid infusion increases risk of precipitous fall in B/P and signs of anaphylaxis (facial flushing, chest tightness, chills, fever, nausea, vomiting, diaphoresis). Assess pt closely during infusion, esp. 1st hour; monitor vital signs continuously. Stop infusion temporarily if above signs noted. For treatment of ITP, monitor platelets.

PATIENT/FAMILY TEACHING:

Explain rationale for therapy. Rapid response, lasts 1–3 mos. Local pain or muscle tenderness may occur at IM injection site.

indapamide

in-**dap**-ah-myd
(Lozol)

CANADIAN AVAILABILITY:
Lozide

CLASSIFICATION

Diuretic: Thiazide

AVAILABILITY (Rx)

Tablets: 1.25 mg, 2.5 mg

PHARMACOKINETICS

	ONSET	PEAK	DURATION
PO	1–2 hrs	<2 hrs	Up to 36 hrs (diuretic)

Completely absorbed from GI tract. Metabolized in liver. Primarily excreted in urine. Half-life: 14–18 hrs.

ACTION/*THERAPEUTIC EFFECT*

Diuretic: Blocks reabsorption of water, electrolytes (sodium, potassium) at cortical diluting segment of distal tubule, *promoting renal excretion. Antihypertensive:* Reduces plasma, extracellular fluid volume, decreases peripheral vascular resistance (PVR) by direct effect on blood vessels, *reducing B/P.*

USES

Treatment of hypertension and edema associated w/CHF. May be used alone or w/antihypertensive agents.

PO ADMINISTRATION

1. Give w/food or milk if GI upset occurs, preferably w/breakfast (may prevent nocturia).
2. Do not crush or break tablets.

INDICATIONS/DOSAGE/ROUTES

Edema:
PO: Adults: Initially, 2.5 mg/day, may increase to 5 mg/day in 1 wk.

Hypertension:
PO: Adults: Initially, 1.25 mg, may increase to 2.5 mg/day in 4 wks or 5 mg/day after additional 4 wks.

Usual elderly dosage:
PO: Initially 1.25 mg/day or every other day. May increase up to 5 mg/day.

PRECAUTIONS

CAUTIONS: History of hypersensitivity to sulfonamides or thiazide diuretics, renal decompensation, anuria. Severe renal disease, impaired hepatic function, diabetes mellitus, elderly/debilitated, thyroid disorders. **PREGNANCY/ LACTATION:** Crosses placenta; small amount distributed in breast milk; nursing not advised. **Pregnancy Category D.**

INTERACTIONS

DRUG INTERACTIONS: May increase risk of digoxin toxicity (due to hypokalemia). May decrease clearance, increase toxicity of lithium. **ALTERED LAB VALUES:** May increase plasma renin activity. May decrease calcium, protein-bound iodine, potassium, sodium.

SIDE EFFECTS

FREQUENT (>5%): Fatigue, numbness of extremities, tension, irritability, agitation, headache, dizziness, lightheadedness, insomnia, muscle cramping. **OCCASIONAL (<5%):** Tingling of extremities, frequent urination, polyuria, hives, rhinorrhea, flushing, weight loss, orthostatic hypotension, depression, blurred vision, nausea, vomiting, diarrhea/constipation, dry mouth, impotence, rash, pruritus.

ADVERSE REACTIONS/TOXIC EFFECTS

Vigorous diuresis may lead to profound water loss and electrolyte depletion, resulting in hypokalemia, hyponatremia, dehydration. Acute hypotensive episodes may occur. Hyperglycemia may be noted during prolonged therapy. GI upset, pancreatitis, dizziness, paresthesias, headache, blood dyscrasias, pulmonary edema, allergic pneumonitis, dermatologic reactions occur rarely. Overdosage can lead to lethargy, coma w/o changes in electrolytes or hydration.

NURSING IMPLICATIONS

Baseline Assessment:

Check vital signs, esp. B/P for hypotension prior to administration. Assess baseline electrolytes, particularly check for low potassium. Assess edema, skin turgor, mucous membranes for hydration status. Assess muscle strength, mental status. Note skin temperature, moisture. Obtain baseline weight. Initiate I&O.

Intervention/Evaluation:

Continue to monitor B/P, vital signs, electrolytes, I&O, weight. Note extent of diuresis. Watch for electrolyte disturbances (hypokalemia may result in weakness, tremor, muscle cramps, nausea, vomiting, change in mental status, tachycardia; hyponatremia may result in confusion, thirst, cold/clammy skin).

Patient/Family Teaching:

Expect increased frequency and volume of urination. To reduce hypotensive effect, rise slowly from lying to sitting position and permit legs to dangle momentarily before standing. Eat foods high in potassium such as whole grains (cereals), legumes, meat, bananas, apricots, orange juice, potatoes (white, sweet), raisins.

---

indinavir

in-**din**-oh-vir
(Crixivan)

CANADIAN AVAILABILITY:
Crixivan

CLASSIFICATION

Antiviral

AVAILABILITY (Rx)

Capsules: 200 mg, 333 mg, 400 mg

PHARMACOKINETICS

Rapidly absorbed following oral administration. Metabolized in liver. Primarily excreted in urine. Half-life: 1.8 hrs (increased in pts w/impaired liver function).

ACTION/*THERAPEUTIC EFFECT*

Suppresses human immunodeficiency virus (HIV) protease, an enzyme necessary for splitting viral polyprotein precursors into mature and infectious virus particles. *Resultant effect interrupts HIV replication, forms immature noninfectious viral particles.*

USES

Treatment of human immunodeficiency virus (HIV) when antiretroviral therapy is warranted.

STORAGE/HANDLING

Store at room temperature. Protect from moisture (capsules sensitive to moisture; keep in original bottle).

PO ADMINISTRATION

1. Best given w/o food but w/water only (optimal absorption) 1 hr before or 2 hrs after a meal but may give w/water, skim milk, juice, coffee or tea, or w/light meal (e.g., dry toast w/jelly, juice and coffee w/skim milk and sugar; or cornflakes, skim milk and sugar). Do not give w/meal high in fat, calories, and protein.

2. If indinavir and didanosine are given concurrently, give at least 1 hr apart on an empty stomach.

INDICATIONS/DOSAGE/ROUTES

HIV infection:
PO: Adults: 800 mg (two 400 mg capsules) q8h.

Dosage w/hepatic insufficiency:
PO: Adults: 600 mg q8h.

PRECAUTIONS

CONTRAINDICATIONS: Hypersensitivity to indinavir; nephrolithiasis. **CAUTIONS:** Renal, hepatic function impairment. **PREGNANCY/LACTATION:** Unknown if excreted in breast milk. HIV-infected women not to breast-feed. **Pregnancy Category C**.

INTERACTIONS

DRUG INTERACTIONS: Avoid concurrent administration of indinavir w/terfenadine, astemizole, cisapride, triazolam, midazolam (potential for arrhythmias, prolonged sedation). **ALTERED LAB VALUES:** May increase bilirubin (occurs in 10% of pts), SGOT (AST), SGPT (ALT).

SIDE EFFECTS

FREQUENT: Nausea **(12%)**, abdominal pain **(9%)**, headache **(6%)**, diarrhea **(5%)**. **OCCASIONAL:** Vomiting, asthenia, fatigue **(4%)**, insomnia, accumulation of fat in waist, abdomen, or back of neck. **RARE:** Abnormal taste sensation, heartburn, symptomatic urinary tract disease, transient kidney dysfunction.

ADVERSE REACTIONS/TOXIC EFFECTS

Nephrolithiasis (flank pain with or without hematuria) occurs in 4% of pts.

NURSING IMPLICATIONS

BASELINE ASSESSMENT:

Offer emotional support. Establish baseline lab values. Emphasize need for close monitoring of renal function (urinalysis, serum creatinine) during therapy.

INTERVENTION/EVALUATION:

Encourage adequate hydration. Pt should drink 48 oz (1.5 L) of liquid for each 24 hrs during therapy. Monitor for evidence of nephrolithiasis (flank pain, hematuria) and contact physician if symptoms occur (therapy should be interrupted for 1–3 days). Monitor stool frequency and consistency (watery, loose, soft). Assess for abdominal discomfort, headache.

PATIENT/FAMILY TEACHING:

Advise that indinavir is not cure for HIV, and condition may progress in spite of treatment. Do not modify or discontinue treatment w/o physician approval. If dose is missed, take next dose at regularly scheduled time (do *not* double the dose). Best taken without food but water only (optimal absorption) 1 hr before or 2 hrs after a meal but may take with water, skim milk, juice, coffee or tea, or w/light meal (e.g., dry toast w/jelly, juice and coffee w/skim milk and sugar; or cornflakes, skim milk and sugar).

indomethacin
in-doe-**meth**-ah-sin
(Indocin, Indocin-SR)

indomethacin sodium trihydrate
(Indocin IV)

CANADIAN AVAILABILITY:
Apo-Indomethacin, Indocid, Indotec, Novomethacin

CLASSIFICATION

Nonsteroidal anti-inflammatory

AVAILABILITY (Rx)

Capsules: 25 mg, 50 mg. **Capsules (sustained-release):** 75 mg. **Oral Suspension:** 25 mg/5 ml. **Suppository:** 50 mg. **Powder for Injection:** 1 mg.

PHARMACOKINETICS

	ONSET	PEAK	DURATION
PO (analgesic)	0.5 hr	—	4–6 hrs
PO (antirheumatic)	7 days	1–2 wks	—

Well absorbed from GI tract. Metabolized in liver. Primarily excreted in urine. Half-life: 4–6 hrs (increased in neonates: 2–60 hrs).

ACTION/ *THERAPEUTIC EFFECT*

Produces analgesic and anti-inflammatory effect by inhibiting prostaglandin synthesis, *reducing inflammatory response and intensity of pain stimulus reaching sensory nerve endings. Patent ductus:* Inhibits prostaglandin synthesis, increases sensitivity of premature ductus to dilating effects of prostaglandins, *causing closure of patent ductus arteriosus.*

USES/ *UNLABELED*

Treatment of active stages of rheumatoid arthritis, osteoarthritis, ankylosing spondylitis, acute gouty arthritis, acute painful shoulder. Relief of acute bursitis and/or tendinitis of shoulder. For closure of hemodynamically significant patent ductus arteriosus of premature infants weighing 500–1,750 g. *Treatment of psoriatic arthritis, rheumatic complications associated w/Paget's disease of bone, fever due to malignancy, vascular headache, pericarditis.*

STORAGE/HANDLING

Store capsules, suppositories, oral suspension at room temperature. IV solutions made w/o preservatives should be used immediately. Use IV immediately after reconstitution. IV solution appears clear; discard if cloudy or if precipitate forms. Discard unused portion.

PO/IV ADMINISTRATION

PO:
1. Give after meals or w/food or antacids.
2. Do not crush sustained-release capsules.

RECTAL:

1. If suppository is too soft, chill for 30 min in refrigerator or run cold water over foil wrapper.

2. Moisten suppository w/cold water before inserting well up into rectum.

IV:

Note: IV injection preferred for patent ductus arteriosus in neonate (may give dose orally via NG tube or rectally).

1. To 1 mg vial, add 1–2 ml preservative-free sterile water for injection or 0.9% NaCl injection to provide concentration of 1 mg or 0.5 mg/ml, respectively. Do not further dilute.

2. Administer over 5–10 secs.

3. Restrict fluid intake.

INDICATIONS/DOSAGE/ROUTES

Moderate to severe rheumatoid arthritis, osteoarthritis, ankylosing spondylitis:
PO: Adults, elderly: Initially, 25 mg 2–3 times/day. Increase by 25–50 mg/wk up to 150–200 mg/day. **Extended-release: Adults, elderly:** Initially, 75 mg/day up to 75 mg two times/day.

Acute gouty arthritis:
PO: Adults, elderly: Initially, 100 mg, then 50 mg three times/day.

Acute painful shoulder:
PO: Adults, elderly: 75–150 mg/day in 3–4 divided doses.

Usual rectal dosage:
Adults, elderly: 50 mg four times/day. **Children:** Initially, 1.5–2.5 mg/kg/day, up to 4 mg/kg/day. Do not exceed 150–200 mg/day.

Patent ductus arteriosus:
Note: May give up to 3 doses at 12–24 hr intervals.

IV: Neonates: Initially, 0.2 mg/kg. **>7 days old:** 0.25 mg/kg for 2nd and 3rd doses. **Age 2–7 days:** 0.2 mg/kg for 2nd and 3rd doses. **<48 hrs old:** 0.1 mg/kg for 2nd and 3rd doses.

PRECAUTIONS

CONTRAINDICATIONS: History of allergic reaction to aspirin or other NSAIDs, history of recurrent or active GI lesions. *Suppositories:* History of proctitis or recent rectal bleeding. **CAUTIONS:** Impaired renal/hepatic function, elderly, volume depletion, CHF, sepsis, epilepsy, parkinsonism, psychiatric disturbances, coagulation defects. **PREGNANCY/LACTATION:** Crosses placenta; distributed in breast milk. Avoid use during third trimester (may adversely affect fetal cardiovascular system: premature closure of ductus arteriosus). **Pregnancy Category B.** (Category D if used >48 hrs after 34 wks gestation, or close to delivery.)

INTERACTIONS

DRUG INTERACTIONS: May increase effects of oral anticoagulants, heparin, thrombolytics. May decrease effect of antihypertensives, diuretics. Salicylates, aspirin may increase risk of GI side effects, bleeding. Bone marrow depressants may increase risk of hematologic reactions. May increase concentration, toxicity of lithium. May increase methotrexate toxicity. Probenecid may increase concentration. May increase concentration of aminoglycosides in neonates. **ALTERED LAB VALUES:** May prolong bleeding time. May alter blood glucose. May increase BUN, creatinine, potassium, liver function tests. May decrease sodium, platelet count.

SIDE EFFECTS

FREQUENT (3–11%): Headache, nausea, vomiting, dyspepsia (heartburn, indigestion, epigastric pain), dizziness. **OCCASIONAL (<3%):** Depression, ringing in ears, increased sweating, drowsiness, constipation, diarrhea. *Patent ductus arteriosus:* Bleeding disturbances. **RARE:** Increased B/P, confusion, hives, itching, rash, blurred vision.

ADVERSE REACTIONS/TOXIC EFFECTS

Ulceration of esophagus, stomach, duodenum, or small intestine, paralytic ileus may occur. In those w/impaired renal function, hyperkalemia along w/worsening of impairment may occur. May aggravate depression or psychiatric disturbances, epilepsy, parkinsonism. Nephrotoxicity (dysuria, hematuria, proteinuria, nephrotic syndrome) occurs rarely.

NURSING IMPLICATIONS
BASELINE ASSESSMENT:

May mask signs of infection. Do not give concurrently w/triamterene (may potentiate acute renal failure). Assess onset, type, location, and duration of pain, fever, or inflammation. Inspect appearance of affected joints for immobility, deformities, and skin condition.

INTERVENTION/EVALUATION:

Monitor for evidence of nausea, dyspepsia. Assist w/ambulation if dizziness occurs. Evaluate for therapeutic response: relief of pain, stiffness, swelling, increase in joint mobility, reduced joint tenderness, improved grip strength.

PATIENT/FAMILY TEACHING:

Avoid aspirin, alcohol during therapy (increases risk of GI bleeding). If GI upset occurs, take w/food, milk. Report headache. Avoid tasks that require alertness, motor skills until response to drug is established. Swallow capsule whole; do not crush or chew.

infliximab
(Remicade)
See Supplement

insulin
in-sull-in

Rapid acting:

INSULIN LISPRO
(Humalog)

INSULIN INJECTION
(Humulin R, Novolin R, Regular, Velosulin)

PROMPT INSULIN ZINC SUSPENSION
(Semilente)

Intermediate acting:

ISOPHANE INSULIN SUSPENSION
(Humulin N, Insulatard, Novolin N, NPH)

INSULIN ZINC SUSPENSION
(Humulin L, Lente, Novolin L)

Long acting:

EXTENDED INSULIN ZINC SUSPENSION
(Humulin U, Ultralente)

FIXED-COMBINATION(S): Isophane Insulin Suspension w/insulin injection: **Humulin 70/30, Mixtard, Novolin 70/30.**

CANADIAN AVAILABILITY:
See above.

CLASSIFICATION

Hypoglycemic

AVAILABILITY (OTC)

Regular, NPH, 70/30, 50/50, Lente, Ultralente: all 100 units/ml

PHARMACOKINETICS

	ONSET (HRS)	PEAK (HRS)	DURATION (HRS)
Regular	0.5–1	—	6–8
Semilente	1–1.5	5–10	12–16
NPH	1–1.5	4–12	24
Lente	1–2.5	7–15	24
Ultralente	4–8	10–30	>36

ACTION/ *THERAPEUTIC EFFECT*

Facilitates passage of glucose, K, Mg across cellular membranes of skeletal and cardiac muscle, adipose tissue; controls storage and metabolism of carbohydrates, protein, fats. Promotes conversion of glucose to glycogen in liver.

USES:

Treatment of insulin-dependent type I diabetes mellitus; noninsulin-dependent type II diabetes mellitus when diet/weight control therapy has failed to maintain satisfactory blood glucose levels or in event of pregnancy, surgery, trauma, infection, fever, severe renal, hepatic, or endocrine dysfunction. Regular insulin used in emergency treatment of ketoacidosis, to promote passage of glucose across cell membrane in hyperalimentation, to facilitate intracellular shift of K+ in hyperkalemia.

STORAGE/HANDLING

Store currently used insulin at room temperature (avoid extreme temperatures, direct sunlight). Store extra vials in refrigerator. Discard unused vials if not used for several weeks. No insulin should have precipitate or discoloration.

SUBQ ADMINISTRATION

1. Give SubQ only. (Regular insulin is the *only* insulin that may be given IV, IM for ketoacidosis or other specific situations.)

2. Do not give cold insulin; warm to room temperature.

3. Rotate vial gently between hands; do not shake. Regular insulin should be clear; no insulin should have precipitate or discoloration.

4. Usually administered approximately 30 min before a meal (Insulin lispro given up to 15 min before meals). Check blood glucose concentration before administration; dosage highly individualized.

5. When insulin is mixed, regular insulin is always drawn up first. Mixtures must be administered at once (binding can occur within 5 min). Humalog may be mixed w/Humulin N, Humulin L.

6. SubQ injections may be given in thigh, abdomen, upper arm, buttocks, or upper back if there is adequate adipose tissue.

7. Rotation of injection sites is essential; maintain careful record.

8. For home situations, prefilled syringes are stable for 1 wk under refrigeration (this includes mixtures once they have stabilized, e.g., 15 min for NPH/Regular, 24 hrs for Lente/Regular). Prefilled syringes should be stored in vertical or oblique position to avoid plugging; plunger should be pulled back slightly and the syringe rocked to remix the solution before injection.

INDICATIONS/DOSAGE/ROUTES

Dosage for insulin is individualized/monitored.

Usual dosage guidelines:
Note: Adjust dosage to achieve premeal and bedtime glucose level of 80–140 mg/dl (children <5 yrs: 100–200 mg/dl).

SubQ: Adults, elderly, children: 0.5–1 unit/kg/day. **Adolescents (during growth spurt):** 0.8–1.2 units/kg/day.

PRECAUTIONS

CONTRAINDICATIONS: Hypersensitivity or insulin resistance may require change of type or species source of insulin. **PREGNANCY/ LACTATION:** Insulin is drug of choice for diabetes in pregnancy; close medical supervision is needed. Following delivery, insulin needs may drop for 24–72 hrs, then rise to prepregnancy levels. Not secreted in breast milk; lactation may decrease insulin requirements. Pregnancy Category B.

INTERACTIONS

DRUG INTERACTIONS: Glucocorticoids, thiazide diuretics may increase blood glucose. Alcohol may increase insulin effect. Beta-adrenergic blockers may increase risk of hypo/hyperglycemia, mask signs of hypoglycemia, prolong period of hypoglycemia. **ALTERED LAB VALUES:** May decrease potassium, magnesium, phosphate concentrations.

SIDE EFFECTS

OCCASIONAL: Local redness, swelling, itching (due to improper injection technique or allergy to cleansing solution or insulin). **INFREQUENT:** Somogyi effect (rebound hyperglycemia) w/chronically excessive insulin doses. Systemic allergic reaction (rash, angioedema, anaphylaxis), lipodystrophy (depression at injection site due to breakdown of adipose tissue), lipohypertrophy (accumulation of SubQ tissue at injection site due to lack of adequate site rotation). **RARE:** Insulin resistance.

ADVERSE REACTIONS/TOXIC EFFECTS

Severe hypoglycemia (due to hy-

perinsulinism) may occur in overdose of insulin, decrease or delay of food intake, excessive exercise, or those w/brittle diabetes. Diabetic ketoacidosis may result from stress, illness, omission of insulin dose, or long-term poor insulin control.

NURSING IMPLICATIONS

BASELINE ASSESSMENT:

Question for allergies. Check blood glucose level. Discuss lifestyle to determine extent of learning, emotional needs.

INTERVENTION/EVALUATION:

Monitor blood glucose and food intake; assure between meal/bedtime nourishments. Assess for hypoglycemia (refer to pharmacokinetics table for peak times/ duration): cool wet skin, tremors, dizziness, headache, anxiety, tachycardia, numbness in mouth, hunger, diplopia. Check sleeping pt for restlessness or diaphoresis. Check for hyperglycemia: polyuria (excessive urine output), polyphagia (excessive food intake), polydipsia (excessive thirst), nausea and vomiting, dim vision, fatigue, deep rapid breathing. Be alert to conditions altering glucose requirements: fever, increased activity or stress, surgical procedure.

PATIENT/FAMILY TEACHING:

Prescribed diet is essential part of treatment; do not skip or delay meals. Diabetes mellitus requires lifelong control. Check blood glucose/urine as ordered. Instruct signs and symptoms, treatment of hypo/hyperglycemia, proper handling, and administration of medication. Carry candy, sugar packets, other sugar supplements for immediate response to hypoglycemia. Wear/carry medical alert identification. Check w/

physician when insulin demands are altered, e.g., fever, infection, trauma, stress, heavy physical activity. Avoid alcoholic beverages. Do not take other medication w/o consulting physician. Weight control, exercise, hygiene (including foot care), and not smoking are integral part of therapy. Protect skin, limit sun exposure. Avoid exposure to infections. Important to keep follow-up appointments. Select clothing, positions that do not restrict blood flow. Inform dentist, physician, or surgeon of medication before any treatment is given. Assure follow-up instruction if pt/family does not thoroughly understand diabetes management or administration techniques.

---

interferon alfacon-1
(Infergen)
See Supplement

---

interferon alfa-2a
inn-ter-**fear**-on
(Roferon-A)

CANADIAN AVAILABILITY:
Roferon-A

CLASSIFICATION
Antineoplastic

AVAILABILITY (Rx)
Injection: 3 million units/ml, 6 million units/ml, 9 million units/ml, 36 million units/ml. **Powder for Injection:** 6 million units/ml (18 million units vial).

PHARMACOKINETICS
Well absorbed after IM, SubQ administration. Undergoes proteolytic degradation during reabsorption in kidney. Half-life: *IM* 6–8 hrs; *IV* 3.7–8.5 hrs.

ACTION/ *THERAPEUTIC EFFECT*
Inhibits viral replication in virus-infected cells, *suppressing cell proliferation, increasing phagocytic action of macrophages; augments specific lymphocytic cell toxicity.*

USES/ *UNLABELED*
Treatment of hairy cell leukemia, AIDS-related Kaposi's sarcoma, chronic myelogenous leukemia (CML), chronic hepatitis C. *Treatment of active, chronic hepatitis; bladder, renal carcinoma, non-Hodgkin's lymphoma, malignant melanoma, multiple myeloma, mycosis fungoides.*

STORAGE/HANDLING
Refrigerate. Do not shake vial. Reconstituted solutions stable for 30 days if refrigerated. Solutions appear colorless. Do not use if precipitate or discoloration occurs.

SUBQ/IM ADMINISTRATION
Note: SubQ preferred for thrombocytopenic pts, those at risk for bleeding.
Reconstitute 18 million unit vial w/3 ml diluent (provided by manufacturer) to provide concentration of 6 million units/ml (3 million units/0.5 ml).

INDICATIONS/DOSAGE/ROUTES
Note: Dosage individualized based on clinical response, tolerance to adverse effects. When used in combination therapy, consult specific protocols for optimum dosage, sequence of drug administration. If severe adverse reactions occur, modify dose or temporarily discontinue medication.

Hairy cell leukemia:
SubQ/IM: Adults: Initially, 3 million

units/day for 16–24 wks. **Maintenance:** 3 million units 3 times/wk. Do not use 36 million unit vial.

CML:
SubQ/IM: Adults: 9 million units daily.

AIDS-related Kaposi's sarcoma:
SubQ/IM: Adults: Initially, 36 million units/day for 10–12 wks (may give 3 million units on day 1; 9 million units on day 2; 18 million units on day 3; then begin 36 million units/day for remainder of 10–12 wks). **Maintenance:** 36 million units/day 3 times/wk.

Chronic hepatitis C:
SubQ/IM: Adults: 3 million units 3 times/wk for 12 months.

PRECAUTIONS

CONTRAINDICATIONS: Hypersensitivity to alpha interferon. **CAUTIONS:** Renal, hepatic impairment, seizure disorders, compromised CNS function, cardiac disease, history of cardiac abnormalities, myelosuppression. **PREGNANCY/LACTATION:** If possible, avoid use during pregnancy. Breast-feeding not recommended. **Pregnancy Category C**.

INTERACTIONS

DRUG INTERACTIONS: Bone marrow depressants may have additive effect. **ALTERED LAB VALUES:** May increase SGOT (AST), SGPT (ALT), alkaline phosphatase, LDH. May decrease Hgb, Hct, leukocyte, platelet counts.

SIDE EFFECTS

FREQUENT (>20%): Flulike symptoms (fever, fatigue, headache, aches, pains, anorexia, chills), nausea, vomiting, coughing, dyspnea, hypotension, edema, chest pain, dizziness, diarrhea, weight loss, taste change, abdominal discomfort, confusion, paresthesia, depression, visual and sleep disturbances, sweating, lethargy. **OCCASIONAL (5–20%):** Partial alopecia, rash, dry throat/skin, pruritus, flatulence, constipation, hypertension, palpitations, sinusitis. **RARE (<5%):** Hot flashes, hypermotility, Raynaud's syndrome, bronchospasm, earache, ecchymosis.

ADVERSE REACTIONS/TOXIC EFFECTS

Arrhythmias, stroke, transient ischemic attacks, CHF, pulmonary edema, myocardial infarction occur rarely.

NURSING IMPLICATIONS
BASELINE ASSESSMENT:

CBC, differential and platelet counts, blood chemistries, urinalysis, renal and liver function tests should be performed prior to initial therapy and routinely thereafter.

INTERVENTION/EVALUATION:

Offer emotional support. Monitor all levels of clinical function (numerous side effects). Encourage ample fluid intake, particularly during early therapy.

PATIENT/FAMILY TEACHING:

Clinical response may take 1–3 mos. Flulike symptoms tend to diminish with continued therapy. Do not have immunizations w/o physician's approval (drug lowers body's resistance). Avoid contact w/those who have recently received live virus vaccine. Contact physician if nausea/vomiting continues at home. Do not change brands w/o consulting physician. Avoid alcohol. Use caution driving, performing tasks requirong mental alertness.

interferon alfa-2b

inn-ter-**fear**-on
(Intron-A)

FIXED-COMBINATION(S):
W/ribavirin, an antiviral (**Rebetron**).

CANADIAN AVAILABILITY:
Intron-A

CLASSIFICATION

Antineoplastic

AVAILABILITY (Rx)

Injection (solution): 5 million units/ml. **Powder for Injection:** 3 million units, 5 million units, 10 million units, 18 million units, 25 million units, 50 million units.

PHARMACOKINETICS

Well absorbed after IM, SubQ administration. Undergoes proteolytic degradation during reabsorption in kidney. Half-life: 2–3 hrs.

ACTION / *THERAPEUTIC EFFECT*

Inhibits viral replication in virus-infected cells, suppresses cell proliferation, *increases phagocytic action of macrophages, augments specific cytotoxicity of lymphocytes.*

USES / *UNLABELED*

Treatment of hairy cell leukemia, condylomata acuminata (genital, venereal warts), AIDS-related Kaposi's sarcoma, chronic hepatitis non-A, non-B/C, chronic hepatitis B (including children ≥1 yr), non-Hodgkin's lymphoma. *Treatment of bladder, cervical, renal carcinoma, chronic myelocytic leukemia, laryngeal papillomatosis, multiple myeloma, mycosis fungoides.*

STORAGE / HANDLING

Refrigerate vial. After reconstitution, solution stable for 1 mo. Solution appears clear, colorless to light yellow.

IM/SUBQ ADMINISTRATION

1. Do not give IM if platelets <50,000/m³; give SubQ.

2. For hairy cell leukemia, reconstitute each 3 million IU vial w/1 ml bacteriostatic water for injection to provide concentration of 3 million IU/ml (1 ml to 5 million IU vial; 2 ml to 10 million IU vial; 5 ml to 25 million IU vial provides concentration of 5 million IU/ml).

3. For condylomata acuminata, reconstitute each 10 million IU vial w/1 ml bacteriostatic water for injection to provide concentration of 10 million IU/ml.

4. For AIDS-related Kaposi's sarcoma, reconstitute 50 million IU vial w/1 ml bacteriostatic water for injection to provide concentration of 50 million IU/ml.

5. Agitate vial gently, withdraw w/sterile syringe.

INDICATIONS / DOSAGE / ROUTES

Note: Dosage individualized based on clinical response, tolerance to adverse effects. When used in combination therapy, consult specific protocols for optimum dosage, sequence of drug administration.

Hairy cell leukemia:
IM/SubQ: Adults: 2 million IU/m² 3 times/wk. If severe adverse reactions occur, modify dose or temporarily discontinue.

Condylomata acuminata:
Intralesional: Adults: 1 million IU/lesion 3 times/wk for 3 wks. Use only 10 million IU vial, reconstitute w/no more than 1 ml diluent. Use TB syringe w/25 or 26 gauge needle. Give in evening w/acetaminophen (alleviates side effects).

AIDS-related Kaposi's sarcoma:
IM/SubQ: Adults: 30 million IU/m² 3 times/wk. Use only 50 million IU

vials. If severe adverse reactions occur, modify dose or temporarily discontinue.

Chronic hepatitis non-A, non-B/C:
IM/SubQ: Adults: 3 million IU 3 times/wk for up to 6 mos (for up to 18–24 months for chronic hepatitis C).

Chronic hepatitis B:
IM/SubQ: Adults: 30–35 million IU/wk (5 million IU/day or 10 million IU 3 times/wk).

Malignant melanoma:
IV: Adults: Initially, 20 million units 5 times/wk × 4 wks. **Maintenance:** 10 million units IM/SubQ for 48 wks.

PRECAUTIONS

CONTRAINDICATIONS: History of hypersensitivity to interferon alfa-2b. **CAUTIONS:** Renal, hepatic impairment, seizure disorders, compromised CNS function, cardiac diseases, history of cardiac abnormalities, myelosuppression. **PREGNANCY/LACTATION:** If possible, avoid use during pregnancy. Breast-feeding not recommended. **Pregnancy Category C**.

INTERACTIONS

DRUG INTERACTIONS: Bone marrow depressants may have additive effect. **ALTERED LAB VALUES:** May increase SGOT (AST), SGPT (ALT), alkaline phosphatase, LDH, prothrombin time, partial thromboplastin time. May decrease Hgb, Hct, leukocyte, platelet counts.

SIDE EFFECTS

Note: Dose-related effects. **FREQUENT:** Flulike symptoms (fever, fatigue, headache, aches, pains, anorexia, chills), rash (hairy cell leukemia, Kaposi's sarcoma only). *Kaposi's sarcoma:* All previously mentioned side effects plus depression, dyspepsia, dry mouth/thirst, alopecia,

rigors. **OCCASIONAL:** Dizziness, pruritus, dry skin, dermatitis, alteration in taste. **RARE:** Confusion, leg cramps, back pain, gingivitis, flushing, tremor, nervousness, eye pain.

ADVERSE REACTIONS/TOXIC EFFECTS

Hypersensitivity reaction occurs rarely. Severe adverse reactions of flulike symptoms appear dose related.

NURSING IMPLICATIONS

BASELINE ASSESSMENT:

CBC, differential and platelet counts, blood chemistries, urinalysis, renal and liver function tests should be performed prior to initial therapy and routinely thereafter.

INTERVENTION/EVALUATION:

Offer emotional support. Monitor all levels of clinical function (numerous side effects). Encourage ample fluid intake, particularly during early therapy.

PATIENT/FAMILY TEACHING:

Clinical response occurs in 1–3 mos. Flulike symptoms tend to diminish w/continued therapy. Some symptoms may be alleviated or minimized by bedtime doses. Do not have immunizations w/o physician's approval (drug lowers body's resistance). Avoid contact w/those who have recently received live virus vaccine.

---

interferon alfa-n1
(Wellferon)
See Supplement

---

interferon alfa-n3
inn-ter-**fear**-on
(Alferon N)

CLASSIFICATION

Antineoplastic

AVAILABILITY (Rx)

Injection: 5 million units

PHARMACOKINETICS

Well absorbed after IM, SubQ administration. Undergoes proteolytic degradation during reabsorption in kidney. Half-life: 6–8 hrs.

ACTION/*THERAPEUTIC EFFECT*

Inhibits viral replication in virus-infected cells, *suppresses cell proliferation, increases phagocytic action of macrophages, augments specific cytotoxicity of lymphocytes.*

USES/*UNLABELED*

Treatment of refractory or recurring condylomata acuminata (genital, venereal warts). Treatment of active chronic hepatitis, *bladder carcinoma, chronic myelocytic leukemia, laryngeal papillomatosis, non-Hodgkin's lymphoma, malignant melanoma, multiple myeloma, mycosis fungoides.*

STORAGE/HANDLING

Refrigerate vial. Do not freeze or shake.

INTRALESIONAL ADMINISTRATION

Inject into base of each wart w/30 gauge needle.

INDICATIONS/DOSAGE/ROUTES

Condylomata acuminata:
Intralesional: Adults >18 yrs: 0.05 ml (250,000 IU) per wart 2 times/wk up to 8 wks. **Maximum dose/treatment session:** 0.5 ml (2.5 million IU). Do not repeat for 3 mos after initial 8 wks unless warts enlarge or new warts appear.

PRECAUTIONS

CONTRAINDICATIONS: Hypersensitivity to interferon alfa, previous history of anaphylactic reaction to mouse immunoglobulin (IgG), egg protein, or neomycin. **CAUTIONS:** Unstable angina, uncontrolled CHF, severe pulmonary disease, diabetes mellitus w/ketoacidosis, thrombophlebitis, pulmonary embolism, hemophilia, severe myelosuppression, seizure disorders. **PREGNANCY/LACTATION:** If possible, avoid use during pregnancy. Breast feeding not recommended. **Pregnancy Category C.**

INTERACTIONS

DRUG INTERACTIONS: Bone marrow depressants may have additive effect. **ALTERED LAB VALUES:** May increase SGOT (AST), SGPT (ALT), alkaline phosphatase, LDH. May decrease Hgb, Hct, leukocyte, platelet counts.

SIDE EFFECTS

FREQUENT: Flulike symptoms (fever, fatigue, headache, aches, pains, anorexia, chills). **OCCASIONAL:** Dizziness, pruritus, dry skin, dermatitis, alteration in taste. **RARE:** Confusion, leg cramps, back pain, gingivitis, flushing, tremor, nervousness, eye pain.

ADVERSE REACTIONS/TOXIC EFFECTS

Hypersensitivity reaction occurs rarely. Severe adverse reactions of flulike symptoms appear dose related.

NURSING IMPLICATIONS

INTERVENTION/EVALUATION:

Monitor all levels of clinical function (numerous side effects). Encourage ample fluid intake, particularly during early therapy.

PATIENT/FAMILY TEACHING:

Clinical response occurs in 1–3 mos. Flulike symptoms tend to diminish w/continued therapy. Some symptoms may be alleviated or minimized by bedtime doses. Do not have immunizations w/o physician's approval (drug lowers body's resistance). Avoid contact w/those who have recently received live virus vaccine.

interferon beta 1a

inn-ter-**fear**-on
(Avonex)

CANADIAN AVAILABILITY:
Rebif

CLASSIFICATION

Interferon

AVAILABILITY (Rx)

Powder for Injection: 33 mcg (6.6 million units)

PHARMACOKINETICS

Following IM administration, peak serum levels attained in 3–15 hrs. Biological markers increase within 12 hrs and remain elevated for 4 days. Half-life: 10 hrs (IM).

ACTION/THERAPEUTIC EFFECT

Interacts w/specific cell receptors found on surface of human cells. *Possesses antiviral and immunoregulatory activities.*

USES/UNLABELED

Treatment of relapsing multiple sclerosis to slow progression of physical disability, decrease frequency of clinical exacerbations. *Treatment of AIDS, AIDS-related Kaposi's sarcoma, renal cell carcinoma, malignant melanoma, acute non-A, non-B hepatitis.*

STORAGE/HANDLING

Refrigerate vials. Following reconstitution, use within 6 hrs if refrigerated. Discard if discolored, contains a precipitate.

IM ADMINISTRATION

1. Reconstitute 33 mcg (6.6 million IU) vial w/1.1 ml diluent (supplied by manufacturer).
2. Gently swirl to dissolve medication; do not shake.
3. Discard if discolored, contains particulate matter.
4. Discard unused portion (contains no preservative).

INDICATIONS/DOSAGE/ROUTES

Relapsing-remitting multiple sclerosis:
IM: Adults: 30 mcg once weekly.

PRECAUTIONS

CONTRAINDICATIONS: Hypersensitivity to interferon, albumin. **CAUTIONS:** Chronic progressive multiple sclerosis, children <18 yrs. **PREGNANCY/LACTATION:** Interferon beta 1a has abortifacient potential. Unknown whether distributed in breast milk. **Pregnancy Category C.**

INTERACTIONS

DRUG INTERACTIONS: None significant. **ALTERED LAB VALUES:** May increase SGOT (AST), SGPT (ALT), bilirubin, alkaline phosphatase, BUN, calcium, glucose. May decrease Hgb, platelets, WBCs, neutrophils.

SIDE EFFECTS

FREQUENT: Headache (67%), flu-like symptoms (61%), myalgia (34%), upper respiratory infection (31%), pain (24%), asthenia, chills (21%), sinusitis (18%), infection (11%). **OCCASIONAL:** Abdominal pain, arthralgia (9%), chest pain, dyspnea (6%), malaise, syncope (4%). **RARE:** Injection site reaction, hypersensitivity reaction (3%).

ADVERSE REACTIONS/TOXIC EFFECTS

Anemia occurs in 8% of pts.

NURSING IMPLICATIONS

BASELINE ASSESSMENT:

Obtain Hgb, CBC and differential, platelet count, blood chemistries including liver function tests. Assess home situation for support of therapy.

INTERVENTION/EVALUATION:

Assess for headache, flulike symptoms, muscle ache (see Side Effects). Periodically monitor lab results and reevaluate injection technique. Assess for depression and suicidal ideation.

PATIENT/FAMILY TEACHING:

Do not change schedule or dosage w/o consultation w/ physician. Instruct on correct reconstitution of product and administration, including aseptic technique. Provide puncture-resistant container for used needles, syringes, and explain proper disposal. Explain that injection site reactions may occur. These do not require discontinuation of therapy, but note type and extent carefully. Depression or suicidal ideation must be reported immediately.

interferon beta 1b

inn-ter-**fear**-on
(Betaseron)

CANADIAN AVAILABILITY:
Betaseron

CLASSIFICATION

Interferon

AVAILABILITY (Rx)

Powder for Injection: 0.3 mg (9.6 million units)

PHARMACOKINETICS

Half-life: 8 min–4.3 hrs.

ACTION/*THERAPEUTIC EFFECT*

Interacts w/specific cell receptors found on surface of human cells. *Possesses antiviral and immunoregulatory activities.*

USES/*UNLABELED*

Reduces frequency of clinical exacerbations w/pts w/relapsing-remitting multiple sclerosis (recurrent attacks of neurologic dysfunction). *Treatment of AIDS, AIDS-related Kaposi's sarcoma, renal cell carcinoma, malignant melanoma, acute non-A, non-B hepatitis.*

STORAGE/HANDLING

Refrigerate vials. After reconstitution, stable for 3 hrs if refrigerated. Use within 3 hrs of reconstitution. Discard if discolored, contains a precipitate.

SUBQ ADMINISTRATION

1. Reconstitute 0.3 mg (9.6 million IU) vial w/1.2 ml diluent (supplied by manufacturer) to provide concentration of 0.25 mg/ml (8 million U/ml).

2. Gently swirl to dissolve medication; do not shake.

3. Discard if discolored, contains particulate matter.

4. Withdraw 1 ml solution and inject SubQ into arms, abdomen, hips, or thighs using 27 gauge needle.

5. Discard unused portion (contains no preservative).

INDICATIONS/DOSAGE/ROUTES

Relapsing-remitting multiple sclerosis:
SubQ: Adults: 0.25 mg (8 million IU) every other day.

PRECAUTIONS

CONTRAINDICATIONS: Hypersensitivity to interferon, albumin. **CAUTIONS:** Chronic progressive multiple sclerosis, children <18 yrs of age. **PREGNANCY/LACTATION:** Unknown whether distributed in breast milk. **Pregnancy Category C**.

INTERACTIONS

DRUG INTERACTIONS: None significant. **ALTERED LAB VALUES:** May increase SGOT (AST), SGPT (ALT), bilirubin, alkaline phosphatase, BUN, calcium, glucose, WBC's. May decrease Hgb, platelets, WBCs, neutrophils.

SIDE EFFECTS

FREQUENT: Injection site reaction (85%), headache (84%), flulike symptoms (76%), fever (59%), pain (52%), asthenia (49%), myalgia (44%), sinusitis (36%), diarrhea, dizziness (35%), mental symptoms (29%), constipation (24%), diaphoresis (23%), vomiting (21%). **OCCASIONAL:** Malaise (15%), somnolence (6%), alopecia (4%).

ADVERSE REACTIONS/TOXIC EFFECTS

Seizures occur rarely.

NURSING IMPLICATIONS

BASELINE ASSESSMENT:

Obtain Hgb, CBC and differential, platelet count, blood chemistries including liver function tests. Assess home situation for support of therapy.

INTERVENTION/EVALUATION:

Periodically monitor lab results and reevaluate injection technique. Assess for nausea (high incidence). Monitor sleep pattern. Monitor stool frequency and consistency (watery, loose, soft). Assist w/ambulation if dizziness occurs. Question for evidence of heartburn, epigastric discomfort. Monitor food intake. Assess for depression and suicidal ideation.

PATIENT/FAMILY TEACHING:

Do not change schedule or dosage w/o consultation w/physician. Instruct on correct reconstitution of product and administration, including aseptic technique. Provide puncture-resistant container for used needles, syringes, and explain proper disposal. Explain that injection site reactions may occur. These do not require discontinuation of therapy, but note type and extent carefully. Depression or suicidal ideation must be reported immediately. Inform physician of flulike symptoms (occur commonly but decrease over time). Wear sunscreens, protective clothing if exposed to ultraviolet light or sunlight until tolerance known. Interferon beta 1b has abortifacient potential.

interferon gamma-1b

inn-ter-**fear**-on
(Actimmune)

CLASSIFICATION

Biologic response modifier

AVAILABILITY (Rx)

Injection: 100 mcg (3 million units)

PHARMACOKINETICS

Slowly absorbed following SubQ administration. Metabolic fate unknown.

ACTION/*THERAPEUTIC EFFECT*

Induces activation of macrophages in blood monocytes to phagocytes (necessary in cellular immune response to intracellular and extracellular pathogens). *Enhances phagocytic function, antimicrobial activity of monocytes.*

USES

Reduces frequency, severity of serious infections due to chronic granulomatous disease.

STORAGE/HANDLING

Refrigerate vials. Do not freeze. Do not keep at room temperature >12 hrs; discard if left out longer. Vials are single dose; discard unused portion. Clear, colorless solution. Do not use if discolored, precipitate formed.

SUBQ ADMINISTRATION

Note: Avoid excessive agitation of vial; do not shake.
SubQ: When given 3 times/week.

Give in left deltoid, right deltoid, and anterior thigh.

INDICATIONS/DOSAGE/ROUTES

Chronic granulomatous disease:
SubQ: Adults, children >1 yr: 50 mcg/m^2 (1.5 million units/m^2) in pts with body surface area (BSA) >0.5 m^2; 1.5 mcg/kg/dose in pts with ≤BSA 0.5 m^2. Give 3 times/wk.

PRECAUTIONS

CONTRAINDICATIONS: Hypersensitivity to *Escherichia coli* products. **CAUTIONS:** Seizure disorders, compromised CNS function, preexisting cardiac disease (including ischemia, CHF, arrhythmia), myelosuppression. **PREGNANCY/LACTATION:** Unknown if drug crosses placenta or is distributed in breast milk. **Pregnancy Category C.**

INTERACTIONS

DRUG INTERACTIONS: Bone marrow depressants may increase bone marrow depression. **ALTERED LAB VALUES:** None significant.

SIDE EFFECTS

FREQUENT (>15%): Fever, headache, rash, chills, fatigue, diarrhea. **OCCASIONAL (4–14%):** Nausea, vomiting, muscle aches. **RARE (1–3%):** Anorexia, hypersensitivity reaction.

ADVERSE REACTIONS/TOXIC EFFECTS

May exacerbate preexisting CNS, cardiac abnormalities demonstrated as decreased mental status, gait disturbance, dizziness.

NURSING IMPLICATIONS

BASELINE ASSESSMENT:

CBC, differential and platelet counts, blood chemistries, urinalysis, renal and liver function tests should be performed prior to initial therapy and at 3 mo intervals during course of treatment.

INTERVENTION/EVALUATION:

Monitor for flulike symptoms (fever, chills, fatigue, muscle aches). Assess for evidence of hypersensitivity reaction. Check for gait disturbance, dizziness. Assist with walking if these symptoms appear.

PATIENT/FAMILY TEACHING:

Flulike symptoms (fever, chills, fatigue, muscle aches) are generally mild and tend to disappear as treatment continues. Symptoms may be minimized by bedtime administration. Avoid tasks that require alertness, motor skills until response to drug is established. If home use prescribed, instruct in proper technique of administration, care in proper disposal of needles, syringes. Vial should remain refrigerated.

---

interleukin-2
(Proleukin)
See Supplement

---

ipecac syrup
ip-eh-kak

CANADIAN AVAILABILITY:
PMS Ipecac Syrup

CLASSIFICATION

Antidote

AVAILABILITY (OTC)

Syrup: 15 ml, 30 ml

PHARMACOKINETICS

	ONSET	PEAK	DURATION
PO	<30 min	—	—

After administration, vomiting occurs within 20–30 min.

ACTION/*THERAPEUTIC EFFECT*

Acts centrally by stimulating medullary chemoreceptor trigger zone and locally by irritating gastric mucosa, *producing emesis.*

USES

Induces vomiting in early treatment of unabsorbed oral poisons, drug overdosage.

STORAGE/HANDLING

Store syrup at room temperature.

PO ADMINISTRATION

1. Before administering, instruct pt to sit upright before drinking syrup (enhances emetic effect).
2. Do not confuse ipecac fluid extract w/ipecac syrup (fluid extract is 14 times more potent and may cause death if given inadvertently at syrup dosage).
3. Emetic action may be facilitated if 200–300 ml water or clear liquid is given immediately following ipecac.

INDICATIONS/DOSAGE/ROUTES

Note: If vomiting has not occurred within 20 min after first dose, repeat w/15 ml. If vomiting has not occurred within 30 min after last dose, initiate gastric lavage, activated charcoal.

Emetic:
PO: Adults, elderly, children >12 yrs: 15–30 ml; give w/3–4 glasses water immediately following administration. **Children 1–12 yrs:** 15 ml; follow w/1–2 glasses water. **Children 6 mos–1 yr:** 5–10 ml; follow w/1 glass water. If vomiting has not occurred within 30 min, repeat initial dosage.

PRECAUTIONS

CONTRAINDICATIONS: Ingestion of petroleum distillates (paint thinner, gasoline, kerosene), alkali (lye), acids, strychnine. **CAUTIONS:** Impaired cardiac function, pathologic blood vessel disease. **PREGNANCY/LACTATION:** Unknown if drug crosses placenta or is distributed in breast milk. **Pregnancy Category C**.

INTERACTIONS

DRUG INTERACTIONS: Antiemetics may decrease effect. Avoid carbonated beverages (causes stomach distention), milk or milk products (decreases effectiveness). **ALTERED LAB VALUES:** None significant.

SIDE EFFECTS

EXPECTED RESPONSE: Nausea, vomiting. After vomiting, diarrhea and CNS symptoms (drowsiness, mild CNS depression) commonly occur.

ADVERSE REACTIONS/TOXIC EFFECTS

Cardiotoxicity may occur if ipecac syrup is not vomited (noted as hypotension, tachycardia, precordial chest pain, pulmonary congestion, dyspnea, ventricular tachycardia and fibrillation, cardiac arrest). Overdose may produce diarrhea, fast/irregular heartbeat, nausea continuing >30 min, stomach pain, respiratory difficulty, unusually tired, aching/stiff muscles.

NURSING IMPLICATIONS

BASELINE ASSESSMENT:

Do not administer to semiconscious, unconscious, or convulsing pt. Gastric lavage, activated charcoal is necessary if vomiting does not occur within 30 min of second dosage to avoid drug toxicity (bloody stools, vomitus, abdominal pain, hypotension, dyspnea, shock, cardiac disturbances, seizures, coma). Maintain pt in upright position to enhance emetic effect.

INTERVENTION/EVALUATION:

Closely monitor vital signs, EKG during and after drug is administered. Watch for changes from initial assessment. Check for reversal of poisoning or overdosage symptoms. Monitor daily bowel activity and stool consistency (watery, loose, soft, semisolid, solid) and record time of evacuation. Assess for dehydration in excessive vomiting: poor skin turgor, dry mucous membranes, longitudinal furrows in tongue.

---

ipratropium bromide

ih-prah-**trow**-pea-um
(Atrovent)

FIXED-COMBINATION(S):
W/albuterol, a bronchodilator
(**Combivent**).

CANADIAN AVAILABILITY:
Atrovent

CLASSIFICATION

Bronchodilator

AVAILABILITY (Rx)

Aerosol Solution for Inhalation: 0.02% (500 mcg). **Nasal Spray:** 0.03%, 0.06%

PHARMACOKINETICS

	ONSET	PEAK	DURATION
Inhalation	<15 min	1–2 hrs	3–4 hrs

Minimal systemic absorption. Metabolized in liver (systemic absorption). Primarily eliminated in feces. Half-life: 1.5–4 hrs.

ACTION / *THERAPEUTIC EFFECT*

Inhibits vagal mediated response by reversing action of acetylcholine, *producing smooth muscle relaxation, bronchodilating response*. Produces significant increase in forced vital lung capacity.

USES

Maintenance treatment of bronchospasm due to chronic obstructive airway disease, including bronchitis, emphysema. Adjunct to bronchodilators for maintenance treatment of bronchial asthma. Not to be used for immediate bronchospasm relief. *Nasal spray:* Rhinorrhea (0.03% associated w/perineal rhinitis, 0.06% associated w/common cold).

INHALATION ADMINISTRATION

1. Shake container well, exhale completely, then holding mouthpiece 1 inch away from lips, inhale and hold breath as long as possible before exhaling.

2. Wait 1–10 min before inhaling second dose (allows for deeper bronchial penetration).

3. Rinse mouth w/water immediately after inhalation (prevents mouth/throat dryness).

INDICATIONS / DOSAGE / ROUTES

Bronchospasm:
Inhalation: Adults, elderly: 2 inhalations 4 times/day. Wait 1–10 min before administering second inhalation. **Maximum:** 12 inhalations/24 hrs.
Nebulization: Adults, elderly: 500 mcg 3–4 times/day.

Rhinorrhea:
Intranasal: Adults, children >6 yrs: *0.03%:* 2 sprays 2–3 times/day; **Adults, children >12 yrs:** *0.06%:* 2 sprays 3–4 times/day.

PRECAUTIONS

CONTRAINDICATIONS: History of hypersensitivity to atropine. **CAUTIONS:** Narrow-angle glaucoma, prostatic hypertrophy, bladder neck obstruction. **PREGNANCY/LACTATION:** Unknown if distributed in breast milk. **Pregnancy Category B**.

INTERACTIONS

DRUG INTERACTIONS: Avoid mixing w/cromolyn inhalation solution (forms precipitate). **ALTERED LAB VALUES:** None significant.

SIDE EFFECTS

FREQUENT: *Inhalation (3–6%):* Cough, dry mouth, headache, nausea. *Nasal:* Dry nose/mouth, headache, nasal irritation. **OCCASIONAL:** *Inhalation (2%):* Dizziness, transient increased bronchospasm. **RARE (<1%):** Hypotension, insomnia, metallic/unpleasant taste, palpitations, urinary retention. *Nasal:* Diarrhea/constipation, dry throat, stomach pain, stuffy nose.

ADVERSE REACTIONS / TOXIC EFFECTS

Worsening of narrow-angle glaucoma, acute eye pain, hypotension occur rarely.

NURSING IMPLICATIONS
BASELINE ASSESSMENT:

Offer emotional support (high incidence of anxiety due to difficulty in breathing and sympathomimetic response to drug).

INTERVENTION/EVALUATION:

Monitor rate, depth, rhythm, type of respiration; quality and rate of pulse. Assess lung sounds for rhonchi, wheezing, rales. Monitor arterial blood gases. Observe lips, fingernails for blue or dusky color in light-skinned pts; gray in dark-skinned pts. Observe for clavicular retractions, hand tremor. Evaluate for clinical improvement (quieter, slower respirations, relaxed facial expression, cessation of clavicular retractions).

PATIENT/FAMILY TEACHING:

Increase fluid intake (decreases lung secretion viscosity). Do not take more than 2 inhalations at any one time (excessive use may produce paradoxical bronchoconstriction or a decreased bronchodilating effect). Rinsing mouth with water immediately after inhalation may prevent mouth/throat dryness. Avoid excessive use of caffeine derivatives (chocolate, coffee, tea, cola, cocoa).

---

irbesartan
(Avapro)
See Supplement

---

irinotecan
eye-rin-**oh**-teh-can
(Camptosar)

CANADIAN AVAILABILITY:
Camptosar

CLASSIFICATION

Antineoplastic

AVAILABILITY (Rx)

Injection: 20 mg/ml vial

PHARMACOKINETICS

Following IV administration, metabolized to active metabolite in liver. Excreted in urine and eliminated via biliary route. Half-life: 6 hrs (metabolite: 10 hrs).

ACTION/*THERAPEUTIC EFFECT*

Interacts w/topoisomerase I, an enzyme, which relieves torsional strain in DNA by inducing reversible single-strand breaks. Binds to topoisomerase-DNA complex preventing relegation of these single-strand breaks. *Produces cytotoxic effect due to double-strand DNA damage produced during DNA synthesis.*

USES/*UNLABELED*

Treatment of metastatic carcinoma of colon/rectum in pts whose disease has recurred or progressed following 5-fluorouracil–based therapy.

STORAGE/HANDLING

Store vials at room temperature, protect from light. Solution diluted in 5% dextrose stable for 48 hrs if refrigerated. Use within 24 hrs if refrigerated or 6 hrs if kept at room temperature. Do not refrigerate solution if diluted w/0.9% NaCl.

IV ADMINISTRATION

1. Dilute in 5% dextrose (preferred) or 0.9% NaCl to concentration of 0.12 to 1.1 mg/ml.
2. Administer all doses as IV solution over 90 min.
3. Assess for extravasation (flush site w/sterile water, apply ice if extravasation occurs).

INDICATIONS/DOSAGE/ROUTES

Carcinoma of colon/rectum:
IV Infusion: Adults, elderly: Initially, 125 mg/m^2 once weekly for 4

wks. Rest 2 wks. Additional courses may be repeated q6 wks. Subsequent doses adjusted in 25–50 mg/m^2 increments as high as 150 mg/m^2, as low as 50 mg/m^2.

Note: Do not begin a new course until granulocyte count recovered to >1,500/mm^3, platelet count recovered to >100,000/mm^3, and treatment-related diarrhea fully resolved.

PRECAUTIONS

CONTRAINDICATIONS: Hypersensitivity to irinotecan. **CAUTIONS:** Pt previously receiving pelvic/abdominal irradiation (increased risk of myelosuppression, elderly >65 yrs). **PREGNANCY/ LACTATION:** May cause fetal harm. Unknown if distributed in breast milk; discontinue nursing. **Pregnancy Category D**.

INTERACTIONS

DRUG INTERACTIONS: Other myelosuppressants may increase risk of myelosuppression. May increase akathisia w/prochlorperazone. Laxatives may increase severity of diarrhea. Diuretics may increase risk of dehydration (due to vomiting/diarrhea w/irinotecan therapy). Live virus vaccines may potentiate virus replication, increase vaccine side effects, decrease antibody response to vaccine. **ALTERED LAB VALUES:** May increase SGOT (AST), alkaline phosphatase.

SIDE EFFECTS

COMMON (>80%): Diarrhea, nausea, asthenia (loss of strength). **FREQUENT (60–80%):** Vomiting, anorexia, fever, abdominal pain/ cramps, alopecia. **OCCASIONAL (15–60%):** Constipation, flatulence, stomatitis (erythema of oral mucosa, glossitis, gingivitis), dyspepsia, headache, back pain, edema, decreased body weight, dehydration, rash, sweating, dyspnea, increased cough, rhinitis, insomnia, dizziness.

ADVERSE REACTIONS/TOXIC EFFECTS

Myelosuppression: neutropenic fever, neutrophil count <500/mm^3, leukopenia.

NURSING IMPLICATIONS

BASELINE ASSESSMENT:

Question if hypersensitive to irinotecan. Offer emotional support to pt and family. Assess hydration status, electrolytes, CBC w/differential hemoglobin, and platelet count before each dose. Premedicate w/antiemetics on day of treatment, starting at least 30 min prior to administration.

INTERVENTION/EVALUATION:

Assess for early signs of diarrhea (preceded by c/o diaphoresis and abdominal cramping). Treat w/loperamide, give fluids/ electrolyte replacement if dehydrated. Monitor hydration status, I/O electrolytes, CBC w/differential, Hgb, platelets. Monitor infusion site for signs of inflammation (flush site w/sterile water, apply ice if extravasation occurs).

PATIENT/FAMILY TEACHING:

Inform pt of possible late diarrhea causing dehydration, electrolyte depletion. Provide antiemetic/antidiarrheal regimen for subsequent use. Notify physician if diarrhea, vomiting continues at home. Do not have immunizations without physician's approval (drug lowers body's resistance). Avoid contact with those who have recently received live virus vaccine.

iron dextran

iron **dex**-tran
(Infed)

CANADIAN AVAILABILITY:
Dexiron, Infufer

CLASSIFICATION

Hematinic

AVAILABILITY (Rx)

Injection: 50 mg/ml

PHARMACOKINETICS

Readily absorbed after IM administration. Major portion of absorption occurs within 72 hrs; remainder within 3–4 wks. Iron is bound to protein to form hemosiderin, ferritin, or transferrin. No physiologic system of elimination. Small amounts lost daily in shedding of skin, hair, and nails, and in feces, urine, and perspiration. Half-life: 5–20 hrs.

ACTION/*THERAPEUTIC EFFECT*

Essential component of formation of hemoglobin, *replenishes hemoglobin and depleted iron stores*. Necessary for effective erythropoiesis and oxygen transport capacity of blood. Serves as cofactor of several essential enzymes.

USES

Treatment of established iron deficiency anemia. Use only when oral administration is not feasible or when rapid replenishment of iron is warranted.

STORAGE/HANDLING

Store at room temperature. Dark brown, slightly viscous liquid.

IM/IV ADMINISTRATION

Note: Test doses are generally given before the full dosage; stay w/pt for several minutes after injection due to potential for anaphylactic reaction and keep epinephrine and resuscitative equipment available.

IM:

1. Draw up medication w/one needle, use new needle for injection (minimizes skin staining).
2. Administer deep IM in upper outer quadrant of buttock only.
3. Use Z-tract technique (displacement of SubQ tissue lateral to injection site before inserting needle) to minimize skin staining.

IV:

Note: A too rapid IV rate may produce flushing, chest pain, shock, hypotension, tachycardia.

1. May give undiluted or diluted in normal saline for infusion.
2. Do not exceed IV administration rate of 50 mg/min (1 ml/min).
3. Pt must remain recumbent 30–45 min following IV administration (avoid postural hypotension).

INDICATIONS/DOSAGE/ROUTES

Note: Discontinue oral iron form before administering iron dextran. Dosage expressed in terms of milligrams of elemental iron. Dosage individualized based on degree of anemia, pt weight, presence of any bleeding. Use periodic hematologic determinations as guide to therapy.

Iron deficiency anemia (no blood loss):
IM/IV: Adults, elderly: Mg iron = $0.66 \times$ weight (kg) $\times$ (100−Hgb <g/dl>/14.8).

Replacement secondary to blood loss:
IM/IV: Adults, elderly: Replacement iron (mg) = blood loss (ml) × hematocrit.

PRECAUTIONS

CONTRAINDICATIONS: All anemias except iron deficiency anemia (eliminates pernicious, aplastic, normocytic, refractory). **EXTREME CAUTION:** Serious liver impairment. **CAUTIONS:** History of allergies, bronchial asthma, rheumatoid arthritis. **PREGNANCY/LACTATION:** May cross placenta in some form (unknown); trace distributed in breast milk. **Pregnancy Category C**.

INTERACTIONS

DRUG INTERACTIONS: None significant. **ALTERED LAB VALUES:** None significant.

SIDE EFFECTS

FREQUENT: Allergic reaction (rash, itching), backache, muscle pain, chills, dizziness, headache, fecer, nausea, vomiting, flushed skin, pain or redness at injection site, brown discoloration of skin, metallic taste.

ADVERSE REACTIONS/TOXIC EFFECTS

Anaphylaxis has occurred during the first few minutes after injection, causing death on rare occasions. Leukocytosis, lymphadenopathy occur rarely.

NURSING IMPLICATIONS

BASELINE ASSESSMENT:

Do not give concurrently w/oral iron form (excessive iron may produce excessive iron storage [hemosiderosis]). Be alert to those w/rheumatoid arthritis or iron deficiency anemia (acute exacerbation of joint pain and swelling may occur). Inguinal lymphadenopathy may occur w/IM injection. Assess for adequate muscle mass before injecting medication.

INTERVENTION/EVALUATION:

Monitor IM site for abscess formation, necrosis, atrophy, swelling, brownish color to skin. Question pt regarding soreness, pain, inflammation at or near IM injection site. Check IV site for phlebitis. Monitor serum ferritin levels.

PATIENT/FAMILY TEACHING:

Pain and brown staining may occur at injection site. Oral iron should not be taken when receiving iron injections. Stools frequently become black w/iron therapy; this is harmless unless accompanied by red streaking, sticky consistency of stool, abdominal pain or cramping, which should be reported to physician. Oral hygiene, hard candy, or gum may reduce metallic taste. Notify physician immediately if fever, back pain, headache occur.

isoetharine hydrochloride

eye-sew-**eth**-ah-reen
(Bronkosol, Dey-Dose)

isoetharine mesylate

(Bronkometer)

CLASSIFICATION

Bronchodilator

AVAILABILITY (Rx)

Aerosol Solution for Inhalation:
0.062%, 0.08%, 0.1%, 0.125%,
0.167%, 0.17%, 0.2%, 0.25%, 1%

PHARMACOKINETICS

	ONSET	PEAK	DURATION
Aerosol			
	1–6 min	5–15 min	1–4 hrs
Nebulization			
	1–6 min	5–15 min	1–4 hrs
IPPB	1–6 min	5–15 min	1–4 hrs

Inhaled medication rapidly absorbed from respiratory tract. Metabolized in GI tract, lungs, liver; excreted in urine.

ACTION/*THERAPEUTIC EFFECT*

Stimulates beta$_2$-adrenergic receptors in lungs, resulting in relaxation of bronchial smooth muscle, *relieving bronchospasm; reduces airway resistance.*

USES

Relief of acute bronchial asthma, bronchospasm associated w/chronic bronchitis, emphysema.

STORAGE/HANDLING

Store at room temperature. Do not use if solution is pink to brown, contains a precipitate, or becomes cloudy.

PO ADMINISTRATION

**METERED DOSE AEROSOL
(I. mesylate):**

1. Shake container well, exhale completely, then holding mouthpiece 1 inch away from lips, inhale and hold breath as long as possible before exhaling.
2. Wait 1–10 min before inhaling 2nd dose (allows for deeper bronchial penetration).
3. Rinse mouth w/water immediately after inhalation (prevents mouth/throat dryness).

**NEBULIZATION, IPPB
(I. hydrochloride):**

1. Dilute 0.5 or 1% solution with sterile water, sterile purified water, or 0.45 or 0.9% NaCl solution at 1:3 ratio (0.125, 0.2, or 0.25% may be given undiluted).
2. Adjust oxygen flow rate at 4–6 L/min over 120 min.
3. For IPPB, adjust at 15 L/min at cycling pressure of 15 cm water (allowing for adjustment of flow rate, cycling pressure, further dilution).

INDICATIONS/DOSAGE/ROUTES

Bronchospasm:
Hand-bulb Nebulizer: Adults, elderly: 4 inhalations (range: 3–7 inhalations) undiluted. May be repeated up to 5 times/day.
Metered Dose Inhalation: Adults, elderly: 1–2 inhalations q4h. Wait 1 min before administering 2nd inhalation.
IPPB, Oxygen Aerolization: Adults, elderly: 0.5–1 ml of a 0.5% or 0.5 ml of a 1% solution diluted 1:3.

PRECAUTIONS

CONTRAINDICATIONS: History of hypersensitivity to sympathomimetics. **CAUTIONS:** Hypertension, cardiovascular disease, hyperthyroidism, diabetes mellitus. **PREGNANCY/LACTATION:** Unknown if drug crosses placenta or is distributed in breast milk. May inhibit uterine contractility. **Pregnancy Category C.**

INTERACTIONS

DRUG INTERACTIONS: May decrease effects of beta blockers. Digoxin may increase risk of arrhythmias. **ALTERED LAB VAL-UES:** May decrease serum potassium levels.

SIDE EFFECTS

OCCASIONAL: Tremor, nausea, nervousness, palpitations, tachycardia, peripheral vasodilation, dryness of mouth, throat, dizziness, vomiting, wakness, headache, increased B/P, insomnia.

ADVERSE REACTIONS/TOXIC EFFECTS

Excessive sympathomimetic stimulation may cause palpitations, extrasystoles, tachycardia, chest pain, slight increase in B/P followed by a substantial decrease, chills, sweating, and blanching of skin. Too frequent or excessive use may lead to loss of bronchodilating effectiveness and/or severe, paradoxical bronchoconstriction.

NURSING IMPLICATIONS
BASELINE ASSESSMENT:

Offer emotional support (high incidence of anxiety due to difficulty in breathing and sympathomimetic response to drug).

INTERVENTION/EVALUATION:

Monitor rate, depth, rhythm, type of respiration; quality and rate of pulse. Assess lung sounds for rhonchi, wheezing, rales. Monitor arterial blood gases. Observe lips, fingernails for blue or dusky color in light-skinned pts; gray in dark-skinned pts. Observe for clavicular retractions, hand tremor. Evaluate for clinical improvement (quieter, slower respirations, relaxed facial expression, cessation of clavicular retractions).

PATIENT/FAMILY TEACHING:

Increase fluid intake (decreases lung secretion viscosity). Do not take more than 2 inhalations at any one time (excessive use may produce paradoxical bronchoconstriction or a decreased bronchodilating effect). Rinsing mouth with water immediately after inhalation may prevent mouth/throat dryness. Avoid excessive use of caffeine derivatives (chocolate, coffee, tea, cola, cocoa).

---

isoflurophate
(Floropryl)
See Classification section under:
Antiglaucoma

---

isoniazid
eye-sew-**nye**-ah-zid
(INH, Laniazid, Nydrazid)

FIXED-COMBINATION(S):
W/rifampin, an antitubercular **(Rifamate)**; w/pyrazinamide and rifampin, antituberculars **(Rifater).**

CANADIAN AVAILABILITY:
Isotamine, PMS Isoniazid

CLASSIFICATION

Antitubercular

AVAILABILITY (Rx)

Tablets: 50 mg, 100 mg, 300 mg. **Syrup:** 50 mg/5 ml. **Injection:** 100 mg/ml.

PHARMACOKINETICS

Readily absorbed from GI tract. Widely distributed (including CSF). Metabolized in liver. Primarily excreted in urine. Removed by hemodialysis. Half-life: 0.5–5 hrs.

ACTION/*THERAPEUTIC EFFECT*

Inhibits mycolic acid synthesis that causes disruption of bacterial cell wall and loss of acid-fast properties in susceptible mycobacteria. Active only during cell division. *Bactericidal.*

USES

Drug of choice in tuberculosis prophylaxis. Used in combination w/one or more other antitubercular agents for treatment of all forms of active tuberculosis.

PO ADMINISTRATION

1. Give 1 hr before or 2 hrs after meals (may give w/food to decrease GI upset, but will delay absorption).

2. Administer at least 1 hr before antacids, esp. those containing aluminum.

INDICATIONS/DOSAGE/ROUTES

Tuberculosis (treatment):
PO/IM: Adults, elderly: 5 mg/kg/day (maximum 300 mg/day) as single dose. **Children:** 10–20 mg/kg/day (maximum 300 mg/day) as single dose.

Tuberculosis (prevention):
PO/IM: Adults, elderly: 300 mg/day as single dose. **Children:** 10 mg/kg/day (maximum 300 mg/day) as single dose.

PRECAUTIONS

CONTRAINDICATIONS: Acute liver disease, history of hypersensitivity reactions or hepatic injury w/previous isoniazid therapy. **CAUTIONS:** Chronic liver disease or alcoholism, severe renal impairment. May be cross sensitive w/nicotinic acid or other chemically related medications. **PREGNANCY/LACTATION:** Prophylaxis usually postponed until after delivery. Crosses placenta; distributed in breast milk. **Pregnancy Category C**.

INTERACTIONS

DRUG INTERACTIONS: Alcohol may increase hepatotoxicity, metabolism. May increase toxicity of carbamazepine, phenytoin. May decrease ketoconazole concentrations. Disulfiram may increase CNS effects. Hepatotoxic medications may increase hepatotoxicity. **ALTERED LAB VALUES:** May increase SGOT (AST), SGPT (ALT), bilirubin.

SIDE EFFECTS

FREQUENT: Nausea, vomiting, diarrhea, stomach pain.. **RARE:** Pain at injection site, hypersensitivity reaction, optic neuritis.

ADVERSE REACTIONS/TOXIC EFFECTS

Neurotoxicity (clumsy or unsteadiness, numbness, tingling, burning or pain in hands/feet), hepatotoxicity occur rarely. Hepatitis (dark urine, yellow eyes or skin, loss of appetite, unusually tired).

NURSING IMPLICATIONS
Baseline Assessment:

Question for history of hypersensitivity reactions or hepatic injury from isoniazid, sensitivity to nicotinic acid or chemically related medications. Assure collection of specimens for culture, sensitivity. Evaluate initial hepatic function results.

INTERVENTION/EVALUATION:

Monitor hepatic function test results and assess for hepatitis: anorexia, nausea, vomiting, weakness, fatigue, dark urine, jaundice (hold INH and inform physician promptly). Check for tingling, numbness, or burning of extremities (those esp. at risk for neuropathy may be given pyridoxine prophylactically: malnourished, elderly, diabetics, those w/chronic liver disease, including alcoholics). Be alert for fever, skin eruptions (hypersensitivity reaction). Report vision difficulties at once. Evaluate mental status. Check for dizziness; assist w/ambulation as needed. Monitor CBC results and blood sugar.

PATIENT/FAMILY TEACHING:

Do not skip doses; continue taking isoniazid for full length of therapy (6 to 24 mos). Office visits, vision and lab tests are important part of treatment. Take preferably 1 hr before or 2 hrs after meals (w/food if GI upset). Avoid alcohol during treatment. Do not take any other medications w/o consulting physician, including antacids; must take isoniazid at least 1 hr before antacid. Avoid tuna, sauerkraut, aged cheeses, smoked fish (provide list of tyramine-containing foods) that may cause reaction such as red/itching skin, pounding heartbeat, lightheadedness, hot or clammy feeling, headache; contact physician. Be certain pt not experiencing vision difficulty, dizziness, or other impairment before driving, using machinery. Notify physician of any new symptom immediately for vision difficulties, nausea/vomiting, dark urine, yellowing of skin/eyes, fatigue, numbness or tingling of hands or feet.

isoproterenol hydrochloride

eye-sew-pro-**tear**-en-all
(**Isuprel, Dey-Dose**)

isoproterenol sulfate

(**Medihaler-Iso**)

FIXED-COMBINATION(S):
W/phenylephrine, a vasoconstrictor (**Duo-Medihaler**).

CANADIAN AVAILABILITY:
Isuprel

CLASSIFICATION

Cardiac stimulant, bronchodilator

AVAILABILITY (Rx)

Injection: 1:5,000 (0.2 mg/ml). **Tablets (sublingual):** 10 mg, 15 mg. **Solution for Inhalation:** 0.25%, 0.5%, 1%. **Aerosol.**

PHARMACOKINETICS

	ONSET	PEAK	DURATION
Inhalation	2–5 min	—	0.5–2 hrs
Sublingual	15–30 min	—	1–2 hrs
SubQ, IM	Prompt	—	1–2 hrs
IV	Immediate	—	Length of infusion

Rapidly absorbed after inhalation/parenteral administration. Metabolized in liver. Primarily ex-

creted in urine. Half-life: 2.5–5
minutes.

ACTION / *THERAPEUTIC EFFECT*

Stimulates beta$_1$-adrenergic receptors, *increasing myocardial
contractility, stroke volume, cardiac
output.* Also stimulates beta$_2$-
adrenergic receptors, resulting in
relaxation of bronchial smooth
muscle, *relieving bronchospasm;
reduces airway resistance.*

USES

Treatment of carotid sinus hypersensitivity, Adams-Stokes syndrome, ventricular arrhythmias
due to AV nodal block, reversible
bronchospasm, diagnosis of coronary artery disease; adjunct in
treatment of shock. Treatment of
bronchospasm due to bronchial
asthma, emphysema, bronchitis,
bronchiectasis.

STORAGE / HANDLING

Do not use if solution is pink to
brown, contains a precipitate, or
appears cloudy.

PO / INHALATION / IV
ADMINISTRATION

SUBLINGUAL:

1. Dissolve sublingual tablet
under tongue (do not chew or
swallow tablet).
2. Do not swallow saliva until
tablet is dissolved.

INHALATION:

1. Shake container well, exhale completely, then holding
mouthpiece 1 inch away from lips,
inhale and hold breath as long as
possible before exhaling.
2. Wait 1–10 min before inhaling second dose (allows for deeper bronchial penetration).
3. Rinse mouth w/water immediately after inhalation (prevents
mouth/throat dryness).

IV:

Note: May also be given SubQ,
IM, intracardiac.
1. For IV injection, dilute 0.2
mg (1 ml) of 1:5,000 solution to a
volume of 10 ml 0.9% NaCl injection or 5% dextrose injection.
2. Administer IV injection at
rate of 1 ml/min, regulated by EKG
monitoring.
3. For IV infusion, dilute 0.2–2
mg (1–10 ml) of 1:5,000 solution in
500 ml of 5% dextrose in water to
provide a solution of 0.4–4
mcg/ml.
4. Rate of IV infusion determined by pt's heart rate, central
venous pressure, systemic B/P, and
urine flow measurements.
5. Use microdrip (60 drops/
ml) or infusion pump to administer
drug.
6. If EKG changes occur, heart
rate exceeds 110 beats/min, or
premature beats occur, consider
reducing rate of infusion or temporarily stopping infusion.

INDICATIONS / DOSAGE / ROUTES

Arrhythmias:
IV Bolus: Adults, elderly: Initially,
0.02–0.06 mg (1–3 ml of diluted
solution). Subsequent dose range:
0.01–0.2 mg (0.5–10 ml of diluted
solution).
IV Infusion: Adults, elderly: Initially, 5 mcg/min (1.25 ml/min of
diluted solution). Subsequent
dose range: 2–20 mcg/min. **Children:** 2.5 mcg/min or 0.1 mcg/kg
per min.
IM/SubQ: Adults, elderly: 0.2
mg, then 0.02–1 mg, as needed.

Mild arrhythmias:
Sublingual: Adults, elderly:
10–30 mg 4–6 times/day.

Complete heart block following closure of ventricular septal defects:

IV: Adults, elderly: 0.04–0.06 mg (2–3 ml of diluted solution). **Infants:** 0.01–0.03 (0.5–1.5 ml of diluted solution).

Shock:

IV Infusion: Adults, elderly: Rate of 0.5–5 mcg/min (0.25–2.5 ml of 1:500,000 dilution); rate of infusion based on clinical response (heart rate, central venous pressure, systemic B/P, urine flow measurements).

Bronchospasm:

Metered Dose Inhalation: Adults, elderly, children >6 yrs: 1–2 inhalations 4–6 times/day at no less than 3–4 hr intervals. Wait 1–5 min before administering second inhalation.

IPPB: Adults, elderly: 2 ml (0.125%) or 2.5 ml (0.1%) up to 5 times/day. Flow rate adjusted to administer dose over 15–20 min IPPB: 10–20 min via nebulization. **Children:** 2 ml (0.0625%) or 2.5 ml (0.05%) up to 5 times/day.

Nebulization Solution: Adults, elderly, children: 6–12 inhalations (0.025%). Repeat at 5–15 min intervals (maximum 3 treatments). **Maximum:** 8 treatments/24 hrs.

Sublingual: Adults, elderly: 10–20 mg q6–8h. **Children >6 yrs:** 5–10 mg q6–8h.

IV Infusion: Adults, elderly: 0.01–0.02 mg (0.5–1 ml of a diluted solution). **Children:** $1/10$–$1/12$ adult dose.

PRECAUTIONS

CONTRAINDICATIONS: Tachycardia due to digitalis toxicity, preexisting arrhythmias, angina, precordial distress. **CAUTIONS:** Hypersensitivity to sulfite, elderly/debilitated, hypertension, cardiovascular disease, impaired renal function, hyperthyroidism, diabetes mellitus, prostatic hypertrophy, glaucoma. Safety and efficacy in children not established. **PREGNANCY/LACTATION:** Unknown if drug crosses placenta or is distributed in breast milk. May inhibit uterine contractility. **Pregnancy Category C.**

INTERACTIONS

DRUG INTERACTIONS: Tricyclic antidepressants may increase cardiovascular effects. May decrease effects of beta blockers. Digoxin may increase risk of arrhythmias. **ALTERED LAB VALUES:** May decrease serum potassium levels.

SIDE EFFECTS

FREQUENT: (10–20%): Palpitations, tachycardia, restlessness, nervousness, tremor, insomnia, anxiety. **OCCASIONAL: (<10%):** Increased sweating, headache, nausea, flushed skin, dizziness, coughing.

ADVERSE REACTIONS/TOXIC EFFECTS

Excessive sympathomimetic stimulation may cause palpitations, extrasystoles, tachycardia, chest pain, slight increase in B/P followed by a substantial decrease, chills, sweating, and blanching of skin. Ventricular arrhythmias may occur if heart rate is above 130 beats/min. When used for bronchospasm, too frequent or excessive use may lead to loss of bronchodilating effectiveness and/or severe, paradoxical bronchoconstriction. Parotid gland swelling may occur w/prolonged use.

NURSING IMPLICATIONS

BASELINE ASSESSMENT:

Be alert to anginal pain or precordial distress, pulse rate exceeding 110 beats/min.

INTERVENTION/EVALUATION:

Cardiac stimulant: Monitor EKG,

blood PCO_2 or bicarbonate and blood pH, central venous pressure, pulse, systemic B/P, urine output. *Bronchospasm:* Monitor rate, depth, rhythm, type of respiration; quality and rate of pulse. Assess lung sounds for rhonchi, wheezing, rales. Monitor arterial blood gases. Observe lips, fingernails for blue or dusky color in light-skinned pts; gray in dark-skinned pts. Observe for clavicular retractions, hand tremor. Evaluate for clinical improvement (quieter, slower respirations, relaxed facial expression, cessation of clavicular retractions).

PATIENT/FAMILY TEACHING:

Bronchospasm: Increase fluid intake (decreases lung secretion viscosity). Do not take more than 2 inhalations at any one time (excessive use may produce paradoxical bronchoconstriction or a decreased bronchodilating effect). Rinsing mouth with water immediately after inhalation may prevent mouth/throat dryness. Saliva may turn pink after sublingual administration. Due to acidity of drug, frequent sublingual use may damage teeth. Avoid excessive use of caffeine derivatives (chocolate, coffee, tea, cola, cocoa).

isosorbide dinitrate
eye-sew-**sore**-bide
(Dilatrate, Isordil, Sorbitrate)

isosorbide mononitrate
(Imdur, ISMO, Monoket)

CANADIAN AVAILABILITY:
Apo-ISDN, Cedocard, Isordil, Imdur, Ismo

CLASSIFICATION
Nitrate

AVAILABILITY (Rx)
Dinitrate: **Tablets:** 5 mg, 10 mg, 20 mg, 30 mg, 40 mg. **Tablets (sublingual):** 2.5 mg, 5 mg, 10 mg. **Tablets (chewable):** 5 mg, 10 mg. **Tablets (sustained-release):** 40 mg. **Capsules (sustained-release):** 40 mg.

Mononitrate: **Tablets:** 10 mg, 20 mg. **Tablets (extended-release):** 60 mg.

PHARMACOKINETICS

	ONSET	PEAK	DURATION
Chewable			
	5–20 min	15–60 min	1–4 hrs
Sublingual			
	5–20 min	15–60 min	1–4 hrs
Extended-release			
	up to 4 hrs	—	6–8 hrs
Tablets, capsules			
	20–40 min	45–120 min	4–6 hrs
Mononitrate			
	30–60 min	—	—

Poorly absorbed from GI tract; well absorbed after sublingual administration. Metabolized in liver (undergoes first-pass effect). Primarily excreted in urine. Half-life: *oral:* 4 hrs, *sublingual:* 1 hr. *Mononitrate:* Not subjected to first-pass metabolism in liver.

ACTION/ *THERAPEUTIC EFFECT*

Decreases myocardial O_2 demand, increases myocardial O_2 supply, reducing wall tension by venous dilation (preload) and arterial dilation (afterload). *Dilates coronary arteries; improves collateral blood flow to ischemic areas within myocardium.*

USES

Treatment and prevention of

angina pectoris. Chronic prophylaxis of angina. *Mononitrate:* Prevention of angina pectoris due to coronary artery disease.

PO/SUBLINGUAL ADMINISTRATION

PO:

1. Best if taken on an empty stomach.

2. Oral tablets may be crushed.

3. Do not crush or break sublingual or extended-release form.

4. Do not crush chewable form before administering.

SUBLINGUAL:

1. Do not crush/chew sublingual tablets.

2. Dissolve tablets under tongue; do not swallow.

INDICATIONS/DOSAGE/ROUTES

Note: Drug-free interval at least 14 hrs. Patch: Allow 10–12 hr drug-free interval.

Acute angina, prophylactic management in situations likely to provoke attack:
Sublingual/Chewable: Adults, elderly: Initially, 2.5–5 mg. Repeat at 5–10 min intervals. No more than 3 doses in 15–30 min period.

Acute prophylactic management of angina:
Sublingual/Chewable: Adults, elderly: 5–10 mg q2–3h.

Long-term prophylaxis of angina:
PO: Adults, elderly: Initially, 5–20 mg 3–4 times/day. **Maintenance:** 10–40 mg q6h. Consider 2–3 times/day, last dose no later than 7 PM to minimize intolerance.
Mononitrate: Adults, elderly: 20 mg 2 times/day, 7 hrs apart. First dose upon awakening in morning.
Extended-Release: Adults, elderly: Initially, 40 mg. **Maintenance:** 40–80 mg 2–3 times/day. Consider 1–2 times/day, last dose at 2 PM to minimize intolerance.
Imdur: 60–120 mg/day as single dose.

PRECAUTIONS

CONTRAINDICATIONS: Hypersensitivity to nitrates, severe anemia, closed-angle glaucoma, postural hypotension, head trauma, increased intracranial pressure. *Extended-release:* GI hypermotility/malabsorption, severe anemia. **CAUTIONS:** Acute MI, hepatic/renal disease, glaucoma (contraindicated in closed-angle glaucoma), blood volume depletion from diuretic therapy, systolic B/P below 90 mm Hg. **PREGNANCY/LACTATION:** Unknown if drug crosses placenta or is distributed in breast milk. **Pregnancy Category C**.

INTERACTIONS

DRUG INTERACTIONS: Alcohol, antihypertensives, vasodilators may increase risk of orthostatic hypotension. **ALTERED LAB VALUES:** May increase urine catecholamines, urine VMA (vanilmandelic acid).

SIDE EFFECTS

FREQUENT: Headache (may be severe) occurs mostly in early therapy, diminishes rapidly in intensity, usually disappears during continued treatment; transient flushing of face and neck, dizziness (esp. if pt is standing immobile or is in a warm environment), weakness, postural hypotension, nausea, vomiting, restlessness. *Sublingual:* Burning, tingling sensation at oral point of dissolution. **OCCASIONAL:** GI upset, blurred vision, dry mouth.

ADVERSE REACTIONS/TOXIC EFFECTS

Drug should be discontinued if blurred vision, dry mouth occurs. Severe postural hypotension manifested by fainting, pulselessness, cold/clammy skin, profuse sweating. Tolerance may occur w/repeated, prolonged therapy (minor tolerance w/intermittent use of sublingual tablets). Tolerance may not occur w/extended-release form. High dose tends to produce severe headache.

NURSING IMPLICATIONS

BASELINE ASSESSMENT:

Record onset, type (sharp, dull, squeezing), radiation, location, intensity, and duration of anginal pain, and precipitating factors (exertion, emotional stress). If headache occurs during management therapy, administer medication w/meals.

INTERVENTION/EVALUATION:

Assist w/ambulation if lightheadedness, dizziness occurs. Assess for facial/neck flushing. Monitor B/P for hypotension.

PATIENT/FAMILY TEACHING:

Rise slowly from lying to sitting position and dangle legs momentarily before standing. Take oral form on empty stomach (however, if headache occurs during management therapy, take medication w/meals). Dissolve sublingual tablet under tongue; do not swallow. Take at first signal of angina. If not relieved within 5 min, dissolve second tablet under tongue. Repeat if no relief in another 5 min. If pain continues, contact physician. Expel from mouth any remaining sublingual tablet after pain is completely relieved. Do not change from one brand of drug to another. Avoid alcohol (intensifies hypotensive effect). If alcohol is ingested soon after taking nitroglycerin, possible acute hypotensive episode (marked drop in B/P, vertigo, pallor) may occur.

isotretinoin

eye-sew-**tret**-ih-noyn
(Accutane)

CANADIAN AVAILABILITY:
Accutane, Isotrex

CLASSIFICATION

Acne aid

AVAILABILITY (Rx)

Capsules: 10 mg, 20 mg, 40 mg

PHARMACOKINETICS

Rapidly absorbed from GI tract. Protein binding: 99.9%. Metabolized in liver. Excreted in urine via biliary system. Half-life: 10–20 hrs.

ACTION/*THERAPEUTIC EFFECT*

Reduces sebaceous gland size, inhibiting its activity. *Produces anti-keratinizing, anti-inflammatory effects.*

USES/*UNLABELED*

Treatment of severe, recalcitrant cystic acne that is unresponsive to conventional acne therapies. *Treatment of gram-negative folliculitis, severe rosacea, correcting severe keratinization disorders.*

PO ADMINISTRATION

1. Administer whole; do not crush.

2. Give w/food to facilitate absorption.

INDICATIONS/DOSAGE/ROUTES

Recalcitrant cystic acne:
PO: Adults: Initially, 0.5–2 mg/kg/day divided in 2 doses for 15–20 wks. May repeat after at least 2 mos of therapy.

PRECAUTIONS

CONTRAINDICATIONS: Hypersensitivity to isotretinoin or parabens (component of capsules). **CAUTIONS:** Renal, hepatic dysfunction. Safety in children not established. **PREGNANCY/LACTATION:** Contraindicated in females who are or may become pregnant while undergoing treatment. Extremely high risk of major deformities in infant if pregnancy occurs while taking any amount of isotretinoin, even for short periods. Pt must be capable of understanding and carrying out instructions and of complying w/ mandatory contraception. Excretion in milk unknown; due to potential for serious adverse effects, not recommended during nursing. **Pregnancy Category X.**

INTERACTIONS

DRUG INTERACTIONS: Etretinate, tretinoin, vitamin A may increase toxic effects. Tetracycline may increase potential of pseudotumor cerebri. **ALTERED LAB VALUES:** May increase triglycerides, cholesterol, SGPT (ALT), SGOT (AST), alkaline phosphatase, LDH, sedimentation rate, fasting blood glucose, uric acid; may decrease HDL.

SIDE EFFECTS

FREQUENT: Cheilitis (inflammation of lips) (90%); skin/mucous membrane dryness (80%); skin fragility, pruritus, epistaxis, dry nose/mouth; conjunctivitis (40%); hypertriglyceridemia (25%); nausea, vomiting, abdominal pain (20%). **OCCASIONAL:** Musculoskeletal symptoms (16%) including bone or joint pain, arthralgia, generalized muscle aches; photosensitivity (5–10%). **RARE:** Decreased night vision, depression.

ADVERSE REACTIONS/TOXIC EFFECTS

Inflammatory bowel disease and pseudotumor cerebri (benign intracranial hypertension) have been temporarily associated w/isotretinoin therapy.

NURSING IMPLICATIONS

BASELINE ASSESSMENT:

Question for hypersensitivity to isotretinoin or parabens. Assess baselines for blood lipids and glucose.

INTERVENTION/EVALUATION:

Assess acne for decreased cysts. Evaluate skin and mucous membranes for excessive dryness. Monitor blood glucose, lipids.

PATIENT/FAMILY TEACHING:

A transient exacerbation of acne may occur during initial period. May have decreased tolerance to contact lenses during and after therapy. Topical acne agents should not be used w/o physician approval. Do not take vitamin supplements w/vitamin A because of additive effects. Notify physician immediately of onset of abdominal pain, severe diarrhea, rectal bleeding (possible inflammatory bowel disease), or headache, nausea and vomiting, visual disturbances (possible pseudotumor cerebri).

Decreased night vision may occur suddenly; take caution w/night driving. Minimize or eliminate alcohol consumption (may potentiate serum triglyceride elevation). Avoid prolonged exposure to sunlight; use sunscreens, protective clothing until sunlight or ultraviolet light tolerance established. Do not donate blood during or for 1 mo after treatment. *Women:* Explain the serious risk to fetus if pregnancy occurs (both oral and written warnings are given, w/pt acknowledging in writing that she understands the warnings and consents to treatment). Must have a negative serum pregnancy test within 2 wks prior to starting therapy; therapy will begin on the second or third day of the next normal menstrual period. Effective contraception (using 2 reliable forms of contraception simultaneously) must be used for at least 1 mo before, during, and for at least 1 mo after therapy w/isotretinoin.

isradipine

iss-**ray**-dih-peen
(DynaCirc, DynaCirc CR)

CLASSIFICATION

Calcium channel blocker

AVAILABILITY (Rx)

Capsules: 2.5 mg, 5 mg. **Extended-Release Capsules:** 5 mg, 10 mg.

PHARMACOKINETICS

	ONSET	PEAK	DURATION
PO	2–3 hrs	—	—

Well absorbed from GI tract. Metabolized in liver (undergoes first-pass effect). Primarily excreted in urine. Half-life: 8 hrs.

ACTION / *THERAPEUTIC EFFECT*

Inhibits calcium movement across cardiac, vascular smooth muscle. Potent peripheral vasodilator (does not depress SA, AV nodes). *Increases myocardial contractility, heart rate, cardiac output; decreases peripheral vascular resistance.*

USES / *UNLABELED*

Management of hypertension. May be used alone or w/thiazide-type diuretics. *Treatment of chronic angina pectoris, Raynaud's phenomena.*

PO ADMINISTRATION

Do not crush or break capsule.

INDICATIONS / DOSAGE / ROUTES

Hypertension:
PO: Adults, elderly: Initially, 2.5 mg 2 times/day. May increase by 5 mg q2–4 wks. **Maximum:** 20 mg/day.

PRECAUTIONS

CONTRAINDICATIONS: Sick-sinus syndrome/second- or third-degree AV block (except in presence of pacemaker). **CAUTIONS:** Impaired renal/hepatic function, CHF. **PREGNANCY/LACTATION:** Unknown if drug crosses placenta or is distributed in breast milk. **Pregnancy Category C**.

INTERACTIONS

DRUG INTERACTIONS: Beta blockers may have additive effect. **ALTERED LAB VALUES:** None significant.

SIDE EFFECTS

FREQUENT (4–7%): Peripheral edema, palpitations (higher in females). **OCCASIONAL (3%):** Palpitations, facial flushing, cough. **RARE (1–2%):** Angina, tachycardia, rash, pruritus.

ADVERSE REACTIONS/TOXIC EFFECTS

CHF occurs rarely. Overdosage produces nausea, drowsiness, confusion, slurred speech.

NURSING IMPLICATIONS
BASELINE ASSESSMENT:

Assess baseline renal/liver function tests. Assess B/P, apical pulse immediately before drug is administered (if pulse is 60/min or below, or systolic B/P is below 90 mm Hg, withhold medication, contact physician).

INTERVENTION/EVALUATION:

Assist w/ambulation if light-headedness, dizziness occurs. Assess for peripheral edema behind medial malleolus (sacral area in bedridden pts). Monitor pulse rate for bradycardia. Assess skin for flushing. Monitor liver enzyme tests.

PATIENT/FAMILY TEACHING:

Do not abruptly discontinue medication. Compliance w/therapy regimen is essential to control hypertension. To avoid hypotensive effect, rise slowly from lying to sitting position, wait momentarily before standing. Avoid tasks that require alertness, motor skills until response to drug is established. Contact physician/nurse if irregular heartbeat, shortness of breath, pronounced dizziness, or nausea occurs.

itraconazole
eye-tra-**con**-ah-zoll
(Sporanox)

CANADIAN AVAILABILITY:
Sporanox

CLASSIFICATION
Antifungal

AVAILABILITY (Rx)
Capsules: 100 mg. **Oral Solution:** 10 mg/ml. **Injection.**

PHARMACOKINETICS

Moderately absorbed from GI tract (increased w/food). Widely distributed (primarily in liver, kidney, fatty tissue). Metabolized in liver to active metabolite. Primarily excreted in urine. Not removed by hemodialysis. Half-life: 21 hrs; metabolite: 12 hrs.

ACTION/*THERAPEUTIC EFFECT*

Inhibits synthesis of ergosterol (vital component of fungal cell formation), damaging fungal cell membrane. *Fungistatic.*

USES/*UNLABELED*

Treatment of blastomycosis (pulmonary, extrapulmonary), histoplasmosis, aspergillosis, onychomycosis, dermatophyte skin infections, tinea pedis in pts unable to take topical therapy. Solution: Oral, esophageal candidiasis. *Suppresses histoplasmosis; treatment of fungal pneumonia/septicemia, disseminated sporotrichosis, ringworm of hand.*

PO ADMINISTRATION
Take w/food (increases absorption).

INDICATIONS/DOSAGE/ROUTES
Note: Doses >200 mg given in 2 divided doses.

Blastomycosis, histoplasmosis:
PO: Adults, elderly: Initially, 200 mg/day w/food. May increase in 100 mg increments. **Maximum:** 400 mg/day.

Aspergillosis:
PO: Adults, elderly: 200–400 mg/day.

Onychomycosis:
PO: Adults, elderly: 200 mg/day for 12 consecutive wks or 200 mg twice daily for 1 wk; 3 wk rest period; repeat.

Life-threatening infection:
PO: Adults, elderly: Initially, 200 mg 3 times/day for 3 days as loading dose.

Oral candidiasis:
PO: Adults: 200 mg daily for 1–2 wks.

Esophageal candidiasis:
PO: Adults: 100–200 mg daily for 3 wks.

Usual IV dosage:
IV: Adults: 200 mg 2 times/day × 4 doses; then 200 mg once daily. Infuse over 1 hr.

PRECAUTIONS

CONTRAINDICATIONS: Coadministration of terfenadine. Hypersensitivity to itraconazole, fluconazole, ketoconazole, miconazole. **CAUTIONS:** Hepatitis, HIV-infected pts, pts w/achlorhydria, hypochlorhydria (decreases absorption), impaired liver function. **PREGNANCY/LACTATION:** Distributed in breast milk. **Pregnancy Category C.**

INTERACTIONS

DRUG INTERACTIONS: May increase buspirone, cyclosporine, digoxin, lovastatin, simvastatin concentrations. May increase cisapride, terfenadine, astemizole concentration, increasing risk of cardiac dysrhythmias. May increase effect of oral anticoagulants. Phenytoin, rifampin may decrease concentrations. Antacids, H₂ antagonists, didanosine may decrease absorption. **ALTERED LAB VALUES:** May increase SGOT (AST), SGPT (ALT), alkaline phosphatase, LDH, bilirubin. May decrease potassium.

SIDE EFFECTS

FREQUENT (11%): Nausea, rash, constipation, headache. **OCCASIONAL (3–5%):** Vomiting, diarrhea, hypertension, headache, peripheral edema, fatigue. **RARE (≤2%):** Abdominal pain, anorexia, pruritus, fever).

ADVERSE REACTIONS/TOXIC EFFECTS

Hepatitis (anorexia, abdominal pain, unusual tiredness/weakness, jaundice, dark urine) occurs rarely.

NURSING IMPLICATIONS

BASELINE ASSESSMENT:

Obtain specimens for fungal cultures and other lab studies before first dose. Therapy may begin before results are known. Determine baseline temperature, liver function tests. Assess allergies.

INTERVENTION/EVALUATION:

Assess for signs and symptoms of liver dysfunction and monitor hepatic enzyme test results in pts w/preexisting liver dysfunction. Check temperature.

PATIENT/FAMILY TEACHING:

Take w/food. Therapy will continue for at least 3 mos and until lab tests and clinical presentation indicate infection is controlled. Report the following at once: unusual fatigue, yellow skin, dark urine, pale stool, anorexia/nausea/vomiting.

ivermectin
(Stromectol)
See Supplement

kanamycin sulfate

can-ah-**my**-sin
(Kantrex)

CLASSIFICATION

Antibiotic: Aminoglycoside

AVAILABILITY (Rx)

Injection: 75 mg/2 ml, 500 mg/2 ml, 1 g/3 ml. **Capsules:** 500 mg.

PHARMACOKINETICS

Rapid, complete absorption after IM administration. Widely distributed (does not cross blood-brain barrier; low concentrations in CSF). Excreted unchanged in urine. Removed by hemodialysis. Half-life: 2–4 hrs (increased in decreased renal function, neonates; decreased in cystic fibrosis, burn or febrile pts).

ACTION/THERAPEUTIC EFFECT

Irreversibly binds to protein on bacterial ribosome, *interfering in protein synthesis of susceptible microorganisms.*

USES

Treatment of skin/skin structure, bone, joint, respiratory tract, intra-abdominal and complicated urinary tract infections; wound and surgical site irrigation, burns, septicemia, hepatic encephalopathy. Adjunctive therapy for tuberculosis; before operation for intestinal antisepsis.

STORAGE/HANDLING

Store parenteral form, capsules at room temperature. Solutions appear clear, colorless to pale yellow. Darkening of solution does not indicate loss of potency. Intermittent IV infusion (piggy-back) stable for 24 hrs at room temperature. Discard if precipitate forms.

PO/IM/IV ADMINISTRATION

Note: Coordinate peak and trough lab draws w/administration times.

PO:

1. Give w/o regard to meals.
2. If GI upset occurs, give w/food or milk.

IM:

To minimize discomfort, give deep IM slowly. Less painful to inject into gluteus maximus rather than lateral aspect of thigh.

IV:

1. Dilute each 500 mg w/100–200 ml 5% dextrose, 0.9% NaCl, or other compatible IV fluid. Amount of diluent for infants, children depends on individual needs.
2. Administer IV infusion (piggyback) over 30–60 min.
3. Alternating IV sites, use large veins to reduce risk of phlebitis.

INDICATIONS/DOSAGE/ROUTES

Space doses evenly around the clock.

Mild to moderate infections:
IM/IV: Adults, children: 15 mg/kg/day in divided doses q8–12h (IM doses may be given q6h). **Elderly:** 5–7.5 mg/kg/dose q12–24h.

Hepatic encephalopathy (adjunctive treatment):
PO: Adults, elderly: 8–12 g/day in 4 divided doses.

Preop intestinal antisepsis:
PO: Adults, elderly: 1 g every hour for 4 doses, then 1 g q6h for up to 3 days.

Intraperitoneal instillation:
Adults: 500 mg dissolved in 20 ml sterile water, instilled via catheter into wound.

Irrigation:
Adults: 0.25% solution to irrigate pleural space, ventricular or abscess cavities, wounds, or surgical sites.

Inhalation:
Adults: 250 mg diluted w/3 ml 0.9% NaCl and nebulized 2–4 times/day.

Dosage in renal impairment:
Dose and/or frequency is modified based on degree of renal impairment, serum concentration of drug.

PRECAUTIONS

CONTRAINDICATIONS: Hypersensitivity to kanamycin, other aminoglycosides (cross-sensitivity). Oral administration contraindicated in intestinal obstruction. **CAUTIONS:** Elderly, neonates (due to renal insufficiency or immaturity); neuromuscular disorders (potential for respiratory depression), prior hearing loss, vertigo, renal impairment. Not for long-term therapy due to associated toxicities. Cumulative effects may occur when given via more than one route. **PREGNANCY/LACTATION:** Readily crosses placenta; distributed in breast milk. May cause fetal nephrotoxicity. **Pregnancy Category D**.

INTERACTIONS

DRUG INTERACTIONS: Other aminoglycosides, nephrotoxic, ototoxic medications may increase toxicity. May increase effects of neuromuscular blocking agents. **ALTERED LAB VALUES:** May increase BUN, SGPT (ALT), SGOT (AST), bilirubin, creatinine, LDH concentrations; may decrease serum calcium, magnesium, potassium, sodium concentrations.

SIDE EFFECTS

FREQUENT: *Oral:* Nausea, vomiting, diarrhea. **OCCASIONAL:** *IM:* Pain, irritation at injection site. *IV:* Phlebitis; hypersensitivity reactions: rash, fever, urticaria, pruritus. **RARE:** Headache.

ADVERSE REACTIONS/TOXIC EFFECTS

Nephrotoxicity (evidenced by increased BUN and serum creatinine, decreased creatinine clearance) may be reversible if drug stopped at first sign of symptoms; irreversible ototoxicity (tinnitus, dizziness, ringing/roaring in ears, reduced hearing) and neurotoxicity (headache, dizziness, lethargy, tremors, visual disturbances) occur occasionally. Risk is greater w/higher dosages, prolonged therapy. Superinfections, particularly w/fungi, may result from bacterial imbalance. Severe respiratory depression, anaphylaxis occur rarely.

NURSING IMPLICATIONS
BASELINE ASSESSMENT:

Dehydration must be treated before aminoglycoside therapy. Establish pt's baseline hearing acuity before beginning therapy. Question for history of allergies, esp. to aminoglycosides. Obtain specimens for culture, sensitivity before giving first dose (therapy may begin before results are known). Maintain adequate hydration.

INTERVENTION/EVALUATION:

Monitor I&O (maintain hydration), urinalysis (casts, RBCs, WBCs, decrease in specific

gravity). Monitor results of peak/trough blood tests. Be alert to ototoxic and neurotoxic symptoms (see Adverse Reactions/Toxic Effects). Check IM injection site for pain, induration. Evaluate IV site for phlebitis (heat, pain, red streaking over vein). Assess for rash. Be alert to respiratory depression. Assess for superinfection, particularly genital/anal pruritus, changes of oral mucosa, diarrhea.

PATIENT/FAMILY TEACHING:

Continue antibiotic for full length of treatment. Space doses evenly. Discomfort may occur w/IM injection. Notify physician in event of headache, shortness of breath, dizziness, hearing or urinary problem even after therapy is completed. Do not take other medication w/o consulting physician. Lab tests are an essential part of therapy.

kaolin/pectin

kay-oh-lyn
(Kaopectate, Kapectolin)

FIXED-COMBINATION(S):
W/atropine, hyoscyamine, scopolamine, belladonna alkaloids, opium (Donnagel PG, Kapectolin PG); w/opium (Parepectolin).

CANADIAN AVAILABILITY:
Kaopectate

CLASSIFICATION

Antidiarrheal

AVAILABILITY (OTC)

Suspension

PHARMACOKINETICS

Not absorbed orally. Up to 90% of pectin decomposed in GI tract.

ACTION/*THERAPEUTIC EFFECT*

Adsorbent, protectant *(adsorbs bacteria, toxins, reduces water loss)*.

USES

Symptomatic treatment of mild to moderate acute diarrhea.

PO ADMINISTRATION

Shake suspension well before administration.

INDICATIONS/DOSAGE/ROUTES

Antidiarrheal:
PO: Adults, elderly: 60–120 ml after each loose bowel movement (LBM). **Children >12 yrs:** 60 ml after each LBM; **6–12 yrs:** 30–60 ml after each LBM; **3–6 yrs:** 15–30 ml after each LBM.

PRECAUTIONS

CONTRAINDICATIONS: None significant. **CAUTIONS:** None significant. **PREGNANCY/LACTATION:** Unknown if drug crosses placenta or is distributed in breast milk. **Pregnancy Category C**.

INTERACTIONS

DRUG INTERACTIONS: May decrease absorption of digoxin. **ALTERED LAB VALUES:** None significant.

SIDE EFFECTS

RARE: Constipation.

ADVERSE REACTIONS/TOXIC EFFECTS

None significant.

NURSING IMPLICATIONS
INTERVENTION/EVALUATION:

Encourage adequate fluid intake. Assess bowel sounds for

peristalsis. Assess stools for frequency and consistency (watery, loose, soft, semisolid, solid).

PATIENT/FAMILY TEACHING:

Do not use for more than 2 days or w/high fever. Not for children under 3 yrs of age w/o physician direction.

ketamine hydrochloride
(Ketalar)
See Classification section under: Anesthetics: general

ketoconazole
keet-oh-**con**-ah-zol
(Nizoral, Nizoral AD)

CANADIAN AVAILABILITY:
Apo-Ketocomazole, Nizoral

CLASSIFICATION

Antifungal

AVAILABILITY (Rx)

Tablets: 200 mg. **Cream:** 2%. **Shampoo:** 2%, 1% (OTC).

PHARMACOKINETICS

Oral: Readily absorbed from GI tract. Widely distributed. Metabolized in liver. Primarily excreted via biliary elimination. Half-life: 8 hrs. *Topical:* Minimal systemic absorption.

ACTION/THERAPEUTIC EFFECT

Inhibits synthesis of ergosterol (vital component of fungal cell formation), damaging fungal cell membrane. *Fungistatic.*

USES/UNLABELED

Treatment of histoplasmosis, blastomycosis, candidiasis, chronic mucocutaneous candidiasis, coccidioidomycosis, paracoccidioidomycosis, chromomycosis, seborrheic dermatitis, tineas (ringworm): corporis, capitis, manus, cruris, pedis, unguium (onychomycosis), oral thrush, candiduria. *Shampoo:* Reduces scaling due to dandruff. Treatment of tinea versicolor. *Topical:* Treatment of tineas, pityriasis versicolor, cutaneous candidiasis, seborrhea dermatitis, dandruff. *Systemic:* Treatment of fungal pneumonia, septicemia, prostate cancer.

PO ADMINISTRATION

1. Give w/food to minimize GI irritation.
2. Tablets may be crushed.
3. Ketoconazole requires acidity; give antacids, anticholinergics, H_2 blockers *at least* 2 hrs after dosing.

INDICATIONS/DOSAGE/ROUTES

Mild to moderate infections:
PO: Adults, elderly: 200 mg/day. **Children >2 yrs:** 3.3–6.6 mg/kg/day as single dose.

Severe infections:
PO: Adults, elderly: 400 mg/day.

Cutaneous fungal infections:
Topical: Adults, elderly: Apply 1–2 times/day for 2–4 wks.

Dandruff:
Shampoo: Adults, elderly: 2 times/wk for 4 wks, allowing at least 3 days between shampooing. Intermittent use to maintain control.

Tinea versicolor:
Shampoo: Adults: Apply to damp skin w/wide margin around it, lather, leave 5 mins, rinse.

PRECAUTIONS

CONTRAINDICATIONS: Hypersensitivity to ketoconazole, children <2 yrs. **CAUTIONS:** Hepatic impairment. **PREGNANCY/LACTA-TION:** Unknown if crosses placenta; probably distributed in breast milk. **Pregnancy Category C**.

INTERACTIONS

DRUG INTERACTIONS: Alcohol, hepatotoxic medications may increase hepatotoxicity. Antacids, anticholinergics, H_2 antagonists, omeprazole may decrease absorption (allow 2 hr interval). May increase concentration, toxicity of cyclosporine, lovastatin, simvastatin. Isoniazid, rifampin may decrease concentration. May increase concentration of cisapride, terfenadine causing cardiotoxicity. **ALTERED LAB VALUES:** May increase SGOT (AST), SGPT (ALT), alkaline phosphatase, bilirubin. May decrease corticosteroid, testosterone concentrations.

SIDE EFFECTS

OCCASIONAL (3–10%): Nausea, vomiting. **RARE (<2%):** Abdominal pain, diarrhea, headache, dizziness, photophobia, pruritus. Topical application may cause itching, burning, irritation.

ADVERSE REACTIONS/TOXIC EFFECTS

Hematologic toxicity occurs occasionally (thrombocytopenia, hemolytic anemia, leukopenia). Hepatotoxicity may occur within first week to several months of therapy. Anaphylaxis occurs rarely.

NURSING IMPLICATIONS

BASELINE ASSESSMENT:

Question for history of allergies, esp. to ketoconazole (sulfite when using topical cream). Confirm that a culture or histologic test was done for accurate diagnosis; therapy may begin before results known.

INTERVENTION/EVALUATION:

Monitor hepatic function tests; be alert for hepatotoxicity: dark urine, pale stools, fatigue, anorexia/nausea/vomiting (unrelieved by giving medication w/food). Determine pattern of bowel activity, stool consistency, check for blood in stool. Assess mental status (dizziness, somnolence) and provide assistance as needed. Evaluate skin for rash, urticaria, itching. Check sleep pattern. Topical: Check for local burning, itching, irritation.

PATIENT/FAMILY TEACHING:

Prolonged therapy (weeks or months) is usually necessary. Do not miss a dose; continue therapy as long as directed. Avoid alcohol (due to potential liver problem). Wear sunglasses and avoid bright light in event of photophobia. Do not drive car, machinery if dizziness occurs. Take any antacids/anti-ulcer medications at least 2 hrs after ketoconazole. Notify physician of dark urine, pale stool, yellow skin/eyes, increased irritation in topical use, or onset of other new symptom. Consult physician before taking any other medication. Topical: Rub well into affected areas. Avoid contact w/eyes. Keep skin clean, dry; wear light clothing for ventilation. Separate personal items in direct contact w/affected area. Do not use other preparations or occlusive covering w/o consulting physician. Shampoo: Apply shampoo to wet hair to produce enough lather to wash hair and scalp. Leave in place about 1 min, then rinse. Apply shampoo and lather a second time, leaving on scalp 3 min, then rinse again thoroughly. Initially use twice weekly for 4 wks w/at least 3 days between shampooing; frequency then will be determined by response.

ketoprofen

key-toe-**pro**-fen
(Actron, Orudis, Orudis KT, Oruvail)

CANADIAN AVAILABILITY:
Apo-Keto, Orafen, Orudis, Rhodis

CLASSIFICATION

Nonsteroidal anti-inflammatory

AVAILABILITY (Rx)

Tablets: (OTC) 12.5 mg. **Capsules:** 25 mg, 50 mg, 75 mg. **Capsules (extended-release):** 100 mg, 150 mg, 200 mg.

PHARMACOKINETICS

Rapid, complete absorption from GI tract. Primarily metabolized in liver, excreted in urine. Removed by hemodialysis. Half-life: 1.5–4 hrs.

ACTION/ *THERAPEUTIC EFFECT*

Produces analgesic and anti-inflammatory effect by inhibiting prostaglandin synthesis, *reducing inflammatory response and intensity of pain stimulus reaching sensory nerve endings.*

USES/ *UNLABELED*

Symptomatic treatment of acute and chronic rheumatoid arthritis and osteoarthritis. Relief of mild to moderate pain, primary dysmenorrhea. *Treatment of ankylosing spondylitis, psoriatic arthritis, acute gouty arthritis, vascular headache.*

PO ADMINISTRATION

1. May give w/food, milk, or full glass (8 oz) water (minimizes potential GI distress).

2. Do not break, chew extended-release capsules.

INDICATIONS/DOSAGE/ROUTES

Note: Do not exceed 300 mg/day. Oruvail not recommended as initial therapy in pts who are small, >75 yrs of age, or renally impaired.

Acute and chronic rheumatoid arthritis, osteoarthritis:
PO: Adults: Initially, 75 mg three times/day or 50 mg four times/day. **Elderly:** Initially, 25–50 mg 3–4 times/day. **Maintenance:** 150–300 mg/day in 3–4 divided doses. *Extended-release:* 100–200 mg/day as single dose.

Mild to moderate pain, dysmenorrhea:
PO: Adults: 25–50 mg q6–8h.

PRECAUTIONS

CONTRAINDICATIONS: Active peptic ulcer, GI ulceration, chronic inflammation of GI tract, GI bleeding disorders, history of hypersensitivity to aspirin or NSAIDs. **CAUTIONS:** Impaired renal/hepatic function, history of GI tract disease, predisposition to fluid retention. **PREGNANCY/ LACTATION:** Unknown if drug is distributed in breast milk. Avoid use during third trimester (may adversely affect fetal cardiovascular system: premature closure of ductus arteriosus). **Pregnancy Category B**. (Category D if used in 3rd trimester or near delivery.)

INTERACTIONS

DRUG INTERACTIONS: May increase effects of oral anticoagulants, heparin, thrombolytics. May decrease effect of antihypertensives, diuretics. Salicylates, aspirin may increase risk of GI side effects, bleeding. Bone marrow depressants may increase risk of hematologic reactions. May increase concentration, toxicity of lithium. May increase methotrexate toxicity. Probenecid may increase concentration. **ALTERED LAB VALUES:** May prolong bleeding time. May increase alkaline phosphatase, LDH, liver function tests. May decrease sodium, Hgb, Hct.

SIDE EFFECTS

FREQUENT (11%): Dyspepsia (heartburn, indigestion, epigastric pain). **OCCASIONAL (>3%):** Nausea, diarrhea/constipation, flatulence, abdominal cramping, headache. **RARE (<2%):** Anorexia, vomiting, visual disturbances, fluid retention.

ADVERSE REACTIONS/TOXIC EFFECTS

Peptic ulcer, GI bleeding, gastritis, severe hepatic reaction (cholestasis, jaundice) occur rarely. Nephrotoxicity (dysuria, hematuria, proteinuria, nephrotic syndrome) and severe hypersensitivity reaction (bronchospasm, angiofacial edema) occur rarely.

NURSING IMPLICATIONS
BASELINE ASSESSMENT:

Assess onset, type, location, and duration of pain or inflammation. Inspect appearance of affected joints for immobility, deformities, skin condition.

INTERVENTION/EVALUATION:

Monitor for evidence of nausea, dyspepsia. Monitor pattern of daily bowel activity and stool consistency. Assist w/ambulation if dizziness occurs. Check behind medial malleolus for fluid retention (usually first area noted). Evaluate for therapeutic response: relief of pain, stiffness, swelling, increase in joint mobility, reduced joint tenderness, improved grip strength.

PATIENT/FAMILY TEACHING:

Avoid aspirin, alcohol during therapy (increases risk of GI bleeding). If GI upset occurs, take w/food, milk. Avoid tasks that require alertness, motor skills until response to drug is established. Swallow capsule whole; do not crush or chew.

ketorolac tromethamine

key-**tore**-oh-lack
(Toradol, Acular, Acular PF)

CANADIAN AVAILABILITY:
Acular, Toradol

CLASSIFICATION

Nonsteroidal anti-inflammatory

AVAILABILITY (Rx)

Tablets: 10 mg. **Injection:** 15 mg/ml, 30 mg/ml. **Ophthalmic Solution:** 0.5%.

PHARMACOKINETICS

	ONSET	PEAK	DURATION
IM	10 min	1–2 hrs	4–6 hrs
IV	10 min	1–2 hrs	4–6 hrs

Readily absorbed from GI tract, after IM administration. Partially metabolized primarily in kidneys. Primarily excreted in urine. Half-life: 3.8–6.3 hrs (increased in decreased renal function, elderly).

ACTION/ *THERAPEUTIC EFFECT*

Produces analgesic effect by inhibiting prostaglandin synthesis, *reducing intensity of pain stimulus reaching sensory nerve endings.* Reduces prostaglandin levels in aqueous humor, *reducing intraocular inflammation.*

USES/ *UNLABELED*

Short-term relief of mild to moderate pain. Ophthalmic: Relief of ocular itching due to seasonal allergic conjunctivitis. Treatment postop for inflammation following cataract extraction, pain following incisional refractive surgery. *Ophthalmic: Prophylaxis/treatment of ocular inflammation.*

STORAGE/HANDLING

Store oral, parenteral form at room temperature.

PO/IM/IV/OPHTHALMIC ADMINISTRATION

PO:

May give w/food, milk, or antacids if GI distress occurs.

IM:

Give slowly, deeply into muscle.

IV:

Give over at least 15 secs.

OPHTHALMIC:

1. Place finger on lower eyelid and pull out until pocket is formed between eye and lower lid. Hold dropper above pocket and place prescribed number of drops in pocket.

2. Close eye gently. Apply digital pressure to lacrimal sac for 1–2 min (minimized drainage into nose and throat, reducing risk of systemic effects).

3. Remove excess solution w/tissue.

INDICATIONS/DOSAGE/ROUTES

Note: Combined duration of IM/IV and oral not to exceed 5 days. May give as single dose, regular, or as needed schedule.

Analgesic (multiple dosing):
PO: Adults, elderly: 10 mg q4–6h. **Maximum:** 40 mg/24 hrs.
IV/IM: Adults <65 yrs: 30 mg q6h. **Maximum:** 120 mg/24 hrs. **>65 yrs, renally impaired, <50 kg:** 15 mg q6h. **Maximum:** 60 mg/24 hrs.

Analgesic (single dose):
IM: Adults <65 yrs: 60 mg; **>65 yrs, renally impaired, <50 kg:** 30 mg.
IV: Adults <65 yrs: 30 mg; **>65 yrs, renally impaired, <50 kg:** 15 mg.

Usual ophthalmic dosage:
Adults, elderly: 1 drop 4 times/day.

PRECAUTIONS

CONTRAINDICATIONS: Active peptic ulcer, GI ulceration, chronic inflammation of GI tract, GI bleeding disorders, history of hypersensitivity to aspirin or NSAIDs. **CAUTIONS:** Impaired renal/hepatic function, history of GI tract disease, predisposition to fluid retention. **PREGNANCY/LACTATION:** Unknown if drug is excreted in breast milk. Avoid use during third trimester (may adversely affect fetal cardiovascular system: premature closure of ductus arteriosus). **Pregnancy Category C.** (Category D if used in 3rd trimester.)

INTERACTIONS

DRUG INTERACTIONS: May increase effects of oral anticoagulants, heparin, thrombolytics. Salicylates, aspirin may increase risk of GI side effects, bleeding. May increase concentration, toxicity of lithium. May increase methotrexate toxicity. Probenecid may increase concentration. **ALTERED LAB VALUES:** May prolong bleeding time. May increase liver function tests.

SIDE EFFECTS

Note: Age increases possibility of side effects.
FREQUENT (12–17%): Headache, nausea, abdominal cramping/pain, dyspepsia (heartburn, indigestion, epigastric pain). **OCCASIONAL (3–9%):** Diarrhea. *Ophthalmic:* Transient stinging and burning. **RARE (1–3%):** Constipation, vomiting, flatulence, stomatitis. *Ophthalmic:* Ocular irritation, allergic reactions, superficial ocular infection, keratitis.

ADVERSE REACTIONS/TOXIC EFFECTS

GI bleeding, peptic ulcer occur infrequently. Nephrotoxicity (glomerular nephritis, interstitial nephritis, and nephrotic syndrome) may occur in those with preexisting impaired renal function. Acute hypersensitivity reaction (fever, chills, joint pain) occurs rarely.

NURSING IMPLICATIONS
BASELINE ASSESSMENT:

Assess onset, type, location, and duration of pain.

INTERVENTION/EVALUATION:

Assist with ambulation if dizziness occurs. Monitor stool frequency, consistency. Assess for evidence of rash. Evaluate for therapeutic response: relief of pain, stiffness, swelling, increase in joint mobility, reduced joint tenderness, improved grip strength. Be alert to signs of bleeding (may also occur w/ophthalmic due to systemic absorption).

PATIENT/FAMILY TEACHING:

Avoid aspirin, alcohol during therapy w/oral or ophthalmic ketorolac (increases tendency to bleed). If GI upset occurs, take with food, milk. Avoid tasks that require alertness, motor skills until response to drug is established. *Ophthalmic:* Transient stinging and burning may occur upon instillation. Do not administer while wearing soft contact lenses.

ketotifen
(Zaditor)
See Supplement

labetolol hydrochloride

lah-**bet**-ah-lol
(Normodyne, Trandate)

FIXED-COMBINATION(S):
W/hydrochlorothiazide, a diuretic
(Normozide)

CANADIAN AVAILABILITY:
Trandate

CLASSIFICATION

Beta-adrenergic blocker

AVAILABILITY (Rx)

Tablets: 100 mg, 200 mg, 300 mg. **Injection:** 5 mg/ml.

PHARMACOKINETICS

	ONSET	PEAK	DURATION
PO	0.5–2 hrs	2–4 hrs	8–12 hrs
IV	2–5 min	5–15 min	2–4 hrs

Completely absorbed from GI

tract. Undergoes first-pass metabolism. Metabolized in liver. Primarily excreted in urine. Half-life: oral: 6–8 hrs; IV: 5.5 hrs.

ACTION/ *THERAPEUTIC EFFECT*

Selectively blocks beta$_1$-adrenergic receptors, *slowing sinus heart rate, decreasing cardiac output, decreasing B/P* (exact mechanism unknown but may block peripheral adrenergic receptors, decrease sympathetic outflow from CNS or decrease renin release from kidney). Large dose may block beta$_2$-adrenergic receptors, *increasing airway resistance.* Alpha blockage causes *vasodilation, decreased peripheral vascular resistance.*

USES/ *UNLABELED*

Management of mild, moderate, severe hypertension. May be used alone or in combination w/other antihypertensives. *Treatment of chronic angina pectoris; produces controlled hypotension during surgery.*

STORAGE/HANDLING

Store oral, parenteral form at room temperature. After dilution, IV solution is stable for 24 hrs. Solution appears clear, colorless to light yellow. Discard if precipitate forms or discoloration occurs.

PO/IV ADMINISTRATION

PO:

1. May give w/o regard to food.
2. Tablets may be crushed.

IV:

Note: Pt must be in supine position for IV administration and for 3 hrs after receiving medication (substantial drop in B/P on standing should be expected).

1. For IV injection, give over 2 min at 10 min intervals.
2. For IV infusion, dilute 200 mg in 160 ml 5% dextrose, 0.9% NaCl, or other compatible IV fluid to provide concentration of 1 mg/ml.
3. Administer at rate of 2 mg/min (2 ml/min) initially. Rate is adjusted according to B/P.
4. Monitor B/P immediately before, and every 5–10 min during IV administration (maximum effect occurs within 5 min).

INDICATIONS/DOSAGE/ROUTES

Hypertension:
PO: Adults: Initially, 100 mg 2 times/day adjusted in increments of 100 mg 2 times/day every 2–3 days. **Maintenance:** 200–400 mg 2 times/day. **Maximum:** 2.4 g/day.

Usual elderly dosage:
PO: Initially, 100 mg 1–2 times/day. May increase as needed.

Severe hypertension, hypertensive emergency:
IV: Adults: Initially, 20 mg. Additional doses of 20–80 mg may be given at 10 min intervals, up to total dose of 300 mg.
IV Infusion: Adults: Initially, 2 mg/min up to total dose of 300 mg.
PO: Adults: (After IV therapy): Initially, 200 mg; then, 200–400 mg in 6–12 hrs. Increase dose at 1 day intervals to desired level.

PRECAUTIONS

CONTRAINDICATIONS: Bronchial asthma, uncontrolled CHF, second- or third-degree heart block, severe bradycardia, cardiogenic shock. **CAUTIONS:** Drug-controlled CHF, nonallergic bronchospastic disease (chronic bronchitis, emphysema), impaired hepatic, cardiac function, pheochromocytoma, diabetes mellitus. **PREGNANCY/LACTATION:** Drug crosses placenta; small amount distributed in breast milk. **Pregnancy Category C**. (Category D if used in 2nd or 3rd trimester.)

INTERACTIONS

DRUG INTERACTIONS: Diuretics, other hypotensives may increase hypotensive effect; sympathomimetics, xanthines may mutually inhibit effects; may mask symptoms of hypoglycemia, prolong hypoglycemic effect of insulin, oral hypoglycemics. MAO inhibitors may produce hypertension. **ALTERED LAB VALUES:** May increase ANA titer, SGOT (AST), SGPT (ALT), alkaline phosphatase, LDH, bilirubin, BUN, creatinine, potassium uric acid, lipoproteins, triglycerides.

SIDE EFFECTS

FREQUENT: Drowsiness, trouble sleeping, unusually tired or weak, decreased sexual ability. **OCCASIONAL:** Dizziness, difficulty breathing, swelling of hands/feet, depression, anxiety, constipation, diarrhea, nasal congestion, nausea, vomiting, stomach discomfort. **RARE:** Altered taste, dry eyes, increased urination, numbness or tingling in fingers, toes, or scalp.

ADVERSE REACTIONS/TOXIC EFFECTS

May precipitate or aggravate CHF (due to decreased myocardial stimulation). Abrupt withdrawal may precipitate ischemic heart disease, producing sweating, palpitations, headache, tremulousness. Beta blockers may mask signs, symptoms of acute hypoglycemia (tachycardia, B/P changes) in diabetic pts.

NURSING IMPLICATIONS
BASELINE ASSESSMENT:

Assess baseline renal/liver function tests. Assess B/P, apical pulse immediately before drug is administered (if pulse is 60/min or below, or systolic B/P is below 90 mm Hg, withhold medication, contact physician).

INTERVENTION/EVALUATION:

Monitor B/P for hypotension, respiration for shortness of breath. Assess pulse for strength/weakness, irregular rate, bradycardia. Monitor EKG for cardiac arrhythmias. Monitor stool frequency and consistency. Assist w/ambulation if dizziness occurs. Assess for evidence of CHF: dyspnea (particularly on exertion or lying down), night cough, peripheral edema, distended neck veins. Monitor I&O (increase in weight, decrease in urine output may indicate CHF). Assess for nausea, diaphoresis, headache, fatigue.

PATIENT/FAMILY TEACHING:

Do not discontinue drug except upon advice of physician (abrupt discontinuation may precipitate heart failure). Transient scalp tingling may occur, esp. when drug is initiated. Compliance w/therapy regimen is essential to control hypertension, arrhythmias. Avoid tasks that require alertness, motor skills until response to drug is established. Report shortness of breath, excessive fatigue, weight gain, prolonged dizziness or headache. Do not use nasal decongestants, OTC cold preparations (stimulants) w/o physician approval. Outpatients should monitor B/P, pulse before taking medication. Restrict salt, alcohol intake.

lactulose
lack-tyoo-lows
(Chronulac, Evalose, Heptalac)

CANADIAN AVAILABILITY:
Acilac, Duphalac, Laxilose

CLASSIFICATION

Laxative: Osmotic

AVAILABILITY (Rx)

Syrup: 10 g/15 ml

PHARMACOKINETICS

	ONSET	PEAK	DURATION
PO	24–48 hrs	—	—
Rectal	30–60 min	—	—

Poorly absorbed from GI tract. Acts in colon.

ACTION/*THERAPEUTIC EFFECT*

Retains ammonia in colon (decreases blood ammonia concentration), producing osmotic effect. *Promotes increased peristalsis, bowel evacuation (expelling ammonia from colon).*

USES

Prevention/treatment of portal systemic encephalopathy (including hepatic precoma, coma); treatment of constipation.

STORAGE/HANDLING

Store solution at room temperature. Solution appears pale yellow to yellow, sweet, viscous liquid. Cloudiness, darkened solutions do not indicate potency loss.

PO/RECTAL ADMINISTRATION

PO:

Drink water, juice, or milk w/each dose (aids stool softening, increases palatability).

RECTALLY:

1. Lubricate anus w/petroleum jelly before enema insertion.

2. Insert carefully (prevents damage to rectal wall) w/nozzle toward navel.

3. Squeeze container until entire dose expelled.

4. Retain until definite lower abdominal cramping felt.

INDICATIONS/DOSAGE/ROUTES

Constipation:
PO: Adults, elderly: 15–30 ml/day up to 60 ml/day.

Portal-systemic encephalopathy:
PO: Adults, elderly: Initially, 30–45 ml every hour. Then, 30–45 ml 3–4 times/day. Adjust dose every 1–2 days to produce 2–3 soft stools/day. **Children:** 40–90 ml/day in divided doses. **Infants:** 2.5–10 ml/day in divided doses.

Usual rectal dosage (as retention enema):
Adults, elderly: 300 ml w/700 ml water or saline; retain 30–60 min; repeat every 4–6 hrs. (If evacuation occurs too promptly, repeat immediately.)

PRECAUTIONS

CONTRAINDICATIONS: Those on galactose-free diet, abdominal pain, nausea, vomiting, appendicitis. **CAUTIONS:** Diabetes mellitus. **PREGNANCY/LACTATION:** Unknown if drug crosses placenta or is distributed in breast milk. **Pregnancy Category B.**

INTERACTIONS

DRUG INTERACTIONS: May decrease transit time of concurrently administered oral medication, decreasing absorption. **ALTERED LAB VALUES:** May decrease potassium concentration.

SIDE EFFECTS

OCCASIONAL: Cramping, diarrhea, flatulence, increased thirst, abdominal discomfort. **RARE:** Nausea, vomiting.

574 / **lamivudine**

ADVERSE REACTIONS/TOXIC EFFECTS

Diarrhea indicates overdosage. Long-term use may result in laxative dependence, chronic constipation, loss of normal bowel function.

NURSING IMPLICATIONS

INTERVENTION/EVALUATION:

Encourage adequate fluid intake. Assess bowel sounds for peristalsis. Monitor daily bowel activity and stool consistency (watery, loose, soft, semisolid, solid) and record time of evacuation. Assess for abdominal disturbances. Monitor serum electrolytes in those exposed to prolonged, frequent, or excessive use of medication.

PATIENT/FAMILY TEACHING:

Evacuation occurs in 24–48 hrs of initial dose. Institute measures to promote defecation: Increase fluid intake, exercise, high-fiber diet. Cola, unsalted crackers, dry toast may relieve nausea.

lamivudine

lah-**mih**-view-deen
(Epivir)

FIXED-COMBINATION(S):
w/zidovudine, an antiviral (**Combivir**)

CANADIAN AVAILABILITY:
3TC

CLASSIFICATION

Antiviral

AVAILABILITY (Rx)

Tablets: 100 mg, 150 mg. **Oral Solution:** 5 mg/ml, 10 mg/ml

PHARMACOKINETICS

Rapidly, completely absorbed from GI tract. Widely distributed (crosses blood-brain barrier). Primarily excreted unchanged in urine. Unknown if removed by hemo/peritoneal dialysis. Half-life: 11–15 hrs (intracellular); serum (adults) 2–11 hrs, (children) 1.7–2 hrs. Half-life increases w/diminished renal function.

ACTION/THERAPEUTIC EFFECT

Inhibits HIV reverse transcriptase via viral DNA chain termination. Also inhibits RNA- and DNA-dependent DNA polymerase, an enzyme necessary for viral HIV replication, *slowing HIV replication, reducing progression of HIV infection.*

USES/UNLABELED

Used in combination w/zidovudine for treatment of HIV infection when therapy is necessary based on clinical or immunologic evidence of disease. Treatment for chronic hepatitis B. *Prophylaxis in health-care workers at risk of acquiring HIV after occupational exposure to virus.*

PO ADMINISTRATION

May give w/o regard to meals.

INDICATIONS/DOSAGE/ROUTES

Note: Complete prescribing information for zidovudine should be consulted before concurrent therapy w/lamivudine and zidovudine is begun.

HIV infection:
PO: Adults, children 12–16 yrs, >50 kg (>100 lbs): 150 mg twice daily in combination w/zidovudine. **Adults <50 kg:** 2 mg/kg twice daily in combination w/zidovudine. **Children 3 mos–12 yrs:** 4 mg/kg twice daily (up to 150 mg) in combination w/zidovudine.

Chronic hepatitis B:
PO: Adults: 100 mg daily.

Dosage in renal impairment:
Dose and/or frequency is modified based on creatinine clearance.

CREATININE CLEARANCE	DOSAGE
≤ 50	150 mg twice daily
30–49	150 mg once daily
15–29	150 mg first dose, then 100 mg once daily
5–14	150 mg first dose, then 50 mg once daily
< 5	50 mg first dose, then 25 mg once daily

PRECAUTIONS

CONTRAINDICATIONS: None sig-nif-icant. **CAUTIONS:** Peripheral neuropathy or history of peripheral neuropathy, history of pancreatitis in children, impaired renal function. **PREGNANCY/LACTATION:** Drug crosses placenta; unknown if distributed in breast milk. Breast-feeding not recommended (possibility of HIV transmission). **Pregnancy Category C**.

INTERACTIONS

DRUG INTERACTIONS: Trimethoprim-sulfamethoxazole increases lamivudine concentration. **ALTERED LAB VALUES:** May increase neutrophil count, SGOT (AST), SGPT (ALT), amylase serum level, Hgb.

SIDE EFFECTS

FREQUENT: Headache (35%), nausea (33%), malaise/fatigue (27%), nasal disturbances (20%), diarrhea, cough (18%), musculoskeletal pain, neuropathy (12%), insomnia (11%), anorexia, dizziness, fever/chills (10%). **OCCASIONAL:** Depression, (9%), myalgia (8%), abdominal cramps (6%), dyspepsia, arthralgia (5%).

ADVERSE REACTIONS/TOXIC EFFECTS

Pancreatitis occurs in 13% of pediatric pts. Anemia, neutropenia, thrombocytopenia occur rarely.

NURSING IMPLICATIONS
BASELINE ASSESSMENT:

Offer emotional support. Estab-lish baseline lab values, esp. renal function. Advise parents to closely monitor pediatric pts for symptoms of pancreatitis (severe, steady abdominal pain often radiating to the back, clammy skin, reduced B/P; nausea and vomiting may accompany abdominal pain). Question for hypersensitivity to lamivudine, pregnancy.

INTERVENTION/EVALUATION:

Monitor amylase, lipase, BUN, serum creatinine. Assess for headache, nausea, cough. Determine pattern of bowel activity and stool consistency. Modify diet, or administer laxative as needed. Assess for dizziness, sleep pattern. If pancreatitis in children occurs, movement aggravates abdominal pain; sitting up or flexion at the waist relieves the pain.

PATIENT/FAMILY TEACHING:

Continue therapy for full length of treatment. Doses should be evenly spaced. Do not take any medications w/o consulting physician. Inform pt lamivudine is not a cure and pt may continue to experience illnesses, including opportunistic infections. Do not drive, use machinery, or engage in other activities that require mental acuity if experiencing dizziness.

lamotrigine
lam-**oh**-trih-geen
(Lamictal)

CANADIAN AVAILABILITY:
Lamictal

CLASSIFICATION

Anticonvulsant

AVAILABILITY (Rx)

Tablets: 25 mg, 100 mg, 150 mg, 200 mg. **Chewable Tablets:** 5 mg, 25 mg.

PHARMACOKINETICS

Rapidly, completely absorbed following oral administration (not affected by food). Binds to melanin-containing tissue (e.g., eye, pigmented skin). Metabolized in liver. Primarily excreted unchanged in urine. Partially removed by hemodialysis. Half-life: 7.5–12.5 hrs (increased in pts receiving other anticonvulsants).

ACTION / THERAPEUTIC EFFECT

Exact mechanism unknown. May be due to inhibition of voltage-sensitive sodium channels, stabilizing neuronal membranes and regulating presynaptic transmitter release of excitatory amino acids, *producing anticonvulsant activity.*

USES / UNLABELED

Adjunctive therapy in adults w/partial seizures, adults and children in treatment of generalized seizures of Lennox-Gastaut syndrome. Conversion to monotherapy in adults treated w/another enzyme-inducing antiepileptic drug (EIAED).

INDICATIONS / DOSAGE / ROUTES

Note: If pt currently on valproic acid, reduce lamotrigine dosage to less than half the normal dosage.

Seizure control in pts receiving enzyme-inducing antiepileptic drugs (AEDs), but not valproate:
PO: Adults, elderly, children >12 yrs: Recommended as add-on therapy: 50 mg once/day for 2 wks, followed by 100 mg/day in 2 divided doses for 2 wks. **Maintenance:** Dose may be increased by 100 mg/day every week, up to 300–500 mg/day in 2 divided doses.

Addition for without valproic acid:
Children (2–12 yrs): 0.6 mg/kg/day in 2 divided doses for 2 wks; then 1.2 mg/kg/day in 2 divided doses for wks 3 and 4. **Maintenance:** 5–15 mg/kg/day. **Maximum:** 400 mg/day.

Seizure control in pts receiving combination therapy of valproic acid and enzyme-inducing antiepileptic drugs (AEDs):
PO: Adults, elderly, children >12 yrs: 25 mg every other day for 2 wks, followed by 25 mg once/day for 2 wks. **Maintenance:** Dose may be increased by 25–50 mg/day every 1–2 wks, up to 150 mg/day in 2 divided doses.

Addition for with valproic acid:
Children (2–12 yrs): 0.15 mg/kg/day in 2 divided doses for 2 wks; then 0.3 mg/kg/day in 2 divided doses for wks 3 and 4. **Maintenance:** 1–5 mg/kg/day in 2 divided doses. **Maximum:** 200 mg/day.

Conversion to monotherapy:
PO: Adults, children >12 yrs: Add lamotrigine 50 mg/day for 2 wks; then 100 mg/day during wks 3 and 4; then increase by 100 mg/day q1–2 wks until maintenance dosage achieved (300–500 mg/day in 2 divided doses/day). Gradually discontinue other EIAED over 4 wks once maintenance dose achieved.

Renal function impairment:
Note: Same dosage as combination therapy (see above).

Discontinuation therapy:
Note: A reduction in dosage over at least 2 wks (approx. 50% per week) is recommended.

PRECAUTIONS

CONTRAINDICATIONS: None significant. **CAUTIONS:** Renal/hepatic function impairment, cardiac function impairment. **PREGNANCY/ LACTATION:** Reduced fetal weight, delayed ossification noted in animals. Distributed in breast milk. Breast-feeding not recommended. **Pregnancy Category C**.

INTERACTIONS

DRUG INTERACTIONS: Lamotrigine may increase carbamazepine, valproic acid serum levels. Phenobarbital, primidone, phenytoin, carbamazepine, valproic acid decreases lamotrigine concentration. **ALTERED LAB VALUES:** None significant.

SIDE EFFECTS

FREQUENT: Dizziness (38%), double vision (28%), headache (29%), ataxia [muscular incoordination] (22%), nausea (19%), blurred vision (16%), somnolence, rhinitis (14%). **OCCASIONAL:** Rash (10%), pharyngitis, vomiting (9%), cough (8%), flu syndrome (7%), diarrhea, dysmenorrhea, fever, insomnia (6%), dyspepsia (5%). **RARE:** Constipation, tremor, anxiety, pruritus, vaginitis.

ADVERSE REACTIONS/TOXIC EFFECTS

Abrupt withdrawal may increase seizure frequency. Severe, potentially life threatening rash.

NURSING IMPLICATIONS
BASELINE ASSESSMENT:

Review history of seizure disorder (type, onset, intensity, frequency, duration, level of consciousness), drug history (esp. other anticonvulsants), other medical conditions (e.g., renal function impairment). Provide safety precautions, quiet, dark environment. Obtain vital signs.

INTERVENTION/EVALUATION:

Report to physician promptly if evidence of rash occurs (drug discontinuation may be necessary). Assist w/ambulation if dizziness, ataxia occurs. Observe frequently for recurrence of seizure activity. Assess for clinical improvement (decrease in intensity/frequency of seizures). Assess for visual abnormalities, headache.

PATIENT/FAMILY TEACHING:

Take lamotrigine only as prescribed; do not abruptly withdraw medication after long-term therapy. Avoid tasks that require alertness, motor skills until response to drug is established. Avoid alcohol. Carry identification card/bracelet to note anticonvulsant therapy. Strict maintenance of drug therapy is essential for seizure control. If noncompliance is an issue in causing acute seizures, discuss reasons for noncompliance and address it. Report first sign of rash to physician.

lansoprazole

lan-sew-**prah**-zoll
(Prevacid)

CANADIAN AVAILABILITY:
Prevacid

CLASSIFICATION

Gastric acid pump inhibitor

AVAILABILITY (Rx)

Capsules (extended-release): 15 mg, 30 mg

PHARMACOKINETICS

	ONSET	PEAK	DURATION
15 mg	2–3 hrs	—	24 hrs
30 mg	1–2 hrs	—	>24 hrs

Once leaving stomach, rapid and complete absorption (food may decrease absorption). Distributed primarily to gastric parietal cells, converted to two active metabolites.

Extensively metabolized in liver. Eliminated from body in bile and urine. Half-life: 1.5 hrs (increased in elderly, pts w/liver impairment).

ACTION/*THERAPEUTIC EFFECT*

Converted to active metabolites that irreversibly bind to and inhibit H+/K+ ATPase (an enzyme on surface of gastric parietal cells). Inhibits hydrogen ion transport into gastric lumen, *increasing gastric pH, reducing gastric acid production.*

USES/*UNLABELED*

Short-term treatment (up to 4 wks) for healing and symptomatic relief of active duodenal ulcer, short-term treatment (up to 8 wks) for healing and symptomatic relief of erosive esophagitis. Long-term treatment of pathologic hypersecretory conditions including Zollinger-Ellison syndrome. Short-term treatment (up to 8 wks) of active gastric ulcer. *H. pylori*-associated duodenal ulcer, maintenance treatment for healed duodenal ulcer. Treatment for gastroesophageal reflux disease (GERD).

PO ADMINISTRATION

1. Give while fasting or before meals (food diminishes absorption).
2. Do not chew or crush delayed-release capsules.
3. If pt has difficulty swallowing capsules, open capsules and sprinkle granules on 1 tablespoon of applesauce and swallow immediately.

INDICATIONS/DOSAGE/ROUTES

Duodenal ulcer:
PO: Adults, elderly: 15–30 mg/day, before eating, preferably in AM, for up to 4 wks.

Erosive esophagitis:
PO: Adults, elderly: 30 mg/day, before eating, for up to 8 wks. If healing does not occur within 8 wks (5–10%), may give for additional 8 wks.

Gastric ulcer:
PO: Adults: 30 mg/day for up to 8 wks.

Healed duodenal ulcer, GERD:
PO: Adults: 15 mg/day

H. pylori:
PO: Adults: 30 mg 2 times/day for 10 days (w/amoxicillin, clarithromycin).

Pathologic hypersecretory conditions (including Zollinger-Ellison syndrome):
PO: Adults, elderly: 60 mg/day. Individualize dosage according to pt needs and for as long as clinically indicated. May increase to >120 mg/day in divided doses.

PRECAUTIONS

CONTRAINDICATIONS: None significant. **CAUTIONS:** Impaired hepatic function. **PREGNANCY/LACTATION:** Unknown if distributed in breast milk. **Pregnancy Category B.**

INTERACTIONS

DRUG INTERACTIONS: May interfere with ketoconazole, ampicillin, iron salts, digoxin absorption. Sucralfate may delay lansoprazole absorption (give lansoprazole 30 min before sucralfate). **ALTERED LAB VALUES:** May increase SGOT (AST), SGPT (ALT), serum creatinine, alkaline phosphatase, bilirubin, triglycerides, uric acid, LDH, cholesterol. May produce abnormal WBC, RBC and platelet counts, albumin/globulin ratio, electrolyte balance. May increase Hct, Hgb.

SIDE EFFECTS

OCCASIONAL (2–3%): Diarrhea, abdominal pain, rash, pruritus, altered appetite. **RARE (1%):** Nausea, headache.

ADVERSE REACTIONS/TOXIC EFFECTS

Bilirubinemia, eosinophilia, hyperlipemia occur rarely.

NURSING IMPLICATIONS
BASELINE ASSESSMENT:

Obtain baseline lab values. Assess drug history, esp. use of sucralfate.

INTERVENTION/EVALUATION:

Monitor ongoing laboratory results. Assess for therapeutic response, i.e., relief of GI symptoms. Question if diarrhea, abdominal pain, nausea occur.

PATIENT/FAMILY TEACHING:

Do not chew or crush delayed-release capsules. For those who have difficulty swallowing capsules, open capsules and sprinkle granules on 1 tablespoon of applesauce and swallow immediately. Report any adverse reactions.

---

latanoprost

lah-**tan**-oh-prost
(Xalatan)

CANADIAN AVAILABILITY:
Xalatan

CLASSIFICATION

Anti-glaucoma (prostaglandin)

AVAILABILITY (Rx)

Solution: 0.005% (50 mcg/ml)

PHARMACOKINETICS

	ONSET	PEAK	DURATION
Ophthalmic	3–4 hrs	8–12 hrs	24 hrs

A prodrug, rapidly hydrolyzed to active latanoprost acid in the cornea/plasma. Only minimal amount penetrates the eye (balance absorbed into systemic circulation, which is metabolized in liver and primarily excreted in urine). Half-life: 17 min.

ACTION/*THERAPEUTIC EFFECT*

Increases uveoscleral (iris, ciliary body, choroid, sclera) outflow of aqueous humor, *decreasing intraocular pressure (IOP), ocular hypertension.*

USES

Reduces intraocular pressure (IOP) in management of chronic open-angle glaucoma, ocular hypertension in pts intolerant of other IOP-lowering medications or insufficiently responsive to another IOP-lowering medication.

STORAGE/HANDLING

Refrigerate unopened bottle. Once opened, may store container at room temperature for up to 6 wks.

OPHTHALMIC ADMINISTRATION

1. Instruct pt to lie down or tilt head backward and look up.
2. Gently pull lower eyelid down to form pocket between eye and lower lid. Hold dropper above pocket and place prescribed number of drops in pocket (do not touch tip of applicator to any surface).
3. Close eye gently. Apply gentle finger pressure to lacrimal sac (bridge of nose, inside corner of eye) for 1–2 min (minimizes drainage into nose and throat, reducing risk of systemic effects).
4. Remove excess solution around eye w/tissue.
5. Tell pt not to close eyes tightly or blink more often than necessary.
6. Never rinse dropper.

INDICATIONS/DOSAGE/ROUTES

Note: May be used concurrently w/other topical ophthalmics to lower IOP, but administer the medications at least 5 min apart (may cause precipitate).

Glaucoma:
PO: Adults, elderly: One drop

(1.5 mcg) in affected eye(s) once daily in the evening.

PRECAUTIONS

CONTRAINDICATIONS: Hypersensitivity to latanoprost or any component of medication. **CAUTIONS:** None significant. **PREGNANCY/LACTATION:** Unknown if distributed in breast milk. **Pregnancy Category C**.

INTERACTIONS

DRUG INTERACTIONS: None significant. **ALTERED LAB VALUES:** None significant.

SIDE EFFECTS

FREQUENT (5–15%): Transient blurred vision, burning/stinging, foreign body sensation, conjunctival hyperemia (excess blood), change in eye color (increase in amount of brown pigment), itching. **OCCASIONAL (<4%):** Dry eye, eye pain, lid crusting, excessive tearing, lid edema, lid erythema, lid discomfort/pain, photophobia. **RARE:** Conjunctivitis, blurred vision, eye discharge, darkened eyelids/eyelashes; increased growth of eyelashes.

ADVERSE REACTIONS/TOXIC EFFECTS

Systemic events produce upper respiratory tract infection/cold/flu (4%), and rarely, musculoskeletal pain, chest pain, angina pectoris, allergic skin reaction (1–2%).

NURSING IMPLICATIONS

BASELINE ASSESSMENT:

Question for hypersensitivity to latanoprost or any component of medication. Assess physical appearance of eye and pt's perception of vision.

INTERVENTION/EVALUATION:

Monitor for potential systemic reaction.

PATIENT/FAMILY TEACHING:

Inform pt of possibility of iris color change, darkened eyelids/eyelashes, longer eyelashes, increased amount of brown pigment (more noticeable w/green-brown, blue/gray-brown or yellow-brown iris). Change may be permanent. Remove contact lenses prior to administration. Lenses may be inserted 15 min following administration. Instruct pt on proper administration of drops, particularly to avoid allowing tip of container to contact eye or surrounding area (increased risk of ocular infections due to contamination). If more than one ophthalmic drug is being used, administer drugs at least 5 min apart. Transient stinging, transient blurred vision, or foreign body sensation is common; notify physician if conjunctivitis or lid reaction occurs.

leflunomide
(Atrava)
See Supplement

lepirudin
(Refludan)
See Supplement

letrozole
(Femara)
See Supplement

leucovorin calcium (folinic acid, citrovorum factor)
lou-**koe**-vor-in
(Wellcovorin)

CANADIAN AVAILABILITY:
Lederle, Leucovorin

CLASSIFICATION

Folic acid antagonist

AVAILABILITY (Rx)

Tablets: 5 mg, 15 mg, 25 mg.
Injection: 3 mg/ml. **Powder for Injection:** 50 mg, 100 mg, 350 mg.

PHARMACOKINETICS

Readily absorbed from GI tract. Widely distributed. Primarily concentrated in liver. Metabolized in liver, intestinal mucosa to active metabolite. Primarily excreted in urine. Half-life: 6.2 hrs.

ACTION/*THERAPEUTIC EFFECT*

Competes w/methotrexate for same transport processes into cells (limits methotrexate action on normal cells). *Allows purine, DNA, RNA, protein synthesis.*

USES

Antidote (diminishes toxicity, counteracts effect of unintentional overdose of folic acid antagonists [e.g., methotrexate]); prevention/treatment of undesired hematopoietic effects of folic acid antagonists (e.g., rescue w/high-dose methotrexate therapy); treatment of megaloblastic anemias due to folic acid deficiency. Palliative treatment of advanced colorectal cancer (in combination w/5-fluorouracil).

STORAGE/HANDLING

Store tablets/vials for parenteral use at room temperature. Injection is clear, yellowish solution.

IM/IV ADMINISTRATION

PO:

Scored tablets may be crushed.

IV:

1. Reconstitute each 50 mg vial w/5 ml sterile water for injection or bacteriostatic water for injection containing benzyl alcohol to provide concentration of 10 mg/ml. Due to benzyl alcohol in 1 mg ampule and in bacteriostatic water, reconstitute doses >10 mg/m² w/sterile water.

2. Use immediately if reconstituted w/sterile water; stable for 7 days if reconstituted w/bacteriostatic water for injection.

3. Further dilute w/5% dextrose or 0.9% NaCl.

4. Do not exceed 160 mg/min if given by IV infusion (because of calcium content).

INDICATIONS/DOSAGE/ROUTES

Antidote, prevention/treatment of hematopoietic effects of folic acid antagonists:
Note: For rescue therapy in cancer chemotherapy, refer to specific protocol being used for optimal dosage and sequence of leucovorin administration.
Conventional Rescue Dosage: 10 mg/m² parenterally one time then q6h orally until serum methotrexate <10⁻⁸M. If 24 hr serum creatinine increased by 50% or more over baseline or methotrexate >5 × 10⁻⁶M or 48 hr level >9 × 10⁻⁷M, increase to 100 mg/m² IV q3h until methotrexate level <10⁻⁸M.

Megaloblastic anemia:
IM: Adults: Up to 1 mg/day.

Advanced colorectal cancer:
IV: Adults: 200 mg/m² over minimum of 3 min (follow w/5-fluorouracil 370 mg/m² by IV injection) or 20 mg/m² (follow w/5-fluorouracil 425 mg/m²). Repeat daily for 5 days; repeat cycle at 4 wk intervals for 2 cycles; then, at 4–5 wk intervals. **Note:** Do not start next cycle until pt recovered from prior treatment course (until WBC is 4,000/mm³ and platelets are 130,000/mm³).

PRECAUTIONS

CONTRAINDICATIONS: Pernicious anemia, other megaloblastic anemias secondary to vitamin B$_{12}$ deficiency. **CAUTIONS:** History of allergies, bronchial asthma. *W/5-fluorouracil:* Pts w/GI toxicities (more common/severe). **PREGNANCY/ LACTATION:** Unknown if drug crosses placenta or is distributed in breast milk. **Pregnancy Category C**.

INTERACTIONS

DRUG INTERACTIONS: May decrease effect of anticonvulsants. May increase effect, toxicity of 5-fluorouracil. **ALTERED LAB VALUES:** None significant.

SIDE EFFECTS

FREQUENT: *W/5-fluorouracil:* Diarrhea, stomatitis, nausea, vomiting, lethargy/malaise/fatigue, alopecia, anorexia. **OCCASIONAL:** Urticaria, dermatitis.

ADVERSE REACTIONS/TOXIC EFFECTS

Excessive dosage may negate chemotherapeutic effect of folic acid antagonists. Anaphylaxis occurs rarely. Diarrhea may cause rapid clinical deterioration and death.

NURSING IMPLICATIONS

BASELINE ASSESSMENT:

Give as soon as possible, preferably within 1 hr, for treatment of accidental overdosage of folic acid antagonists.

INTERVENTION/EVALUATION:

Monitor for vomiting—may need to change from oral to parenteral therapy. Observe elderly and debilitated closely because of risk of severe toxicities. Assess CBC, differential, platelet count (also electrolytes and liver function tests for combination w/5-fluorouracil).

PATIENT/FAMILY TEACHING:

Explain purpose of medication in treatment of cancer. Report allergic reaction, vomiting.

leuprolide acetate

leu-pro-lied
(Lupron, Lupron Depot Ped)

CANADIAN AVAILABILITY: Lupron

CLASSIFICATION

Antineoplastic

AVAILABILITY (Rx)

Injection: 5 mg/ml. **Lypholized Microspheres for Injection:** 3.75 mg, 7.5 mg, 11.25 mg, 15 mg, 22.5 mg, 30 mg.

PHARMACOKINETICS

Rapid, well absorbed after SubQ administration. Slow absorption after IM administration. Half-life: 3–4 hrs.

ACTION/ *THERAPEUTIC EFFECT*

Initial or intermittent administration stimulates release of luteinizing hormone (LH) and follicle-stimulating hormone (FSH) from anterior pituitary, increasing (within 1 wk) testosterone level in males, estradiol in premenopausal women. Continuous daily administration suppresses secretion of gonadotropin-releasing hormone, *producing fall (within 2–4 wks) in testosterone levels to castrate level in males, estrogen level in premenopausal women to postmenopausal levels. In central precocious puberty, gonadotropins reduced to prepubertal levels.*

USES

Treatment of advanced prostatic carcinoma, endometriosis, central precocious puberty, uterine fibroid tumors, anemia caused by uterine leiomyomata.

STORAGE/HANDLING

Note: May be carcinogenic, mutagenic, or teratogenic. Handle w/extreme care during preparation/administration.

Injection appears clear, colorless. Refrigerate. Store opened vial at room temperature. Discard if precipitate forms or solution appears discolored. *Depot vials:* Store at room temperature. Reconstitute only w/diluent provided; use immediately. Do not use needles <22 gauge.

SUBQ ADMINISTRATION

Use syringes provided by manufacturer (0.5 ml low-dose insulin syringe may be used as alternative).

INDICATIONS/DOSAGE/ROUTES

Prostatic carcinoma:
SubQ: Adults, elderly: 1 mg daily.
IM: Adults, elderly: *Depot:* 7.5 mg q28–33 days or 22.5 mg q3 mos or 30 mg q4 mos.

Endometriosis, uterine leiomyomata:
IM: Adults: *Depot:* 3.75 mg monthly or 11.25 mg as single injection.

Central precocious puberty:
SubQ: Children: Initially, 50 mcg/kg/day; if down regulation not achieved, titrate upward by 10 mcg/kg/day.
IM: Children: Initially, 0.3 mg/kg/4 wks (minimum: 7.5 mg); if down regulation not achieved, titrate upward in 3.75 mg increments q4 wks.

PRECAUTIONS

CONTRAINDICATIONS: None significant. **EXTREME CAUTION:** Pts w/life-threatening disease when rapid symptomatic relief is necessary. **CAUTIONS:** Hypersensitivity to benzyl alcohol. **PREGNANCY/LACTATION:** *Depot:* Contraindicated in pregnancy. May cause spontaneous abortion. **Pregnancy Category X.**

INTERACTIONS

DRUG INTERACTIONS: None significant. **ALTERED LAB VALUES:** May increase serum acid phosphatase. Initially increases testosterone, then decreases testosterone concentration.

SIDE EFFECTS

FREQUENT: Hot flashes (ranging from mild flushing to sweating). *Females:* Amenorrhea, spotting. **OCCASIONAL:** Arrhythmias/palpitations, blurred vision, dizziness, edema, headache, burning/itching, swelling at injection site, nausea, insomnia, increased weight. *Females:* Deepening voice, increased hair growth, decreased libido, increased breast tenderness, vaginitis, altered mood. *Males:* Constipation, decreased testicle size, gynecomastia, impotence, decreased appetite, angina. **RARE:** *Males:* Thrombophlebitis.

ADVERSE REACTIONS/TOXIC EFFECTS

Occasionally, a worsening of signs/symptoms of prostatic carcinoma occurs 1–2 wks after initial dosing (subsides during continued therapy). Increased bone pain and less frequently dysuria or hematuria, weakness or paresthesia of lower extremities may be noted. Myocardial infarction, pulmonary embolism occur rarely.

NURSING IMPLICATIONS

BASELINE ASSESSMENT:

Question for possibility of pregnancy before initiating therapy (Pregnancy Category X). Obtain serum testosterone, prostatic acid phosphatase (PAP) levels periodically during therapy.

Serum testosterone and PAP levels should increase during first week of therapy. Testosterone level then should decrease to baseline level or less within 2 wks, PAP level within 4 wks.

INTERVENTION/EVALUATION:

Monitor closely for signs/symptoms of worsening of disease.

PATIENT/FAMILY TEACHING:

Hot flashes tend to decrease during continued therapy. A temporary exacerbation of signs/symptoms of disease may occur during first few weeks of therapy.

---

levalbuterol

(Xopenex)
See Supplement
See Classification section under:
Bronchodilators

---

levamisole hydrochloride

lev-**am**-ih-sole
(Ergamisol)

CANADIAN AVAILABILITY:
Ergamisol

CLASSIFICATION

Antineoplastic

AVAILABILITY (Rx)

Tablets: 50 mg

PHARMACOKINETICS

Rapidly absorbed from GI tract. Metabolized in liver. Primarily excreted in urine. Half-life: 3–4 hrs.

ACTION/THERAPEUTIC EFFECT

Stimulates T-cell activation and proliferation; augments monocyte and macrophage activity; increases neutrophil stimulation, mobility. *Restores depressed immune function.*

USES/UNLABELED

Adjunctive treatment with concurrent use of fluorouracil after surgical resection in those with Duke's stage C colon cancer. *Treatment of malignant melanoma.*

INDICATIONS/DOSAGE/ROUTES

Colon cancer:
PO: Adults, elderly: Initially, 50 mg q8h for 3 days (begin 7–30 days postop); repeat 50 mg q8h for 3 days every 2 wks for 1 yr.

PRECAUTIONS

CONTRAINDICATIONS: None significant. **PREGNANCY/LACTATION:** Unknown if drug crosses placenta or is distributed in breast milk. **Pregnancy Category C.**

INTERACTIONS

DRUG INTERACTIONS: Bone marrow depressants may increase bone marrow depression. **ALTERED LAB VALUES:** None significant.

SIDE EFFECTS

FREQUENT (10–20%): Diarrhea, nausea, metallic taste. **OCCASIONAL (3–10%):** Muscle or joint pain, anxiety, dizziness, headache, inability to sleep, unusual tiredness, skin rash, itching, vomiting, alopecia. **RARE (1–3%):** Numbness in hand, face, feet, blurred vision, confusion, ataxia, sezures, tradive dyskinesia, tremors, liver toxicity.

ADVERSE REACTIONS/TOXIC EFFECTS

Earliest sign of toxicity (4–8 days after beginning therapy) is stomatitis (dry mouth, burning sensation, mucosal erythema, ulceration at inner margin of lips). Most common dermatologic toxicity is pruritic rash (generally appears on extremities, less frequently on trunk). Leukopenia generally occurs within 9–14 days after drug administration (may occur as late as 25th day). Thrombocytopenia occasionally occurs within 7–17 days after administration. Hematologic toxicity may also manifest itself as agranulocytosis, evidenced as fever, chills.

NURSING IMPLICATIONS
BASELINE ASSESSMENT:

Give emotional support to pt and family. Perform neurologic function tests prior to chemotherapy. Check blood counts prior to each course of therapy, monthly or as clinically indicated. Drug should be discontinued if intractable vomiting, diarrhea, stomatitis, GI bleeding occurs.

INTERVENTION/EVALUATION:

Monitor for hematologic toxicity (fever, sore throat, signs of local infection, easy bruising, unusual bleeding), symptoms of anemia (excessive tiredness, weakness). Measure all vomitus (general guideline requiring immediate notification of physician: 750 ml/8 hrs, urinary output less than 100 ml/hr). Monitor for rapidly falling WBC and/or intractable diarrhea, GI bleeding (bright red or tarry stool). Assess oral mucosa for mucosal erythema, ulceration at inner margin of lips, sore throat, difficulty swallowing (stomatitis). Assess skin for rash. Assess pattern of daily bowel activity and stool consistency. Be alert to symptoms of chills, fever (may be evidence of agranulocytosis).

PATIENT/FAMILY TEACHING:

Exposure to sunlight may intensify skin reaction. Maintain fastidious oral hygiene. Do not have immunizations w/o physician's approval (drug lowers body's resistance). Avoid contact with those who have recently received live virus vaccine. Promptly report fever, sore throat, signs of local infection, easy bruising, unusual bleeding from any site. Avoid alcohol (disulfiram effect may occur: facial flushing, throbbing headache, extreme nausea, copious vomiting, diaphoresis, marked uneasiness). Contact physician/nurse if chills, fever occur.

levetiracetam
(Keppra)
See Supplement
See Classification section under:
Anticonvulsant

levobunolol hydrochloride
(Betagan Liquifilm)
See Classification section under:
Antiglaucoma agents

levobupivacaine
(Chirocaine)
See Classification section under:
Local anesthetics

levocabastine hydrochloride
lev-oh-cah-**bass**-teen
(Livostin)

CANADIAN AVAILABILITY:
Livostin

CLASSIFICATION
Antiallergic

AVAILABILITY (Rx)
Ophthalmic Suspension: 0.05%. **Nasal Spray.**

PHARMACOKINETICS

	ONSET	PEAK	DURATION
Ophthalmic			
	—	—	2 hrs

Minimal systemic absorption.

ACTION/THERAPEUTIC EFFECT

Selective H₁ receptor antagonist. *Blocks histamine-associated symptoms of allergic conjunctivitis.*

USES

Temporary relief of signs and symptoms of seasonal allergic conjunctivitis.

STORAGE/HANDLING

Store at room temperature, protect from freezing. Discard if suspension is discolored. Keep tightly closed.

OPHTHALMIC ADMINISTRATION

1. Instruct pt to lie down or tilt head backward and look up.
2. Shake suspension well.
3. Gently pull lower lid down to form pouch and instill medication.
4. Do not touch tip of applicator to any surface.
5. When lower lid is released, have pt keep eye open w/o blinking for at least 30 secs.
6. Apply gentle finger pressure to lacrimal sac (bridge of the nose, inside corner of the eye) for 1–2 min.
7. Remove excess solution around eye w/tissue.
8. Tell pt not to close eyes tightly or blink more often than necessary.
9. Never rinse dropper.

INDICATIONS/DOSAGE/ROUTES

Allergic conjunctivitis:
Ophthalmic: Adults, elderly, children >12 yrs: 1 drop 4 times/day, for up to 2 wks.

PRECAUTIONS

CONTRAINDICATIONS: Hypersensitivity. Wearing soft contact lenses (product contains benzalkonium chloride). **CAUTIONS:** For ophthalmic use only. Not for injection. Safety in children <12 years not known. **PREGNANCY/LACTATION:** Excreted in breast milk. **Pregnancy Category C.**

INTERACTIONS

DRUG INTERACTIONS: None significant. **ALTERED LAB VALUES:** None significant.

SIDE EFFECTS

FREQUENT (5–15%): Transient stinging, burning, discomfort, headache. **OCCASIONAL (3–5%):** Dry mouth, fatigue, eye dryness, lacrimation/discharge, eyelid edema. **RARE (<1–3%):** Rash, erythema, nausea, dyspnea.

ADVERSE REACTIONS/TOXIC EFFECTS

None significant.

NURSING IMPLICATIONS

BASELINE ASSESSMENT:

Assess for hypersensitivity to any component of suspension. Evaluate ocular signs and symptoms.

PATIENT/FAMILY TEACHING:

Shake well before using. Do not use if suspension is discolored. Teach correct procedure for administration of drops. Do not wear soft contact lenses during therapy. For ophthalmic use only. May experience mild transitory burning, stinging upon instillation. Therapy may last up to 2 wks. If disorder does not improve or new symptoms develop, notify physician.

levofloxacin

(Levaquin)
See Supplement
See Classification section under:
Antibiotics: fluoroquinolones

levorphanol tartrate

leh-**vor**-phan-ole
(Levo-Dromoran)

CLASSIFICATION

Opioid: Analgesic (Schedule II)

AVAILABILITY (Rx)

Tablets: 2 mg. **Injection:** 2 mg/ml.

PHARMACOKINETICS

	ONSET	PEAK	DURATION
PO	30–45 min	60–120 min	4 hrs (analgesic) 4–6 hrs (antitussive)
IM	10–30 min	30–60 min	4 hrs
SubQ	10–30 min	—	2.5–4 hrs

Well absorbed from GI tract, after IM, SubQ administration. Metabolized in liver. Primarily excreted in urine. Half-life: 11 hrs.

ACTION/ *THERAPEUTIC EFFECT*

Binds w/opioid receptors within CNS, *altering processes affecting pain perception, emotional response to pain.*

USES

Relief of moderate to severe pain. Used preoperatively to produce sedation, and as adjunct w/nitrous oxide/oxygen anesthesia.

STORAGE/HANDLING

Store oral, parenteral forms at room temperature.

PO/SUBQ/IV ADMINISTRATION

PO:

1. May be given w/o regard to meals.
2. Tablets may be crushed.

SubQ:

1. Pt should be in recumbent position before administering.
2. Those w/circulatory impairment may experience overdosage due to delayed absorption of repeated SubQ administration.

IV:

1. Always administer very slowly (over 2–3 min).
2. Rapid IV increases risk of severe adverse reactions (chest wall rigidity, apnea, peripheral circulatory collapse, anaphylactoid effect, cardiac arrest).

INDICATIONS/DOSAGE/ROUTES

Note: Reduce initial dosage in those w/hypothyroidism, Addison's disease, renal insufficiency, elderly/debilitated, those on concurrent CNS depressants.
PO/SubQ: Adults, elderly: 2 mg. May be increased to 3 mg, if needed.
IV: Adults: Optimum dosage not established.

PRECAUTIONS

CONTRAINDICATIONS: None significant. **EXTREME CAUTION:** CNS depression, anoxia, hypercapnia, respiratory depression, seizures, acute alcoholism, shock, untreated myxedema, respiratory dysfunction. **CAUTIONS:** Increased intracranial pressure, impaired hepatic function, acute abdominal conditions, hypothy-

588 / **levorphanol tartrate**

roidism, prostatic hypertrophy, Addison's disease, urethral stricture, COPD. **PREGNANCY/LACTATION:** Readily crosses placenta; unknown if distributed in breast milk. Respiratory depression may occur in neonate if mother received opiates during labor. Regular use of opiates during pregnancy may produce withdrawal symptoms in neonate (irritability, excessive crying, tremors, hyperactive reflexes, fever, vomiting, diarrhea, yawning, sneezing, seizures). **Pregnancy Category B.** (Category D if used for prolonged periods or in high doses at term.)

INTERACTIONS

DRUG INTERACTIONS: Alcohol, CNS depressants may increase CNS or respiratory depression, hypotension. MAO inhibitors may produce severe, fatal reaction (reduce dose to usual 1/4 dose). **ALTERED LAB VALUES:** May increase amylase, lipase plasma concentrations.

SIDE EFFECTS

Note: Effects are dependent on dosage amount, route of administration. Ambulatory pts and those not in severe pain may experience dizziness, nausea, vomiting, hypotension more frequently than those in supine position or having severe pain. **FREQUENT:** Dizziness, drowsiness, hypotension, nausea, vomiting, unusual tiredness. **OCCASIONAL:** Shortness of breath, trouble breathing, confusion, decreased urination, stomach cramps, altered vision, constipation, dry mouth, headache, redness, pain, swelling at injection site, difficult or painful urination. **RARE:** Allergic reaction (rash, itching), histamine reaction (decreased B/P, increased sweating, flushed face, wheezing), paralytic ileus, inability to sleep.

ADVERSE REACTIONS/TOXIC EFFECTS

Overdosage results in respiratory depression, skeletal muscle flaccidity, cold clammy skin, cyanosis, extreme somnolence progressing to convulsions, stupor, coma. Tolerance to analgesic effect, physical dependence may occur w/repeated use.

NURSING IMPLICATIONS
BASELINE ASSESSMENT:

Pt should be in a recumbent position before drug is administered by parenteral route. Assess onset, type, location, and duration of pain. Obtain vital signs before giving medication. If respirations are 12/min or lower (20/min or lower in children), withhold medication, contact physician.

INTERVENTION/EVALUATION:

Monitor vital signs after parenteral administration for decreased B/P, a change in rate or quality of pulse, decreased respirations. Assess for adequate voiding, possible constipation. Initiate deep breathing and coughing exercises, particularly in those w/impaired pulmonary function. Assess therapeutic response and contact physician if pain relief is inadequate.

PATIENT/FAMILY TEACHING:

Promptly report recurrence of pain (effect of medication is reduced if full pain recurs before next dose). Discomfort may occur w/injection. Change positions slowly to avoid orthostatic hypotension. Avoid tasks that require alertness, motor skills until response to drug is established. Tolerance/dependence may occur w/prolonged use of high doses. Avoid alcohol. Report nausea, vomiting, constipation, shortness of breath, difficulty breathing.

levothyroxine

lee-voe-thye-**rox**-een
(Eltroxin, Levothroid, Levoxyl, Synthroid)

FIXED-COMBINATION(S):
W/liothyronine, T_3 (Thyrolar)

CANADIAN AVAILABILITY:
Eltroxin, Levotec, Synthroid

CLASSIFICATION

Thyroid

AVAILABILITY (Rx)

Tablets: 0.025 mg, 0.05 mg, 0.075 mg, 0.088 mg, 0.1 mg, 0.112 mg, 0.125 mg, 0.137 mg, 0.15 mg, 0.175 mg, 0.2 mg, 0.3 mg. **Injection:** 200 mcg, 500 mcg.

PHARMACOKINETICS

Variable, incomplete absorption from GI tract. Widely distributed. Deiodinated in peripheral tissues, minimal metabolism in liver. Eliminated by biliary excretion. Half-life: 6–7 days.

ACTION/ *THERAPEUTIC EFFECT*

Involved in normal metabolism, growth and development (esp. CNS of infants). Possesses catabolic and anabolic effects. *Increases basal metabolic rate, enhances gluconeogenesis, stimulates protein synthesis.*

USES

Replacement in decreased or absent thyroid function (partial or complete absence of gland, primary atrophy, functional deficiency, effects of surgery, radiation or antithyroid agents, pituitary or hypothalamic hypothyroidism); management of simple (nontoxic) goiter and chronic lymphocytic thyroiditis; treatment of thyrotoxicosis (w/antithyroid drugs) to prevent goitrogenesis and hypothyroidism. Management of thyroid cancer. Diagnostic in thyroid suppression tests.

PO/IM/IV ADMINISTRATION

Do not interchange brands because there have been problems w/bioequivalence between manufacturers.

PO:

1. Give at same time each day to maintain hormone levels.
2. Administer before breakfast to prevent insomnia.
3. Tablets may be crushed.

IV:

1. Reconstitute 200 mcg or 500 mcg vial w/5 ml 0.9% NaCl to provide a concentration of 40 or 100 mcg/ml, respectively; shake until clear.
2. Do not use or mix w/other IV solutions.
3. Use immediately and discard unused portions.

INDICATIONS/DOSAGE/ROUTES

Note: Begin therapy w/small doses; gradually increase.

Hypothyroidism:
PO: Adults, elderly: Initially, 0.05 mg/day. Increase by 0.025 mg q2–3 wks. **Maintenance:** 0.1–0.2 mg/day.

Myxedema coma or stupor (medical emergency):
IV: Adults, elderly: Initially, 0.4 mg. Follow w/daily supplements of 0.1–0.2 mg. **Maintenance:** 0.05–0.1 mg/day.

Thyroid suppression therapy:
PO: Adults, elderly: 2.6 mcg/kg/day for 7–10 days.

TSH suppression in thyroid cancer, nodules, euthyroid goiters:

PO: **Adults, elderly:** Use larger doses than that used for replacement therapy.

Congenital hypothyroidism:
PO: Children >12 yrs: >0.15 mg/day; **Children 6–12 yrs:** 0.1–0.15 mg/day; **Children 1–5 yrs:** 0.075–0.1 mg/day; **Children 6–12 mos:** 0.05–0.075 mg/day; **Infants 0–6 mos:** 0.025–0.05 mg/day.

Usual parenteral dosage:
IV: Adults, elderly: Initial dosage approximately $1/2$ the previously established oral dosage.

PRECAUTIONS

CONTRAINDICATIONS: Thyrotoxicosis and myocardial infarction uncomplicated by hypothyroidism, hypersensitivity to any component (w/tablets: tartrazine, allergy to aspirin, lactose intolerance), treatment of obesity. **CAUTIONS:** Elderly, angina pectoris, hypertension or other cardiovascular disease. **PREGNANCY/LACTATION:** Drug does not cross placenta; minimal excretion in breast milk. **Pregnancy Category A**.

INTERACTIONS

DRUG INTERACTIONS: May alter effect of oral anticoagulants. Cholestyramine, colestipol may decrease absorption. Sympathomimetics may increase effects, coronary insufficiency. **ALTERED LAB VALUES:** None significant.

SIDE EFFECTS

OCCASIONAL: Children may have reversible hair loss upon initiation. **RARE:** Dry skin, GI intolerance, skin rash, hives, pseudotumor cerebri (severe headache in children).

ADVERSE REACTIONS/TOXIC EFFECTS

Excessive dosage produces signs/symptoms of hyperthyroidism: weight loss, palpitations, increased appetite, tremors, nervousness, tachycardia, increased B/P, headache, insomnia, menstrual irregularities. Cardiac arrhythmias occur rarely.

NURSING IMPLICATIONS
BASELINE ASSESSMENT:

Question for hypersensitivity to tartrazine, aspirin, lactose. Obtain baseline weight, vital signs. Check results of thyroid function tests. Signs and symptoms of diabetes mellitus, diabetes insipidus, adrenal insufficiency, hypopituitarism may become intensified. Treat w/adrenocortical steroids prior to thyroid therapy in coexisting hypothyroidism and hypoadrenalism.

INTERVENTION/EVALUATION:

Monitor pulse for rate, rhythm (report pulse of 100 or marked increase). Assess for tremors, nervousness. Check appetite and sleep pattern.

PATIENT/FAMILY TEACHING:

Do not discontinue; replacement for hypothyroidism is lifelong. Follow-up office visits and thyroid function tests are essential. Take medication at the same time each day, preferably in morning. Monitor pulse, report marked increase, pulse of 100 or above, change of rhythm. Do not change brands. Take other medications only on advice of physician. Notify physician promptly of chest pain, weight loss, nervousness or tremors, insomnia. Children may have reversible hair loss or increased aggressiveness during the first few months of therapy. Full therapeutic effect may take 1–3 wks.

lidocaine hydrochloride

lie-doe-cane
(LidoPen, Xylocaine)

FIXED-COMBINATION(S):
W/epinephrine, a sympatho-mimetic (**Lidocaine with Epinephrine, Xylocaine with Epinephrine**)

CANADIAN AVAILABILITY:
Xylocaine, Xylocard, Zilactin-L

CLASSIFICATION

Antiarrhythmic, anesthetic

AVAILABILITY (Rx)

Injection: IM: 300 mg/3 ml. **Direct IV:** 10 mg/ml, 20 mg/ml. **IV Admixture:** 40 mg/ml, 100 mg/ml, 200 mg/ml. **IV Infusion:** 2 mg/ml, 4 mg/ml, 8 mg/ml. **Injection (anesthesia):** 0.5%, 1%, 1.5%, 2%, 4%.

Topical: Liquid: 2.5%, 5%. **Ointment:** 2.5%, 5%. **Cream:** 0.5%. **Gel:** 0.5%, 2.5%. **Spray:** 0.5%. **Solution:** 2%, 4%. **Jelly:** 2%. **Dermal Patch:** 5%.

PHARMACOKINETICS

	ONSET	PEAK	DURATION
IV	30–90 secs	—	10–20 min
Local anesthetic	2.5 min	—	30–60 min

Completely absorbed after IM administration. Widely distributed. Metabolized in liver. Primarily excreted in urine. Half-life: 1–2 hrs.

ACTION/THERAPEUTIC EFFECT

Anesthetic: Inhibits conduction of nerve impulses, *causing temporary loss of feeling and sensation.* *Antiarrhythmic:* Decreases depolarization, automaticity, excitability of ventricle during diastole by direct action, *reversing ventricular arrhythmias.*

USES

Antiarrhythmic: Rapid control of acute ventricular arrhythmias following myocardial infarction, cardiac catheterization, cardiac surgery, digitalis-induced ventricular arrhythmias. *Local anesthetic:* Infiltration or nerve block for dental or surgical procedures, childbirth. *Topical anesthetic:* Local skin disorders (minor burns, insect bites, prickly heat, skin manifestations of chicken pox, abrasions). Mucous membranes (local anesthesia of oral, nasal, and laryngeal mucous membranes, respiratory or urinary tracts; relieve discomfort of pruritus ani, hemorrhoids, pruritus vulvae). *Dermal patch:* Treatment of shingles-related skin pain.

IM/IV/INFILTRATION-NERVE BLOCK/TOPICAL ADMINISTRATION

Note: Resuscitative equipment and drugs (including oxygen) must always be readily available when administering lidocaine by any route.

IM:

1. Use 10% (100 mg/ml); clearly identify lidocaine that is *for IM use.*
2. Give in deltoid muscle (blood level is significantly higher than if injection is given in gluteus muscle or lateral thigh).

IV:

Note: Use only lidocaine without preservative, clearly marked *for IV use.*

1. For direct IV, use 1% (10 mg/ml) or 2% (20 mg/ml).
2. Administer for direct IV at rate of 25–50 mg/min.
3. For IV infusion, prepare so-

lution by adding 1 g to 1 L 5% dextrose to provide concentration of 1 mg/ml (0.1%).

4. Commercially available preparations of 0.2%, 0.4%, and 0.8% may be used for IV infusion.

5. Administer for IV infusion at rate of 1–4 mg/min (1–4 ml); use volume control IV set.

6. Monitor EKG constantly during infusion.

7. Terminate IV infusion when cardiac rhythm is stable or toxic effects occur.

8. Monitor pt response during IV administration.

9. If excessive cardiac depression (arrhythmias; prolongation of PR interval, QRS complex) occurs, discontinue medication immediately, institute supportive measures.

10. Unused lidocaine without preservative must be discarded.

INFILTRATION/NERVE BLOCK

Note: Only clinicians skilled in administration of anesthetics may give lidocaine for local anesthesia.

1. For spinal or epidural anesthesia, use only preservative-free solutions.

2. Monitor B/P, pulse, respirations, and pt's state of consciousness throughout regional anesthesia due to potential for cardiovascular or CNS toxicity.

3. Consult standard textbooks for positioning and general care of pts undergoing regional anesthesia.

TOPICAL

1. Not for ophthalmic use.

2. For skin disorders, apply directly to affected area or put on gauze or bandage, which is then applied to the skin.

3. For mucous membrane use, apply to desired area using manufacturer's insert.

4. Administer the lowest dose possible that still provides anesthesia.

INDICATIONS/DOSAGE/ROUTES

Ventricular arrhythmias:
IM: Adults, elderly: 300 mg (or 4.3 mg/kg). May repeat in 60–90 min.
IV: Adults, elderly: Initially, 50–100 mg (1 mg/kg) IV bolus at rate of 25–50 mg/min. May repeat in 5 min. Give no more than 200–300 mg in 1 hr. **Maintenance:** 20–50 mcg/kg/min (1–4 mg/min) as IV infusion. **Children, infants:** Initially, 0.5–1 mg/kg IV bolus; may repeat but total dose not to exceed 3–5 mg/kg. **Maintenance:** 10–50 mcg/kg/min as IV infusion.

Usual local anesthetic dosage:
Note: Do not use any preparation containing preservatives for spinal or epidural anesthesia.
Infiltration: 0.5 or 1% solution.
Epidural (Including Caudal): 1 or 2% solution.
Peripheral Nerve Block: 1 or 1.5% solution.
Sympathetic Nerve Block: 1% solution.
Spinal Anesthesia: 1.5 or 5% solution (with dextrose).

Usual topical dosage:
Topical: Adults, elderly: Apply to affected areas as needed. **Dermal Patch:** Apply to intact skin over most painful area (up to 3 patches once for up to 12 hrs in a 24-hr period).

PRECAUTIONS

CONTRAINDICATIONS: Hypersensitivity to amide-type local anesthetics, Adams-Stokes syndrome, supraventricular arrhythmias, Wolff-Parkinson-White syndrome. Spinal anesthesia contraindicated in septicemia. **CAUTIONS:** Dosage should be reduced for elderly, debilitated, acutely ill; safety in children not established. Severe renal/hepatic disease, hypovolemia, CHF, shock, heart block, marked hypoxia, severe respiratory depression, bradycardia, incomplete heart block. Anesthetic solutions containing epinephrine should be used with caution in peripheral or hypertensive vascular disease, and during or following potent general anesthesia. Sulfite sensitivity or asthma for some local and topical anesthetic preparations. Tartrazine or aspirin sensitivity with some topical preparations. **PREGNANCY/LACTATION:** Crosses placenta; distributed in breast milk. **Pregnancy Category C**.

INTERACTIONS

DRUG INTERACTIONS: May increase cardiac effects w/other antiarrhythmics. Anticonvulsants may increase cardiac depressant effects. Beta-adrenergic blockers may increase risk of toxicity. **ALTERED LAB VALUES:** IM lidocaine may increase CPK level (used in diagnostic test for presence of acute MI).

SIDE EFFECTS

CNS effects generally dose related and of short duration. **OCCASIONAL:** *IM:* pain at injection site. *Topical:* Burning, stinging, tenderness. **RARE:** Generally with high dose: drowsiness, dizziness, disorientation, lightheadedness, tremors, apprehension, euphoria, sensation of heat/cold/numbness, blurred/double vision, ringing/roaring in ears (tinnitus), nausea.

ADVERSE REACTIONS/TOXIC EFFECTS

Although serious adverse reactions to lidocaine are uncommon, high dosage by any route may produce cardiovascular depression: bradycardia, somnolence, hypotension, arrhythmias, heart block, cardiovascular collapse, cardiac arrest. Potential for malignant hyperthermia. CNS toxicity may occur, esp. with regional anesthesia use, progressing rapidly from mild side effects to tremors, convulsions, vomiting, respiratory depression, arrest. Methemoglobinemia (evidenced by cyanosis) has occurred following topical application of lidocaine for teething discomfort and laryngeal anesthetic spray. Overuse of oral lidocaine has caused seizures in children. Allergic reactions are rare.

NURSING IMPLICATIONS
BASELINE ASSESSMENT:

Question for hypersensitivity to lidocaine, amide anesthetics, or components of preparation. Obtain baseline B/P, pulse, respirations, EKG, and electrolytes.

INTERVENTION/EVALUATION:

Monitor EKG, vital signs closely during and after drug is administered for cardiac performance. If EKG shows arrhythmias, prolongation of PR interval or QRS complex, inform physician immediately. Assess pulse for irregularity, strength/weakness, bradycardia. Assess B/P for evidence of hypotension. Monitor I&O, electrolyte serum level. Monitor for therapeutic serum level (1.5–6 mcg/ml). For lidocaine given by all routes, monitor vital signs and pt's state of consciousness. Drowsiness should be considered a warning sign of high blood levels of lidocaine.

PATIENT/FAMILY TEACHING:

Explain action of lidocaine.

Report drowsiness or CNS effects promptly (see Adverse Reactions/Toxic Effects). *Local anesthesia:* Assure that pt understands loss of feeling, sensation and need for protection until anesthetic wears off (e.g., no ambulation, including special positions for some regional anesthesia; not chewing gum, eating, or drinking following administration to oral area, etc.). *Topical anesthesia:* Use only as directed; too frequent use may cause overdosage. Do not eat, drink, or chew gum for 1 hr following application (swallowing reflex may be impaired increasing risk of aspiration; numbness of tongue or buccal mucosa may lead to biting trauma).

liothyronine

lye-oh-**thigh**-roe-neen
(Cytomel)

FIXED-COMBINATION(S): W/levothyroxine, T_4 **(Thyrolar)**

CLASSIFICATION

Thyroid

AVAILABILITY (Rx)

Tablets: 5 mcg, 25 mcg, 50 mcg. **Injection:** 10 mcg/ml.

PHARMACOKINETICS

Almost complete absorption from GI tract. Widely distributed. Deiodinated in peripheral tissues, minimal metabolism in liver. Eliminated by biliary excretion. Half-life: 1 day.

ACTION/*THERAPEUTIC EFFECT*

Involved in normal metabolism, growth and development (esp. CNS of infants). Possesses catabolic and anabolic effects. *Increases basal metabolic rate, enhances gluconeogenesis, stimulates protein synthesis.*

USES

Oral: Replacement in decreased or absent thyroid function (partial or complete absence of gland, primary atrophy, functional deficiency, effects of surgery, radiation or antithyroid agents, pituitary or hypothalamic hypothyroidism). Management of simple (nontoxic) goiter; diagnostically in T_3 suppression test (differentiates hyperthyroidism from euthyroidism). *IV:* Myxedema coma, precoma.

STORAGE/HANDLING

Refrigerate parenteral dosage form; store oral tablets at room temperature.

PO/IV ADMINISTRATION

PO:

1. Give at the same time each day to maintain hormone levels.

2. Administer before breakfast to prevent insomnia.

3. When transferred *from* another thyroid preparation, the other thyroid agent should be discontinued first; begin liothyronine at low dose.

4. When transferring *to* another thyroid preparation, continue liothyronine for several days to prevent relapse (rapid action, short duration).

IV:

1. Do not administer IM or SubQ.

2. Switch to oral as soon as pt stabilized clinically. Initiate oral therapy at low dose, increasing gradually according to pt response.

INDICATIONS/DOSAGE/ROUTES

Hypothyroidism:
PO: Adults: Initially, 25 mcg/day. Increase by 12.5–25 mcg q1–2 wks. **Elderly:** Initially, 5 mcg/day. May increase by 5 mcg/day q1–2 wks. **Maintenance:** 25–75 mcg/day.

Myxedema:
PO: Adults, elderly: Initially, 5 mcg/day. Increase by 5–10 mcg q1–2 wks (after 25 mcg/day reached, may increase by 12.5 mcg increments). **Maintenance:** 50–100 mcg/day.

Nontoxic goiter:
PO: Adults, elderly: Initially, 5 mcg/day. Increase by 5–10 mcg/day q1–2 wks. When 25 mcg/day obtained, may increase by 12.5–25 mcg/day q1–2 wks. **Maintenance:** 75 mcg/day.

Congenital hypothyroidism:
PO: Children: Initially, 5 mcg/day. Increase by 5 mcg/day q3–4 days. **Maintenance: (Infants):** 20 mcg/day. **(1 yr):** 50 mcg/day. **(>3 yrs):** Full adult dosage.

T_3 suppression test:
PO: Adults, elderly: 75–100 mcg/day for 7 days, then repeat I^{131} thyroid uptake test.

Myxedema coma, precoma:
Note: Initial and subsequent dosage based on pt's clinical status, response. Administer IV dose at least 4 hrs but no longer than 12 hrs apart.
IV: Adults, elderly: Initially, 25–50 mcg (10–20 mcg in pts w/cardiovascular disease). Total dose at least 65 mcg/day.

PRECAUTIONS

CONTRAINDICATIONS: Thyrotoxicosis and MI uncomplicated by hypothyroidism, treatment of obesity. **CAUTIONS:** Elderly, angina pectoris, hypertension, or other cardiovascular disease. **PREGNANCY/LACTATION:** Drug does not cross placenta, minimal excretion in breast milk. **Pregnancy Category A.**

INTERACTIONS

DRUG INTERACTIONS: May alter effect of oral anticoagulants. Cholestyramine, colestipol may decrease absorption. Sympathomimetics may increase effects, coronary insufficiency. **ALTERED LAB VALUES:** None significant.

SIDE EFFECTS

OCCASIONAL: Children may have reversible hair loss upon initiation. **RARE:** Dry skin, GI intolerance, skin rash, hives, pseudotumor cerebri (severe headache in children).

ADVERSE REACTIONS/TOXIC EFFECTS

Excessive dosage produces signs/symptoms of hyperthyroidism: weight loss, palpitations, increased appetite, tremors, nervousness, tachycardia, increased B/P, headache, insomnia, menstrual irregularities. Cardiac arrhythmias occur rarely.

NURSING IMPLICATIONS
BASELINE ASSESSMENT:

Question for hypersensitivity to tartrazine, aspirin. Obtain baseline weight, vital signs. Check results of thyroid function tests. Signs and symptoms of diabetes mellitus, diabetes insipidus, adrenal insufficiency, hypopituitarism may become intensified. Treat w/adrenocortical steroids prior to thyroid therapy in coexisting hypothyroidism and hypoadrenalism.

INTERVENTION/EVALUATION:

Monitor pulse for rate, rhythm (report pulse ≥100 or marked increase). Assess for tremors, nervousness. Check appetite and sleep pattern.

PATIENT/FAMILY TEACHING:

Do not discontinue; replacement for hypothyroidism is lifelong. Follow-up office visits and thyroid function tests are essential. Take medication at the same time each day, preferably in morning. Teach pt or family to take pulse correctly, report marked increase, pulse of 100 or above, change of rhythm. Do not change brands (not equivalent). Take other medications only on advice of physician. Notify physician promptly of chest pain, weight loss, nervousness or tremors, insomnia. Children may have reversible hair loss or increased aggressiveness during first few months of therapy.

lisinopril

lih-**sin**-oh-prill
(Prinivil, Zestril)

FIXED-COMBINATION(S):
W/hydrochlorothiazide, a diuretic
(Prinizide, Zestoretic)

CANADIAN AVAILABILITY:
Prinivil, Zestril

CLASSIFICATION

Angiotensin-converting enzyme (ACE) inhibitor

AVAILABILITY (Rx)

Tablets: 2.5 mg, 5 mg, 10 mg, 20 mg, 40 mg

PHARMACOKINETICS

	ONSET	PEAK	DURATION
PO	1 hr	6 hrs	24 hrs

Incompletely absorbed from GI tract. Primarily excreted unchanged in urine. Removed by hemodialysis. Half-life: 12 hrs (prolonged in decreased renal function).

ACTION/THERAPEUTIC EFFECT

Suppresses renin-angiotensin-aldosterone system (prevents conversion of angiotensin I to angiotensin II, a potent vasoconstrictor; may also inhibit angiotensin II at local vascular and renal sites). Decreases plasma angiotensin II, increases plasma renin activity, decreases aldosterone secretion. *Reduces peripheral arterial resistance, B/P (afterload), pulmonary capillary wedge pressure (preload), pulmonary vascular resistance.* In those w/heart failure, *also decreases heart size, increases cardiac output, exercise tolerance time.*

USES/UNLABELED

Treatment of hypertension. Used alone or in combination w/other antihypertensives. Adjunctive therapy in management of heart failure. Improves survival in pts who had myocardial infarction. *Treatment of hypertension/renal crises w/scleroderma.*

PO ADMINISTRATION

1. May give w/o regard to food.
2. Tablets may be crushed.

INDICATIONS/DOSAGE/ROUTES

Hypertension (used alone):
PO: Adults: Initially, 10 mg/day.

Maintenance: 20–40 mg/day as single dose.

Hypertension (combination therapy):
Note: Discontinue diuretic 2–3 days prior to initiating lisinopril therapy.
PO: Adults: Initially, 5 mg/day titrated to pt's needs.

Heart failure:
PO: Adults: Initially, 5 mg/day (2.5 mg/day in pts w/hyponatremia). **Range:** 5–20 mg/day.

Myocardial infarction:
PO: Adults, elderly: Initially, 5 mg, then 5 mg after 24 hrs, 10 mg after 48 hrs, then 10 mg/day × 6 wks. (Pts w/low systolic B/P: 2.5 mg/day for 3 days, then 2.5–5 mg/day.

Usual elderly dosage:
PO: Initially, 2.5–5 mg/day. May increase by 2.5–5 mg/day at 1–2 wk intervals. **Maximum:** 40 mg/day.

Dosage in renal impairment:
Titrate to pt's needs after giving the following initial dose:

CREATININE CLEARANCE	INITIAL DOSE
>30 ml/min	10 mg
10–30 ml/min	5 mg
<10 ml/min	2.5 mg

PRECAUTIONS

CONTRAINDICATIONS: MI, coronary insufficiency, angina, evidence of coronary artery disease, hypersensitivity to phentolamine, history of angioedema w/previous treatment w/ACEIs. **CAUTIONS:** Renal impairment, those w/sodium depletion or on diuretic therapy, dialysis, hypovolemia, coronary or cerebrovascular insufficiency. **PREGNANCY/LACTATION:** Crosses placenta; unknown if distributed in breast milk. **Pregnancy**

Category D. Has caused fetal/neonatal mortality, morbidity.

INTERACTIONS

DRUG INTERACTIONS: Alcohol, diuretics, hypotensive agents may increase effects. NSAIDs may decrease effect. Potassium-sparing diuretics, potassium supplements may cause hyperkalemia. May increase lithium concentration, toxicity. **ALTERED LAB VALUES:** May increase potassium, SGOT (AST), SGPT (ALT), alkaline phosphatase, bilirubin, BUN, creatinine. May decrease sodium. May cause positive ANA titer.

SIDE EFFECTS

FREQUENT (5–12%): Headache, dizziness, postural hypotension. **OCCASIONAL (2–4%):** Chest discomfort, fatigue, rash, abdominal pain, nausea, diarrhea, upper respiratory infection. **RARE (≤1%):** Palpitations, tachycardia, peripheral edema, insomnia, paresthesia, confusion, constipation, dry mouth, muscle cramps.

ADVERSE REACTIONS/TOXIC EFFECTS

Excessive hypotension ("first-dose syncope") may occur in those w/CHF, severely salt/volume depleted. Angioedema (swelling of face/lips), hyperkalemia occurs rarely. Agranulocytosis, neutropenia may be noted in those w/impaired renal function or collagen vascular disease (systemic lupus erythematosus, scleroderma). Nephrotic syndrome may be noted in those w/history of renal disease.

NURSING IMPLICATIONS
BASELINE ASSESSMENT:

Obtain B/P and apical pulse immediately before each dose, in addition to regular monitoring (be alert to fluctuations). If excessive reduction in B/P occurs, place pt in supine position, feet slightly elevated. Renal function tests should be performed before therapy begins. In those w/renal impairment, autoimmune disease, or taking drugs that affect leukocytes or immune response, CBC and differential count should be performed before therapy begins and q2 wks for 3 mos, then periodically thereafter.

INTERVENTION/EVALUATION:

Assess for edema; check lungs for rales. Monitor I&O; weigh daily. Assess stools for frequency and consistency; prevent constipation. Assist w/ambulation if dizziness occurs.

PATIENT/FAMILY TEACHING:

To reduce hypotensive effect, rise slowly from lying to sitting position and permit legs to dangle from bed momentarily before standing. Full therapeutic effect may take 2–4 wks. Report any sign of infection (sore throat, fever), swelling of hands or feet or face, chest pain, difficulty breathing or swallowing. Skipping doses or voluntarily discontinuing drug may produce severe, rebound hypertension. Do not take cold preparations, nasal decongestants. Restrict sodium and alcohol as ordered.

lithium carbonate

lith-ee-um
(Eskalith, Lithane, Lithobid)

lithium citrate
(Cibalith-S)

CANADIAN AVAILABILITY:
Carbolith, Duralith, Lithane,

CLASSIFICATION

Antimanic

AVAILABILITY (Rx)

Capsules: 150 mg, 300 mg, 600 mg. **Tablets:** 300 mg. **Tablets (slow-release):** 300 mg, 450 mg. **Syrup:** 300 mg/5 ml.

PHARMACOKINETICS

Rapid, complete absorption from GI tract. Primarily excreted unchanged in urine. Half-life: 18–24 hrs (increased in elderly).

ACTION/*THERAPEUTIC EFFECT*

Alters ion transport at cellular sites in body tissue. Cations necessary in synthesis, storage, release, reuptake of neurotransmitters involved in *producing antimanic, antidepressant effects.*

USES/*UNLABELED*

Prophylaxis, treatment of acute mania, manic phase of bipolar disorder (manic-depressive illness). *Treatment of mental depression, prophylaxis of vascular headache, treatment of neutropenia.*

STORAGE/HANDLING

Store all forms at room temperature.

PO ADMINISTRATION

1. Preferable to administer w/meals or milk.
2. Do not crush, chew, or break extended-release or film-coated tablets.

INDICATIONS/DOSAGE/ROUTES

Note: During acute phase, therapeutic serum lithium concentration of 1–1.4 mEq/L is required. Desired level during long-term control: 0.5–1.3 mEq/L.

Acute manic phase:
PO: Adults: Initially, 1.8 g (or 20–30 mg/kg) lithium carbonate or 30 ml lithium citrate/day, in 2–3 divided doses. **Elderly:** 600–900 mg/day.

Long-term control:
PO: Adults: 900 mg–1.2 g lithium carbonate or 15–20 ml lithium citrate, daily, in 2–4 divided doses.

Usual elderly dosage:
PO: Initially, 300 mg 2 times/day. May increase by 300 mg/day at weekly intervals. **Maintenance:** 900–1,200 mg/day.

PRECAUTIONS

CONTRAINDICATIONS: Severe cardiovascular disease, severe renal disease, severe dehydration/sodium depletion, debilitated patients. **CAUTIONS:** Cardiovascular disease, thyroid disease, elderly. **PREGNANCY/LACTATION:** Freely crosses placenta; distributed in breast milk. **Pregnancy Category D**.

INTERACTIONS

DRUG INTERACTIONS: May increase effects of antithyroid medication, iodinated glycerol, potassium iodide. NSAIDs may increase concentration, toxicity. May decrease absorption of phenothiazines. Phenothiazines may increase intracellular concentration, increase renal excretion, extrapyramidal symptoms (EPS), delirium, mask early signs of lithium toxicity. Diuretics may increase concentration, toxicity. Haloperidol may increase EPS, neurologic toxicity. Molindone may increase risk of neurotoxic symptoms. **ALTERED LAB VALUES:** May increase blood glucose, calcium, immunoreactive parathyroid hormone.

SIDE EFFECTS

Note: Effects are dose-related and seldom occur at serum lithium levels <1.5 mEq/L.
OCCASIONAL: Fine hand tremor, polydipsia (excessive thirst), polyuria (increased urination), mild nausea. **RARE:** Weight gain, fast/slow heartbeat, acne, rash, muscle twitching, blue hue in fingers/toes, coldness in arms/legs, pseudotumor cerebri (eye pain, headache, vision problems, noises in ears).

ADVERSE REACTIONS/TOXIC EFFECTS

Serum lithium concentration of 1.5–2.0 mEq/L may produce vomiting, diarrhea, drowsiness, incoordination, coarse hand tremor, muscle twitching, EKG T-wave depression, mental confusion. Serum lithium concentration of 2.0–2.5 mEq/L may result in ataxia, giddiness, tinnitus, blurred vision, clonic movements, severe hypotension. Acute toxicity characterized by seizures, oliguria, circulatory failure, coma, death.

NURSING IMPLICATIONS

BASELINE ASSESSMENT:

Serum lithium levels should be tested every 3–4 days during initial phase of therapy, every 1–2 mos thereafter, and weekly if there is no improvement of disorder or adverse effects occur.

INTERVENTION/EVALUATION:

Lithium serum testing should be performed as close as possible to 12th hour after last dose.

Besides serum lithium concentration levels, clinical assessment of therapeutic effect or tolerance to drug effect is necessary for correct dosing-level management. Assess behavior, appearance, emotional status, response to environment, speech pattern, thought content. Monitor serum lithium concentrations, differential count, urinalysis, creatinine clearance. Assess for increased urine output, persistent thirst. Report polyuria, prolonged vomiting, diarrhea, fever to physician (may need to temporarily reduce or discontinue dosage). Monitor for signs of lithium toxicity. Supervise suicidal risk pt closely during early therapy (as depression lessens, energy level improves, and suicide potential increases). Assess for therapeutic response (interest in surroundings, improvement in self-care, increased ability to concentrate, relaxed facial expression).

PATIENT/FAMILY TEACHING:

Take as directed; do not discontinue except on physician's advice. Do not engage in activities requiring alert response until effects of drug are known. Thirst, frequent urination may occur. A fluid intake of 2–3 quarts liquid per day and maintenance of a normal salt intake are necessary during initial phase of treatment to avoid dehydration. Thereafter, 1–1.5 L fluid intake daily is necessary. GI disturbances generally disappear during continued therapy. Thyroid function tests should be performed every 6–12 mos in elderly pts (increased incidence of goiter, hypothyroidism). Therapeutic improvement noted in 1–3 wks. Avoid alcohol and OTC drugs. Consult physician regarding contraception.

Iodoxamide tromethamine

low-**dox**-ah-myd
(Alomide)

CANADIAN AVAILABILITY:
Alomide

CLASSIFICATION

Antiallergic

AVAILABILITY (Rx)

Ophthalmic Solution: 0.1%

PHARMACOKINETICS

Minimal systemic absorption. Primarily excreted in urine. Half-life: 8.5 hrs.

ACTION/*THERAPEUTIC EFFECT*

Mast cell stabilizer. Prevents increase in cutaneous vascular permeability, antigen-stimulated histamine release and may prevent calcium influx into mast cells, *inhibiting hypersensitivity reaction.*

USES

Treatment of vernal keratoconjunctivitis, conjunctivitis, and keratitis.

STORAGE/HANDLING

Keep at room temperature; protect from freezing. Do not use if discolored. Keep tightly closed.

OPHTHALMIC ADMINISTRATION

1. Instruct pt to lie down or tilt head backward and look up.
2. Gently pull lower lid down to form pouch and instill medication.

3. Do not touch tip of applicator to any surface.

4. When lower lid is released, have pt keep eye open w/o blinking for at least 30 secs.

5. Apply gentle finger pressure to lacrimal sac (bridge of the nose, inside corner of the eye) for 1–2 min.

6. Remove excess solution around eye w/tissue.

7. Tell pt not to close eyes tightly or blink more often than necessary.

8. Never rinse dropper.

INDICATIONS/DOSAGE/ROUTES

Usual ophthalmic dosage:
Adults, elderly, children >2 yrs: 1–2 drops 4 times/day, for up to 3 mos.

PRECAUTIONS

CONTRAINDICATIONS: Hypersensitivity. Wearing soft contact lenses (product contains benzalkonium chloride). **CAUTIONS:** For ophthalmic use only. Not for injection. Safety in children <2 yrs not known. **PREGNANCY/LACTATION:** Unknown if excreted in breast milk. **Pregnancy Category B.**

INTERACTIONS

DRUG INTERACTIONS: None significant. **ALTERED LAB VALUES:** None significant.

SIDE EFFECTS

FREQUENT: Transient stinging, burning, instillation discomfort. **OCCASIONAL:** Ocular itching, blurred vision, dry eye, tearing/discharge/foreign body sensation, headache. **RARE:** Scales on lid/lash, ocular swelling, sticky sensation, dizziness, somnolence, nausea, sneezing, dry nose, rash.

ADVERSE REACTIONS/TOXIC EFFECTS

None significant.

NURSING IMPLICATIONS
BASELINE ASSESSMENT:

Assess for hypersensitivity to any component of suspension. Evaluate ocular signs and symptoms.

PATIENT/FAMILY TEACHING:

Teach correct procedure for administration of drops. Do not wear soft contact lenses during therapy. For ophthalmic use only. May experience mild transitory burning, stinging upon instillation; inform physician if continues. Therapy may last up to 3 mos. If disorder does not improve or new symptoms develop, notify physician.

lomefloxacin hydrochloride

low-meh-**flocks**-ah-sin
(Maxaquin)

CLASSIFICATION

Anti-infective: Quinolone

AVAILABILITY (Rx)

Tablets: 400 mg

PHARMACOKINETICS

Well absorbed from GI tract. Widely distributed. Metabolized in liver. Primarily excreted in urine. Minimal removal by hemodialysis. Half-life: 4–6 hrs (increased in decreased renal function, elderly).

ACTION/*THERAPEUTIC EFFECT*

Inhibits the enzyme DNA-gyrase in susceptible microorganisms, *interfering w/bacterial DNA replication and repair. Bactericidal.*

USES

Treatment of infections of urinary tract, lower respiratory tract, postop prophylaxis in pts undergoing transurethral procedures.

PO ADMINISTRATION

1. May be given w/o regard to meals (preferred dosing time: 2 hrs after meals).

2. Do not administer antacids (aluminum, magnesium) within 2 hrs of lomefloxacin.

3. Encourage cranberry juice, citrus fruits (to acidify urine).

INDICATIONS/DOSAGE/ROUTES

Urinary tract infections:
PO: **Adults, elderly:** 400 mg/day for 10–14 days.

Uncomplicated UTI:
PO: **Adults (females):** 400 mg/day for 3 days.

Lower respiratory tract infections:
PO: **Adults, elderly:** 400 mg/day for 10 days.

Postop prophylaxis:
PO: **Adults, elderly:** 400 mg 2–6 hrs prior to surgery.

Dosage in renal impairment:
The dose and/or frequency is modified in pts based on severity of renal impairment.

CREATININE CLEARANCE	DOSAGE
>40 ml/min	No change
10–40 ml/min	400 mg initially, then 200 mg/day for 10–14 days

PRECAUTIONS

CONTRAINDICATIONS: Hypersensitivity to lomefloxacin, quinolones, any component of the preparation. **CAUTIONS:** Renal impairment, CNS disorders, seizures, those taking theophylline or caffeine. **PREGNANCY/LACTATION:** Unknown if distributed in breast milk. If possible, do not use during pregnancy/lactation (risk of arthropathy to fetus/infant). **Pregnancy Category C.**

INTERACTIONS

DRUG INTERACTIONS: Antacids, iron prep, sucralfate may decrease absorption. Decreases clearance, may increase concentration, toxicity of theophylline. May increase effects of oral anticoagulants. **ALTERED LAB VALUES:** May increase SGOT (AST), SGPT (ALT), alkaline phosphatase, LDH, serum bilirubin, BUN, serum creatinine concentration.

SIDE EFFECTS

FREQUENT: Nausea, diarrhea, headache, dizziness, photosensitivity.

ADVERSE REACTIONS/TOXIC EFFECTS

Superinfection (bacterial or fungal overgrowth of nonsusceptible organisms), photosensitivity reaction.

NURSING IMPLICATIONS

BASELINE ASSESSMENT:

Question for history of hypersensitivity to lomefloxacin, quinolones, any component of preparation. Obtain specimen for diagnostic tests before giving first dose (therapy may begin before results are known).

INTERVENTION/EVALUATION:

Evaluate food tolerance. Determine pattern of bowel activity; be alert to blood in feces. Check for dizziness, headache. Monitor B/P at least twice daily. Assess for chest, joint pain.

PATIENT/FAMILY TEACHING:

Do not skip dose; take full

course of therapy. Take w/8 oz water; drink several glasses of water between meals. Eat/drink high sources of ascorbic acid to prevent crystalluria (cranberry juice, citrus fruits). Do not take antacids (reduces/destroys effectiveness). Avoid sunlight/ultraviolet exposure; wear sunscreen, protective clothing if photosensitivity develops. Notify nurse/physician if new symptoms occur. Report inflammation or tendon pain.

lomustine

low-**meuw**-steen
(CeeNU)

CANADIAN AVAILABILITY: CeeNu

CLASSIFICATION

Antineoplastic

AVAILABILITY (Rx)

Capsules: 10 mg, 40 mg, 100 mg

PHARMACOKINETICS

Rapidly, well absorbed from GI tract. Widely distributed. Crosses blood-brain barrier. Metabolized in liver to active metabolite. Primarily excreted in urine. Half-life: 16–48 hrs.

ACTION / *THERAPEUTIC EFFECT*

Acts as alkylating agent. Inhibits DNA, RNA synthesis by cross-linking w/DNA, RNA strands, preventing cellular division, *interfering w/DNA/RNA function.* Cell cyclephase nonspecific.

USES / *UNLABELED*

Treatment of primary and metastatic brain tumors, disseminated Hodgkin's disease. *Treatment of gastrointestinal, lung, renal, breast carcinoma, multiple myeloma, malignant melanoma.*

PO ADMINISTRATION

Note: May be carcinogenic, mutagenic, or teratogenic. Handle w/extreme care during administration.

Give on empty stomach (reduces potential for nausea).

INDICATIONS/DOSAGE/ROUTES

Note: Dosage is individualized based on clinical response and tolerance to adverse effects. When used in combination therapy, consult specific protocols for optimum dosage, sequence of drug administration.

Usual dosage:
PO: Adults, elderly, children: 100–130 mg/m² as single dose. Repeat dose at intervals of at least 6 wks but not until circulating blood elements have returned to acceptable levels. Adjust dose based on hematologic response to previous dose.

PRECAUTIONS

CONTRAINDICATIONS: Previous hypersensitivity to drug. **CAUTIONS:** Depressed platelet, leukocyte, erythrocyte counts. **PREGNANCY/LACTATION:** If possible, avoid use during pregnancy, esp. first trimester. May cause fetal harm. Unknown if distributed in breast milk. Breast-feeding not recommended. **Pregnancy Category D.**

INTERACTIONS

DRUG INTERACTIONS: Bone marrow depressants may increase bone marrow depression. Live virus vaccines may potentiate virus replication, increase vaccine side effects, decrease pt's antibody response to vaccine. **ALTERED LAB VALUES:** May increase liver function tests.

SIDE EFFECTS

FREQUENT: Nausea, vomiting occur 45 min–6 hrs after dosing, lasts 12–24 hrs. Anorexia often follows for 2–3 days. **OCCASIONAL:** Neurotoxicity (confusion, slurred speech), stomatitis, darkening of skin, diarrhea, skin rash, itching, hair loss.

ADVERSE REACTIONS/TOXIC EFFECTS

Bone marrow depression manifested as hematologic toxicity (principally leukopenia, mild anemia, thrombocytopenia). Leukopenia occurs at about 6 wks, thrombocytopenia at about 4 wks, and persists for 1–2 wks. Refractory anemia, thrombocytopenia occur commonly if therapy continued longer than 1 yr. Hepatotoxicity occurs infrequently. Large cumulative doses may result in renal damage.

NURSING IMPLICATIONS

BASELINE ASSESSMENT:

Manufacturer recommends weekly blood counts; experts recommend first blood count obtained 2–3 wks after initial therapy, subsequent blood counts indicated by prior toxicity. Antiemetics can reduce duration, frequency of nausea, vomiting.

INTERVENTION/EVALUATION:

Monitor hematologic status, liver function tests. Monitor for stomatitis (burning/erythema of oral mucosa at inner margin of lips, sore throat, difficulty swallowing). Monitor for hematologic toxicity (fever, sore throat, signs of local infection, easy bruising, unusual bleeding from

any site), symptoms of anemia (excessively tired, weak).

PATIENT/FAMILY TEACHING:

Nausea, vomiting abates generally in <1 day. Fasting prior to therapy can reduce frequency/duration of GI effects. Maintain fastidious oral hygiene. Do not have immunizations w/o physician's approval (drug lowers body's resistance). Avoid crowds and those w/known illness. Promptly report fever, sore throat, signs of local infection, easy bruising or unusual bleeding from any site, swelling of legs and feet, yellow skin. Contact physician if nausea/vomiting continues at home. Avoid alcohol and OTC medications. Contraception is recommended during therapy.

loperamide hydrochloride

low-**pear**-ah-myd
(Imodium, Imodium A-D)

FIXED-COMBINATION(S):
W/simethicone, an antiflatulent (**Imodium Advanced**)

CANADIAN AVAILABILITY:
Apo-Loperamide, Imodium, Loperacap, Novo-Loperamide

CLASSIFICATION

Antidiarrheal

AVAILABILITY (OTC)

Tablets: 2 mg. **Capsules (Rx):** 2 mg. **Liquid:** 1 mg/5 ml.

PHARMACOKINETICS

Poorly absorbed from GI tract. Metabolized in liver. Eliminated in feces, excreted in urine. Half-life: 9.1–14.4 hrs.

ACTION / *THERAPEUTIC EFFECT*

Direct effect on intestinal wall muscles; *slows intestinal motility, prolongs transit time of intestinal contents (reduces fecal volume, diminishes loss of fluid/electrolytes, increases viscosity, bulk).*

USES

Controls, provides symptomatic relief of acute nonspecific diarrhea; chronic diarrhea associated w/inflammatory bowel disease; traveler's diarrhea. Reduces volume of discharge from ileostomy.

INDICATIONS / DOSAGE / ROUTES

Acute diarrhea (capsules):
PO: **Adults, elderly:** Initially, 4 mg, then 2 mg after each unformed stool. **Maximum:** 16 mg/day. **Children, 8–12 yrs, >30 kg:** Initially, 2 mg 3 times/day for 24 hrs; **5–8 yrs, 20–30 kg:** Initially, 2 mg 2 times/day for 24 hrs; **2–5 yrs, 13–20 kg:** Initially, 1 mg 3 times/day for 24 hrs. **Maintenance:** 1 mg/10 kg only after loose stool.

Chronic diarrhea:
PO: **Adults, elderly:** Initially 4 mg, then 2 mg after each unformed stool until diarrhea is controlled.

Traveler's diarrhea:
PO: **Adults, elderly:** Initially, 4 mg, then 2 mg after each loose bowel movement (LBM). **Maximum:** 8 mg/day for 2 days. **Children 9–11 yrs:** Initially 2 mg, then 1 mg after each LBM. **Maximum:** 6 mg/day for 2 days. **Children 6–8 yrs:** Initially, 1 mg, then 1 mg after each LBM. **Maximum:** 4 mg/day for 2 days.

PRECAUTIONS

CONTRAINDICATIONS: Those who must avoid constipation, diarrhea associated w/pseudomembranous enterocolitis due to broad-spectrum antibiotics or w/organisms that invade intestinal mucosa (*Escherichia coli,* shigella, salmonella), acute ulcerative colitis (may produce toxic megacolon). **CAUTIONS:** Those w/ fluid/electrolyte depletion, hepatic impairment. **PREGNANCY/LACTATION:** Unknown if drug crosses placenta or is distributed in breast milk. **Pregnancy Category B**.

INTERACTIONS

DRUG INTERACTIONS: Opioid (narcotic) analgesics may increase risk of constipation. **ALTERED LAB VALUES:** None significant.

SIDE EFFECTS

RARE: Dry mouth, drowsiness, abdominal discomfort, allergic reaction (rash, itching).

ADVERSE REACTIONS / TOXIC EFFECTS

Toxicity results in constipation, GI irritation including nausea, vomiting, CNS depression. Treatment: Activated charcoal.

NURSING IMPLICATIONS

BASELINE ASSESSMENT:

Do not administer in presence of bloody diarrhea or temperature >101°F.

INTERVENTION / EVALUATION:

Encourage adequate fluid intake. Assess bowel sounds for peristalsis. Monitor stool frequency and consistency (watery, loose, soft, semisolid, solid). Withhold drug and notify physician promptly in event of abdominal pain, distension, or fever.

PATIENT/FAMILY TEACHING:

Do not exceed prescribed dose. Avoid tasks that require alertness, motor skills until response to drug is established. Notify physician if diarrhea does not stop within 3 days, if abdominal distention or pain occurs, or if fever develops.

loracarbef

laur-ah-**car**-bef
(Lorabid)

CLASSIFICATION

Antibiotic: Cephalosporin

AVAILABILITY (Rx)

Capsules: 200 mg. **Powder for Oral Suspension:** 100 mg/5 ml.

PHARMACOKINETICS

Well absorbed from GI tract. Widely distributed. Primarily excreted unchanged in urine. Removed by hemodialysis. Half-life: 1 hr (increased in decreased renal function).

ACTION/ THERAPEUTIC EFFECT

Bactericidal. Binds to bacterial membranes, *inhibiting bacterial cell wall synthesis.*

USES

Treatment of bronchitis, otitis media, pharyngitis, pneumonia, sinusitis, skin and soft tissue infections, urinary tract infections (uncomplicated cystitis, pyelonephritis).

STORAGE/HANDLING

After reconstitution, powder for suspension may be kept at room temperature for 14 days. Discard unused portion after 14 days.

PO ADMINISTRATION

1. Give 1 hr before or 2 hrs after meal.

2. Shake oral suspension well before using.

INDICATIONS/DOSAGE/ROUTES

Bronchitis:
PO: Adults, elderly, children >12 yrs: 200–400 mg q12h for 7 days.

Pharyngitis:
PO: Adults, elderly, children >12 yrs: 200 mg q12h for 10 days. **Children 6 mos–12 yrs:** 7.5 mg/kg q12h for 10 days.

Pneumonia:
PO: Adults, elderly, children >12 yrs: 400 mg q12h for 14 days.

Sinusitis:
PO: Adults, elderly, children >12 yrs: 400 mg q12h for 10 days. **Children: 6 mos–12 yrs:** 15 mg/kg q12h for 10 days.

Skin, soft tissue infections:
PO: Adults, elderly, children >12 yrs: 200 mg q12h for 7 days. **Children 6 mos–12 yrs:** 7.5 mg/kg q12h for 7 days.

Urinary tract infections:
PO: Adults, elderly, children 6 mos–12 yrs: 200–400 mg q12h for 7–14 days.

Otitis media:
PO: Children 6 mos–12 yrs: 15 mg/kg q12h for 10 days.

PRECAUTIONS

CONTRAINDICATIONS: History of hypersensitivity to cephalosporins, anaphylactic reaction to penicillins. **CAUTIONS:** Renal impairment. **PREGNANCY/LACTATION:** Unknown whether distributed in breast milk. **Pregnancy Category B.**

INTERACTIONS

DRUG INTERACTIONS: Probenecid increases serum concentrations, half-life of loracarbef. **ALTERED LAB VALUES:** May increase SGOT (AST), SGPT (ALT), alkaline phosphatase, BUN, creatinine. May decrease leukocytes, platelets.

SIDE EFFECTS

FREQUENT: Abdominal pain, anorexia, nausea, vomiting, diarrhea. **OCCASIONAL:** Skin rash, itching. **RARE:** Dizziness, headache, vaginitis.

ADVERSE REACTIONS/TOXIC EFFECTS

Antibiotic-associated colitis, other superinfections may result from altered bacterial balance. Hypersensitivity reactions (ranging from rash, urticaria, fever to anaphylaxis) occur in less than 5%, generally those w/history of allergies, esp. penicillin.

NURSING IMPLICATIONS
BASELINE ASSESSMENT:

Question history of allergies, particularly cephalosporins, penicillins. Obtain culture and sensitivity test before giving first dose (therapy may begin before results are known).

INTERVENTION/EVALUATION:

Assess for nausea, vomiting. Check stool frequency and consistency. Assess skin for rash (diaper area in children). Monitor I&O, urinalysis, renal function reports for nephrotoxicity. Be alert for superinfection: genital/anal pruritus, moniliasis, abdominal pain, sore mouth or tongue, moderate to severe diarrhea.

PATIENT/FAMILY TEACHING:

Continue antibiotic therapy for full length of treatment. Doses should be evenly spaced, given at least 1 hr before or 2 hrs after a meal. Notify physician in event of diarrhea, rash, or onset of other new symptoms.

loratadine
low-**rah**-tah-deen
(Claritin, Claritin Reditabs)

FIXED-COMBINATION(S): W/pseudoephedrine, a sympathomimetic **(Claritin-D)**

CANADIAN AVAILABILITY: Claritin

CLASSIFICATION

Antihistamine

AVAILABILITY (Rx)

Tablets: 10 mg. **Syrup:** 10 mg/10 ml.

PHARMACOKINETICS

	ONSET	PEAK	DURATION
PO	1–3 hrs	8–12 hrs	24 hrs

Rapidly, almost completely absorbed from GI tract. Distributed mainly in liver, lungs, GI tract, bile. Metabolized in liver to active metabolite (undergoes extensive first-pass metabolism). Excreted in urine, eliminated in feces. Half-life: 3–20 hrs; metabolite: 28 hrs (increased in elderly, liver disease).

ACTION/ THERAPEUTIC EFFECT

Long acting w/selective peripheral histamine H-1 receptor antagonist action. Competes w/histamine for receptor site *to prevent allergic responses mediated by histamine (urticaria, pruritus).* Has no significant anticholinergic effects.

USES / *UNLABELED*

Relief of nasal and non-nasal symptoms of seasonal allergic rhinitis (hay fever). Treatment of idiopathic chronic urticaria (hives). *Adjunct treatment of bronchial asthma.*

PO ADMINISTRATION

Preferably give on an empty stomach (food delays absorption).

INDICATIONS / DOSAGE / ROUTES

Allergic rhinitis, hives:
PO: **Adults, elderly, children >6 yrs:** 10 mg once daily. **Hepatic Function Impairment:** 10 mg every other day.

PRECAUTIONS

CONTRAINDICATIONS: Hypersensitivity to loratadine or any ingredient. **CAUTIONS:** Pts w/liver impairment. Safety in children <6 yrs not known. **PREGNANCY/ LACTATION:** Excreted in breast milk. **Pregnancy Category B**.

INTERACTIONS

DRUG INTERACTIONS: Ketoconazole, erythromycin may increase concentrations. **ALTERED LAB VALUES:** May suppress wheal and flare reactions to antigen skin testing, unless antihistamines are discontinued 4 days before testing.

SIDE EFFECTS

FREQUENT (8–12%): Headache, fatigue, drowsiness. **OCCASIONAL (3%):** Dry mouth, nose, throat.

ADVERSE REACTIONS / TOXIC EFFECTS

None significant.

NURSING IMPLICATIONS

BASELINE ASSESSMENT:

Assess lung sounds, rhinitis, urticaria, or other symptoms.

INTERVENTION / EVALUATION:

For upper respiratory allergies, increase fluids to maintain thin secretions and offset thirst, loss of fluids from increased sweating. Monitor symptoms for therapeutic response.

PATIENT / FAMILY TEACHING:

Take loratadine on an empty stomach. Does not cause drowsiness; however, if blurred vision or eye pain occurs, do not drive or perform activities requiring visual acuity. Avoid alcohol during antihistamine therapy.

lorazepam

low-**raz**-ah-pam
(Alzapam, Ativan)

CANADIAN AVAILABILITY:
Apo-Lorazepam, Ativan, Novolorazepam

CLASSIFICATION

Antianxiety

AVAILABILITY (Rx)

Tablets: 0.5 mg, 1 mg, 2 mg. **Injection:** 2 mg/ml, 4 mg/ml.

PHARMACOKINETICS

	ONSET	PEAK	DURATION
IM	15–30 min	—	12–24 hrs
IV	1–5 min	—	12–24 hrs

Well absorbed after oral, IM administration. Widely distributed. Metabolized in liver. Primarily excreted in urine. Half-life: 10–20 hrs.

ACTION/*THERAPEUTIC EFFECT*

Enhances inhibitory neurotransmitter gamma-aminobutyric acid (GABA) neurotransmission at CNS, *producing anxiolytic effect.* Inhibits spinal afferent pathways, *producing skeletal muscle relaxation.* Depressant effects occur at all levels of CNS. Directly depresses motor nerve, muscle function.

USES/*UNLABELED*

Management of anxiety disorders associated w/depressive symptoms. Parenteral form used preoperatively to provide sedation, relieve anxiety, and produce anterograde amnesia. Treatment of status epilepticus. *Treatment of alcohol withdrawal, adjunct to endoscopic procedures (diminishes pt recall), panic disorders, skeletal muscle spasms, cancer chemotherapy–induced nausea/vomiting, tension headache, tremors.*

STORAGE/HANDLING

Refrigerate parenteral form. Do not use if precipitate forms or solution appears discolored. Avoid freezing.

PO/IM/IV ADMINISTRATION

PO:

1. Give w/food.
2. Tablets may be crushed.

IM:

Give deep IM into large muscle mass.

IV:

1. Dilute w/equal volume of sterile water for injection, 0.9% NaCl injection, or 5% dextrose injection.

2. To dilute prefilled syringe, remove air from half-filled syringe, aspirate equal volume of diluent, pull plunger back slightly to allow for mixing, and gently invert syringe several times (do not shake vigorously).

3. Give by direct IV injection or into tubing of free-flowing IV infusion (0.9% NaCl, 5% dextrose) at rate of infusion not to exceed 2 mg/min.

4. Direct IV injection should be made w/repeated aspiration to ensure prevention of intra-arterial administration (produces arteriospasm; may result in gangrene).

INDICATIONS/DOSAGE/ROUTES

Anxiety:
PO: Adults: 1–2 mg daily in 2–3 evenly divided doses. **Elderly:** Initially, 0.5–1 mg/day. May increase gradually.

Insomnia due to anxiety:
PO: Adults: 2–4 mg at bedtime. **Elderly:** 0.5–1 mg at bedtime.

Preop:
IM: Adults, elderly: 0.05 mg/kg given 2 hrs before procedure. Do not exceed 4 mg.
IV: Adults, elderly: 0.044 mg/kg (up to 2 mg total) 15–20 min before surgery.

Status epilepticus:
PO: Adults: 4 mg, may repeat in 10–15 min. Give slowly 2 mg/min.

PRECAUTIONS

CONTRAINDICATIONS: Acute narrow-angle glaucoma, acute alcohol intoxication. **CAUTIONS:** Impaired kidney/liver function. **PREGNANCY/LACTATION:** May cross placenta; may be distributed in breast milk. May increase risk of fetal abnormalities if administered during first trimester of pregnancy. Chronic ingestion during pregnancy may produce fetal toxicity, withdrawal symptoms, CNS depression in neonates. **Pregnancy Category D**.

INTERACTIONS

DRUG INTERACTIONS: Alcohol, CNS depressants may increase CNS depressant effect. **ALTERED LAB VALUES:** None significant.

SIDE EFFECTS

FREQUENT: Drowsiness, dizziness, incoordination. Morning drowsiness may occur initially. **OCCASIONAL:** Blurred vision, slurred speech, hypotension, headache. **RARE:** Paradoxical CNS restlessness, excitement in elderly/debilitated (generally noted during first 2 wks of therapy, particularly noted in presence of uncontrolled pain).

ADVERSE REACTIONS/TOXIC EFFECTS

Abrupt or too rapid withdrawal may result in pronounced restlessness, irritability, insomnia, hand tremors, abdominal/muscle cramps, sweating, vomiting, seizures. Overdosage results in somnolence, confusion, diminished reflexes, coma.

NURSING IMPLICATIONS

BASELINE ASSESSMENT:

Offer emotional support to anxious pt. Pt must remain recumbent for up to 8 hrs (individualized) after parenteral administration to reduce hypotensive effect. Assess motor responses (agitation, trembling, tension) and autonomic responses (cold, clammy hands, sweating).

INTERVENTION/EVALUATION:

For those on long-term therapy, liver/renal function tests, blood counts should be performed periodically. Assess for paradoxical reaction, particularly during early therapy. Assist w/ambulation if drowsiness, lightheadedness occurs. Evaluate for therapeutic response: a calm facial expression, decreased restlessness and/or insomnia.

PATIENT/FAMILY TEACHING:

Drowsiness usually disappears during continued therapy. If dizziness occurs, change positions slowly from recumbent to sitting position before standing. Avoid tasks that require alertness, motor skills until response to drug is established. Smoking reduces drug effectiveness. Do not abruptly withdraw medication after long-term therapy. Do not use alcohol or CNS depressants. Contraception is recommended for long-term therapy. Notify physician at once if pregnancy is suspected.

losartan

loh-**sar**-tan
(Cozaar)

CANADIAN AVAILABILITY:
Cozaar

FIXED-COMBINATION(S):
W/hydrochlorothiazide, a thiazide diuretic **(Hyzaar)**

CLASSIFICATION

Angiotensin II receptor antagonist

AVAILABILITY (Rx)

Tablets: 25 mg, 50 mg

PHARMACOKINETICS

	ONSET	PEAK	DURATION
PO	—	6 hrs	24 hrs

Well absorbed following oral administration. Undergoes first-pass metabolism in liver to active metabolites. Excreted in urine and via biliary system. Not removed by hemodialysis. Half-life: 2 hrs.

ACTION/ *THERAPEUTIC EFFECT*

Potent vasodilator. An angiotensin II receptor (type AT_1) antagonist; blocks vasoconstrictor and aldosterone-secreting effects of angiotensin II, inhibiting the binding of angiotensin II to the AT_1 receptors, *causing vasodilation, decreased peripheral resistance, decrease in B/P.*

USES

Treatment of hypertension. Used alone or in combination w/other antihypertensives.

PO ADMINISTRATION

1. May give w/o regard to food.
2. Do not crush or break tablets.

INDICATIONS/DOSAGE/ROUTES

Note: If antihypertensive effect using once-daily dosing is inadequate, twice-daily regimen at same total daily dose or an increase in dose may provide therapeutic response. May be given concurrently w/other antihypertensives. If B/P not controlled by losartan alone, a low-dose diuretic may be added.

Hypertension:
PO: Adults, elderly: Initially, 50 mg once daily. **Maximum:** May be given once or twice daily w/total daily doses ranging from 25 to 100 mg.

Hypertension (pts treated w/potassium-depleting diuretics, history of hepatic impairment):
PO: Adults, elderly: Initially, 25 mg once daily. **Maximum:** May be given once or twice daily w/total daily doses ranging from 25 to 100 mg.

PRECAUTIONS

CONTRAINDICATIONS: None sig-nificant. **CAUTIONS:** Renal/hepatic function impairment, renal arterial stenosis. **PREGNANCY/LACTATION:** Has caused fetal/neonatal morbidity, mortality. Potential for adverse effects on nursing infant. Do not breast-feed. **Pregnancy Category C:** First trimester. **Pregnancy Category D:** Second and third trimesters (fetal/neonatal morbidity/mortality).

INTERACTIONS

DRUG INTERACTIONS: Cimetidine may increase effects. Phenobarbital, rifampin may decrease effects. May inhibit effects of ketoconazole, troleandomycin, sulfaphenazole. May increase concentration, toxicity of lithium. **ALTERED LAB VALUES:** May increase BUN, serum creatinine, SGOT (AST), SGPT (ALT), alkaline phosphatase, bilirubin. May decrease Hgb, Hct.

SIDE EFFECTS

FREQUENT (8%): Upper respiratory infection. **OCCASIONAL (2–4%):** Dizziness, diarrhea, cough. **RARE (≤1%):** Insomnia, dyspepsia, heartburn, back/leg pain, muscle cramps/ache, nasal congestion, sinusitis.

ADVERSE REACTIONS/TOXIC EFFECTS

Overdosage may manifest as hypotension and tachycardia; bradycardia occurs less often. Institute supportive measurement.

NURSING IMPLICATIONS
BASELINE ASSESSMENT:

Obtain B/P and apical pulse immediately before each dose, in addition to regular monitoring (be alert to fluctuations). If excessive reduction in B/P occurs, place pt in supine position, feet slightly elevated. Question possibility of pregnancy (see Pregnancy/Lactation). Assess medication history (esp. diuretic). Question for history of hepatic/renal impairment, renal artery stenosis.

INTERVENTION/EVALUATION:

Maintain hydration (offer fluids frequently). Assess for evidence of upper respiratory infection, cough. Assist w/ambulation if dizziness occurs. Monitor stool frequency and consistency (watery, loose, soft).

PATIENT/FAMILY TEACHING:

Inform female pt regarding consequences of second- and third-trimester exposure to losartan. Report pregnancy to physician as soon as possible. Avoid tasks that require alertness, motor skills (possible dizziness effect). Report any sign of infection (sore throat, fever), chest pain. Do not take cold preparations, nasal decongestants. Restrict sodium and alcohol as indicated. Follow diet and control weight. Do not take other medications w/o consulting physician. Do not stop taking medication. Need for lifelong control. Caution against exercising during hot weather (risk of dehydration, hypotension).

---

loteprednol
(Lotemax)
See Supplement

---

lovastatin
low-vah-**stah**-tin
(Mevacor)

CANADIAN AVAILABILITY:
Mevacor

CLASSIFICATION

Antihyperlipoproteinemic

AVAILABILITY (Rx)

Tablets: 10 mg, 20 mg, 40 mg

PHARMACOKINETICS

Incompletely absorbed from GI tract (increased on empty stomach). Hydrolyzed in liver to active metabolite. Primarily eliminated in feces. Half-life: 3 hrs.

ACTION/ *THERAPEUTIC EFFECT*

Inhibits HMG-CoA reductase, the enzyme that catalyzes the early step in cholesterol synthesis. *Decreases LDL cholesterol, VLDL cholesterol, plasma triglycerides; increases HDL cholesterol.*

USES

Treatment of hypercholesterolemia and coronary atherosclerosis. Reduces risk of myocardial infarction, unstable angina, need for revascularization procedures in those w/o symptomatic cardiovascular disease, w/average to moderately elevated total cholesterol and LDL cholesterol levels and below average HDL cholesterol levels.

PO ADMINISTRATION

Give w/meals.

INDICATIONS/DOSAGE/ROUTES

Hyperlipoproteinemia:
PO: Adults, elderly: Initially: 20–40 mg/day w/evening meal. Increase at 4 wk intervals up to maximum of 80 mg/day. **Maintenance:** 20–80 mg/day in single or divided doses.

PRECAUTIONS

CONTRAINDICATIONS: Hypersensitivity to lovastatin, active liver disease, unexplained elevated liver function tests. **CAUTIONS:** Anticoagulant therapy, history of liver disease, substantial alcohol consumption. Withholding/discontinuing lovastatin may be necessary when pt is at risk for renal failure (secondary to rhabdomyolysis); major surgery, severe acute infection, trauma, hypotension, severe metabolic, endocrine or electrolyte disorders, or uncontrolled seizures. **PREGNANCY/LACTATION:** Contraindicated in pregnancy (suppression of cholesterol biosynthesis may cause fetal toxicity) and lactation. Unknown if drug is distributed in breast milk. **Pregnancy Category X.**

INTERACTIONS

DRUG INTERACTIONS: Increased risk of rhabdomyolysis, acute renal failure w/cyclosporine, erythromycin, gemfibrozil, niacin, other immunosuppressants. Erythromycin, itraconazole, ketoconazole may increase concentration causing severe muscle pain, inflammation, weakness. **ALTERED LAB VALUES:** May increase creatinine kinase, serum transaminase concentrations. **FOOD:** Large amounts of grapefruit juice may increase risk of side effects (e.g., muscle pain, weakness).

SIDE EFFECTS

Generally well tolerated. Side effects usually mild and transient. **FREQUENT (5–9%):** Headache, flatulence, diarrhea, abdominal pain or cramps, rash/pruritus. **OCCASIONAL (3–4%):** Nausea, vomiting, constipation, dyspepsia. **RARE (1–2%):** Dizziness, heartburn, myalgia, blurred vision, eye irritation.

ADVERSE REACTIONS/TOXIC EFFECTS

Potential for malignancy, cataracts.

NURSING IMPLICATIONS
BASELINE ASSESSMENT:

Question for possibility of pregnancy before initiating therapy (Pregnancy Category X). Question history of hypersensitivity to lovastatin. Assess baseline lab results: cholesterol, triglycerides, liver function tests.

INTERVENTION/EVALUATION:

Evaluate food tolerance. Determine pattern of bowel activity. Check for headache, dizziness, blurred vision. Assess for rash, pruritus. Monitor cholesterol and triglyceride lab results for therapeutic response. Be alert for malaise, muscle cramping or weakness. Monitor temperature at least twice a day.

PATIENT/FAMILY TEACHING:

Take w/meals. Follow special diet (important part of treatment). Periodic lab tests are essential part of therapy. Do not take other medications w/o physician's knowledge. Do not stop medication w/o consulting physician. Report promptly any muscle pain or weakness, esp. if accompanied by fever or malaise. Do not drive or perform activities that require alert response if dizziness occurs. Avoid drinking large amounts of grapefruit juice.

loxapine hydrochloride

lox-ah-peen
(Loxitane)

loxapine succinate

(Loxitane)

CANADIAN AVAILABILITY:
Apo-Loxapine, Loxapac

CLASSIFICATION

Antipsychotic

AVAILABILITY (Rx)

Capsules: 5 mg, 10 mg, 25 mg, 50 mg. **Oral Concentrate:** 25 mg/ml. **Injection:** 50 mg/ml.

PHARMACOKINETICS

	ONSET	PEAK	DURATION
PO (sedation)			
	20–30 min	1.5–3 hrs	12 hrs
IM (sedation)			
	15–30 min	—	12 hrs

Well absorbed after oral, IM administration. Metabolized in liver to active metabolite. Primarily excreted in urine. Half-life: 12–19 hrs.

ACTION/ *THERAPEUTIC EFFECT*

Blocks dopamine at postsynaptic receptor sites in brain. *Suppresses locomotor activity, produces tranquilization.* Strong anticholinergic effects.

USES/ *UNLABELED*

Symptomatic management of psychotic disorders. *Management anxiety associated w/mental depression.*

STORAGE/HANDLING

Store oral, parenteral form at room temperature. Yellow discoloration of solutions does not affect potency, but discard if markedly discolored.

PO/IM ADMINISTRATION

Note: Give by oral or IM route.

PO:

1. Give w/o regard to meals.
2. Dilute oral concentrate w/orange or grapefruit juice.

IM:

Inject slow, deep IM into upper outer quadrant of gluteus maximus.

INDICATIONS/DOSAGE/ROUTES

Psychotic disorders:
PO: Adults: 10 mg 2 times/day. Increase dosage rapidly during first week to 50 mg, if needed. **Usual therapeutic, maintenance range:** 60–100 mg daily in 2–4 divided doses. **Maximum:** 250 mg/day.
IM: Adults: 12.5–50 mg q4–6h.

Usual elderly dosage:
PO: Initially, 5–10 mg 1–2 times/day. May increase by 5–10 mg q4–7 days.
IM: 12.5–25 mg q48h. May increase by 12.5 mg up to 50 mg.

PRECAUTIONS

CONTRAINDICATIONS: Severe CNS depression, comatose states. **EXTREME CAUTION:** History of seizures. **CAUTION:** Cardiovascular disorders, glaucoma, history of urinary retention, prostatic hypertrophy. **PREGNANCY/LACTATION:** Crosses placenta; distributed in breast milk. **Pregnancy Category C.**

INTERACTIONS

DRUG INTERACTIONS: Alcohol, CNS depressants may increase CNS depression. Antacids, antidiarrheals may decrease absorption. Extrapyramidal symptom (EPS)–producing medications may increase risk of EPS. **ALTERED LAB VALUES:** None significant.

SIDE EFFECTS

FREQUENT: Blurred vision, confusion, drowsiness, dry mouth, dizziness, lightheadedness. **OCCASIONAL:** Allergic reaction (rash, itching), decreased urination, constipation, decreased sexual ability, enlarged breasts, headache, increased sensitivity of skin to sunlight, nausea, vomiting, inability to sleep, weight gain.

ADVERSE REACTIONS/TOXIC EFFECTS

Extrapyramidal symptoms frequently noted are akathisia (motor restlessness, anxiety). Less frequently noted are akinesia (rigidity, tremor, salivation, mask-like facial expression, reduced voluntary movements). Infrequently noted dystonias: torticollis (neck muscle spasm), opisthotonos (rigidity of back muscles), and oculogyric crisis (rolling back of eyes). Tardive dyskinesia (protrusion of tongue, puffing of cheeks, chewing/puckering of mouth) occurs rarely but may be irreversible. Risk is greater in female elderly pts. Grand mal seizures may occur in epileptic pts (risk higher w/IM administration).

NURSING IMPLICATIONS
BASELINE ASSESSMENT:

Assess behavior, appearance, emotional status, response to environment, speech pattern, thought content.

INTERVENTION/EVALUATION:

Supervise suicidal risk pt closely during early therapy (as depression lessens, energy level improves, and suicide potential increases). Monitor B/P for hypotension. Assess for peripheral edema behind medial malleolus (sacral area in bedridden pts). Assess stool consistency and frequency. Monitor for rigidity, tremor, mask-like facial expression (esp. in those receiving IM injection). Assess for therapeutic response (interest in surroundings, improvement in self-care, increased ability to concentrate, relaxed facial expression).

PATIENT/FAMILY TEACHING:

Full therapeutic effect may take up to 6 wks. Report visual disturbances. Sugarless gum, sips of tepid water may relieve dry mouth. Drowsiness generally subsides during continued therapy. Avoid tasks that require alertness, motor skills until response to drug is established. Avoid alcohol, CNS depressants, OTC medications. Describe signs and symptoms of extrapyramidal involvement and tardive dyskinesia for pt to report immediately.

mafenide acetate
ma-fe-nide
(Sulfamylon)

CLASSIFICATION

Burn preparation

AVAILABILITY (Rx)

Cream: 85 mg/g. **Topical solution:** 5%.

PHARMACOKINETICS

Absorbed through devascularized areas into systemic circulation. Rapidly metabolized. Primarily excreted in urine.

ACTION/*THERAPEUTIC EFFECT*

Decreases number of bacteria in avascular tissue of second- and third-degree burns. *Bacteriostatic. Promotes spontaneous healing of deep partial-thickness burns.*

USES

Adjunctive therapy for second- and third-degree burns to prevent infection, septicemia; protection against conversion from partial- to full-thickness wounds (infection causes extended tissue destruction). *Solution:* Adjunct agent to control bacterial infection when used under moist dressing over meshed autografts on excised burn wounds.

TOPICAL ADMINISTRATION

1. Apply to cleansed, debrided burns using sterile glove.

2. Keep burn areas covered w/mafenide cream at all times; reapply to any areas where removed (e.g., w/pt activity).

3. Dressings usually not required; if ordered (e.g., when eschar begins to separate), apply thin layer.

INDICATIONS/DOSAGE/ROUTES

Usual topical dosage:
Adults, elderly: Apply 1–2 times/day.

PRECAUTIONS

CONTRAINDICATIONS: Hypersensitivity to mafenide or sulfite. **CAUTIONS:** Impaired renal function that increases risk of metabolic acidosis. Cross-sensitivity to sulfonamides not certain. **PREGNANCY/LACTATION:** Unknown if distributed in breast milk. Safety during lactation unknown; potential for serious adverse effects to neonate. Not recommended during pregnancy unless burn area is >20% of body surface; contraindicated at or near term. **Pregnancy Category C**.

INTERACTIONS

DRUG INTERACTIONS: None significant. **ALTERED LAB VALUES:** None significant.

SIDE EFFECTS

Difficult to distinguish side effects and effects of severe burn. **FREQUENT:** Pain, burning upon application. **OCCASIONAL:** Allergic reaction (usually 10–14 days after initiation of mafenide): itching, rash, facial edema, swelling; unexplained syndrome of marked hyperventilation w/respiratory alkalosis. **RARE:** Delay in eschar separation, excoriation of new skin.

ADVERSE REACTIONS/TOXIC EFFECTS

Hemolytic anemia, porphyria, bone marrow depression, superinfections (esp. w/fungi), metabolic acidosis occurs rarely.

NURSING IMPLICATIONS
BASELINE ASSESSMENT:

Question for hypersensitivity to mafenide, sulfite (more frequent in asthmatics). Evaluate arterial blood gases (ABGs) for acid-base balance, renal function tests and CBCs for baseline.

INTERVENTION/EVALUATION:

Be alert to fluid balance and renal function: Monitor I&O, renal function tests, urinary pH, and promptly report changes. Watch for signs/symptoms of metabolic acidosis: Kussmaul's respirations, nausea, vomiting, diarrhea, headache, tremors, weakness and cardiac arrhythmias (due to associated hyperkalemia), sensorium changes, decreased PCO_2, blood pH, and HCO_3. Monitor vital signs, evaluate ABG results. Assess burns, surrounding skin areas for allergic reaction or superinfection: rash, excoriation, swelling, itching, increased pain, purulent exudate. Monitor hematologic tests.

PATIENT/FAMILY TEACHING:

Application may cause temporary pain or burning; burn areas must be completely covered by cream. Therapy must not be interrupted (attempts will be made to reduce adverse reaction before considering discontinuance of drug). Inform physician if condition worsens, irritation occurs, or hyperventilation occurs. Bathe burn area daily.

magnesium

magnesium chloride
(Slow-Mag)

magnesium citrate
(Citrate of Magnesia, Citroma, Citro-Nesia)

magnesium hydroxide
(MOM)

magnesium oxide
(Mag-Ox 400, Maox)

magnesium protein complex
(Mg-PLUS)

magnesium sulfate
(Epsom salt, Magnesium Sulfate injection)

FIXED-COMBINATION(S):
W/aluminum, an antacid (**Aludrox, Delcid, Gaviscon, Maalox**); w/aluminum and simethicone, an antiflatulent (**Di-Gel, Gelusil, Maalox Plus, Mylanta, Silain-Gel**); w/aluminum and calcium, an antacid (**Camalox**); w/mineral oil, a lubricant laxative (**Haley's MO**); w/magnesium oxide and aluminum oxide, antacids (**Riopan**).

CANADIAN AVAILABILITY:
Citro-Mag, Phillips' Magnesia Tablets, Slow-Mag

CLASSIFICATION
Antacid, anticonvulsant, electrolyte, laxative

AVAILABILITY (OTC)
Tablets: 400 mg, 500 mg. **Tablets (chewable):** 311 mg. **Tablets (sustained-release):** 535 mg. **Capsules:** 140 mg. **Liquid:** 54 mg/5 ml, 400 mg/5 ml, 800 mg/5 ml. **MOM:** 30 ml, 60 ml. **Injection (Rx):** 10%, 12.5%, 20%, 50%.

PHARMACOKINETICS
Antacid, laxative: Minimal absorption through intestine. Absorbed dose primarily excreted in urine. *Systemic:* Widely distributed. Primarily excreted in urine.

ACTION/THERAPEUTIC EFFECT
Antacid: Acts in stomach to neutralize *gastric acid, increase pH.* **Laxative:** Osmotic effect primarily in small intestine. Draws water into intestinal lumen, produces *distention, promotes peristalsis, bowel evacuation.* **Systemic (dietary supplement, replacement):** Found primarily in intracellular fluids. Essential *for enzyme activity, nerve conduction, and muscle contraction.* **Anticonvulsant:** Blocks neuromuscular transmission, amount of acetylcholine released at motor end plate, *producing seizure control.*

USES
Antacid: Symptomatic relief of upset stomach associated w/hyperacidity (heartburn, acid indigestion, sour stomach), gastric, duodenal ulcers. Symptomatic treatment of GERD. Prophylactic treatment of GI bleeding secondary to gastritis and stress ulceration. *Laxative:* Evacuation of colon for rectal and bowel exami-

M

nation, elective colon surgery. Accelerates excretion of various parasites, poisonous substances (except acid or alkali) from GI tract. *Systemic:* Dietary supplement, replacement therapy. Nutritional adjunct in hyperalimentation. *Anticonvulsant:* Immediate control of life-threatening seizures in treatment of severe toxemia of pregnancy, seizures associated w/ acute nephritis in children.

STORAGE/HANDLING

Store oral, parenteral forms at room temperature. Refrigerate citrate of magnesia (retains potency, palatability).

PO/IM/IV ADMINISTRATION

PO (Antacid):

1. Suspensions to be shaken well before use.
2. Chew chewable tablets thoroughly before swallowing and follow w/full glass of water.

PO (Laxative):

1. Drink full glass of liquid (8 oz) w/each dose (prevents dehydration).
2. Flavor improved by following w/fruit juice or citrus carbonated beverage.

IM:

1. For adults, elderly, use 250 mg/ml (25%) or 500 mg/ml (50%) magnesium sulfate concentration.
2. For infants, children, do not exceed 200 mg/ml (20%).

IV:

1. For IV infusion, do not exceed magnesium sulfate concentration 200 mg/ml (20%).
2. Do not exceed IV infusion rate of 150 mg/min.

INDICATIONS/DOSAGE/ROUTES

Note: 1 g = 8.12 mEq as magnesium sulfate.

ANTACID:

Magnesium hydroxide:
PO: Adults, elderly, children >12 yrs: 5–15 ml or 0.65–1.3 g 4 times/day.

Magnesium oxide:
PO: Adults, elderly: 400–840 mg/day.

LAXATIVE:

Citrate of magnesia:
PO: Adults, elderly: 240 ml as needed. Children: $^1/_2$ adult dose, repeat as needed.

Magnesium hydroxide:
PO: Adults, elderly: 30–60 ml/day w/liquids. Children ≥2 yrs: 5–30 ml (dependent on age).

Magnesium sulfate:
PO: Adults, elderly: 10–15 g in glass of water. Children: 5–10 g in glass of water.

DIETARY SUPPLEMENT:

PO: Adults, elderly: 54–483 mg/day (refer to individual products).

MILD DEFICIENCY:

IM: Adults, elderly: 1 g q6h for 4 doses.

SEVERE DEFICIENCY:

IM/IV Infusion: Adults, elderly: 0.5–1 mEq/kg/day (lean body wt) in divided doses.

HYPERALIMENTATION:

IV: Adults, elderly: 1–3 g (8–24 mEq)/day. Children: 0.25–1.25 g (2–10 mEq)/day.

ANTICONVULSANT:

IM: Adults: 4–5 g (32–40 mEq) of 50% solution q4h as needed. Chil-

dren: 20–40 mg/kg of 20% solution, may repeat as needed.
IV: Adults: 4 g (32 mEq) of 10–20% solution (do not exceed rate of 1.5 ml/min of 10% solution).
IV Infusion: Adults: 4–5 g (32–40 mEq)/250 ml 5% dextrose or 0.9% NaCl (do not exceed rate of 3 ml/min).

PRECAUTIONS

CONTRAINDICATIONS: *Antacids:* Severe renal impairment, appendicitis or symptoms of appendicitis, ileostomy, intestinal obstruction. *Laxative:* Appendicitis, undiagnosed rectal bleeding, CHF, intestinal obstruction, hypersensitivity, colostomy, ileostomy. *Systemic:* Heart block, myocardial damage, renal failure. **CAUTIONS:** Safety in children <6 yrs not known. *Antacids:* Undiagnosed gastrointestinal or rectal bleeding, ulcerative colitis, colostomy, diverticulitis, chronic diarrhea. *Laxative:* Diabetes mellitus or pts on low-salt diet (some products contain sugar, sodium). *Systemic:* Severe renal impairment. **PREGNANCY/LACTATION:** *Antacid:* Unknown whether distributed in breast milk. **Pregnancy Category C**. *Parenteral:* Readily crosses placenta; distributed in breast milk for 24 hrs after magnesium therapy is discontinued. Continuous IV infusion increases risk of magnesium toxicity in neonate. IV administration should not be used 2 hrs preceding delivery. **Pregnancy Category B** (anticonvulsant/laxative).

INTERACTIONS

DRUG INTERACTIONS: *Antacids:* May decrease absorption of ketoconazole, tetracyclines. May decrease effect of methenamine. *Antacids, laxatives:* May decrease effects of oral anticoagulants, digoxin, phenothiazines. May form nonabsorbable complex w/tetracyclines. *Systemic:* Calcium may neutralize effects. CNS depression–producing medications may increase CNS depression. May cause changes in cardiac conduction/heart block w/digoxin. **ALTERED LAB VALUES:** *Antacid:* May increase gastrin, pH. *Laxative:* May decrease potassium. *Systemic:* None significant.

SIDE EFFECTS

FREQUENT: *Antacid:* Chalky taste, diarrhea, laxative effect. **OCCASIONAL:** *Antacid:* Nausea, vomiting, stomach cramps. *Antacid, laxative:* Prolonged use or large dose w/renal impairment may cause increased magnesium (dizziness, irregular heartbeat, mental changes, tiredness, weakness). *Laxative:* Cramping, diarrhea, increased thirst, gas. *Systemic:* Reduced respiratory rate, decreased reflexes, flushing, hypotension, decreased heart rate.

ADVERSE REACTIONS/TOXIC EFFECTS

Antacid, laxative: None significant. *Systemic:* May produce prolonged PQ interval, widening of QRS intervals. May cause loss of deep tendon reflexes, heart block, respiratory paralysis, and cardiac arrest. *Antidote:* 10–20 ml 10% calcium gluconate (5–10 mEq of calcium).

NURSING IMPLICATIONS
BASELINE ASSESSMENT:

Assess if pt is sensitive to magnesium. *Antacid:* Assess gastrointestinal pain (duration, location, time of occurrence, relief w/food or caused by food or alcohol, constant or sporadic, worsened when lying down or bending over). *Laxative:* Assess color, amount, consistency of stool. Assess bowel habits (usual pattern), bowel sound for peristalsis. Assess pt for any abdominal pain, weight loss, nausea, vomiting, history of recent abdominal surgery. *Systemic:* Assess renal function, magnesium level.

INTERVENTION/EVALUATION:

Antacid: Assess for relief of gastric distress. Monitor renal function (esp. if dosing is long term or frequent). *Laxative:* Monitor stools for diarrhea or constipation. Maintain adequate fluid intake. *Systemic:* Monitor renal function, magnesium levels, EKG for cardiac function. Test patellar reflex or knee jerk reflexes before giving repeat parenteral doses (used as indication of CNS depression; suppressed reflex may be sign of impending respiratory arrest). Patellar reflex must be present, respiratory rate >16/min before each parenteral dose. Provide seizure precautions.

PATIENT/FAMILY TEACHING:

Antacid: Give at least 2 hrs apart from other medication. Do not take >2 wks unless directed by physician. For peptic ulcer take 1 and 3 hrs after meals and at bedtime for 4–6 wks. Chew tablets thoroughly followed w/glass of water; shake suspensions well. Repeat dosing/large doses may have laxative effect. *Laxative:* Drink full glass (8 oz) liquid to aid stool softening. Use only for short term. Teach other methods of bowel regulation (diet, exercise, increased fluid intake). Do not use if abdominal pain, vomiting, nausea are present. Inform pt of normal bowel

movement range: 3 per day to 3 per week. *Systemic:* Inform physician of any signs of hypermagnesemia (confusion, irregular heartbeat, cramping, unusual tiredness or weakness, lightheadedness, or dizziness).

mannitol
man-ih-toll
(Osmitrol)

CANADIAN AVAILABILITY:
Osmitrol

CLASSIFICATION

Osmotic diuretic

AVAILABILITY (Rx)

Injection: 5%, 10%, 15%, 20%, 25%

PHARMACOKINETICS

Remains in extracellular fluid. Primarily excreted in urine. Half-life: 100 min. Onset diuresis occurs in 1–3 hrs, decreases intraocular pressure in 0.5–1 hr, duration 4–6 hrs. Decreases cerebral spinal fluid pressure in 15 min, duration 3–8 hrs.

ACTION/*THERAPEUTIC EFFECT*

Elevates osmotic pressure of glomerular filtrate, increases flow of water into interstitial fluid and plasma, inhibiting renal tubular reabsorption of sodium, chloride, *producing diuresis.* Enhances flow of water from eye into plasma, *reducing intraocular pressure (IOP).*

USES

Prevention, treatment of oliguric phase of acute renal failure (before evidence of permanent renal failure). Reduces increased intracranial pressure due to cerebral edema, edema of injured spinal cord, intraocular pressure due to acute glaucoma. Promotes urinary excretion of toxic substances (aspirin, bromides, imipramine, barbiturates).

STORAGE/HANDLING

Store at room temperature. Crystallization can occur. Do not use if crystals remain after warming procedure (see IV Administration).

IV ADMINISTRATION

Note: Assess IV site for patency before each dose. Extravasation noted w/pain, thrombosis.
1. Rate of administration should be titrated to promote urinary output of 30–50 ml/hr.
2. If crystals are noted in solution, warm bottle in hot water and shake vigorously at intervals. Cool to body temperature before administration.
3. Use filter for infusion of 20% or more concentration.
4. Do not add KCl or NaCl to mannitol 20% or greater. Do not add to whole blood for transfusion.

INDICATIONS/DOSAGE/ROUTES

Note: Dosage based on pt's condition/fluid requirements, urinary output, concentration and rate of administration.

Test dose for marked oliguria/suspected inadequate renal function:
IV: Adults, elderly: 0.2 g/kg or 12.5 g w/15–20% solution. Infuse over 3–5 min to produce urinary output of 30–50 ml in 2–3 hrs. Test dose may be repeated once.

Oliguria/acute renal failure prevention:
IV: Adults, elderly: 50–100 g of a concentrated solution followed by 5–10% solution.

Treatment of oliguria:
IV: Adults, elderly: 100 g w/ 15–20% solution infused over 90 min to a few hours.

Intracranial/intraocular pressure:
IV: Adults, elderly: 1.5–2 g/kg administered as a 15–20–25% solution, infused over 30–60 min. Rebound increase of intracranial pressure may occur 12 hrs after use. For preop use, administer 1–1½ hrs before surgery.

Treatment of drug intoxications:
IV: Adults, elderly: Loading dose of 25 g followed by dosage titrated to maintain urinary output of 100–500 ml/hr. For barbiturates, 0.5 g/kg w/5–10% solutions titrated to urine output. Dosage and treatment based on fluid balance, urine pH, urine volume.

PRECAUTIONS

CONTRAINDICATIONS: Increasing oliguria or anuria, CHF, pulmonary edema, organic CNS disease, severe dehydration, fluid overload, active intracranial bleeding (except during craniotomy), severe electrolyte depletion. **CAUTIONS:** Impaired renal, hepatic function. **PREGNANCY/LACTATION:** Unknown whether drug crosses placenta or is distributed in breast milk. **Pregnancy Category C**.

INTERACTIONS

DRUG INTERACTIONS: May increase digoxin toxicity (due to hypokalemia). **ALTERED LAB VALUES:** May decrease phosphate, potassium, sodium.

SIDE EFFECTS

FREQUENT: Dry mouth, thirst.

OCCASIONAL: Blurred vision, increased urination, headache, arm pain, backache, nausea, vomiting, urticaria (hives), dizziness, hypotension, hypertension, tachycardia, fever, angina-like chest pain.

ADVERSE REACTIONS/TOXIC EFFECTS

Fluid and electrolyte imbalance may occur because of rapid administration of large doses or inadequate urinary output resulting in overexpansion of extracellular fluid. Circulatory overload may produce pulmonary edema, CHF. Excessive diuresis may produce hypokalemia, hyponatremia. Fluid loss in excess of electrolyte excretion may produce hypernatremia, hyperkalemia.

NURSING IMPLICATIONS
BASELINE ASSESSMENT:

Check B/P, pulse before giving medication. Baseline electrolyte, renal and hepatic function, BUN may be ordered. Assess skin turgor, mucous membranes, mental status, muscle strength. Obtain baseline weight. Initiate I&O. For acute situations, a foley catheter may assist in measuring hourly outputs.

INTERVENTION/EVALUATION:

Monitor urinary output to ascertain therapeutic response. Monitor electrolyte, BUN, renal, hepatic reports. Assess vital signs, skin turgor, mucous membranes. Weigh daily. Signs of hyponatremia include confusion, drowsiness, thirst or dry mouth, cold/clammy skin. Signs of hypokalemia include changes in muscle strength, tremors, muscle cramps, changes in mental status, cardiac arrhythmias.

Signs of hyperkalemia include colic, diarrhea, muscle twitching followed by weakness or paralysis, arrhythmias.

PATIENT/FAMILY TEACHING:

Expect increased frequency and volume of urination.

---

maprotiline hydrochloride

mah-**pro**-tih-leen
(Ludiomil)

CANADIAN AVAILABILITY:
Ludiomil

CLASSIFICATION

Antidepressant

AVAILABILITY (Rx)

Tablets: 25 mg, 50 mg, 75 mg

PHARMACOKINETICS

Slowly, completely absorbed from GI tract. Widely distributed. Metabolized in liver to active metabolites. Primarily excreted in urine. Half-life: 27–58 hrs; metabolite: 60–90 hrs.

ACTION/*THERAPEUTIC EFFECT*

Blocks reuptake of norepinephrine by CNS presynaptic neuronal membranes, increasing availability at postsynaptic neuronal receptor sites. Resulting enhancement of synaptic activity *produces antidepressant effect.* Moderate anticholinergic activity.

USES/*UNLABELED*

Relief of depressive-affective (mood) disorders, including depressive neurosis, major depression. Also used for depression phase of bipolar disorder (manic-depressive illness). *Treatment of neurogenic pain.*

PO ADMINISTRATION

1. Give w/food or milk if GI distress occurs.

2. Do not crush or break enteric-coated tablets.

3. Scored tablets may be crushed.

INDICATIONS/DOSAGE/ROUTES

Mild to moderate depression:
PO: Adults: 75 mg/day to start, in 1–4 divided doses. **Elderly:** 50–75 mg/day. In 2 wks, increase dosage gradually in 25 mg increments until therapeutic response is achieved. Reduce to lowest effective maintenance level.

Severe depression:
PO: Adults: 100–150 mg/day in 1–4 divided doses. May increase gradually to maximum 225 mg/day.

Usual elderly dosage:
PO: Initially, 25 mg at bedtime. May increase by 25 mg q3–7 days. **Maintenance:** 50–75 mg/day.

PRECAUTIONS

CONTRAINDICATIONS: Acute recovery period following MI, within 14 days of MAO inhibitor ingestion, known or suspected seizure disorders. **CAUTIONS:** Prostatic hypertrophy, history of urinary retention or obstruction, glaucoma, diabetes mellitus, history of seizures, hyperthyroidism, cardiac/hepatic/renal disease, schizophrenia, increased intraocular pressure, hiatal hernia. **PREGNANCY/LACTATION:** Crosses placenta; distributed in breast milk. **Pregnancy Category B.**

INTERACTIONS

DRUG INTERACTIONS: Alcohol, CNS depressants may increase effect. MAO inhibitors may increase risk of hypertensive crisis, severe convulsions. Sympathomimetics may increase cardiovascular effects (arrhythmias, tachycardia, severe hypertension). **ALTERED LAB VALUES:** None significant.

SIDE EFFECTS

FREQUENT: Drowsiness, fatigue, dry mouth, blurred vision, constipation, delayed micturition, postural hypotension, excessive sweating, disturbed concentration, increased appetite, urinary retention. **OCCASIONAL:** GI disturbances (nausea, GI distress, metallic taste sensation), increased sensitivity of skin to sunlight. **RARE:** Paradoxical reaction (agitation, restlessness, nightmares, insomnia), extrapyramidal symptoms (particularly fine hand tremor).

ADVERSE REACTIONS/TOXIC EFFECTS

Higher incidence of seizures than w/tricyclic antidepressants (esp. in those w/no previous history of seizures). High dosage may produce cardiovascular effects (severe postural hypotension, dizziness, tachycardia, palpitations, arrhythmias) and seizures. May also result in altered temperature regulation (hyperpyrexia or hypothermia). Abrupt withdrawal from prolonged therapy may produce headache, malaise, nausea, vomiting, vivid dreams.

NURSING IMPLICATIONS
BASELINE ASSESSMENT:

For those on long-term therapy, liver/renal function tests, blood counts should be performed periodically.

INTERVENTION/EVALUATION:

Supervise suicidal risk pt closely during early therapy (as depression lessens, energy level improves, increasing suicide potential). Assess appearance, behavior, speech pattern, level of interest, mood. Monitor bowel activity; avoid constipation. Monitor B/P, pulse for hypotension, arrhythmias. Assess for urinary retention.

PATIENT/FAMILY TEACHING:

Change positions slowly to avoid hypotensive effect. Tolerance to postural hypotension, sedative and anticholinergic effects usually develops during early therapy. Therapeutic effect may be noted within 3–7 days, maximum effect within 2–3 wks. Wear protective clothing, use sunscreen to protect skin from ultraviolet light or sunlight. Dry mouth may be relieved by sugarless gum, sips of tepid water. Report visual disturbances. Do not abruptly discontinue medication. Avoid tasks that require alertness, motor skills until response to drug is established.

---

masoprocol

mass-oh-**pro**-call
(Actinex)

CLASSIFICATION

Topical

AVAILABILITY (Rx)

Cream: 10%

PHARMACOKINETICS

Minimal absorption systemically (<2%).

ACTION/THERAPEUTIC EFFECT

Produces antiproliferative activity against keratinocytes.

USES

Topical treatment for actinic (solar) keratoses.

TOPICAL ADMINISTRATION

1. Wash and dry affected area before application.
2. Apply directly to desired area, massaging gently (avoid eyes and mucous membranes of nose/mouth).
3. Avoid occlusive dressing.
4. If applied w/fingers, wash hands immediately w/soap and water after use.

INDICATIONS/DOSAGE/ROUTES

Actinic (solar) keratoses:
Topical: Adults, elderly: Apply to area topically as needed. Do not cover surface (minimizes irritation). Repeat each morning and evening for 28 days.

PRECAUTIONS

CONTRAINDICATIONS: Hypersensitivity to masoprocol or other components of preparation. **CAUTIONS:** Sulfite sensitivity. For external use only. Avoid occlusive dressings. Safety in children not established. **PREGNANCY/LACTATION:** Unknown whether excreted in breast milk. **Pregnancy Category B.**

INTERACTIONS

DRUG INTERACTIONS: None significant. **ALTERED LAB VALUES:** None significant.

SIDE EFFECTS

FREQUENT (>5%): Erythema, flaking (46%), itching (32%), edema (14%), burning (12%), soreness. **OCCASIONAL (1–5%):** Bleeding, crusting, eye irritation, rash, skin irritation, stinging, tightness, tingling. **RARE (<1%):** Blistering, excoriation, fissuring, skin roughness, wrinkling.

ADVERSE REACTIONS/TOXIC EFFECTS

Allergic contact dermatitis represents sensitization. Discontinue medication, contact physician.

NURSING IMPLICATIONS
BASELINE ASSESSMENT:

Question for hypersensitivity to masoprocol or other components of preparation.

INTERVENTION/EVALUATION:

Assess for irritation.

PATIENT/FAMILY TEACHING:

Use only as directed. For external use only. Take special care to avoid eyes, nose, mouth. If contact w/eyes occurs, rinse promptly and thoroughly w/water. If applied w/fingers, wash hands immediately after application. Do not use occlusive coverings. Do not use other skin products or makeup during therapy w/o advice of physician. May stain clothing, fabrics. Does not cause photosensitivity, but avoid undue sun exposure because of keratoses. May have transient local burning after application. Contact physician if oozing, blistering, or other severe reaction occurs.

---

mebendazole

meh-**ben**-dah-zole
(Vermox)

CANADIAN AVAILABILITY:
Vermox

CLASSIFICATION
Anhelminthic

AVAILABILITY (Rx)
Tablets (chewable): 100 mg

PHARMACOKINETICS
Poorly absorbed from GI tract (absorption increases w/food). Highest concentration in liver. Metabolized in liver. Primarily eliminated in feces. Half-life: 2.5–9 hrs (increased in decreased renal function).

ACTION/*THERAPEUTIC EFFECT*
Vermicidal. Degrades parasite cytoplasmic microtubules, irreversibly blocks glucose uptake in helminths and larvae *(depletes glycogen, decreases ATP, causes helminth death)*.

USES
Treatment of trichuriasis (whipworm), enterobiasis (pinworm), ascariasis (roundworm), hookworm caused by *Ancylostoma duodenale* or *Necator americanus.* Effective in mixed helminthic infections due to broad spectrum of activity.

PO ADMINISTRATION
1. No special fasting is required.
2. Tablet may be crushed, chewed, swallowed, or mixed w/food.
3. For high dosage, best if taken w/food.

INDICATIONS/DOSAGE/ROUTES
Trichuriasis, ascariasis, hookworm:
PO: Adults, elderly, children >2 yrs: 1 tablet in morning and at bedtime for 3 days.

Enterobiasis:
PO: Adults, elderly, children >2 yrs: 1 tablet one time.

PRECAUTIONS

CONTRAINDICATIONS: None significant. **CAUTIONS:** None significant. **PREGNANCY/LACTATION:** Unknown whether drug crosses placenta or is distributed in breast milk. **Pregnancy Category C**.

INTERACTIONS

DRUG INTERACTIONS: Carbamazepine may decrease concentrations. **ALTERED LAB VALUES:** May increase SGOT (AST), SGPT (ALT), alkaline phosphatase, BUN. May decrease Hgb.

SIDE EFFECTS

OCCASIONAL: Nausea, vomiting, headache, dizziness. Transient abdominal pain, diarrhea w/massive infection and expulsion of helminths. **RARE:** Fever.

ADVERSE REACTIONS/TOXIC EFFECTS

High dosage may produce reversible myelosuppression (granulocytopenia, leukopenia, neutropenia).

NURSING IMPLICATIONS
BASELINE ASSESSMENT:

Question for history of hypersensitivity to mebendazole. Obtain specimens to confirm diagnosis: (1) Stool must be collected in clean, dry bedpan or container (parasites may be destroyed by urine, water, or medications). (2) Obtain pinworm specimens early in morning by applying transparent tape to tongue blade and pressing sticky side of tape to perianal area (female pinworms usually deposit eggs in this area during night).

INTERVENTION/EVALUATION:

Encourage intake of fruits, vegetables, fluids to avoid constipation (parasites expelled by normal peristalsis). Collect stool or perianal specimens as required to confirm cure. Monitor CBC w/high dosage. Assess food tolerance. Provide assistance w/ambulation if dizzy.

PATIENT/FAMILY TEACHING:

Complete full course of therapy; may need to repeat. Wash hands thoroughly after toileting, before eating. Keep hands away from mouth, fingernails short. Disinfect toilet facilities daily. Due to high transmission of pinworm infections, all family members should be treated simultaneously; infected person should sleep alone, shower frequently. Do not shake bedding; change and launder underclothing, pajamas, bedding, towels, and washcloths daily. W/hookworm, avoid walking barefoot (larval entry into system). Continue iron supplements as long as ordered (may be 6 mos after treatment) for anemia associated w/whipworm, hookworm. Notify physician if symptoms do not improve in a few days or if they become worse. Follow-up w/office visits, stool collection are important parts of therapy. Don't drive, use machinery if dizzy.

mechlorethamine hydrochloride

meh-klor-**eth**-ah-meen
(Mustargen)

CANADIAN AVAILABILITY:
Mustargen

CLASSIFICATION

Antineoplastic

AVAILABILITY (Rx)

Powder for Injection: 10 mg

PHARMACOKINETICS

Incompletely absorbed after intracavitary administration. Rapidly deactivated in fluids/tissues. Primarily excreted in urine.

ACTION / *THERAPEUTIC EFFECT*

Primarily crosslinks w/DNA, RNA strands, *inhibiting protein synthesis.* Cell cycle-phase nonspecific.

USES

Treatment of advanced Hodgkin's disease, lymphosarcoma, mycosis fungoides, bronchogenic carcinoma, chronic myelocytic and lymphocytic leukemia, polycythemia vera, malignant effusions (pericardial, peritoneal, pleural) by intracavitary administration.

STORAGE/HANDLING

Note: May be carcinogenic, mutagenic, or teratogenic. Handle w/extreme care during preparation/administration.

Prepare solution immediately before use. Use only clear, colorless solutions. Discard if change in color occurs, precipitate forms, or water droplets are noted inside vial prior to reconstitution.

IV ADMINISTRATION

Note: Give by IV injection. Avoid high concentration, prolonged local contact w/drug. Wear gloves when preparing solution. Avoid inhalation of dust or vapors, contact w/skin, mucous membranes. If eye contact occurs, immediately institute copious irrigation w/0.9% NaCl or ophthalmic irrigating solution. If skin contact occurs, wash affected part immediately w/copious amounts of water for 15 min, followed by 2% sodium thiosulfate solution.

1. Reconstitute each 10 mg vial w/10 ml sterile water for injection or 0.9% NaCl injection to provide concentration of 1 mg/ml.

2. Shake vial several times w/needle still in rubber stopper (minimizes risk of skin contact) to ensure complete dissolution.

3. Withdraw dose from vial using one sterile needle; use second sterile needle for injection.

4. Give desired dose over a few minutes directly into suitable vein or tubing of running IV infusion.

5. Flush vein and/or tubing for 2–5 min after administration to remove any remaining drug from tubing.

6. Extravasation produces painful inflammation, induration (may last 4–6 wks). Sloughing may occur. If extravasation occurs, infiltrate the area promptly w/isotonic sodium thiosulfate and apply cold compresses for 6–12 hrs. Vein irritation produces dark bluish gray hyperpigmentation.

INDICATIONS/DOSAGE/ROUTES

Note: Dosage individualized based on clinical response, tolerance to adverse effects. When used in combination therapy, consult specific protocols for optimum dosage, sequence of drug administration. Dosage based on ideal body weight.

Usual dosage:
IV: Adults: 0.4 mg/kg per course as single dose, or 0.1–0.2 mg/kg/day in 2–4 divided doses. Repeat q3–6 wks.

Advanced Hodgkin's disease:
IV: Adults: MOPP regimen: 6

mg/m^2 on days 1 and 8 of 28 day cycle.

PRECAUTIONS

CONTRAINDICATIONS: Acute phase of herpes zoster infection, those w/foci of acute/chronic pustule inflammation, presence of known infectious disease. **EXTREME CAUTION:** Leukopenia, thrombocytopenia, anemia due to infiltration of bone marrow w/malignant cells. **PREGNANCY/LACTATION:** If possible, avoid use during pregnancy, esp. first trimester. Breast-feeding not recommended. **Pregnancy Category D**.

INTERACTIONS

DRUG INTERACTIONS: May decrease effect of antigout medications. Bone marrow depressants may increase bone marrow depression. Live virus vaccines may potentiate virus replication, increase vaccine side effects, decrease pt's antibody response to vaccine. **ALTERED LAB VALUES:** May increase uric acid.

SIDE EFFECTS

FREQUENT: Nausea, vomiting occurs within 1–3 hrs after therapy; vomiting usually stops within 8 hrs but nausea may persist for 24 hrs. Lymphocytopenia occurs within 24 hrs of first dose; anorexia, diarrhea, dehydration secondary to vomiting. **OCCASIONAL:** Weakness, headache, drowsiness, lightheadedness, maculopapular rash. **INFREQUENT:** Alopecia. **RARE:** Tinnitus, fever, metallic taste sensation.

ADVERSE REACTIONS/TOXIC EFFECTS

Severe bone marrow depression manifested as hematologic toxicity (severe leukopenia, anemia, thrombocytopenia, bleeding) may occur, particularly when dose exceeds 0.4 mg/kg for single course. Leukopenia occurs within 6–8 days and persists for 10–21 days, recovery within 2 wks. Risk of neurotoxicity (seizures, paresthesia, vertigo) increases w/age and in those who also receive procarbazine or cyclophosphamide.

NURSING IMPLICATIONS

BASELINE ASSESSMENT:

Check CBC and establish baseline for myelosuppressive action of drug. Antiemetics may be effective in preventing, treating nausea, vomiting.

INTERVENTION/EVALUATION:

Assess for severe thrombocytopenia (bleeding from gums, tarry stool, petechiae, small subcutaneous hemorrhages). Monitor I&O; assess for dehydration. Check stools for frequency, consistency. Monitor Hgb, Hct, WBC, differential, platelet count, serum uric acid level. Monitor for hematologic toxicity (fever, sore throat, signs of local infection, easy bruising, unusual bleeding from any site), symptoms of anemia (excessive tiredness, weakness). Avoid IM injections, rectal temperatures, other traumas that may induce bleeding.

PATIENT/FAMILY TEACHING:

Do not have immunizations w/o physician's approval (drug lowers body's resistance). Avoid crowds and those w/infections. Promptly report fever, sore throat, signs of local infection, easy bruising, or unusual bleeding from any site. Contact physician if nausea/vomiting continues at home. Do not take alcohol or any medication (including OTC drugs) w/o consulting physician. Contraception should be used.

meclizine

mek-lih-zeen
(Antivert, Bonine)

CANADIAN AVAILABILITY: Bonamine

CLASSIFICATION

Antiemetic, antivertigo

AVAILABILITY (Rx)

Tablets: 12.5 mg, 25 mg, 50 mg. **Tablets (chewable):** 25 mg. **Capsules:** 25 mg.

PHARMACOKINETICS

	ONSET	PEAK	DURATION
PO	30–60 min	—	12–24 hrs

Well absorbed from GI tract. Widely distributed. Metabolized in liver. Primarily excreted in urine. Half-life: 6 hrs.

ACTION/ *THERAPEUTIC EFFECT*

Reduces labyrinth excitability, diminishes vestibular stimulation of labyrinth, affecting chemoreceptor trigger zone (CTZ), *reducing nausea, vomiting, vertigo.* Anticholinergic activity.

USES

Prevention and treatment of nausea, vomiting, vertigo due to motion sickness. Treatment of vertigo associated with diseases affecting vestibular system.

PO ADMINISTRATION

1. Give w/o regard to meals.
2. Scored tablets may be crushed.
3. Do not crush or break capsule form.

INDICATIONS/DOSAGE/ROUTES

Motion sickness:
PO: Adults, elderly, children >12 yrs: 25–50 mg 1 hr before exposure to motion. Repeat q24h as needed.

Vertigo:
PO: Adults, elderly, children >12 yrs: 25–100 mg/day in divided doses as needed.

PRECAUTIONS

CONTRAINDICATIONS: None significant. **CAUTIONS:** Narrow-angle glaucoma, prostatic hypertrophy, pyloroduodenal or bladder neck obstruction, asthma, COPD, increased intraocular pressure, cardiovascular disease, hyperthyroidism, hypertension, seizure disorders. **PREGNANCY/LACTATION:** Unknown whether drug crosses placenta or is distributed in breast milk (may produce irritability in nursing infants). **Pregnancy Category B.**

INTERACTIONS

DRUG INTERACTIONS: Alcohol, CNS depression–producing medications may increase CNS depressant effect. **ALTERED LAB VALUES:** May suppress wheal, flare reactions to antigen skin testing, unless meclizine discontinued 4 days before testing.

SIDE EFFECTS

Note: Elderly (>60 yrs) tend to develop sedation, dizziness, hypotension, mental confusion, disorientation, agitation, psychotic-like symptoms. **FREQUENT:** Drowsiness. **OCCASIONAL:** Blurred vision, dry mouth, nose, or throat.

ADVERSE REACTIONS/TOXIC EFFECTS

Children may experience dominant paradoxical reaction (restlessness, insomnia, euphoria, nervousness, tremors). Overdosage in children may result in hallucinations, convulsions, death. Hypersensitivity reaction (eczema, pruritus, rash, cardiac disturbances, photosensitivity) may occur. Overdosage may vary from CNS depression (sedation, apnea, cardiovascular collapse, death) to severe paradoxical reaction (hallucinations, tremor, seizures).

NURSING IMPLICATIONS
INTERVENTION/EVALUATION:

Monitor B/P, esp. in elderly (increased risk of hypotension). Monitor children closely for paradoxical reaction. Monitor serum electrolytes in those with severe vomiting. Assess skin turgor, mucous membranes to evaluate hydration status.

PATIENT/FAMILY TEACHING:

Tolerance to sedative effect may occur. Avoid tasks that require alertness, motor skills until response to drug is established. Dry mouth, drowsiness, dizziness may be an expected response of drug. Avoid alcoholic beverages during therapy. Sugarless gum, sips of tepid water may relieve dry mouth. Coffee or tea may help reduce drowsiness.

meclofenamate sodium
(Meclodium, Meclomen)
See Classification section under: Nonsteroidal Anti-Inflammatory Drugs (NSAIDs)

medroxyprogesterone acetate
meh-drocks-ee-pro-**jes**-ter-own
(**Amen, Curretab, Depo-Provera, Provera**)

FIXED-COMBINATION(S): W/conjugated estrogens (**Lunelle, Premphase, Prempro**)

CANADIAN AVAILABILITY: Depo-Provera, Novo-Medrone, Provera

CLASSIFICATION
Progestin, antineoplastic

AVAILABILITY (Rx)
Tablets: 2.5 mg, 5 mg, 10 mg. **Injection:** 100 mg/ml, 150 mg/ml, 400 mg/ml.

PHARMACOKINETICS
Slow absorption after IM administration. Metabolized in liver. Primarily excreted in urine.

ACTION/THERAPEUTIC EFFECT
Transforms endometrium from proliferative to secretory (in an estrogen-primed endometrium); inhibits secretion of pituitary gonadotropins, *preventing follicular maturation and ovulation.* Stimulates growth of mammary alveolar tissue; relaxes uterine smooth muscle. *Restores hormonal imbalance.*

USES / UNLABELED

Oral: Prevention of endometrial hyperplasia (concurrently given w/estrogen to women with intact uterus), treatment of secondary amenorrhea, abnormal uterine bleeding. *IM:* Adjunctive therapy, palliative treatment of inoperable, recurrent, metastatic endometrial carcinoma, renal carcinoma; prevention of pregnancy. *Treatment of endometriosis, hormonal replacement therapy in estrogen-treated menopausal women.*

PO / IM ADMINISTRATION

PO:

   Give w/o regard to meals.

IM:

   1. Shake vial immediately before administering (ensures complete suspension).
   2. Rarely, a residual lump, change in skin color, or sterile abscess occurs at injection site.

INDICATIONS / DOSAGE / ROUTES

Endometrial hyperplasia:
PO: Adults: 2–10 mg/day for 14 days.

Secondary amenorrhea:
PO: Adults: 5–10 mg/day for 5–10 days (begin at any time during menstrual cycle).

Abnormal uterine bleeding:
PO: Adults: 5–10 mg/day for 5–10 days (begin on calculated day 16 or day 21 of menstrual cycle).

Endometrial, renal carcinoma:
IM: Adults, elderly: Initially, 400–1,000 mg, repeat at 1 wk intervals. If improvement occurs, disease stabilized, begin maintenance w/as little as 400 mg/mo.

Pregnancy prevention:
IM: Adults: 150 mg q3 mos.

PRECAUTIONS

CONTRAINDICATIONS: History of or active thrombotic disorders (cerebral apoplexy, thrombophlebitis, thromboembolic disorders), hypersensitivity to progestins, severe liver dysfunction, estrogen-dependent neoplasia, undiagnosed abnormal genital bleeding, missed abortion, use as pregnancy test, undiagnosed vaginal bleeding, carcinoma of breast, known or suspected pregnancy. **CAUTIONS:** Those w/conditions aggravated by fluid retention (asthma, seizures, migraine, cardiac or renal dysfunction), diabetes, history of mental depression. **PREGNANCY/LACTATION:** Avoid use during pregnancy, esp. first 4 mos (congenital heart, limb reduction defects may occur). Distributed in breast milk. **Pregnancy Category D**.

INTERACTIONS

DRUG INTERACTIONS: May interfere w/effects of bromocriptine. **ALTERED LAB VALUES:** May increase alkaline phosphatase, LDL. May decrease HDL cholesterol.

SIDE EFFECTS

   FREQUENT: Transient menstrual abnormalities (spotting, change in menstrual flow or cervical secretions, amenorrhea) at initiation of therapy. **OCCASIONAL:** Edema, weight change, breast tenderness, nervousness, insomnia, fatigue, dizziness. **RARE:** Alopecia, mental depression, dermatologic changes, headache, fever, nausea.

M

ADVERSE REACTIONS/TOXIC EFFECTS

Thrombophlebitis, pulmonary or cerebral embolism, retinal thrombosis occurs rarely.

NURSING IMPLICATIONS

BASELINE ASSESSMENT:

Question for hypersensitivity to progestins, possibility of pregnancy before initiating therapy (Pregnancy Category X). Obtain baseline weight, blood glucose, B/P.

INTERVENTION/EVALUATION:

Check weight daily; report weekly gain of 5 lbs or more. Check B/P periodically. Assess skin for rash, hives. Report immediately the development of chest pain, sudden shortness of breath, sudden decrease in vision, migraine headache, pain (esp. w/swelling, warmth, and redness) in calves, numbness of an arm or leg (thrombotic disorders). Monitor I&O in those with renal carcinoma or those experiencing weight gain. Note medroxyprogesterone therapy on pathology specimens.

PATIENT/FAMILY TEACHING:

Importance of medical supervision. Do not take other medications w/o physician approval. Use sunscreens, protective clothing to protect from sunlight or ultraviolet light until tolerance determined. Notify physician of abnormal vaginal bleeding or other symptoms. Teach how to perform Homans' test and the signs and symptoms of blood clots (report these to physician immediately). Teach breast self-exam. Stop taking medication and contact physician at once if pregnancy is suspected.

medrysone

med-rih-sohn
(HMS Liquifilm)

CLASSIFICATION

Corticosteroid, ophthalmic

AVAILABILITY (Rx)

Ophthalmic Suspension: 1%

PHARMACOKINETICS

Absorbed into conjunctival sac, systemically absorbed.

ACTION/ *THERAPEUTIC EFFECT*

Produces vasoconstriction, inhibits edema, fibrin deposition, and migration of leukocytes and phagocytes due to inflammatory response to mechanical, chemical, or immunologic agents.

USES

Symptomatic relief of inflammatory conditions of the conjunctiva, cornea, lid, and anterior segment of the globe (e.g., allergic conjunctivitis, superficial punctate keratitis, herpes zoster keratitis and cyclitis). Also used to help prevent fibrosis, scarring and potential visual impairment caused by chemical, radiation, or thermal burns or penetration of foreign bodies.

OPHTHALMIC ADMINISTRATION

1. For topical ophthalmic use only.
2. Position pt w/head tilted back, looking up.

3. Gently pull lower lid down to form pouch and instill drops.

4. Do not touch tip of applicator to lids or any surface.

5. When lower lid is released, have pt keep eye open w/o blinking for at least 30 secs.

6. Apply gentle finger pressure to lacrimal sac (bridge of the nose, inside corner of the eye) for 1–2 min after administration of solution.

7. Remove excess solution around eye with a tissue. Wash hands immediately to remove medication.

INDICATIONS/DOSAGE/ROUTES

Usual ophthalmic dosage:
Adults, elderly: Instill 1 drop into conjunctival sac q4h; may increase to 1 drop q1–2h for severe cases. Gradually taper dosage when discontinuing medication.

PRECAUTIONS

CONTRAINDICATIONS: Hypersensitivity to any component of preparation, acute superficial herpes simplex keratitis, fungal diseases of ocular structure. In pts w/vaccinia, varicella, or most other viral diseases of the cornea and conjunctiva; ocular tuberculosis. Not for use in iritis or uveitis. **CAUTIONS:** Safety and efficacy in children not established. **PREGNANCY/LACTATION:** Safety during pregnancy, lactation not established. **Pregnancy Category C**.

INTERACTIONS

DRUG INTERACTIONS: None significant. **ALTERED LAB VALUES:** None significant.

SIDE EFFECTS

OCCASIONAL: Transient stinging, burning on instillation. High doses may slow corneal healing. **RARE:** Filtering blebs after cataract surgery; hypersensitivity.

ADVERSE REACTIONS/TOXIC EFFECTS

Systemic reactions occur rarely with extensive use.

NURSING IMPLICATIONS
BASELINE ASSESSMENT:

Question for hypersensitivity to any components of preparation.

INTERVENTION/EVALUATION:

Assess for therapeutic response, superinfection, delayed healing or irritation.

PATIENT/FAMILY TEACHING:

Explain possible burning or stinging upon application. Visual acuity may be decreased after administration; avoid driving or operating machinery if vision decreases. Do not discontinue use w/o consulting physician. Notify physician if no improvement in 7–8 days, if condition worsens, or if pain, itching, or swelling of eye occurs. Sensitivity to bright light may occur; wear sunglasses to minimize discomfort.

megestrol acetate

meh-**jes**-troll
(Megace)

CANADIAN AVAILABILITY:
Megace

CLASSIFICATION

Antineoplastic

AVAILABILITY (Rx)

Tablets: 20 mg, 40 mg. **Suspension:** 40 mg/ml.

PHARMACOKINETICS

Well absorbed from GI tract. Metabolized in liver; excreted in urine.

ACTION/*THERAPEUTIC EFFECT*

Suppresses release of luteinizing hormone from anterior pituitary by inhibiting pituitary function, *regressing tumor size. Increases appetite* (mechanism unknown).

USES/*UNLABELED*

Palliative management of recurrent, inoperable, or metastatic endometrial or breast carcinoma. Treatment of anorexia, cachexia, or unexplained significant weight loss in pts w/AIDS. *Treatment of hormonally dependent/advanced prostate carcinoma.*

INDICATIONS/DOSAGE/ROUTES

Palliative treatment of advanced breast cancer:
PO: Adults, elderly: 160 mg/day in 4 equally divided doses.

Palliative treatment of advanced endometrial carcinoma:
PO: Adults, elderly: 40–320 mg/day in divided doses. **Maximum:** 800 mg/day.

Anorexia, cachexia, weight loss:
PO: Adults, elderly: 800 mg (20 ml)/day.

PRECAUTIONS

CONTRAINDICATIONS: None significant. **CAUTIONS:** History of thrombophlebitis. **PREGNANCY/ LACTATION:** If possible, avoid use during pregnancy, esp. first 4 mos. Breast-feeding not recommended. **Pregnancy Category N/A.**

INTERACTIONS

DRUG INTERACTIONS: None significant. **ALTERED LAB VALUES:** May increase serum glucose levels.

SIDE EFFECTS

FREQUENT: Weight gain secondary to increased appetite. **OCCASIONAL:** Nausea, breakthrough bleeding, backache, headache, breast tenderness, carpal tunnel syndrome. **RARE:** Feeling of coldness.

ADVERSE REACTIONS/TOXIC EFFECTS

Thrombophlebitis, pulmonary embolism occurs rarely.

NURSING IMPLICATIONS

BASELINE ASSESSMENT:

Question for possibility of pregnancy before initiating therapy (Pregnancy Category X). Provide support to pt, family, recognizing this drug is palliative, not curative.

PATIENT/FAMILY TEACHING:

Importance of contraception. Notify physician if headache, nausea, breast tenderness, or other symptom persists.

melphalan

mel-fah-lan
(Alkeran)

CANADIAN AVAILABILITY:
Alkeran

CLASSIFICATION

Antineoplastic

AVAILABILITY (Rx)

Tablets: 2 mg

PHARMACOKINETICS

Variably, incompletely absorbed from GI tract. Deactivated in body fluids, tissues. Excreted in urine, eliminated in feces. Half-life: 90 min.

ACTION/*THERAPEUTIC EFFECT*

Primarily cross-links strands of DNA, RNA, *inhibiting protein synthesis*. Cell cycle-phase nonspecific.

USES/*UNLABELED*

Treatment of multiple myeloma, nonresectable epithelial carcinoma of ovary. *Treatment of breast, testicular carcinoma.*

INDICATIONS/DOSAGE/ROUTES

Note: May be carcinogenic, mutagenic, or teratogenic. Handle w/extreme care during administration. Dosage individualized based on clinical response, tolerance to adverse effects. When used in combination therapy, consult specific protocols for optimum dosage, sequence of drug administration. Leukocyte count usually maintained between 3,000–4,000/mm^3.

Ovarian carcinoma:
PO: Adults, elderly: 0.2 mg/kg/day for 5 successive days. Repeat at 4–6 wk intervals.

Multiple myeloma:
PO: Adults, elderly: Initially, 6 mg/day as single dose for 2–3 wks. Discontinue drug for up to 4 wks.

Maintenance: 2 mg/day when leukocytes, platelets increase.

PRECAUTIONS

CONTRAINDICATIONS: Known hypersensitivity to drug, resistance to previous therapy w/drug. **CAUTIONS:** Bone marrow depression, chickenpox (present or recent), herpes zoster, infection, decreased renal function, history of gout. **PREGNANCY/LACTATION:** If possible, avoid use during pregnancy, esp. first trimester. May cause fetal harm. Unknown whether drug crosses placenta or is distributed in breast milk. Breast-feeding not recommended. **Pregnancy Category D**.

INTERACTIONS

DRUG INTERACTIONS: May decrease effect of antigout medications. Bone marrow depressants may increase bone marrow depression. Live virus vaccines may potentiate virus replication, increase vaccine side effects, decrease pt's antibody response to vaccine. **ALTERED LAB VALUES:** May increase uric acid.

SIDE EFFECTS

FREQUENT: Severe nausea, vomiting (large dose). **OCCASIONAL:** Diarrhea, stomatitis, mild nausea, vomiting (usual dose), rash, itching, temporary alopecia.

ADVERSE REACTIONS/TOXIC EFFECTS

Bone marrow depression manifested as hematologic toxicity (principally leukopenia, thrombocytopenia, and to lesser extent, anemia, pancytopenia,

M

agranulocytosis). Leukopenia may occur as early as 5 days. WBC, platelet counts return to normal levels during fifth wk, but leukopenia or thrombocytopenia may last more than 6 wks after discontinuing drug. Hyperuricemia noted by hematuria, crystalluria, flank pain.

NURSING IMPLICATIONS
BASELINE ASSESSMENT:

Obtain blood counts weekly. Dosage may be decreased or discontinued if WBC falls below 3,000/mm^3 or platelet count falls below 100,000/mm^3. Antiemetics may be effective in preventing, treating nausea, vomiting.

INTERVENTION/EVALUATION:

Monitor Hgb, Hct, WBC, differential, platelet count, urinalysis, serum uric acid level. Monitor for stomatitis (burning/erythema of oral mucosa at inner margin of lips, sore throat, difficulty swallowing, oral ulceration). Monitor for hematologic toxicity (fever, sore throat, signs of local infection, easy bruising, unusual bleeding from any site), symptoms of anemia (excessive tiredness, weakness), signs of hyperuricemia (hematuria, flank pain). Avoid IM injections, rectal temperatures, other traumas that may induce bleeding.

PATIENT/FAMILY TEACHING:

Increase fluid intake (may protect against hyperuricemia). Maintain fastidious oral hygiene. Alopecia is reversible, but new hair growth may have different color or texture. Do not have immunizations w/o physician's approval (drug lowers body's resistance). Avoid crowds and those w/infections. Promptly report fever, sore throat, signs of local infection, easy bruising, or unusual bleeding from any site, yellow discoloration of eyes or skin, black tarry stools. Contact physician if nausea/vomiting continues at home. Contraceptives are recommended during therapy.

menotropins

men-oh-**troe**-pins
(Humegon, Pergonal, Repronex)

CANADIAN AVAILABILITY:
Pergonal

CLASSIFICATION

Gonadotropin

AVAILABILITY (Rx)

Powder for Injection: 75 IU FSH/LH, 150 IU FSH/LH activity

PHARMACOKINETICS

Well absorbed after IM administration. Excreted in urine. Half-life: *FSH:* 70 hrs; *LH:* 4 hrs.

ACTION/*THERAPEUTIC EFFECT*

Gonadotropic agent w/follicle-stimulating hormone (FSH) and luteinizing hormone (LH) actions. *Promotes ovarian follicular growth and maturation in women; stimulates spermatogenesis in men.*

USES

Treatment of infertility in conjunction w/chorionic gonadotropin (HCG) to stimulate ovulation and pregnancy in women w/secondary ovarian dysfunction and to stimulate spermatogenesis in men w/primary or secondary hypogonadotropic hypogonadism.

STORAGE/HANDLING

Powder for reconstitution may be refrigerated or kept at room temperature.

IM ADMINISTRATION

1. Reconstitute w/1–2 ml 0.9% NaCl injection.

2. Administer immediately after reconstitution; discard unused portion.

3. Give IM only.

INDICATIONS/DOSAGE/ROUTES

Induction ovulation/pregnancy:
IM: Adults: Initially, 75 IU FSH/75 IU LH per day for 9–12 days. Follow w/10,000 IU HCG 1 day after last dose menotropin. May repeat at least 2 courses before increasing dose to 150 IU FSH/150 IU LH if evidence of ovulation, but no pregnancy.
Note: Omit HCG if hyperstimulation syndrome likely to occur (total estrogen excretion >100 mcg/24 hrs or estradiol excretion >50 mcg/24 hrs) or ovaries abnormally enlarged on last day of menotropin therapy.

Stimulation of spermatogenesis:
Note: Pretreat w/HCG alone (5,000 IU 3 times/wk) until normal serum testosterone level and masculinization. May take 4–6 mos.
IM: Adults: Initially, 75 IU FSH/75 IU LH 3 times/wk and HCG 2,000 IU 2 times/wk for at least 4 mos. If no response, may increase dose to 150 IU FSH/150 IU LH w/same HCG dose.

PRECAUTIONS

CONTRAINDICATIONS: Prior hypersensitivity to menotropins; primary ovarian failure; thyroid or adrenal dysfunction; organic intracranial lesion (e.g., pituitary tumor); ovarian cysts or enlargement not due to polycystic ovary syndrome; abnormal vaginal bleeding of undetermined origin; men w/normal urinary gonadotropin concentrations, primary testicular failure or infertility problems other than hypogonadotropic hypogonadism. **PREGNANCY/LACTATION:** Excretion in breast milk unknown. **Pregnancy Category X.**

INTERACTIONS

DRUG INTERACTIONS: None significant. **ALTERED LAB VALUES:** None significant.

SIDE EFFECTS

FREQUENT: Irritation, pain, swelling at injection site, rash. *Females:* Ovarian enlargement/ovarian cysts w/abdominal distention. **OCCASIONAL:** *Males:* Erythrocytosis (shortness of breath, irregular heartbeat, dizziness, anorexia, headache, fainting), gynecomastia.

ADVERSE REACTIONS/TOXIC EFFECTS

Risk of atelectasis and acute respiratory distress syndrome, intravascular thrombosis and embolism, ovarian hyperstimulation syndrome (OHSS), high incidence (20%) of multiple births (premature deliveries and neonatal prematurity), ruptured ovarian cysts.

NURSING IMPLICATIONS

BASELINE ASSESSMENT:

Question for prior allergic reaction to drug.

INTERVENTION/EVALUATION:

Monitor carefully for OHSS; early signs include weight gain, severe pelvic pain, nausea, vomiting progressing to ascites, dyspnea; report immediately. (Ascitic, pleural, or pericardial fluids should not be removed unless absolutely necessary because of potential injury to the ovary. Pelvic examination should be avoided due to potential rupture of an ovarian cyst.)

PATIENT/FAMILY TEACHING:

Importance of close physician supervision during treatment. Promptly report abdominal pain/distention, vaginal bleeding or signs of edema (weigh 2–3 times/week; report >5 lbs/wk gain or swelling of fingers or feet). In anovulation treatment, teach proper method of taking/recording daily basal temperature; advise intercourse daily beginning the day preceding HCG treatment. Intercourse should be discontinued w/significant ovarian enlargement. Possibility of multiple births.

meperidine hydrochloride

meh-**pear**-ih-deen
(Demerol)

CANADIAN AVAILABILITY:
Demerol

CLASSIFICATION

Opiate analgesic (**Schedule II**)

AVAILABILITY (Rx)

Tablets: 50 mg, 100 mg. **Syrup:** 50 mg/5 ml. **Injection:** 10 mg/ml, 25 mg/ml, 50 mg/ml, 75 mg/ml, 100 mg/ml.

PHARMACOKINETICS

	ONSET	PEAK	DURATION
PO	15 min	60 min	2–4 hrs
SubQ	10–15 min	30–50 min	2–4 hrs
IM	10–15 min	30–50 min	2–4 hrs
IV	1 min	5–7 min	2–4 hrs

Variably absorbed from GI tract, well absorbed after IM administration. Widely distributed. Metabolized in liver to active metabolite. Primarily excreted in urine. Half-life: 2.4–4 hrs (increased in elderly).

ACTION/ *THERAPEUTIC EFFECT*

Binds w/opioid receptors within CNS, *altering processes affecting pain perception, emotional response to pain.*

USES

Relief of moderate to severe pain, preop sedation, obstetrical support, anesthesia adjunct.

STORAGE/HANDLING

Store oral, parenteral form at room temperature. Do not use if solution appears cloudy or contains a precipitate.

PO/SUBQ/IM/IV ADMINISTRATION

PO:

1. May give w/o regard to meals.

2. Dilute syrup in glass H_2O (prevents anesthetic effect on mucous membranes).

SubQ/IM:

Note: IM preferred over SubQ route (SubQ produces pain, local irritation, induration).

1. Administer slowly.
2. Those with circulatory impairment experience higher risk of overdosage due to delayed absorption of repeated administration.

IV:

Note: Give by slow IV injection or IV infusion. Physically incompatible with amobarbital, aminophylline, ephedrine, heparin, hydrocortisone, methicillin, methylprednisolone, morphine, nitrofurantoin, oxytetracycline, pentobarbital, phenobarbital, secobarbital, sodium bicarbonate, sodium iodide, tetracycline, thiamylal, thiopental, solutions containing potassium iodide, aminosalicylic acid, salicylamide.

1. Dilute in 5% dextrose and lactated Ringer's, dextrose-saline combination, 2.5%, 5%, or 10% dextrose in water, Ringer's, lactated Ringer's, 0.45% or 0.9% NaCl, or molar sodium lactate diluent for IV injection or infusion.
2. IV dosage must always be administered very slowly, over 2–3 min.
3. Rapid IV increases risk of severe adverse reactions (chest wall rigidity, apnea, peripheral circulatory collapse, anaphylactoid effects, cardiac arrest).

INDICATIONS/DOSAGE/ROUTES

Pain:
PO/IM/SubQ: Adults: 50–150 mg q3–4h. **Children:** 1.1–1.8 mg/kg q3–4h. Do not exceed single pediatric dose 100 mg.
IV: Adults: 15–35 mg/hr.

Usual elderly dosage:
PO: 50 mg q4h as needed.
IM: 25 mg q4h as needed.

Preop:
IM/SubQ: Adults: 50–100 mg given as single dose 30–90 min before induction of anesthesia. **Children:** 1–2 mg/kg 30–90 min before anesthesia.

Labor:
IM: Adults: 50–100 mg when labor pains are regular. Repeat at 1–3 hr intervals.

PRECAUTIONS

CONTRAINDICATIONS: Those receiving MAO inhibitors in past 14 days, diarrhea due to poisoning, delivery of premature infant. **EXTREME CAUTION:** Impaired renal, hepatic function, elderly/debilitated, supraventricular tachycardia, cor pulmonale, history of seizures, acute abdominal conditions, increased intracranial pressure, respiratory abnormalities. **PREGNANCY/LACTATION:** Crosses placenta; distributed in breast milk. Respiratory depression may occur in neonate if mother received opiates during labor. Regular use of opiates during pregnancy may produce withdrawal symptoms in neonate (irritability, excessive crying, tremors, hyperactive reflexes, fever, vomiting, diarrhea, yawning, sneezing, seizures). **Pregnancy Category B.** (Category D if used for prolonged periods or in high doses at term.)

INTERACTIONS

DRUG INTERACTIONS: Alcohol, CNS depressants may increase CNS or respiratory depression, hypotension. MAO inhibitors may produce severe, fatal reaction (reduce dose to 1/4 usual dose). **ALTERED LAB VALUES:** May increase amylase, lipase.

SIDE EFFECTS

Note: Effects are dependent on dosage amount, route of administration. Ambulatory pts and those not in severe pain may experience dizziness, nausea, vomiting more frequently than those in supine position or having severe pain. **FREQUENT:** Sedation, decreased B/P, diaphoresis, flushed face, dizziness, nausea, vomiting, constipation. **OCCASIONAL:** Confusion, irregular heartbeat, tremors, decreased urination, abdominal pain, dry mouth, headache, irritation at injection site, euphoria, dysphoria. **RARE:** Allergic reaction (rash, itching), insomnia.

ADVERSE REACTIONS/TOXIC EFFECTS

Overdosage results in respiratory depression, skeletal muscle flaccidity, cold clammy skin, cyanosis, extreme somnolence progressing to convulsions, stupor, coma. Antidote: 0.4 mg naloxone (Narcan). Tolerance to analgesic effect, physical dependence may occur with repeated use.

NURSING IMPLICATIONS
BASELINE ASSESSMENT:

Pt should be in recumbent position before drug is administered by parenteral route. Assess onset, type, location, duration of pain. Obtain vital signs before giving medication. If respirations are 12/min or lower (20/min or lower in children), withhold medication, contact physician. Effect of medication is reduced if full pain recurs before next dose.

INTERVENTION/EVALUATION:

Monitor vital signs 15–30 min after SubQ/IM dose, 5–10 min after IV dose (monitor for decreased B/P, change in rate/quality of pulse). Monitor stools; avoid constipation. Check for ad-

equate voiding. Initiate deep breathing and coughing exercises, particularly in those with impaired pulmonary function.

PATIENT/FAMILY TEACHING:

Medication should be taken before pain fully returns, within ordered intervals. Discomfort may occur with injection. Change positions slowly to avoid orthostatic hypotension. Avoid tasks that require alertness, motor skills until response to drug is established. Increase fluids, bulk to prevent constipation. Tolerance/dependence may occur with prolonged use of high doses. Avoid alcohol and other CNS depressants.

mepivacaine hydrochloride
(Carbocaine, Polocaine)

FIXED-COMBINATION(S):
W/levonordefrin, a vasoconstrictor (Isocaine)
See Classification section under: Anesthetics: local

mequinol/tretinoin
(Solage)
See Supplement

mercaptopurine
mur-cap-toe-**pure**-een
(Purinethol)

CANADIAN AVAILABILITY:
Purinethol

CLASSIFICATION

Antineoplastic

AVAILABILITY (Rx)

Tablets: 50 mg

PHARMACOKINETICS

Variably, incompletely absorbed from GI tract. Crosses blood-brain barrier. Metabolized in liver. Primarily excreted in urine. Removed by hemodialysis. Half-life: 45 min.

ACTION / *THERAPEUTIC EFFECT*

After activation in tissue, *inhibits DNA, RNA synthesis.* Cell cycle-specific for S phase of cell division.

USES / *UNLABELED*

Treatment of acute lymphatic (lymphocytic, lymphoblastic) leukemia, acute myelogenous leukemia, acute myelomonocytic leukemia. *Treatment of chronic myelocytic leukemia, non-Hodgkin's lymphoma, polycythemia vera, Crohn's disease, ulcerative colitis, psoriatic arthritis.*

INDICATIONS / DOSAGE / ROUTES

Note: May be carcinogenic, mutagenic, or teratogenic. Handle w/extreme care during administration. Dosage individualized based on clinical response, tolerance to adverse effects. When used in combination therapy, consult specific protocols for optimum dosage, sequence of drug administration. Reduce dose in those w/renal impairment.

Induction remission:
PO: Adults, elderly, children: 2.5 mg/kg/day as single dose (100–200 mg in average adults, 50 mg in average children). Increase dose up to 5 mg/kg/day after 4 wks if no improvement and no toxicity.

Maintenance:
PO: Adults, elderly, children: 1.5–2.5 mg/kg/day as single dose.

PRECAUTIONS

CONTRAINDICATIONS: Previous therapy resistance to drug. **CAUTIONS:** Bone marrow depression, existing or recent chickenpox, herpes zoster, infection decreased liver or renal function. **PREGNANCY/LACTATION:** If possible, avoid use during pregnancy, esp. first trimester. May cause fetal harm. Unknown if distributed in breast milk. Breast-feeding not recommended. **Pregnancy Category D**.

INTERACTIONS

DRUG INTERACTIONS: May decrease effect of antigout medications. Bone marrow depressants may increase bone marrow depression. Hepatotoxic medications may increase risk of hepatotoxicity. Immunosuppressants may increase risk of infection, develop neoplasms. Live virus vaccines may potentiate virus replication, increase vaccine side effects, decrease pt's antibody response to vaccine. **ALTERED LAB VALUES:** May increase uric acid.

SIDE EFFECTS

FREQUENT: Bone marrow depression. **OCCASIONAL:** Nausea, vomiting, darkening of skin, diarrhea, headache, skin rash, itching, weakness, decreased appetite. **RARE:** Stomach pain, stomatitis.

ADVERSE REACTIONS / TOXIC EFFECTS

Hepatotoxicity manifested by jaundice, ascites, cholestasis, elevated hepatic enzyme concentrations, severe fibrosis, necrosis, and bone marrow depression manifested as hematologic toxicity (principally leukopenia, anemia, thrombocytopenia, and to lesser extent, pancytopenia, agranulocytosis). Hyperuricemia results in

M

hematuria, crystalluria, and flank pain.

NURSING IMPLICATIONS

BASELINE ASSESSMENT:

Risk of hepatic injury increases when dosage exceeds 2.5 mg/kg/day. Hematology tests should be performed weekly. Therapy may be discontinued if large or rapid decrease in WBC or abnormal bone marrow depression occurs, and resumed when WBC or platelet count increases or remains constant for 2–3 days. Liver function tests should be performed weekly during initial therapy, monthly thereafter.

INTERVENTION/EVALUATION:

Monitor hepatic function tests, hemoglobin/hematocrit, WBC, differential, platelet count, urinalysis. Monitor for hematologic toxicity (fever, sore throat, signs of local infection, easy bruising, unusual bleeding from any site), symptoms of anemia (excessive tiredness, weakness), signs of hyperuricemia (hematuria, flank pain). Avoid IM injections, rectal temperatures, or other traumas that may induce bleeding.

PATIENT/FAMILY TEACHING:

Increase fluid intake (may protect against hyperuricemia). Do not have immunizations w/o physician's approval (drug lowers body's resistance). Avoid crowds and those w/infection. Promptly report fever, sore throat, signs of local infection, easy bruising, unusual bleeding from any site, yellow skin or eyes, dark urine, pale stools. Contact physician if nausea/vomiting continues at home. Do not take alcohol or medications w/o consulting physician.

Contraception should be practiced during therapy.

meropenem

murr-**oh**-pen-em
(Merrem IV)

CANADIAN AVAILABILITY:
Merrem IV

CLASSIFICATION

Antibiotic

AVAILABILITY (Rx)

Powder for Injection: 500 mg, 1 g

PHARMACOKINETICS

Following IV administration, widely distributed into tissues/fluid including cerebrospinal fluid. Primarily excreted unchanged in urine. Removed by hemodialysis. Half-life: 1 hr.

ACTION/*THERAPEUTIC EFFECT*

Penetrates most gram-positive and gram-negative cell walls, *inhibiting bacterial cell wall synthesis. Bactericidal.*

USES/*UNLABELED*

Treatment of intra-abdominal infections, bacterial meningitis (pediatric pts ≥3 mos only). *Lowers respiratory infections, febrile neutropenia, obstetric/gynecologic infections, sepsis.*

STORAGE/HANDLING

Store vials at room temperature. After reconstitution w/0.9% NaCl, stable for 4 hrs at room temperature, 24 hrs if refrigerated (w/5% dextrose, stable for 1 hr at room temperature, 4 hrs if refrigerated).

IV ADMINISTRATION

IV:

1. May give by IV bolus injection or IV intermittent infusion (piggyback).

2. If administering as IV intermittent infusion (piggyback), give over 15–30 min; if administered by IV bolus injection (5–20 ml), give over 3–5 min.

INDICATIONS/DOSAGE/ROUTES

Note: Space doses evenly around the clock.

Usual parenteral dosage:
IV: Adults, elderly: 1 g q8h.

Intra-abdominal (pediatric):
IV: Children ≥3 mos: 20 mg/kg q8h. **Children >50 kg:** 1 g q8h. **Maximum:** 2 g q8h.

Meningitis (pediatric):
IV: Children ≥3 mos: 40 mg/kg q8h. **Children >50 kg:** 2 g q8h. **Maximum:** 2 g q8h.

Dosage in renal impairment:
Reduce dosage in pts w/creatinine clearance <50 ml/min.

CREATININE CLEARANCE	DOSAGE	DOSING INTERVAL
26–50 ml/min	Recommended dose (1,000 mg)	q12h
10–25 ml/min	½ recommended dose	q12h
<10 ml/min	½ recommended dose	q24h

PRECAUTIONS

CONTRAINDICATIONS: Hypersensitivity to meropenem, other beta lactams. **CAUTIONS:** Hypersensitivity to penicillins, cephalosporins, other allergens; renal function impairment, CNS disorders, particularly w/history of seizures. **PREGNANCY/LACTATION:** Un-

known if distributed in breast milk. **Pregnancy Category B.**

INTERACTIONS

DRUG INTERACTIONS: Probenecid inhibits renal excretion of meropenem (do not use concurrently). **ALTERED LAB VALUES:** May increase SGOT (AST), SGPT (ALT), alkaline phosphatase, LDH, bilirubin, BUN, creatinine. May decrease Hgb, Hct, potassium.

SIDE EFFECTS

FREQUENT: Diarrhea (5%), nausea, vomiting (4%), headache, inflammation at injection site (3%). **OCCASIONAL:** Oral moniliasis, rash, pruritus (2%). **RARE:** Constipation, glossitis.

ADVERSE REACTIONS/TOXIC EFFECTS

Antibiotic-associated colitis, other superinfections may occur. Anaphylactic reactions in those receiving beta lactams have occurred. Seizures may occur in those w/CNS disorders (brain lesions, history of seizures) or w/bacterial meningitis or impaired renal function.

NURSING IMPLICATIONS

BASELINE ASSESSMENT:

Question pt for history of allergies, particularly to meropenem, other beta lactams, penicillins, cephalosporins. Inquire about history of seizures. Obtain culture and sensitivity tests before giving first dose (therapy may begin before results are known).

INTERVENTION/EVALUATION:

Monitor daily bowel activity and stool consistency (watery, loose, soft). Monitor for nausea, vomiting. Evaluate hydration status. Evaluate for inflammation at IV injection site. Assess skin for rash. Monitor I&O, renal function tests. Check mental status; be alert to tremors and possible seizures. Assess temperature, B/P twice daily, more often if necessary. Monitor electrolytes, esp. potassium.

PATIENT/FAMILY TEACHING:

Continue therapy for full length of treatment. Doses should be evenly spaced. Do not take any other medication unless approved by physician. Notify physician in event of tremors, seizures, rash, diarrhea, or other new symptom.

mesalamine (5-aminosalicylic acid, 5-ASA)

mess-**al**-ah-meen
(Asacol, Fiv-ASA, Pentasa, Rowasa)

CANADIAN AVAILABILITY:
Asacol, Mesasal, Pentasa, Quintasa, Salofalk

CLASSIFICATION

Anti-inflammatory agent

AVAILABILITY (Rx)

Tablets (delayed-release): 400 mg. **Capsules (control-release):** 250 mg. **Suppository:** 500 mg. **Rectal Suspension:** 4 g/60 ml.

PHARMACOKINETICS

Poorly absorbed from colon. Moderately absorbed from GI tract. Metabolized in liver to active metabolite. Unabsorbed portion eliminated in feces; absorbed portion excreted in urine. Half-life: 0.5–1.5 hrs; metabolite: 5–10 hrs.

ACTION/*THERAPEUTIC EFFECT*

Produces local inhibitory effect on arachidonic acid metabolite production (increased in pts w/chronic inflammatory bowel disease). *Blocks prostaglandin production, diminishes inflammation in colon.*

USES

Treatment of active mild to moderate distal ulcerative colitis, proctosigmoiditis, or proctitis. Asacol: Maintenance of remission of ulcerative colitis.

STORAGE/HANDLING

Store rectal suspension, suppository, oral forms at room temperature.

PO/RECTAL ADMINISTRATION

PO:

1. Have pt swallow whole; do not break outer coating of tablet.
2. May take w/o regard to food.

RECTAL:

1. Shake bottle well.
2. Instruct pt to lie on left side with lower leg extended, upper leg flexed forward.
3. Knee-chest position may also be used.
4. Insert applicator tip into rectum, pointing toward umbilicus.
5. Squeeze bottle steadily until contents are emptied.

INDICATIONS/DOSAGE/ROUTES

Ulcerative colitis, proctosigmoiditis, proctitis:
PO: Adults, elderly: *(Asacol):* 800 mg 3 times/day for 6 wks; *(Pentasa):* 1 g 4 times/day for 8 wks.
Rectal: Adults, elderly: (suppository) 500 mg 2 times/day. Retain

1–3 hrs. (suspension) 4 g (60 ml) daily, preferably at bedtime.

Maintenance of remission, ulcerative colitis:
PO: Adults, elderly: 1.6 g/day in divided doses.

PRECAUTIONS

CONTRAINDICATIONS: None significant. **CAUTIONS:** Preexisting renal disease, sulfasalazine sensitivity. **PREGNANCY/LACTATION:** Unknown whether drug crosses placenta or is distributed in breast milk. **Pregnancy Category B.**

INTERACTIONS

DRUG INTERACTIONS: None significant. **ALTERED LAB VALUES:** May increase SGOT (AST), SGPT (ALT), alkaline phosphatase, BUN, serum creatinine.

SIDE EFFECTS

Note: Generally well tolerated, with only mild and transient effects. **FREQUENT (>6%):** *Oral:* Abdominal cramps/pain, diarrhea, dizziness, headache, nausea, vomiting, rhinitis, unusual tiredness. *Rectal:* Abdominal/stomach cramps, flatulence, headache, nausea. **OCCASIONAL (2–6%):** *Oral:* Hair loss, decreased appetite, back/joint pain, flatulence, acne. *Rectal:* Hair loss. **RARE (<2%):** *Rectal:* Anal irritation.

ADVERSE REACTIONS/TOXIC EFFECTS

Sulfite sensitivity in susceptible pts noted as cramping, headache, diarrhea, fever, rash, hives, itching, wheezing. Discontinue drug immediately. Hepatitis, pancreatitis, pericarditis occur rarely w/oral dosage.

NURSING IMPLICATIONS
INTERVENTION/EVALUATION:

Encourage adequate fluid in-take. Assess bowel sounds for peristalsis. Monitor daily bowel activity and stool consistency (watery, loose, soft, semisolid, solid) and record time of evacuation. Assess for abdominal disturbances. Assess skin for rash, hives. Discontinue medication if rash, fever, cramping, or diarrhea occurs.

PATIENT/FAMILY TEACHING:

Avoid tasks that require alertness, motor skills until response to drug is established.

M

mesna
mess-nah
(Mesnex)

CANADIAN AVAILABILITY:
Uromitexan

CLASSIFICATION
Antidote

AVAILABILITY (Rx)
Injection: 100 mg/ml

PHARMACOKINETICS
Rapidly metabolized after IV administration to mesna disulfide, which is reduced to mesna in kidney. Excreted in urine. Half-life: 0.36 hrs.

ACTION/*THERAPEUTIC EFFECT*
Reduced to free thiol compound, mesna, which reacts with urotoxic ifosfamide metabolites (detoxification). *Inhibits ifosfamide-induced hemorrhagic cystitis.*

USES
Decreased incidence of ifosfamide-induced hemorrhagic cystitis.

STORAGE/HANDLING

Store parenteral form at room temperature. After dilution, stable for 24 hrs at room temperature (recommended use within 6 hrs). Discard unused medication.

IV ADMINISTRATION

1. Dilute each 100 mg with 5% dextrose or 0.9% NaCl to provide concentration of 20 mg/ml.
2. Administer direct IV injection.

INDICATIONS/DOSAGE/ROUTES

Hemorrhagic cystitis:
IV: Adults, elderly: 20% of ifosfamide dose at time of ifosfamide administration and 4 and 8 hrs after each dose of ifosfamide. Total dose: 60% of ifosfamide dosage.

PRECAUTIONS

CONTRAINDICATIONS: None significant. **CAUTIONS:** None significant. **PREGNANCY/LACTATION:** Unknown whether drug crosses placenta or is distributed in breast milk. **Pregnancy Category B.**

INTERACTIONS

DRUG INTERACTIONS: None significant. **ALTERED LAB VALUES:** May produce false-positive test for urinary ketones.

SIDE EFFECTS

FREQUENT (>17%): Bad taste in mouth, soft stools. *Large doses:* Diarrhea, limb pain, headache, fatigue, nausea, hypotension, allergic reaction.

ADVERSE REACTIONS/TOXIC EFFECTS

Hematuria occurs occasionally.

NURSING IMPLICATIONS

BASELINE ASSESSMENT:

Each dose must be administered with ifosfamide.

INTERVENTION/EVALUATION:

Assess morning urine specimen for hematuria. If such occurs, dosage reduction or discontinuation may be necessary. Monitor daily bowel activity and stool consistency (watery, loose, soft, semisolid, solid) and record time of evacuation. Monitor B/P for hypotension.

PATIENT/FAMILY TEACHING:

Inform physician/nurse if headache, limb pain, or nausea occurs.

---

mesoridazine besylate

mess-oh-**rid**-ah-zeen
(Serentil)

CANADIAN AVAILABILITY:
Serentil

CLASSIFICATION

Antipsychotic

AVAILABILITY (Rx)

Tablets: 10 mg, 25 mg, 50 mg, 100 mg. **Oral Concentrate:** 25 mg/ml. **Injection:** 25 mg/ml.

PHARMACOKINETICS

Variably absorbed from GI tract. Metabolized in liver to some active metabolites. Primarily excreted in urine. Half-life: 20–40 hrs.

ACTION/THERAPEUTIC EFFECT

Blocks dopamine at postsynaptic receptor sites in brain. *Suppresses behavioral response in psychosis.* Strong anticholinergic, sedative effects.

USES

Symptomatic management of psychotic disorders, treatment of hyperactivity, uncooperativeness associated w/mental deficiency, chronic brain syndrome; as adjunctive treatment of alcohol dependence, management of anxiety/tension associated w/neurosis.

STORAGE/HANDLING

Store oral, parenteral form at room temperature. Yellow discoloration of solution does not affect potency, but discard if markedly discolored or if precipitate forms.

PO/IM ADMINISTRATION

PO:

Dilute oral solution w/water, orange or grape juice.

IM:

Note: Pt must remain recumbent for 30–60 min in head-low position w/legs raised, to minimize hypotensive effect.
1. Inject slow, deep IM into upper outer quadrant of gluteus maximus. If irritation occurs, further injections may be diluted w/0.9% NaCl or 2% procaine hydrochloride.
2. Massage IM injection site to reduce discomfort.

INDICATIONS/DOSAGE/ROUTES

Note: Increase dosage gradually to optimum response, then decrease to lowest effective level for maintenance. Replace parenteral therapy w/oral therapy as soon as possible.

Usual parenteral dosage:
IM: Adults, children >12 yrs: 25 mg given as single dose. May repeat in 30–60 min, if needed. **Maximum dose:** 200 mg/day.

Psychotic disorders:
PO: Adults, children >12 yrs: Initially, 50 mg 3 times/day. **Maintenance:** 100–400 mg/day.

Hyperactivity:
PO: Adults, children >12 yrs: 25 mg 3 times/day. **Maintenance:** 75–300 mg/day.

Alcohol dependence:
PO: Adults, children >12 yrs: 25 mg twice/day. **Maintenance:** 50–200 mg/day.

Anxiety/tension:
PO: Adults, children >12 yrs: 10 mg 3 times/day. **Maintenance:** 30–150 mg/day.

Usual elderly dosage (nonpsychotic):
PO: Initially, 10 mg 1–2 times/day. May increase by 10–25 mg/day every 7–10 days. **Maximum:** 250 mg/day.

PRECAUTIONS

CONTRAINDICATIONS: Severe CNS depression, comatose states, severe cardiovascular disease, bone marrow depression, subcortical brain damage. **CAUTIONS:** Impaired respiratory/hepatic/renal/cardiac function, alcohol withdrawal, history of seizures, urinary retention, glaucoma, prostatic hypertrophy. **PREGNANCY/LACTATION:** Crosses placenta, distributed in breast milk. **Pregnancy Category C.**

INTERACTIONS

DRUG INTERACTIONS: Alcohol, CNS depressants may increase CNS, respiratory depression, hypotensive effects. Tricyclic antidepressants, MAO inhibitors may increase sedative, anticholinergic effects. Antithyroid agents may increase risk of agranulocytosis. Extrapyramidal symptoms (EPS) may increase w/EPS-producing medications. Hypotensives may increase hypotension. May decrease levodopa effects. Lithium may decrease absorption, produce adverse neurologic effects. **ALTERED LAB VALUES:** May produce false-positive pregnancy test, PKU. EKG changes may occur, including Q and T wave disturbances.

SIDE EFFECTS

FREQUENT: Orthostatic hypotension, dizziness, and fainting occur frequently after first injection, occasionally after subsequent injections, and rarely w/oral dosage. **OCCASIONAL:** Drowsiness during early therapy, dry mouth, blurred vision, lethargy, constipation or diarrhea, nasal congestion, peripheral edema, urinary retention. **RARE:** Ocular changes, skin pigmentation (those on high doses for prolonged periods).

ADVERSE REACTIONS/TOXIC EFFECTS

Abrupt withdrawal following long-term therapy may precipitate nausea, vomiting, gastritis, dizziness, tremors. Blood dyscrasias, particularly agranulocytosis, mild leukopenia (sore mouth/gums/throat) may occur. May lower seizure threshold.

NURSING IMPLICATIONS
BASELINE ASSESSMENT:

Avoid skin contact w/solution (contact dermatitis). Assess behavior, appearance, emotional status, response to environment, speech pattern, thought content.

INTERVENTION/EVALUATION:

Assess for orthostatic hypotension. Monitor stool frequency and consistency (watery, loose, soft, semisolid, solid). Monitor WBC, differential count for blood dyscrasias. Supervise suicidal risk pt closely during early therapy (as depression lessens, energy level improves, increasing suicide potential). Assess for therapeutic response (interest in surroundings, improvement in self-care, increased ability to concentrate, relaxed facial expression).

PATIENT/FAMILY TEACHING:

Full therapeutic effect may take up to 6 wks. Urine may become pink, reddish brown. Do not abruptly withdraw from long-term drug therapy. Report visual disturbances. Sugarless gum, sips of tepid water may relieve dry mouth. Drowsiness generally subsides during continued therapy. Avoid tasks that require alertness, motor skills until response to drug is established. Do not use alcohol or other CNS depressants. Use sunscreen, protective clothing for possible photosensitivity.

---

metaproterenol sulfate
met-ah-pro-**tair**-in-all
(Alupent, Metaprel)

CANADIAN AVAILABILITY:
Alupent

CLASSIFICATION

Bronchodilator

AVAILABILITY (Rx)

Tablets: 10 mg, 20 mg. **Syrup:** 10 mg/5 ml. **Aerosol Solution for Inhalation:** 0.4%, 0.6%, 5%.

PHARMACOKINETICS

	ONSET	PEAK	DURATION
Aerosol			
	1 min	1 hr	4 hrs
PO	15 min	1 hr	4 hrs
Nebulization			
	5–30 min	1 hr	3–4 hrs

Partially absorbed from GI tract, minimal after inhalation. Metabolized in liver. Primarily excreted in urine.

ACTION/*THERAPEUTIC EFFECT*

Stimulates beta$_2$-adrenergic receptors resulting in relaxation of bronchial smooth muscle, *relieving bronchospasm; reduces airway resistance.*

USES

Relief of reversible bronchospasm due to bronchial asthma, bronchitis, emphysema.

STORAGE/HANDLING

Do not use solution for nebulization if brown in color or contains a precipitate.

PO/INHALATION ADMINISTRATION

AEROSOL:

1. Shake container well, exhale completely, then holding mouthpiece 1 inch away from lips, inhale and hold breath as long as possible before exhaling.
2. Wait 1–10 min before inhaling second dose (allows for deeper bronchial penetration).
3. Rinse mouth w/water immediately after inhalation (prevents mouth/throat dryness).

PO:

1. Give w/o regard to meals.
2. Tablets may be crushed.

NEBULIZATION:

Administer undiluted solution in hand nebulizer.
IPPB: Dilute in 2.5 ml saline solution.

INDICATIONS/DOSAGE/ROUTES

Bronchospasm:
Metered-Dose Inhalation: Adults, elderly, children >12 yrs: 2–3 inhalations as single dose. Wait 2 min before administering second dose. Do not repeat for 3–4 hrs. **Maximum:** 12 inhalations/day.
PO: Adults, children >9 yrs or weigh >60 lbs: 20 mg 3–4 times/day. **Children 6–9 yrs or weigh <60 lbs:** 10 mg 3–4 times/day.
Nebulization: Adults, elderly, children >12 yrs: 10 inhalations (range 5–15 inhalations) of undiluted 5% solution, up to 3–4 times/day.
IPPB: Adults, elderly: 0.3 ml 3–4 times/day. May repeat no more often than q4h.

Usual elderly dosage:
PO: Initially, 10 mg 3–4 times/day. May increase up to 20 mg 3–4 times/day.

PRECAUTIONS

CONTRAINDICATIONS: Preexisting arrhythmias. **CAUTIONS:** Impaired cardiac function, diabetes mellitus, hypertension, hyperthyroidism. **PREGNANCY/LACTATION:** Unknown whether drug crosses placenta or is distributed in breast milk. May inhibit uterine contractility. **Pregnancy Category C.**

INTERACTIONS

DRUG INTERACTIONS: Tricyclic antidepressants may increase cardiovascular effects. MAO inhibitors may increase risk of hypertensive crises. May decrease effects of beta blockers. Digoxin, sympathomimetics may increase risk of arrhythmias. **ALTERED LAB VALUES:** May decrease serum potassium levels.

SIDE EFFECTS

FREQUENT (>10%): Tremors, tachycardia, shakiness, nervousness, nausea, vomiting, dry mouth. **OCCASIONAL (1–10%):** Palpitations, dizziness, vertigo, weakness, headache, GI distress, cough, dry throat. **RARE (<1%):** Changes in B/P, drowsiness, diarrhea, unusual taste.

ADVERSE REACTIONS/TOXIC EFFECTS

Excessive sympathomimetic stimulation may cause palpitations, extrasystoles, tachycardia, chest pain, slight increase in B/P followed by a substantial decrease, chills, sweating, and blanching of skin. Too frequent or excessive use may lead to loss of bronchodilating effectiveness and/or severe, paradoxical bronchoconstriction.

NURSING IMPLICATIONS

BASELINE ASSESSMENT:

Offer emotional support (high incidence of anxiety because of difficulty in breathing and sympathomimetic response to drug).

INTERVENTION/EVALUATION:

Monitor rate, depth, rhythm, type of respiration; quality and rate of pulse. Assess lung sounds for rhonchi, wheezing, rales. Monitor arterial blood gases. Observe lips, fingernails for blue or dusky color in light-skinned pts; gray in dark-skinned pts. Observe for clavicular retractions, hand tremor. Evaluate for clinical improvement (quieter, slower respirations, relaxed facial expression, cessation of clavicular retractions).

PATIENT/FAMILY TEACHING:

Increase fluid intake (decreases lung secretion viscosity). Do not take more than 2 inhalations at any one time (excessive use may produce paradoxical bronchoconstriction or a decreased bronchodilating effect). Rinsing mouth w/water immediately after inhalation may prevent mouth/throat dryness. Avoid excessive use of caffeine derivatives (chocolate, coffee, tea, cola, cocoa).

---

metaraminol bitartrate
(Aramine)
See Classification section under: Sympathomimetics

---

metformin
met-**for**-min
(Glucophage)

CANADIAN AVAILABILITY
Glucophage, Novo-Metformin

CLASSIFICATION
Antidiabetic (antihyperglycemic)

AVAILABILITY (Rx)
Tablets: 500 mg, 850 mg

PHARMACOKINETICS
Slowly, incompletely absorbed following oral administration (food delays/decreases extent of absorption). Primarily distributed to intestinal mucosa, salivary glands. Primarily excreted unchanged in urine. Removed by hemodialysis. Half-life: 8.9–19 hrs.

ACTION/*THERAPEUTIC EFFECT*

Lowers both basal and postprandial plasma glucose by decreasing hepatic glucose production, intestinal absorption of glucose and improves insulin sensitivity. *Provides improvement in glycemic control, stabilizes or decreases body weight, improves lipid profile.*

USES/*UNLABELED*

Adjunct to diet in management of noninsulin-dependent diabetes mellitus (type II, NIDDM) whose hyperglycemia cannot be managed by diet alone. May be used concurrently with a sulfonylurea antidiabetic agent or insulin when diet and metformin or a sulfonylurea alone do not result in adequate glycemic control. *Treatment of metabolic complications of AIDS.*

PO ADMINISTRATION

1. When transferring pts from oral hypoglycemic agents other than chlorpropamide, no transition period necessary. When transferring from chlorpropamide, exercise care during first 2 wks (prolonged retention of chlorpropamide) as overlapping drug effects, possible hypoglycemia may occur.

2. If no adequate response to maximum dose of metformin within 4 wks, gradually add oral sulfonylurea antidiabetic agent while continuing metformin at maximum dose.

3. Do not crush film-coated tablets.

4. Give w/meals.

INDICATIONS/DOSAGE/ROUTES

Diabetes mellitus (500 mg tablet):
PO: Adults, elderly: Initially, 500 mg twice daily (w/morning and evening meals). May increase dosage in 500 mg increments every week, in divided doses. Can be given twice daily up to 2,000 mg/day (e.g., 1,000 mg twice daily w/morning and evening meals). If 2,500 mg/day dose is required, give t.i.d. w/meals. **Maximum dose/day:** 2500 mg/day.

Diabetes mellitus (850 mg tablet):
PO: Adults, elderly: Initially, 850 mg/day, w/morning meal. May increase dosage in 850 mg increments every *other* week, in divided doses. **Maintenance:** 850 mg twice daily (w/morning and evening meals). **Maximum dose/day:** 2,550 mg (850 mg t.i.d.).

PRECAUTIONS

CONTRAINDICATIONS: History of lactic acidosis, conditions associated w/hypoxemia (e.g., CHF), hypersensitivity to metformin, renal disease or dysfunction (serum creatinine >1.5 mg/dl [males], >1.4 mg/dl [females]) or abnormal creatinine clearance (Ccr), acute or chronic metabolic acidosis, including diabetic ketoacidosis, with or w/o coma. Temporarily withhold metformin therapy in pts undergoing radiologic studies involving parenteral iodinated contrast material (alters renal function). **CAUTIONS:** Conditions delaying food absorption (e.g., diarrhea, gastroparesis, vomiting), causing hyperglycemia (e.g., high fever) or hypoglycemia (e.g., malnutrition), uncontrolled hypo/hyperthyroidism, cardiovascular pts, concurrent drugs that effect renal function, hepatic impairment, elderly, malnourished, or debilitated, pts w/decreased renal function, CHF, excessive alcohol intake, chronic respiratory difficulty. **PREGNANCY/LACTATION:** Insulin is drug of choice during pregnancy. Distributed in breast milk in animals. **Pregnancy Category B**.

INTERACTIONS

DRUG INTERACTIONS: Alcohol, amiloride, digoxin, morphine, procainamide, quinidine, quinine, ranitidine, triamterene, trimethoprim, vancomycin, cimetidine, furosemide, nifedipine increases metformin concentration. Furosemide, hypoglycemia-causing medication may decrease dosage of metformin needed. Iodinated contrast studies may produce acute renal failure (increases risk of lactic acidosis). **ALTERED LAB VALUES:** None significant.

SIDE EFFECTS

FREQUENT (>3%): GI disturbances are transient and resolve spontaneously during therapy (diarrhea, nausea, vomiting, abdominal bloating, flatulence, anorexia). **OCCASIONAL (1–3%):** Unpleasant or metallic taste (resolves spontaneously during therapy).

ADVERSE REACTIONS/TOXIC EFFECTS

Lactic acidosis occurs rarely (0.03 cases/1,000 pts) but is a serious, often fatal (50%) complication. Characterized by increase in blood lactate levels (>5 mmol/L), decrease in blood pH, electrolyte disturbances. Symptoms include unexplained hyperventilation, myalgia, malaise, somnolence. May advance to cardiovascular collapse (shock), acute CHF, acute MI, prerenal azotemia.

NURSING IMPLICATIONS
BASELINE ASSESSMENT:

Inform pt of potential risks and advantages of therapy (see Adverse Reactions/Toxic Effects) and of alternative modes of therapy. Before initiation of therapy and annually thereafter, assess hgb, hct, RBC, and renal function (serum creatinine) tests. Discuss lifestyle to determine extent of learning, emotional needs. Assure follow-up instruction if pt/family do not thoroughly understand diabetes management or glucose-testing technique.

INTERVENTION/EVALUATION:

Encourage adequate hydration, particularly if diarrhea or vomiting occurs. Monitor folic acid, renal function tests for evidence of early lactic acidosis. Monitor serum B_{12} levels. If low, encourage parenteral B_{12} supplementation. Monitor blood glucose and glycosylated hemoglobin. If pt is on concurrent oral sulfonylureas, assess for hypoglycemia (cool wet skin, tremors, dizziness, anxiety, headache, tachycardia, numbness in mouth, hunger, diplopia). Monitor serum electrolytes, ketones, blood glucose, blood pH, lactate, pyruvate and metformin levels. Fasting glucose should be obtained to assess therapeutic response. Be alert to conditions that alter glucose requirements: fever, increased activity or stress, surgical procedure. Withhold medication, contact physician in presence of hypoxemia or dehydration (may potentiate acute renal impairment).

PATIENT/FAMILY TEACHING:

Discontinue metformin and contact physician immediately if evidence of lactic acidosis appears (unexplained hyperventilation, muscle aches, extreme tiredness, unusual sleepiness). Contact physician if significant diarrhea and vomiting continue. Prescribed diet is principal part of treatment; do not skip or delay meals. Diabetes mellitus requires lifelong control. Check blood glucose/urine as ordered. Wear medical alert identification. Check w/physician when glucose demands are altered (e.g., fever, infection, trauma, stress, heavy physical activity). Avoid excessive alcoholic beverages. Do not take other medication w/o consulting physician. Weight control, exercise, hygiene (including foot care) and nonsmoking are essential part of therapy. Inform dentist, physician, or surgeon of this medication before any treatment.

methadone hydrochloride

meth-ah-doan
(Dolophine)

CLASSIFICATION

Opioid analgesic **(Schedule II)**

AVAILABILITY (Rx)

Tablets: 5 mg, 10 mg. **Tablets (dispersable):** 40 mg. **Oral Solution:** 5 mg/5 ml, 10 mg/5 ml. **Oral Concentrate:** 10 mg/ml. **Injection:** 10 mg/ml.

PHARMACOKINETICS

	ONSET	PEAK	DURATION
PO	30–60 min	0.5–1 hr	4–6 hrs
SubQ	10–15 min	—	4–6 hrs
IM	10–15 min	—	4–6 hrs

Well absorbed after IM injection.

Metabolized in liver. Primarily excreted in urine. Half-life: 15–25 hrs.

ACTION / THERAPEUTIC EFFECT

Binds w/opioid receptors within CNS, *altering processes affecting analgesia, emotional response to acute withdrawal syndrome.*

USES

Relief of severe pain, detoxification, and temporary maintenance treatment of narcotic abstinence syndrome.

STORAGE/HANDLING

Store oral, parenteral form at room temperature. Do not use if solution appears cloudy or contains a precipitate.

PO/SUBQ/IM ADMINISTRATION

PO:

1. May give w/o regard to meals.
2. Dilute syrup in glass of H_2O (prevents anesthetic effect on mucous membranes).

SubQ/IM:

Note: IM preferred over SubQ route (SubQ produces pain, local irritation, induration).
1. Administer slowly.
2. Those w/circulating impairment experience higher risk of overdosage because of delayed absorption of repeated administration.

INDICATIONS/DOSAGE/ROUTES

Pain:
PO/SubQ/IM: Adults: 2.5–10 mg q3–4h as necessary. **Elderly:** 2.5 mg q8–12h.

Detoxification:
Note: Refer to local FDA-approved methadone programs.

PO: Adults: 15–40 mg/day until suppression of withdrawal symptoms. **Maintenance:** 20–100 mg/day.

PRECAUTIONS

CONTRAINDICATIONS: Hypersensitivity to narcotics, diarrhea due to poisoning, delivery of premature infant, during labor. **EXTREME CAUTION:** Impaired renal, hepatic function, elderly/debilitated, supraventricular tachycardia, cor pulmonale, history of seizures, acute abdominal conditions, increased intracranial pressure, respiratory abnormalities. **PREGNANCY/LACTATION:** Crosses placenta; distributed in breast milk. Respiratory depression may occur in neonate if mother received opiates during labor. Regular use of opiates during pregnancy may produce withdrawal symptoms in neonate (irritability, excessive crying, tremors, hyperactive reflexes, fever, vomiting, diarrhea, yawning, sneezing, seizures). **Pregnancy Category B**. (Category D if used for prolonged periods or in high doses at term.)

INTERACTIONS

DRUG INTERACTIONS: Alcohol, CNS depressants may increase CNS, respiratory depression, hypotension. MAO inhibitors may produce severe, fatal reaction (reduce dose to $1/4$ usual dose). Effects may be decreased w/buprenorphine. **ALTERED LAB VALUES:** May increase amylase, lipase.

SIDE EFFECTS

Note: Effects are dependent on dosage amount, route of administration. Ambulatory pts and those not in severe pain may experience dizziness, nausea, vomiting more frequently than those in supine position or having severe pain. **FREQUENT:** Sedation, decreased B/P, increased sweating, flushed face, constipation, dizziness, nausea, vomiting. **OCCASIONAL:** Confusion, decreased urination, pounding heartbeat, stomach cramps, visual changes, dry mouth, headache, decreased appetite, nervousness, inability to sleep. **RARE:** Allergic reaction (rash, itching), paralytic ileus.

ADVERSE REACTIONS/TOXIC EFFECTS

Overdosage results in respiratory depression, skeletal muscle flaccidity, cold clammy skin, cyanosis, extreme somnolence progressing to convulsions, stupor, coma. *Antidote:* 0.4 mg naloxone (Narcan). Tolerance to analgesic effect, physical dependence may occur w/repeated use.

NURSING IMPLICATIONS

BASELINE ASSESSMENT:

Pt should be in recumbent position before drug is administered by parenteral route. Assess onset, type, location, duration of pain. Obtain vital signs before giving medication. If respirations are 12/min or lower (20/min or lower in children), withhold medication, contact physician. Effect of medication is reduced if full pain recurs before next dose.

INTERVENTION/EVALUATION:

Monitor vital signs 15–30 min after SubQ/IM dose, 5–10 min after IV dose (monitor for decreased B/P and/or respirations, change in rate or quality of pulse). Oral medication is one-half as potent as parenteral. Assess for adequate voiding. Monitor stools; avoid constipation with increased fluids, bulky foods, and exercise. Initiate deep breathing and coughing exercises, particularly in those w/impaired pulmonary function. Assess for clinical improvement and record onset of relief of pain. Provide support to pt in detoxification program; monitor for withdrawal symptoms.

PATIENT/FAMILY TEACHING:

Discomfort may occur with injection. Change positions slowly to avoid orthostatic hypotension. Avoid tasks that require alertness, motor skills until response to drug is established. Tolerance/dependence may occur w/prolonged use of high doses. Do not take alcohol or other CNS depressants.

methicillin sodium
meth-ih-sill-in
(Staphcillin)

CLASSIFICATION

Antibiotic: Penicillin

AVAILABILITY (Rx)

Powder for Injection: 1 g, 4 g, 6 g, 10 g

PHARMACOKINETICS

Widely distributed. Partially metabolized in liver. Primarily excreted in urine. Half-life: 0.4–0.8 hrs (increased in decreased renal function).

ACTION/THERAPEUTIC EFFECT

Binds to bacterial membranes, *inhibiting cell wall synthesis. Bactericidal.*

USES

Treatment of respiratory tract, skin/skin structure infections, osteomyelitis, meningitis, endocardi-

tis, perioperatively, esp. cardiovascular, orthopedic procedures. Predominantly treatment of infections caused by penicillinase-producing staphylococci.

STORAGE/HANDLING

Solution for IM injection is stable for 24 hrs at room temperature, 96 hrs if refrigerated; IV infusion (piggyback) is stable for 8 hrs at room temperature. Discard if precipitate forms.

IM/IV ADMINISTRATION

Note: Space doses evenly around the clock for full effectiveness.

IM:

1. Reconstitute 500 mg vial w/1.5 ml sterile water for injection or 0.9% NaCl injection to provide concentration of 500 mg/ml.
2. Inject IM deeply into gluteus maximus.
3. Administer IM injection slowly.

IV:

1. For IV injection, further dilute w/20–25 ml sterile water for injection or 0.9% NaCl injection; administer at rate of 10 ml/min.
2. For intermittent IV infusion (piggyback), infuse over 20–30 min.
3. Alternating IV sites, use large veins to reduce risk of phlebitis.
4. Because of potential for hypersensitivity/anaphylaxis, start initial dose at few drops per minute, increase slowly to ordered rate; stay w/pt first 10–15 min, then check q10 min.

INDICATIONS/DOSAGE/ROUTES

Usual adult dosage:
IM/IV: Adults, elderly: 1–2 g q4–6h.

Usual pediatric dosage:
IM/IV: Children >1 mo: 100–300 mg/kg/day in divided doses q4–6h.

Usual dosage (neonates):
IM/IV: Neonates 0–7 days, <2 kg: 50–100 mg/kg/day in divided doses q12h. **Neonates 7–28 days, <2 kg or 0–7 days, >2 kg:** 75–150 mg/kg/day in divided doses q8h. **Neonates 7–28 days, >2 kg:** 100–200 mg/kg/day in divided doses q6h.

PRECAUTIONS

CONTRAINDICATIONS: Hypersensitivity to any penicillin. **CAUTIONS:** Renal impairment, history of allergies, particularly cephalosporins. **PREGNANCY/LACTATION:** Readily crosses placenta, appears in cord blood, amniotic fluid. Distributed in breast milk in low concentrations. May lead to allergic sensitization, diarrhea, candidiasis, skin rash in infant. **Pregnancy Category B.**

INTERACTIONS

DRUG INTERACTIONS: Probenecid may increase concentration, toxicity risk. **ALTERED LAB VALUES:** May increase SGOT (AST). May cause positive Coombs' test.

SIDE EFFECTS

FREQUENT: Mild hypersensitivity reaction (fever, rash, pruritus), nausea, vomiting, diarrhea more common w/oral therapy. **OCCASIONAL:** Phlebitis, thrombophlebitis (more common in elderly). **RARE:** Sterile abscess at IM injection site.

ADVERSE REACTIONS/TOXIC EFFECTS

Superinfections, potentially fatal antibiotic-associated colitis may result from bacterial imbalance. Neurotoxicity w/IV methicillin. Adverse hematologic effects, severe hypersensitivity reactions, rarely anaphylaxis. Acute interstitial nephritis occurs occasionally.

NURSING IMPLICATIONS

BASELINE ASSESSMENT:

Question history of allergies, esp. penicillins, cephalosporins. Obtain specimen for culture and sensitivity before giving first dose (therapy may begin before results are known).

INTERVENTION/EVALUATION:

Hold medication and promptly report rash (possible hypersensitivity) or diarrhea (w/fever, abdominal pain, mucus and blood in stool may indicate antibiotic-associated colitis). Assess food tolerance. Evaluate IV site for phlebitis (heat, pain, red streaking over vein). Monitor I&O; check for hematuria. Assess IM injection sites for pain, induration. Be alert for superinfection: increased fever, onset sore throat, nausea, vomiting, diarrhea, ulceration or changes of oral mucosa, anal/genital pruritus. Check hematology reports (esp. WBCs), periodic renal or hepatic reports in prolonged therapy.

PATIENT/FAMILY TEACHING:

Space doses evenly. Continue antibiotic for full length of treatment. Discomfort may occur w/IM injection. Notify physician in event of diarrhea, rash, blood in urine, or other new symptom.

methimazole

meth-**im**-ah-zole
(Tapazole)

CANADIAN AVAILABILITY:
Tapazole

CLASSIFICATION

Antithyroid

AVAILABILITY (Rx)

Tablets: 5 mg, 10 mg

PHARMACOKINETICS

Readily absorbed from GI tract (food may alter absorption). Primarily concentrated in thyroid gland. Metabolized in liver. Primarily excreted in urine. Minimally removed by hemodialysis. Half-life: 5–6 hrs.

ACTION/ *THERAPEUTIC EFFECT*

Inhibits thyroid hormone synthesis, *effective in treatment of hyperthyroidism.*

USES

Palliative treatment of hyperthyroidism; adjunct to relieve hyperthyroidism in preparation for surgical treatment or radioactive iodine therapy.

PO ADMINISTRATION

Space doses evenly, usually at 8 hr intervals.

INDICATIONS/DOSAGE/ROUTES

Hyperthyroidism:
PO: Adults, elderly: Initially, 15–60 mg/day. **Maintenance:** 5–15 mg/day. **Children:** Initially, 0.4 mg/kg/day. **Maintenance:** $1/2$ the initial dose.

PRECAUTIONS

CONTRAINDICATIONS: Hypersensitivity to the drug. **CAUTIONS:** Pts >40 yrs or in combination w/other agranulocytosis-inducing drugs, impaired liver function. **PREGNANCY/ LACTATION:** Readily crosses placenta, distributed in breast milk. Contraindicated in nursing mothers (can induce goiter, cretinism in neonate). **Pregnancy Category D**.

INTERACTIONS

DRUG INTERACTIONS: Amiodarone, iodinated glycerol, iodine, potassium iodide may decrease response. May decrease effect of oral anticoagulants. May increase concentration of digoxin (as pt becomes euthyroid). May decrease thyroid uptake of I^{131}. **ALTERED LAB VALUES:** May increase SGOT (AST), SGPT (ALT), alkaline phosphatase, LDH, bilirubin, prothrombin time. May decrease prothrombin level.

SIDE EFFECTS

FREQUENT (3–5%): Fever, rash, itching. **OCCASIONAL (1–3%):** Dizziness, loss of taste, nausea, vomiting, stomach pain, peripheral neuropathy (numbness in fingers, toes, face). **RARE (<1%):** Swollen lymph nodes/salivary glands.

ADVERSE REACTIONS/TOXIC EFFECTS

Agranulocytosis (which may occur as long as 4 mos after therapy); pancytopenia and fatal hepatitis have occurred.

NURSING IMPLICATIONS

BASELINE ASSESSMENT:

Question for hypersensitivity. Obtain baseline weight, pulse.

INTERVENTION/EVALUATION:

Monitor pulse and weight daily. Assess food tolerance. Check for skin eruptions, itching, swollen lymph glands. Be alert to hepatitis: nausea, vomiting, drowsiness, jaundice. Monitor hematology results for bone marrow suppression; check for signs of infection or bleeding.

PATIENT/FAMILY TEACHING:

Do not exceed ordered dose; follow-up w/physician is essential. Space evenly around the clock. Take resting pulse (teach pt/family) daily to monitor therapeutic results and report as directed. Do not take other medications w/o approval of physician. Seafood and iodine products may be restricted. Report illness, unusual bleeding, or bruising immediately. Inform physician of sudden or continuous weight gain, cold intolerance or depression.

---

methocarbamol
(Robaxin)

FIXED-COMBINATION(S):
W/aspirin, a salicylate (Robaxisal)
*See Classification section under:
Skeletal muscle relaxants*

---

methohexital sodium
(Brevital)
*See Classification section under:
Anesthetics: general*

---

methotrexate sodium

meth-oh-**trex**-ate
(Folex, Mexate, Rheumatrex)

CANADIAN AVAILABILITY:
Rheumatrex

CLASSIFICATION

Antineoplastic, antiarthritic, antipsoriatic

AVAILABILITY (Rx)

Tablets: 2.5 mg. **Powder for Injection:** 20 mg, 50 mg, 100 mg, 1 g. **Injection:** 2.5 mg/ml, 25 mg/ml. **Injection (preservative-free):** 25 mg/ml.

PHARMACOKINETICS

Variably absorbed from GI tract. Widely distributed. Metabolized in liver, intracellularly. Primarily excreted in urine. Half-life: 3–10 hrs (high doses: 8–15 hrs).

ACTION/*THERAPEUTIC EFFECT*

Inhibits DNA, RNA, protein synthesis by competing w/enzyme necessary to reduce folic acid to tetrahydrofolic acid, a component essential to DNA, RNA, protein synthesis. Cell cycle-specific for S phase of cell division. Mild immunosuppressant activity.

USES/*UNLABELED*

Treatment of trophoblastic neoplasms (gestational choriocarcinoma, chorioadenoma destruens, hydatidiform mole), acute leukemias, breast cancer, epidermoid cancers of head and neck, lung cancer, advanced stages of lymphosarcoma, mycosis fungoides, meningeal leukemia, severe psoriasis, rheumatoid arthritis. *Treatment of cervical, ovarian, bladder, renal, prostatic, testicular carcinoma, acute myelocytic leukemia, psoriatic arthritis, systemic dermatomyositis.*

STORAGE/HANDLING

Note: May be carcinogenic, mutagenic, or teratogenic. Handle w/extreme care during preparation/administration.

Solutions w/o preservatives should be prepared immediately before use.

IM/IV ADMINISTRATION

Note: May give IM, IV, intra-arterially, intrathecally. Wear gloves when preparing solution. If powder or solution comes in contact w/skin, wash immediately, thoroughly w/soap, water.

1. Reconstitute vial w/2–10 ml sterile water for injection or 0.9% NaCl injection.

2. May further dilute w/5% dextrose or 0.9% NaCl.

3. For intrathecal use, dilute w/preservative-free 0.9% NaCl to provide a 1 mg/ml concentration.

INDICATIONS/DOSAGE/ROUTES

Note: Dosage individualized based on clinical response, tolerance to adverse effects. When used in combination therapy, consult specific protocols for optimum dosage, sequence of drug administration.

Trophoblastic neoplasms, choriocarcinoma:
PO/IM: Adults: 15–30 mg/day for 5 days. Repeat 3–5 times w/rest periods of 1–2 wks between courses.

Leukemia:
PO: Adults, children: (Combined w/prednisone): *Induction:* 3.3 mg/m^2/day produces remission within 4–6 wks.
PO/IM: Adults, children: Maintenance: 30 mg/m^2/wk in divided doses 2 times/wk.
IV: Adults, children: Maintenance: 2.5 mg/kg every 14 days.

Meningeal leukemia:
Intrathecal: Adults, children >2 yrs: 12 mg/m^2 every 2–5 days until CSF normal, then give one additional dose. **Children 2 yrs:** 10 mg/m^2. **Children 1–2 yrs:** 8 mg/m^2. **Children <1 yr:** 6 mg/m^2.

Burkitt's lymphoma, stage I or II:
PO: Adults: 10–25 mg/day for 4–8 days. Repeat in 7–10 days.

Stage III lymphosarcoma:
PO: Adults: 0.625–2.5 mg/kg/day.

Osteosarcoma:
IV Infusion: Adults: (Combination therapy): Initially, 12 g/m^2 over 4 hrs. May increase to 15 g/m^2 w/subsequent treatments. Give w/leucovorin 15 mg orally q6h for 10 doses, begin 24 hrs after start of methotrexate (MTX) infusion. Give IM/IV if pt vomiting or unable to tolerate oral medication. Dosage may vary based upon serum (MTX) levels, impairment of liver function.
Note: Delay MTX therapy w/leucovorin rescue until recovery if WBCs <1,500/mm^3, neutrophil count <200/mm^3, platelet count <75,000mm^3, serum bilirubin >1.2 mg/dl, SGPT (ALT) level >450 units. If mucositis present, delay until evidence of healing. If persistent pleural effusion, drain prior to infusion. Serum creatinine must be normal, creatinine clearance >60 ml/min before initiation of therapy. Pt must be well hydrated.

Mycosis fungoides:
PO: Adults: 2.5–10 mg/day.
IM: Adults: 50 mg once/wk or 25 mg 2 times/wk.

Psoriasis:
IM/IV: Adults: 5–10 mg 1 wk prior to initiation of therapy to detect idiosyncratic reaction.
PO: Adults: *Divided doses:* 2.5–5 mg q12h for 3 doses or q8h for 4 doses each wk. Increase dose by 2.5 mg/wk. Do not exceed 25–30

mg/wk. **Daily dose:** 2.5 mg/day for 5 days. Rest 2 days. Repeat. **Maximum daily dose:** 6.25 mg. **PO/IM/IV: Adults:** *Weekly single dose:* 10–25 mg/wk up to 50 mg/wk.

Rheumatoid arthritis:
PO: Adults: Initially: 7.5 mg/wk as single dose or 2.5 mg q12h × 3 doses. Adjust dose gradually to achieve optimal response, usually not >20 mg/wk.

Usual elderly dose (rheumatoid arthritis/psoriasis):
PO: Initially, 5 mg/wk as single or divided doses. May increase up to 7.5 mg/wk. **Maximum:** 20 mg/wk.

PRECAUTIONS

CONTRAINDICATIONS: Impaired renal function. *Psoriasis:* Poor nutritional status, severe renal/hepatic disease, preexisting blood dyscrasias. **EXTREME CAUTION:** Infection, peptic ulcer, ulcerative colitis, very young, elderly, debilitated, preexisting liver damage, impaired hepatic function, preexisting bone marrow depression. **CAUTIONS:** Impaired renal, hepatic function, peptic ulcer, ulcerative colitis. **PREGNANCY/LACTATION:** Avoid pregnancy during MTX therapy and minimum 3 mos after therapy in males or at least one ovulatory cycle after therapy in females. May cause fetal death, congenital anomalies. Drug is distributed in breast milk. Breast-feeding not recommended. **Pregnancy Category D.**

INTERACTIONS

DRUG INTERACTIONS: Parenteral acyclovir may increase neurotoxicity. Alcohol, hepatotoxic medications may increase hepatotoxicity. NSAIDs may increase toxicity. Asparaginase may decrease effects of methotrexate. Bone marrow depressants may increase bone marrow depression. Probenecid, salicylates may increase concentration, toxicity. Live virus vaccines may potentiate virus replication, increase vaccine side effects, decrease pt's antibody response to vaccine. **ALTERED LAB VALUES:** May increase uric acid, SGOT (AST).

SIDE EFFECTS

FREQUENT (3–10%): Nausea, vomiting, stomatitis. In psoriatic pts, burning, erythema at psoriatic site. **OCCASIONAL (1–3%):** Diarrhea, rash, dermatitis, pruritis, alopecia, dizziness, anorexia, malaise, headache, drowsiness, blurred vision.

ADVERSE REACTIONS/TOXIC EFFECTS

High potential for various, severe toxicity. GI toxicity may produce oral ulcers of mouth, gingivitis, glossitis, pharyngitis, stomatitis, enteritis, hematemesis. Hepatotoxicity occurs more frequently w/frequent, small doses than w/large, intermittent doses. Pulmonary toxicity characterized as interstitial pneumonitis. Hematologic toxicity resulting from marked bone marrow depression may be manifested as leukopenia, thrombocytopenia, anemia, hemorrhage (may develop rapidly). Skin toxicity produces rash, pruritus, urticaria, pigmentation, photosensitivity, petechiae, ecchymosis, pustules. Severe nephropathy produces azotemia, hematuria, renal failure.

NURSING IMPLICATIONS
BASELINE ASSESSMENT:

Question for possibility of pregnancy before initiating therapy (Pregnancy Category X) in those w/psoriasis or rheumatoid arthritis. Obtain all functional tests before therapy and repeat throughout therapy. Antiemetics may prevent nausea, vomiting.

INTERVENTION/EVALUATION:

Monitor hepatic and renal function tests, Hgb, Hct, WBC, differential, platelet count, urinalysis, chest radiographs, serum uric acid level. Monitor for hematologic toxicity (fever, sore throat, signs of local infection, easy bruising, unusual bleeding from any site), symptoms of anemia (excessive tiredness, weakness). Assess skin for evidence of dermatologic toxicity. Keep pt well hydrated, urine alkaline. Avoid IM injections, rectal temperatures, traumas that induce bleeding. Apply 5 full min of pressure to IV sites.

PATIENT/FAMILY TEACHING:

Maintain fastidious oral hygiene. Do not have immunizations w/o physician's approval (drug lowers body's resistance). Avoid crowds, those w/infection. Avoid alcohol, salicylates. Avoid sunlamp and sunlight exposure. Use contraceptive measures during therapy and for 3 mos (males) or one ovular cycle (females) after therapy. Promptly report fever, sore throat, signs of local infection, easy bruising, unusual bleeding from any site. Alopecia is reversible, but new hair growth may have different color or texture. Contact physician if nausea/vomiting continues at home.

methylcellulose

meth-ill-**cell**-you-los
(Citrucel, Cologel)

CLASSIFICATION

Laxative: Bulk-forming

AVAILABILITY (OTC)

Powder

PHARMACOKINETICS

	ONSET	PEAK	DURATION
PO	12–24 hrs	—	—

Full effect may not be evident for 2–3 days. Acts in small/large intestine.

ACTION/*THERAPEUTIC EFFECT*

Dissolves and expands in water, *providing increased bulk, moisture content in stool, increasing peristalsis, bowel motility.*

USES

Prophylaxis in those who should not strain during defecation. Facilitates defecation in those w/diminished colonic motor response.

PO ADMINISTRATION

1. Instruct pt to drink 6–8 glasses of water/day (aids stool softening).
2. Not to be swallowed in dry form; mix w/at least 1 full glass (8 oz) liquid.

INDICATIONS/DOSAGE/ROUTES

Laxative:
PO: Adults, elderly: 1 tbsp (15 ml) in 8 oz water 1–3 times/day. **Children 6–12 yrs:** 1 tsp (5 ml) in 4 oz water 3–4 times/day.

PRECAUTIONS

CONTRAINDICATIONS: Abdominal pain, nausea, vomiting, symptoms of appendicitis, partial bowel obstruction, dysphagia. **CAUTIONS:** None significant. **PREGNANCY/LACTATION:** Safe for use in pregnancy. **Pregnancy Category C**.

INTERACTIONS

DRUG INTERACTIONS: May interfere w/effects of potassium-sparing diuretics, potassium supplements. May decrease effect of oral anticoagulants, digoxin, salicylates by decreasing absorption. **ALTERED LAB VALUES:** May increase glucose. May decrease potassium.

SIDE EFFECTS

RARE: Some degree of abdominal discomfort, nausea, mild cramps, griping, faintness.

ADVERSE REACTIONS/TOXIC EFFECTS

Esophageal or bowel obstruction may occur if administered with insufficient liquid (less than 250 ml or 1 full glass).

NURSING IMPLICATIONS
INTERVENTION/EVALUATION:

Encourage adequate fluid intake. Assess bowel sounds for peristalsis. Monitor daily bowel activity and stool consistency (watery, loose, soft, semisolid, solid) and record time of evacuation. Monitor serum electrolytes in those exposed to prolonged, frequent, or excessive use of medication.

PATIENT/FAMILY TEACHING:

Institute measures to promote defecation: increase fluid intake, exercise, high-fiber diet.

methyldopa

meth-ill-**doe**-pah
(Aldomet)

methyldopate hydrochloride

FIXED-COMBINATION(S):

W/hydrochlorothiazide, a diuretic **(Aldoril)**; w/chlorothiazide, a diuretic **(Aldoclor).**

CANADIAN AVAILABILITY:

Aldomet, Apo-Methyldopa, Novo-medopa

CLASSIFICATION

Antihypertensive

AVAILABILITY (Rx)

Tablets: 125 mg, 250 mg, 500 mg. **Oral Suspension:** 250 mg/5 ml. **Injection:** 250 mg/5 ml.

PHARMACOKINETICS

	ONSET	PEAK	DURATION
PO	—	4–6 hrs	—
IV	—	4–6 hrs	10–16 hrs

Variably absorbed from GI tract. Metabolized in liver. Primarily excreted in urine. Removed by hemodialysis. Half-life: 1.7 hrs (increased in decreased renal function).

ACTION/*THERAPEUTIC EFFECT*

Stimulates central inhibitory alpha-adrenergic receptors (lowers arterial pressure, reduces plasma renin activity). *Reduces standing and supine B/P.*

USES

Management of moderate to severe hypertension.

STORAGE/HANDLING

Store tablets at room temperature. IV solution is stable for 24 hrs at room temperature.

PO/IV ADMINISTRATION

PO:

1. May give w/o regard to food. If GI upset occurs, give w/food.
2. Tablets may be crushed.

IV:

1. Give by IV infusion (piggyback). Avoid SubQ, IM (unpredictable absorption).
2. For IV infusion, dilute 250 or 500 mg vial w/50 or 100 ml 5% dextrose.
3. Infuse slowly over 30–60 min.

INDICATIONS/DOSAGE/ROUTES

Hypertension:
PO: Adults: Initially, 250 mg 2–3 times/day for 2 days. Adjust dosage at intervals of 2 days (minimum). **Elderly:** Initially, 125 mg 1–2 times/day. May increase by 125 mg q2–3 days. **Maintenance:** 500 mg to 2 g/day in 2–4 divided doses. **Children:** Initially, 10 mg/kg/day in 2–4 divided doses. Adjust dose at intervals of 2 days (minimum). **Maximum:** 65 mg/kg/day or 3 g/day, whichever is less.
IV: Adults: 250–500 mg q6h up to 1 g q6h. **Children:** 20–40 mg/kg/day in divided doses q6h. **Maximum:** 65 mg/kg/day or 3 g/day, whichever is less.

PRECAUTIONS

CONTRAINDICATIONS: Acute hepatitis, active cirrhosis. **CAUTIONS:** Impaired hepatic function. **PREGNANCY/LACTATION:** Crosses placenta; distributed in breast milk. Reduction of neonate systolic B/P (4–5 mm Hg) has occurred for 2–3 days after delivery; tremors reported. **Pregnancy Category C**.

INTERACTIONS

DRUG INTERACTIONS: Tricyclic antidepressants, NSAIDs may decrease effect. Hypotensive-producing medications may increase effect. May increase risk of toxicity of lithium. May cause hyperexcitability w/MAO inhibitors. Sympathomimetics may decrease effects. **ALTERED LAB VALUES:** May increase SGOT (AST), SGPT (ALT), alkaline phosphatase, bilirubin, BUN, creatinine, potassium, sodium, prolactin, uric acid. May produce false positive Coombs' test, prolong prothrombin time.

SIDE EFFECTS

FREQUENT: Peripheral edema, drowsiness, headache, dry mouth. **OCCASIONAL:** Mental changes (e.g., anxiety, depression), decreased sexual ability or interest, diarrhea, swelling of breasts, nausea, vomiting, lightheadedness, numbness in hands/feet, rhinitis.

ADVERSE REACTIONS/TOXIC EFFECTS

Hepatotoxicity (abnormal liver function tests, jaundice, hepatitis), hemolytic anemia, unexplained fever and flulike symptoms: Discontinue medication, contact physician.

NURSING IMPLICATIONS

BASELINE ASSESSMENT:

Obtain baseline B/P, pulse, weight.

INTERVENTION/EVALUATION:

Monitor B/P, pulse closely q30 min until stabilized. Monitor weight daily during initial therapy. Monitor liver function tests. Assess for peripheral edema of hands, feet (usually, first area of low extremity swelling is behind medial malleolus in ambulatory, sacral area in bedridden).

PATIENT/FAMILY TEACHING:

Urine may darken in color. To reduce hypotensive effect, rise slowly from lying to sitting position and permit legs to dangle from bed momentarily before standing. Avoid sudden or prolonged standing, exercise, hot environment or hot shower, alcohol ingestion, particularly in morning (may aggravate orthostatic hypotension). Full therapeutic effect of oral administration may take 2–3 days. Drowsiness usually disappears during continued therapy. Sugarless gum, sips of tepid water may relieve dry mouth.

methylergonovine

meth-ill-er-go-**noe**-veen
(Methergine)

CLASSIFICATION

Oxytocic

AVAILABILITY (Rx)

Tablets: 0.2 mg. **Injection:** 0.2 mg/ml.

PHARMACOKINETICS

	ONSET	PEAK	DURATION
PO	5–10 min	—	—
IM	2–5 min	—	—
IV	Immediate	—	3 hrs

Rapidly absorbed from GI tract, after IM administration. Distributed rapidly to plasma, extracellular fluid, tissues. Metabolized in liver (undergoes first-pass effect). Primarily excreted in urine.

ACTION/*THERAPEUTIC EFFECT*

Stimulates alpha-adrenergic, serotonin receptors, producing arterial vasoconstriction. Causes vasospasm of coronary arteries. Directly stimulates uterine muscle *(increases strength, frequency of contractions, decreases uterine bleeding).*

USES/*UNLABELED*

To prevent and treat postpartum, postabortion hemorrhage due to atony or involution (not for induction or augmentation of labor). *Treatment of incomplete abortion.*

PO/IM/IV ADMINISTRATION

1. Initial dose may be given parenterally, followed by oral regimen.

2. IV use in life-threatening emergencies only; dilute to volume of 5 ml w/0.9% NaCl injection and give over at least 1 min, carefully monitoring B/P.

INDICATIONS/DOSAGE/ROUTES

Usual oral dosage:
PO: Adults: 0.2 mg 3–4 times/day for maximum of 7 days.

Usual parenteral dosage:
IM/IV: Adults: Initially, 0.2 mg. May repeat no more often than q2–4h for no more than 5 doses total.

PRECAUTIONS

CONTRAINDICATIONS: Hypersensitivity to ergot, hypertension, pregnancy, toxemia, untreated hypocalcemia. **CAUTIONS:** Renal or hepatic impairment, coronary artery disease, occlusive peripheral vascular disease, sepsis. **PREGNANCY/LACTATION:** Contraindicated during pregnancy. Small amounts in breast milk. **Pregnancy Category C**.

INTERACTIONS

DRUG INTERACTIONS: Vasoconstrictors, vasopressors may increase effect. **ALTERED LAB VALUES:** May decrease prolactin concentration.

SIDE EFFECTS

FREQUENT: Nausea, uterine cramping, vomiting. **OCCASIONAL:** Abdominal/stomach pain, diarrhea, dizziness, sweating, ringing in ears, bradycardia, chest pain. **RARE:** Allergic reaction (rash, itching), dyspnea, sudden/severe hypertension.

ADVERSE REACTIONS/TOXIC EFFECTS

Severe hypertensive episodes may result in cerebrovascular accident, serious arrhythmias, seizures; hypertensive effects more frequent w/pt susceptibility, rapid IV administration, concurrent regional anesthesia or vasoconstrictors. Peripheral ischemia may lead to gangrene.

NURSING IMPLICATIONS

BASELINE ASSESSMENT:

Question for hypersensitivity to any ergot derivatives. Determine calcium, B/P, and pulse baselines. Assess bleeding prior to administration.

INTERVENTION/EVALUATION:

Monitor uterine tone, bleeding, B/P, and pulse every 15 min until stable (about 1–2 hrs). Assess extremities for color, warmth, movement, pain. Report chest pain promptly. Provide support w/ambulation if dizziness occurs.

PATIENT/FAMILY TEACHING:

Avoid smoking because of added vasoconstriction. Report increased cramping, bleeding, or foul-smelling lochia. Pale, cold hands or feet should be reported because may mean decreased circulation.

methylphenidate hydrochloride

meh-thyl-**fen**-ih-date
(Ritalin)

CANADIAN AVAILABILITY:
Ritalin

CLASSIFICATION

CNS stimulant

AVAILABILITY (Rx)

Tablets: 5 mg, 10 mg, 20 mg. **Tablets (sustained-release):** 20 mg.

PHARMACOKINETICS

	ONSET	PEAK	DURATION
PO (tablets)	—	—	3–6 hrs
PO (extended-release)	—	—	8 hrs

Slowly, incompletely absorbed from GI tract. Metabolized in liver. Excreted in urine, eliminated in feces via biliary system. Half-life: 2–4 hrs.

ACTION/THERAPEUTIC EFFECT

Blocks reuptake mechanisms of dopaminergic neurons. *Decreases motor restlessness, enhances ability to pay attention. Increases motor activity, mental alertness; diminish-*

es sense of fatigue, enhances spirit, produces mild euphoria.

USES/UNLABELED

Adjunct to treatment of attention deficit disorder with moderate to severe distractability, short attention spans, hyperactivity, emotional impulsivity in children >6 yrs. Management of narcolepsy in adults. Treatment of secondary mental depression.

PO ADMINISTRATION

1. Do not give drug in afternoon or evening (drug causes insomnia).

2. Do not crush or break sustained-release capsules.

3. Tablets may be crushed.

4. Give dose 30–45 min before meals.

INDICATIONS/DOSAGE/ROUTES

Note: Do not use extended release for initial therapy.

Attention deficit disorder:
PO: Children >6 yrs: Initially, 5 mg before breakfast and lunch. May increase dosage by 5–10 mg/day at weekly intervals. **Maximum:** 60 mg/day. Therapy usually discontinued when adolescence reached.

Narcolepsy:
PO: Adults, elderly: 10 mg 2–3 times/day. **Range:** 10–60 mg/day.

PRECAUTIONS

CONTRAINDICATIONS: History of marked anxiety, tension, agitation; glaucoma, those with motor tics, family history of Tourette's disorder. **CAUTIONS:** History of seizures, hypertension, history of drug dependence. **PREGNANCY/LACTATION:** Unknown whether drug crosses placenta or is distributed in breast milk. **Pregnancy Category C**.

INTERACTIONS

DRUG INTERACTIONS: CNS stimulants may have additive effect. MAO inhibitors may increase effects. **ALTERED LAB VALUES:** None significant.

SIDE EFFECTS

FREQUENT: Nervousness, insomnia, anorexia. **OCCASIONAL:** Dizziness, drowsiness, headache, nausea, stomach pain, fever, rash, joint pain. **RARE:** Blurred vision, Tourette's syndrome (uncontrolled vocal outbursts, repeated body movements).

ADVERSE REACTIONS/TOXIC EFFECTS

Prolonged administration to children w/attention deficit disorder may produce a temporary suppression of normal weight gain pattern. Overdose may produce tachycardia, palpitations, cardiac irregularities, chest pain, psychotic episode, seizures, coma. Hypersensitivity reactions, blood dyscrasias occur rarely.

NURSING IMPLICATIONS
INTERVENTION/EVALUATION:

CBC, differential, and platelet count should be performed routinely during therapy. If paradoxical return of attention deficit occurs, dosage should be reduced or discontinued.

PATIENT/FAMILY TEACHING:

Avoid tasks that require alertness, motor skills until response to drug is established. Dry mouth may be relieved by sugarless gum, sips of tepid water. Report any increase in seizures. Take last dose early in evening to avoid insomnia. Report nervousness, palpitations, fever, vomiting, skin rash.

methylprednisolone

meth-ill-pred-**niss**-oh-lone
(Medrol)

methylprednisolone sodium succinate

(Solu-Medrol, A-Methapred)

methylprednisolone acetate

(Depo-Medrol, Duralone)

FIXED-COMBINATIONS:
Methylprednisolone acetate w/Neomycin, an anti-infective **(Neo-Medrol)**

CANADIAN AVAILABILITY:
Medrol, Depo-Medrol, Solu-Medrol

CLASSIFICATION

Corticosteroid

AVAILABILITY (Rx)

Tablets: 2 mg, 4 mg, 8 mg, 16 mg, 24 mg, 32 mg
Succinate: Powder for Injection: 40 mg, 125 mg, 500 mg, 1 g, 2 g
Acetate: Injection: 20 mg/ml, 40 mg/ml, 80 mg/ml

PHARMACOKINETICS

Well absorbed from GI tract, after IM administration. Widely distributed. Metabolized in liver. Excreted in urine. Half-life: >3.5 hrs.

ACTION / *THERAPEUTIC EFFECT*

Inhibits accumulation of inflammatory cells at inflammation sites,

phagocytosis, lysosomal enzyme release and synthesis and/or release of mediators of inflammation. *Prevents/suppresses cell-mediated immune reactions. Decreases/prevents tissue response to inflammatory process.*

USES

Substitution therapy of deficiency states: acute/chronic adrenal insufficiency, congenital adrenal hyperplasia, adrenal insufficiency secondary to pituitary insufficiency. Nonendocrine disorders: arthritis, rheumatic carditis, allergic, collagen, intestinal tract, liver, ocular, renal, and skin diseases, bronchial asthma, cerebral edema, malignancies.

PO/IM/IV ADMINISTRATION

PO:

1. Give w/food or milk.
2. Give single doses before 9 AM; give multiple doses at evenly spaced intervals.

IM:

1. Methylprednisolone acetate should not be further diluted.
2. Methylprednisolone sodium succinate should be reconstituted w/bacteriostatic water.
3. Give deep IM in gluteus maximus.

IV:

1. For infusion, add to 5% dextrose, 0.9% NaCl, or 5% dextrose in 0.9% NaCl.
2. Do *not* give methylprednisolone acetate IV.

INDICATIONS/DOSAGE/ROUTES

Note: Individualize dose based on disease, pt, and response.

ORAL METHYLPREDNISOLONE:

PO: Adults, elderly: Initially, 4–48 mg/day.

M

METHYLPREDNISOLONE SODIUM SUCCINATE:

IV: Adults, elderly: (High dose): 30 mg/kg over at least 30 min. Repeat q4–6h for 48–72 hrs.
IV: Adults, elderly: Initially, 10–40 mg q4–6h, may give subsequent doses IM. **Children, infants:** Not less than 0.5 mg/kg/day.

METHYLPREDNISOLONE ACETATE:

Adrenogenital syndrome:
IM: Adults, elderly: 40 mg q2 wks.

Rheumatoid arthritis:
IM: Adults: 40–120 mg/wk.

Dermatologic lesions:
IM: Adults, elderly: 40–120 mg/wk for 1–4 wks.

Asthma, allergic rhinitis:
IM: Adults, elderly: 80–120 mg/wk.

PRECAUTIONS

CONTRAINDICATIONS: Hypersensitivity to any corticosteroid, systemic fungal infection, peptic ulcers (except life-threatening situations). Avoid immunizations, smallpox vaccination. **CAUTIONS:** History of tuberculosis (may reactivate disease), hypothyroidism, cirrhosis, nonspecific ulcerative colitis, CHF, hypertension, psychosis, renal insufficiency. Prolonged therapy should be discontinued slowly. **PREGNANCY/LACTATION:** Drug crosses placenta, distributed in breast milk. May cause cleft palate (chronic use first trimester). Nursing contraindicated. **Pregnancy Category C**.

INTERACTIONS

DRUG INTERACTIONS: Amphotericin may increase hypokalemia. May decrease effect of oral hypoglycemics, insulin, diuretics, potassium supplements. May increase digoxin toxicity (due to hypokalemia). Hepatic enzyme inducers may decrease effect. Live virus vaccines may potentiate virus replication, increase vaccine side effects, decrease pt's antibody response to vaccine. **ALTERED LAB VALUES:** May decrease calcium, potassium, thyroxine. May increase cholesterol, lipids, glucose, sodium, amylase.

SIDE EFFECTS

FREQUENT: Insomnia, heartburn, nervousness, abdominal distension, increased sweating, acne, mood swings, increased appetite, facial flushing, GI distress, delayed wound healing, increased susceptibility to infection, diarrhea/constipation. **OCCASIONAL:** Headache, edema, tachycardia, change in skin color, frequent urination, depression. **RARE:** Psychosis, increased blood coagulability, hallucinations.

ADVERSE REACTIONS/TOXIC EFFECTS

Long-term therapy: Muscle wasting (esp. arms, legs), osteoporosis, spontaneous fractures, amenorrhea, cataracts, glaucoma, peptic ulcer, CHF. *Abrupt withdrawal following long-term therapy:* Anorexia, nausea, fever, headache, severe joint pain, rebound inflammation, fatigue, weakness, lethargy, dizziness, orthostatic hypotension.

NURSING IMPLICATIONS
BASELINE ASSESSMENT:

Question for hypersensitivity to any of the corticosteroids, components. Obtain baselines for height, weight, B/P, glucose, electrolytes. Check results of initial tests, e.g., TB skin test, x-rays, EKG.

INTERVENTION/EVALUATION:

Monitor I&O, weight; assess for edema. Evaluate food tolerance and bowel activity; report hyperacidity promptly. Check B/P, TPR at least 2 times/day. Be alert to infection: sore throat, fever, or vague symptoms. Monitor electrolytes. Watch for hypocalcemia (muscle twitching, cramps, positive Trousseau's or Chvostek's signs) or hypokalemia (weakness and muscle cramps, numbness/tingling [esp. lower extremities], nausea and vomiting, irritability, EKG changes). Assess emotional status, ability to sleep. Check lab results for blood coagulability and clinical evidence of thromboembolism. Provide assistance w/ambulation.

PATIENT/FAMILY TEACHING:

Take oral dose w/food or milk. For those on long-term therapy, carry identification of drug and dose, physician name and phone number. Do not change dose/schedule or stop taking drug; must taper off gradually under medical supervision. Notify physician of fever, sore throat, muscle aches, sudden weight gain/swelling. Obtain instructions for prescribed diet (usually sodium restricted w/high vitamin D, protein, and potassium). Maintain careful personal hygiene, avoid exposure to disease or trauma. Severe stress (serious infection, surgery or trauma) may require increased dosage. Do not take any other medication w/o consulting physician. Follow-up visits, lab tests are necessary; children must be assessed for growth retardation. Inform dentist or other physicians of methylprednisolone therapy now or within past 12 mos.

methysergide maleate
meth-i-**sir**-guide
(Sansert)

CANADIAN AVAILABILITY:
Sansert

CLASSIFICATION

Antimigraine

AVAILABILITY (Rx)

Tablets: 2 mg

PHARMACOKINETICS

Rapidly absorbed from GI tract. Widely distributed. Metabolized in liver to active metabolite. Primarily excreted in urine. Half-life: 10 hrs.

ACTION/THERAPEUTIC EFFECT

Directly stimulates smooth muscle leading to vasoconstriction, *preventing or aborting vascular headaches.*

USES

Treatment of vascular headaches (e.g., migraine, cluster headaches).

PO ADMINISTRATION

Give w/meals to avoid GI upset.

INDICATIONS/DOSAGE/ROUTES

Vascular headaches:
PO: Adults: 4–8 mg/day in divided doses. Do not give continuously >6 mos w/o 3–4 wk drug-free interval between courses of therapy. Discontinue gradually over 2–3 wks (avoids rebound headaches).

PRECAUTIONS

CONTRAINDICATIONS: Hypersensitivity to ergot alkaloids, peripheral vascular disease (thromboangiitis obliterans, leutic arteritis, severe arteriosclerosis, Raynaud's disease), phlebitis or cellulitis of lower limbs, pulmonary disease, collagen diseases, fibrotic disease, impaired renal or hepatic function, severe pruritus, valvular heart disease, coronary artery disease, severe hypertension, debilitated, malnutrition. **CAUTIONS:** None significant. **PREGNANCY/LACTATION:** Contraindicated in pregnancy (produces uterine stimulant action, resulting in possible fetal death or retarded fetal growth; increases vasoconstriction of placental vascular bed). Drug distributed in breast milk. May produce diarrhea, vomiting in neonate. May inhibit lactation. **Pregnancy Category X.**

INTERACTIONS

DRUG INTERACTIONS: Ergot alkaloids, systemic vasoconstrictors (e.g., norepinephrine) may increase vasoconstrictor effect. **ALTERED LAB VALUES:** May increase BUN.

SIDE EFFECTS

FREQUENT: Dizziness, lightheadedness, diarrhea, drowsiness, nausea, vomiting, stomach pain, numbness in fingers, toes, face, pain, cold hands/feet, weakness in legs. **OCCASIONAL:** Changes in vision, clumsiness, peripheral edema, fast/slow heartbeat, flushed face, rash, constipation, inability to sleep, heartburn. **RARE:** Pulmonary fibrosis.

ADVERSE REACTIONS/TOXIC EFFECTS

Prolonged administration or excessive dosage may produce ergotamine poisoning: nausea, vomiting, weakness of legs, pain in limb muscles, numbness and tingling of fingers/toes, precordial pain, tachycardia or bradycardia, hyper/hypotension. Localized edema, itching due to vasoconstriction of peripheral arteries and arterioles. Feet and hands will become cold, pale, numb. Muscle pain occurs when walking and, later, even at rest. Gangrene may occur. Occasionally, confusion, depression, drowsiness, convulsions may appear.

NURSING IMPLICATIONS

BASELINE ASSESSMENT:

Question pt regarding history of peripheral vascular disease, renal or hepatic impairment, or possibility of pregnancy. Contact physician with findings before administering drug. Question pt regarding onset, location, and duration of migraine, and possible precipitating symptoms.

INTERVENTION/EVALUATION:

Monitor closely for evidence of ergotamine overdosage as result of prolonged administration or excessive dosage (see Adverse Reactions/Toxic Effects). Contact physician if any signs and symptoms of ergotamine poisoning present.

PATIENT/FAMILY TEACHING:

Initiate therapy at first sign of

migraine attack. Inform physician if need to progressively increase dose in order to relieve vascular headaches or if irregular heartbeat, nausea, vomiting, numbness or tingling of fingers or toes or if pain or weakness of extremities is noted. Contraindicated in pregnancy; use nonhormonal contraception.

metipranolol
(OptiPranolol)
See Classification section under: Antiglaucoma agents

metoclopramide
meh-tah-**klo**-prah-myd
(Reglan)

CANADIAN AVAILABILITY:
Apo-Metoclop, Maxeran, Reglan

CLASSIFICATION

GI stimulant, antiemetic

AVAILABILITY (Rx)

Tablets: 5 mg, 10 mg. **Syrup:** 5 mg/5 ml. **Injection:** 5 mg/ml.

PHARMACOKINETICS

Well absorbed from GI tract. Metabolized in liver. Primarily excreted in urine. Half-life: 4–6 hrs.

ACTION/*THERAPEUTIC EFFECT*

Stimulates motility of upper GI tract, *accelerates intestinal transit and gastric emptying.* Decreases reflux into esophagus. Raises threshold activity of chemorecep-

tor trigger zone, *producing antiemetic activity.*

USES/*UNLABELED*

To facilitate small-bowel intubation, stimulate gastric emptying, intestinal transit. Relieves symptoms of acute, recurrent gastroparesis (nausea, vomiting, persistent fullness after meals). Prevents nausea, vomiting associated w/cancer chemotherapy. Treatment of heartburn, delayed gastric emptying secondary to reflux esophagitis. *Treatment of slow gastric emptying, vascular headaches, persistent hiccups, drug-related postop nausea/vomiting. Prophylaxis of aspiration pneumonia.*

STORAGE/HANDLING

Store tablets, syrup at room temperature. After reconstitution, IV infusion (piggyback) is stable for 48 hrs.

PO/IV ADMINISTRATION

PO:

1. Give 30 min before meals and at bedtime.
2. Tablets may be crushed.

IV:

1. For IV infusion (piggyback), may dilute w/5% dextrose or 0.9% NaCl.
2. Infuse >15 min.
3. May give slow IV push at rate of 10 mg over 1–2 min.
4. A too rapid IV injection may produce intense feeling of anxiety or restlessness, followed by drowsiness.

INDICATIONS/DOSAGE/ROUTES

Note: May give PO, IM, direct IV, IV infusion.

Diabetic gastroparesis:
PO/IV: Adults: 10 mg 4 times/day for 2–8 wks.

PO: Elderly: Initially, 5 mg 30 min before meals and at bedtime. May increase to 10 mg for 2–8 wks.
IV: Elderly: 5 mg over 1–2 min. May increase to 10 mg.

Symptomatic gastroesophageal reflux:
PO: Adults: 10–15 mg up to 4 times/day; single doses up to 20 mg, as needed. **Elderly:** Initially, 5 mg 4 times/day. May increase to 10 mg.

Prevent cancer chemotherapy–induced nausea and vomiting:
IV: Adults, elderly, children: 1–2 mg/kg 30 min prior to chemotherapy; repeat q2h for 2 doses, then q3h, as needed.

To facilitate small-bowel intubation (single dose):
IV: Adults, elderly: 10 mg. **Children 6–14 yrs:** 2.5–5 mg. **Children <6 yrs:** 0.1 mg/kg.

PRECAUTIONS

CONTRAINDICATIONS: Pheochromocytoma, history of seizure disorders, concurrent use of medications likely to produce extrapyramidal reactions, GI obstruction or perforation, GI hemorrhage. **CAUTIONS:** Impaired renal function, CHF, cirrhosis. **PREGNANCY/LACTATION:** Crosses placenta; distributed in breast milk. **Pregnancy Category B**.

INTERACTIONS

DRUG INTERACTIONS: Alcohol may increase CNS depressant effect. CNS depressants may increase sedative effect. **ALTERED LAB VALUES:** May increase aldosterone, prolactin concentrations.

SIDE EFFECTS

Note: Doses of 2 mg/kg or higher or length of therapy may result in a greater incidence of side effects. **FREQUENT (10%):** Drowsiness, restlessness, fatigue, lassitude. **OCCASIONAL (3%):** Dizziness, anxiety, headache, insomnia, breast tenderness, altered menstruation, constipation, rash, dry mouth, galactorrhea, gynecomastia. **RARE:** Hypotension, hypertension, tachycardia.

ADVERSE REACTIONS/TOXIC EFFECTS

Extrapyramidal reactions occur most frequently in children and young adults (age 18–30) receiving high doses (2 mg/kg) during cancer chemotherapy, and is usually limited to akathisia (motor restlessness), involuntary limb movement, and facial grimacing.

NURSING IMPLICATIONS
BASELINE ASSESSMENT:

Antiemetic: Assess for dehydration (poor skin turgor, dry mucous membranes, longitudinal furrows in tongue).

INTERVENTION/EVALUATION:

Monitor for anxiety, restlessness, extrapyramidal symptoms during IV administration. Monitor pattern of daily bowel activity and stool consistency. Assess for periorbital edema. Assess skin for rash, hives. Evaluate for therapeutic response from gastroparesis (nausea, vomiting, persistent fullness after meals).

PATIENT/FAMILY TEACHING:

Avoid tasks that require alertness, motor skills until drug response is established. Report involuntary eye, facial, or limb movement (extrapyramidal reaction). Avoid alcohol.

metolazone

me-**toh**-lah-zone
(Diulo, Mykrox, Zaroxolyn)

CANADIAN AVAILABILITY:
Zaroxolyn

CLASSIFICATION

Diuretic: Thiazide

AVAILABILITY (Rx)

Tablets: 2.5 mg, 5 mg, 10 mg.
Tablets (Mykrox): 0.5 mg

PHARMACOKINETICS

	ONSET	PEAK	DURATION
PO **(diuretic)**	1 hr	2 hrs	12–24 hrs

Incompletely absorbed from GI tract. Primarily excreted unchanged in urine. Half-life: 14 hrs.

ACTION/*THERAPEUTIC EFFECT*

Diuretic: Blocks reabsorption of sodium, potassium, chloride at distal convoluted tubule, promoting delivery of sodium to potassium side, increasing potassium excretion (Na-K) exchange, *producing renal excretion. Antihypertensive:* Reduces plasma, extracellular fluid volume. *Decreases peripheral vascular resistance, reduced B/P by direct effect on blood vessels.*

USES

Diulo, Zaroxolyn: Treatment of mild to moderate essential hypertension, edema of renal disease, edema due to CHF. *Mykrox:* Treatment of mild to moderate hypertension.

PO ADMINISTRATION

May give w/food or milk if GI upset occurs, preferably w/breakfast (may prevent nocturia).

INDICATIONS/DOSAGE/ROUTES
DIULO, ZAROXOLYN:

Edema due to CHF:
PO: Adults: 5–10 mg once daily in morning. Reduce dose to lowest maintenance level when dry weight is achieved (nonedematous state).

Edema due to renal disease:
PO: Adults: 5–20 mg once daily in morning. Reduce dose to lowest maintenance level when dry weight is achieved (nonedematous state).

Hypertension:
PO: Adults: 2.5–5 mg once daily in morning.

Usual elderly dosage (Diulo, Zaroxolyn):
PO: Initially, 2.5 mg/day or every other day.

MYKROX:

Hypertension:
PO: Adults: 0.5 mg once daily in morning. Dose may be increased to 1 mg once daily if B/P response is insufficient.

PRECAUTIONS

CONTRAINDICATIONS: History of hypersensitivity to sulfonamides or thiazide diuretics, renal decompensation, anuria, hepatic coma or precoma. **CAUTIONS:** Severe renal disease, impaired hepatic function, diabetes mellitus, elderly/debilitated, thyroid disorders. **PREGNANCY/LACTATION:** Crosses placenta; small amount distributed in breast milk—nursing not advised. **Pregnancy Category D.**

INTERACTIONS

DRUG INTERACTIONS: Cholestyramine, colestipol may decrease absorption, effects. May increase digoxin toxicity (due to hypokalemia). May increase lithium toxicity. **ALTERED LAB VALUES:** May increase bilirubin, serum calcium, LDL, cholesterol, triglycerides, creatinine, glucose, uric acid. May decrease urinary calcium, magnesium, potassium, sodium.

SIDE EFFECTS

EXPECTED: Increase in urine frequency/volume. **FREQUENT (9–10%):** Dizziness, lightheadedness, headache. **OCCASIONAL (4–6%):** Muscle cramps/spasm, fatigue, lethargy. **RARE (<2%):** Weakness, palpitations, depression, nausea, vomiting, abdominal bloating, constipation, diarrhea, urticaria.

ADVERSE REACTIONS/TOXIC EFFECTS

Vigorous diuresis may lead to profound water loss and electrolyte depletion, resulting in hypokalemia, hyponatremia, dehydration. Acute hypotensive episodes may occur. Hyperglycemia may be noted during prolonged therapy. GI upset, pancreatitis, dizziness, paresthesias, headache, blood dyscrasias, pulmonary edema, allergic pneumonitis, dermatologic reactions occur rarely. Overdosage can lead to lethargy, coma w/o changes in electrolytes or hydration.

NURSING IMPLICATIONS
BASELINE ASSESSMENT:

Check vital signs, esp. B/P for hypotension prior to administration. Assess baseline electrolytes, particularly check for low potassium. Assess edema, skin turgor, mucous membranes for hydration status. Assess muscle strength, mental status. Note skin temperature, moisture. Obtain baseline weight. Initiate I&O.

INTERVENTION/EVALUATION:

Continue to monitor B/P, vital signs, electrolytes, I&O, weight. Note extent of diuresis. Watch for electrolyte disturbances (hypokalemia may result in weakness, tremor, muscle cramps, nausea, vomiting, change in mental status, tachycardia; hyponatremia may result in confusion, thirst, cold/clammy skin).

PATIENT/FAMILY TEACHING:

Expect increased frequency and volume of urination. To reduce hypotensive effect, rise slowly from lying to sitting position and permit legs to dangle momentarily before standing. Eat foods high in potassium such as whole grains (cereals), legumes, meat, bananas, apricots, orange juice, potatoes (white, sweet), raisins.

metoprolol tartrate

meh-**toe**-pro-lol
(Lopressor, Toprol XL)

FIXED-COMBINATION(S):
W/hydrochlorothiazide, a diuretic **(Lopressor HCT)**

CANADIAN AVAILABILITY:
Apo-Metoprolol, Betaloc, Lopressor, Novometoprol

CLASSIFICATION

Beta-adrenergic blocker

AVAILABILITY (Rx)

Tablets: 50 mg, 100 mg. **Tablets (extended-release):** 50 mg, 100 mg, 200 mg. **Injection:** 1 mg/ml.

PHARMACOKINETICS

	ONSET	PEAK	DURATION
PO	10–15 min	—	6 hrs
IV	—	20 min	5–8 hrs

Well absorbed from GI tract. Widely distributed. Metabolized in liver (undergoes significant first-pass metabolism). Primarily excreted in urine. Half-life: 3–7 hrs.

ACTION/*THERAPEUTIC EFFECT*

Selectively blocks beta$_1$-adrenergic receptors, *slowing sinus heart rate, decreasing cardiac output, decreasing B/P* (exact mechanism unknown but may block peripheral adrenergic receptors, decrease sympathetic outflow from CNS, or decrease renin release from kidney). Large dose may block beta$_2$-adrenergic receptors, *increasing airway resistance. Decreases myocardial ischemia* severity by decreasing oxygen requirements.

USES/*UNLABELED*

Management of mild to moderate hypertension. Used alone or in combination with diuretics, esp. thiazide type. Management of chronic stable angina pectoris. Reduces cardiovascular mortality in those with definite or suspected acute MI. *Extended-release:* Management of hypertension, long-term treatment of angina pectoris. *Treatment/prophylaxis of cardiac arrhythmias, hypertrophic cardiomyopathy, pheochromocytoma, vascular headache, tremors, anxiety, thyrotoxicosis, mitral valve prolapse syndrome.* Increases survival rate in diabetics w/heart disease.

STORAGE/HANDLING

Store parenteral form at room temperature.

PO/IV ADMINISTRATION

PO:

1. Tablets may be crushed; do not crush or break extended-release tablets.
2. Give at same time each day.
3. May be given w/or immediately after meals (enhances absorption).

IV:

1. Administer IV injection rapidly.
2. Monitor EKG during administration.

INDICATIONS/DOSAGE/ROUTES

Hypertension, angina pectoris:
PO: Adults: Initially, 100 mg/day as single or divided dose. Increase at weekly (or longer) intervals. **Maintenance:** 100–450 mg/day.

Usual elderly dosage:
PO: Initially, 25 mg/day. **Range:** 25–300 mg/day.

Usual dosage for extended-release tablets:
PO: Adults: *Hypertension:* 50–100 mg/day as single dose. May increase at least at weekly intervals until optimum B/P attained. *Angina:* Initially, 100 mg/day as single dose. May increase at least at weekly intervals until optimum clinical response achieved.

Myocardial infarction (early treatment):
IV: Adults: 5 mg q2 min for 3 doses, followed by 50 mg orally q6h for 48 hrs. Begin oral dose 15 min after last IV dose. Alternatively, in those who do not tolerate full IV dose, give 25–50 mg orally q6h, 15 min after last IV dose.

Myocardial infarction (late treatment, maintenance):
PO: Adults: 100 mg 2 times/day for at least 3 mos.

PRECAUTIONS

CONTRAINDICATIONS: Overt cardiac failure, cardiogenic shock, heart block greater than first degree, sinus bradycardia. *MI:* Heart rate <45 beats/min, systolic B/P <100 mm Hg. **CAUTIONS:** Bronchospastic disease, impaired renal function, peripheral vascular disease, hyperthyroidism, diabetes, inadequate cardiac function. **PREGNANCY/LACTATION:** Crosses placenta; distributed in breast milk. Avoid use during first trimester. May produce bradycardia, apnea, hypoglycemia, hypothermia during delivery, small birth weight infants. **Pregnancy Category C.** (Category D if used in 2nd or 3rd trimester.)

INTERACTIONS

DRUG INTERACTIONS: Diuretics, other hypotensives may increase hypotensive effect; sympathomimetics, xanthines may mutually inhibit effects; may mask symptoms of hypoglycemia, prolong hypoglycemic effect of insulin, oral hypoglycemics; NSAIDs may decrease antihypertensive effect; cimetidine may increase concentration. **ALTERED LAB VALUES:** May increase ANA titer, SGOT (AST), SGPT (ALT), alkaline phosphatase, LDH, bilirubin, BUN, creatinine, potassium, uric acid, lipoproteins, triglycerides.

SIDE EFFECTS

Generally well tolerated, w/transient and mild side effects. **FREQUENT:** Decreased sexual ability, drowsiness, insomnia, unusual tiredness/weakness. **OCCASION-AL:** Anxiety, nervousness, diarrhea, constipation, nausea, vomiting, nasal congestion, stomach discomfort, dizziness, difficulty breathing, cold hands/feet. **RARE:** Altered taste, dry eyes, nightmares, numbness in fingers/feet, allergic reaction (rash, pruritus).

ADVERSE REACTIONS/TOXIC EFFECTS

Excessive dosage may produce profound bradycardia, hypotension, bronchospasm. Abrupt withdrawal may result in sweating, palpitations, headache, tremulousness, exacerbation of angina, MI, ventricular arrhythmias. May precipitate CHF, MI in those with cardiac disease, thyroid storm in those with thyrotoxicosis, peripheral ischemia in those w/existing peripheral vascular disease. Hypoglycemia may occur in previously controlled diabetics.

NURSING IMPLICATIONS

BASELINE ASSESSMENT:

Assess baseline renal/liver function tests. Assess B/P, apical pulse immediately before drug is administered (if pulse is 60/min or below, or systolic B/P is below 90 mm Hg, withhold medication, contact physician). *Antianginal:* Record onset, type (sharp, dull, squeezing), radiation, location, intensity, and duration of anginal pain, and precipitating factors (exertion, emotional stress).

INTERVENTION/EVALUATION:

Measure B/P near end of dosing interval (determines if B/P is controlled throughout day). Monitor B/P for hypotension, respiration for shortness of breath. Assess pulse for strength/weakness, irregular rate, bradycardia. Assist w/ambulation if dizziness occurs. Check skin for evidence of rash.

Assess for evidence of CHF: dyspnea (particularly on exertion or lying down), night cough, peripheral edema, distended neck veins. Monitor I&O (increase in weight, decrease in urine output may indicate CHF). Therapeutic response to hypertension noted in 1–2 wks.

PATIENT/FAMILY TEACHING:

Do not abruptly discontinue medication. Compliance w/therapy regimen is essential to control hypertension, arrhythmias. If a dose is missed, take next scheduled dose (do not double dose). To avoid hypotensive effect, rise slowly from lying to sitting position, wait momentarily before standing. Avoid tasks that require alertness, motor skills until response to drug is established. Report excessive fatigue, dizziness. Do not use nasal decongestants, OTC cold preparations (stimulants) w/o physician approval. Outpatients should monitor B/P, pulse before taking medication. Restrict salt, alcohol intake.

metronidazole hydrochloride

meh-trow-**nye**-dah-zoll
(Flagyl, MetroCream, MetroGel, MetroLotion, Noritate, Protostat, Satric)

FIXED-COMBINATION(S):

W/bismuth subsalicylate and tetracycline, an anti-infective (**Helidac, Noritate**)

CANADIAN AVAILABILITY:

Apo-Metronidazole, Flagyl, MetroCream, Metrogel, NidaGel, Noritate, Novonidazol

CLASSIFICATION

Antibacterial, antiprotozoal

AVAILABILITY (Rx)

Tablets: 250 mg, 500 mg. **Extended-Release Tablet:** 750 mg. **Capsules:** 375 mg. **Powder for Injection:** 500 mg. **Injection (infusion):** 500 mg/100 ml. **Lotion:** 0.75% **Vaginal Gel:** 0.75%. **Topical Gel:** 0.75%. **Topical Cream:** 1%.

PHARMACOKINETICS

Well absorbed from GI tract, minimal absorption after topical application. Widely distributed, crosses blood-brain barrier. Metabolized in liver to active metabolite. Primarily excreted in urine; partially eliminated in feces. Removed by hemodialysis. Half-life: 8 hrs (increased in alcoholic liver disease, neonates).

ACTION/*THERAPEUTIC EFFECT*

Taken up by cells in susceptible microorganisms. Disrupts DNA, inhibits nucleic acid synthesis *producing bactericidal, amebicidal, trichomonacidal effects*. Produces anti-inflammatory, immunosuppressive effects when applied topically.

USES/*UNLABELED*

Treatment of anaerobic infections (skin/skin structure, CNS, lower respiratory tract, bone and joints, intra-abdominal, gynecologic, endocarditis, septicemia). Treatment of trichomoniasis, amebiasis, perioperatively for contaminated/potentially contaminated intra-abdominal surgery, antibiotic-associated pseudomembranous colitis. Treatment of *H. pylori*–associated gastritis/duodenal ulcer. Topical application in treatment of acne rosacea. Also used in treatment of grade III, IV decubitus ulcers w/anaerobic infection. Treatment of bacterial vaginosis.

M

Treatment of inflammatory bowel disease.

PO/IV ADMINISTRATION

PO:

May give w/o regard to meals. Give w/food to decrease GI irritation.

IV:

1. Infuse >30–60 min. Do not give bolus.
2. Avoid prolonged use of indwelling catheters.

INDICATIONS/DOSAGE/ROUTES

Anaerobic bacterial infections:
IV: Adults, elderly: Initially, 1 g, then 500 mg q6–8h.
PO: Adults, elderly: 500 mg q6–8h. **Maximum:** 4 g/24 hrs.

Antibiotic-associated pseudomembranous colitis:
PO: Adults, elderly: 750 mg to 2 g/day in 3–4 divided doses for 7–14 days.

Trichomoniasis:
PO: Adults: 2 g as single or in 2 divided doses for 1 day or 250 mg 3 times/day for 7 days or 375 mg 2 times/day for 7 days. **Children:** 15 mg/kg in 3 divided doses for 7–10 days. **Infants:** 10–30 mg/kg/day for 5–8 days.

Bacterial vaginosis:
Intravaginally: Adults: One applicatorful 2 times/day or once daily at bedtime for 5 days.
PO: Adults: 750 mg at bedtime for 7 days.

Amebiasis:
PO: Adults, elderly: 500–750 mg 3 times/day for 5–10 days. **Children:** 35–50 mg/kg/day in 3 divided doses for 5 days.

Perioperative prophylaxis:
IV: Adults, elderly: 1 g 1 hr before surgery and 500 mg 6 and 12 hrs after initial dose.

Rosacea:
Topical: Adults: Thin application 2 times/day to affected area. **Cream:** Once daily. **Lotion:** Apply twice daily.

PRECAUTIONS

CONTRAINDICATIONS: Hypersensitivity to metronidazole or other nitroimidazole derivatives (also parabens w/topical application). **CAUTIONS:** Blood dyscrasias, severe hepatic dysfunction, CNS disease, predisposition to edema, concurrent corticosteroid therapy. Safety and efficacy of topical administration in those <21 yrs of age not established. **PREGNANCY/LACTATION:** Readily crosses placenta; distributed in breast milk. Contraindicated during first trimester in those w/trichomoniasis. Topical use during pregnancy or lactation discouraged. **Pregnancy Category B.**

INTERACTIONS

DRUG INTERACTIONS: Alcohol may cause disulfiram-type reaction. May increase effect of oral anticoagulants. May increase toxicity w/disulfiram. **ALTERED LAB VALUES:** May increase SGOT (AST), SGPT (ALT), LDH.

SIDE EFFECTS

FREQUENT: Anorexia, nausea, dry mouth, metallic taste. *Vaginal:* Symptomatic cervicitis/vaginitis, abdominal cramps, uterine pain. **OCCASIONAL:** Diarrhea or constipation, vomiting, dizziness, erythematous rash, urticaria, reddish brown or dark urine. *Topical:* Transient redness, mild dryness, burning, irritation, stinging (also tearing when applied too close to eyes). *Vaginal:* Vaginal, perineal, vulvar itching, vulvar swelling. **RARE:** Mild, transient leukopenia, thrombophlebitis w/IV therapy.

ADVERSE REACTIONS/TOXIC EFFECTS

Oral therapy may result in furry tongue, glossitis, cystitis, dysuria, pancreatitis, flattening of T waves w/EKG readings. Peripheral neuropathy (numbness, tingling, paresthesia) is usually reversible if treatment is stopped immediately upon appearance of neurologic symptoms. Seizures occur occasionally.

NURSING IMPLICATIONS

BASELINE ASSESSMENT:

Question for history of hypersensitivity to metronidazole or other nitroimidazole derivatives (and parabens w/topical). Obtain specimens for diagnostic tests before giving first dose (therapy may begin before results are known).

INTERVENTION/EVALUATION:

Evaluate food tolerance. Determine pattern of bowel activity. Check leukocyte counts frequently. Monitor I&O and assess for urinary problems. Be alert to neurologic symptoms: dizziness, numbness, tingling or paresthesia of extremities. Assess for rash, urticaria. Watch for onset of superinfection: ulceration or change of oral mucosa, furry tongue, vaginal discharge, genital/anal pruritus.

PATIENT/FAMILY TEACHING:

Urine may be red-brown or dark because of metabolism of drug. Avoid alcohol and alcohol-containing preparations, e.g., cough syrups, elixirs. Hard candy, gum, or tepid water may help w/dry mouth. If dizziness occurs, do not drive or use machines that require alertness. If taking metronidazole for trichomoniasis, refrain from sexual intercourse until physician advises. Report any new symptom to physician, esp. dizziness, numbness, tingling. For amebiasis, frequent stool specimen checks will be necessary. *Topical:* Avoid contact w/eyes. May apply cosmetics after application. Metronidazole acts on redness, papules, and pustules but has no effect on rhinophyma (hypertrophy of nose), telangiectasia, or ocular problems (conjunctivitis, keratitis, blepharitis). Other recommendations for rosacea include avoidance of hot or spicy foods, alcohol, extremes of hot or cold temperatures, excessive sunlight.

mexiletine hydrochloride

mex-**ill**-eh-teen
(Mexitil)

CANADIAN AVAILABILITY:
Mexitil

CLASSIFICATION

Antiarrhythmic

AVAILABILITY (Rx)

Capsules: 150 mg, 200 mg, 250 mg

PHARMACOKINETICS

	ONSET	PEAK	DURATION
PO	0.5–2 hrs	2–3 hrs	8–12 hrs

Well absorbed from upper intestinal section of GI tract. Metabolized in liver (undergoes first-pass effect). Excreted via biliary system. Removed by hemodialysis. Half-life: 10–12 hrs (increase in liver disease, decreased renal function).

ACTION/*THERAPEUTIC EFFECT*

Shortens duration of action potential, decreases effective refractory period in His-Purkinje system of myocardium by blocking sodium transport across myocardial cell membranes, *suppressing ventricular arrhythmias.*

USES/*UNLABELED*

Suppress symptomatic ventricular arrhythmias (PVCs, unifocal or multifocal, couplets, and ventricular tachycardia). *Diabetic neuropathy.*

PO ADMINISTRATION

1. Do not crush or break capsules.
2. Give w/food or antacid to reduce GI distress.

INDICATIONS/DOSAGE/ROUTES

Usual dosage for arrhythmias:
PO: Adults, elderly: Initially, 200 mg q8h. Adjust dose by 50–100 mg at 2–3 day intervals. **Maintenance:** 200–300 mg q8h. **Maximum:** 1,200 mg/day. **Note:** If 300 mg q8h or less controls arrhythmias, may give dose q12h. **Maximum:** 450 mg q12h.

Rapid control of arrhythmias:
PO: Adults, elderly: Initially, 400 mg, then 200 mg q8h.

PRECAUTIONS

CONTRAINDICATIONS: Cardiogenic shock, preexisting second- or third-degree AV block (w/o presence of pacemaker). **CAUTIONS:** Impaired myocardial function, second- or third-degree AV block (w/pacemaker), CHF, sick-sinus syndrome (bradycardia/tachycardia). **PREGNANCY/LACTATION:** Unknown whether drug crosses placenta; distributed in breast milk. **Pregnancy Category C**.

INTERACTIONS

DRUG INTERACTIONS: Urinary acidifiers may increase excretion, urinary alkalizers may decrease excretion. Hepatic enzyme inducers may decrease concentrations. Metoclopramide may increase absorption. **ALTERED LAB VALUES:** May cause positive ANA titers. May increase SGOT (AST).

SIDE EFFECTS

FREQUENT (>10%): GI distress (nausea, vomiting, heartburn), dizziness, lightheadedness, tremor. **OCCASIONAL (1–10%):** Nervousness, change in sleep habits, headache, visual disturbances, paresthesia, diarrhea/constipation, palpitations, chest pain, rash, respiratory difficulty, edema. **RARE (<1%):** Dry mouth, weakness, fatigue, tinnitus, depression, speech difficulties.

ADVERSE REACTIONS/TOXIC EFFECTS

Has ability to worsen existing arrhythmias or produce new ones. May produce or worsen CHF.

NURSING IMPLICATIONS

INTERVENTION/EVALUATION:

Monitor EKG, vital signs closely during and after drug administration for cardiac performance. Assess pulse for irregular rate, strength/weakness. Observe for GI disturbances (high incidence). Monitor pattern of daily bowel activity and stool consistency. Assess for dizziness, syncope. Evaluate hand movement for tremor. Check for evidence of CHF (cough, dyspnea [particularly on exertion], rales at base of lungs, fatigue). Monitor fluid and electrolyte serum levels. Check for therapeutic serum level (0.5–2 mcg/ml).

PATIENT/FAMILY TEACHING:

Compliance w/therapy regimen is essential to control cardiac arrhythmias. Report shortness of breath, cough, unexplained sore throat or fever, generalized fatigue. Do not use nasal decongestants, OTC cold preparations (stimulants) w/o physician approval. Restrict salt, alcohol intake.

mezlocillin sodium

mezz-low-**sill**-in
(Mezlin)

CLASSIFICATION

Antibiotic: Penicillin

AVAILABILITY (Rx)

Powder for Injection: 1 g, 2 g, 3 g, 4 g, 10 g

PHARMACOKINETICS

Well absorbed after IM administration. Widely distributed. Primarily excreted unchanged in urine. Removed by hemodialysis. Half-life: 50–70 min.

ACTION/THERAPEUTIC EFFECT

Binds to bacterial membranes, *inhibiting cell wall synthesis. Bactericidal.*

USES

Treatment of gynecologic, skin/skin structure, respiratory, urinary tract, bone and joint, intra-abdominal infections, septicemia, gonorrhea (w/probenecid), perioperative prophylaxis, esp. in abdominal surgery.

STORAGE/HANDLING

Solution appears clear, colorless to pale yellow; may darken slightly (does not indicate loss of potency). If precipitate forms, redissolve in warm water, agitate. IV infusion (piggyback) is stable for 24 hrs at room temperature.

IM/IV ADMINISTRATION

Note: Space doses evenly around the clock.

IM:

1. For IM injection, inject slowly and deeply into gluteus maximus.

2. Avoid IM injections >2 g.

IV:

1. For IV injection, administer over 3–5 min.

2. For intermittent IV infusion (piggyback), infuse over 30 min.

3. Because of potential for hypersensitivity/anaphylaxis, start initial dose at few drops per minute, increase slowly to ordered rate; stay w/pt first 10–15 min, then check q10 min.

4. Alternating IV sites, use large veins to reduce risk of phlebitis.

INDICATIONS/DOSAGE/ROUTES

Uncomplicated UTI:
IM/IV: Adults, elderly: 1.5–2 g q6h.

Complicated UTI:
IM/IV: Adults, elderly: 3 g q6h.

Lower respiratory tract, intra-abdominal, gynecologic, skin/skin structure infections, septicemia:
IV: Adults, elderly: 4 g q6h or 3 g q4h.

Life-threatening infections:
IV: Adults, elderly: Up to 4 g q4h.
Maximum: 24 g/day.

Acute, uncomplicated gonococcal urethritis:
IM/IV: Adults: 1–2 g one time w/1 g probenecid.

Perioperative prophylaxis:
IV: Adults, elderly: 4 g 30–90 min before surgery and 6 and 12 hrs after first dose.

Cesarean section:
IV: Adults: 4 g after umbilical cord clamped, then 4 and 8 hrs after first dose.

Usual dosage (children):
IM/IV: Children 1 mo–12 yrs: 50 mg/kg q4h.

Usual dosage (neonates):
IM/IV: Neonates 0–7 days: 75 mg/kg q8–12h. **Neonates 7–28 days:** 75 mg/kg q6–12h.

Dosage in renal impairment:
Dose and/or frequency modified on basis of creatinine clearance and/or severity of infection.

CREATININE CLEARANCE	
10–30 ml/min	<10 ml/min
Uncomplicated UTI	
1.5 g q8h	1.5 g q8h
Complicated UTI	
1.5 g q6h	1.5 g q8h
Serious infections	
3 g q8h	2 g q8h
Life-threatening infections	
3 g q6h	2 g q6h

PRECAUTIONS

CONTRAINDICATIONS: Hypersensitivity to any penicillin. **CAUTIONS:** History of allergies, esp. cephalosporins. **PREGNANCY/LACTATION:** Readily crosses placenta, appears in cord blood, amniotic fluid. Distributed in breast milk in low concentrations. May lead to allergic sensitization, diarrhea, candidiasis, skin rash in infant. **Pregnancy Category B**.

INTERACTIONS

DRUG INTERACTIONS: Probenecid may increase concentration, toxicity risk. **ALTERED LAB VALUES:** May increase SGOT (AST), SGPT (ALT), alkaline phosphatase, bilirubin, creatinine, sodium. May cause positive Coombs' test. May decrease potassium.

SIDE EFFECTS

FREQUENT: Rash, urticaria, pain, and induration at IM injection site; phlebitis, thrombophlebitis w/IV doses. **OCCASIONAL:** Nausea, vomiting, diarrhea, hypernatremia. **RARE:** Bleeding may occur w/high IV dosage; hypokalemia, headache, fatigue, dizziness.

ADVERSE REACTIONS/TOXIC EFFECTS

Superinfections, potentially fatal antibiotic-associated colitis may result from altered bacterial balance. Seizures, neurologic reactions may occur w/overdosage (most often w/renal impairment). Acute interstitial nephritis, severe hypersensitivity reactions occur rarely.

NURSING IMPLICATIONS
BASELINE ASSESSMENT:

Question for history of allergies, esp. penicillins, cephalosporins. Obtain specimen for culture and sensitivity before giving first dose (therapy may begin before results are known).

INTERVENTION/EVALUATION:

Hold medication and promptly report rash (hypersensitivity) or diarrhea (w/fever, abdominal pain, mucus and blood in stool may indicate antibiotic-associated colitis). Assess food tolerance. Evaluate IV site for phlebitis (heat, pain, red streaking over vein). Check IM injection sites for pain, induration. Monitor I&O, urinalysis, renal function tests. Assess for bleeding: overt bleeding, bruising or tissue swelling; check hematology reports. Monitor electrolytes, particularly sodium, potassium. Be alert for superinfection: increased fever, onset sore throat, diarrhea, vomiting, ulceration or other oral changes, anal/genital pruritus.

PATIENT/FAMILY TEACHING:

Continue antibiotic for full length of treatment. Space doses evenly. Discomfort may occur at IM injection site. Notify physician in event of rash, diarrhea, bleeding, bruising, other new symptom.

---

miconazole nitrate

mih-**kon**-nah-zoll
(Micatin, Monistat 3, 7, Monistat-Derm, M-Zole 3)

miconazole

(Monistat IV)

CANADIAN AVAILABILITY:
Micatin, Micozole, Monistat

CLASSIFICATION

Antifungal

AVAILABILITY (Rx)

Injection: 10 mg/ml. **Vaginal Suppository:** 100 mg, 200 mg. **Topical Cream:** 2%. **Vaginal Cream:** 2%. **Topical Powder:** 2%. **Topical Spray:** 2%.

PHARMACOKINETICS

Parenteral: Widely distributed in tissues. Metabolized in liver. Primarily excreted in urine. Half-life: 24 hrs. *Topical:* No systemic absorption following application to intact skin. *Intravaginally:* Small amount absorbed systemically.

ACTION/*THERAPEUTIC EFFECT*

Inhibits synthesis of ergosterol (vital component of fungal cell formation), damaging fungal cell membrane. *Fungistatic; may be fungicidal, depending on concentration.*

USES

Treatment of coccidioidomycosis, paracoccidioidomycosis, cryptococcosis, petriellidiosis (allescheriosis), disseminated candidiasis, chronic mucocutaneous candidiasis. Fungal meningitis usually treated intrathecally as well as IV; urinary bladder infections w/installations as well as IV miconazole. *Vaginally:* Vulvovaginal candidiasis. *Topical:* Cutaneous candidiasis, tinea cruris, t. corporis, t. pedis, t. versicolor.

STORAGE/HANDLING

After reconstitution, IV solution is stable for 24 hrs at room temperature w/5% dextrose or 0.9% NaCl.

IV ADMINISTRATION

1. Dilute each 200 mg ampoule w/at least 200 ml 5% dextrose or 0.9% NaCl to provide maximum concentration of 1 mg/ml.

2. Give IV infusion (piggyback) over at least 30–60 min (rapid administration may cause arrhythmias).

3. Because of incidence of phlebitis, central venous catheters are recommended.

4. Initial treatment should be performed in hospital w/physician in attendance for first 200 mg dose.

INDICATIONS/DOSAGE/ROUTES

Note: IV doses may be divided over 3 IV infusions.

Coccidioidomycosis:
IV: Adults, elderly: 1.8–3.6 g/day for 3–20 wks or longer.

Cryptococcosis:
IV: Adults, elderly: 1.2–2.4 g/day for 3–12 wks or longer.

Petriellidiosis:
IV: Adults, elderly: 0.6–3.0 g/day for 5–20 wks or longer.

Candidiasis:
IV: Adults, elderly: 0.6–1.8 g/day for 1–20 wks or longer.

Paracoccidioidomycosis:
IV: Adults, elderly: 0.2–1.2 g/day for 2–16 wks or longer.

Usual dosage for children:
IV: 20–40 mg/kg/day in 3 divided doses. (Do not exceed 15 mg/kg for any 1 infusion.)

Vulvovaginal candidiasis:
Intravaginally: Adults, elderly: One 200 mg suppository at bedtime for 3 days; one 100 mg suppository or one applicatorful at bedtime for 7 days.

Topical fungal infections, cutaneous candidiasis:
Topical: Adults, elderly: Apply liberally 2 times/day, morning and evening.

PRECAUTIONS

CONTRAINDICATIONS: Hypersensitivity to miconazole. Children <1 yr; topically, children <2 yrs. **CAUTIONS:** Hepatic insufficiency. **PREGNANCY/LACTATION:** Unknown whether drug crosses placenta or is distributed in breast milk. **Pregnancy Category C**.

INTERACTIONS

DRUG INTERACTIONS: May increase effects of oral anticoagulants, oral hypoglycemics. Isoniazid, rifampin may decrease concentrations. May increase cisapride concentration, risk of cardiotoxicity. **ALTERED LAB VALUES:** None significant.

SIDE EFFECTS

FREQUENT (>5%): Phlebitis, fever, chills, rash, itching, nausea, vomiting. **OCCASIONAL (1–5%):** Dizziness, drowsiness, headache, flushed face, abdominal pain, constipation, diarrhea, decreased appetite. *Topical:* Itching, burning, stinging, erythema, urticaria. *Vaginal (2%):* Vulvovaginal burning, itching, irritation, headache, skin rash.

ADVERSE REACTIONS/TOXIC EFFECTS

Anemia, thrombocytopenia, liver toxicity occur rarely.

NURSING IMPLICATIONS

BASELINE ASSESSMENT:

Question for history of allergies, esp. to miconazole. Confirm that cultures or histologic tests were done. Check for/obtain orders for antiemetics, antihistamines (given before infusion to reduce nausea, vomiting).

INTERVENTION/EVALUATION:

Check for nausea, vomiting (administer medication for symptomatic relief; avoid dosing at mealtimes, slow infusion rate). Assess skin for rash. Evaluate IV site for phlebitis. Determine pattern of bowel activity, stool consistency. Assess mental status (dizziness, drowsiness), provide assistance as needed. Monitor Hgb/Hct results, be alert for bleeding, bruising. *Topical/vaginal:* Assess for burning, itching, irritation.

PATIENT/FAMILY TEACHING:

Continue full length of treatment; prolonged therapy (weeks or months) may be necessary for some conditions. Discomfort may occur at IV site. Notify physician in event of bleeding, bruising, soft tissue swelling, or other new symptom. Do not ambulate w/o assistance or use any machinery if dizziness, drowsiness occur. Consult physician before taking any other medication. *Vaginal preparations:* Base interacts w/certain latex products such as contraceptive diaphragm. Ask physician about douching, sexual intercourse. *Topical:* Rub well into affected areas. Avoid getting in eyes. Do not apply any other preparations or occlusive covering w/o consulting physician. Use ointment (sparingly) or lotion in intertriginous areas. Keep areas clean, dry; wear light clothing for ventilation. Separate personal items in contact w/affected areas.

---

midazolam hydrochloride

my-**day**-zoe-lam
(Versed)

CANADIAN AVAILABILITY:
Versed

CLASSIFICATION

Sedative (Schedule IV)

AVAILABILITY (Rx)

Injection: 1 mg/ml, 2 mg/ml, 5 mg/ml. **Syrup:** 2 mg/ml.

PHARMACOKINETICS

	ONSET	PEAK	DURATION
IM	5–15 min	45 min	1–6 hrs
IV	1–5 min	—	Dose related

Well absorbed after IM administration. Metabolized in liver to active metabolite. Primarily excreted in urine. Half-life: 1–5 hrs.

ACTION / *THERAPEUTIC EFFECT*

Enhances action of gamma-aminobutyric acid (GABA) neurotransmission at CNS, *producing sedative, anxiolytic effect due to CNS depressant action.* Inhibits spinal afferent pathways, *producing skeletal muscle relaxation.* Directly depresses motor nerve, muscle function effects.

USES / *UNLABELED*

IM: Preop for sedation, relief of anxiety; produces anterograde amnesia. *IV:* Sedation (w/o loss of consciousness) to relieve anxiety; produces anterograde amnesia for short diagnostic, endoscopic procedures, intubated/mechanical ventilator pts. *Adjunct to local anesthesia.*

STORAGE / HANDLING

Store at room temperature. Although undiluted solution should be protected from light, it is unnecessary to protect diluted solution from light.

IM / IV ADMINISTRATION

Note: Compatible w/5% dextrose, 0.9% NaCl, lactated Ringer's. Compatible for 30 min w/atropine, meperidine, morphine, scopolamine, low doses of opiate agonists.

IM:

Give deep IM into large muscle mass.

IV:

1. Oxygen, resuscitative equipment must be readily available before IV is administered.
2. Administer by slow IV injection, in incremental dosages: Give each incremental dose over 2 or more minutes at intervals of at least 2 min.

3. Reduce IV rate in those >60 yrs, and/or debilitated, those w/chronic disease states, and/or impaired pulmonary function.

4. A too rapid IV rate, excessive doses, or a single large dose increases risk of respiratory depression/arrest.

INDICATIONS/DOSAGE/ROUTES

Preop:
IM: Adults >18 yrs: 70–80 mcg/kg (0.07–0.08 mg/kg) 30–60 min before surgery. **Elderly/debilitated:** Dosage should be lowered. **Children:** Individualized.

Conscious sedation:
IV: Adults: Initially, up to 2.5 mg. May further titrate in small increments to desired effect. Total dose rarely >5 mg. **Elderly:** Initially, up to 1.5 mg. May further titrate to desired effect. Total dose rarely >3.5 mg. **Children:** Individualized.

Adjunct to anesthesia:
IV: Adults: Initially, 150–350 mcg/kg. **Elderly:** Initially, 150–300 mcg/kg. Additional doses, 25% of initial dose. **Note:** Dosage in children individualized.

Usual oral dosage:
Children: 0.25–1 mg/kg. **Maximum:** 20 mg.

PRECAUTIONS

CONTRAINDICATIONS: Shock, comatose pts, acute alcohol intoxication, acute narrow-angle glaucoma. **CAUTIONS:** Acute illness, severe fluid/electrolyte imbalance, impaired renal function, CHF, treated open-angle glaucoma. **PREGNANCY/LACTATION:** Crosses placenta; unknown whether drug is distributed in breast milk. **Pregnancy Category D.**

INTERACTIONS

DRUG INTERACTIONS: Alcohol, CNS depressants may increase CNS, respiratory depression, hypotensive effects. Hypotension-producing medications may increase hypotensive effects. Grapefruit juice increases oral absorption. **ALTERED LAB VALUES:** None significant.

SIDE EFFECTS

FREQUENT (4–10%): Decreased respiratory rate, tenderness at IM/IV injection site, pain during injection, desaturation, hiccups. **OCCASIONAL (2–3%):** Pain at IM injection site, hypotension, paradoxical reaction. **RARE (<2%):** Nausea, vomiting, headache, coughing, hypotensive episodes.

ADVERSE REACTIONS/TOXIC EFFECTS

Too much or too little dosage, improper administration, or cerebral hypoxia may result in agitation, involuntary movements, hyperactivity, combativeness. Underventilation/apnea may produce hypoxia, cardiac arrest. A too rapid IV rate, excessive doses, or a single large dose increases risk of respiratory depression/arrest.

NURSING IMPLICATIONS

BASELINE ASSESSMENT:

Resuscitative equipment, endotracheal tube, suction, oxygen must be available. Obtain vital signs before administration.

INTERVENTION/EVALUATION:

Monitor respiratory rate continuously during parenteral administration for underventilation, apnea. Monitor vital signs q3–5 min during recovery period.

PATIENT/FAMILY TEACHING:

Discomfort may occur w/IM injection.

midodrine
(ProAmatine)
See Supplement

miglitol
(Glyset)
See Supplement
See Classification section under:
Antidiabetics

milrinone lactate
mill-rih-known
(Primacor)

CANADIAN AVAILABILITY:
Primacor

CLASSIFICATION

Cardiotonic

AVAILABILITY (Rx)

Injection: 1 mg/ml. **Injection (premix):** 200 mcg/ml.

PHARMACOKINETICS

	ONSET	PEAK	DURATION
IV	5–15 min	—	—

Metabolized in liver; excreted in urine. Half-life: 2.4 hrs.

ACTION/THERAPEUTIC EFFECT

Possesses positive inotropic effect (increases force of myocardial contraction), direct arterial vasodilation. Reduces preload and afterload by direct effect on vascular smooth muscle. *Increases cardiac output, decreases pulmonary capillary wedge pressure and vascular resistance.*

USES

Short-term management of congestive heart failure (CHF).

STORAGE/HANDLING

Store parenteral form at room temperature.

IV ADMINISTRATION

1. Avoid furosemide injection into tubing of milrinone IV infusion (precipitate forms immediately).
2. For IV injection (loading dose) administer slowly over 10 min.
3. For IV infusion, dilute 20 mg (20 ml) vial with 80 or 180 ml diluent (0.9% NaCl, 5% dextrose) to provide concentration of 200 or 100 mcg/ml, respectively.
4. Monitor for arrhythmias, hypotension during IV therapy. Reduce or temporarily discontinue infusion until condition stabilizes.

INDICATIONS/DOSAGE/ROUTES

Congestive heart failure:
IV: Adults: Initially, give 50 mcg/kg over 10 min. Continue w/maintenance infusion rate of 0.375–0.75 mcg/kg/min based on hemodynamic and clinical response (total daily dose: 0.59–1.13 mg/kg). Reduce dose to 0.2–0.43 mcg/kg/min in pts w/severe renal impairment.

PRECAUTIONS

CONTRAINDICATIONS: Severe obstructive aortic or pulmonic valvular disease. **CAUTIONS:** Impaired renal, hepatic function. **PREGNANCY/LACTATION:** Unknown whether drug crosses placenta or is distributed in breast milk. **Pregnancy Category C**.

INTERACTIONS

DRUG INTERACTIONS: Produces additive inotropic effects w/cardiac glycosides. **ALTERED LAB VALUES:** None significant.

SIDE EFFECTS

OCCASIONAL (1–3%): Headache, hypotension. **RARE (<1%):** Angina, chest pain.

ADVERSE REACTIONS/TOXIC EFFECTS

Supraventricular and ventricular arrhythmias occur in 12%; nonsustained ventricular tachycardia occurs in 2%, sustained ventricular tachycardia in 1% of those treated.

NURSING IMPLICATIONS

BASELINE ASSESSMENT:

Offer emotional support (difficulty breathing may produce anxiety). Assess B/P, apical pulse rate before treatment begins and during IV therapy. Assess lung sounds, check edema.

INTERVENTION/EVALUATION:

Monitor for hypotension during administration (discontinue or slow IV rate until condition stabilizes). Assess heart rate, serum electrolytes, I&O, renal function studies. Monitor CHF symptoms.

minocycline hydrochloride

min-know-**sigh**-clean
(Dynacin, Minocin)

CANADIAN AVAILABILITY:
Minocin, Novo Minocycline

CLASSIFICATION

Antibiotic: Tetracycline

AVAILABILITY (Rx)

Capsules: 50 mg, 75 mg, 100 mg. **Tablets:** 50 mg, 100 mg. **Oral Suspension:** 50 mg/5 ml. **Powder for Injection:** 100 mg.

PHARMACOKINETICS

Well absorbed from GI tract. Widely distributed. Partially inactivated in liver. Excreted in urine, eliminated in feces via biliary secretion. Minimally removed by hemodialysis. Half-life: 11–23 hrs.

ACTION/*THERAPEUTIC EFFECT*

Binds to ribosomes, *inhibiting protein synthesis. Bacteriostatic.*

USES/*UNLABELED*

Treatment of prostate, urinary tract, CNS infections (not meningitis), uncomplicated gonorrhea, inflammatory acne, brucellosis, skin granulomas, cholera, trachoma, nocardiasis, yaws, and syphilis when penicillins are contraindicated. *Treatment of atypical mycobacterial infections, rheumatoid arthritis, scleroderma*

STORAGE/HANDLING

Store capsules, oral suspension at room temperature. IV solution stable for 24 hrs at room temperature. Use IV infusion (piggyback) immediately after reconstitution. Discard if precipitate forms.

PO/IV ADMINISTRATION

PO:

Give oral capsules, tablets w/full glass of water.

IV:

1. For intermittent IV infusion (piggyback), reconstitute each 100 mg vial w/5–10 ml sterile water for injection to provide concentration of 20 or 10 mg/ml respectively.

2. Further dilute w/500–1,000 ml 5% dextrose or 0.9% NaCl. Infuse over 6 hrs.

3. Alternating IV sites, use large veins to reduce risk of phlebitis.

INDICATIONS/DOSAGE/ROUTES

Note: Space doses evenly around the clock.

Mild to moderate to severe infections:
PO: Adults, elderly: Initially,

100–200 mg, then 100 mg q12h or 50 mg q6h.
IV: Adults, elderly: Initially, 200 mg, then 100 mg q12h up to 400 mg/day.
PO/IV: Children >8 yrs: Initially, 4 mg/kg, then 2 mg/kg q12h.

PRECAUTIONS

CONTRAINDICATIONS: Hypersensitivity to tetracyclines, last half of pregnancy, children <8 yrs. **CAUTIONS:** Renal impairment, sun or ultraviolet exposure (severe photosensitivity reaction). **PREGNANCY/LACTATION:** Readily crosses placenta; distributed in breast milk. Avoid use in women during last half of pregnancy. May produce permanent teeth discoloration, enamel hypoplasia, inhibit fetal skeletal growth in children <8 yrs. **Pregnancy Category D.**

INTERACTIONS

DRUG INTERACTIONS: Cholestyramine, colestipol may decrease absorption. May decrease effect of oral contraceptives. Carbamazepine, phenytoin may decrease concentrations. **ALTERED LAB VALUES:** May increase SGOT (AST), SGPT (ALT), alkaline phosphatase, amylase, bilirubin concentrations.

SIDE EFFECTS

FREQUENT: Dizziness, lightheadedness, diarrhea, nausea, vomiting, stomach cramps, increased sensitivity of skin to sunlight. **OCCASIONAL:** Pigmentation of skin, mucus membranes, itching in rectal/genital area, sore mouth/tongue.

ADVERSE REACTIONS/TOXIC EFFECTS

Superinfection (esp. fungal), anaphylaxis, increased intracranial pressure, bulging fontanelles occur rarely in infants.

NURSING IMPLICATIONS
BASELINE ASSESSMENT:

Question for history of allergies, esp. tetracyclines, sulfite. Obtain culture and sensitivity test before giving first dose (therapy may begin before results are known).

INTERVENTION/EVALUATION:

Check IV site for phlebitis (heat, pain, red streaking over vein). Assess ability to ambulate: drowsiness, vertigo, dizziness. Determine pattern of bowel activity and stool consistency. Monitor food intake, tolerance. Assess skin for rash. Check B/P and level of consciousness for increased intracranial pressure. Be alert for superinfection: diarrhea, ulceration or changes of oral mucosa, anal/genital pruritus.

PATIENT/FAMILY TEACHING:

Continue antibiotic for full length of treatment. Space doses evenly. Drink full glass of water w/capsules, tablets and avoid bedtime doses. Avoid tasks that require alertness, motor skills until response to drug is established. Notify physician if diarrhea, rash, other new symptom occurs. Protect skin from sun exposure. Consult physician before taking any other medication.

minoxidil

min-**ox**-ih-dill
(Loniten, Rogaine, Rogaine Extra Strength)

CANADIAN AVAILABILITY:
Loniten, Rogaine

CLASSIFICATION

Antihypertensive

M

AVAILABILITY (Rx)

Tablets: 2.5 mg, 10 mg. **Topical Solution (OTC):** 20 mg/ml, 50 mg/ml.

PHARMACOKINETICS

	ONSET	PEAK	DURATION
PO	0.5 hrs	2–8 hrs	2–5 days

Well absorbed from GI tract, minimal absorption after topical application. Widely distributed. Metabolized in liver to active metabolite. Primarily excreted in urine. Removed by hemodialysis. Half-life: 4.2 hrs.

ACTION/*THERAPEUTIC EFFECT*

Direct action of vascular smooth muscle, producing vasodilation of arterioles, *decreasing peripheral vascular resistance, B/P.* Topical: Vasodilatory action *increases cutaneous blood flow, stimulates hair follicle epithelium, hair follicle growth.*

USES

Treatment of severe symptomatic hypertension, or hypertension associated w/organ damage. Used for those who fail to respond to maximal therapeutic dosages of diuretic and two other antihypertensive agents. Treatment of alopecia androgenetica (males: baldness of vertex of scalp; females: diffuse hair loss or thinning of frontoparietal areas).

PO/TOPICAL ADMINISTRATION

PO:

1. Give w/o regard to food (w/food if GI upset occurs).
2. Tablets may be crushed.

TOPICAL:

1. Shampoo and dry hair before applying medication.

2. Wash hands immediately after application.
3. Do not use hair dryer after application (reduces effectiveness).

INDICATIONS/DOSAGE/ROUTES

Hypertension:
PO: Adults: Initially, 5 mg/day. Increase w/at least 3 day intervals to 10 mg, 20 mg, up to 40 mg/day in 1–2 doses. **Elderly:** Initially, 2.5 mg/day. May increase gradually. **Maintenance:** 10–40 mg/day. **Maximum:** 100 mg/day. **Children:** Initially, 0.2 mg/kg (5 mg maximum) daily. Gradually increase at minimum 3 day intervals of 0.1–2 mg/kg. **Maintenance:** 0.25–1 mg/kg/day in 1–2 doses. **Maximum:** 50 mg/day.

Hair regrowth:
Topical: Adults: 1 ml to total affected areas of scalp 2 times/day. Total daily dose not to exceed 2 ml.

PRECAUTIONS

CONTRAINDICATIONS: Pheochromocytoma. **CAUTIONS:** Severe renal impairment, chronic CHF, coronary artery disease, recent MI (1 mo). **PREGNANCY/LACTATION:** Crosses placenta; distributed in breast milk. **Pregnancy Category C**.

INTERACTIONS

DRUG INTERACTIONS: Parenteral antihypertensives may increase hypotensive effect. NSAIDs may decrease effect. **ALTERED LAB VALUES:** May increase BUN, creatinine, plasma renin activity, alkaline phosphatase, sodium. May decrease Hgb, Hct, erythrocyte count.

SIDE EFFECTS

FREQUENT: *Oral:* Edema with concurrent weight gain, hypertrichosis (elongation, thickening, increased pigmentation of fine body hair) develops in 80% of pts within 3–6 wks after beginning therapy. **OCCASIONAL:** T wave changes but usually these revert to pretreatment state with continued therapy or drug withdrawal. *Topical:* Itching, skin rash, dry/flaking skin, erythema. **RARE:** Rash, pruritus, breast tenderness in male and female, headache. *Topical:* Allergic reaction, alopecia, burning scalp, soreness at hair root, headache, visual disturbances.

ADVERSE REACTIONS/TOXIC EFFECTS

Tachycardia and angina pectoris may occur because of increased oxygen demands associated w/increased heart rate, cardiac output. Fluid and electrolyte imbalance, CHF may be observed (esp. if diuretic is not given concurrently). Too rapid reduction in B/P may result in syncope, cerebral vascular accident, MI, ischemia of special sense organs (vision, hearing). Pericardial effusion and tamponade may be seen in those w/impaired renal function not on dialysis.

NURSING IMPLICATIONS

BASELINE ASSESSMENT:

Assess B/P on both arms and take pulse for 1 full min immediately before giving medication. If pulse increases 20 beats/min or more over baseline, or systolic or diastolic B/P decreases more than 20 mm Hg, withhold drug, contact physician.

INTERVENTION/EVALUATION:

Assess for peripheral edema of hands, feet (usually, first area of low extremity swelling is be-hind medial malleolus in ambulatory, sacral area in bedridden). Assess for signs of CHF (cough, rales at base of lungs, cool extremities, dyspnea on exertion). Monitor fluid and electrolyte serum levels. Assess for distant or muffled heart sounds by auscultation (pericardial effusion, tamponade).

PATIENT/FAMILY TEACHING:

Maximum B/P response occurs in 3–7 days. Reversible growth of fine body hair may begin 3–6 wks after treatment is initiated. When used topically for stimulation of hair growth, treatment must continue on a permanent basis—cessation of treatment will begin reversal of new hair growth.

mirtazapine

murr-**taz**-ah-peen
(Remeron)

CLASSIFICATION

Antidepressant

AVAILABILITY (Rx)

Tablets: 15 mg, 30 mg

PHARMACOKINETICS

Rapidly, completely absorbed following oral administration (not affected by food). Metabolized in liver. Primarily excreted in urine. Half-life: 20–40 hrs (longer in males than females [37 hrs vs. 26 hrs]).

ACTION/*THERAPEUTIC EFFECT*

Acts as antagonist at presynaptic alpha$_2$-adrenergic receptors, increasing both norepinephrine and serotonin neurotransmission.

Produces antidepressant effect. Prominent sedative effects, low anticholinergic activity.

USES

Treatment of depression.

PO ADMINISTRATION

1. Give w/o regard to food.
2. May crush or break scored tablets.

INDICATIONS/DOSAGE/ROUTES

Note: At least 14 days should elapse between discontinuing MAO inhibitors and instituting mirtazapine therapy. Also, allow at least 14 days after discontinuing mirtazapine therapy and instituting MAO inhibitor therapy.

Depression:
PO: Adults, elderly: 15 mg/day as single dose, preferably in evening prior to sleep (high sedative effect). **Range:** 15–45 mg/day. Dose adjustment should be no sooner than at 1–2 wk intervals.

PRECAUTIONS

CONTRAINDICATIONS: Within 14 days of MAO inhibitor ingestion. **CAUTIONS:** History of MI, angina, hypotensive episodes, history of mania/hypomania, hepatic/renal function impairment, elderly. **PREGNANCY/LACTATION:** Unknown if distributed in breast milk. **Pregnancy Category C.**

INTERACTIONS

DRUG INTERACTIONS: Alcohol, diazepam may increase impairment of cognition, motor skills. MAO inhibitors may increase risk of hypertensive crisis, severe convulsions. **ALTERED LAB VALUES:** May increase cholesterol, triglycerides, SGOT (ALT), SGPT (AST).

SIDE EFFECTS

FREQUENT: Somnolence (54%), dry mouth (25%), increase in appetite (17%), constipation (13%), weight gain (12%). **OCCASIONAL:** Asthenia (8%), dizziness (7%), flu syndrome (5%), abnormal dreams (4%). **RARE:** Abdominal discomfort, vasodilation, paresthesia, acne, dry skin, thirst, arthralgia.

ADVERSE REACTIONS/TOXIC EFFECTS

Higher incidence of seizures than w/tricyclic antidepressants (esp. in those w/no previous history of seizures). High dosage may produce cardiovascular effects (severe postural hypotension, dizziness, tachycardia, palpitations, arrhythmias). Abrupt withdrawal from prolonged therapy may produce headache, malaise, nausea, vomiting, vivid dreams. Agranulocytosis occurs rarely.

NURSING IMPLICATIONS

BASELINE ASSESSMENT:

For those on long-term therapy, liver/renal function tests, blood counts should be performed periodically.

INTERVENTION/EVALUATION:

Supervise suicidal risk pt closely during early therapy (as depression lessens, energy level improves, increasing suicide potential). Assess appearance, behavior, speech pattern, level of interest, mood. Monitor B/P, pulse for hypotension, arrhythmias.

PATIENT/FAMILY TEACHING:

Avoid tasks that require alertness, motor skills until response to drug is established. Change positions slowly to avoid hypotensive effect. Tolerance to postural hypotension, sedative effects usually develops during early therapy. Do not abruptly discontinue medication. Report any sign of infection. Notify physician if pregnancy is planned or if pregnancy occurs.

misoprostol

mis-oh-**pros**-toll
(Cytotec)

FIXED-COMBINATION(S):
W/diclofenac, a NSAID (**Arthrotec**)

CANADIAN AVAILABILITY:
Cytotec

CLASSIFICATION

Antisecretory, gastric protectant

AVAILABILITY (Rx)

Tablets: 100 mcg, 200 mcg

PHARMACOKINETICS

	ONSET	PEAK	DURATION
PO	30 min	—	3–6 hrs

Rapidly absorbed from GI tract. Rapidly converted to active metabolite. Primarily excreted in urine. Half-life: 20–40 min.

ACTION/ *THERAPEUTIC EFFECT*

Inhibits basal, nocturnal gastric acid secretion via direct action on parietal cells. *Increases production of protective gastric mucus.*

USES/ *UNLABELED*

Prevention of NSAID-induced gastric ulcers and in those at high risk of developing gastric ulcer or gastric ulcer complication. *Treatment of duodenal ulcer.*

PO ADMINISTRATION

Give with or after meals (minimizes diarrhea).

INDICATIONS/DOSAGE/ROUTES

Prevention of NSAID-induced gastric ulcer:
PO: **Adults:** 200 mcg 4 times/day w/food (last dose at bedtime). Continue for duration of NSAID therapy. May reduce dosage to 100 mcg if 200 mcg dose is not tolerable. **Elderly:** 100–200 mcg 4 times/day w/food.

PRECAUTIONS

CONTRAINDICATIONS: Pregnancy (produces uterine contractions), history of allergy to prostaglandins. **CAUTIONS:** Impaired renal function. **PREGNANCY/LACTATION:** Unknown whether distributed in breast milk. Produces uterine contractions, uterine bleeding, expulsion of products of conception (abortifacient property). **Pregnancy Category X.**

INTERACTIONS

DRUG INTERACTIONS: None significant. **ALTERED LAB VALUES:** None significant.

SIDE EFFECTS

FREQUENT (20–40%): Abdominal pain, diarrhea. **OCCASIONAL (2–3%):** Nausea, flatulence, dyspepsia, headache. **RARE (1%):** Vomiting, constipation.

ADVERSE REACTIONS/TOXIC EFFECTS

Overdosage may produce sedation, tremor, convulsions, dyspnea, palpitations, hypotension, bradycardia.

NURSING IMPLICATIONS

BASELINE ASSESSMENT:

Question for possibility of pregnancy before initiating therapy (Pregnancy Category X).

M

PATIENT/FAMILY TEACHING:

Avoid magnesium-containing antacids (minimizes potential for diarrhea). Women of childbearing potential must not be pregnant before or during medication therapy (may result in hospitalization, surgery, infertility, fetal death).

mitomycin

my-toe-**my**-sin
(Mutamycin)

CANADIAN AVAILABILITY:
Mutamycin

CLASSIFICATION

Antineoplastic

AVAILABILITY (Rx)

Powder for Injection: 5 mg, 20 mg, 40 mg

PHARMACOKINETICS

Widely distributed. Does not cross blood-brain barrier. Primarily metabolized in liver and excreted in urine. Half-life: 50 min.

ACTION/THERAPEUTIC EFFECT

Causes cross-linking of DNA strands, inhibiting DNA synthesis and, to a lesser extent, RNA and protein synthesis, *preventing cellular division.* Cell cycle-phase nonspecific (most active in G and S phase of cell division).

USES/UNLABELED

Treatment of disseminated adenocarcinoma of stomach, pancreas. *Treatment of colorectal, breast, head/neck, bladder, lung, biliary, cervical carcinoma, chronic myelocytic leukemia.*

STORAGE/HANDLING

Note: May be carcinogenic, mutagenic, or teratogenic. Handle w/extreme care during preparation/administration.

Use only clear, blue-gray solutions. Concentrations of 0.5 mg/ml are stable for 7 days at room temperature or 2 wks if refrigerated. Further diluted solutions w/5% dextrose are stable for 3 hrs, 24 hrs if diluted w/0.9% NaCl.

IV ADMINISTRATION

Note: Give IV via IV catheter, IV infusion. Extremely irritating to vein. May produce pain on injection, w/induration, thrombophlebitis, paresthesia.

1. Reconstitute 5 mg vial w/10 ml sterile water for injection (40 ml for 20 mg vial) to provide solution containing 0.5 mg/ml.

2. Do not shake vial to dissolve. Allow vial to stand at room temperature until complete dissolution occurs.

3. Give IV through tubing of functional IV catheter or running IV infusion.

4. For IV infusion, further dilute w/50–100 ml 5% dextrose or 0.9% NaCl injection.

5. Extravasation may produce cellulitis, ulceration, tissue sloughing. Terminate immediately, inject ordered antidote. Apply ice intermittently for up to 72 hrs; keep area elevated.

INDICATIONS/DOSAGE/ROUTES

Note: Dosage individualized based on clinical response, tolerance to adverse effects. When used in combination therapy, consult specific protocols for optimum dosage, sequence of drug administration.

Initial dosage:
IV: Adults, elderly: 20 mg/m^2 as single dose. Repeat q6–8 wks. Give additional courses only after circulating blood elements (platelets, WBC) are within acceptable levels.

PRECAUTIONS

CONTRAINDICATIONS: Platelet count less than 75,000/mm^3, WBC less than 3,000/mm^3, serum creatinine greater than 1.7 mg/dl, coagulation disorders/bleeding tendencies, serious infection. **CAUTIONS:** Impaired renal function, pulmonary disorders. **PREGNANCY/LACTATION:** If possible, avoid use during pregnancy, esp. first trimester. Breast-feeding not recommended. Safety in pregnancy not established.

INTERACTIONS

DRUG INTERACTIONS: Bone marrow depressants may increase bone marrow depression. Live virus vaccines may potentiate virus replication, increase vaccine side effects, decrease pt's antibody response to vaccine. **ALTERED LAB VALUES:** May increase BUN, creatinine.

SIDE EFFECTS

FREQUENT (>10%): Fever, anorexia, nausea, vomiting. **OCCASIONAL (2–10%):** Stomatitis, numbness of fingers/toes, purple color bands on nails, skin rash, loss of hair, unusual tiredness. **RARE (<1%):** Bloody vomiting, thrombophlebitis, cellulitis, extravasation (pain at injection site).

ADVERSE REACTIONS/TOXIC EFFECTS

Marked bone marrow depression results in hematologic toxicity manifested as leukopenia, thrombocytopenia and, to a lesser extent, anemia (generally occurs within 2–4 wks after initial therapy). Renal toxicity may be evidenced by rise in BUN and/or serum creatinine. Pulmonary toxicity manifested as dyspnea, cough, hemoptysis, pneumonia. Long-term therapy may produce hemolytic-uremic syndrome (HUS), characterized by hemolytic anemia, thrombocytopenia, renal failure, hypertension.

NURSING IMPLICATIONS

BASELINE ASSESSMENT:

Obtain WBC, platelet, differential, prothrombin, bleeding time, Hgb before and periodically during therapy. Antiemetics before and during therapy may alleviate nausea/vomiting.

INTERVENTION/EVALUATION:

Monitor hematologic status, BUN, serum creatinine, kidney function studies. Assess IV site for phlebitis, extravasation. Monitor for hematologic toxicity (fever, sore throat, signs of local infection, easy bruising, unusual bleeding from any site), symptoms of anemia (excessive tiredness, weakness). Assess for renal toxicity (foul odor, rise in BUN, serum creatinine).

PATIENT/FAMILY TEACHING:

Maintain fastidious oral hygiene. Immediately report any stinging, burning at injection site. Do not have immunizations w/o physician's approval (drug lowers body's resistance). Avoid contact w/those who have recently received live virus vaccine. Promptly report fever, sore throat, signs of local infection, easy bruising, unusual bleeding from any site, burning on urination, increased frequency. Alopecia is reversible, but new hair growth may have different color or texture. Contact physician if nausea/vomiting continues at home.

mitotane

my-tow-tain
(Lysodren)

CANADIAN AVAILABILITY:
Lysodren

CLASSIFICATION

Antineoplastic

AVAILABILITY (Rx)

Tablets: 500 mg

PHARMACOKINETICS

Partially absorbed from GI tract. Widely distributed. Metabolized in liver/kidney. Primarily excreted in urine. Half-life: 18–159 days.

ACTION/*THERAPEUTIC EFFECT*

Inhibits activity of the adrenal cortex, *suppressing functional and nonfunctional adrenocortical neoplasms by direct cytoxic effect.*

USES/*UNLABELED*

Treatment of inoperable functional and nonfunctional adrenocortical carcinomas. *Treatment of Cushing's syndrome.*

INDICATIONS/DOSAGE/ROUTES

Note: May be carcinogenic, mutagenic, or teratogenic. Handle w/extreme care during administration.

Adrenocortical carcinomas:
PO: Adults: Initially, 2–6 g/day in 3–4 divided doses. Increase by 2–4 g/day q3–7 days, up to 9–10 g/day. **Range:** 2–16 g/day.

PRECAUTIONS

CONTRAINDICATIONS: Known hypersensitivity to drug. **CAUTIONS:** Hepatic disease. **PREGNANCY/ LACTATION:** If possible, avoid use during pregnancy, esp. first trimester. Breast-feeding not recommended. **Pregnancy Category C**.

INTERACTIONS

DRUG INTERACTIONS: CNS depressants may increase CNS depression. **ALTERED LAB VALUES:** May decrease plasma cortisol, urinary 17-OH, PBI, uric acid.

SIDE EFFECTS

FREQUENT (>15%): Anorexia, nausea, vomiting, diarrhea, lethargy, somnolence, adrenocortical insufficiency, dizziness, vertigo, maculopapular rash, hypouricemia. **OCCASIONAL (<15%):** Blurred or double vision, retinopathy, decreased hearing, excess salivation, urine abnormalities (hematuria, cystitis, albuminuria), hypertension, orthostatic hypotension, flushing, wheezing, shortness of breath, generalized aching, fever.

ADVERSE REACTIONS/TOXIC EFFECTS

Brain damage, functional impairment may occur w/long-term, high-dosage therapy.

NURSING IMPLICATIONS
BASELINE ASSESSMENT:

Therapy should be discontinued immediately following shock, trauma (drug produces adrenal suppression). Steroid replacement therapy generally necessary during therapy.

INTERVENTION/EVALUATION:

Monitor uric acid serum levels, hepatic function studies, urine tests. Perform neurologic and behavioral assessments periodically in those receiving prolonged therapy (over 2 yrs). Assess pattern of daily bowel activity and stool consistency. Assess skin for maculopapular rash.

PATIENT/FAMILY TEACHING:

Immediately report injury, infection, other illnesses. Do not have immunizations w/o physician's approval (drug lowers body resistance). Increase fluid intake (may protect against urine abnormalities). Contact physician if nausea/vomiting continues at home. Do not drive or perform tasks requiring alert response if dizziness, drowsiness occur. Contraception is recommended during therapy. Report loss of appetite, diarrhea, depression, rash, darkening of skin.

mitoxantrone
my-toe-**zan**-trone
(Novantrone)

CANADIAN AVAILABILITY:
Novantrone

CLASSIFICATION

Antineoplastic

AVAILABILITY (Rx)

Injection: 2 mg/ml

PHARMACOKINETICS

Widely distributed. Metabolized in liver. Primarily eliminated in feces via biliary system. Half-life: 2.3–13 days.

ACTION/*THERAPEUTIC EFFECT*

Inhibits DNA synthesis, *resulting in cell death.* Cell cycle-phase nonspecific. Most active in late S phase of cell division.

USES/*UNLABELED*

Treatment of acute, nonlymphocytic leukemia (monocytic, myelogenous, promyelocytic), late-stage hormone-resistant prostate cancer. *Treatment of breast, liver carcinoma, non-Hodgkin's lymphoma.*

IV ADMINISTRATION

Note: May be carcinogenic, mutagenic, or teratogenic. Handle w/extreme care during preparation/administration. Give by IV injection, IV infusion. Must dilute before administration.

1. Dilute w/at least 50 ml 5% dextrose or 0.9% NaCl. Infuse into freely running IV over at least 3 min.
2. Do not mix w/heparin in same IV solution (precipitate forms).

INDICATIONS/DOSAGE/ROUTES

Note: Dosage individualized based on clinical response, tolerance to adverse effects. When used in combination therapy, consult specific protocols for optimum dosage, sequence of drug administration.

Usual dosage:
IV: Adults: Combined w/cytosine: *Induction:* 12 mg/m^2/day on days 1–3. *Second course (for incomplete response):* 12 mg/m^2/day on days 1 and 2.

PRECAUTIONS

CONTRAINDICATIONS: None significant. **CAUTIONS:** None significant. **PREGNANCY/LACTATION:** If possible, avoid use during pregnancy, esp. first trimester. May cause fetal harm. Breastfeeding not recommended. **Pregnancy Category D**.

INTERACTIONS

DRUG INTERACTIONS: May decrease effect of antigout medications. Bone marrow depressants may increase bone marrow depression. Live virus vaccines may potentiate virus replication, increase vaccine side effects, decrease pt's antibody response to vaccine. **ALTERED LAB VALUES:** May increase SGOT (AST), SGPT (ALT), bilirubin, uric acid.

SIDE EFFECTS

FREQUENT (>10%): Nausea, vomiting, diarrhea, cough, headache, inflammation of mucous membranes, abdominal discomfort, fever, alopecia. **OCCASIONAL (4–10%):** Easy bruising, fungal infection, conjunctivitis, urinary tract infection. **RARE (3%):** Arrhythmias.

ADVERSE REACTIONS/TOXIC EFFECTS

Bone marrow suppression may be severe, resulting in GI bleeding, sepsis, pneumonia. Renal failure, seizures, jaundice, CHF may occur.

NURSING IMPLICATIONS

BASELINE ASSESSMENT:

Offer emotional support. Establish baseline for CBC, temperature, rate and quality of pulse, lung status.

INTERVENTION/EVALUATION:

Monitor lung sounds for pulmonary toxicity (dyspnea, fine lung rales). Monitor hematologic status, pulmonary function studies, hepatic and renal function tests. Monitor for stomatitis (burning/erythema of oral mucosa at inner margin of lips), fever, sore throat, signs of local infection, easy bruising, or unusual bleeding from any site.

PATIENT/FAMILY TEACHING:

Urine will appear blue/green 24 hrs after administration. Blue tint to sclera may also appear. Maintain adequate daily fluid intake (may protect against renal impairment). Do not have immunizations w/o physician's approval (drug lowers body's resistance). Avoid contact w/those who have recently received live virus vaccine. Contact physician if nausea/vomiting continues at home.

mivacurium chloride
(Mivacron)
See Classification section under: Neuromuscular blocking agents

moexipril hydrochloride

mow-**ex**-ih-prill
(Univasc)

FIXED-COMBINATION(S)
W/hydrochlorothiazide, a diuretic
(Uniretic)

CLASSIFICATION

Angiotensin-converting enzyme (ACE) inhibitor

AVAILABILITY (Rx)

Tablets: 7.5 mg, 15 mg

PHARMACOKINETICS

	ONSET	PEAK	DURATION
PO	1 hr	3–6 hrs	24 hrs

Incompletely absorbed from GI tract (food decreases absorption). Rapidly converted to active metabolite. Primarily recovered in feces, partially excreted in urine. Unknown if removed by dialysis. Half-life: 1 hr (metabolite 2–9 hrs).

ACTION/*THERAPEUTIC EFFECT*

Suppresses renin-angiotensin-aldosterone system (prevents conversion of angiotensin I to angiotensin II, a potent vasoconstrictor; may also inhibit angiotensin II at local vascular and renal sites). *Reduces peripheral arterial resistance, B/P.*

USES

Treatment of hypertension. Used alone or in combination w/thiazide diuretics.

PO ADMINISTRATION

1. Give 1 hr before meals.
2. Tablets may be crushed.

INDICATIONS/DOSAGE/ROUTES

Hypertension (used alone):
PO: Adults, elderly: Initially, 7.5 mg once daily 1 hr before meals. Adjust according to B/P effect. **Maintenance:** 7.5–30 mg/daily in 1–2 divided doses 1 hr before meals.

Hypertension (concurrent diuretic therapy):
Note: To reduce risk of hypotension, discontinue diuretic 2–3 days before initiating moexipril therapy. If B/P not controlled, resume diuretic. If diuretic cannot be discontinued, give initial dose of 3.75 mg moexipril.

Renal function impairment:
PO: Adults, elderly: 3.75 mg once daily in pts w/creatinine clearance of ≤40 ml/min/1.73m^2. **Maximum:** May titrate up to 15 mg/day.

PRECAUTIONS

CONTRAINDICATIONS: History of angioedema w/previous treatment w/ACE inhibitors. **CAUTIONS:** Renal impairment, those w/sodium depletion or on diuretic therapy, dialysis, hypovolemia, coronary or cerebrovascular insufficiency, hyperkalemia, aortic stenosis, ischemic heart disease, angina, severe CHF, cerebrovascular disease. **PREGNANCY/LACTATION:** Crosses placenta; unknown if distributed in breast milk. **Pregnancy Category C:** First trimester. **Pregnancy Category D:** Second and third trimesters. Has caused fetal/neonatal mortality, morbidity.

INTERACTIONS

DRUG INTERACTIONS: Alcohol, diuretics, hypotensive agents may increase effects. NSAIDs may decrease effect. Potassium-sparing diuretics, potassium supplements may cause hyperkalemia. May increase lithium concentration, toxicity. **ALTERED LAB VALUES:** May increase potassium, SGOT (AST), SGPT (ALT), alkaline phosphatase, bilirubin, BUN, creatinine. May decrease sodium. May cause positive ANA titer.

SIDE EFFECTS

OCCASIONAL: Cough, headache (6%), dizziness (4%), nausea, fatigue (3%). **RARE:** Flushing, rash, myalgia, nausea, vomiting.

ADVERSE REACTIONS/TOXIC EFFECTS

Excessive hypotension ("first-dose syncope") may occur in those w/CHF, severely salt/volume depleted. Angioedema (swelling of face/lips), hyperkalemia occur rarely. Agranulocytosis, neutropenia may be noted in those w/impaired renal function or collagen vascular disease (systemic lupus erythematosus, scleroderma). Nephrotic syndrome may be noted in those w/history of renal disease.

NURSING IMPLICATIONS
BASELINE ASSESSMENT:

Obtain B/P and apical pulse immediately before each dose, in addition to regular monitoring (be alert to fluctuations). If excessive reduction in B/P occurs, place pt in supine position, feet slightly elevated. Renal function tests should be performed before therapy begins. In those w/renal impairment, autoimmune disease, or taking drugs that affect leukocytes or immune response, CBC and differential count should be performed before therapy begins and q2 wks for 3 mos, then periodically thereafter.

INTERVENTION/EVALUATION:

Monitor B/P, WBC count, serum potassium. Monitor for cough, question for headache. Assist w/ambulation if dizziness occurs.

PATIENT/FAMILY TEACHING:

To reduce hypotensive effect, rise slowly from lying to sitting position and permit legs to dangle from bed momentarily before standing. Full therapeutic effect may take 2–4 wks. Report any sign of infection (sore throat, fever), swelling of hands or feet or face, chest pain, difficulty breathing or swallowing. Skipping doses or voluntarily discontinuing drug may produce severe, rebound hypertension. Do not take cold preparations, nasal decongestants. Restrict sodium and alcohol as ordered.

molindone hydrochloride

mole-**in**-doan
(Moban)

CLASSIFICATION

Antipsychotic

AVAILABILITY (Rx)

Tablets: 5 mg, 10 mg, 25 mg, 50 mg, 100 mg. **Oral Concentrate:** 20 mg/ml.

PHARMACOKINETICS

	ONSET	PEAK	DURATION
PO	—	—	36 hrs

Rapidly absorbed from GI tract. Widely distributed. Metabolized in liver to active metabolite. Primarily excreted in urine.

ACTION/*THERAPEUTIC EFFECT*

Acts on dopamine receptors in reticular activating, limbic systems in brain, decreases dopamine activity. *Suppresses locomotor activity, aggressiveness, suppresses conditioned responses. Produces tranquilization w/o compromising alertness.*

USES

Symptomatic management of schizophrenic disorders.

PO ADMINISTRATION

1. Give w/o regard to meals.
2. Give oral concentrate alone

or mix w/water, milk, fruit juice, or carbonated beverages.

INDICATIONS/DOSAGE/ROUTES

Management of schizophrenia:
PO: Adults: Initially, 50–75 mg/day in 3–4 divided doses. Increase to 100 mg/day in 3–4 days, if needed.

Maintenance (mild symptoms):
PO: Adults: 5–15 mg 3–4 times/day.

Maintenance (moderate symptoms):
PO: Adults: 10–25 mg 3–4 times/day.

Maintenance (severe symptoms):
PO: Adults: Up to 225 mg may be needed.

Usual elderly dosage (nonpsychotic):
PO: Initially, 5–10 mg 1–2 times/day. May increase by 5–10 mg every 4–7 days. **Maximum:** 112 mg/day.

PRECAUTIONS

CONTRAINDICATIONS: Severe CNS depression, comatose states. **CAUTIONS:** Severe cardiovascular disorders, history of seizures. **PREGNANCY/LACTATION:** Unknown whether drug crosses placenta or is distributed in breast milk. **Pregnancy Category C.**

INTERACTIONS

DRUG INTERACTIONS: Alcohol, CNS depression–producing medications may prolong CNS effects. Anticholinergics, antihistamines, MAO inhibitors, maprotiline, tricyclic antidepressants may increase anticholinergic, sedative effects. Extrapyramidal symptoms (EPS) may increase in severity, frequency w/EPS-producing medications. May cause neurotoxic symptoms w/lithium. **ALTERED LAB VALUES:** May alter BUN, RBCs, glucose values. May increase prolactin concentration, WBCs.

SIDE EFFECTS

FREQUENT: Transient drowsiness, dry mouth, constipation, blurred vision, nasal congestion. **OCCASIONAL:** Diarrhea, peripheral edema, rash, urinary retention, nausea, mild/transient postural hypotension, tachycardia. **RARE:** Skin pigmentation, ocular changes.

ADVERSE REACTIONS/TOXIC EFFECTS

Frequently noted extrapyramidal symptom is akathisia (motor restlessness, anxiety). Occurring less frequently is akinesia (rigidity, tremor, salivation, mask-like facial expression, reduced voluntary movements). Infrequently noted are dystonias: torticollis (neck muscle spasm), opisthotonos (rigidity of back muscles), and oculogyric crisis (rolling back of eyes). Tardive dyskinesia (protrusion of tongue, puffing of cheeks, chewing/puckering of mouth) occurs rarely but may be irreversible. Risk is greater in female geriatric pts. Potentially fatal neuroleptic malignant syndrome (NMS) requires immediate discontinuation of the drug.

NURSING IMPLICATIONS

BASELINE ASSESSMENT:

Assess behavior, appearance, emotional status, response to environment, speech pattern, thought content.

INTERVENTION/EVALUATION:

Supervise suicidal risk pt closely during early therapy (as depression lessens, energy level improves, increasing suicide potential). Monitor B/P for hypotension. Assess for peripheral edema behind medial malleolus (sacral area in bedridden pts). Monitor stools; avoid constipation. Assess for extrapyramidal symptoms (see Adverse Reactions/Toxic Effects), hyperthermia, altered mental status or level of consciousness, and autonomic instability (NMS); evaluate for evidence of tardive dyskinesia. Assess for therapeutic response (interest in surroundings, improvement in self-care, increased ability to concentrate, relaxed facial expression).

PATIENT/FAMILY TEACHING:

Full therapeutic effects may take up to 6 wks. Report visual disturbances. Sugarless gum, sips of tepid water may relieve dry mouth. Drowsiness generally subsides during continued therapy. Avoid tasks that require alertness, motor skills until response to drug is established. Avoid alcohol and CNS depressants.

---

mometasone
(Elocon)
See Classification section under: Corticosteroids: topical

---

montelukast
(Singulair)
See Supplement
See Classification section under: Bronchodilators

---

moricizine hydrochloride

mor-ih-**see**-zeen
(Ethmozine)

CLASSIFICATION

Antiarrhythmic

AVAILABILITY (Rx)

Tablets: 200 mg, 250 mg, 300 mg

PHARMACOKINETICS

	ONSET	PEAK	DURATION
PO	—	2–4 hrs	—

Well absorbed from GI tract. Undergoes significant first-pass metabolism. Metabolized in liver (induces own metabolism). Primarily eliminated in feces via biliary system. Minimal removal by hemodialysis. Half-life: 1.5–3.5 hrs.

ACTION/THERAPEUTIC EFFECT

Prevents sodium current across myocardial cell membranes. Has potent local anesthetic activity and membrane stabilizing effects. Slows AV, Purkinje conduction, decreases action potential duration, effective refractory period, *suppressing ventricular arrhythmias.*

USES

Treatment of documented, life-threatening ventricular arrhythmias (e.g., sustained ventricular tachycardia).

PO ADMINISTRATION

1. May be given w/o regard to food but give w/food if GI upset occurs.
2. Monitor EKG for cardiac changes, particularly increase in PR and QRS intervals. Notify physician of any significant interval changes.

INDICATIONS/DOSAGE/ROUTES

Usual dosage for arrhythmias:
PO: Adults, elderly: 200–300 mg q8h; may increase by 150 mg/day at 3 day intervals until desired effect achieved.

Dosage in hepatic/renal impairment:

Initially, 600 mg or less/day.

PRECAUTIONS

CONTRAINDICATIONS: Preexisting second- or third-degree AV block or right bundle-branch block associated w/left hemiblock (bifascicular block), w/o pacemaker; cardiogenic shock. **CAUTIONS:** CHF, electrolyte imbalance, sick-sinus syndrome (bradycardia-tachycardia), impaired hepatic/renal function. **PREGNANCY/LACTATION:** Unknown if drug crosses placenta; distributed in breast milk. **Pregnancy Category B.**

INTERACTIONS

DRUG INTERACTIONS: Cimetidine may increase concentrations; moricizine may decrease theophylline concentrations. **ALTERED LAB VALUES:** May cause EKG changes (prolong PR, QT intervals).

SIDE EFFECTS

FREQUENT (5–15%): Dizziness, nausea, headache, fatigue, dyspnea. **OCCASIONAL (2–5%):** Nervousness, paresthesia, sleep disturbances, dyspepsia, vomiting, diarrhea. **RARE (<2%):** Urinary retention/frequency, sweating, dry mouth, swelling of lips/tongue, periorbital edema, impotence, decreased libido, generalized body aches.

ADVERSE REACTIONS/TOXIC EFFECTS

Has ability to worsen existing arrhythmias or produce new ones. Jaundice w/hepatitis occurs rarely. Overdosage produces emesis, lethargy, syncope, hypotension, conduction disturbances, exacerbation of CHF, MI, sinus arrest.

NURSING IMPLICATIONS
BASELINE ASSESSMENT:

Correct electrolyte imbalance before administering medication.

INTERVENTION/EVALUATION:

Monitor EKG for cardiac changes, particularly increase in PR and QRS intervals. Notify physician of any significant interval changes. Assess pulse for strength/weakness, irregular rate. Question for headache, GI upset, dizziness, nausea. Monitor fluid and electrolyte serum levels. Monitor pattern of daily bowel activity and stool consistency. Assess for dizziness, unsteadiness. Monitor liver enzyme results.

PATIENT/FAMILY TEACHING:

Do not abruptly discontinue medication. Compliance w/therapy regimen is essential to control arrhythmias.

morphine sulfate
(Astramorph, Duramorph, Kadian, MS Contin, MSIR, RMS, Roxanol, Roxanol-T)

CANADIAN AVAILABILITY:
Kadian MSIR, M.O.S., MSContin, Oramorph

CLASSIFICATION

Opioid: Analgesic **(Schedule II)**

AVAILABILITY (Rx)

Injection: 0.5 mg/ml, 1 mg/ml, 2 mg/ml, 3 mg/ml, 4 mg/ml, 5 mg/ml, 8 mg/ml, 10 mg/ml, 15 mg/ml. **Tablets:** 15 mg, 30 mg. **Tablets (soluble):** 10 mg, 15 mg, 30 mg. **Tablets (controlled-release):** 30 mg, 60 mg. **Oral Solu-**

tion: 10 mg/5 ml, 20 mg/5 ml, 20 mg/ml, 100 mg/5 ml. **Suppositories:** 5 mg, 10 mg, 20 mg, 30 mg.

PHARMACOKINETICS

	ONSET	PEAK	DURATION
PO	Variable	60–120 min	4–5 hrs
Extended release			
	—	60–120 min	8–12 hrs
SubQ	5–30 min	50–90 min	4–5 hrs
IM	5–30 min	30–60 min	3–7 hrs
IV	Rapid	20 min	4–5 hrs
Rectal			
	20–60 min	—	4–5 hrs
Epidural			
	15–60 min	—	16–24 hrs
Intrathecal			
	15–60 min	—	16–24 hrs

Variably absorbed from GI tract. Readily absorbed after SubQ, IM administration. Widely distributed. Metabolized in liver. Primarily excreted in urine. Half-life: 2–3 hrs.

ACTION / THERAPEUTIC EFFECT

Binds w/opioid receptors within CNS, *altering processes affecting pain perception, emotional response to pain. Decreases intestinal motility* by local, central actions.

USES

Relief of severe, acute, chronic pain, preop sedation, anesthesia supplement, analgesia during labor. Drug of choice for pain due to myocardial infarction, dyspnea from pulmonary edema not resulting from chemical respiratory irritant.

STORAGE / HANDLING

Store suppositories, parenteral, oral form at room temperature. Discard unused portion from pt-controlled IV infusion.

PO/SUBQ/IM/IV/RECTAL ADMINISTRATION

Note: Give by IM injection if repeated doses necessary (repeated SubQ may produce local tissue irritation, induration). May also be given slow IV injection or IV infusion. Incompatible w/aminophylline, amobarbital, chlorothiazide, phenytoin, heparin, meperidine, methicillin, nitrofurantoin, pentobarbital, phenobarbital, sodium bicarbonate, sodium iodide, thiopental.

PO:

1. Mix liquid form w/fruit juice to improve taste.

2. Do not crush or break extended-release capsule.

3. Kadian: May mix w/applesauce immediately prior to administration.

SubQ/IM:

1. Administer slowly, rotating injection sites.

2. Pts with circulatory impairment experience higher risk of overdosage because of delayed absorption of repeated administration.

IV:

1. For IV injection, dilute 2.5–15 mg morphine in 4–5 ml sterile water for injection.

2. Always administer very slowly, over 4–5 min. Rapid IV increases risk of severe adverse reactions (apnea, chest wall rigidity, peripheral circulatory collapse, cardiac arrest, anaphylactoid effects).

3. For multiple IV injections, may give pt-controlled analgesia, using pt-controlled infusion device.

4. For continuous IV infusion, dilute to concentration of 0.1–1 mg/ml in 5% dextrose and give through controlled infusion device.

RECTAL:

1. If suppository is too soft, chill for 30 min in refrigerator or run cold water over foil wrapper.

2. Moisten suppository w/cold water before inserting well up into rectum.

INDICATIONS/DOSAGE/ROUTES

Note: Reduce dosage in elderly/debilitated, those on concurrent CNS depressants.

Pain:
PO: Adults, elderly: 10–30 mg q4h. **Extended-release:** 30 mg q8–12h.
Rectal: Adults, elderly: 10–30 mg q4h.
SubQ/IM: Adults, elderly: 10 mg q4h, as needed. **Usual dosage range:** 5–20 mg q4h. **Children:** 0.1–0.2 mg/kg per dose. Give q4h, as needed. Do not exceed single dose of 15 mg.
IV: Adults, elderly: 4–10 mg, given very slowly.

Severe, chronic pain associated w/cancer:
IV Infusion: Adults, elderly: 0.8–10 mg/hr. Increase to effective dosage level, as needed. **Maintenance:** 0.8–80 mg/hr. **Children (Maintenance):** 0.025–2.6 mg/kg/hr.
Epidural: Adults, elderly: Initially, 5 mg. If pain relief not obtained in 1 hr, may give additional doses in increments of 1–2 mg at sufficient intervals. **Maximum total daily dose:** 10 mg.
Continuous Epidural Infusion: Adults, elderly: Initially, 2–4 mg/day. May be increased by 1–2 mg/day if needed.
Intrathecal: Adults, elderly: 0.2–1 mg.
SubQ: Children: Usual maintenance level: 0.025–1.79 mg/kg/hr.

Myocardial infarction pain:
SubQ/IM/IV: Adults, elderly: 8–15 mg. Give additional smaller doses q3–4h.

Analgesia during labor:
SubQ/IM: Adults: 10 mg.

PRECAUTIONS

CONTRAINDICATIONS: Postop biliary tract surgery, surgical anastomosis. **EXTREME CAUTION:** CNS depression, anoxia, hypercapnia, respiratory depression, seizures, acute alcoholism, shock, untreated myxedema, respiratory dysfunction. **CAUTIONS:** Toxic psychoses, increased intracranial pressure, impaired hepatic function, acute abdominal conditions, hypothyroidism, prostatic hypertrophy, Addison's disease, urethral stricture, COPD. **PREGNANCY/LACTATION:** Crosses placenta; distributed in breast milk. May prolong labor if administered in latent phase of first stage of labor or before cervical dilation of 4–5 cm has occurred. Respiratory depression may occur in neonate if mother received opiates during labor. Regular use of opiates during pregnancy may produce withdrawal symptoms in neonate (irritability, excessive crying, tremors, hyperactive reflexes, fever, vomiting, diarrhea, yawning, sneezing, seizures). **Pregnancy Category B.** (Category D if used for prolonged periods or in high doses at term.)

INTERACTIONS

DRUG INTERACTIONS: Alcohol, CNS depressants may increase CNS or respiratory depression, hypotension. MAO inhibitors may produce severe, fatal reaction (reduce dose to $\frac{1}{4}$ usual dose). **ALTERED LAB VALUES:** May increase amylase, lipase.

M

SIDE EFFECTS

Note: Effects dependent on dosage amount, route of administration. Ambulatory pts, those not in severe pain may experience dizziness, nausea, vomiting, hypotension more frequently than those in supine position or who have severe pain.
FREQUENT: Sedation, decreased B/P, increased sweating, flushed face, constipation, dizziness, drowsiness, nausea, vomiting. **OCCASIONAL:** Allergic reaction (rash, itching), difficulty breathing, confusion, pounding heartbeat, tremors decreased urination, stomach cramps, vision changes, dry mouth, headache, decreased appetite, pain/burning at injection site. **RARE:** Paralytic ileus.

ADVERSE REACTIONS/TOXIC EFFECTS

Overdosage results in respiratory depression, skeletal muscle flaccidity, cold clammy skin, cyanosis, extreme somnolence progressing to convulsions, stupor, coma. Tolerance to analgesic effect, physical dependence may occur w/repeated use. Prolonged duration of action, cumulative effect may occur in those w/impaired hepatic, renal function.

NURSING IMPLICATIONS
BASELINE ASSESSMENT:

Pt should be in a recumbent position before drug is given by parenteral route. Assess onset, type, location, and duration of pain. Obtain vital signs before giving medication. If respirations are 12/min or lower (20/min or lower in children), withhold medication, contact physician. Effect of medication is reduced if full pain recurs before next dose.

INTERVENTION/EVALUATION:

Monitor vital signs 5–10 min after IV administration, 15–30 min after SubQ or IM. Be alert for decreased respirations or B/P. Check for adequate voiding; palpate bladder if output questionable. Monitor stools; avoid constipation. Initiate deep breathing and coughing exercises, particularly in those w/impaired pulmonary function. Assess for clinical improvement and record onset of pain relief. Consult physician if pain relief is not adequate.

PATIENT/FAMILY TEACHING:

Discomfort may occur w/injection. Change positions slowly to avoid orthostatic hypotension. Avoid tasks that require alertness, motor skills until response to drug is established. Avoid alcohol and CNS depressants. Tolerance/dependence may occur with prolonged use of high doses.

---

moxifloxacin
(Avelox)
See Supplement
See Classification section under:
Antibiotics: quinolones

---

mupirocin

mew-pee-ro-sin
(Bactroban)

CANADIAN AVAILABILITY:
Bactroban

CLASSIFICATION

Topical antibacterial

AVAILABILITY (Rx)

Ointment: 2%. Nasal Ointment: 2%.

PHARMACOKINETICS

Metabolized in skin to inactive metabolite. Transported to skin surface; removed by normal skin desquamation.

ACTION/THERAPEUTIC EFFECT

Inhibits bacterial protein, RNA synthesis. Less effective on DNA synthesis. *Nasal:* Eradicates nasal colonization of MRSA. *Prevents bacterial growth and replication. Bacteriostatic.*

USES/UNLABELED

Topical treatment of impetigo, infected traumatic skin lesions. *Nasal:* Reduces spread of MRSA (methicillin-resistant *S. aureus*). *Treatment of infected eczema, folliculitis, minor bacterial skin infections.*

TOPICAL ADMINISTRATION

1. Gown and gloves are to be worn until 24 hrs after therapy is effective. Disease is spread by direct contact w/moist discharges.

2. Apply small amount to affected areas.

3. Cover affected areas w/ gauze dressing if desired.

INDICATIONS/DOSAGE/ROUTES

Usual topical dosage:
Topical: Adults, elderly, children: Apply 3 times/day (may cover w/gauze).

Usual nasal dosage:
Intranasal: Adults, elderly, children: Apply 2 times/day for 5 days.

PRECAUTIONS

CONTRAINDICATIONS: Hypersensitivity to any of the components. CAUTIONS: Impaired renal function. Safety of nasal preparation not established in children <12 yrs. PREGNANCY/LACTATION: Not known whether present in breast milk; temporarily discontinue nursing while using mupirocin. Pregnancy Category B.

INTERACTIONS

DRUG INTERACTIONS: None significant. ALTERED LAB VALUES: None significant.

SIDE EFFECTS

FREQUENT: *Nasal (3–9%):* Headache, rhinitis, upper respiratory congestion, pharyngitis, altered taste. OCCASIONAL: *Nasal (2%):* Burning, stinging, cough. *Topical (1–2%):* Pain, burning, stinging, itching. RARE: *Nasal (<1%):* Pruritis, diarrhea, dry mouth, epistaxis, nausea, rash. *Topical (<1%):* Rash, nausea, dry skin, contact dermatitis.

ADVERSE REACTIONS/TOXIC EFFECTS

Superinfection may result in bacterial or fungal infections, esp. w/prolonged or repeated therapy.

NURSING IMPLICATIONS

BASELINE ASSESSMENT:

Question for hypersensitivity to components. Assess skin for type and extent of lesions.

INTERVENTION/EVALUATION:

Keep neonates or pts w/poor hygiene isolated. Wear gloves and gown if necessary when contact w/discharges is likely; continue until 24 hrs after therapy is effective. Cleanse/dispose of articles soiled with discharge according to institutional guidelines. In event of skin reaction, stop applications, cleanse area gently, and notify physician.

PATIENT/FAMILY TEACHING:

For external use only. Avoid contact w/eyes. Explain precautions to avoid spread of infection; teach how to apply medication. If skin reaction, irritation develops, notify physician. If there is no improvement in 3–5 days, pt should be reevaluated.

muromonab-CD3

meur-oh-**mon**-ab
(Orthoclone, OKT3)

CANADIAN AVAILABILITY:
Orthoclone

CLASSIFICATION

Immunosuppressant

AVAILABILITY (Rx)

Injection: 1 mg/ml

ACTION / THERAPEUTIC EFFECT

Antibody (purified IgG_2 immune globulin) that reacts with T3 (CD3) antigen of human T-cell membranes. Blocks function of T-cells (has major role in acute renal rejection). *Reverses graft rejection.*

USES

Treatment of acute allograft rejection in renal transplant pts, steroid-resistant acute allograft rejection in cardiac, hepatic transplant pts.

STORAGE / HANDLING

Refrigerate ampule. Do not shake ampule before using. Fine translucent particles may develop; does not affect potency.

IV ADMINISTRATION

IV:

1. Administer direct IV over <1 min.

2. Give methylprednisolone 1 mg/kg before and 100 mg hydrocortisone 30 min after dose (decreases adverse reaction to first dose).

3. Draw solution into syringe through 0.22 micron filter. Discard filter; use needle for IV administration.

INDICATIONS / DOSAGE / ROUTES

Prevention of allograft rejection:
IV: Adults, elderly: 5 mg/day for 10–14 days. Begin when acute renal rejection is diagnosed.

PRECAUTIONS

CONTRAINDICATIONS: History of hypersensitivity to muromonab-CD3 or any murine origin product, those in fluid overload evidenced by chest x-ray or >3% weight gain within the week before initial treatment. **CAUTIONS:** Impaired hepatic, renal, cardiac function. **PREGNANCY/LACTATION:** Unknown whether drug crosses placenta or is distributed in breast milk. Avoid nursing. **Pregnancy Category C**.

INTERACTIONS

DRUG INTERACTIONS: Other immunosuppressants may increase risk of infection or development of lymphoproliferative disorders. Live virus vaccines may potentiate virus replication, increase vaccine side effects, decrease pt's antibody response to vaccine. **ALTERED LAB VALUES:** None significant.

SIDE EFFECTS

FREQUENT: First-dose reaction: Fever, chills, dyspnea, malaise occurs 30 min to 6 hrs after first dose (reaction markedly reduced w/subsequent dosing after first 2 days of treatment). **OCCASIONAL:** Chest pain, nausea, vomiting, diarrhea, tremor.

ADVERSE REACTIONS / TOXIC EFFECTS

Cytokine release syndrome (CRS) may range from flulike illness to life-threatening shock-like reaction. Occasionally fatal hypersensitivity reactions. Severe pulmonary edema occurs in <2% of those treated w/muromonab-CD3. Infection (due to immunosuppression) generally occurs within 45 days after initial treatment; cytomegalovirus occurs in 19%, herpes simplex in 27%. Severe and life-threatening infection occurs in <4.8%.

NURSING IMPLICATIONS
BASELINE ASSESSMENT:

Chest x-ray must be taken within 24 hrs of initiation of therapy and be clear of fluid. Weight should be ≤3% above minimum weight the week before treatment begins (pulmonary edema occurs where fluid overload is present before treatment). Have resuscitative drugs and equipment immediately available.

INTERVENTION/EVALUATION:

Monitor WBC, differential, platelet count, renal and hepatic function tests, and immunologic tests (plasma levels or quantitative T lymphocyte surface phenotyping) before and during therapy. If fever exceeds 100°F, antipyretics should be instituted. Monitor for fluid overload by chest x-ray and weight gain of >3% over weight before treatment began. Assess lung sounds for evidence of fluid overload. Monitor I&O. Assess stool frequency and consistency.

PATIENT/FAMILY TEACHING:

Inform pt of first-dose reaction prior to treatment; headache, tremor may occur as a response to medication. Avoid crowds, those w/infections. Do not receive immunizations.

mycophenolate mofetil

my-koe-**phen**-oh-late
(CellCept)

CANADIAN AVAILABILITY:
CellCept

CLASSIFICATION

Immunosuppressant

AVAILABILITY (Rx)

Capsules: 250 mg. **Tablets:** 500 mg. **Oral Suspension, Injection.**

PHARMACOKINETICS

Rapidly, extensively absorbed following oral administration (food does not alter the extent of absorption but plasma concentration decreased in presence of food). Completely hydrolyzed to active metabolite, mycophenolic acid (MPA). Primarily excreted in urine. Usually not removed by hemodialysis. Half-life: 17.9 hrs.

ACTION

Inhibits inosine monophosphate dehydrogenase, an enzyme that deprives lymphocytes of nucleotides necessary for DNA and RNA synthesis. Inhibits proliferation of T- and B-lymphocytes. Suppresses immunologically mediated inflammatory response. *Prevents renal transplant rejection.*

USES/ UNLABELED

Prophylaxis of organ rejection in pts receiving allogeneic renal/ cardiac transplants. Should be used concurrently w/cyclosporine and corticosteroids. *Prevents organ rejection in pts undergoing heart transplants.*

PO ADMINISTRATION

1. Give on an empty stomach.
2. Do not open or crush capsules. Avoid inhalation of powder in capsules and avoid direct contact of powder on skin or mucous membranes. If contact occurs, wash thoroughly w/soap and water; rinse eyes profusely w/plain water.

INDICATIONS/DOSAGE/ROUTES

Kidney transplantation:
PO: Adults, elderly: 1 g twice/day (2 g/day) w/initial dose given within 72 hrs after transplant. Give in combination w/corticosteroids and cyclosporine.

Cardiac transplant:
PO: Adults, elderly: 1.5 g twice/day.

PRECAUTIONS

CONTRAINDICATIONS: Hypersensitivity to mycophenolate, mycophenolic acid, or any component of drug product. **CAUTIONS:** Immunosuppressed pts, pts w/active, serious digestive system disease; renal function impairment. **PREGNANCY/LACTATION:** Unknown if distributed in breast milk. If at all possible, avoid use. **Pregnancy Category C.**

INTERACTIONS

DRUG INTERACTIONS: Acyclovir, ganciclovir compete w/MPA (active metabolite) for renal excretion; may increase plasma concentration of each in presence of renal impairment. Antacids (magnesium, aluminum-containing), cholestyramine may decrease absorption. Other immunosuppressants may increase risk of infection or development of lymphomas. Live virus vaccines may potentiate virus replication, increase vaccine side effects, decrease pt's antibody response to vaccine. Probenecid may increase concentration. **ALTERED LAB VAL-**UES: May increase alkaline phosphatase, creatinine, SGOT (AST), SGPT (ALT). Alters calcium, glucose protein, uric acid, lipids levels.

SIDE EFFECTS

FREQUENT (>15%): Diarrhea/constipation, fever, headache, hypertension, UTI, peripheral edema, nausea, dyspepsia. **OCCASIONAL (10–15%):** Asthenia, hematuria, vomiting, oral moniliasis, dyspnea, cough, acne, tremor, insomnia, pharyngitis. **RARE (<10%):** Dizziness, rash, back pain.

ADVERSE REACTIONS/TOXIC EFFECTS

Sepsis, infection occur occasionally, GI tract hemorrhage rarely. There is an increased risk of neoplasia (new, abnormal growth tumors). Significant anemia, leukopenia, thrombocytopenia, neutropenia, leukocytosis may occur, particularly in those undergoing kidney rejection.

NURSING IMPLICATIONS

BASELINE ASSESSMENT:

Women of childbearing potential should have a negative serum or urine pregnancy test within 1 wk prior to initiation of drug therapy. A negative pregnancy test report should be obtained before therapy is initiated. Assess medical history, esp. renal function, existence of active digestive system disease, drug history, esp. other immunosuppressants.

INTERVENTION/EVALUATION:

CBC should be performed weekly during first month of therapy, twice monthly during second and third months of treatment, then monthly throughout the first year. If rapid fall in WBC occurs, dosage should be reduced or discontinued. Assess particularly for delayed bone marrow suppression. Report any major change in assessment of pt. Routinely watch for any change from normal.

PATIENT/FAMILY TEACHING:

Effective contraception should be used before, during, and for 6 wks after discontinuing therapy, even if there has been a history of infertility, other than hysterectomy. Two forms of contraception must be used concurrently unless abstinence is absolute. Contact physician if unusual bleeding or bruising, sore throat, mouth sores, abdominal pain, or fever occurs. Inform pts of need for laboratory tests while taking medication. Inform pts of risk of malignancies that may occur.

---

nabumetone

nah-**byew**-meh-tone
(Relafen)

CANADIAN AVAILABILITY:
Relafen

CLASSIFICATION

Nonsteroidal anti-inflammatory

AVAILABILITY (Rx)

Tablets: 500 mg, 750 mg

PHARMACOKINETICS

Readily absorbed from GI tract. Widely distributed. Metabolized in liver to active metabolite. Primarily excreted in urine. Half-life: 22–30 hrs.

ACTION/*THERAPEUTIC EFFECT*

Produces analgesic and anti-inflammatory effect by inhibiting prostaglandin synthesis, *reducing inflammatory response and intensi-*

ty of pain stimulus reaching sensory nerve endings.

USES

Acute and chronic treatment of osteoarthritis, rheumatoid arthritis.

PO ADMINISTRATION

1. Give w/food, milk, or antacids if GI distress occurs.
2. Do not crush; swallow whole.

INDICATIONS/DOSAGE/ROUTES

Rheumatoid arthritis, osteoarthritis:
PO: Adults, elderly: Initially, 1,000 mg as single dose or in 2 divided doses. May increase up to 2,000 mg/day as single or in 2 divided doses.

PRECAUTIONS

CONTRAINDICATIONS: Active peptic ulcer, GI ulceration, chronic inflammation of GI tract, GI bleeding disorders, history of hypersensitivity to aspirin or NSAIDs, history of significantly impaired renal function. **CAUTIONS:** Impaired renal/hepatic function, history of GI tract disease, predisposition to fluid retention. **PREGNANCY/LACTATION:** Distributed in low concentration in breast milk. Avoid use during last trimester (may adversely affect fetal cardiovascular system: premature closing of ductus arteriosus). **Pregnancy Category C.** (Category D if used in 3rd trimester or near delivery.)

INTERACTIONS

DRUG INTERACTIONS: May increase effects of oral anticoagulants, heparin, thrombolytics. May decrease effect of antihypertensives, diuretics. Salicylates, aspirin may increase risk of GI side effects, bleeding. Bone marrow depressants may increase risk of hematologic reactions. May increase concentration, toxicity of lithium. May increase methotrexate toxicity. Probenecid may increase concentration. **ALTERED LAB VALUES:** May increase alkaline phosphatase, LDH, serum transaminase, potassium, urine protein, BUN, serum creatinine. May decrease uric acid.

SIDE EFFECTS

FREQUENT (12–14%): Diarrhea, abdominal cramping/pain, dyspepsia. **OCCASIONAL (3–9%):** Nausea, constipation, flatulence, dizziness, headache. **RARE (1–3%):** Vomiting, stomatitis.

ADVERSE REACTIONS/TOXIC EFFECTS

Overdose may result in acute hypotension, tachycardia. Peptic ulcer, GI bleeding, nephrotoxicity (dysuria, cystitis, hematuria, proteinuria, nephrotic syndrome), gastritis, severe hepatic reaction (cholestasis, jaundice), severe hypersensitivity reaction (bronchospasm, angiofacial edema) occur rarely.

NURSING IMPLICATIONS

BASELINE ASSESSMENT:

Assess onset, type, location, and duration of pain or inflammation. Inspect appearance of affected joints for immobility, deformities, and skin condition.

INTERVENTION/EVALUATION:

Assist w/ambulation if somnolence/drowsiness/dizziness occurs. Monitor for evidence of dyspepsia. Monitor pattern of daily bowel activity and stool consistency. Check behind medial malleolus for fluid retention (usually first area noted). Evaluate for therapeutic response: relief of pain,

stiffness, swelling, increase in joint mobility, reduced joint tenderness, improved grip strength.

PATIENT/FAMILY TEACHING:

Swallow capsule whole; do not crush or chew. Avoid tasks that require alertness, motor skills until response to drug is established. If GI upset occurs, take w/food, milk. Avoid aspirin, alcohol during therapy (increases risk of GI bleeding). Report headache, GI distress, visual disturbances, edema. Report skin rash, itching, visual disturbances, weight gain, black stools, persistent headache.

nadolol

nay-**doe**-lol
(Corgard)

FIXED-COMBINATION(S):
W/bendroflumethiazide, a diuretic **(Corzide)**

CANADIAN AVAILABILITY:

Apo-Nadol, Corgard, Novo-Nadolol

CLASSIFICATION

Beta-adrenergic blocker

AVAILABILITY (Rx)

Tablets: 20 mg, 40 mg, 80 mg, 120 mg, 160 mg

PHARMACOKINETICS

	ONSET	PEAK	DURATION
PO	—	—	24 hrs

Partially absorbed from GI tract. Primarily excreted unchanged in urine. Moderately removed by hemodialysis. Half-life: 20–24 hrs (increased in decreased renal function).

ACTION / *THERAPEUTIC EFFECT*

Nonselective beta blocker. Blocks beta$_1$-adrenergic receptors, *slowing sinus heart rate, decreasing cardiac output, decreasing B/P.* Blocks beta$_2$-adrenergic receptors, *increasing airway resistance. Decreases myocardial ischemia severity* by decreasing oxygen requirements.

USES / *UNLABELED*

Management of mild to moderate hypertension. Used alone or in combination w/diuretics, esp. thiazide type. Management of chronic stable angina pectoris. *Treatment of cardiac arrhythmias, hypertrophic cardiomyopathy, myocardial infarction, pheochromocytoma, vascular headaches, tremors, thyrotoxicosis, mitral valve prolapse syndrome, neuroleptic-induced akathisia.*

PO ADMINISTRATION

1. May be given w/o regard to meals.
2. Tablets may be crushed.

INDICATIONS / DOSAGE / ROUTES

Hypertension:
PO: Adults: Initially, 40 mg/day. Increase by 40–80 mg/day at 7 day intervals. **Maintenance:** 40–80 mg/day up to 240–320 mg/day.

Angina pectoris:
PO: Adults: Initially, 40 mg/day. Increase by 40–80 mg/day at 3–7 day intervals. **Maintenance:** 40–80 mg/day up to 160–240 mg/day.

Usual elderly dosage:
PO: Initially, 20 mg/day for angina/hypertension.

Dosage in renal impairment:
Dose is modified based on creatinine clearance.

CREATININE CLEARANCE	DOSAGE INTERVAL
>50 ml/min	q24h
31–50 ml/min	q24–36h
10–30 ml/min	q24–48h
<10 ml/min	q40–60h

PRECAUTIONS

CONTRAINDICATIONS: Bronchial asthma, COPD, uncontrolled cardiac failure, sinus bradycardia, heart block greater than first degree, cardiogenic shock, CHF unless secondary to tachyarrhythmias, those on MAO inhibitors. **CAUTIONS:** Inadequate cardiac function, impaired renal/hepatic function, diabetes mellitus, hyperthyroidism. **PREGNANCY/LACTATION:** Crosses placenta; distributed in breast milk. Avoid use during first trimester. May produce bradycardia, apnea, hypoglycemia, hypothermia during delivery, small birth weight infants. **Pregnancy Category C.** (Category D if used in 2nd or 3rd trimester.)

INTERACTIONS

DRUG INTERACTIONS: Diuretics, other hypotensives may increase hypotensive effect; sympathomimetics, xanthines may mutually inhibit effects; may mask symptoms of hypoglycemia, prolong hypoglycemic effect of insulin, oral hypoglycemics; NSAIDs may decrease antihypertensive effect; cimetidine may increase concentration. **ALTERED LAB VALUES:** May increase ANA titer, SGOT (AST), SGPT (ALT), alkaline phosphatase, LDH, bilirubin, BUN, creatinine, potassium, uric acid, lipoproteins, triglycerides.

SIDE EFFECTS

Generally well tolerated, w/ transient and mild side effects. **FREQUENT:** Decreased sexual

N

ability, drowsiness, unusual tired-ness/weakness. **OCCASIONAL:** Bradycardia, difficulty breathing, depression, cold hands/feet, diar-rhea, constipation, anxiety, nasal congestion, nausea, vomiting. **RARE:** Altered taste, dry eyes, itching.

ADVERSE REACTIONS/TOXIC EFFECTS

Excessive dosage may pro-duce profound bradycardia, hy-potension. Abrupt withdrawal may result in sweating, palpitations, headache, tremulousness, exacer-bation of angina, MI, ventricular arrhythmias. May precipitate CHF, MI in those w/cardiac disease, thyroid storm in those w/thyrotoxi-cosis, peripheral ischemia in those w/existing peripheral vas-cular disease. Hypoglycemia may occur in previously controlled diabetics.

NURSING IMPLICATIONS

BASELINE ASSESSMENT:

Assess baseline renal/liver function tests. Assess B/P, apical pulse immediately before drug is administered (if pulse is 60/min or below, or systolic B/P is below 90 mm Hg, withhold medication, contact physician). *Antianginal:* Record onset, type (sharp, dull, squeezing), radiation, location, intensity, and duration of anginal pain, and precipitating factors (exertion, emotional stress).

INTERVENTION/EVALUATION:

Monitor B/P for hypotension, respiration for shortness of breath. Assess pulse for strength/weakness, irregular rate, brady-cardia. Assess fingers for color, numbness (Raynaud's). Assist w/ambulation if dizziness occurs.

Assess for evidence of CHF: dys-pnea (particularly on exertion or lying down), night cough, periph-eral edema, distended neck veins. Monitor I&O (increase in weight, decrease in urine output may indicate CHF).

PATIENT/FAMILY TEACHING:

Do not abruptly discontinue medication. Compliance w/ther-apy regimen is essential to con-trol hypertension, arrhythmias. To avoid hypotensive effect, rise slowly from lying to sitting posi-tion; wait momentarily before standing. Avoid tasks that require alertness, motor skills until re-sponse to drug is established. Report excessive fatigue, dizzi-ness. Do not use nasal deconges-tants, OTC cold preparations (stimulants) w/o physician ap-proval. Outpatients should moni-tor B/P, pulse before taking med-ication. Restrict salt, alcohol intake.

---

nafarelin acetate

naf-ah-**rell**-in
(Synarel)

CANADIAN AVAILABILITY:
Synarel

CLASSIFICATION

Gonadotropin inhibitor

AVAILABILITY (Rx)

Nasal Solution: 2 mg/ml

PHARMACOKINETICS

Well absorbed after intranasal administration. Primarily eliminat-ed in feces. Half-life: 3 hrs.

ACTION/THERAPEUTIC EFFECT

Initially stimulates the release of the pituitary gonadotropins, luteinizing hormone and follicle-stimulating hormone, *resulting in temporary increase of ovarian steroidogenesis.* Continued dosing *abolishes the stimulatory effect on the pituitary gland* and, after about 4 wks, leads to *decreased secretion of gonadal steroids.*

USES

Management of endometriosis, including dysmenorrhea, dyspareunia, pelvic pain. Treatment of central precocious puberty.

INTRANASAL ADMINISTRATION

1. Use metered spray pump to administer correct dose.
2. When dose is given 2 times/day, alternate nostrils.
3. When a topical nasal decongestant is necessary, do not use until at least 30 min after nafarelin dose.

INDICATIONS/DOSAGE/ROUTES

Endometriosis:
Note: Initiate treatment between days 2 and 4 of menstrual cycle. Duration of therapy is 6 mos.
Intranasal: Adults: 400 mcg/day: 200 mcg (1 spray) into 1 nostril in morning, 1 spray into other nostril in evening. For pts w/persistent regular menstruation after months of treatment, increase dose to 800 mcg/day (1 spray into each nostril in morning and evening).

Central precocious puberty:
Intranasal: Children: 1,600 mcg/day: 400 mcg (2 sprays into each nostril in morning and evening; total 8 sprays).

PRECAUTIONS

CONTRAINDICATIONS: Hypersensitivity to nafarelin, other agonist analogues and components of the preparation; undiagnosed abnormal vaginal bleeding. **CAUTIONS:** History of osteoporosis, chronic alcohol or tobacco use, intercurrent rhinitis. **PREGNANCY/LACTATION:** Contraindicated during pregnancy or breast-feeding. **Pregnancy Category X**.

INTERACTIONS

DRUG INTERACTIONS: None significant. **ALTERED LAB VALUES:** None significant.

SIDE EFFECTS

FREQUENT (>10%): Hot flashes (90%), nasal irritation, decreased libido, vaginal dryness, headache, acne, muscle pain, decreased breast size. **OCCASIONAL (1–10%):** Insomnia, edema, weight gain, depression, hair growth. **RARE (<1%):** Palpitations, eye pain, hypersensitivity reaction (rash, itching).

ADVERSE REACTIONS/TOXIC EFFECTS

None significant.

NURSING IMPLICATIONS

BASELINE ASSESSMENT:

Question for hypersensitivity to any agonist analogue ingredients. Inquire about menstrual cycle; therapy should begin between days 2 and 4 of cycle.

INTERVENTION/EVALUATION:

Check for pain relief as result of therapy. Inquire about menstrual cessation and other decreased estrogen effects.

PATIENT/FAMILY TEACHING:

Pt should use nonhormonal contraceptive during therapy. Do not take drug, check w/physician if pregnancy is suspected (risk to fetus). Importance of full length of therapy, regular visits to physician's office. Notify physician if regular menstruation continues (menstruation should stop w/therapy).

nafcillin sodium

naph-**sill**-in
(Nafcil, Nallpen, Unipen)

CLASSIFICATION

Antibiotic: Penicillin

AVAILABILITY (Rx)

Tablets: 500 mg. **Capsules:** 250 mg. **Powder for Injection:** 1 g, 2 g, 10 g.

PHARMACOKINETICS

Poorly absorbed from GI tract (food decreases absorption). Metabolized in liver. Primarily excreted in urine. Not removed by hemodialysis. Half-life: 0.5–1 hr (increased in decreased renal function, neonates).

ACTION/ *THERAPEUTIC EFFECT*

Binds to bacterial membranes, *inhibiting cell wall synthesis. Bactericidal.*

USES

Treatment of respiratory tract, skin/skin structure infections, osteomyelitis, endocarditis, meningitis; perioperatively, esp. in cardiovascular, orthopedic procedures. Predominantly treatment of infections caused by penicillinase-producing staphylococci.

STORAGE/HANDLING

Store capsules, tablets at room temperature. *Oral solution:* After reconstitution, stable for 7 days if refrigerated. *IV infusion (piggyback):* Stable for 24 hrs at room temperature, 96 hrs if refrigerated. Discard if precipitate forms.

PO/IM/IV ADMINISTRATION

Note: Space doses evenly around the clock.

PO:

Give 1 hr before or 2 hrs after food/beverages.

IM:

1. Reconstitute each 500 mg w/1.7 ml sterile water for injection or 0.9% NaCl injection to provide concentration of 250 mg/ml.
2. Inject IM into large muscle mass.

IV:

1. For IV injection, reconstitute as above, then further dilute each vial w/15–30 ml sterile water for injection or 0.9% NaCl injection. Administer over 5–10 min.
2. For intermittent IV infusion (piggyback), further dilute with 50–100 ml 5% dextrose, 0.9% NaCl, or other compatible IV fluid. Infuse over 30–60 min.
3. Because of potential for hypersensitivity/anaphylaxis, start initial dose at few drops per minute, increase slowly to ordered rate; stay w/pt first 10–15 min, then check q10 min.
4. Limit IV therapy to <48 hrs, if possible. Alternating IV sites, use large veins to reduce risk of phlebitis.
5. Stop infusion if pt complains of pain.

INDICATIONS/DOSAGE/ROUTES

Usual dosage:
IV: Adults, elderly: 3–6 g/24 hrs in divided doses.
IM: Adults, elderly: 500 mg q4–6h.
PO: Adults, elderly: 250 mg to 1 g q4–6h.

Usual pediatric dosage:
IM/IV: 25 mg/kg 2 times/day.
PO: 25–50 mg/kg/day in 4 divided doses.

Usual neonate dosage:
IM/IV: Neonates <7 days: 50 mg/kg/day in 2–3 divided doses. **>7 days:** 75 mg/kg/day in 4 divided doses.

PRECAUTIONS

CONTRAINDICATIONS: Hypersensitivity to any penicillin. **CAUTIONS:** History of allergies, particularly cephalosporins. **PREGNANCY/LACTATION:** Readily crosses placenta, appears in cord blood, amniotic fluid. Distributed in breast milk in low concentrations. May lead to allergic sensitization, diarrhea, candidiasis, skin rash in infant. **Pregnancy Category B**.

INTERACTIONS

DRUG INTERACTIONS: Probenecid may increase concentration, toxicity risk. **ALTERED LAB VALUES:** May cause positive Coombs' test.

SIDE EFFECTS

FREQUENT: Mild hypersensitivity reaction (fever, rash, pruritus), GI effects (nausea, vomiting, diarrhea) more frequent w/oral administration. **OCCASIONAL:** Hypokalemia w/high IV doses, phlebitis, thrombophlebitis (more common in elderly). **RARE:** Extravasation w/IV administration.

ADVERSE REACTIONS/TOXIC EFFECTS

Superinfections, potentially fatal antibiotic-associated colitis may result from altered bacterial balance. Hematologic effects (esp. involving platelets, WBCs), severe hypersensitivity reactions, rarely anaphylaxis.

NURSING IMPLICATIONS

BASELINE ASSESSMENT:

Question for history of allergies, esp. penicillins, cephalosporins. Obtain specimen for culture and sensitivity before giving first dose (therapy may begin before results are known).

INTERVENTION/EVALUATION:

Hold medication and promptly report rash (possible hypersensitivity) or diarrhea (w/fever, abdominal pain, mucus and blood in stool may indicate antibiotic-associated colitis). Assess food tolerance. Evaluate IV site frequently for phlebitis (heat, pain, red streaking over vein) and infiltration (potential extravasation). Check IM injection sites for pain, induration. Monitor potassium. Be alert for superinfection: increased fever, onset sore throat, vomiting, diarrhea, ulceration/changes of oral mucosa, anal/genital pruritus. Check hematology reports (esp. WBCs), periodic renal or hepatic reports in prolonged therapy.

PATIENT/FAMILY TEACHING:

Continue antibiotic for full length of treatment. Doses should be evenly spaced. Discomfort may occur w/IM injection. Report IV discomfort immediately. Notify physician in event of diarrhea, rash, other new symptom.

N

naftifine hydrochloride
(Naftin)
See Classification section under:
Antifungals, topical

nalbuphine hydrochloride

nail-**byew**-phin
(Nubain)

CANADIAN AVAILABILITY:
Nubain

CLASSIFICATION

Opioid analgesic

AVAILABILITY (Rx)

Injection: 10 mg/ml, 20 mg/ml

PHARMACOKINETICS

	ONSET	PEAK	DURATION
SubQ	<15 min	—	3–6 hrs
IM	<15 min	60 min	3–6 hrs
IV	2–3 min	30 min	3–6 hrs

Well absorbed after SubQ, IM administration. Metabolized in liver. Primarily eliminated in feces via biliary secretion. Half-life: 3.5–5 hrs.

ACTION/*THERAPEUTIC EFFECT*

Binds w/opioid receptors within CNS, *altering pain perception, emotional response to pain.* May displace opioid agonists and competitively inhibit their action (may precipitate withdrawal symptoms).

USES

Relief of moderate to severe pain, preop sedation, obstetrical analgesia, adjunct to anesthesia.

STORAGE/HANDLING

Store parenteral form at room temperature.

SUBQ/IM/IV ADMINISTRATION

IM:
    Rotate IM injection sites.

IV:
    For IV injection, administer each 10 mg >3–5 min.

INDICATIONS/DOSAGE/ROUTES

Note: Dosage based on severity of pain, physical condition of pt, concurrent use of other medications.

Analgesia:
SubQ/IM/IV: Adults, elderly: 10 mg q3–6h, as necessary. Do not exceed maximum single dose of 20 mg, maximum daily dose of 160 mg. In pts chronically receiving narcotic analgesics of similar duration of action, give 25% of usual dosage.

Supplement to anesthesia:
IV: Adults, elderly: Induction: 0.3–3 mg/kg over 10–15 min. **Maintenance:** 0.25–0.5 mg/kg as necessary.

PRECAUTIONS

CONTRAINDICATIONS: Respirations <12/min. **CAUTIONS:** Impaired hepatic/renal function, elderly, debilitated, head injury, increased intracranial pressure, MI w/nausea, vomiting, respiratory disease, hypertension, before biliary tract surgery (produces spasm of sphincter of Oddi). **PREGNANCY/LACTATION:** Readily crosses placenta; distributed in breast milk (breast feeding not recommended). **Pregnancy Category B**. (Category D if used for prolonged periods or in high doses at term.)

INTERACTIONS

DRUG INTERACTIONS: Alcohol, CNS depressants may increase CNS or respiratory depression, hypotension. MAO inhibitors may produce severe, fatal reaction (reduce dose to 1/4 usual dose). Effects may be decreased w/buprenorphine. **ALTERED LAB VALUES:** May increase amylase, lipase, serum levels.

SIDE EFFECTS

FREQUENT (35%): Sedation. **OCCASIONAL (3–9%):** Sweaty/clammy feeling, nausea, vomiting, dizziness, vertigo, dry mouth, headache. **RARE (≤1%):** Restlessness, crying, euphoria, hostility, confusion, numbness, tingling, flushing, paradoxical reaction.

ADVERSE REACTIONS/TOXIC EFFECTS

Abrupt withdrawal after prolonged use may produce symptoms of narcotic withdrawal (abdominal cramping, rhinorrhea, lacrimation, anxiety, increased temperature, piloerection [goose bumps]). Overdose results in severe respiratory depression, skeletal muscle flaccidity, cyanosis, extreme somnolence progressing to convulsions, stupor, coma. Tolerance to analgesic effect, physical dependence may occur w/chronic use.

NURSING IMPLICATIONS

BASELINE ASSESSMENT:

Raise bed rails. Obtain vital signs before giving medication. If respirations are 12/min or lower (20/min or lower in children), withhold medication, contact physician. Assess onset, type, location, and duration of pain. Effect of medication is reduced if full pain recurs before next dose. Low abuse potential.

INTERVENTION/EVALUATION:

Increase fluid intake and environmental humidity to improve viscosity of lung secretions. Monitor for change in respirations, B/P, change in rate or quality of pulse. Monitor pattern of daily bowel activity and stool consistency. Initiate deep breathing and coughing exercises, particularly in those w/impaired pulmonary function. Change pt's position q2–4h. Assess for clinical improvement and record onset of relief of pain. Consult physician if pain relief is not adequate.

PATIENT/FAMILY TEACHING:

Change positions slowly to avoid dizziness. Avoid tasks that require alertness, motor skills until response to drug is established. Note effects of abrupt withdrawal following long-term use. Avoid alcohol and CNS depressants.

---

nalmefene
(Revex)
See Supplement

---

naloxone hydrochloride

nay-**lox**-own
(Narcan)

CANADIAN AVAILABILITY:
Narcan

CLASSIFICATION

Opioid antagonist

AVAILABILITY (Rx)

Injection: 0.02 mg/ml, 0.4 mg/ml, 1 mg/ml

PHARMACOKINETICS

	ONSET	PEAK	DURATION
SubQ	2–5 min	—	1–4 hrs
IM	2–5 min	—	1–4 hrs
IV	1–2 min	—	1–4 hrs

Well absorbed after SubQ, IM administration. Metabolized in liver. Primarily excreted in urine. Half-life: 60–100 min.

ACTION/ *THERAPEUTIC EFFECT*

Displaces opiates at opiate-occupied receptor sites in CNS, *blocking narcotic effects. Reverses opiate-induced sleep or sedation. Increases respiratory rate, returns depressed B/P to normal rate.*

USES

Diagnosis and treatment of opioid toxicity, treatment of opiod induced respiratory depression, and other effects (e.g., sedation, coma, convulsions). Used in neonates to reverse respiratory depression caused by opioids given to mother during labor and delivery. Adjunctive therapy to treat hypotension in management of septic shock.

STORAGE/HANDLING

Store parenteral form at room temperature. Use mixture within 24 hrs; discard unused solution.

IM/IV ADMINISTRATION

IM:

Give in upper, outer quadrant of buttock.

IV:

1. May dilute 1 mg/ml with 50 ml sterile water for injection to provide a concentration of 0.02 mg/ml.

2. Use the 0.4 mg/ml and 1 mg/ml for injection for adults, the 0.02 mg/ml concentration for neonates.

3. For continuous IV infusion, dilute each 2 mg of naloxone with 500 ml of 5% dextrose in water or 0.9% NaCl, producing solution containing 0.004 mg/ml.

INDICATIONS/DOSAGE/ROUTES

Opioid toxicity (IV route preferred):
IM/IV/SubQ: Adults: 0.4–2 mg as single dose. May repeat at 2–3 min intervals. **Children:** 0.01 mg/kg. May repeat w/0.1 mg/kg. **Note:** AAP recommends initial dose of 0.1 mg/kg for infants and children up to 5 yrs and weighing <20 kg. Children >5 yrs or >20 kg recommended initial dose is 2 mg.

Opioid respiratory depression:
IV: Adults: 0.1–0.2 mg q2–3 min until adequate ventilation and alertness w/o pain are obtained. May repeat dose at 1–2 hr intervals. **Children:** 5–10 mcg (0.005–0.01 mg) q2–3 min. **Neonates:** 10 mcg (0.01 mg)/kg. May repeat q2–3 min.

Septic shock:
IV: Adults: 0.03–0.2 mg/kg initially, then IV infusion of 0.03–0.3 mg/kg/hr for 1–20 hrs.

PRECAUTIONS

CONTRAINDICATIONS: Respiratory depression due to nonopiate drugs. **CAUTIONS:** Opiate-dependent pt, cardiovascular disorders. **PREGNANCY/LACTATION:** Unknown whether drug crosses placenta or is distributed in breast milk. **Pregnancy Category B**.

INTERACTIONS

DRUG INTERACTIONS: Reverses analgesic/side effects, may precipitate withdrawal symptoms of butorphanol, nalbuphine, pentazocine, opioid agonist analgesics. **ALTERED LAB VALUES:** None significant.

SIDE EFFECTS

None significant (little or no

pharmacologic effect in absence of narcotics).

ADVERSE REACTIONS/TOXIC EFFECTS

Too rapid reversal of narcotic depression may result in nausea, vomiting, tremulousness, sweating, increased B/P, tachycardia. Excessive dosage in postop pts may produce significant reversal of analgesia, excitement, tremulousness. Hypotension or hypertension, ventricular tachycardia and fibrillation, pulmonary edema may occur in those w/cardiovascular disease.

NURSING IMPLICATIONS
BASELINE ASSESSMENT:

Maintain clear airway. Obtain weight of children to calculate drug dosage.

INTERVENTION/EVALUATION:

Monitor vital signs esp. rate, depth, and rhythm of respiration during and frequently after administration. Carefully observe pt after satisfactory response (duration of opiate may exceed duration of naloxone, resulting in recurrence of respiratory depression). Assess for increased pain w/reversal of opiate.

---

naltrexone hydrochloride

nal-**trex**-own
(ReVia)

CANADIAN AVAILABILITY:
ReVia

CLASSIFICATION

Opioid antagonist

AVAILABILITY (Rx)

Tablets: 50 mg

PHARMACOKINETICS

	ONSET	PEAK	DURATION
PO	—	—	24–72 hrs

Rapid, complete absorption following oral administration. Undergoes extensive first-pass hepatic metabolism. Metabolized in liver to active metabolite. Excreted in urine. Half-life: 4–13 hrs.

ACTION/*THERAPEUTIC EFFECT*

Opioid antagonist: Binds to opioid receptors, *blocking physical effects of morphine, heroin, other opioids.* Alcohol deterrent: Exact mechanism unknown. *Decreases craving, drinking days, relapse rate.*

USES/*UNLABELED*

Blockade of effects of exogenously administered opioids. Treatment of alcohol dependence. *Treatment of postconcussional syndrome unresponsive to other treatments; eating disorders.*

SUBQ/IV ADMINISTRATION

1. In those w/narcotic dependence, do not attempt treatment until pt has remained opioid free for 7–10 days. Test urine for opioids for verification. Pt should not be experiencing withdrawal symptoms.

2. Administer a naloxone challenge test (see Indications/Dosage/Routes). If pt experiences any signs/symptoms of withdrawal, withhold treatment (challenge test can be repeated in 24 hrs). Naloxone challenge test must be negative before naltrexone therapy is initiated.

INDICATIONS/DOSAGE/ROUTES

Naloxone challenge test:
IV: Adults, elderly: Draw 2 am-

pules naloxone, 2 ml (0.8 mg) into syringe. Inject 0.5 ml (0.2 mg); while needle is still in vein, observe for 30 secs for withdrawal signs/symptoms (see Adverse Reactions/Toxic Effects). If no evidence of withdrawal, inject remaining 1.5 ml (0.6 mg); observe for additional 20 min for withdrawal signs/symptoms.

SubQ: Adults, elderly: Give 2 ml (0.8 mg); observe for 45 min for withdrawal signs/symptoms.

Opioid-free state:
PO: Adults, elderly: Initially, 25 mg. Observe pt for 1 hr. If no withdrawal signs appear, give another 25 mg. May be given as 100 mg q.o.d. or 150 mg every 3 days.

Adjunct in treatment of alcohol dependence:
PO: Adults, elderly: 50 mg once daily.

PRECAUTIONS

CONTRAINDICATIONS: Pts experiencing opiate withdrawal, opioid dependent, acute opioid withdrawal, failed naloxone challenge, positive urine screen for opioids, history of sensitivity to naltrexone, acute hepatitis, liver failure. **CAUTIONS:** Active liver disease. **PREGNANCY/LACTATION:** Unknown whether drug crosses placenta or is distributed in breast milk. **Pregnancy Category C**.

INTERACTIONS

DRUG INTERACTIONS: Concurrent use w/thioridazine may produce lethargy, somnolence. Benefits of opioid-containing products (cough and cold preparations, antidiarrheal preparations, opioid analgesics) are negated. **ALTERED LAB VALUES:** May increase serum transaminase, SGOT (AST), SGPT (ALT).

SIDE EFFECTS

FREQUENT: *Alcoholism:* Nausea (10%), headache (7%), depression (5–7%). *Narcotic addiction:* Insomnia, anxiety, nervousness, headache, low energy, abdominal cramps, nausea, vomiting, joint/muscle pain (>10%). **OCCASIONAL:** *Alcoholism:* Dizziness, nervousness, fatigue (4%), insomnia, vomiting (3%), anxiety, suicidal ideation (2%). *Narcotic addiction:* Irritability, increased energy, dizziness, anorexia, diarrhea or constipation, rash, chills, increased thirst.

ADVERSE REACTIONS/TOXIC EFFECTS

Signs and symptoms of opioid withdrawal include stuffy or runny nose, tearing, yawning, sweating, tremor, vomiting, piloerection (goose bumps), feeling of temperature change, joint/bone/muscle pain, abdominal cramps, feeling of skin crawling. May cause hepatocellular injury if given in large doses. Accidental naltrexone overdosage produces withdrawal symptoms within 5 min of ingestion, lasts up to 48 hrs. Symptoms present as confusion, visual hallucinations, somnolence, significant vomiting and diarrhea.

NURSING IMPLICATIONS
BASELINE ASSESSMENT:

If there is any question of opioid dependence, a naloxone challenge test (see Indications/Dosage/Routes) should be performed. Treatment w/naltrexone should not be instituted unless pt is opioid free for 7–10 days before therapy begins. Pt should wear identification indicating naltrexone therapy. Obtain medication history (esp. opioids), other medical conditions (esp. hepatitis, other liver disease).

INTERVENTION/EVALUATION:

Monitor closely for evidence of hepatotoxicity (abdominal pain that lasts longer than a few days, white bowel movements, dark urine, jaundice), SGOT, SGPT, bilirubin, creatinine clearance lab values.

PATIENT/FAMILY TEACHING

If heroin or other opiates are self-administered, there will be no effect. However, any attempt to overcome naltrexone's prolonged 24–72 hr blockade of opioid effect by taking large amounts of opioids is very dangerous and may result in coma, serious injury, or fatal overdose. Naltrexone also blocks effects of opioid-containing medicine (cough and cold preparations, antidiarrheal preparations, opioid analgesics). Contact physician if abdominal pain that lasts longer than 3 days, white bowel movements, dark-colored urine, yellow eyes occurs. Periodic blood testing should be performed to detect liver toxicity. Stress importance of compliance/support groups/counseling. Carry identification card indicating use of naltrexone.

naphazoline

na-**faz**-oh-leen
(Albalon, Estivin, Naphcon, Vasocon)

FIXED-COMBINATION(S):

W/pheniramine maleate, an antihistamine **(Naphcon-A)**

CANADIAN AVAILABILITY:
Albalon, Naphcon, Vasocon

CLASSIFICATION

Sympathomimetic, decongestant

AVAILABILITY (OTC)

Nasal Solution: 0.05%. **Ophthalmic Solution:** 0.012%, 0.02%, 0.03%, 0.1% **(Rx)**.

ACTION/*THERAPEUTIC EFFECT*

Directly acts on alpha-adrenergic receptors in arterioles of conjunctiva, *causing vasoconstriction, w/subsequent decreased congestion to area.*

USES

Ophthalmic: Relief of itching, congestion, and minor irritation; to control hyperemia in pts with superficial corneal vascularity. Occasionally may be used during some ocular diagnostic procedures. *Intranasal:* Relief of nasal congestion due to common cold, acute or chronic rhinitis, hay fever or other allergies.

STORAGE/HANDLING

Do not store in aluminum containers (degraded by aluminum). Do not use if cloudy or discolored solution.

OPHTHALMIC/INTRANASAL ADMINISTRATION

OPHTHALMIC:

1. Follow manufacturer's directions regarding contact lenses.
2. Tilt pt's head back; place solution in conjunctival sac.
3. Have pt close eyes; press gently on lacrimal sac for 1 min.
4. Take care not to touch any area w/the applicator.

5. Remove excess solution by gently blotting w/tissue.

INTRANASAL:

Note: Applicator should not touch any surface; rinse tip of dispenser or dropper w/hot water following use. Use for only 1 person.

Drops:

1. Position pt in lateral, head-low position or reclining w/head tilted as far back as possible.

2. Apply drops to one nostril and maintain position for 5 min. Then apply drops to second nostril and maintain position for 5 min.

Spray:

1. Administer spray into each nostril w/pt's head erect so that excess solution is not released.

2. After 2–3 min, have pt blow nose thoroughly.

INDICATIONS/DOSAGE/ROUTES

Usual nasal dosage:
Intranasal: Adults, elderly, children >12 yrs: 2 drops/sprays (0.05%) in each nostril q3–6h.

Usual ophthalmic dosage:
Ophthalmic: Adults, elderly: 1–2 drops q3–4h for 3–4 days.

PRECAUTIONS

CONTRAINDICATIONS: Hypersensitivity to naphazoline or any component of the preparation; narrow-angle glaucoma or those w/a narrow angle who do not have glaucoma; before peripheral iridectomy; eyes capable of angle closure. **CAUTIONS:** Hypertension, diabetes, hyperthyroidism, heart disease, hypertensive cardiovascular disease, coronary artery disease, cerebral arteriosclerosis, long-standing bronchial asthma. Consider precautions for individual

components. **PREGNANCY/LACTATION:** Safety during pregnancy and lactation not established. **Pregnancy Category C**.

INTERACTIONS

DRUG INTERACTIONS: Tricyclic antidepressants, maprotiline may increase effect. **ALTERED LAB VALUES:** None significant.

SIDE EFFECTS

OCCASIONAL: *Nasal:* Burning, stinging, drying nasal mucosa, sneezing, rebound congestion. *Ophthalmic:* Blurred vision, large pupils, increased eye irritation. **Note:** *Systemic absorption:* Fast/irregular/pounding heartbeat, headache, lightheadedness, nervousness, trembling, insomnia, nausea.

ADVERSE REACTIONS/TOXIC EFFECTS

Large doses may produce tachycardia, palpitations, lightheadedness, nausea, vomiting. Overdosage in pts >60 yrs: hallucinations, CNS depression, seizures.

NURSING IMPLICATIONS

BASELINE ASSESSMENT:

Question for hypersensitivity to naphazoline or any component of preparation.

PATIENT/FAMILY TEACHING:

Teach correct application (see Ophthalmic/Intranasal Administration). Do not use beyond 72 hrs w/o consulting a physician. Use caution w/activities that require visual acuity. Discontinue and consult physician if the following occur: vision changes, headache, eye pain, floating spots, pain w/light exposure, acute eye redness, insomnia, dizziness, weakness, tremor, irregular heartbeat. Too frequent use may result in rebound effect.

---

naproxen
nah-**prox**-en
(EC-Naprosyn, Naprelan, Naprosyn)

naproxen sodium
(Aleve, Anaprox)

CANADIAN AVAILABILITY:
Anaprox, Apo-Napro, Naprosyn, Naxen, Novonaprox, Synflex

CLASSIFICATION
Nonsteroidal anti-inflammatory

AVAILABILITY (Rx)
Gelcap: 200 mg (OTC). **Tablets:** 200 mg **(OTC)**, 250 mg, 375 mg, 500 mg. **Tablets (delayed-release):** 375 mg, 500 mg. **Oral Suspension:** 125 mg/5 ml.

PHARMACOKINETICS

	ONSET	PEAK	DURATION
PO: (analgesic)	<1 hr	—	Up to 7 hrs
PO: (anti-rheumatic)	Up to 14 days	2–4 wks	—

Completely absorbed from GI tract. Metabolized in liver. Primarily excreted in urine. Half-life: 13 hrs.

ACTION/ *THERAPEUTIC EFFECT*
Produces analgesic and anti-inflammatory effect by inhibiting prostaglandin synthesis, *reducing inflammatory response and intensity of pain stimulus reaching sensory nerve endings.*

USES/ *UNLABELED*
Treatment of acute or long-term mild to moderate pain, primary dysmenorrhea, mild to moderately severe pain, rheumatoid arthritis, juvenile rheumatoid arthritis, osteoarthritis, ankylosing spondylitis, acute gouty arthritis, bursitis, tendinitis. *Treatment of vascular headaches.*

PO ADMINISTRATION
1. Do not crush or break enteric-coated form.
2. May give with food, milk, or antacids if GI distress occurs.

INDICATIONS/DOSAGE/ROUTES
Note: Each 275 or 550 mg tablet of naproxen sodium equals 250 or 500 mg naproxen, respectively.

Rheumatoid arthritis, osteoarthritis, ankylosing spondylitis:
PO: Adults, elderly: 250–500 mg (275–550 mg) 2 times/day or 250 mg (275 mg) in morning and 500 mg (550 mg) in evening. *Naprelan:* 750–1,000 mg daily as single dose.

Juvenile rheumatoid arthritis (naproxen only):
PO: Children: 10 mg/kg/day in 2 divided doses.

Acute gouty arthritis:
PO: Adults, elderly: Initially, 750 (825) mg, then 250 (275) mg q8h until attack subsides. *Naprelan:* Initially, 1,000–1,500 mg, then 1,000 mg/day as single dose until attack subsides.

Mild to moderate pain, dysmenorrhea, bursitis, tendinitis:
PO: Adults, elderly: Initially, 500 (550) mg, then 250 (275) mg q6–8h

as needed. Total daily dose not to exceed 1.25 (1.375) g. *Naprelan:* 1,000 mg/day as single dose.

PRECAUTIONS

CONTRAINDICATIONS: GI ulceration, chronic inflammation of GI tract, bleeding disorders, history of hypersensitivity to aspirin or NSAIDs. **CAUTIONS:** Impaired renal/hepatic function, history of GI tract disease, predisposition to fluid retention. **PREGNANCY/ LACTATION:** Crosses placenta; distributed in breast milk. Avoid use during third trimester (may adversely affect fetal cardiovascular system: premature closing of ductus arteriosus). **Pregnancy Category B**. (Category D if used in 3rd trimester or near delivery.)

INTERACTIONS

DRUG INTERACTIONS: May increase effects of oral anticoagulants, heparin, thrombolytics. May decrease effect of antihypertensives, diuretics. Salicylates, aspirin may increase risk of GI side effects, bleeding. Bone marrow depressants may increase risk of hematologic reactions. May increase concentration, toxicity of lithium. May increase methotrexate toxicity. Probenecid may increase concentration. **ALTERED LAB VALUES:** May prolong bleeding time, alter blood glucose levels. May increase liver function tests. May decrease sodium, uric acid.

SIDE EFFECTS

FREQUENT (3–9%): Nausea, constipation, abdominal cramps/ pain, heartburn, dizziness, headache, drowsiness. **OCCASIONAL (<3%):** Stomatitis, diarrhea, indigestion. **RARE (<1%):** Vomiting, confusion.

ADVERSE REACTIONS/TOXIC EFFECTS

Peptic ulcer, GI bleeding, gastritis, severe hepatic reaction (cholestasis, jaundice) occur rarely. Nephrotoxicity (dysuria, hematuria, proteinuria, nephrotic syndrome) and severe hypersensitivity reaction (fever, chills, bronchospasm) occur rarely.

NURSING IMPLICATIONS

BASELINE ASSESSMENT:

Assess onset, type, location, and duration of pain or inflammation. Inspect appearance of affected joints for immobility, deformities, and skin condition.

INTERVENTION/EVALUATION:

Assist w/ambulation if dizziness occurs. Monitor pattern of daily bowel activity and stool consistency. Check behind medial malleolus for fluid retention (usually first area noted). Evaluate for therapeutic response: relief of pain, stiffness, swelling, increase in joint mobility, reduced joint tenderness, improved grip strength.

PATIENT/FAMILY TEACHING:

Avoid tasks that require alertness, motor skills until response to drug is established. If GI upset occurs, take w/food, milk. Avoid aspirin, alcohol during therapy (increases risk of GI bleeding). Report headache, rash, visual disturbances, weight gain, black stools, persistent headache. Scored tablets may be broken or crushed; swallow enteric-coated form whole.

---

naratriptan
(Amerge)
See Supplement

natamycin
(Natacyn)
See Classification section under:
Antifungals: topical

nedocromil sodium
ned-oh-**crow**-mul
(Tilade)

CANADIAN AVAILABILITY:
Mireze, Tilade

CLASSIFICATION
Anti-inflammatory

AVAILABILITY (Rx)
Inhalation Aerosol: 1.75 mg/activation

PHARMACOKINETICS

	ONSET	PEAK	DURATION
Inhalation	30 min	—	—

Minimal absorption from GI tract after inhalation. Distributed to plasma. Primarily excreted unchanged in urine or via biliary system. Half-life: 1.5–3.3 hrs.

ACTION/*THERAPEUTIC EFFECT*
Prevents activation, release of mediators of inflammation (e.g., histamine, leukotrienes, mast cells, eosinophils, monocytes). *Prevents both early and late asthmatic responses.*

USES/*UNLABELED*
Maintenance therapy for preventing airway inflammation, bronchoconstriction in pts w/mild to moderate bronchial asthma. *Prevents bronchospasm in pts w/reversible obstructive airway disease.*

INHALATION ADMINISTRATION
1. Shake container well, then remove cap from mouthpiece.
2. Position mouthpiece to bottom, tilt head back.
3. Breathe out through mouth to functional volume.
4. Place mouthpiece in mouth or hold 1–2 inches away from open mouth.
5. Activate inhaler while breathing in slowly and deeply.
6. Hold breath 5–10 secs (or as long as possible).
7. Remove inhaler from mouth and breathe out slowly.
8. Wait 1–10 min before second inhalation.

INDICATIONS/DOSAGE/ROUTES
Asthma:
Oral Inhalation: Adults, elderly, children >6 yrs: Two inhalations (4 mg) 4 times/day. May decrease to 3 times/day then 2 times/day as control of asthma occurs. **Maximum:** 16 mg/24 hrs.

PRECAUTIONS
CONTRAINDICATIONS: Hypersensitivity to nedocromil. **CAUTIONS:** Not for reversing acute bronchospasm. **PREGNANCY/LACTATION:** Unknown whether drug crosses placenta or is distributed in breast milk. **Pregnancy Category B.**

INTERACTIONS
DRUG INTERACTIONS: None significant. **ALTERED LAB VALUES:** None significant.

SIDE EFFECTS
FREQUENT (5–10%): Cough, pharyngitis, bronchospasm, headache, unpleasant taste. **OCCASIONAL (1–5%):** Rhinitis, upper respiratory tract infection, abdominal pain, fatigue. **RARE (<1%):** Diarrhea, dizziness.

ADVERSE REACTIONS/TOXIC EFFECTS

None significant.

NURSING IMPLICATIONS
BASELINE ASSESSMENT:

Assess sensitivity to nedocromil.

INTERVENTION/EVALUATION:

Evaluate therapeutic response: reduced dependence on antihistamine, less frequent/less severe asthmatic attacks.

PATIENT/FAMILY TEACHING:

Increase fluid intake (decreases lung secretion viscosity). Must be administered at regular intervals (even when symptom free) to achieve optimal results of therapy. Proper inhalation technique is essential (illustrated pt information leaflet accompanies medication). Do not increase or decrease dosage w/o consulting physician. Unpleasant taste after inhalation may be relieved by rinsing mouth w/water immediately, using sugarless hard candy or gum.

nefazodone hydrochloride

nef-**ah**-zoh-doan
(Serzone)

CANADIAN AVAILABILITY:
Serzone

CLASSIFICATION

Antidepressant

AVAILABILITY (Rx)

Tablets: 100 mg, 150 mg, 200 mg, 250 mg

PHARMACOKINETICS

Rapidly, completely absorbed from GI tract. Food delays absorption. Widely distributed in body tissues, including CNS. Extensively metabolized to active metabolites. Excreted in urine and eliminated in feces. Half-life: 2–4 hrs.

ACTION/ THERAPEUTIC EFFECT

Exact mechanism unknown. Appears to inhibit neuronal uptake of serotonin and norepinephrine, antagonize alpha$_1$-adrenergic receptors, *producing antidepressant effect.*

USES

Treatment of depression exhibited as persistent, prominent dysphoria (occurring nearly every day for at least 2 wks) manifested by 4 of 8 symptoms: change in appetite, change in sleep pattern, increased fatigue, impaired concentration, feelings of guilt or worthlessness, loss of interest in usual activities, psychomotor agitation or retardation, or suicidal tendencies. Maintenance treatment for prevention of relapse of acute depressive episode.

PO ADMINISTRATION

Give w/o regard to meals.

INDICATIONS/DOSAGE/ROUTES

Note: At least 14 days should elapse between discontinuing MAO inhibitors and initiation of nefazodone therapy. At least 7 days should elapse after discontinuing nefazodone and initiation of MAO inhibitor therapy.

Depression, prevention of relapse of acute episode:
PO: Adults: Initially, 200 mg/day, given in two divided doses. Gradually increase dose in increments of 100–200 mg/day on a twice daily schedule, at intervals of at least 1 wk. **Elderly:** Initially, 100 mg/day

on a twice daily schedule. Adjust the rate of subsequent dose titration based on clinical response. **Range:** 300–600 mg/day.

PRECAUTIONS

CONTRAINDICATIONS: Within 14 days of MAO inhibitor ingestion, coadministration w/astemizole, cisapride, or terfenadine therapy, hypersensitivity to nefazodone. **CAUTIONS:** Recent MI, unstable heart disease, hepatic cirrhosis, dehydration, hypovolemia, cerebrovascular disease, history of mania/hypomania, history of seizures. **PREGNANCY/LACTATION:** Not known whether drug crosses placenta or is distributed in breast milk. **Pregnancy Category C.**

INTERACTIONS

DRUG INTERACTIONS: Cisapride may increase risk of arrythmias. May increase concentration, toxicity of alprazolam triazolam (dosage reduction advised). Blocks metabolism, increases concentration, possible cardiovascular effects of astemizole, terfenadine. MAOIs may produce severe reactions (see Adverse Reactions/Toxic Effects). At least 14 days should elapse between discontinuing MAO inhibitors and initiation of nefazodone therapy. At least 7 days should elapse after discontinuing nefazodone and initiation of MAO inhibitor therapy. **ALTERED LAB VALUES:** None significant.

SIDE EFFECTS

Elderly/debilitated experience increased susceptibility to side effects. **FREQUENT:** Headache (36%), dry mouth, somnolence (25%), nausea (22%), dizziness (17%), constipation (14%), insomnia, asthenia (loss of strength, energy) (10%), lightheadedness (10%). **OCCASIONAL:** Dyspepsia, blurred vision (9%), diarrhea, infection (8%), confusion, abnormal vision (7%), pharyngitis (6%), increased appetite (5%), postural hypotension, vasodilation (flushing, feeling of warmth) (4%), peripheral edema, cough, flu syndrome (3%).

ADVERSE REACTIONS/TOXIC EFFECTS

Concurrent MAO inhibitor administration or if time frame between discontinuation and initiation of drug therapy (see Indications/Dosage/Routes) is not followed, serious reactions (hyperthermia, rigidity, myoclonus, extreme agitation, delirium, coma) occur. Coadministration w/astemizole or terfenadine therapy may produce serious cardiovascular abnormalities.

NURSING IMPLICATIONS
BASELINE ASSESSMENT:

Question for history of sensitivity to nefazodone or trazodone, other medication (esp. alprazolam, astemizole, MAOIs, terfenadine, triazolam). Obtain history of cardiovascular or cerebrovascular disease, mania/hypomania, seizures.

INTERVENTION/EVALUATION:

Supervise suicidal risk pt closely during early therapy (as energy level improves, suicide potential increases). Assess appearance, behavior, speech pattern, level of interest, mood. Assist w/ambulation if dizziness, lightheadedness occurs. Monitor stool frequency and consistency.

PATIENT/FAMILY TEACHING:

Maximum therapeutic response may require several weeks of therapy. If orthostatic hypotension occurs, rise very slowly from lying to sitting, sitting to standing position. Dry mouth may be relieved by sugarless gum, sips of tepid water. Report headache, nausea, visual disturbances. Avoid tasks that require alertness, motor skills until response to drug is established. Avoid alcohol.

nelfinavir
(Viracept)
See Supplement
See Classification section under:
Human immunodeficiency virus
(HIV) infection

neomycin sulfate

ne-oh-**my**-sin
(Mycifradin, Myciguent)

FIXED-COMBINATION(S):
W/polymyxin B, an anti-infective **(Neosporin, Neosporin G.U. Irrigant)**; w/polymyxin B and bacitracin, an antibiotic **(Mycitracin, Neosporin, Neo-Polycin)**; w/polymyxin B and hydrocortisone, a steroid **(Cortisporin)**; w/gramicidin, an anti-infective **(Spectrocin)**.

CANADIAN AVAILABILITY:
Mycifradin, Myciguent

CLASSIFICATION

Antibiotic: Aminoglycoside

AVAILABILITY (Rx)

Tablets: 500 mg. **Oral Solution:** 125 mg/5 ml. **Ointment. Cream. Ophthalmic (combination).**

PHARMACOKINETICS

Minimal absorption from GI tract, after ophthalmic, topical administration. Primarily eliminated unchanged in feces. Half-life: 2–3 hrs.

ACTION/*THERAPEUTIC EFFECT*

Irreversibly binds to protein on bacterial ribosome, *interfering in protein synthesis of susceptible microorganisms.* Decreases ammonia production in intestine (inhibits bacteria from ammonia synthesis), *suppressing bacterial growth in bowel.*

USES/*UNLABELED*

Irrigation of wounds, surgical sites, bladder; preop use for intestinal antisepsis; diarrhea due to enteropathogenic *Escherichia coli,* adjunctive therapy for hepatic encephalopathy. *Ophthalmic:* Ointment/solution for superficial eye infections. *Topical:* Prevention or treatment of superficial skin infections. Not for long-term therapy due to associated toxicities. *Topical: Treatment of minor bacterial skin infections, dermal ulcer.*

PO/OPHTHALMIC ADMINISTRATION

Note: Given orally, as retention enema, bladder irrigation, ophthalmic, otic, or topical. Neomycin frequently combined w/corticosteroids, anesthetics, other anti-infectives when applied in topical/ophthalmic form.

PO:

1. Give w/o regard to meals.
2. If GI upset occurs, give w/food or milk.
3. Tablets may be crushed.

OPHTHALMIC:

1. Place finger on lower eyelid and pull out until a pocket is formed between eye and lower lid.
2. Hold dropper above pocket and place correct number of drops ($1/4$–$1/2$ inch ointment) into pocket.
3. Close eye gently.
4. *Solution:* Apply digital pres-

sure to lacrimal sac for 1–2 min (minimizes drainage into nose and throat, reducing risk of systemic effects). *Ointment:* Close eye for 1–2 min, rolling eyeball (increases contact area of drug to eye).

5. Remove excess solution or ointment around eye w/tissue.

INDICATIONS/DOSAGE/ROUTES

Hepatic encephalopathy, adjunctive therapy:
PO: Adults, elderly: 4–12 g/day in 4 divided doses.

Preop intestinal antisepsis:
PO: Adults, elderly: 1 g every hours for 4 doses; then 1 g q4h for balance of 24 hrs, or 1 g at 1, 2, and 11 PM on day before surgery (w/erythromycin).

Continuous bladder irrigation:
Adults, elderly: 1 ml of urogenital concentrate (contains 200,000 units polymyxin B and 57 mg neomycin) added to 1,000 ml 0.9% NaCl given over 24 hrs for up to 10 days (may increase to 2,000 ml/day).

Usual ophthalmic dosage:
Ointment: Adults, elderly, children: Thin strip to conjunctiva q3–4h.
Liquid: Adults, elderly, children: 1 drop to conjunctiva q3–4h.

Usual topical dosage:
Topical: Adults, elderly, children: Apply gently 1–3 times/day up to 5 times/day. Apply no more than once daily in pts w/>20% burns.

PRECAUTIONS

CONTRAINDICATIONS: Hypersensitivity to neomycin, other aminoglycosides (cross-sensitivity). Oral administration contraindicated in intestinal obstruction.
CAUTIONS: Elderly, infants w/ renal insufficiency/immaturity; neuromuscular disorders (potential for respiratory depression), prior hearing loss, vertigo, renal impairment. **PREGNANCY/LACTATION:** Unknown whether drug crosses placenta or is distributed in breast milk. **Pregnancy Category C.**

INTERACTIONS

DRUG INTERACTIONS: If significant systemic absorption occurs, may increase nephrotoxicity, ototoxicity w/aminoglycosides, other nephrotoxic, ototoxic medications. **ALTERED LAB VALUES:** None significant.

SIDE EFFECTS

FREQUENT: *Systemic:* Nausea, vomiting, diarrhea, irritation of mouth/rectal area. *Ophthalmic:* Hypersensitivity (itching, rash, redness, swelling). *Ophthalmic/Topical:* Itching, redness, swelling, rash. **OCCASIONAL:** *Ophthalmic:* Itching, burning, redness. **RARE:** *Systemic:* Malabsorption syndrome, neuromuscular blockade (drowsiness, weakness, difficulty breathing).

ADVERSE REACTIONS/TOXIC EFFECTS

Nephrotoxicity (evidenced by increased BUN and serum creatinine, decreased creatinine clearance) may be reversible if drug stopped at first sign of symptoms; irreversible ototoxicity (tinnitus, dizziness, ringing/roaring in ears, reduced hearing) and neurotoxicity (headache, dizziness, lethargy, tremors, visual disturbances) occur occasionally. Risk is greater with higher dosages, prolonged therapy, or if preparation applied directly to mucosa (particularly extensive areas). Severe respiratory depression, anaphylaxis occur rarely. Superinfections, particularly w/fungi, may result from bacterial imbalance following administration via any route.

NURSING IMPLICATIONS

BASELINE ASSESSMENT:

Dehydration must be treated before aminoglycoside therapy. Establish pt's baseline hearing acuity before beginning therapy. Cumulative effects may occur when given via more than one route. Question for history of allergies, esp. aminoglycosides. Obtain specimens for culture, sensitivity before giving first dose (therapy may begin before results are known).

INTERVENTION/EVALUATION:

Monitor I&O (maintain hydration), urinalysis (casts, RBCs, WBCs, decrease in specific gravity). Monitor results of peak/trough blood tests. Be alert to ototoxic and neurotoxic symptoms (see Adverse Reactions/ Toxic Effects). Assess for rash (*ophthalmic*—assess for redness, burning, itching, tearing; *topical*—assess for redness, itching). Be alert for superinfection, particularly genital/anal pruritus, changes of oral mucosa, diarrhea. When treating pts w/neuromuscular disorders, assess respiratory response carefully.

PATIENT/FAMILY TEACHING:

Continue antibiotic for full length of treatment. Space doses evenly. Notify physician in event of hearing, visual, balance, urinary problems, even after therapy is completed. Do not take other medication w/o consulting physician. Lab tests are an essential part of therapy. *Ophthalmic:* Blurred vision or tearing may occur briefly after application. Contact physician if tearing, redness, irritation continue. *Topical:* Cleanse area gently before application; report redness, itching.

---

neostigmine bromide

nee-oh-**stig**-meen
(Prostigmin [oral])

neostigmine methylsulfate

(Prostigmin [parenteral])

CANADIAN AVAILABILITY:
Prostigmin

CLASSIFICATION

Anticholinesterase agent

AVAILABILITY (Rx)

Tablets: 15 mg. **Injection:** 1:1,000, 1:2,000, 1:4,000.

PHARMACOKINETICS

	ONSET	PEAK	DURATION
PO	2–4 hrs	—	—
IM	10–30 min	20–30 min	2.5–4 hrs

Poorly absorbed from GI tract. Rapid absorption following IM administration. Metabolized in liver, plasma. Primarily excreted in urine. Half-life: 24–79 min.

ACTION / *THERAPEUTIC EFFECT*

Prevents destruction of acetylcholine by attaching to enzyme, anticholinesterase. *Improves intestinal/skeletal muscle tone, increases secretions, salivation.*

USES

Improvement of muscle strength in control of myasthenia gravis, to diagnose myasthenia gravis, prevention/treatment of postop distention and urinary retention, as antidote for reversal of effects of nondepolarizing neuromuscular blocking agents after surgery.

STORAGE / HANDLING

Store parenteral, oral form at room temperature.

PO / SUBQ / IM / IV ADMINISTRATION

PO:

For those w/difficulty chewing, give dose 30–45 min before meals, preferably w/milk (drug produces fewer cholinergic effects if taken w/milk or food).

SubQ/IM/IV:

Note: May be given undiluted. Do not add to IV solutions.

1. When given as curariform block antidote following surgery (unless tachycardia is present), give 0.6–1.2 mg atropine concurrently w/neostigmine to prevent bradycardia.

2. If bradycardia is present, increase pulse rate to 80/min w/atropine before administering neostigmine.

3. Administer IV very slowly (0.5 mg or less over 1 min).

INDICATIONS / DOSAGE / ROUTES

Note: Dosage, frequency of administration dependent on daily clinical pt response (remissions, exacerbations, physical and emotional stress).

Myasthenia gravis:
PO: Adults, elderly: Initially, 15–30 mg 3–4 times/day. Increase dose gradually until therapeutic response achieved. **Usual maintenance dose:** 150 mg/day w/range of 15–375 mg. **Children:** Initially, 2 mg/kg/day divided q3–4h. **Neonatal:** 1–4 mg q2–3h.
SubQ/IM/IV: Adults: 0.5–2.5 mg as needed. **Neonatal:** 0.1–0.2 mg SubQ or 0.03 mg/kg IM q2–4h.

Diagnosis of myasthenia gravis:
Note: Discontinue all anticholinesterase therapy at least 8 hrs before testing. Give 0.011 mg/kg atropine sulfate IV simultaneously w/neostigmine or IM 30 min before administering neostigmine (prevents adverse effects).
IM: Adults, elderly: 0.022 mg/kg. If cholinergic reaction occurs, discontinue tests and administer 0.4–0.6 mg or more atropine sulfate IV. **Children:** 0.025–0.04 mg/kg IM preceded by atropine sulfate 0.011 mg/kg SubQ.

Prevention of postop urinary retention:
SubQ/IM: Adults, elderly: 0.25 mg q4–6h for 2–3 days.

Postop distention, urinary retention:
SubQ/IM: Adults, elderly: 0.5–1 mg. Catheterize if voiding does not occur within 1 hr. After voiding, continue 0.5 mg q3h for 5 injections.

Reversal of neuromuscular blockade:
IV: Adults, elderly: 0.5–2.5 mg given slowly.

PRECAUTIONS

CONTRAINDICATIONS: Concurrent use of high doses of halothane, cyclopropane, mechanical GI or GU obstruction, peritonitis, doubtful bowel viability. **CAUTIONS:** Bronchial asthma, bradycardia, epilepsy, coronary occlusion, vagotonia, hyperthyroidism, cardiac arrhythmias, peptic ulcer. **PREGNANCY/LACTATION:** Transient muscular weakness occurs in 10–20% of neonates born to mothers treated w/drug therapy for myasthenia gravis during pregnancy. May produce uterine irritability, induce premature labor if administered IV near term. **Pregnancy Category C**.

INTERACTIONS

DRUG INTERACTIONS: Anticholinergics reverse/prevent effects. Cholinesterase inhibitors may increase toxicity. Antagonizes neuromuscular blocking agents. Quinidine, procainamide may antagonize action. **ALTERED LAB VALUES:** None significant.

SIDE EFFECTS

FREQUENT: Muscarinic effects (diarrhea, increased sweating/watering of mouth, nausea, vomiting, stomach cramps/pain). **OCCASIONAL:** Muscarinic effects (increased frequency/urge to urinate, increased bronchial secretions, unusually small pupils/watering of eyes).

ADVERSE REACTIONS/TOXIC EFFECTS

Overdose produces a cholinergic reaction manifested as abdominal discomfort/cramping, nausea, vomiting, diarrhea, flushing, feeling of warmth/heat about face, excessive salivation and sweating, lacrimation, pallor, bradycardia/tachycardia, hypotension, urinary urgency, blurred vision, bronchospasm, pupillary contraction, involuntary muscular contraction visible under the skin (fasciculation).

Overdose may also produce *cholinergic crisis,* manifested by increasingly severe muscle weakness (appears first in muscles involving chewing, swallowing, followed by muscular weakness of shoulder girdle and upper extremities), respiratory muscle paralysis followed by pelvic girdle and leg muscle paralysis. Requires a withdrawal of all cholinergic drugs and immediate use of 0.6–1.2 mg atropine sulfate IV for adults, 0.01 mg/kg in infants, children under 12 yrs.

Myasthenic crisis (due to underdose) also produces extreme muscle weakness but requires a *more* intensive drug therapy program (differentiation between the two crises is imperative for accurate treatment). Weakness beginning 1 hr after drug administration suggests overdosage; weakness occurring 3 hrs or more after administration suggests underdosage or resistance to anticholinesterase drugs. Extremely high doses may produce CNS stimulation followed by CNS depression.

NURSING IMPLICATIONS
BASELINE ASSESSMENT:

Larger doses should be given at time of greatest fatigue. Assess muscle strength before testing for diagnosis of myasthenia gravis, as well as after drug administration. Avoid large doses in those w/megacolon or reduced GI motility. Have tissues readily available at pt's bedside.

INTERVENTION/EVALUATION:

Monitor vital capacity during myasthenia gravis testing or if dosage is increased. Distinguish carefully between cholinergic crisis and myasthenic crisis (see Adverse Reactions/Toxic Effects). Monitor for therapeutic response to medication (increased muscle strength, decreased fatigue, improved chewing, swallowing functions).

PATIENT/FAMILY TEACHING:

Report nausea, vomiting, diarrhea, sweating, increased salivary secretions, irregular heartbeat, muscle weakness, severe abdominal pain, or difficulty in breathing.

netilmicin sulfate

neh-till-**my**-sin
(Netromycin)

CANADIAN AVAILABILITY:
Netromycin

CLASSIFICATION

Antibiotic: Aminoglycoside

AVAILABILITY (Rx)

Injection: 100 mg/ml

PHARMACOKINETICS

Rapid, complete absorption after IM administration. Widely distributed (does not cross blood-brain barrier, low concentrations in CSF). Excreted unchanged in urine. Removed by hemodialysis. Half-life: 2–4 hrs (increased in decreased renal function, neonates; decreased in cystic fibrosis, burn or febrile pts).

ACTION/ *THERAPEUTIC EFFECT*

Irreversibly binds to protein on bacterial ribosome, *interfering in protein synthesis of susceptible microorganisms.*

USES

Treatment of skin/skin structure, bone, joint, lower respiratory tract, intra-abdominal, complicated urinary tract infections; burns, septicemia.

STORAGE/HANDLING

Store parenteral form at room temperature. Solutions appear clear, colorless to pale yellow. May be discolored by light, air (does not affect potency). Intermittent IV infusion (piggyback) stable for 72 hrs at room temperature, or refrigerated. Discard if precipitate forms.

IM/IV ADMINISTRATION

Note: Coordinate peak and trough lab draws w/administration times.

IM:

To minimize discomfort, give deep IM slowly. Less painful if injected into gluteus maximus rather than lateral aspect of thigh.

IV:

1. Dilute with 50–200 ml 5% dextrose, 0.9% NaCl, or other compatible IV fluid.
2. Infuse over 30–60 min for adults, older children, and over 60–120 min for infants, young children.
3. Alternating IV sites, use large veins to reduce risk of phlebitis.

INDICATIONS/DOSAGE/ROUTES

Note: Space doses evenly around the clock. Dosage based on ideal body weight. Peak, trough serum concentrations determined periodically to maintain desired serum concentrations (minimizes risk of toxicity). *Recommended peak level:* 6–12 mcg/ml; *trough level:* 0.5–2 mcg/ml.

Complicated urinary tract infections:
IM/IV: Adults, elderly: 3–4 mg/kg/day in divided doses q12h.

Septicemia, skin/skin structure, intra-abdominal, lower respiratory infections:
IM/IV: Adults, elderly: 4–6.5 mg/kg/day in divided doses q8–12h. **Children >6 wks:** 5.5–8 mg/kg/day in divided doses q8–12h. **Neonates:** 4–6.5 mg/kg/day in divided doses q12h.

Dosage in renal impairment:
Dose and/or frequency is modified based on degree of renal impairment, serum concentration of drug. After loading dose of 1.3–2.2 mg/kg, maintenance doses, intervals are based on serum creatinine or creatinine clearance.

PRECAUTIONS

CONTRAINDICATIONS: Hypersensitivity to netilmicin, other aminoglycosides (cross-sensitivity). Sulfite sensitivity may result in anaphylaxis, esp. in asthmatics. **CAUTIONS:** Elderly, neonates w/renal insufficiency/immaturity; neuromuscular disorders (potential for respiratory depression), prior hearing loss, vertigo, renal impairment. **PREGNANCY/LACTATION:** Readily crosses placenta; distributed in breast milk. May produce fetal nephrotoxicity. **Pregnancy Category D**.

INTERACTIONS

DRUG INTERACTIONS: Other aminoglycosides, nephrotoxic, ototoxic-producing medications may increase toxicity. May increase effects of neuromuscular blocking agents. **ALTERED LAB VALUES:** May increase BUN, SGPT (ALT), SGOT (AST), bilirubin, creatinine, LDH concentrations; may decrease serum calcium, magnesium, potassium, sodium concentrations.

SIDE EFFECTS

OCCASIONAL: Pain, induration at IM injection site; phlebitis, thrombophlebitis w/IV administration; hypersensitivity reactions: Rash, fever, urticaria, pruritus. **RARE:** Headache.

ADVERSE REACTIONS/TOXIC EFFECTS

Nephrotoxicity (evidenced by increased BUN and serum creatinine, decreased creatinine clearance) may be reversible if drug stopped at first sign of symptoms; irreversible ototoxicity (tinnitus, dizziness, ringing/roaring in ears, reduced hearing) and neurotoxicity (headache, dizziness, lethargy, tremors, visual disturbances) occur occasionally. Risk is greater w/higher dosages, prolonged therapy. Superinfections, particularly w/fungi, may result from bacterial imbalance.

NURSING IMPLICATIONS

BASELINE ASSESSMENT:

Dehydration must be treated before aminoglycoside therapy. Establish pt's baseline hearing acuity before beginning therapy. Question for history of allergies, esp. aminoglycosides, sulfite. Obtain specimens for culture, sensitivity before giving first dose (therapy may begin before results are known).

INTERVENTION/EVALUATION:

Monitor I&O (maintain hydration), urinalysis (casts, RBCs, WBCs, decrease in specific gravity). Monitor results of peak/trough blood tests. Be alert to ototoxic and neurotoxic symptoms (see Adverse Reactions/Toxic Effects). Check IM injection site for pain, induration. Evaluate IV site for phlebitis (heat, pain, red streaking over vein). Assess for rash. Assess for superinfection, particularly genital/anal pruritus, changes of oral mucosa, diarrhea.

PATIENT/FAMILY TEACHING:

Continue antibiotic for full length of treatment. Space doses evenly. Discomfort may occur with IM injection. Notify physician in event of headache, shortness of breath, dizziness, hearing, urinary problem even after therapy is completed. Do not take other medication w/o consulting physician. Lab tests are an essential part of therapy.

nevirapine

neh-**vear**-ah-peen
(Viramune)

CLASSIFICATION

Antiviral

AVAILABILITY (Rx)

Tablets: 200 mg. **Oral Suspension:** 50 mg/5 ml.

PHARMACOKINETICS

Readily absorbed following oral administration (unaffected by food). Widely distributed. Extensively metabolized in liver; primarily excreted in urine.

ACTION/THERAPEUTIC EFFECT

Binds directly to virus type 1 (HIV-1) reverse transcriptase (RT), blocking RNA and DNA-dependent DNA polymerase activity (changes the shape of RT enzyme), *slowing HIV replication, reducing progression of HIV infection.*

USES/UNLABELED

Used in combination w/nucleoside analogues or protease inhibitors for treatment of HIV-1 infected adults who have experienced clinical and immunologic deterioration. *Reduces risk of transmitting HIV from infected mother to newborn.*

PO ADMINISTRATION

May give w/o regard to meals.

INDICATIONS/DOSAGE/ROUTES

Note: Always administer nevirapine in combination with at least one additional antiretroviral agent (resistant HIV virus appears rapidly when nevirapine is given as monotherapy).

HIV-1 infection:
PO: Adults: 200 mg daily for 14 days (reduces risk of rash). **Maintenance:** 200 mg twice daily in combination w/nucleoside analogue antiretroviral agents. **Children, 2 mos–8 yrs:** 4 mg/kg once daily for 14 days; then 7 mg/kg 2 times/day. **Children >8 yrs:** 4 mg/kg once daily for 14 days; then 4 mg/kg 2 times/day. **Maximum:** 400 mg/day

PRECAUTIONS

CONTRAINDICATIONS: None significant. **CAUTIONS:** Renal or hepatic function impairment. **PREGNANCY/LACTATION:** Drug crosses placenta, distributed in breast milk. Breast-feeding not recommended (possibility of HIV transmission). **Pregnancy Category C.**

INTERACTIONS

DRUG INTERACTIONS: May decrease protease inhibitors, oral contraceptives, plasma concentration. **ALTERED LAB VALUES:** May significantly increase SGPT (ALT), SGOT (AST), bilirubin, GGT. May significantly decrease Hgb, platelets, neutrophil count.

SIDE EFFECTS

FREQUENT (3–8%): Rash (may become severe), fever, headache, nausea. **OCCASIONAL (1–3%):** Stomatitis (erythema/irritation of oral mucous membranes, gingivitis, glossitis). **RARE (<1%):** Paresthesia, myalgia, abdominal pain.

ADVERSE REACTIONS/TOXIC EFFECTS

Rash may become severe and life threatening. Hepatitis occurs rarely.

NURSING IMPLICATIONS
BASELINE ASSESSMENT:

Offer emotional support. Establish baseline lab values, esp. liver function tests, prior to initiating therapy and at intervals during therapy. Obtain medication history (esp. use of oral contraceptives).

INTERVENTION/EVALUATION:

Closely monitor for evidence of rash (usually appears on trunk, face, and extremities; occurs within first 6 wks of drug initiation). Observe for rash accompanied by fever, blistering, oral lesions, conjunctivitis, swelling, muscle or joint aches, general malaise. Monitor clinical chemistry tests for marked laboratory abnormalities. Assess for fever, headache, nausea.

PATIENT/FAMILY TEACHING:

If nevirapine therapy is missed for more than 7 days, restart by using one 200 mg tablet daily for first 14 days, followed by one 200 mg tablet twice daily. Continue therapy for full length of treatment. Doses should be evenly spaced. Do not take any medications w/o consulting physician. Nevirapine is not a cure for HIV infection, nor does it reduce risk of transmission to others. If rash appears, contact physician before continuing therapy.

niacin, nicotinic acid
(Niaspan, Nicobid, Nico-400, Nicotinex)

CLASSIFICATION

Antihyperlipoproteinemic

AVAILABILITY (OTC)

Tablets: 25 mg, 50 mg, 100 mg, 250 mg, 500 mg. **Tablets (timed-release):** 250 mg, 500 mg, 750 mg. **Capsules (timed-release):** 125 mg, 250 mg, 300 mg, 400 mg, 500 mg. **Elixir:** 50 mg/5 ml. **Injection:** (Rx) 100 mg/ml.

PHARMACOKINETICS

Readily absorbed from GI tract. Widely distributed. Metabolized in liver. Primarily excreted in urine. Half-life: 45 min.

ACTION/ *THERAPEUTIC EFFECT*

Inhibits free fatty acid release in fat tissue, decreases rate of VLDL, LDL synthesis in liver, increases lipoprotein lipase activity. Component of coenzymes that are necessary for *lipid metabolism, tissue respiration, and glycogenolysis. Lowers serum cholesterol and triglycerides (decreases LDL, VLDL, increases HDL).*

USES

Adjunct to diet therapy to decrease elevated serum cholesterol and triglyceride concentrations (elevated LDL, VLDL in treatment of Type II, III, IV, or V hyperlipoproteinemia). Extended release tablets: Increase HDL cholesterol. Prevention and treatment of vitamin B_3 deficiency states (i.e., pellagra).

PO ADMINISTRATION

Preferably given w/or after meals (decreases GI upset).

INDICATIONS/DOSAGE/ROUTES

Hyperlipoproteinemia:
PO: Adults, elderly: Initially, 100 mg 3 times/day. Increase by 300 mg/day at 4–7 day intervals. **Maintenance:** 1–2 g 3 times/day. **Maximum:** 8 g/day. **Extended-Release:** Initially, 500 mg/day. **Maintenance:** 1,000–2,000 mg/day at bedtime.

Nutritional supplement:
PO: Adults, elderly: 10–20 mg/day.

PRECAUTIONS

CONTRAINDICATIONS: Hypersensitivity to niacin or tartrazine (frequently seen in pts sensitive to aspirin), active peptic ulcer, severe hypotension, hepatic dysfunction, arterial hemorrhaging. **CAUTIONS:** Diabetes mellitus, gallbladder disease, gout, history of jaundice or liver disease. **PREGNANCY/LACTATION:** Not recommended for use during pregnancy/lactation. Distributed in breast milk. **Pregnancy Category A.** (Category C if used in doses above RDA.)

INTERACTIONS

DRUG INTERACTIONS: Lovastatin, pravastatin, simvastatin may increase risk of rhabdomyolysis and acute renal failure. **ALTERED LAB VALUES:** May increase uric acid.

SIDE EFFECTS

FREQUENT: Flushing (esp. of face, neck) occurring within 20 min of administration and lasting for 30–60 min, GI upset, pruritus. **OCCASIONAL:** Dizziness, hypotension, headache, blurred vision, burning or tingling of skin, flatulence, nausea, vomiting, diarrhea. **RARE:** Hyperglycemia, glycosuria, rash, hyperpigmentation, dry skin.

ADVERSE REACTIONS/TOXIC EFFECTS

Cardiac arrhythmias, particularly in those w/CHD, occur rarely.

NURSING IMPLICATIONS
BASELINE ASSESSMENT:

Question for history of hypersensitivity to niacin, tartrazine, or aspirin. Assess baselines: cholesterol, triglyceride, blood glucose, liver function tests.

INTERVENTION/EVALUATION:

Evaluate flushing and degree of discomfort. Check for headache, dizziness, blurred vision. Monitor B/P at least 2 times/day. Assess food tolerance. Determine pattern of bowel activity. Monitor liver function test results, cholesterol and triglyceride. Check blood glucose levels carefully in those on insulin or oral antihyperglycemics. Assess skin for rash, dryness.

PATIENT/FAMILY TEACHING:

Take w/meals to decrease GI upset. Follow special diet (important part of treatment). Do not alter dosage. Consult physician before taking other medication. In event of new symptoms, notify physician. If dizziness occurs, avoid sudden posture changes and activities that require steady/alert response. Flushing may decrease w/continued therapy; however, discuss considerable discomfort w/ physician.

nicardipine hydrochloride

nigh-**car**-dih-peen
(Cardene, Cardene SR)

CANADIAN AVAILABILITY:
Cardene

CLASSIFICATION

Calcium channel blocker

AVAILABILITY (Rx)

Capsules: 20 mg, 30 mg. **Capsules (sustained-release):** 30 mg, 45 mg, 60 mg. **Injection:** 2.5 mg/ml.

PHARMACOKINETICS

	ONSET	PEAK	DURATION
PO	—	1–2 hrs	8 hrs

Rapidly, completely absorbed from GI tract. Undergoes first-pass metabolism in liver. Metabolized in liver. Primarily excreted in urine. Half-life: 8.6 hrs.

ACTION/ THERAPEUTIC EFFECT

Inhibits calcium ion movement across cell membrane, depressing contraction of cardiac and vascular smooth muscle. *Increases heart rate, cardiac output. Decreases systemic vascular resistance, B/P.*

USES/ UNLABELED

Oral: Treatment of chronic stable (effort-associated) angina or essential hypertension. *Sustained-release:* Treatment of essential hypertension. *Parenteral:* Short-term treatment of hypertension when oral therapy not feasible or desirable. *Treatment of vasospastic angina, Raynaud's phenomenon, subarachnoid hemorrhage, associated neurologic deficits.*

STORAGE/ HANDLING

Store oral, parenteral forms at room temperature. Diluted IV solution is stable for 24 hrs at room temperature.

PO/IV ADMINISTRATION

PO:

1. Do not crush or break oral, sustained-release capsules.
2. May take w/o regard to food.

IV:

1. Dilute each 25 mg ampule w/240 ml 5% dextrose, 0.9% NaCl, or other compatible IV to provide a concentration of 1 mg/10 ml.
2. Change IV site q12h if administered peripherally.

INDICATIONS/ DOSAGE/ ROUTES

Chronic stable angina:
PO: **Adults, elderly:** Initially, 20 mg 3 times/day. **Range:** 20–40 mg 3 times/day.

Essential hypertension:
PO: **Adults, elderly:** Initially, 20 mg 3 times/day. **Range:** 20–40 mg 3 times/day.
Sustained-release: Adults, elderly: Initially, 30 mg 2 times/day. **Range:** 30–60 mg 2 times/day.

Dosage in liver impairment:
Initially, 20 mg 2 times/day, then titrate.

Dosage in renal impairment:

Initially, 20 mg q8h (30 mg 2 times/day sustained-release), then titrate.

Usual parenteral dosage: Substitute for oral nicardipine:
IV: Adults, elderly: 0.5 mg/hr (20 mg q8h); 1.2 mg/hr (30 mg q8h); 2.2 mg/hr (40 mg q8h).

Drug-free pt:
IV: Adults, elderly: *(Gradual B/P decrease):* Initially, 5 mg/hr. May increase by 2.5 mg/hr q15 min. *(Rapid B/P decrease):* Initially, 5 mg/hr. May increase by 2.5 mg/hr q5 min. **Maximum:** 15 mg/hr until desired B/P attained.
Note: After B/P goal achieved, decrease rate to 3 mg/hr.

Changing to oral antihypertensive therapy:

Begin 1 hr after IV discontinued; for nicardipine, give first dose 1 hr before discontinuing IV.

PRECAUTIONS

CONTRAINDICATIONS: Severe hypotension, advanced aortic stenosis. **CAUTIONS:** Impaired renal, hepatic function. **PREGNANCY/LACTATION:** Unknown whether distributed in breast milk. **Pregnancy Category C.**

INTERACTIONS

DRUG INTERACTIONS: Beta blockers may have additive effect. May increase digoxin concentration. Procainamide, quinidine may increase risk of QT interval prolongation. Hypokalemia-producing agents may increase risk of arrhythmias. **ALTERED LAB VALUES:** None significant.

SIDE EFFECTS

FREQUENT (7–10%): Headache, flushing of skin, peripheral edema, lightheadedness, dizziness. **OCCASIONAL (3–6%):** Asthenia (loss of strength, energy), palpitations, angina, tachycardia. **RARE (<2%):** Nausea, abdominal cramps, dyspepsia, dry mouth, rash.

ADVERSE REACTIONS/TOXIC EFFECTS

Marked hypotension, CHF.

NURSING IMPLICATIONS
BASELINE ASSESSMENT:

Concurrent therapy of sublingual nitroglycerin may be used for relief of anginal pain. Record onset, type (sharp, dull, squeezing), radiation, location, intensity, and duration of anginal pain, and precipitating factors (exertion, emotional stress).

INTERVENTION/EVALUATION:

Monitor B/P during and after IV infusion. Assist w/ambulation if dizziness occurs. Assess for peripheral edema behind medial malleolus (sacral area in bedridden pts). Assess skin for facial flushing, dermatitis, rash. Question for asthenia, headache. Monitor liver enzyme results. Assess EKG, pulse for tachycardia, palpitations.

PATIENT/FAMILY TEACHING:

Do not abruptly discontinue medication. Compliance w/therapy regimen is essential to control anginal pain. To avoid hypotensive effect, rise slowly from lying to sitting position; wait momentarily before standing. Avoid tasks that require alertness, motor skills until response to drug is established. Contact physician/nurse if irregular heartbeat, shortness of breath, pronounced dizziness, or nausea occurs.

nicotine polacrilex

nick-oh-teen
(Nicorette)

nicotine transdermal system

(Habitrol, Nicoderm, Nicotrol)

CANADIAN AVAILABILITY:
Habitrol, Nicoderm, Nicorette, Nicotrol

CLASSIFICATION

Smoking deterrent

AVAILABILITY (OTC)

Transdermal: Habitrol (Rx): 7 mg/day, 14 mg/day, 21 mg/day. **Nicoderm (OTC):** 7 mg/day, 14 mg/day, 21 mg/day. **Nicotrol (Rx):** 5 mg/day, 10 mg/day; **(OTC)** 15 mg/day.

Chewing Gum (OTC): 2 mg, 4 mg squares

Nasal Spray (Rx). Inhaler (Rx).

PHARMACOKINETICS

Not absorbed from GI tract. Absorption increased from buccal mucosa, well absorbed after topical administration. Metabolized in liver. Primarily excreted in urine. Half-life: 1–2 hrs.

ACTION

Nicotine, a cholinergic-receptor agonist, produces autonomic effects by binding to acetylcholine receptors. Produces both stimulating and depressant effects on peripheral and central nervous systems; respiratory stimulant; low amounts increase heart rate, B/P; high doses may decrease B/P; may increase motor activity of GI smooth muscle. Nicotine produces psychological and physical dependence.

USES

An alternative, less potent form of nicotine (w/o tar, carbon monoxide, carcinogenic substances of tobacco) used as part of a smoking cessation program.

TRANSDERMAL/GUM ADMINISTRATION

TRANSDERMAL:

1. Apply promptly upon removal from protective pouch (prevents evaporation, loss of nicotine). Use only intact pouch.
2. Apply only once/day to hairless, clean, dry skin on upper body or outer arm.
3. Replace daily at different sites; do not use same site within 7 days; do not use same patch >24 hrs.
4. Wash hands after applying patch. Wash w/water alone (soap may increase nicotine absorption).
5. Discard used patch by folding patch in half (sticky side together), placing in pouch of new patch, and throwing away in such a way as to prevent child/pet accessibility.

GUM:

1. Do not swallow.
2. Chew 1 piece whenever urge to smoke present.
3. Chew slowly/intermittently for 30 min.
4. Chew until distinctive nicotine taste (peppery) or slight tingling in mouth perceived, then stop; when tingling almost gone (about 1 min) repeat chewing procedure (this allows constant slow buccal absorption).
5. Too rapid chewing may cause excessive release of nicotine, resulting in adverse effects similar to oversmoking (e.g., nausea, throat irritation).

INHALER:

    1. Insert cartridge into mouthpiece.

    2. Vigorously puff for 20 min.

INDICATIONS/DOSAGE/ROUTES

Smoking deterrent:
Note: Individualize dose; stop smoking immediately.
Transdermal: Adults, elderly: (Habitrol/Nicoderm): 21 mg/day for 6 wks; then 14 mg/day for 2 wks; then 7 mg/day for 2 wks.
Gum: Adults, elderly: Usually, 10–12 pieces/day. **Maximum:** 30 pieces/day.
Nasal Spray: Adults, elderly: (1 dose = 2 sprays = 1 mg) 1–2 doses/hr up to 40 doses/day.
Inhaler: Adults, elderly: Puff on nicotine cartridge mouthpiece for about 20 min as needed.

PRECAUTIONS

CONTRAINDICATIONS: During immediate post-MI period, life-threatening arrhythmias, severe or worsening angina, active temporomandibular joint disease. **CAUTIONS:** Hyperthyroidism, pheochromocytoma, insulin-dependent diabetes mellitus, severe renal impairment, eczematous dermatitis, oral or pharyngeal inflammation, esophagitis, peptic ulcer (delays healing in peptic ulcer disease). **PREGNANCY/LACTATION:** Passes freely into breast milk. Use of cigarettes or nicotine gum associated w/decrease in fetal breathing movements. **Pregnancy Category X:** Nicotine polacrilex; **Pregnancy Category D:** Transdermal nicotine.

INTERACTIONS

DRUG INTERACTIONS: Smoking cessation may increase effects of beta-adrenergic blockers, bronchodilators (e.g., theophylline), insulin, propoxyphene. **ALTERED LAB VALUES:** None significant.

SIDE EFFECTS

FREQUENT: Hiccups, nausea. *Gum:* Mouth or throat soreness, nausea, hiccups. *Transdermal:* Erythema, pruritus, burning at application site. **OCCASIONAL:** Eructation, GI upset, dry mouth, insomnia, sweating, irritability. *Gum:* Hiccups, hoarseness. *Inhaler:* Mouth/throat irritation, cough. **RARE:** Dizziness, muscle/joint pain.

ADVERSE REACTIONS/TOXIC EFFECTS

    Overdose produces palpitations, tachyarrhythmias, convulsions, depression, confusion, profuse diaphoresis, hypotension, rapid/weak pulse, difficulty breathing. Lethal dose, adults: 40–60 mg. Death results from respiratory paralysis.

NURSING IMPLICATIONS

BASELINE ASSESSMENT:

    Screen, evaluate those w/coronary heart disease (history of MI, angina pectoris), serious cardiac arrhythmias, Buerger's disease, Prinzmetal's variant angina.

INTERVENTION/EVALUATION:

    If increase in cardiovascular symptoms occurs, discontinue use. Assess all symptoms carefully w/regard to method of medication (see Side Effects).

PATIENT/FAMILY TEACHING:

    Give instruction sheet to pt; review proper application and disposal of transdermal system. Gradually withdraw or stop nicotine gum usage <3 mos, transdermal nicotine after 4–8 wks of use, progressively decreasing dose q2–4 wks. Do not eat or drink anything during or immediately before nicotine gum use (reduces salivary pH). Use contraceptive measures during therapy.

nifedipine

nye-**fed**-ih-peen
(Adalat, Procardia)

CANADIAN AVAILABILITY:
Adalat, Apo-Nifed, Novonifedin

CLASSIFICATION

Calcium channel blocker

AVAILABILITY (Rx)

Capsules: 10 mg, 20 mg.
Tablets (extended-release): 30 mg, 60 mg, 90 mg.

PHARMACOKINETICS

	ONSET	PEAK	DURATION
PO	20 min	30–60 min	—

Rapidly, completely absorbed from GI tract. Undergoes first-pass metabolism in liver. Metabolized in liver. Primarily excreted in urine. Half-life: 2–5 hrs.

ACTION/ *THERAPEUTIC EFFECT*

Inhibits calcium ion movement across cell membrane, depressing contraction of cardiac and vascular smooth muscle. *Increases heart rate, cardiac output. Decreases systemic vascular resistance, B/P.*

USES/ *UNLABELED*

Treatment of angina due to coronary artery spasm (Prinzmetal's variant angina), chronic stable angina (effort-associated angina). *Extended-release:* Treatment of essential hypertension. *Treatment of Raynaud's phenomena.*

PO/SUBLINGUAL ADMINISTRATION

PO:

1. Do not crush or break film-coated tablet or sustained-release capsule.
2. May give w/o regard to meals.
3. Grapefruit juice may alter absorption.

SUBLINGUAL:

Capsule must be punctured, chewed, and/or squeezed to express liquid into mouth.

INDICATIONS/DOSAGE/ROUTES

Note: May give 10–20 mg sublingual as needed for acute attacks of angina.

Prinzmetal's variant angina, chronic stable angina:
PO: Adults, elderly: Initially, 10 mg 3 times/day. Increase at 7–14 day intervals. **Maintenance:** 10 mg 3 times/day up to 30 mg 4 times/day.
Extended-release: Adults, elderly: Initially, 30–60 mg/day. **Maintenance:** Up to 120 mg/day.

Hypertension:
Extended-release: Adults, elderly: Initially, 30–60 mg/day. **Maintenance:** Up to 120 mg/day.

PRECAUTIONS

CONTRAINDICATIONS: Severe hypotension, advanced aortic stenosis. **CAUTIONS:** Impaired renal/hepatic function. **PREGNANCY/LACTATION:** Insignificant amount distributed in breast milk. **Pregnancy Category C**.

INTERACTIONS

DRUG INTERACTIONS: Beta blockers may have additive effect. May increase digoxin concentration. Hypokalemia-producing agents may increase risk of arrhythmias. **ALTERED LAB VALUES:** May cause positive ANA, direct Coombs' test.

SIDE EFFECTS

FREQUENT (>10%): Peripheral edema (swelling of ankles/feet), headache, flushed skin, nausea, dizziness. **OCCASIONAL (3–10%):** Constipation, unusual tiredness, muscle cramps/pain, shortness of breath, wheezing, cough, palpitations, nasal congestion. **RARE (<3%):** Allergic reaction (rash, hives), arthritis, gingival hyperplasia.

ADVERSE REACTIONS/TOXIC EFFECTS

May precipitate CHF, MI in those w/cardiac disease, peripheral ischemia. Overdose produces nausea, drowsiness, confusion, slurred speech.

NURSING IMPLICATIONS
BASELINE ASSESSMENT:

Concurrent therapy of sublingual nitroglycerin may be used for relief of anginal pain. Record onset, type (sharp, dull, squeezing), radiation, location, intensity, and duration of anginal pain, and precipitating factors (exertion, emotional stress). Check B/P for hypotension immediately before giving medication.

INTERVENTION/EVALUATION:

Observe for giddiness (common effect). Assist w/ambulation if lightheadedness, dizziness occurs. Assess for peripheral edema behind medial malleolus (sacral area in bedridden pts). Assess skin for flushing. Monitor liver enzyme tests.

PATIENT/FAMILY TEACHING:

Rise slowly from lying to sitting position and permit legs to dangle from bed momentarily before standing to reduce hypotensive effect. Contact physician/nurse if irregular heartbeat, shortness of breath, pronounced dizziness, or nausea occurs. Avoid concomitant grapefruit/juice use.

nilutamide
nih-**lute**-ah-myd
(Nilandron)

CANADIAN AVAILABILITY
Anandron

CLASSIFICATION
Antineoplastic: hormone

AVAILABILITY (Rx)
Tablets: 50 mg, 100 mg

PHARMACOKINETICS
Rapidly, completely absorbed following oral administration. Extensively metabolized in liver to inactive metabolites. Primarily excreted in urine. Half-life: 23–72 hrs.

ACTION/*THERAPEUTIC EFFECT*
Competitively inhibits androgen action by binding to androgen receptors in target tissue. *Decreases growth of prostatic carcinoma.*

USES

Treatment of metastatic prostatic carcinoma (stage D_2) in combination w/surgical castration. For maximum benefit, begin on same day or day after surgical castration.

PO ADMINISTRATION

1. May be given with or without food.
2. Take at same time each day.

INDICATIONS/DOSAGE/ROUTES

Prostatic carcinoma:
PO: Adults, elderly: 300 mg once a day for 30 days, then 150 mg once a day. Begin on same day or day after surgical castration.

PRECAUTIONS

CONTRAINDICATIONS: Hypersensitivity to nilutamide, severe liver impairment, severe respiratory insufficiency. **CAUTIONS:** Hepatitis, marked increase in liver enzymes. **PREGNANCY/LACTATION:** Pregnancy Category C.

INTERACTIONS

DRUG INTERACTIONS: None significant. **ALTERED LAB VALUES:** May increase SGOT (AST), SGPT (ALT), bilirubin, creatinine.

SIDE EFFECTS

FREQUENT (>10%): Hot flashes, delay in recovering vision after bright illumination (sun, television, bright lights), loss of libido, sexual potency, mild nausea, gynecomastia, alcohol intolerance. **OCCASIONAL (<10%):** Constipation, hypertension, dizziness, dyspnea, urinary tract infections.

ADVERSE REACTIONS/TOXIC EFFECTS

Interstitial pneumonitis may occur.

NURSING IMPLICATIONS

BASELINE ASSESSMENT:

Baseline chest x-ray, hepatic enzyme levels should be obtained before therapy begins. Question for hypersensitivity to nilutamide. Assess medical condition (esp. liver function).

INTERVENTION/EVALUATION:

Monitor B/P periodically and hepatic function tests in long-term therapy.

PATIENT/FAMILY TEACHING:

Do not stop taking medication. Contact physician if any side effects occur at home, esp. signs of liver toxicity (jaundice, dark urine, fatigue, abdominal pain). Explain side effects and action on carcinoma. Report any dyspnea or aggravation of preexisting dyspnea. Caution about driving at night (tinted glasses may help). Avoid alcohol.

nimodipine

nih-**moad**-ih-peen
(Nimotop)

CANADIAN AVAILABILITY:
Nimotop

CLASSIFICATION

Calcium channel blocker

AVAILABILITY (Rx)

Capsules: 30 mg

PHARMACOKINETICS

Rapidly absorbed from GI tract. Metabolized in liver. Excreted in urine, eliminated in feces. Half-life: (terminal) 8–9 hrs.

ACTION / *THERAPEUTIC EFFECT*

Inhibits movement of calcium ions across cellular membranes in vascular smooth muscle. *Produces favorable effect on severity of neurologic deficits due to cerebral vasospasm. Greatest effect on cerebral arteries; may prevent cerebral spasm.*

USES / *UNLABELED*

Improvement of neurologic deficits due to spasm following subarachnoid hemorrhage from ruptured congenital intracranial aneurysms in pts in good neurologic condition. *Treatment of chronic and classic migraine, chronic cluster headaches.*

PO ADMINISTRATION

1. If pt unable to swallow, place hole in both ends of capsule with 18 gauge needle to extract contents into syringe.
2. Empty into nasogastric tube; wash tube w/30 ml normal saline.

INDICATIONS / DOSAGE / ROUTES

Subarachnoid hemorrhage:
PO: Adults, elderly: 60 mg q4h for 21 days. Begin within 96 hrs of subarachnoid hemorrhage.

PRECAUTIONS

CONTRAINDICATIONS: Severe hypotension. CAUTIONS: Impaired renal/hepatic function. PREGNANCY/LACTATION: Unknown whether drug crosses placenta or is distributed in breast milk. Pregnancy Category C.

INTERACTIONS

DRUG INTERACTIONS: None significant. ALTERED LAB VALUES: None significant.

SIDE EFFECTS

OCCASIONAL (2–6%): Hypotension, peripheral edema, diarrhea, headache. RARE (<2%): Allergic reaction (rash, hives), tachycardia, flushing of skin.

ADVERSE REACTIONS / TOXIC EFFECTS

Overdosage produces nausea, weakness, dizziness, drowsiness, confusion, slurred speech.

NURSING IMPLICATIONS

BASELINE ASSESSMENT:

Assess level of consciousness, neurologic response, initially and throughout therapy. Monitor baseline liver function tests. Assess B/P, apical pulse immediately before drug is administered (if pulse is 60/min or below, or systolic B/P is below 90 mm Hg, withhold medication, contact physician).

INTERVENTION / EVALUATION:

Monitor pulse rate for bradycardia. Assess skin for dermatitis, rash, flushing. Monitor daily bowel activity and stool consistency. Assess for headache.

PATIENT / FAMILY TEACHING:

To avoid hypotensive effect, rise slowly from lying to sitting position; wait momentarily before standing. Avoid tasks that require alertness, motor skills until response to drug is established. Contact physician/nurse if irregular heartbeat, shortness of breath, pronounced dizziness, or nausea occurs.

nisoldipine

nye-**soul**-dih-peen
(Sular)

CLASSIFICATION

Calcium channel blocker

AVAILABILITY (Rx)

Tablets (extended-release): 10 mg, 20 mg, 30 mg, 40 mg

PHARMACOKINETICS

	ONSET	PEAK	DURATION
PO	—	1–2 hrs	8 hrs

Rapidly, completely absorbed from GI tract. Undergoes first-pass metabolism in liver. Metabolized in liver. Primarily excreted in urine. Half-life: 7–12 hrs.

ACTION/*THERAPEUTIC EFFECT*

Inhibits calcium ion movement across cell membrane, depressing contraction of cardiac and vascular smooth muscle. *Increases heart rate, cardiac output. Decreases systemic vascular resistance, B/P.*

USES/*UNLABELED*

Treatment of hypertension, alone or in combination w/other antihypertensive agents, *stable angina pectoris, CHF.*

PO ADMINISTRATION

1. Do not crush or break sustained-release capsule.
2. May give w/o regard to meals.
3. Avoid grapefruit products before or after giving medication.

INDICATIONS/DOSAGE/ROUTES

Hypertension:
Extended-Release: Adults: Initially, 20 mg once daily, then increase by 10 mg per week, or longer intervals until therapeutic B/P response is attained. **Elderly:** Initially, 10 mg once daily. Increase by 10 mg per week to therapeutic response. **Maintenance:** 20–40 mg once daily. **Maximum:** 60 mg once daily.

PRECAUTIONS

CONTRAINDICATIONS: Sick-sinus syndrome/second- or third-degree AV block (except in presence of pacemaker). **CAUTIONS:** Impaired renal/hepatic function, aortic stenosis, elderly, cirrhosis. **PREGNANCY/LACTATION:** Insignificant amount distributed in breast milk. **Pregnancy Category C.**

INTERACTIONS

DRUG INTERACTIONS: None significant. **ALTERED LAB VALUES:** None significant.

SIDE EFFECTS

FREQUENT: Giddiness, dizziness, lightheadedness, peripheral edema, headache, flushing, weakness, nausea. **OCCASIONAL:** Transient hypotension, heartburn, muscle cramps, nasal congestion, cough, wheezing, sore throat, palpitations, nervousness, mood changes. **RARE:** Increase in frequency, intensity, duration of anginal attack during initial therapy.

ADVERSE REACTIONS/TOXIC EFFECTS

May precipitate CHF, MI in those w/cardiac disease, peripheral ischemia. Overdose produces nausea, drowsiness, confusion, slurred speech.

NURSING IMPLICATIONS

BASELINE ASSESSMENT:

Concurrent therapy of sublingual nitroglycerin may be used for relief of anginal pain. Record onset, type (sharp, dull, squeezing), radiation, location, intensity, and duration of anginal pain, and precipitating factors (exertion, emotional stress). Check B/P for hypotension immediately before giving medication.

INTERVENTION/EVALUATION:

Monitor B/P closely during dosage adjustment. Observe for giddiness (common effect). Assist w/ambulation if lightheadedness, dizziness occurs. Assess for peripheral edema behind medial malleolus (sacral area in bedridden pts). Assess skin for flushing. Monitor liver enzyme tests.

PATIENT/FAMILY TEACHING:

Avoid eating grapefruit, high-fat meal before and after taking medication. Swallow capsule whole; do not chew, divide, or crush. Rise slowly from lying to sitting position and permit legs to dangle from bed momentarily before standing to reduce hypotensive effect. Contact physician/nurse if irregular heartbeat, shortness of breath, pronounced dizziness, or nausea occurs.

---

nitric oxide
(INOmax)
See Supplement

---

nitrofurantoin sodium

ny-tro-feur-**an**-twon
(Furadantin, Furalan, Macrodantin)

CANADIAN AVAILABILITY:
Apo-Nitrofurantoin, Macrodantin

CLASSIFICATION

Antibacterial

AVAILABILITY (Rx)

Capsules: 25 mg, 50 mg, 100 mg. **Capsules:** 100 mg (25 mg as macrocrystals/75 mg as microcrystals). **Oral Suspension:** 25 mg/5 ml.

PHARMACOKINETICS

Microcrystalline: rapidly, completely absorbed; macrocrystalline: more slowly absorbed. Food increases absorption. Primarily concentrated in urine, kidneys. Metabolized in most body tissues. Primarily excreted in urine. Half-life: 20–60 min.

ACTION/*THERAPEUTIC EFFECT*

Bactericidal. Inactivates or alters bacterial ribosomal proteins, *producing bacteriostatic activity; bactericidal at high concentrations.*

USES/*UNLABELED*

Treatment of urinary tract infections, initial and chronic. *Prophylaxis of bacterial UTIs.*

PO ADMINISTRATION

Give w/food, milk to enhance absorption, reduce GI upset.

INDICATIONS/DOSAGE/ROUTES

Initial or recurrent urinary tract infection (UTI):
PO: Adults, elderly: 50–100 mg 4 times/day. **Maximum:** 400 mg/day. **Children >1 mo:** 5–7 mg/kg in 4 divided doses.

Long-term prophylactic therapy of UTI:
PO: Adults, elderly: 50–100 mg as single evening dose. **Children:** 1–2 mg/kg in 1–2 divided doses.

PRECAUTIONS

CONTRAINDICATIONS: Hypersensitivity to nitrofurantoin, infants <1 mo of age because of hemolytic anemia, anuria, oliguria, substantial renal impairment (creatinine clearance <40 ml/min). **CAUTIONS:** Renal impairment, diabetes mellitus, electrolyte imbalance, anemia, vitamin B deficiency, debilitated (greater risk of peripheral neuropathy), glucose 6-phosphate dehydrogenase (G-6-PD) deficiency (greater risk of hemolytic anemia). **PREGNANCY/LACTATION:** Readily crosses placenta; distributed in breast milk. Contraindicated at term and during lactation when infant suspected of having G-6-PD deficiency. **Pregnancy Category B**.

INTERACTIONS

DRUG INTERACTIONS: Hemolytics may increase risk of toxicity. Neurotoxic medications may increase risk of neurotoxicity. Probenecid may increase concentration, toxicity. **ALTERED LAB VALUES:** None significant.

SIDE EFFECTS

FREQUENT: Anorexia, nausea, vomiting. **OCCASIONAL:** Abdominal pain, diarrhea, rash, pruritus, urticaria, hypertension, headache, dizziness, drowsiness. **RARE:** Photosensitivity, transient alopecia, asthmatic attack in those with history of asthma.

ADVERSE REACTIONS/TOXIC EFFECTS

Superinfection, hepatotoxicity, peripheral neuropathy (may be irreversible), Stevens-Johnson syndrome, permanent pulmonary function impairment (rarely respiratory failure, death), anaphylaxis occur rarely.

NURSING IMPLICATIONS

BASELINE ASSESSMENT:

Question for history of asthma, hypersensitivity to nitrofurantoin. Obtain urine specimens for culture and sensitivity before giving first dose (therapy may begin before results are known). Evaluate lab test results for renal and hepatic baselines.

INTERVENTION/EVALUATION:

Monitor I&O, renal function results. Evaluate food tolerance. Determine pattern of bowel activity. Assess skin for rash, urticaria. Be alert for numbness or tingling, esp. of lower extremities (may signal onset of peripheral neuropathy). Watch for signs of hepatotoxicity: fever, rash, arthralgia, hepatomegaly. Check B/P at least 2 times/day. Perform respiratory assessment: Auscultate lungs, check for cough, chest pain, difficulty breathing.

PATIENT/FAMILY TEACHING:

Urine may become dark yellow or brown. Take with food or milk for best results and to reduce GI upset. Complete full course of therapy. Avoid sun and ultraviolet light; use sunscreens, wear protective clothing. Notify physician if cough, fever, chest pain, difficult breathing, numbness/tingling of fingers or toes occurs. Rare occurrence of alopecia is transient.

nitroglycerin intravenous

nigh-trow-**glih**-sir-in

(Nitro-Bid, Nitrostat, Tridil)

nitroglycerin sublingual

(Nitrostat)

nitroglycerin sustained-release

(Nitro-Bid, Nitroglyn)

nitroglycerin topical

(Nitro-Bid, Nitrol)

nitroglycerin transdermal

(Minitran, Nitrek, Nitro-Dur, Transderm Nitro, Nitrodisc)

nitroglycerin translingual

(Nitrolingual)

nitroglycerin transmucosal

(Nitrogard)

CANADIAN AVAILABILITY:
Minitran, Nitro-Dur, Nitrol, Nitrolingual, Nitrong, Nitrostat, Trans-Derm-Nitro, Trinipatch

CLASSIFICATION

Nitrate

AVAILABILITY (Rx)

Tablets (sublingual): 0.4 mg. **Spray:** 0.4 mg/dose. **Tablets (buccal, controlled-release):** 1 mg, 2 mg, 3 mg. **Tablets (sustained-release):** 2.6 mg, 6.5 mg, 9 mg. **Capsules (sustained-release):** 2.5 mg, 6.5 mg, 9 mg, 13 mg. **Transdermal:** 0.1 mg/hr, 0.2 mg/hr, 0.3 mg/hr, 0.4 mg/hr, 0.6 mg/hr, 0.8 mg/hr. **Topical Ointment:** 2%. **Injection:** 0.5 mg/ml, 5 mg/ml. **Injection Solution:** 100 mcg/ml, 200 mcg/ml.

PHARMACOKINETICS

	ONSET	PEAK	DURATION
Sublingual			
	2–5 min	4–8 min	30–60 min
Transmucosal tablet			
	2–5 min	4–10 min	3–5 hrs
Extended-release			
	20–45 min	—	3–8 hrs
Topical			
	15–60 min	0.5–2 hrs	3–8 hrs
Patch			
	30–60 min	1–3 hrs	8–12 hrs
IV	1–2 min	—	3–5 min

Well absorbed after oral, sublingual, topical administration. Undergoes extensive first-pass metabolism. Metabolized in liver, enzymes in bloodstream. Primarily excreted in urine. Half-life: 1–4 min.

ACTION/*THERAPEUTIC EFFECT*

Decreases myocardial oxygen demand. Reduces left ventricular preload and afterload. *Dilates coronary arteries, improves collateral blood flow to ischemic areas within myocardium.* **Intravenous:** *Produces peripheral vasodilation.*

USES

Lingual/sublingual/buccal dose used for acute relief of angina pectoris. Extended-release, topical forms used for prophylaxis, long-term angina management. IV form used in treatment of CHF associated w/acute MI.

STORAGE/HANDLING

Store tablets/capsules at room temperature. Keep sublingual tablets in original container.

PO/TOPICAL/IV ADMINISTRATION

PO:

1. Do not chew extended-release form.

2. Do not shake oral aerosol canister before lingual spraying.

SUBLINGUAL:

1. Do not swallow; dissolve under the tongue.

2. Administer while seated.

3. Slight burning sensation under tongue may be lessened by placing tablet in buccal pouch.

TOPICAL:

Spread thin layer on clean/dry/hairless skin of upper arm or body (not below knee or elbow), using applicator or dose-measuring papers. Do not use fingers; do not rub or massage into skin.

TRANSDERMAL:

Apply patch on clean/dry/hairless skin of upper arm or body (not below knee or elbow).

IV:

1. Dilute in given amount of 5% dextrose in water or 0.9% NaCl.

2. Use microdrop or infusion pump.

INDICATIONS/DOSAGE/ROUTES

Acute angina, acute prophylaxis:
Lingual Spray: Adults, elderly: 1 spray onto or under tongue q3–5 min until relief is noted (no more than 3 sprays in 15 min period).
Sublingual: Adults, elderly: 0.4 mg q5 min until relief is noted (no more than 3 doses in 15 min period). Use prophylactically 5–10 min before activities that may cause an acute attack.

Long-term prophylaxis of angina:
PO (Extended-Release): Adults, elderly: Initially, 2.5 mg 3–4 times/day. Increase by 2.5 mg 2–4 times/day at intervals of several days or weeks.

Topical: Adults, elderly: Initially, $1/2$ inch q8h. Increase by $1/2$ inch w/each application. **Range:** 1–2 inches q8h up to 4–5 inches q4h.
Transdermal Patch: Adults, elderly: Initially, 0.2–0.4 mg/hr. **Maintenance:** 0.4–0.8 mg/hr. Consider patch on 12–14 hrs, patch off 10–12 hrs (prevents tolerance).

Usual parenteral dosage:
IV: Adults, elderly: Initially, 5 mcg/min via infusion pump. Increase in 5 mcg/min increments at 3–5 min intervals until B/P response is noted or until dosage reaches maximum of 20 mcg/min. Dosage may be further titrated according to pt, therapeutic response.

PRECAUTIONS

CONTRAINDICATIONS: Hypersensitivity to nitrates, severe anemia, closed-angle glaucoma, postural hypotension, head trauma, increased intracranial pressure. *Sublingual:* Early MI. *Transdermal:* Allergy to adhesives. *Extended-release:* GI hypermotility/malabsorption, severe anemia. *IV:* Uncorrected hypovolemia, hypotension, inadequate cerebral circulation, constrictive pericarditis, pericardial tamponade. **CAUTIONS:** Acute MI, hepatic/renal disease, glaucoma (contraindicated in closed-angle glaucoma), blood volume depletion from diuretic therapy, systolic B/P below 90 mm Hg. **PREGNANCY/LACTATION:** Unknown whether drug crosses placenta or is distributed in breast milk. **Pregnancy Category B**.

INTERACTIONS

DRUG INTERACTIONS: Alcohol,

antihypertensives, vasodilators may increase risk of orthostatic hypotension. **ALTERED LAB VALUES:** May increase methemoglobin, urine catecholamines, urine VMA.

SIDE EFFECTS

FREQUENT: Headache (may be severe) occurs mostly in early therapy, diminishes rapidly in intensity, usually disappears during continued treatment; transient flushing of face and neck, dizziness (esp. if pt is standing immobile or is in a warm environment), weakness, postural hypotension. *Sublingual:* Burning, tingling sensation at oral point of dissolution. *Ointment:* Erythema, pruritus. **OCCASIONAL:** GI upset. *Transdermal:* Contact dermatitis.

ADVERSE REACTIONS/TOXIC EFFECTS

Drug should be discontinued if blurred vision, dry mouth occurs. Severe postural hypotension manifested by fainting, pulselessness, cold/clammy skin, profuse sweating. Tolerance may occur w/repeated, prolonged therapy (minor tolerance w/intermittent use of sublingual tablets). High dose tends to produce severe headache.

NURSING IMPLICATIONS
BASELINE ASSESSMENT:

Record onset, type (sharp, dull, squeezing), radiation, location, intensity, and duration of anginal pain, and precipitating factors (exertion, emotional stress). Assess B/P and apical pulse before administration and periodically after dose. Pt must have continuous EKG monitoring for IV administration.

INTERVENTION/EVALUATION:

Assist w/ambulation if lightheadedness, dizziness occurs. Assess for facial/neck flushing. Cardioverter/defibrillator must not be discharged through paddle electrode overlying nitroglycerin system (may cause burns to pt or damage to paddle via arcing).

PATIENT/FAMILY TEACHING:

Rise slowly from lying to sitting position and dangle legs momentarily before standing. Take oral form on empty stomach (however, if headache occurs during therapy, take medication w/meals). Use inhalants only when lying down. Dissolve sublingual tablet under tongue; do not swallow. Take at first sign of angina. If not relieved within 5 min, dissolve second tablet under tongue. Repeat if no relief in another 5 min. If pain continues, contact physician or go immediately to emergency room. Do not change brands. Keep container away from heat, moisture. Do not inhale lingual aerosol but spray onto or under tongue (avoid swallowing after spray is administered). Expel from mouth any remaining lingual/sublingual/intrabuccal tablet after pain is completely relieved. Place transmucosal tablets under upper lip or buccal pouch (between cheek and gum); do not chew or swallow tablet. Avoid alcohol (intensifies hypotensive effect). If alcohol is ingested soon after taking nitroglycerin, possible acute hypotensive episode (marked drop in B/P, vertigo, pallor) may occur.

N

nitroprusside sodium

nigh-troe-**pruss**-eyd
(Nipride, Nitropress)

CANADIAN AVAILABILITY:
Nipride

CLASSIFICATION

Antihypertensive

AVAILABILITY (Rx)

Powder for Injection: 50 mg

PHARMACOKINETICS

	ONSET	PEAK	DURATION
IV	1–2 min	Dependent on infusion rate	Dissipates rapidly after stopping IV

Reacts w/hemoglobin in erythrocytes, producing cyanmethemoglobin, cyanide ions. Primarily excreted in urine. Half-life: 2 min.

ACTION/ *THERAPEUTIC EFFECT*

Direct vasodilating action on arterial, venous smooth muscle. Decreases peripheral vascular resistance, preload, afterload, improves cardiac output. *Dilates coronary arteries, decreases oxygen consumption, relieves persistent chest pain.*

USES/ *UNLABELED*

Immediate reduction of B/P in hypertensive crisis. Produces controlled hypotension in surgical procedures to reduce bleeding. Treatment of acute CHF. *Controls paroxysmal hypertension prior to/during surgery for pheochromocytoma; treatment adjunct for myocardial infarction, valvular regurgitation, peripheral vasospasm caused by ergot alkaloid overdose.*

STORAGE/HANDLING

Protect solution from light. Solution should appear very faint brown in color. Use only freshly prepared solution. Once prepared, do not keep or use longer than 24 hrs. Deterioration evidenced by color change from brown to blue, green, or dark red. Discard unused portion.

IV ADMINISTRATION

1. Give by IV infusion only.
2. Reconstitute 50 mg vial with 2–3 ml 5% dextrose or sterile water for injection w/o preservative.
3. Further dilute w/250–1,000 ml of 5% dextrose to provide concentration of 200 mcg, 50 mcg/ml, respectively.
4. Wrap infusion bottle in aluminum foil immediately after mixing.
5. Administer using IV infusion pump or microdrip (60 gtt/ml).
6. Be alert for extravasation (produces severe pain, sloughing).

INDICATIONS/DOSAGE/ROUTES

Usual parenteral dosage:
IV: Adults, elderly, children: Initially, 0.3 mcg/kg/min. **Range:** 0.5–10 mcg/kg/min. Do not exceed 10 mcg/kg/min (risk of precipitous drop in B/P).

PRECAUTIONS

CONTRAINDICATIONS: Compensatory hypertension (arteriovenous shunt or coarctation of aorta), inadequate cerebral circulation, moribund pts. **CAUTIONS:** Severe hepatic, renal impairment, hypothyroidism, hyponatremia, elderly. Except at low concentrations or brief use, may cause increased quantities of cyanide ion (may be toxic, lethal). **PREGNANCY/LACTATION:** Unknown whether drug crosses placenta or is distributed in breast milk. **Pregnancy Category C**.

INTERACTIONS

DRUG INTERACTIONS: Dobutamine may increase cardiac output, decrease pulmonary wedge pressure. Hypotensive-producing medications may increase hypotensive effect. **ALTERED LAB VALUES:** None significant.

SIDE EFFECTS

OCCASIONAL: Flushing of skin, increased intracranial pressure, rash, pain/redness at injection site.

ADVERSE REACTIONS/TOXIC EFFECTS

A too rapid IV rate reduces B/P too quickly. Nausea, retching, diaphoresis (sweating), apprehension, headache, restlessness, muscle twitching, dizziness, palpitation, retrosternal pain, and abdominal pain may occur. Symptoms disappear rapidly if rate of administration is slowed or temporarily discontinued. Overdosage produces metabolic acidosis, tolerance to therapeutic effect.

NURSING IMPLICATIONS

BASELINE ASSESSMENT:

Pt must have continuous EKG monitoring and B/P monitoring (using either continually reinflated sphygmomanometer or an intra-arterial pressure sensor). Check w/physician for desired B/P level (B/P is normally maintained about 30–40% below pretreatment levels). Medication should be discontinued if therapeutic response is not achieved within 10 min following IV infusion at 10 mcg/kg/min.

INTERVENTION/EVALUATION:

Assess IV site for extravasation. Monitor rate of infusion frequently. Monitor blood acid-base balance, electrolytes, laboratory results, I&O. Assess for metabolic acidosis (weakness, disorientation, headache, nausea, hyperventilation, vomiting). Assess for therapeutic response to medication. Monitor B/P for potential rebound hypertension after infusion is discontinued.

nizatidine

nye-**zaye**-tih-deen
(Axid, Axid AR)

CANADIAN AVAILABILITY:
Axid

CLASSIFICATION

H_2 receptor antagonist

AVAILABILITY (Rx)

Capsules: 75 mg **(OTC)**, 150 mg, 300 mg

PHARMACOKINETICS

Rapidly, well absorbed from GI tract. Metabolized in liver. Primarily excreted in urine. Half-life: 1–2 hrs (increased in decreased renal function).

ACTION/ *THERAPEUTIC EFFECT*

Inhibits histamine action at H_2 receptors of parietal cells, *inhibiting basal and nocturnal gastric acid secretion.*

USES/ *UNLABELED*

Short-term treatment of active duodenal ulcer, active benign gastric ulcer. Prevention of duodenal ulcer recurrence. Treatment of gastroesophageal reflux disease (GERD) including erosive esophagitis. *Treatment of gastric hypersecretory conditions, Zollinger-Ellison syndrome, multiple endocrine adenoma.*

PO ADMINISTRATION

1. Give w/o regard to meals.

Best given after meals or at bedtime.

2. Do not administer within 1 hr of magnesium or aluminum-containing antacids (decreases absorption).

3. May give right before eating for heartburn prevention.

INDICATIONS/DOSAGE/ROUTES

Active duodenal ulcer:
PO: Adults, elderly: 300 mg at bedtime or 150 mg 2 times/day.

Maintenance of healed ulcer:
PO: Adults, elderly: 150 mg at bedtime.

GERD:
PO: Adults, elderly: 150 mg 2 times/day.

Active benign gastric ulcer:
PO: Adults, elderly: 150 mg 2 times/day or 300 mg at bedtime.

Dosage in renal impairment:

CREATININE CLEARANCE	ACTIVE ULCER	MAINTENANCE THERAPY
20–50 ml/min	150 mg at bedtime	150 mg every other day
<20 ml/min	150 mg every other day	150 mg every 3 days

PRECAUTIONS

CONTRAINDICATIONS: None significant. **CAUTIONS:** Impaired renal/hepatic function. **PREGNANCY/LACTATION:** Unknown whether drug crosses placenta or is distributed in breast milk. **Pregnancy Category B**.

INTERACTIONS

DRUG INTERACTIONS: Antacids may decrease absorption (do not give within 1 hr). May decrease absorption of ketoconazole (give at least 2 hrs after). **ALTERED LAB VALUES:** Interferes w/skin tests using allergen extracts. May increase SGOT (AST), SGPT (ALT), alkaline phosphatase.

SIDE EFFECTS

OCCASIONAL (2%): Somnolence, fatigue. **RARE (<1%):** Sweating, rash.

ADVERSE REACTIONS/TOXIC EFFECTS

Asymptomatic ventricular tachycardia, hyperuricemia (not associated w/gout), nephrolithiasis occur rarely.

NURSING IMPLICATIONS

INTERVENTION/EVALUATION:

Assess for abdominal pain, GI bleeding (overt blood in emesis or stool, tarry stools). Monitor blood tests for elevated SGOT (AST), SGPT (ALT), alkaline phosphatase (hepatocellular injury).

PATIENT/FAMILY TEACHING:

Avoid tasks that require alertness, motor skills until drug response is established. Avoid alcohol, aspirin, and smoking.

norepinephrine bitartrate

nor-eh-pih-**nef**-rin
(Levophed)

CANADIAN AVAILABILITY:
Levophed

CLASSIFICATION

Sympathomimetic

AVAILABILITY (Rx)

Injection: 1 mg/ml

PHARMACOKINETICS

	ONSET	PEAK	DURATION
IV	Rapid	1–2 min	—

Localized in sympathetic tissue. Metabolized in liver. Primarily excreted in urine.

ACTION / *THERAPEUTIC EFFECT*

Stimulates beta$_1$-adrenergic receptors, *enhancing contractile myocardial force, increasing cardiac output.* Stimulates alpha-adrenergic receptors, *constricting resistance and capacitance vessels, resulting in increased systemic B/P, coronary artery blood flow.* Pressor effect primarily due to increased peripheral resistance.

USES

Corrects hypotension unresponsive to adequate fluid volume replacement, as part of shock syndrome, caused by myocardial infarction, bacteremia, open heart surgery, renal failure.

STORAGE / HANDLING

Do not use if brown in color or contains precipitate.

IV ADMINISTRATION

Note: Blood, fluid volume depletion should be corrected before drug is administered.

1. Add 4 ml to 250 ml (16 mcg base/ml)–1,000 ml (4 mcg base/ml) of D$_5$W.

2. Infuse through plastic catheter, using antecubital vein of arm.

3. Avoid catheter tie-in technique (encourages stasis, increases local drug concentration).

4. Closely monitor IV infusion flow rate (use microdrip or infusion pump).

5. Monitor B/P q2 min during IV infusion until desired therapeutic response is achieved, then q5 min during remaining IV infusion. Never leave pt unattended.

6. Maintain B/P at 80–100 mm Hg in previously normotensive pts, and 30–40 mm Hg below preexisting B/P in previously hypertensive pts.

7. Reduce IV infusion gradually. Avoid abrupt withdrawal.

8. It is imperative to check the IV site frequently for free flow and infused vein for blanching, hardness to vein, coldness, pallor to extremity.

9. If extravasation occurs, area should be infiltrated w/10–15 ml sterile saline containing 5–10 mg phentolamine (does not alter pressor effects of norepinephrine).

INDICATIONS / DOSAGE / ROUTES

Acute hypotension:
IV: Adults, elderly: Initially, administer at 8–12 mcg/min. Adjust rate of flow to establish, maintain normal B/P (40 mm Hg below preexisting systolic pressure). **Average maintenance dose:** 2–4 mcg/min. **Children:** Administer at rate of 2 mcg/min.

PRECAUTIONS

CONTRAINDICATIONS: Hypovolemic states (unless an emergency measure), mesenteric/peripheral vascular thrombosis, profound hypoxia. **CAUTIONS:** Severe cardiac disease, hypertensive and hypothyroid pts, those on MAO inhibitors. **PREGNANCY/LACTATION:** Readily crosses placenta. May produce fetal anoxia due to uterine contraction, constriction of uterine blood vessels. **Pregnancy Category C.**

INTERACTIONS

DRUG INTERACTIONS: Tricyclic antidepressants, maprotiline may increase cardiovascular effects. May decrease effect of methyldopa. May have mutually inhibitory effects w/beta blockers. May increase risk of arrhythmias w/ digoxin. Ergonovine, oxytocin may increase vasoconstriction. **ALTERED LAB VALUES:** None significant.

SIDE EFFECTS

Norepinephrine produces less pronounced and less frequent side effects than epinephrine. **OCCASIONAL (3–5%):** Anxiety, bradycardia, awareness of slow, forceful heartbeat. **RARE (1–2%):** Nausea, anginal pain, shortness of breath, fever.

ADVERSE REACTIONS/TOXIC EFFECTS

Extravasation may produce tissue necrosis, sloughing. Overdosage manifested as severe hypertension w/violent headache (may be first clinical sign of overdosage), arrhythmias, photophobia, retrosternal/pharyngeal pain, pallor, excessive sweating, vomiting. Prolonged therapy may result in plasma volume depletion. Hypotension may recur if plasma volume is not maintained.

NURSING IMPLICATIONS

BASELINE ASSESSMENT:

Assess EKG and B/P continuously (be alert to precipitous B/P drop). Never leave pt alone during IV infusion. Be alert to pt complaint of headache.

INTERVENTION/EVALUATION:

Monitor IV flow rate diligently.

Assess for extravasation characterized by blanching of skin over vein, coolness (results from local vasoconstriction); color and temperature of IV site extremity (pallor, cyanosis, mottling). Assess nailbed capillary refill. Monitor I&O; measure output hourly and report <30 cc. IV should not be reinstated unless systolic B/P falls below 70–80 mm Hg.

norfloxacin

nor-**flocks**-ah-sin
(Chibroxin, Noroxin)

CANADIAN AVAILABILITY:
Noroxin

CLASSIFICATION

Anti-infective: Quinolone

AVAILABILITY (Rx)

Tablets: 400 mg. **Ophthalmic Solution:** 3 mg/ml.

PHARMACOKINETICS

Rapidly, incompletely absorbed from GI tract. Widely distributed. Possibly metabolized in liver. Primarily excreted in urine. Half-life: 3–4 hrs (increased in decreased renal function).

ACTION/THERAPEUTIC EFFECT

Inhibits DNA replication and repair by interfering w/DNA-gyrase in susceptible microorganisms, *producing bactericidal activity.*

USES

Treatment of complicated and

uncomplicated urinary tract infections, uncomplicated gonococcal infections, acute/chronic prostatitis. *Ophthalmic:* Conjunctival keratitis, keratoconjunctivitis, corneal ulcers, blepharitis, blepharoconjunctivitis, acute meibomianitis, dacryocystitis.

PO/OPHTHALMIC ADMINISTRATION

PO:

1. Give 1 hr before or 2 hrs after meals, w/8 oz water.

2. Encourage additional glasses of water between meals.

3. Do not administer antacids w/or within 2 hrs of norfloxacin dose.

4. Encourage cranberry juice, citrus fruits (to acidify urine).

OPHTHALMIC:

1. Tilt pt's head back; place solution in conjunctival sac.

2. Have pt close eyes; press gently on lacrimal sac for 1 min.

3. Do not use ophthalmic solutions for injection.

INDICATIONS/DOSAGE/ROUTES

Complicated or uncomplicated urinary tract infections:
PO: **Adults, elderly:** 400 mg 2 times/day for 7–21 days.

Prostatitis:
PO: **Adults:** 400 mg 2 times/day for 28 days.

Uncomplicated gonococcal infections:
PO: **Adults:** 800 mg as single dose.

Dosage in renal impairment:
The dose and/or frequency is modified based on degree of renal impairment.

CREATININE CLEARANCE	DOSAGE
>30 ml/min	400 mg 2 times/day
<30 ml/min	400 mg once daily

Usual ophthalmic dosage:
Ophthalmic: Adults, elderly: 1–2 drops 4 times/day up to 7 days. For severe infections, may give 1–2 drops q2h while awake the first day.

PRECAUTIONS

CONTRAINDICATIONS: Hypersensitivity to norfloxacin, quinolones, or any component of preparation. Do not use in children <18 yrs of age—produces arthropathy. *Ophthalmic:* Epithelial herpes simplex, keratitis, vaccinia, varicella, mycobacterial infection, fungal disease of ocular structure. Do not use after uncomplicated removal of foreign body. **CAUTIONS:** Impaired renal function; any predisposition to seizures. **PREGNANCY/LACTATION:** Crosses placenta; distributed into cord blood, amniotic fluid. Unknown if distributed in breast milk. Should not be used in pregnant women. **Pregnancy Category C.**

INTERACTIONS

DRUG INTERACTIONS: Antacids, sucralfate may decrease absorption. Decrease clearance, may increase concentration, toxicity of theophylline. May increase effects of oral anticoagulants. **ALTERED LAB VALUES:** May increase SGOT (AST), SGPT (ALT), alkaline phosphatase, LDH, bilirubin, BUN, creatinine.

SIDE EFFECTS

FREQUENT: Nausea, headache, dizziness. *Ophthalmic:* Bad taste in mouth. **OCCASIONAL:** *Ophthalmic:* Temporary blurring of vision, irritation, burning, stinging, itching. **RARE:** Vomiting, diarrhea, dry mouth, bitter taste, nervousness, drowsiness, insomnia, photosensitivity, tinnitus, crystalluria, rash, fever, seizures. *Ophthalmic:* Conjunctival hyperemia, photophobia, decreased vision, pain.

ADVERSE REACTIONS/TOXIC EFFECTS

Superinfection, anaphylaxis, Stevens-Johnson syndrome, arthropathy (joint disease) occurs rarely.

NURSING IMPLICATIONS
BASELINE ASSESSMENT:

Question for history of hypersensitivity to norfloxacin, quinolones, any component of preparation. Obtain specimens for diagnostic tests before giving first dose (therapy may begin before results are known).

INTERVENTION/EVALUATION:

Evaluate food tolerance, taste sensation, and dryness of mouth. Determine pattern of bowel activity. Assess skin for rash. Check for headache, dizziness. Monitor level of consciousness, pattern of sleep. Assess temperature at least 2 times/day. *Ophthalmic:* Check for therapeutic response, side effects (see Side Effects).

PATIENT/FAMILY TEACHING:

Take 1 hr before or 2 hrs after meals. Complete full course of therapy. Take w/8 oz of water, drink several glasses of water between meals. Eat/drink high sources of ascorbic acid, e.g., cranberry juice, citrus fruits. Do not take antacids w/or within 2 hrs of norfloxacin dose. Avoid sunlight/ultraviolet exposure; wear sunscreen and protective clothing if photosensitivity develops. Avoid tasks that require alert response if dizziness/drowsiness occur. Sugarless gum or hard candy, ice chips may help dry mouth and bitter taste. Notify nurse/physician if headache, dizziness, or other symptom occur. Report inflammation or tendon pain. *Ophthalmic:* Report any increased burning, itching, or other discomfort promptly.

nortriptyline hydrochloride

nor-**trip**-teh-leen
(Aventyl, Pamelor)

CANADIAN AVAILABILITY:
Aventyl

CLASSIFICATION

Antidepressant: Tricyclic

AVAILABILITY (Rx)

Capsules: 10 mg, 25 mg, 50 mg, 75 mg. **Oral Solution:** 10 mg/ 5 ml.

PHARMACOKINETICS

Rapidly, well absorbed from GI tract. Metabolized in liver, undergoes first-pass metabolism. Primarily excreted in urine. Minimal removal by hemodialysis. Half-life: 18–44 hrs.

ACTION/*THERAPEUTIC EFFECT*

Blocks reuptake of neurotransmitters (norepinephrine, serotonic) at neuronal presynaptic membranes, increasing availability at postsynaptic receptor sites. *Result-*

ing enhancements of synaptic activity produces antidepressant effect.

USES / *UNLABELED*

Treatment of various forms of depression, often in conjunction w/psychotherapy. *Treatment of panic disorder, neurogenic pain, prophylaxis of headache.*

PO ADMINISTRATION

Give w/food or milk if GI distress occurs.

INDICATIONS/DOSAGE/ROUTES

PO: Adults: 75–100 mg/day in 1–4 divided doses until therapeutic response achieved. Reduce dosage gradually to effective maintenance level. **Elderly:** Initially, 10–25 mg at bedtime. May increase by 25 mg q3–7 days. **Maximum:** 150 mg/day.

PRECAUTIONS

CONTRAINDICATIONS: Acute recovery period following MI, within 14 days of MAO inhibitor ingestion. **CAUTIONS:** Prostatic hypertrophy, history of urinary retention or obstruction, glaucoma, diabetes mellitus, history of seizures, hyperthyroidism, cardiac/hepatic/renal disease, schizophrenia, increased intraocular pressure, hiatal hernia. **PREGNANCY/LACTATION:** Crosses placenta; distributed in breast milk. **Pregnancy Category D.**

INTERACTIONS

DRUG INTERACTIONS: Alcohol, CNS depressants may increase CNS, respiratory depression, hypotensive effects. Antithyroid agents may increase risk of agranulocytosis. Phenothiazines may increase sedative, anticholinergic effects. Cimetidine may increase concentration, toxicity. May decrease effects of clonidine, guanadrel. May increase cardiac effects w/sympathomimetics. May increase risk of hypertensive crisis, hyperpyretic convulsions w/MAOIs. **ALTERED LAB VALUES:** May alter EKG readings, glucose.

SIDE EFFECTS

FREQUENT: Drowsiness, fatigue, dry mouth, blurred vision, constipation, delayed micturition, postural hypotension, excessive sweating, disturbed concentration, increased appetite, urinary retention. **OCCASIONAL:** GI disturbances (nausea, GI distress, metallic taste sensation). **RARE:** Paradoxical reaction (agitation, restlessness, nightmares, insomnia), extrapyramidal symptoms (particularly fine hand tremor).

ADVERSE REACTIONS/TOXIC EFFECTS

High dosage may produce cardiovascular effects (severe postural hypotension, dizziness, tachycardia, palpitations, arrhythmias) and seizures. May also result in altered temperature regulation (hyperpyrexia or hypothermia). Abrupt withdrawal from prolonged therapy may produce headache, malaise, nausea, vomiting, vivid dreams.

NURSING IMPLICATIONS

BASELINE ASSESSMENT:

For those on long-term therapy, liver/renal function tests, blood counts should be performed periodically.

INTERVENTION/EVALUATION:

Supervise suicidal risk pt closely during early therapy (as depression lessens, energy level improves, increasing suicide potential). Assess appearance, behavior, speech pattern, level of interest, mood. Monitor stools; avoid constipation w/increased fluids, bulky foods. Monitor B/P, pulse for hypotension, arrhythmias. Assess for urinary retention including output estimate and bladder palpation if indicated.

PATIENT/FAMILY TEACHING:

Change positions slowly to avoid hypotensive effect. Tolerance to postural hypotension, sedative, and anticholinergic effects usually develops during early therapy. Therapeutic effect may be noted in 2 or more wks. Photosensitivity to sun may occur. Use sunscreens, protective clothing. Dry mouth may be relieved by sugarless gum, sips of tepid water. Report visual disturbances. Do not abruptly discontinue medication. Avoid tasks that require alertness, motor skills until response to drug is established.

nystatin

nigh-**stat**-in
(Mycostatin, Nilstat, Nystop)

FIXED-COMBINATION(S):
W/triamcinolone, a steroid (**Mycolog II, Myco-Triacet II, Mykacet, Mytrex F**)

CANADIAN AVAILABILITY:
Mycostatin, Nadostine, Nilstat

CLASSIFICATION

Antifungal

AVAILABILITY (Rx)

Tablets: 500,000 units. Oral Suspension: 100,000 units/ml. Troches: 200,000 units. Vaginal Tablets: 100,000 units. Cream. Ointment. Powder.

PHARMACOKINETICS

Oral: Poorly absorbed from GI tract. Eliminated unchanged in feces. *Topical:* Not absorbed systemically from intact skin.

ACTION/*THERAPEUTIC EFFECT*

Binds to sterols in cell membrane increasing permeability, permitting loss of potassium, other cell components. *Fungistatic.*

USES/*UNLABELED*

Treatment of intestinal and oral candidiasis, cutaneous/mucocutaneous mycotic infections caused by *Candida albicans* (oral thrush, paronychia, vulvovaginal candidiasis, diaper rash, perleche). *Prophylaxis/treatment of oropharyngeal candidiasis, tinea barbae, capitis.*

PO ADMINISTRATION

1. Dissolve lozenges (troches) slowly/completely in mouth (optimal therapeutic effect). Do not chew or swallow lozenges whole.
2. Shake suspension well before administration.
3. Place and hold suspension in mouth or swish throughout mouth as long as possible before swallowing.

INDICATIONS/DOSAGE/ROUTES

Intestinal candidiasis:
PO: Adults, elderly: 500,000–1,000,000 units 3 times/day. **Children:** 500,000 units 4 times/day.

Oral candidiasis:
PO: Adults, elderly, children: Oral suspension: 400,000–600,000 units 4 times/day. **Infants:** 100,000–200,000 units 4 times/day.

PO: Adults, elderly, children:
Troches: 200,000–400,000 units 4–5 times/day up to 14 days.

Vulvovaginal candidiasis:
Intravaginally: Adults, elderly: 1 tablet high in vagina 1–2 times/day for 14 days.

Topical fungal infections:
Topical: Adults, elderly: Apply 2–3 times/day.

PRECAUTIONS

CONTRAINDICATIONS: Hypersensitivity to nystatin or components of preparation. **PREGNANCY/LACTATION:** Unknown if distributed in breast milk. Vaginal applicators may be contraindicated, requiring manual insertion of tablets during pregnancy. **Pregnancy Category A.**

INTERACTIONS

DRUG INTERACTIONS: None significant. **ALTERED LAB VALUES:** None significant.

SIDE EFFECTS

OCCASIONAL: *Oral:* None significant. *Topical:* Skin irritation. *Vaginal:* Vaginal irritation.

ADVERSE REACTIONS/TOXIC EFFECTS

High dosage with oral form may produce nausea, vomiting, diarrhea, GI distress.

NURSING IMPLICATIONS
BASELINE ASSESSMENT:

Question for history of allergies, esp. to nystatin. Confirm that cultures or histologic tests were done for accurate diagnosis.

INTERVENTION/EVALUATION:

Evaluate food intake, tolerance. Determine pattern of bowel activity and stool consistency. Assess for increased irritation w/topical, increased vaginal discharge with vaginal application.

PATIENT/FAMILY TEACHING:

Do not miss dose; complete full length of treatment (continue vaginal use during menses). Notify physician if nausea, vomiting, diarrhea, stomach pain develop. *Vaginal:* Insert high in vagina. Check w/physician regarding douching, sexual intercourse. *Topical:* Rub well into affected areas. Must not contact eyes. Do not apply any other preparations or occlusive covering w/o consulting physician. Use cream (sparingly)/powder on erythematous areas. Keep areas clean, dry; wear light clothing for ventilation. Separate personal items in contact w/affected areas.

octreotide acetate

ock-**tree**-oh-tide
(Depot, Sandostatin, Sandostatin LAR)

CANADIAN AVAILABILITY:
Sandostatin

CLASSIFICATION

Secretory inhibitor

AVAILABILITY (Rx)

Injection: 0.05 mg/ml, 0.1 mg/ml, 0.2 mg/ml, 0.5 mg/ml, 1 mg/ml. **Suspension for Injection.**

PHARMACOKINETICS

	ONSET	PEAK	DURATION
SubQ	—	—	Up to 12 hrs

Rapidly, completely absorbed from injection site. Excreted in urine. Half-life: 1.5 hrs.

ACTION/ THERAPEUTIC EFFECT

Suppresses secretion of serotonin, gastroenteropancreatic peptides. Enhances fluid/electrolyte absorption from GI tract; *prolongs intestinal transit time.*

USES/ UNLABELED

Symptomatic treatment of pts w/metastatic carcinoid tumors or vasoactive intestinal peptide tumors. Treatment of acromegaly. *Treatment of hypotension due to carcinoid crises during anesthesia induction, adjunct in treatment of symptoms of hyperinsulinemia from severe refractory metastatic insulinoma, AIDS-associated diarrhea.*

STORAGE/HANDLING

Refrigerate ampules. Ampules may be kept at room temperature on day to be used. Do not use if discolored, contains particulates.

SUBQ ADMINISTRATION

1. Recommended route of administration is SubQ (IV bolus has been given in emergency conditions).

2. Do not use if particulates and/or discoloration are noted.

3. Avoid multiple injections at the same site within short periods.

INDICATIONS/DOSAGE/ROUTES

Note: Initial dose is 50 mcg 1–2 times/day; then dose is increased based on response/tolerability of pt to medication.

Carcinoid tumors:
SubQ: Adults, elderly: 100–600 mcg/day in 2–4 divided doses during first 2 wks of therapy. **Maintenance:** 450 mcg/day (range: 50–750 mcg).

Vasoactive intestinal peptide tumors:
SubQ: Adults, elderly: 200–300 mcg/day in 2–4 divided doses during first 2 wks of therapy (range: 150–750 mcg/day). Dosage adjusted to achieve therapeutic response, usually not above 450 mcg/day.

Acromegaly:
SubQ: Adults, elderly: Initially, 50 mcg 3 times/day. Up to 100 mcg 3 times/day.

Usual maintenance dosage:
IM: Adults, elderly: 20 mg q4wks for 2 mos. May increase to 30 mg q4wks.

PRECAUTIONS

CONTRAINDICATIONS: Hypersensitivity to drug or any of its components. **CAUTIONS:** Insulin-dependent diabetes, renal failure. **PREGNANCY/LACTATION:** Excretion in breast milk unknown. **Pregnancy Category B.**

INTERACTIONS

DRUG INTERACTIONS: May alter glucose concentrations w/insulin, oral hypoglycemics, glucagon, growth hormone. **ALTERED LAB VALUES:** May decrease T_4 concentration.

SIDE EFFECTS

FREQUENT (>10%): Diarrhea, nausea, abdominal discomfort, increased glucose. **OCCASIONAL (1–10%):** Vomiting, flatulence, constipation, headache, alopecia, flushing, itching, dizziness, fatigue, arrhythmias, pain at injection site, bruising, blurred vision. **RARE (<1%):** Depression, decreased libido, vertigo, palpitations, shortness of breath.

ADVERSE REACTIONS/TOXIC EFFECTS

Increased risk of cholelithiasis. Potential for hypothyroidism w/prolonged high therapy. Hepatitis, GI bleeding, seizures occur rarely.

NURSING IMPLICATIONS

BASELINE ASSESSMENT:

Question for hypersensitivity to drug, components. Establish baseline B/P, weight, blood glucose, electrolytes.

INTERVENTION/EVALUATION:

Evaluate blood glucose levels (esp. w/diabetics), electrolytes (therapy generally reduces abnormalities). Weigh every 2–3 days, report >5 lbs gain/week. Monitor B/P, pulse, respirations periodically during treatment. Be alert for decreased urinary output, swelling of ankles, fingers. Check food tolerance. Monitor stools for frequency, consistency.

PATIENT/FAMILY TEACHING:

Careful instruction on SubQ injection. Follow-up by physician and tests are essential. Report jaundice (yellow eyes or skin, dark urine, clay-colored stools), abdominal pain, edema. Therapy should provide significant improvement of symptoms.

ocular lubricant

ock-you-lar **lube**-rih-cant
(Hypotears, Lacrilube)

CANADIAN AVAILABILITY:
Tears Naturale

CLASSIFICATION

Ophthalmic lubricant

AVAILABILITY (OTC)

Ophthalmic Ointment. Solution.

ACTION/*THERAPEUTIC EFFECT*

Maintains ocular tonicity (0.9% NaCl equivalent); buffers to adjust pH, viscosity agents to prolong eye contact time. *Protects and lubricates eye.*

USES

Protection and lubrication of the eye in exposure keratitis, decreased corneal sensitivity, recurrent corneal erosions, keratitis sicca (particularly for nighttime use), after removal of a foreign body, during and following surgery.

OPHTHALMIC ADMINISTRATION

1. Do not use w/contact lenses.
2. *Ointment:* Hold tube in hand for a few minutes to warm ointment.
3. Avoid touching tip of tube or dropper to any surface.
4. Gently pull lower lid down to form pouch.
5. Have pt tilt head backward and look up.
6. *Ointment:* Place ordered amount of ointment in pouch w/a sweeping motion. Instruct pt to close the eye for 1–2 min and roll the eyeball around in all directions.
7. *Drops:* Instill drop(s); have pt close eye gently for 1–2 min. Apply gentle pressure w/fingers to bridge of nose (inside corner of eye).
8. Wipe away excess around eye w/a tissue.

INDICATIONS/DOSAGE/ROUTES

Usual ophthalmic dosage:
Ophthalmic: Adults, elderly: Small amount in conjunctival cul-de-sac.

PRECAUTIONS

CONTRAINDICATIONS: Hypersensitivity to any component of preparation. **CAUTIONS:** None. **PREGNANCY/LACTATION:** Pregnancy Category Unknown.

INTERACTIONS

DRUG INTERACTIONS: None significant. **ALTERED LAB VALUES:** None significant.

SIDE EFFECTS

FREQUENT: Temporary blurring after administration, esp. w/ointment.

ADVERSE REACTIONS/TOXIC EFFECTS

None significant.

NURSING IMPLICATIONS

PATIENT/FAMILY TEACHING:

Teach proper application. Do not use contact lenses. Temporary blurring will occur esp. w/administration of ointment. Avoid activities requiring visual acuity until blurring clears. If eye pain, change of vision, or worsening of condition occurs, or if condition is unchanged after 72 hrs, notify physician. Do not touch to any surface (may contaminate).

ofloxacin

oh-**flocks**-ah-sin
(Floxin, Floxin Otic, Ocuflox)

CANADIAN AVAILABILITY:
Apo-Oflox, Floxin, Ocuflox

CLASSIFICATION

Anti-infective: Quinolone

AVAILABILITY (Rx)

Tablets: 200 mg, 300 mg, 400 mg. **Injection:** 200 mg, 400 mg.

Ophthalmic Solution: 3 mg/ml. **Otic Solution:** 0.3%.

PHARMACOKINETICS

Rapidly, well absorbed from GI tract. Widely distributed (penetrates CSF). Metabolized in liver. Primarily excreted in urine. Minimally removed by hemodialysis. Half-life: 4.7–7 hrs (increased in decreased renal function, elderly, cirrhosis).

ACTION/THERAPEUTIC EFFECT

Inhibits DNA-gyrase in susceptible microorganisms, *interfering w/bacterial DNA replication and repair.* Bactericidal.

USES

Treatment of infections of urinary tract, skin/skin structure, sexually transmitted diseases, lower respiratory tract, prostatitis due to *Escherichia coli,* PID. *Ophthalmic:* Bacterial conjunctivitis, corneal ulcers. **Otic:** Otitis externa, acute/chronic otitis media.

STORAGE/HANDLING

Store oral, parenteral forms at room temperature. After dilution, IV stable for 72 hrs at room temperature; 14 days refrigerated. Discard unused portions.

PO/IV/OPHTHALMIC ADMINISTRATION

PO:

1. Do not give w/food; preferred dosing time: 1 hr before or 2 hrs after meals.

2. Do not administer antacids (aluminum, magnesium) or iron-/zinc-containing products within 2 hrs of ofloxacin.

3. Encourage cranberry juice, citrus fruits (to acidify urine).

4. Give w/8 oz water and encourage fluid intake.

IV:

1. Give only by IV infusion; avoid rapid or bolus IV administration. Must dilute the 20 mg/ml or 40 mg/ml vial.

2. Infuse over at least 60 min.

3. Must dilute each 200 mg w/50 ml 5% dextrose or 0.9% NaCl (400 mg w/100 ml) to provide concentration of 4 mg/ml.

4. Do not add or infuse other medication through same IV line at same time.

OPHTHALMIC:

1. Tilt pt's head back; place solution in conjunctival sac.

2. Have pt close eyes; press gently on lacrimal sac for 1 min.

3. Do not use ophthalmic solutions for injection.

4. Unless infection very superficial, systemic administration generally accompanies ophthalmic.

INDICATIONS/DOSAGE/ROUTES

Urinary tract infection:
PO/IV Infusion: Adults: 200 mg q12h.

Lower respiratory tract, skin/skin structure infections:
PO/IV Infusion: Adults: 400 mg q12h for 10 days.

Prostatitis, sexually transmitted diseases (cervicitis, urethritis):
PO: Adults: 300 mg q12h.

PID:
PO: Adults: 400 mg q12h for 10–14 days.

Prostatitis:
IV Infusion: Adults: 300 mg q12h.

Sexually transmitted diseases:
IV Infusion: Adults: 400 mg as single dose.

Acute, uncomplicated gonorrhea:
PO: Adults: 400 mg 1 time.

Usual elderly dosage:
PO: 200–400 mg q12–24h for 7 days up to 6 wks.

Dosage in renal impairment:
After a normal initial dose, dosage/interval based on creatinine clearance.

CREATININE CLEARANCE	ADJUSTED DOSE	DOSAGE INTERVAL
>50 ml/min	none	12 hrs
10–50 ml/min	none	24 hrs
<10 ml/min	½	24 hrs

Bacterial conjunctivitis:
Ophthalmic: Adults, elderly: 1–2 drops q2–4h for 2 days, then 4 times/day for 5 days.

Corneal ulcers:
Ophthalmic: Adults: 1–2 drops q30 min while awake for 2 days, then q60 min while awake for 5–7 days, then 4 times/day.

Usual otic dosage:
Adults, elderly, children: Twice daily. Warm drops before administering.

PRECAUTIONS

CONTRAINDICATIONS: Syphilis, hypersensitivity to ofloxacin or any quinolones. Children <18 yrs. **CAUTIONS:** Renal impairment, CNS disorders, seizures, those taking theophylline or caffeine. May mask or delay symptoms of syphilis; serologic test for syphilis should be done at diagnosis and 3 mos after treatment. **PREGNANCY/LACTATION:** Distributed in breast milk; potentially serious adverse reactions in nursing infants. Risk of arthropathy to fetus. **Pregnancy Category C**.

INTERACTIONS

DRUG INTERACTIONS: Antacids, sucralfate may decrease absorption, effect of ofloxacin. May increase theophylline concentrations, toxicity. **ALTERED LAB VALUES:** None significant.

SIDE EFFECTS

FREQUENT (7–10%): Nausea, headache, insomnia. **OCCASIONAL (3–5%):** Abdominal pain, diarrhea, vomiting, dry mouth, flatulence, dizziness, fatigue, drowsiness, rash, pruritis, fever. **RARE (<1%):** Constipation, numbness of hands/feet.

ADVERSE REACTIONS/TOXIC EFFECTS

Superinfection, severe hypersensitivity reaction occur rarely. Arthropathy (joint disease w/ swelling, pain, clubbing of fingers and toes, degeneration of stress-bearing portion of a joint) may occur if given to children.

NURSING IMPLICATIONS
BASELINE ASSESSMENT:

Question for history of hypersensitivity to ofloxacin or any quinolones. Obtain specimen for diagnostic tests before giving first dose (therapy may begin before results are known).

INTERVENTION/EVALUATION:

Assess skin and discontinue medication at first sign of rash or other allergic reaction. Evaluate food tolerance. Determine pattern of bowel activity, stool consistency. Assess during the night for sleeplessness, restlessness, complaint of dreaming. Check for dizziness, headache, visual difficulties, tremors; provide ambulation assistance as needed. Monitor TPR, B/P at least 2 times/day. Be alert for superinfection, e.g., genital pruritus, vaginitis, fever, sores, and discomfort in mouth.

PATIENT/FAMILY TEACHING:

Do not skip dose; take full course of therapy. Take w/8 oz water; drink several glasses of water between meals. Eat/drink high sources of ascorbic acid (cranberry juice, citrus fruits). Do not take antacids (reduces/destroys effectiveness). Avoid tasks that require alertness, motor skills until response to drug is established. Avoid sunlight/ultraviolet exposure; wear sunscreen, protective clothing if photosensitivity develops. Notify physician if new symptoms occur. Report inflammation or tendon pain. Otic: Warm drops in hands 1–2 min before administering (prevents dizziness).

olanzapine

oh-**lan**-sah-peen
(Zyprexa)

CANADIAN AVAILABILITY: Zyprexa

CLASSIFICATION

Antipsychotic

AVAILABILITY (Rx)

Tablets: 5 mg, 7.5 mg, 10 mg

PHARMACOKINETICS

Well absorbed following oral administration. Extensively distributed throughout body. Extensively metabolized by first-pass liver metabolism. Excreted in urine, w/lesser amount eliminated in feces. Not removed by dialysis. Half-life: 21–54 hrs.

ACTION/ *THERAPEUTIC EFFECT*

Antagonizes dopamine, serotonin, muscarinic, histamine, and

alpha$_1$-adrenergic receptors, *diminishing psychotic disorders*. Produces anticholinergic, histaminic, CNS depressant effects.

USES

Management of manifestations of psychotic disorders. Treatment of acute mania associated w/bipolar disorder.

PO ADMINISTRATION

May give w/o regard to meals.

INDICATIONS/DOSAGE/ROUTES

Psychotic disorders:
PO: Adults, elderly: Initially, 5–10 mg once daily w/target dose of 10 mg/day within several days after initiation. If needed, dose increments/decrements of 5 mg once daily but not less than 1 wk intervals.

Debilitated, predisposition to hypotensive reactions, elderly >65 yrs:
PO: Adults, elderly: Initially, 5 mg/day.

PRECAUTIONS

CONTRAINDICATIONS: Hypersensitivity to olanzapine. **CAUTIONS:** Hypersensitivity to clozapine, pts who should avoid anticholinergics (e.g., pts w/benign prostatic hypertrophy), hepatic function impairment, elderly, concurrent potentially hepatotoxic drugs, dose escalation, known cardiovascular disease (history of MI or ischemia, heart failure, conduction abnormalities), cerebrovascular disease, conditions predisposing pts to hypotension (dehydration, hypovolemia, hypertensive medications), history of seizures, conditions lowering seizure threshold (e.g., Alzheimer's dementia), those at risk of aspiration pneumonia. **PREGNANCY/LACTATION:** Unknown if drug crosses placenta or is distributed in breast milk. **Pregnancy Category C**.

INTERACTIONS

DRUG INTERACTIONS: Alcohol, CNS depressants may increase CNS depressant effects. Antihypertensive agents increase risk of hypotensive effect. May inhibit metabolism of theophylline, imipramine. Fluvoxamine; ciprofloxacin (quinolone) may increase olanzapine blood levels. Antagonizes effects of levodopa, dopamine agonists. Carbamazepine increases olanzapine clearance. **ALTERED LAB VALUES:** May significantly increase SGPT (ALT), SGOT (AST), GGT levels, prolactin levels.

SIDE EFFECTS

FREQUENT: Somnolence (26%), agitation (23%), insomnia (20%), headache (17%), nervousness (16%), hostility (15%), dizziness (11%), rhinitis (10%). **OCCASIONAL:** Anxiety, constipation (9%), nonaggressive objectionable behavior (8%), dry mouth (7%), weight gain (6%), postural hypotension, fever, joint pain, restlessness, cough, pharyngitis, dimness of vision (5%). **RARE:** Tachycardia, back/chest/abdominal pain, tremor, extremity pain.

ADVERSE REACTIONS/TOXIC EFFECTS

Seizures occur rarely. Neuroleptic malignant syndrome (NMS), a potentially fatal syndrome, occurs rarely and may present as hyperpyrexia, muscle rigidity, irregular pulse or B/P, tachycardia, diaphoresis, cardiac dysrhythmias. Extrapyramidal symptoms may occur. Dysphagia (esophageal dysmotility, aspiration) may be noted. Overdosage (300 mg) produces drowsiness, slurred speech.

NURSING IMPLICATIONS

BASELINE ASSESSMENT:

Obtain baseline hepatic function lab values before initiating treatment. Assess behavior, appearance, emotional status, response to environment, speech pattern, thought content.

INTERVENTION/EVALUATION:

Supervise suicidal risk pt closely during early therapy (as depression lessens, energy level improves, increasing suicide potential). Periodically reassess need for maintenance treatment. Assess for therapeutic response (interest in surroundings, improvement in self-care, increased ability to concentrate, relaxed facial expression). Question bowel activity for evidence of constipation. Assist w/ambulation if dizziness occurs. Notify physician if extrapyramidal symptoms occur. Monitor liver function tests.

PATIENT/FAMILY TEACHING:

Avoid dehydration, particularly during exercise, exposure to extreme heat, concurrent medication causing dry mouth, other drying effects. Notify physician if pregnancy occurs or if there is intention to become pregnant during olanzapine therapy. Take medication as ordered; do not stop taking or increase dosage. Report visual disturbances. Sugarless gum, sips of tepid water may relieve dry mouth. Drowsiness generally subsides during continued therapy. Avoid driving or performing tasks that require alertness, motor skills until response to drug is established. Avoid alcohol. Change positions slowly to reduce hypotensive effect.

olopatidine
(Patanol)
See Supplement

olsalazine sodium
ol-**sal**-ah-zeen
(Dipentum)

CANADIAN AVAILABILITY:
Dipentum

CLASSIFICATION

Anti-inflammatory agent

AVAILABILITY (Rx)

Capsules: 250 mg

PHARMACOKINETICS

Minimally absorbed from GI tract (99% reaches colon). Converted to mesalamine in colon. Primarily eliminated in feces. Half-life: 0.9 hrs.

ACTION/*THERAPEUTIC EFFECT*

Converted in colon by bacterial action to mesalamine, *reducing colonic inflammation* by blocking prostaglandin production in bowel mucosa.

USES/*UNLABELED*

Maintenance of remission of ulcerative colitis in those intolerant of sulfasalazine medication. *Treatment of inflammatory bowel disease.*

PO ADMINISTRATION

Give w/food in evenly divided doses.

INDICATIONS/DOSAGE/ROUTES

Maintenance of controlled ulcerative colitis:
PO: Adults, elderly: 1 g/day in 2 divided doses (preferably q12h).

PRECAUTIONS

CONTRAINDICATIONS: History

of hypersensitivity to salicylates. **CAUTIONS:** Preexisting renal disease. **PREGNANCY/LACTATION:** Unknown whether drug crosses placenta or is distributed in breast milk. **Pregnancy Category C**.

INTERACTIONS

DRUG INTERACTIONS: None significant. **ALTERED LAB VALUES:** May increase SGOT (AST), SGPT (ALT).

SIDE EFFECTS

FREQUENT (5–10%): Headache, diarrhea, abdominal pain/cramps, nausea. **OCCASIONAL (1–5%):** Depression, fatigue, dyspepsia, upper respiratory infrection, decreased appetite, rash, itching, arthralgia. **RARE (<1%):** Dizziness, vomiting, stomatitis.

ADVERSE REACTIONS/TOXIC EFFECTS

Sulfite sensitivity in susceptible pts noted as cramping, headache, diarrhea, fever, rash, hives, itching, wheezing. Discontinue drug immediately. Excessive diarrhea associated w/extreme fatigue noted rarely.

NURSING IMPLICATIONS

BASELINE ASSESSMENT:

Discontinue medication if rash, fever, cramping, or diarrhea occurs.

INTERVENTION/EVALUATION:

Encourage adequate fluid intake. Assess bowel sounds for peristalsis. Monitor daily bowel activity and stool consistency (watery, loose, soft, semisolid, solid) and record time of evacuation. Assess for abdominal disturbances. Assess skin for rash, hives.

PATIENT/FAMILY TEACHING:

Notify physician if diarrhea continues or increases, rash or pruritus occurs.

omeprazole

oh-**mep**-rah-zole
(Prilosec)

CANADIAN AVAILABILITY:
Losec

CLASSIFICATION

Gastric acid pump inhibitor

AVAILABILITY (Rx)

Capsules (delayed-release): 10 mg, 20 mg, 40 mg.

PHARMACOKINETICS

Rapidly absorbed from GI tract. Primarily distributed into gastric parietal cells. Metabolized extensively in liver. Primarily excreted in urine. Half-life: 0.5–1 hr (increased in decreased liver function).

ACTION/*THERAPEUTIC EFFECT*

Converted to active metabolites that irreversibly bind to and inhibit H+/K+ ATPase (an enzyme on surface of gastric parietal cells). Inhibits hydrogen ion transport into gastric lumen, *increasing gastric pH, reducing gastric acid production.*

USES

Short-term treatment (4–8 wks) of erosive esophagitis (diagnosed by endoscopy); symptomatic gastroesophageal reflux disease (GERD) poorly responsive to other treatment. Long-term treatment of pathologic hypersecretory conditions; treatment of active duodenal ulcer. Maintenance healing of erosive esophagitis. Treatment of *H. Pylori*–associated duodenal ulcer (w/clarithromycin), active benign gastric ulcers. Prevention/treatment of NSAID-induced ulcers.

PO ADMINISTRATION

1. Give before meals.

2. Do not crush or chew capsule; swallow whole.

INDICATIONS/DOSAGE/ROUTES

Erosive esophagitis, poorly responsive GERD, active duodenal ulcer, prevention/treatment of NSAID-induced ulcers:
PO: Adults, elderly: 20 mg/day.

Maintenance healing of erosive esophagitis:
PO: Adults, elderly: 20 mg/day.

Pathologic hypersecretory conditions:
PO: Adults, elderly: Initially, 60 mg/day up to 120 mg, 3 times/day.

H. Pylori duodenal ulcer:
PO: Adults, elderly: 20 mg 2 times/day for 10 days.

Active benign gastric ulcer:
PO: Adults, elderly: 40 mg/day for 4–8 wks.

PRECAUTIONS

CONTRAINDICATIONS: None significant. CAUTIONS: None significant. PREGNANCY/LACTATION: Unknown whether drug crosses placenta or is distributed in breast milk. Pregnancy Category C.

INTERACTIONS

DRUG INTERACTIONS: May increase concentration of oral anticoagulants, diazepam, phenytoin. ALTERED LAB VALUES: May increase SGOT (AST), SGPT (ALT), alkaline phosphatase.

SIDE EFFECTS

FREQUENT (7%): Headache. OCCASIONAL (2–3%): Diarrhea, abdominal pain, nausea. RARE (<2%): Dizziness, asthenia (loss of strength), vomiting, constipation, upper respiratory infection, back pain, rash, cough.

ADVERSE REACTIONS/TOXIC EFFECTS

None significant.

NURSING IMPLICATIONS
INTERVENTION/EVALUATION:

Evaluate for therapeutic response, i.e., relief of GI symptoms. Question if GI discomfort, nausea, diarrhea occurs.

PATIENT/FAMILY TEACHING:

Report headache. Swallow capsules whole; do not chew or crush. Take prior to eating.

ondansetron hydrochloride
on-**dan**-sah-tron
(Zofran)

CANADIAN AVAILABILITY:
Zofran

CLASSIFICATION

Antiemetic

AVAILABILITY: (Rx)

Tablets: 4 mg, 8 mg, 24 mg. Oral Disintegrating Tablets: 4 mg, 8 mg. Oral Solution: 4 mg/5 ml. Injection: 2 mg/ml. Injection (Premix): 32 mg/50 ml.

PHARMACOKINETICS

Readily absorbed from GI tract. Metabolized in liver. Primarily excreted in urine. Half-life: 4 hrs.

ACTION/*THERAPEUTIC EFFECT*

Exhibits selective 5-HT$_3$ receptor antagonism for *preventing nausea/vomiting associated w/cancer chemotherapy.* Action may be central (CTZ) or peripheral (vagus nerve terminal).

USES/*UNLABELED*

Prevention, treatment of nausea and vomiting due to cancer chemotherapy, including high-dose cisplatin. Prevention of postop nausea, vomiting. Prevention of radiation-induced nausea, vomiting. *Treatment of postop nausea/vomiting.*

PO/IM/IV ADMINISTRATION

PO:

May give w/o regard to food.

IM:

Inject into large muscle mass.

IV:

1. For IV infusion, dilute w/50 ml 5% dextrose or 0.9% NaCl before administration.

2. Infuse over 15 min.

STORAGE/HANDLING

Store parenteral form at room temperature. After dilution, stable at room temperature for 48 hrs.

INDICATIONS/DOSAGE/ROUTE

Nausea, vomiting: Chemotherapy
IV: Adults, elderly, children (4–18 yrs): 3 doses 0.15 mg/kg. First dose given 30 min before chemotherapy; then 4 and 8 hrs after first dose of ondansetron.
PO: Adults, elderly: 24 mg once a day; 8 mg 30 min before start of chemotherapy, then 4 and 8 hrs after first dose; then, 8 mg q8h for 1–2 days after completion of chemotherapy. **Children:** 4 mg using same regimen as for adults.

Nausea, vomiting: Postop
IM/IV: Adults, elderly: 4 mg undiluted over 2–5 min. **Children <40 kg:** 0.1 mg/kg. **>40 kg:** 4 mg.

Nausea, vomiting: Radiation
PO: Adults, elderly: 8 mg 3 times/day.

PRECAUTIONS

CONTRAINDICATIONS: None significant. **CAUTIONS:** None significant. **PREGNANCY/LACTATION:** Unknown whether drug crosses placenta or is distributed in breast milk. **Pregnancy Category B.**

INTERACTIONS

DRUG INTERACTIONS: None sig-

nificant. **ALTERED LAB VALUES:** May transiently increase SGOT (AST), SGPT (ALT), bilirubin.

SIDE EFFECTS

FREQUENT (5–13%): Anxiety, dizziness, drowsiness, headache, fatigue, constipation, diarrhea, hypoxia, urinary retention. **OCCASIONAL (2–4%):** Abdominal pain, xerostomia (diminished saliva secretion), fever, feeling of cold, redness/pain at injection site, paresthesia, weakness. **RARE (<1%):** Hypersensitivity reaction (rash, itching), blurred vision.

ADVERSE REACTIONS/TOXIC EFFECTS

Overdose may produce combination of CNS stimulation and depressant effects.

NURSING IMPLICATIONS

BASELINE ASSESSMENT:

Assess for dehydration if excessive vomiting occurs (poor skin turgor, dry mucous membranes, longitudinal furrows in tongue). Provide emotional support.

INTERVENTION/EVALUATION:

Monitor pt in environment. Assess bowel sounds for peristalsis. Provide supportive measures. Assess mental status. Monitor daily bowel activity and stool consistency (watery, loose, soft, semisolid, solid) and record time of evacuation.

PATIENT/FAMILY TEACHING:

Relief from nausea/vomiting generally occurs shortly after drug administration. Avoid alcohol, barbiturates. Report persistent vomiting.

oprelvekin

(Neumega)
See Supplement

orlistat
(Xenical)
See Supplement

orphenadrine citrate
(Norflex)

FIXED-COMBINATION(S):

W/aspirin, nonnarcotic analgesic
and caffeine, a stimulant (Nor-
gesic)
See Classification section under:
Skeletal Muscle Relaxants

oseltamivir
(Tamiflu)
See Supplement

oxacillin sodium
ox-ah-sill-in
(Bactocill, Prostaphlin)

CLASSIFICATION

Antibiotic: Penicillin

AVAILABILITY (Rx)

Capsules: 250 mg, 500 mg.
Oral Suspension: 250 mg/5 ml.
Powder for Injection: 250 mg,
500 mg, 1 g, 2 g, 4 g, 10 g.

PHARMACOKINETICS

Moderately absorbed from GI
tract (food decreases absorption).
Widely distributed. Metabolized in
liver. Primarily excreted in urine.
Half-life: 0.5–0.7 hrs (increased in
decreased renal function, neonates).

ACTION/ *THERAPEUTIC EFFECT*

Binds to bacterial membranes, *in-*
hibiting cell wall synthesis. Bactericidal.

USES

Treatment of respiratory tract,
skin/skin structure infections, osteomyelitis, endocarditis, meningitis, perioperatively, esp. in cardiovascular, orthopedic procedures.
Predominantly used in treatment
of infections caused by penicillinase-producing staphylococci.

STORAGE/HANDLING

Store capsules at room temperature. After reconstitution, oral solution is stable for 3 days at room
temperature, 14 days if refrigerated; IV infusion (piggyback) is stable for at least 6 hrs at room temperature, 8 days if refrigerated.
Discard if precipitate forms.

PO/IM/IV ADMINISTRATION

Note: Space doses evenly around
the clock.

PO:

Give 1 hr before or 2 hrs after
food.

IM:

1. Dilute 250 mg vial w/1.4 ml
(500 mg with 2.7 ml, 1 g w/5.7 ml,
2 g w/11.4 ml, or 4 g w/21.8 ml)
sterile water for injection or 0.9%
NaCl injection to provide concentration of 250 mg/1.5 ml.

2. Inject IM into large muscle
mass.

IV:

1. For IV injection, dilute each
250 or 500 mg vial w/5 ml (1 g
w/10 ml, 2 g w/20 ml) sterile water
for injection or 0.9% NaCl injection. Administer over 10 min.

2. For intermittent IV infusion
(piggyback), further dilute w/50–
100 ml 5% dextrose, 0.9% NaCl,
or other compatible IV fluid. Infuse over 30–60 min.

3. Because of potential for hy-
persensitivity/anaphylaxis, start
initial dose at few drops per
minute, increase slowly to ordered
rate; stay w/pt first 10–15 min, then
check q10 min.

4. Alternating IV sites, use large veins to reduce risk of phlebitis.

INDICATIONS/DOSAGE/ROUTES

Mild to moderate infections of upper respiratory tract, skin/skin structure infections:
PO: Adults, elderly, children >20 kg: 500 mg q4–6h. **Children <20 kg:** 50 mg/kg/day in divided doses q6h.
IM/IV: Adults, elderly, children >40 kg: 250–500 mg q4–6h. **Children <40 kg:** 50 mg/kg/day in divided doses q6h.

Lower respiratory tract, disseminated infections, serious infections:
PO: Adults, elderly: 1 g q4–6h. **Children:** 100 mg/kg/day in divided doses q4–6h.
IM/IV: Adults, elderly, children >40 kg: 1 g q4–6h. **Maximum:** 12 g/day. **Children <40 kg:** 100 mg/kg/day in divided doses q4–6h. **Maximum:** 300 mg/kg/day.

Usual dosage (neonates):
IM/IV: Neonates 0–7 days: 50–75 mg/kg/day in 2–3 divided doses. **Neonates 7–28 days:** 100–150 mg/kg/day in 3–4 divided doses.

PRECAUTIONS

CONTRAINDICATIONS: Hypersensitivity to any penicillin. **CAUTIONS:** History of allergies, esp. cephalosporins. **PREGNANCY/LACTATION:** Readily crosses placenta, appears in cord blood, amniotic fluid. Distributed in breast milk in low concentrations. May lead to allergic sensitization, diarrhea, candidiasis, skin rash in infant. **Pregnancy Category B**.

INTERACTIONS

DRUG INTERACTIONS: Probenecid may increase concentration,

toxicity risk. **ALTERED LAB VALUES:** May increase SGOT (AST). May cause positive Coombs' test.

SIDE EFFECTS

FREQUENT: Mild hypersensitivity reaction (fever, rash, pruritus), GI effects (nausea, vomiting, diarrhea) more frequent w/oral administration. **OCCASIONAL:** Phlebitis, thrombophlebitis (more common in elderly), hepatotoxicity w/high IV dosage.

ADVERSE REACTIONS/TOXIC EFFECTS

Superinfections, antibiotic-associated colitis may result from altered bacteria balance; hypersensitivity reaction ranging from mild to severe may occur in those allergic to penicillin.

NURSING IMPLICATIONS
BASELINE ASSESSMENT:

Question for history of allergies, esp. penicillins, cephalosporins. Obtain specimen for culture and sensitivity before giving first dose (therapy may begin before results are known).

INTERVENTION/EVALUATION:

Hold medication and promptly report rash (possible hypersensitivity) or diarrhea (w/fever, abdominal pain, blood and mucus in stool may indicate antibiotic-associated colitis). Assess food tolerance. Evaluate IV site frequently for phlebitis (heat, pain, red streaking over vein). Monitor I&O, urinalysis, renal function tests. Be alert for superinfection: vomiting, diarrhea, black/hairy tongue, ulceration/changes of oral mucosa, anal/genital pruritus. Check hematology reports (esp. WBCs), periodic renal or hepatic reports in prolonged therapy.

PATIENT/FAMILY TEACHING:

Continue antibiotic for full length of treatment. Space doses evenly. Discomfort may occur w/IM injection. Notify physician in event of diarrhea, rash, or other new symptom.

oxaprozin

ox-ah-**pro**-zin
(Daypro)

CANADIAN AVAILABILITY: Daypro

CLASSIFICATION

Nonsteroidal anti-inflammatory

AVAILABILITY (Rx)

Tablets: 600 mg

PHARMACOKINETICS

Well absorbed from GI tract. Widely distributed. Metabolized in liver. Primarily excreted in urine; partially eliminated in feces. Half-life: 42–50 hrs.

ACTION/THERAPEUTIC EFFECT

Produces analgesic and anti-inflammatory effect by inhibiting prostaglandin synthesis, *reducing inflammatory response and intensity of pain stimulus reaching sensory nerve endings.*

USES

Acute and chronic treatment of osteoarthritis, rheumatoid arthritis.

PO ADMINISTRATION

May give w/food, milk, or antacids if GI distress occurs.

INDICATIONS/DOSAGE/ROUTES

Osteoarthritis:
PO: Adults, elderly: 1,200 mg once daily; 600 mg in pts w/low body weight, mild disease. **Maximum:** 1,800 mg/day.

Rheumatoid arthritis:
PO: Adults, elderly: 1,200 mg once daily. **Range:** 600–1,800 mg/day.

PRECAUTIONS

CONTRAINDICATIONS: Active peptic ulcer, GI ulceration, chronic inflammation of GI tract, GI bleeding disorders, history of hypersensitivity to aspirin or NSAIDs. **CAUTIONS:** Impaired renal/hepatic function, history of GI tract disease, predisposition to fluid retention. **PREGNANCY/LACTATION:** Unknown whether drug is excreted in breast milk. Avoid use during third trimester (may adversely affect fetal cardiovascular system: premature closure of ductus arteriosus). **Pregnancy Category C**. (Category D if used 3rd trimester or near delivery.)

INTERACTIONS

DRUG INTERACTIONS: May increase effects of oral anticoagulants, heparin, thrombolytics. May decrease effect of antihypertensives, diuretics. Salicylates, aspirin may increase risk of GI side effects, bleeding. Bone marrow depressants may increase risk of hematologic reactions. May increase concentration, toxicity of lithium. May increase methotrexate toxicity. Probenecid may increase concentration. **ALTERED LAB VALUES:** May increase SGOT (AST), SGPT (ALT), serum creatinine, BUN.

SIDE EFFECTS

OCCASIONAL (3–9%): Nausea, diarrhea, constipation, dyspepsia (heartburn, indigestion, epigastric pain). **RARE (<3%):** Vomiting, abdominal cramping/pain, flatulence, anorexia, confusion, ringing in ears, insomnia, drowsiness.

ADVERSE REACTIONS/TOXIC EFFECTS

GI bleeding, coma may occur. Hypertension, acute renal failure, respiratory depression occur rarely.

NURSING IMPLICATIONS

BASELINE ASSESSMENT:

Assess onset, type, location, and duration of pain or inflammation.

INTERVENTION/EVALUATION:

Assist w/ambulation if dizziness occurs. Monitor stools; avoid constipation through high-fiber diet, appropriate exercise, and increased fluids. Check for rash. Evaluate for therapeutic response: relief of pain, stiffness, swelling, increase in joint mobility, reduced joint tenderness, improved grip strength.

PATIENT/FAMILY TEACHING:

Avoid aspirin, alcohol during therapy (increases risk of GI bleeding). Report tarry stools. If GI upset occurs, take w/food, milk. Avoid tasks that require alertness, motor skills until response to drug is established.

---

oxazepam

ox-**az**-eh-pam
(Serax)

CANADIAN AVAILABILITY:
Apo-Oxazepam, Serax

CLASSIFICATION

Antianxiety: Benzodiazepine

AVAILABILITY (Rx)

Capsules: 10 mg, 15 mg, 30 mg. **Tablets:** 15 mg.

PHARMACOKINETICS

Well absorbed from GI tract. Metabolized in liver. Primarily excreted in urine. Half-life: 5–15 hrs.

ACTION/*THERAPEUTIC EFFECT*

Enhances inhibitory gamma-aminobutyric acid (GABA) neurotransmission at CNS, *producing anxiolytic effect.* Inhibits spinal afferent pathways, *producing skeletal muscle relaxation.* Depressant effects occur at all levels of CNS. Directly depresses motor nerve, muscle function.

USES

Management of acute alcohol withdrawal symptoms (tremulousness, anxiety on withdrawal). Treatment of anxiety associated w/depressive symptoms.

PO ADMINISTRATION

1. Give w/o regard to meals.
2. Capsules may be emptied and mixed w/food.

INDICATIONS/DOSAGE/ROUTES

Note: Use smallest effective dose in elderly, debilitated, those w/liver disease, low serum albumin.

Mild to moderate anxiety:
PO: Adults: 10–15 mg 3–4 times/day.

Severe anxiety:
PO: Adults: 15–30 mg 3–4 times/day.

Alcohol withdrawal:
PO: Adults: 15–30 mg 3–4 times/day.

Usual elderly dosage:
PO: Initially, 10 mg 2–3 times/day. May gradually increase up to 30–45 mg/day.

PRECAUTIONS

CONTRAINDICATIONS: Acute

narrow-angle glaucoma. **CAUTIONS:** Impaired renal/hepatic function. **PREGNANCY/LACTATION:** May cross placenta; may be distributed in breast milk. Chronic ingestion during pregnancy may produce withdrawal symptoms, CNS depression in neonates. **Pregnancy Category D.**

INTERACTIONS

DRUG INTERACTIONS: Potentiated effects when used w/other CNS depressants, including alcohol. **ALTERED LAB VALUES:** May produce abnormal renal function tests, elevate SGOT (AST), SGPT (ALT), LDH, alkaline phosphatase, serum bilirubin.

SIDE EFFECTS

FREQUENT: Mild, transient drowsiness at beginning of therapy. **OCCASIONAL:** Dizziness, headache. **RARE:** Paradoxical CNS hyperactivity/nervousness in children, excitement/restlessness in elderly/debilitated (generally noted during first 2 wks of therapy, particularly noted in presence of uncontrolled pain).

ADVERSE REACTIONS/TOXIC EFFECTS

Abrupt or too rapid withdrawal may result in pronounced restlessness, irritability, insomnia, hand tremors, abdominal/muscle cramps, sweating, vomiting, seizures. Overdose results in somnolence, confusion, diminished reflexes, coma.

NURSING IMPLICATIONS
BASELINE ASSESSMENT:

Offer emotional support to anxious pt. Assess motor responses (agitation, trembling, tension) and autonomic responses (cold, clammy hands, sweating).

INTERVENTION/EVALUATION:

For those on long-term therapy, liver/renal function tests, blood counts should be performed periodically. Assess for paradoxical reaction, particularly during early therapy. Assist w/ambulation if drowsiness, lightheadedness occur. Evaluate for therapeutic response: a calm facial expression, decreased restlessness, and/or insomnia.

PATIENT/FAMILY TEACHING:

Drowsiness usually disappears during continued therapy. If dizziness occurs, change positions slowly from recumbent to sitting position before standing. Avoid tasks that require alertness, motor skills until response to drug is established. Smoking reduces drug effectiveness. Do not abruptly withdraw medication after long-term therapy.

---

oxiconazole
(Oxistat)
See Classification section under: Antifungals: Topical

---

oxybutynin chloride
ox-ee-**byoo**-tih-nin
(Ditropan)

CANADIAN AVAILABILITY:
Ditropan

CLASSIFICATION

Antispasmodic

AVAILABILITY (Rx)

Tablets: 5 mg. **Syrup:** 5 mg/5 ml. **Extended Release Tablets:** 5 mg, 10 mg, 15 mg.

PHARMACOKINETICS

	ONSET	PEAK	DURATION
PO	0.5–1 hr	3–6 hrs	6–10 hrs

Rapid absorption from GI tract. Metabolized in liver. Primarily excreted in urine. Half-life: 1–2.3 hrs.

ACTION/*THERAPEUTIC EFFECT*

Exerts antispasmodic (papaverinelike) and antimuscarinic (atropinelike) action on detrusor smooth muscle of bladder. *Increases bladder capacity, diminishes frequency of uninhibited detrusor muscle contraction, delays desire to void.*

USES

Relief of symptoms (urgency, incontinence, frequency, nocturia, urge incontinence) associated w/uninhibited neurogenic bladder or reflex neurogenic bladder.

PO ADMINISTRATION

Give w/o regard to meals.

INDICATIONS/DOSAGE/ROUTES

Neurogenic bladder:
PO: Adults: 5 mg 2–3 times/day. **Maximum:** 5 mg 4 times/day. **Children >5 yrs:** 5 mg 2 times/day. **Maximum:** 5 mg 3 times/day.

Usual elderly dosage:
PO: Initially, 2.5–5 mg/day. May increase by 2.5 mg q1–2 days.

Usual dosage extended release:
PO: Adults, elderly: 5–30 mg/day as single daily dose.

PRECAUTIONS

CONTRAINDICATIONS: Angle-closure glaucoma, GI obstruction, myasthenia gravis, paralytic ileus, megacolon, ulcerative colitis, intestinal atony, unstable cardiovascular disease. **CAUTIONS:** Impaired renal or hepatic function, elderly, autonomic neuropathy.

PREGNANCY/LACTATION: Unknown whether drug crosses placenta or is distributed in breast milk. **Pregnancy Category B**.

INTERACTIONS

DRUG INTERACTIONS: Medication w/anticholinergic effects (e.g., antihistamines) may increase effects. **ALTERED LAB VALUES:** None significant.

SIDE EFFECTS

FREQUENT: Constipation, dry mouth, drowsiness, decreased sweating. **OCCASIONAL:** Decreased lacrimation, salivary/sweat gland secretion, sexual ability. Urinary hesitancy/retention, suppressed lactation, blurred vision, mydriasis, nausea or vomiting, insomnia.

ADVERSE REACTIONS/TOXIC EFFECTS

Overdosage produces CNS excitation (nervousness, restlessness, hallucinations, irritability), hypo/hypertension, confusion, fast heartbeat or tachycardia, flushed or red face, respiratory depression (shortness of breath or troubled breathing).

NURSING IMPLICATIONS
INTERVENTION/EVALUATION:

Assess pulse periodically. Monitor I&O; palpate bladder for retention. Monitor stools; avoid constipation w/fluids, bulk, and exercise. Hold medication and notify physician of diarrhea at once.

PATIENT/FAMILY TEACHING:

May cause dry mouth. Avoid alcohol and sedatives. Report diarrhea promptly (may be early symptom of incomplete intestinal obstruction, esp. those w/ileostomy or colostomy). Do not take medication in high environmental temperature (heat prostration may occur due to decreased sweating). Avoid tasks that require alertness, motor skills until response to drug is established.

oxycodone

ox-ih-**koe**-doan
(Oxycontin, Perolone, Roxicodone)

FIXED-COMBINATION(S): W/acetaminophen **(Percocet, Roxicet, Tylox)**; w/aspirin **(Percodan, Roxiprin)**

CANADIAN AVAILABILITY: OxyContin, Supeudol

CLASSIFICATION

Opioid analgesic **(Schedule II)**

AVAILABILITY (Rx)

Tablets: 5 mg. **Tablets (controlled-release):** 10 mg, 20 mg, 40 mg, 80 mg. **Oral Solution:** 5 mg/5 ml. **Oral Concentrate:** 20 mg/ml.

PHARMACOKINETICS

	ONSET	PEAK	DURATION
PO	10–15 min	30–60 min	3–6 hrs

Moderately absorbed from GI tract. Widely distributed. Metabolized in liver. Excreted in urine. Half-life: 2–3 hrs.

ACTION / THERAPEUTIC EFFECT

Binds w/opioid receptors within CNS, *altering processes affecting pain perception, emotional response to pain.*

USES

Relief of mild to moderately severe pain.

PO ADMINISTRATION

1. Give w/o regard to meals.
2. Tablets may be crushed.
3. *Controlled-Release:* Swallow whole; do not crush, break, chew.

INDICATIONS / DOSAGE / ROUTES

Note: Reduce initial dosage in those w/hypothyroidism, concurrent CNS depressants, Addison's disease, renal insufficiency, elderly/debilitated.

Analgesia:
PO: Adults: 5 mg q6h as needed. **Elderly:** 2.5–5 mg q6h as needed. **Controlled-Release:** 10–30 mg q12h.

PRECAUTIONS

CONTRAINDICATIONS: None significant. **EXTREME CAUTION:** CNS depression, anoxia, hypercapnia, respiratory depression, seizures, acute alcoholism, shock, untreated myxedema, respiratory dysfunction. **CAUTIONS:** Increased intracranial pressure, impaired hepatic function, acute abdominal conditions, hypothyroidism, prostatic hypertrophy, Addison's disease, urethral stricture, COPD. **PREGNANCY/LACTATION:** Readily crosses placenta; distributed in breast milk. Respiratory depression may occur in neonate if mother received opiates during labor. Regular use of opiates during pregnancy may produce withdrawal symptoms in neonate (irritability, excessive crying, tremors, hyperactive reflexes, fever, vomiting, diarrhea, yawning, sneezing, seizures). **Pregnancy Category B.** (Category D if used for prolonged periods or in high doses at term.)

INTERACTIONS

DRUG INTERACTIONS: Alcohol, CNS depressants may increase

CNS or respiratory depression, hypotension. MAO inhibitors may produce severe, fatal reaction (reduce dose to ¼ usual dose). **ALTERED LAB VALUES:** May increase amylase, lipase.

SIDE EFFECTS

Note: Effects are dependent on dosage amount. Ambulatory pts and those not in severe pain may experience dizziness, nausea, vomiting, hypotension more frequently than those in supine position or having severe pain.
FREQUENT: Drowsiness, dizziness, hypotension, anorexia. **OCCASIONAL:** Confusion, diaphoresis, facial flushing, urinary retention, constipation, dry mouth, nausea, vomiting, headache. **RARE:** Allergic reaction, depression.

ADVERSE REACTIONS/TOXIC EFFECTS

Overdose results in respiratory depression, skeletal muscle flaccidity, cold, clammy skin, cyanosis, extreme somnolence progressing to convulsions, stupor, coma. Hepatotoxicity may occur w/overdosage of acetaminophen component. Tolerance to analgesic effect, physical dependence may occur w/repeated use.

NURSING IMPLICATIONS
BASELINE ASSESSMENT:

Assess onset, type, location, and duration of pain. Effect of medication is reduced if full pain recurs before next dose. Obtain vital signs before giving medication. If respirations are 12/min or lower (20/min or lower in children), withhold medication, contact physician.

INTERVENTION/EVALUATION:

Palpate bladder for urinary retention. Monitor pattern of daily bowel activity and stool consistency. Initiate deep breathing and coughing exercises, particularly in those w/impaired pulmonary function. Assess for clinical improvement and record onset of relief of pain.

PATIENT/FAMILY TEACHING:

Change positions slowly to avoid orthostatic hypotension. Avoid tasks that require alertness, motor skills until response to drug is established. Tolerance/dependence may occur w/prolonged use of high doses. Avoid alcohol and CNS depressants.

oxytocin
ox-ih-**toe**-sin
(Pitocin)

CLASSIFICATION
Oxytocic

AVAILABILITY (Rx)
Injection: 10 units/ml. **Nasal Spray:** 40 units/ml.

PHARMACOKINETICS

	ONSET	PEAK	DURATION
IM	3–5 min	—	2–3 hrs
IV	Immediate	—	1 hr
Intranasal			
	Few minutes	—	20 min

Rapidly absorbed through nasal mucous membranes. Distributed in extracellular fluid. Metabolized in liver, kidney. Primarily excreted in urine.

ACTION/THERAPEUTIC EFFECT

Acts on uterine myofibril activity, *stimulates contraction of uterine smooth muscle* (augments number of contracting myofibrils). Stimulates mammary smooth muscle to *enhance milk ejection from breasts.*

USES

Parenteral (Antepartum): To initiate or improve uterine contraction to achieve early vaginal delivery; stimulate or reinforce labor; management of incomplete or inevitable abortion. *(Postpartum):* To produce uterine contractions during third stage of labor; control uterine bleeding. *Nasal:* To promote breast milk ejection.

IV/NASAL ADMINISTRATION

IV:

1. Requires qualified personnel, hospitalization w/availability of surgical facilities and intensive care.
2. Continuous monitoring of uterine contractions, fetal and maternal heart rates, maternal B/P, and, if possible, intrauterine pressure.
3. Dilute 10 units (1 ml) in 1,000 ml of 0.9% NaCl, lactated Ringer's, or 5% dextrose injection to provide a concentration of 10 milliunits/ml solution.
4. Give by IV infusion (use infusion device to carefully control rate of flow).

NASAL SPRAY:

1. W/pt in sitting position, spray in one or both nostrils.
2. Give 2–3 min before nursing or pumping breasts.

INDICATIONS/DOSAGE/ROUTES

Induction/stimulation of labor:
IV Infusion: Adults: Initially, 1–2 milliunits/min; gradually increase in increments of 1–2 milliunits/min q15–30 min (until contraction pattern similar to spontaneous labor reached). **Maximum:** Rarely >20 milliunits/min.

Incomplete/inevitable abortion:
IV Infusion: Adults: 10 units in 500 ml (20 milliunits/ml) 5% dextrose in water or 0.9% NaCl infused at 10–20 milliunits/min.

Control postpartum bleeding:
IV Infusion: Adults: 10–40 units (**maximum:** 40 units/1,000 ml) infused at rate of 20–40 milliunits/min after delivery of infant.
IM: Adults: 10 units after delivery of placenta.

Promote milk ejection:
Nasal: Adults: 1 spray to one or both nostrils 2–3 min before nursing or pumping breasts.

PRECAUTIONS

CONTRAINDICATIONS: Hypersensitivity to oxytocin, cephalopelvic disproportion, unfavorable fetal position or presentation, unengaged fetal head, fetal distress w/o imminent delivery, prematurity, when vaginal delivery is contraindicated (e.g., active genital herpes infection, placenta previa, cord presentation), obstetric emergencies that favor surgical intervention, grand multiparity, hypertonic or hyperactive uterus, adequate uterine activity that fails to progress. Nasal spray during pregnancy. **CAUTIONS:** Induction should be for medical, not elective reasons. **PREGNANCY/LACTATION:** Used as indicated, not expected to present risk of fetal abnormalities. Small amounts in breast milk; nursing not recommended.

INTERACTIONS

DRUG INTERACTIONS: Caudal block anesthetics, vasopressors may increase pressor effects. Other oxytocics may cause uterine hypertonus, uterine rupture, or cervical lacerations. **ALTERED LAB VALUES:** None significant.

SIDE EFFECTS

OCCASIONAL: Tachycardia, PVCs, hypotension, nausea, vomiting. **RARE:** *Nasal:* Lacrimation (tearing), nasal irritation, rhinorrhea, unexpected uterine bleeding or contractions.

ADVERSE REACTIONS/TOXIC EFFECTS

Hypertonicity with tearing of uterus, increased bleeding, abruptio placenta, cervical and vaginal lacerations. *Fetal:* Bradycardia, CNS or brain damage, trauma due to rapid propulsion, low Apgar at 5 min, retinal hemorrhage occur rarely.

Prolonged IV infusion of oxytocin w/excessive fluid volume has caused severe water intoxication w/seizures, coma, and death.

NURSING IMPLICATIONS

BASELINE ASSESSMENT:

Question for hypersensitivity to oxytocin. Assess baselines for TPR, B/P, and fetal heart rate. Determine frequency, duration, and strength of contractions.

INTERVENTION/EVALUATION:

Monitor B/P, pulse, respirations, fetal heart rate, intrauterine pressure, contractions (duration, strength, frequency) every 15 min. Notify physician of contractions that last >1 min, occur more frequently than every 2 min, or stop. Maintain careful I/O; be alert to potential water intoxication. Check for blood loss.

PATIENT/FAMILY TEACHING:

Keep pt, family informed of labor progress. *Nasal spray:* Teach proper use.

paclitaxel

pass-leh-**tax**-ell
(Paxene, Taxol)

CANADIAN AVAILABILITY: Taxol

CLASSIFICATION

Antineoplastic

AVAILABILITY (Rx)

Injection: 30 mg, 100 mg

PHARMACOKINETICS

Does not readily cross blood-brain barrier. Metabolized in liver (active metabolites); eliminated via bile. Half-life: 1.3–8.6 hrs.

ACTION/THERAPEUTIC EFFECT

Binds to fully assembled microtubules, stabilizes microtubules, prevents depolymerization, *resulting in halting mitosis and cell death.* May also interrupt mitosis by distorting mitotic spindles. Cell cycle-specific for G_2, M phases.

USES/UNLABELED

Initial treatment of advanced ovarian cancer, treatment for metastatic ovarian cancer following failure of first-line or subsequent chemotherapy. Treatment of breast carcinoma. Treatment of AIDS-related Kaposi's sarcoma. Treatment of non-small cell lung carcinoma.

STORAGE/HANDLING

Refrigerate unopened vials. Prepared solutions stable at room temperature for 24 hrs. Wear gloves during handling; if contact w/skin, wash hands thoroughly w/soap and water. If in contact w/mucous membranes, flush w/water.

IV ADMINISTRATION

1. Must dilute before administration w/0.9% NaCl, 5% dextrose to final concentration of 0.3–1.2 mg/ml.

2. Store diluted solutions in bottles or plastic bags and administer through polyethylene-lined administration sets (avoid plasticized PVC equipment or devices).

3. Administer through in-line filter not greater than 0.22 microns.

4. Monitor vital signs during infusion, esp. during first hour.

5. Discontinue administration if severe hypersensitivity reaction occurs.

INDICATIONS/DOSAGE/ROUTES

Note: Pretreat w/corticosteroids, diphenhydramine, and H_2 antagonists.

Ovarian cancer:
IV Infusion: Adults: 175 mg/m^2 over 3 hrs q3 wks.

Breast carcinoma:
IV Infusion: Adults, elderly: 175 mg/m^2 over 3 hrs q3 wks.

PRECAUTIONS

CONTRAINDICATIONS: Baseline neutropenia <1,500 cells/mm^3, hypersensitivity to drugs developed w/Cremophor EL (polyoxyethylated castor oil). **CAUTIONS:** History of CHF, cardiac conduction abnormalities, existing/recent chickenpox, infection, herpes zoster. **PREGNANCY/LACTATION:** May produce fetal harm. Unknown whether distributed in breast milk. Avoid pregnancy. **Pregnancy Category D.**

INTERACTIONS

DRUG INTERACTIONS: Bone marrow depressants may increase bone marrow depression. Live virus vaccines may potentiate virus replication, increase vaccine side effects, decrease pt's antibody response to vaccine. **ALTERED LAB VALUES:** May elevate alkaline phosphatase, SGOT (AST), SGPT (ALT), bilirubin.

SIDE EFFECTS

FREQUENT (>10%): Alopecia, pain in joints/muscles (especially arms/legs), diarrhea, nausea, vomiting, peripheral neuropathy, (numbness in hands/feet), hypotension, abnormal ECG, pain/redness at injection site, mucositis. **OCCASIONAL (3–10%):** Bradycardia.

ADVERSE REACTIONS/TOXIC EFFECTS

Severe hypersensitivity reaction (dyspnea, severe hypotension, angioedema, generalized urticaria), myelosuppression (neutropenia and leukopenia).

NURSING IMPLICATIONS

BASELINE ASSESSMENT:

Give emotional support to pt and family. Use strict asepsis and protect pt from infection. Check blood counts, particularly neutrophil, platelet count before each course of therapy, monthly, or as clinically indicated.

INTERVENTION/EVALUATION:

Monitor for hematologic toxicity (fever, sore throat, signs of local infections, easy bruising, unusual bleeding), symptoms of anemia (excessive tiredness, weakness). Assess response to medication; monitor and report for diarrhea. Avoid IM injections, rectal temperatures, other traumas that may induce bleeding. Put pressure to injection sites for full 5 min.

PATIENT/FAMILY TEACHING:

Explain that alopecia is reversible, but new hair may have different color, texture. Do not have immunizations w/o physician's approval (drug lowers body's resistance). Avoid crowds, persons w/known infections. Report signs of infection at once (fever, flulike symptoms). Contact physician if nausea/vomiting continue at home. Teach signs of peripheral neuropathy. Avoid pregnancy during therapy.

palivizumab
(Synagis)
See Supplement

pamidronate disodium

pam-ih-**drow**-nate
(Aredia)

CANADIAN AVAILABILITY:
Aredia

CLASSIFICATION

Hypocalcemic

AVAILABILITY (Rx)

Powder for Injection: 30 mg, 60 mg, 90 mg

PHARMACOKINETICS

After IV administration, rapidly absorbed by bone. Slowly excreted unchanged in urine.

ACTION/*THERAPEUTIC EFFECT*

Decreases release of phosphates, calcium from bone and increases renal excretion as parathyroid levels (usually suppressed in hypercalcemia in malignancy) return to normal levels. *Inhibits accelerated bone resorption* (bone formation and mineralization not inhibited).

USES

Treatment of moderate to severe hypercalcemia associated w/malignancy (w/o or w/bone metastases). Treatment of moderate to severe Paget's disease, osteolytic bone lesions of multiple myeloma, breast cancer.

STORAGE/HANDLING

Store parenteral form at room temperature. Reconstituted vials stable for 24 hrs refrigerated; IV solution stable for 24 hrs after dilution.

IV ADMINISTRATION

1. Adequate hydration is essential in conjunction w/pamidronate therapy (avoid overhydration in pts w/potential for cardiac failure).
2. Reconstitute each 30 mg vial w/10 ml sterile water for injection to provide concentration of 3 mg/ml.
3. Allow drug to dissolve before withdrawing.
4. Further dilute w/1,000 ml sterile 0.45% or 0.9% NaCl or 5% dextrose.
5. Administer IV infusion over 24 hrs.
6. Do not mix w/Ringer's solution or other calcium-containing solutions.

INDICATIONS/DOSAGE/ROUTES

Hypercalcemia:
IV Infusion: Adults, elderly: Moderate (corrected serum calcium 12–13.5 mg/dl): 60–90 mg over 24

hrs. Severe (corrected serum calcium >13.5 mg/dl): 90 mg over 24 hrs.

Paget's disease:
IV Infusion: Adults, elderly: 30 mg/day for 3 days.

Osteolytic bone lesion:
IV Infusion: Adults, elderly: 90 mg over 24 hours.

PRECAUTIONS

CONTRAINDICATIONS: Hypersensitivity to biphosphonates. **CAUTIONS:** Safety and efficacy in children not established. Cardiac failure, renal function impairment. **PREGNANCY/LACTATION:** There are no adequate and well-controlled studies in pregnant women; not known whether fetal harm can occur. Excretion in breast milk unknown. **Pregnancy Category C**.

INTERACTIONS

DRUG INTERACTIONS: Calcium-containing medications, vitamin D may antagonize effects in treatment of hypercalcemia. **ALTERED LAB VALUES:** May decrease phosphate, potassium, magnesium, calcium levels.

SIDE EFFECTS

FREQUENT (>10%): 27% of pts have temperature elevation (at least 1° C) 24–48 hrs after administration. Drug-related redness, swelling, induration, pain at catheter site (18% of pts receiving 90 mg). Anorexia, nausea, fatigue, hypophosphatemia, hypokalemia, hypomagnesemia, hypocalcemia occur more frequently w/higher dosage. **OCCASIONAL (1–10%):** Constipation, GI hemorrhage, rales, rhinitis, anemia, hypertension, tachycardia, atrial fibrillation, somnolence occur more often w/90 mg dosages.

ADVERSE REACTIONS/TOXIC

EFFECTS

None significant.

NURSING IMPLICATIONS

BASELINE ASSESSMENT:

Obtain electrolyte and CBC levels; check B/P, pulse, temperature. Assess lungs for rales, dependent parts of the body for edema.

INTERVENTION/EVALUATION:

Provide adequate hydration; avoid overhydration. Monitor I&O carefully; check lungs for rales, dependent body parts for edema. Monitor B/P, temperature, pulse. Assess catheter site for redness, swelling, pain. Check electrolytes (esp. calcium and potassium) and CBC results. Monitor food intake and stool frequency. Be alert for potential GI hemorrhage w/90 mg dosage.

PATIENT/FAMILY TEACHING:

Explain the rationale for the therapy and how to assist in maintaining an accurate I&O.

---

pancreatin

pan-kree-**ah**-tin
(Pancreatin)

pancrelipase

pan-kree-**lie**-pace
(Cotazym, Creon, Ilozyme, Pancrease MT, Ultrase, Viokase)

CANADIAN AVAILABILITY:
Cotazym, Creon, Pancrease, Ultrase, Viokase

CLASSIFICATION

Digestive enzyme

AVAILABILITY (Rx)

Tablets. Capsules.

ACTION / *THERAPEUTIC EFFECT*

Aids in digestion of protein, carbohydrate, fat in GI tract (primarily in duodenum, upper jejunum).

USES

Pancreatic enzyme replacement/supplement when enzymes are absent or deficient (i.e., chronic pancreatitis, cystic fibrosis, ductal obstruction from pancreatic cancer, common bile duct). Treatment of steatorrhea associated w/postgastrectomy syndrome, bowel resection; reduces malabsorption.

PO ADMINISTRATION

Give before or w/meals. Tablets may be crushed. Do not crush enteric-coated tablets. Instruct pt not to chew (minimizes irritation to mouth, lips, tongue).

INDICATIONS / DOSAGE / ROUTES

Usual oral dosage:
PO: **Adults, elderly:** 1–3 capsules or tablets before or w/meals, snacks. May increase up to 8 tablets/dose.

PRECAUTIONS

CONTRAINDICATIONS: Hypersensitivity to pork protein. **CAUTIONS:** None significant. **PREGNANCY/LACTATION:** Unknown whether drug crosses placenta or is distributed in breast milk. **Pregnancy Category C**.

INTERACTIONS

DRUG INTERACTIONS: Antacids may decrease effect. May decrease absorption of iron supplements. **ALTERED LAB VALUES:** May increase uric acid.

SIDE EFFECTS

RARE: Allergic reaction, mouth irritation, shortness of breath, wheezing.

ADVERSE REACTIONS / TOXIC EFFECTS

Excessive dosage may produce nausea, cramping, and/or diarrhea. Hyperuricosuria, hyperuricemia reported w/extremely high doses.

NURSING IMPLICATIONS

BASELINE ASSESSMENT:

Spilling powder on hands (Viokase) may irritate skin. Inhaling powder may irritate mucous membranes, produce bronchospasm.

INTERVENTION / EVALUATION:

Question for therapeutic relief from GI symptoms. Take before or w/meals. Do not change brands w/o consulting physician.

---

pancuronium bromide
(Pavulon)
See Classification section under:
Neuromuscular blockers

---

paroxetine hydrochloride

pear-**ox**-eh-teen
(Paxil, Paxil CR)

CANADIAN AVAILABILITY:
Paxil

CLASSIFICATION

Antidepressant

AVAILABILITY (Rx)

Tablets: 10 mg, 20 mg, 30 mg, 40 mg. **Controlled Release Tablets:** 12.5 mg, 25 mg.

PHARMACOKINETICS

Well absorbed from GI tract. Widely distributed. Metabolized in liver; excreted in urine. Half-life: 24 hrs.

ACTION/ THERAPEUTIC EFFECT

Selectively blocks uptake of neurotransmitter, serotonin, at CNS neuronal presynaptic membranes, thereby increasing availability at postsynaptic neuronal receptor sites. Resulting enhancement of synaptic activity *produces antidepressant effect, reduces obsessive-compulsive behavior, decreases anxiety.*

USES

Treatment of major depression exhibited as persistent, prominent dysphoria (occurring nearly every day for at least 2 wks) manifested by 4 of 8 symptoms: change in appetite, change in sleep pattern, increased fatigue, impaired concentration, feelings of guilt or worthlessness, loss of interest in usual activities, psychomotor agitation or retardation, or suicidal tendencies. Treatment of panic disorder, obsessive-compulsive disorder manifested as repetitive tasks producing marked distress, time-consuming, or significantly interfering w/social or occupational behavior. Treatment of social anxiety disorder.

PO ADMINISTRATION

1. Give w/food or milk if GI distress occurs.

2. Scored tablet may be crushed.

3. Best if given as single morning dose.

INDICATIONS/DOSAGE/ROUTES

Note: Reduce dosage in elderly, pts w/severe renal, hepatic impairment. Dose changes should occur at 1 wk intervals.

Depression:
PO: Adults: Initially, 20 mg/day, usually in morning. Dosage may be gradually increased in 10 mg/day increments to 50 mg/day. **Extended Release:** Initially, 12.5 mg. **Maximum:** 60 mg/day. **Elderly, debilitated, those w/severe hepatic, renal impairment:** Initially, 10 mg/day. Do not exceed maximum 40 mg/day. **Extended Release:** Initially, 12.5 mg. **Maximum:** 60 mg/day.

Panic disorder:
PO: Adults: Initially, 10 mg/day; increase 10 mg/day at intervals of at least 1 wk up to 40 mg/day. **Maximum:** 60 mg/day. **Elderly:** Initially 10 mg/day. **Maximum:** 40 mg/day.

Obsessive-compulsive disorder:
PO: Adults: Initially, 20 mg/day; increase 10 mg/day at intervals of at least 1 wk. **Elderly:** Initially, 10 mg/day. **Maximum:** 40 mg/day.

Social anxiety disorder:
PO: Adults, elderly: 20 mg/day.

PRECAUTIONS

CONTRAINDICATIONS: Within 14 days of MAO inhibitor therapy. **CAUTIONS:** Severe renal, hepatic impairment. History of mania, seizures, those w/metabolic or hemodynamic disease, history of drug abuse. **PREGNANCY/LACTATION:** May impair reproductive function. Distributed in breast milk. **Pregnancy Category B**.

INTERACTIONS

DRUG INTERACTIONS: MAO inhibitors may cause serotonergic syndrome (excitement, diaphoresis, rigidity, hyperthermia, autonomic hyperactivity, coma). Cimetidine may increase concentrations; phenytoin may decrease concentrations. **ALTERED LAB VALUES:** May increase liver enzymes. May decrease Hb, Hct, WBC.

SIDE EFFECTS

FREQUENT: Nausea (26%), somnolence (23%), headache, dry mouth (18%), weakness (15%), constipation (15%), dizziness, insomnia (13%), diarrhea (12%), excessive sweating (11%), tremor (8%). **OCCASIONAL:** Decreased appetite, respiratory disturbance (6%), anxiety, nervousness (5%), flatulence, paresthesia, yawning (4%), decreased libido/sexual dysfunction, abdominal discomfort (3%). **RARE:** Palpitations, vomiting, blurred vision, taste change, confusion.

ADVERSE REACTIONS/TOXIC EFFECTS

None significant.

NURSING IMPLICATIONS
BASELINE ASSESSMENT:

Assess appearance, behavior, speech pattern, level of interest, mood. Assess for history of drug abuse.

INTERVENTION/EVALUATION:

For those on long-term therapy, liver/renal function tests, blood counts should be performed periodically. Supervise suicidal risk pt closely during early therapy (as depression lessens, energy level improves, increasing suicide potential). Assess appearance, behavior, speech pattern, level of interest, mood.

PATIENT/FAMILY TEACHING:

Therapeutic effect may be noted within 1–4 wks. Dry mouth may be relieved by sugarless gum, sips of tepid water. Do not abruptly discontinue medication. Avoid tasks that require alertness, motor skills until response to drug is established. Inform physician if intention of pregnancy or if pregnancy occurs. Avoid alcohol.

pegasparagase

peg-ah-spa-**raj**-ace
(Oncaspar)

CANADIAN AVAILABILITY:
Oncaspar

CLASSIFICATION

Antineoplastic

AVAILABILITY (Rx)

Injection: 750 IU/ml vial

PHARMACOKINETICS

Half-life: 1.4–5.2 days in pts previously hypersensitive to L-asparaginase (2.5–7.9 days in pts nonhypersensitive).

ACTION/THERAPEUTIC EFFECT

Breaks down extracellular supplies of the amino acid asparagine (necessary for survival of leukemic cells). Normal cells produce own asparagine. Binding to polyethylene glycol causes asparaginase to be less antigenic, less likely to cause hypersensitive reaction, *interfering w/DNA, RNA, protein synthesis in leukemic cells.* Cell cycle-specific for G_1 phase of cell division.

USES

Treatment of acute lymphoblastic leukemia (in combination therapy) in pts who require L-asparaginase in treatment program but have developed hypersensitivity to native forms of L-asparaginase.

STORAGE/HANDLING

Refrigerate (do *not* freeze). Discard if cloudy, if precipitate is present, if stored at room temperature for >48 hrs, or if vial has been previously frozen (freezing destroys activity). Use one dose per vial; do not reenter vial. Discard unused portion.

IM/IV ADMINISTRATION

Note: Wear gloves (drug is contact irritant). Avoid inhalation of vapors, contact w/skin or mucous membranes. In case of contact, wash w/copious amount of water for at least 15 min. Avoid excessive agitation of vial; do *not* shake. IM route preferred (decreased risk of hepatotoxicity, coagulopathy, GI and renal disorders).

IM:

Administer no more than 2 ml at any one IM site. Use multiple injection sites if more than 2 ml is administered.

IV:

1. Add 100 ml NaCl or dextrose injection 5% and administer through an infusion that is already running.

2. Administer over 1–2 hrs.

INDICATIONS/DOSAGE/ROUTES

Acute lymphocytic leukemia:
IM/IV: Adults, elderly: 2,500 IU/m^2 every 14 days. **Children, body surface area ≥0.6 m^2:** 2,500 IU/m^2 every 14 days. **Children, body surface area <0.6 m^2:** 82.5 IU/kg every 14 days.

PRECAUTIONS

CONTRAINDICATIONS: Previous anaphylactic reaction or significant hemorrhagic event associated w/prior L-asparaginase therapy, pancreatitis, history of pancreatitis. **CAUTIONS:** Concurrent anticoagulant therapy, aspirin, or NSAID use. **PREGNANCY/LACTATION:** If possible, avoid use during pregnancy. Breast-feeding not recommended. **Pregnancy Category C**.

INTERACTIONS

DRUG INTERACTIONS: Steroids, vincristine may increase hyperglycemia, risk of neuropathy, disturbances of erythropoiesis. May decrease effect of antigout medications. May block effects of methotrexate. Live virus vaccines may potentiate virus replication, increase vaccine side effects, decrease pt's antibody response to vaccine. **ALTERED LAB VALUES:** May increase blood ammonia, BUN, uric acid, glucose, partial thromboplastin time (PTT), platelet count, prothrombin time (PT), thrombin time (TT), SGOT (AST), SGPT (ALT), alkaline phosphatase, bilirubin. May decrease blood clotting factors (plasma fibrinogen, antithrombin, plasminogen), albumin, calcium, cholesterol.

SIDE EFFECTS

FREQUENT: Allergic reaction (rash, urticaria, arthralgia, facial edema, hypotension, respiratory distress), pancreatitis (severe stomach pain w/nausea/vomiting). **OCCASIONAL:** CNS effects (confusion, drowsiness, depression, nervousness, tiredness), stomatitis (sores in mouth/lips), hypoalbuminemia/uric acid nephropathy (swelling of feet or lower legs), hyperglycemia. **RARE:** Hyperthermia (fever or chills), thrombosis, seizures.

ADVERSE REACTIONS/TOXIC EFFECTS

Risk of hypersensitivity reaction, including anaphylaxis, following drug administration. Increased risk of blood coagulopathies occurs occasionally.

NURSING IMPLICATIONS
BASELINE ASSESSMENT:

Before giving medication, agents for adequate airway and

allergic reaction (antihistamine, epinephrine, oxygen, IV corticosteroid) should be readily available (an abrupt fall in serum asparaginase generally precedes allergic reaction). Keep pt under observation for 1 hr after drug administration. Skin testing, hepatic, renal, pancreatic (including blood glucose), CBC, differential, PT, PTT, fibrinogen, bone marrow tests should be performed before therapy begins and when a week or more has elapsed between doses.

INTERVENTION/EVALUATION:

Monitor and adjust therapeutic regimen according to response and toxicity. Determine serum amylase concentration frequently during therapy (detects early pancreatitis). Discontinue medication at first sign of renal failure, pancreatitis (abdominal pain, nausea, vomiting). Monitor for hematologic toxicity (fever, sore throat, signs of local infection, easy bruising, unusual bleeding), symptoms of anemia (excessive tiredness, weakness), evidence of infection.

PATIENT/FAMILY TEACHING:

Increase fluid intake (protects against renal impairment). Nausea may decrease during therapy. Do not have immunizations w/o physician's approval (drug lowers body's resistance). Avoid contact w/those who have recently taken live virus vaccine. Contact physician if nausea/vomiting continues at home.

---

pemirolast
(Alamast)
See Supplement

---

pemoline
pem-oh-leen
(Cylert)

CANADIAN AVAILABILITY:
Cylert

CLASSIFICATION

CNS stimulant

AVAILABILITY (Rx)

Tablets: 18.75 mg, 37.5 mg, 75 mg. **Tablets (chewable):** 37.5 mg.

PHARMACOKINETICS

	ONSET	PEAK	DURATION
PO (adults)			
	Gradual	4 hrs	8 hrs
PO (children)			
	Gradual	—	—

Readily absorbed from GI tract. Metabolized in liver. Primarily excreted in urine. Half-life: 12 hrs.

ACTION/*THERAPEUTIC EFFECT*

Appears to act through dopaminergic receptor sites. In children, *appears to reduce motor restlessness, increases mental alertness, provides mood elevation, reduces sense of fatigue.*

USES

Treatment of attention deficit disorder in children w/moderate to severe distraction, short attention span, hyperactivity, emotional impulsiveness.

PO ADMINISTRATION

1. Do not administer in afternoon or evening (to avoid insomnia).
2. Tablets may be crushed.

INDICATIONS/DOSAGE/ROUTES

Attention deficit disorder:
PO: Children >6 yrs: Initially, 37.5 mg/day given as single dose in morning. May increase by 18.75 mg at weekly intervals until therapeutic response is achieved. **Range:** 56.25–75 mg/day. **Maximum:** 112.5 mg/day.

PRECAUTIONS

CONTRAINDICATIONS: Impaired hepatic function, pts w/motor tics, family history of Tourette's disorder. **CAUTIONS:** Impaired renal function. **PREGNANCY/LACTATION:** Unknown whether drug crosses placenta or is distributed in breast milk. **Pregnancy Category B**.

INTERACTIONS

DRUG INTERACTIONS: CNS-stimulating medications may increase CNS stimulation. **ALTERED LAB VALUES:** May increase SGOT (AST), SGPT (ALT), LDH.

SIDE EFFECTS

FREQUENT: Anorexia, insomnia. **OCCASIONAL:** Nausea, abdominal discomfort, diarrhea, headache, dizziness, drowsiness.

ADVERSE REACTIONS/TOXIC EFFECTS

Dyskinetic movements of tongue, lips, face, and extremities, and visual disturbances, rash have occurred. Large doses may produce extreme nervousness, tachycardia. Hepatic effects (hepatitis, jaundice) appear to be reversible when drug is discontinued. Prolonged administration to children w/attention deficit disorder may produce a temporary suppression of weight and/or height patterns.

NURSING IMPLICATIONS

BASELINE ASSESSMENT:

Liver function tests should be performed before therapy begins and periodically during therapy.

PATIENT/FAMILY TEACHING:

Therapeutic response to medication may take 3–4 wks. Insomnia, anorexia usually disappear during continued therapy. Anorexia usually accompanied by weight loss. Return to normal weight usually occurs within 3–6 mos.

---

penbutolol

pen-**beaut**-oh-lol
(Levatol)

CLASSIFICATION

Beta-adrenergic blocker

AVAILABILITY (Rx)

Tablets: 20 mg

PHARMACOKINETICS

	ONSET	PEAK	DURATION
PO	—	1 hr	24 hrs

Completely absorbed from GI tract. Metabolized in liver. Primarily excreted in urine. Half-life: 5 hrs (increased in decreased renal function).

ACTION/ *THERAPEUTIC EFFECT*

Nonselective beta blocker. Blocks beta$_1$-adrenergic receptors, *slowing sinus heart rate, decreasing cardiac output, decreasing B/P.* Blocks beta$_2$-adrenergic receptors, *increasing airway resistance. Decreases myocardial ischemia severi-*

ty by decreasing oxygen requirements. Has moderate intrinsic sympathomimetic activity.

USES/*UNLABELED*

Treatment of mild to moderate hypertension. *Treatment of chronic angina pectoris.*

PO ADMINISTRATION

1. May give w/o regard to food.
2. Tablets may be crushed.

INDICATIONS/DOSAGE/ROUTES

Hypertension:
PO: Adults: Initially, 20 mg/day as single dose. May increase to 40–80 mg/day. **Elderly:** Initially, 10 mg/day.

PRECAUTIONS

CONTRAINDICATIONS: Bronchial asthma, COPD, sinus bradycardia, heart block greater than first degree, cardiogenic shock, CHF (unless secondary to tachyarrhythmias), overt cardiac failure. **CAUTIONS:** Inadequate cardiac function, impaired renal/hepatic function, diabetes mellitus, hyperthyroidism. **PREGNANCY/LACTATION:** Crosses placenta; distributed in breast milk. Avoid use during first trimester. May produce bradycardia, apnea, hypoglycemia, hypothermia during delivery, small birth weight infants. **Pregnancy Category C**. (Category D if used in 2nd or 3rd trimester.)

INTERACTIONS

DRUG INTERACTIONS: Diuretics, other hypotensives may increase hypotensive effect; sympathomimetics, xanthines may mutually inhibit effects; may mask symptoms of hypoglycemia, prolong hypoglycemic effect of insulin, oral hypoglycemics; NSAIDs may decrease antihypertensive effect; cimetidine may increase concentration. **ALTERED LAB VALUES:** May increase ANA titer, SGOT (AST), SGPT (ALT), alkaline phosphatase, LDH, bilirubin, BUN, creatinine, potassium, uric acid, lipoproteins, triglycerides.

SIDE EFFECTS

FREQUENT: Decreased sexual ability, drowsiness, trouble sleeping, unusual tiredness/weakness. **OCCASIONAL:** Bradycardia, difficulty breathing, CHF (swelling of feet, shortness of breath), depression, cold hands/feet, diarrhea, constipation, anxiety, nasal congestion, nausea, vomiting. **RARE:** Altered taste, dry eyes, itching, numbness of fingers, toes, scalp.

ADVERSE REACTIONS/TOXIC EFFECTS

Abrupt withdrawal (particularly in those w/coronary artery disease) may produce angina or precipitate MI. May precipitate thyroid crisis in those w/thyrotoxicosis.

NURSING IMPLICATIONS
BASELINE ASSESSMENT:

Assess baseline renal/liver function tests. Assess B/P, apical pulse immediately before drug is administered (if pulse is 60/min or below or systolic B/P is below 90 mm Hg, withhold medication, contact physician).

INTERVENTION/EVALUATION:

Assess pulse for strength/weakness, irregular rate, bradycardia. Monitor EKG for cardiac changes. Assist w/ambulation if dizziness occurs. Assess for peripheral edema of hands, feet (usually, first area of low extremity swelling is behind medial malleolus in ambulatory, sacral area in bedridden). Monitor pattern of daily bowel activity, stool consistency. Assess skin for development of rash. Monitor any unusual changes in pt.

PATIENT/FAMILY TEACHING:

Do not abruptly discontinue medication. Compliance w/therapy regimen is essential to control hypertension. If dizziness occurs, sit or lie down immediately. Full therapeutic response may not occur for up to 2 wks. Avoid tasks that require alertness, motor skills until response to drug is established. Report excessively slow pulse rate (<60 beats/min), peripheral numbness, dizziness. Do not use nasal decongestants, OTC cold preparations (stimulants) w/o physician approval. Outpatients should monitor B/P, pulse before taking medication. Restrict salt, alcohol intake.

penciclovir

pen-**sigh**-klo-vear
(Denavir)

CLASSIFICATION

Antiviral

AVAILABILITY (Rx)

Cream: 1%

PHARMACOKINETICS

Not detected in plasma or urine.

ACTION/THERAPEUTIC EFFECT

Inhibits antiviral activity against herpes simplex virus (HSV). *DNA synthesis and, therefore, HSV replication, is prevented.*

USES

Treatment of recurrent herpes labialis (cold sores).

STORAGE/HANDLING

Store at room temperature. Do not freeze.

INDICATIONS/DOSAGE/ROUTES

Note: Begin treatment as soon as possible (as soon as symptom indicating immediate onset of virus is evident or when lesions appear).

Herpes labialis (cold sores):
Topical: **Adults, elderly:** Apply q2h during waking hours for 4 days.

PRECAUTIONS

CONTRAINDICATIONS: Known hypersensitivity to product. **CAUTIONS:** None significant. **PREGNANCY/LACTATION:** Excreted in breast milk of animals. **Pregnancy Category B**.

INTERACTIONS

DRUG INTERACTIONS: None significant. **ALTERED LAB VALUES:** None significant.

SIDE EFFECTS

FREQUENT (>5%): Headache, mild erythema. **OCCASIONAL (1–5%):** Application site reaction. **RARE (<1%):** Altered taste rash.

ADVERSE REACTIONS/TOXIC EFFECTS

None significant.

NURSING IMPLICATIONS

BASELINE ASSESSMENT:

Use only on lips or face. Do not apply to oral mucous membranes. Avoid application in or near eyes (produces irritation).

PATIENT/FAMILY TEACHING:

Observe precautions to avoid exposure of cold sores to direct sunlight.

---

penicillamine

pen-ih-**sill**-ah-mine
(Cuprimine, Depen)

CANADIAN AVAILABILITY:
Cuprimine, Depen

CLASSIFICATION

Chelating agent, anti-inflammatory

AVAILABILITY (Rx)

Capsules: 125 mg, 250 mg.
Tablets: 250 mg.

PHARMACOKINETICS

Well absorbed from GI tract. Metabolized in liver. Primarily excreted in urine. Half-life: 1.7–3.2 hrs.

ACTION/ *THERAPEUTIC EFFECT*

Chelates copper, iron, mercury, lead to form complexes, *promoting excretion of copper.* Combines with cystine-forming complex, thus reducing concentration of cystine to below levels for formation of cystine stones. *Prevents renal calculi. May dissolve existing stones. Rheumatoid arthritis:* Exact mechanism unknown. May decrease cell-mediated immune response; *acts as anti-inflammatory drug;* may inhibit collagen formation.

USES/ *UNLABELED*

Promotes excretion of copper in treatment of Wilson's disease; decreases excretion of cystine, prevents renal calculi in cystinuria associated w/nephrolithiasis; treatment of active rheumatoid arthritis not controlled w/conventional therapy. *Treatment of rheumatoid vasculitis, heavy metal toxicity.*

PO ADMINISTRATION

1. Preferably give on empty stomach (1 hr before or 2 hrs after meals) or at least 1 hr from any drug, food, or milk.
2. Take w/large amounts of water when treating cystinuria.
3. Largest single dose is 500 mg; give larger amounts in divided doses.
4. Tablets may be crushed; do not crush or break capsules.

INDICATIONS/DOSAGE/ROUTES

Wilson's disease:
Note: Base dosage on urinary copper excretion, serum-free copper concentration that produces/ maintains negative copper balance. Give w/10–40 mg sulfurated potash at each meal for 6–12 mos.
PO: Adults, elderly, children: Initially, 250 mg 4 times/day (some pts may begin at 250 mg/day; gradually increase). Dosages of 750–1,500 mg/day that produce initial 24 hr cupruresis >2 mg should be continued for 3 mos. **Maintenance:** Based on serum-free copper concentration (<10 mcg/dl indicative of adequate maintenance). **Maximum:** 2 g/day.

Cystinuria:
Note: Give in 4 equal doses; if not feasible, give larger dose at bedtime. Dose based on urinary cystine excretion. Maintain high fluid intake.
PO: Adults, elderly: Initially, 250 mg/day. Gradually increase dose.

Maintenance: 2 g/day. **Range:** 1–4 g/day. **Children:** 30 mg/kg/day.

Rheumatoid arthritis:
PO: Adults, elderly: Initially, 125–250 mg/day. May increase by 125–250 mg/day at 1–3 mo intervals. **Maintenance:** 500–750 mg/day. After 2–3 mos w/no improvement or toxicity, may increase by 250 mg/day at 2–3 mo intervals until remission or toxicity. **Maximum:** 1 g up to 1.5 g/day.

PRECAUTIONS

CONTRAINDICATIONS: History of penicillamine-related aplastic anemia or agranulocytosis, rheumatoid arthritis pts w/history or evidence of renal insufficiency, pregnancy, breastfeeding. **CAUTIONS:** Elderly, debilitated, impaired renal/hepatic function, penicillin allergy. **PREGNANCY/LACTATION:** Birth defects noted (pyloric stenosis, hypotonia, perforated bowel, growth retardation, vein fragility, hypertrophy of skin and subcutaneous tissues). Pregnancy, lactation contraindicated. **Pregnancy Category D.**

INTERACTIONS

DRUG INTERACTIONS: Iron supplements, antacids, food may decrease absorption. Bone marrow depressants, gold compounds, immunosuppressants may increase risk of hematologic, renal adverse effects. **ALTERED LAB VALUES:** None significant.

SIDE EFFECTS

FREQUENT: Rash (pruritic, erythematous, maculopapular, morbilliform), reduced/altered sense of taste (hypogeusia), GI disturbances (anorexia, epigastric pain, nausea, vomiting, diarrhea), oral ulcers, glossitis. **OCCASIONAL:** Proteinuria, hematuria, hot flashes, drug fever. **RARE:** Alopecia, tinnitus, pemphigoid rash (water blisters).

ADVERSE REACTIONS/TOXIC EFFECTS

Aplastic anemia, agranulocytosis, thrombocytopenia, leukopenia, myasthenia gravis, bronchiolitis, erythematouslike syndrome, evening hypoglycemia, skin friability at sites of pressure/trauma producing extravasation or white papules at venipuncture, surgical sites reported. Iron deficiency (particularly children, menstruating women) may develop.

NURSING IMPLICATIONS

BASELINE ASSESSMENT:

Baseline WBC, differential, hemoglobin, platelet count should be performed before therapy begins, every 2 wks thereafter for first 6 mos, then monthly during therapy. Liver function tests (GGT, SGOT, SGPT, LDH) and x-ray for renal stones should also be ordered. A 2 hr interval is necessary between iron and penicillamine therapy. In event of upcoming surgery, dosage should be reduced to 250 mg/day until wound healing is complete.

INTERVENTION/EVALUATION:

Encourage copious amounts of water in those w/cystinuria. Monitor WBC, differential, platelet count. If WBC <3,500, neutrophils <2,000/mm³, monocytes >500/mm³, or platelet counts <100,000, or if a progressive fall in either platelet count or WBC in three successive determinations noted, inform physician (drug withdrawal necessary). Assess for evidence of hematuria. Monitor urinalysis for hematuria, proteinuria (if proteinuria exceeds 1 g/24 hrs, inform physician).

PATIENT/FAMILY TEACHING:

Promptly report any missed menstrual periods/other indications of pregnancy, fever, sore throat, chills, bruising, bleeding, difficulty breathing on exertion, unexplained cough or wheezing. Take medication 1 hr before or 2 hrs after meals or at least 1 hr from any other drug, food, or milk.

penicillin G benzathine

pen-ih-**sil**-lin G **benz**-ah-thene **(Bicillin)**

FIXED COMBINATION(S):
W/penicillin G procaine, an antibiotic **(Bicillin CR)**

CANADIAN AVAILABILITY:
Bicillin

penicillin G potassium, sodium

(Pentids, Pfizerpen)

CANADIAN AVAILABILITY:
Crystapen

penicillin G procaine

(Crystacillin, Duracillin, Pfizerpen, Wycillin)

FIXED-COMBINATION(S):
W/probenecid, a renal tubular blocking agent **(Wycillin & Probenecid);** w/penicillin G benzathine, an antibiotic **(Bicillin-CR)**

CLASSIFICATION

Antibiotic: Penicillin

AVAILABILITY (Rx)

Benzathine: 300,000 units/ml, 600,000 units/ml
PCN-G Potassium: Powder for Injection: 1 million units, 5 million units, 10 million units, 20 million units
PCN-G Sodium: Powder for Injection: 5 million units
Procaine: 300,000 units/ml, 500,000 units/ml, 600,000 units/ml

PHARMACOKINETICS

Slowly absorbed after IM administration. Widely distributed. Metabolized in liver. Primarily excreted in urine. Moderately removed by hemodialysis. Half-life: 0.5–0.7 hrs (increased in decreased renal function).

ACTION/ *THERAPEUTIC EFFECT*

Binds to bacterial membranes, *inhibiting cell wall synthesis. Bactericidal.*

USES

Benzathine, procaine: Mild to moderate infections of respiratory tract, skin and skin structure, rheumatic fever prophylaxis, early syphilis, yaws, bejel, pinta. Follow-up to IM/IV therapy w/penicillin G potassium, sodium. *PCN-G:* Treatment of infections of respiratory tract, skin and skin structure, bone and joints; septicemia, meningitis, endocarditis, pericarditis, diphtheria, Listeria, clostridium, disseminated gonococcal infections, actinomycosis, rheumatic fever prophylaxis, syphilis, necrotizing ulcerative gingivitis, anthrax, Lyme disease.

STORAGE/HANDLING

Benzathine, procaine: Refrigerate. *PCN-G:* IV infusion (piggyback) is stable for 24 hrs at room temperature, 7 days if refrigerated. Discard if precipitate forms.

IM/IV ADMINISTRATION

Note: *Benzathine, procaine:* Do not give IV, intra-arterially, intravascularly, or SubQ. Space doses evenly around the clock.

IM:

1. Give IM injection deeply into gluteus maximus or midlateral thigh.

2. Do not administer if blood is aspirated; draw up new dose; select another site.

3. Avoid areas of nerves, repeated IM injections into anterolateral thigh.

4. Administer IM injection slowly; stop if pt complains of severe pain.

IV:

1. After reconstitution, dilute w/50–100 ml 5% dextrose, 0.9% NaCl, or other compatible IV fluid. Infuse over 1–2 hrs in adults, 15–30 min in neonates, children.

2. Because of potential for hypersensitivity/anaphylaxis, start initial dose at few drops/min, increase slowly to ordered rate; stay w/pt first 10–15 min, then check q10 min.

3. Alternating IV sites, use large veins to reduce risk of phlebitis.

INDICATIONS/DOSAGE/ROUTES

Usual parenteral dosage (benzathine):
IM: Adults, elderly: 1.2 million units one time. **Children >27 kg:** 900,000–1.2 million units one time. **Children <27 kg, infants:** 300,000–600,000 units/kg one time. **Neonates:** 50,000 units/kg one time.

Usual parenteral dosage (PCN-G):
IV: Adults, elderly: 5 million units/day minimum. **Children:** 100,000–250,000 units/kg/day in divided doses q4h. **Infants:** 50,000–100,000 units/kg/day in divided doses q6–12h.

Penicillin G Procaine

Moderate to severe upper respiratory tract, otitis media, tonsillitis, pharyngitis, skin/skin structure infections, uncomplicated pneumonia:
IM: Adults, elderly, children: 600,000–1.2 million units/day. **Children <60 lbs:** 300,000 units/day.

Acute uncomplicated gonorrhea:
IM: Adults, elderly: 4.8 million units one time in divided doses (w/1 g probenecid 30 min before penicillin).

Syphilis:
IM: Adults, elderly: 600,000 units/ day for 8 days.

Neurosyphilis:
IM: Adults, elderly: 2.4 million units/day and probenecid 500 mg 4 times/day for 10 days; follow w/penicillin G benzathine 2.4 million units weekly × 3 wks.

Congenital syphilis:
IM: Children <70 lbs, neonates: 50,000 units/kg/day for 10–14 days.

PRECAUTIONS

CONTRAINDICATIONS: Hypersensitivity to any penicillin. **CAUTIONS:** Renal impairment, history of allergies, particularly cephalosporins, aspirin (tartrazine reaction may occur in those sensitive to aspirin). **PREGNANCY/LACTATION:** Readily crosses placenta, appears in cord blood, amniotic fluid. Distributed in breast milk in low concentrations. May lead to allergic sensitization, diarrhea, candidiasis, skin rash in infant. **Pregnancy Category B.**

INTERACTIONS

DRUG INTERACTIONS: Probenecid may increase concentration, toxicity risk. Angiotensin-converting enzyme inhibitors, potassium-sparing diuretics, potassium supplements may increase risk of hyperkalemia. **ALTERED LAB VALUES:** May cause positive Coombs' test.

SIDE EFFECTS

FREQUENT: GI reactions (nausea, vomiting, diarrhea). **OCCASIONAL:** Pain, induration at IM injection site. *PCN-G potassium, sodium:* High IV dosage may cause electrolyte imbalance, phlebitis, thrombophlebitis. **RARE:** Bleeding.

ADVERSE REACTIONS/TOXIC EFFECTS

Hypersensitivity reactions occur frequently, ranging from rash, fever/chills to anaphylaxis. Nephrotoxicity may occur w/high parenteral dosages, preexisting renal disease. Superinfections, potentially fatal antibiotic-associated colitis may result from altered bacterial balance. Toxic reaction to procaine (confusion, combativeness, seizures) w/large doses.

NURSING IMPLICATIONS

BASELINE ASSESSMENT:

Question for history of allergies, particularly penicillins, cephalosporins, aspirin, procaine. Obtain specimen for culture and sensitivity before giving first dose (therapy may begin before results are known).

INTERVENTION/EVALUATION:

Hold medication and promptly report rash (hypersensitivity) or diarrhea (w/fever, abdominal pain, mucus and blood in stool may indicate antibiotic-associated colitis). Assess for food tolerance. Check IM injection sites for induration, tenderness. Check for wheezing, respiratory difficulty due to tartrazine sensitivity. Monitor I&O, urinalysis, renal function tests for nephrotoxicity. Be alert for superinfection: increased fever, sore throat, nausea, vomiting, diarrhea, ulceration or changes of oral mucosa, vaginal discharge, anal/genital pruritus. Evaluate hemoglobin levels and assess for signs of bleeding: overt bleeding, bruising/swelling of tissue.

PATIENT/FAMILY TEACHING:

Continue antibiotic for full length of treatment. Space doses evenly. Discomfort may occur w/IM injection. Notify physician in event of rash, diarrhea, bleeding, bruising, other new symptom. Sodium content of penicillin G sodium must be considered for those on sodium-restricted diets.

P

penicillin V potassium
(Pen Vee K, V-Cillin-K, Veetids)

CANADIAN AVAILABILITY:
Apo-Pen VK, Nadopen-V, Novopen VK

CLASSIFICATION
Antibiotic: Penicillin

AVAILABILITY (Rx)
Tablets: 125 mg, 250 mg, 500 mg. **Powder for Oral Solution:** 125 mg/5 ml, 250 mg/5 ml.

PHARMACOKINETICS
Moderately absorbed from GI tract. Widely distributed. Metabolized in liver. Primarily excreted in urine. Half-life: 1 hr (increased in decreased renal function).

ACTION/THERAPEUTIC EFFECT
Binds to bacterial membranes, *inhibiting cell wall synthesis. Bactericidal.*

USES
Treatment of mild to moderate infections of respiratory tract and skin/skin structure, otitis media, necrotizing ulcerative gingivitis, prophylaxis for rheumatic fever, dental procedures.

STORAGE/HANDLING
Store tabs at room temperature. Oral solution, after reconstitution, is stable for 14 days if refrigerated.

PO ADMINISTRATION
1. Space doses evenly around the clock.
2. Give w/o regard to meals.

INDICATIONS/DOSAGE/ROUTES
Usual adult, elderly dosage:
PO: 125–500 mg 4 times/day.

Usual children's dosage:
PO: 15–50 mg/kg/day in divided doses q6–8h.

PRECAUTIONS
CONTRAINDICATIONS: Hypersensitivity to any penicillin. **CAUTIONS:** Renal impairment, history of allergies, particularly cephalosporins, aspirin. **PREGNANCY/LACTATION:** Readily crosses placenta; appears in cord blood, amniotic fluid. Distributed in breast milk in low concentrations. May lead to allergic sensitization, diarrhea, candidiasis, skin rash in infant. **Pregnancy Category B**.

INTERACTIONS
DRUG INTERACTIONS: Probenecid may increase concentration, toxicity risk. **ALTERED LAB VALUES:** May cause positive Coombs' test.

SIDE EFFECTS
FREQUENT: Mild hypersensitivity reaction (rash, fever/chills), nausea, vomiting, diarrhea. **RARE:** Bleeding, allergic reaction.

ADVERSE REACTIONS/TOXIC EFFECTS
Severe hypersensitivity reaction, including anaphylaxis, may occur. Nephrotoxicity, superinfections (including potentially fatal antibiotic-associated colitis) may result from high dosages, prolonged therapy.

NURSING IMPLICATIONS
BASELINE ASSESSMENT:
Question for history of allergies, particularly penicillins, cephalosporins. Obtain specimen for culture and sensitivity before

giving first dose (therapy may begin before results are known).

INTERVENTION/EVALUATION:

Hold medication and promptly report rash (hypersensitivity) or diarrhea (w/fever, abdominal pain, mucus and blood in stool may indicate antibiotic-associated colitis). Assess food tolerance. Monitor I&O, urinalysis, renal function tests for nephrotoxicity. Be alert for superinfection: increased fever, sore throat, nausea, vomiting, diarrhea, ulceration or changes of oral mucosa, vaginal discharge, anal/genital pruritus. Review hemoglobin levels; check for bleeding: overt bleeding, bruising or swelling of tissue.

PATIENT/FAMILY TEACHING:

Continue antibiotic for full length of treatment. Space doses evenly. Notify physician immediately in event of rash, diarrhea, bleeding, bruising, or other new symptom.

---

pentaerythritol tetranitrate (P.E.T.N.)
(Duotrate, Peritrate)
See Classification section under: Nitrates

---

pentamidine isethionate
pen-**tam**-ih-deen
(NebuPent, Pentam-300)

CANADIAN AVAILABILITY:
Pentacarinat

CLASSIFICATION
Anti-infective

AVAILABILITY (Rx)
Injection: 300 mg. **Aerosol:** 300 mg.

PHARMACOKINETICS
Minimal absorption following inhalation, well absorbed after IM administration. Widely distributed. Primarily excreted in urine. Minimally removed by hemodialysis. Half-life: 6.5 hrs (increased in decreased renal function).

ACTION/*THERAPEUTIC EFFECT*
Exact mechanism unknown. May interfere w/incorporation of nucleotides; *inhibits DNA, RNA, phospholipid, protein synthesis.*

USES/*UNLABELED*
Treatment of pneumonia caused by *Pneumocystis carinii* (PCP). Prevention of PCP in high-risk HIV-infected pts. *Treatment of visceral/cutaneous Leishmaniasis, African Trypanosomiasis.*

STORAGE/HANDLING
Store vials at room temperature. After reconstitution, IV solution and aerosol are stable for 48 hrs at room temperature. Use freshly prepared aerosol solution. Discard unused portion.

IM/IV/INHALATION ADMINISTRATION
Note: Pt must be in supine position during administration w/frequent B/P checks until stable (potential for life-threatening hypotensive reaction). Have resuscitative equipment nearby.

IM:
Reconstitute 300 mg vial w/3 ml

sterile water for injection to provide concentration of 100 mg/ml.

IV:

1. For intermittent IV infusion (piggyback), reconstitute each vial w/3–5 ml 5% dextrose or sterile water for injection.

2. Withdraw desired dose and further dilute w/50–250 ml 5% dextrose; infuse over 60 min.

3. Do not give by IV injection or rapid IV infusion (increases potential for severe hypotension).

AEROSOL (NEBULIZER):

1. Reconstitute 300 mg vial w/6 ml sterile water for injection. Avoid saline (may cause precipitate).

2. Do not mix w/other medication in nebulizer reservoir.

INDICATIONS/DOSAGE/ROUTES

Pneumocystis carinii pneumonia: **IM/IV: Adults, elderly, children:** 4 mg/kg/day once daily for 14 days.

Prevention P. carinii pneumonia: **Aerosol (Nebulizer): Adults, elderly:** 300 mg once q4 wks via nebulizer.

PRECAUTIONS

CONTRAINDICATIONS: When PCP has been firmly established, there are no absolute contraindications. Inhalation of drug is contraindicated in those w/history of severe asthma or anaphylactic reaction to drug by any route. **CAUTIONS:** Hyper/hypotension, hepatic/renal dysfunction, hyper/hypoglycemia, hypocalcemia, thrombocytopenia, leukopenia, anemia. **PREGNANCY/LACTATION:** Unknown whether crosses placenta or is distributed in breast milk. **Pregnancy Category C**.

INTERACTIONS

DRUG INTERACTIONS: Blood dyscrasias–producing medication, bone marrow depressants may increase abnormal hematologic effects. Didanosine may increase risk of pancreatitis. Foscarnet may increase hypocalcemia, hypomagnesemia, nephrotoxicity. Nephrotoxic medications may increase risk of nephrotoxicity. **ALTERED LAB VALUES:** May increase SGOT (AST), SGPT (ALT), alkaline phosphatase, bilirubin, BUN, creatinine. May decrease calcium, magnesium. May alter glucose levels.

SIDE EFFECTS

FREQUENT: *(Injection >10%):* Abscess, pain at injection site. *(Inhalation >5%):* Fatigue, metallic taste, shortness of breath, decreased appetite, dizziness, rash, cough, nausea, vomiting, chills. **OCCASIONAL:** *(Injection 1–10%):* Nausea, decreased appetite, hypotension, fever, rash, bad taste, confusion. *(Inhalation 1–5%):* Diarrhea, headache, anemia, muscle pain. **RARE:** *(Injection <1%):* Neuralgia, thrombocytopenia, phlebitis, dizziness.

ADVERSE REACTIONS/TOXIC EFFECTS

Life-threatening/fatal hypotension, arrhythmias, hypoglycemia, or leukopenia; nephrotoxicity and renal failure; anaphylactic shock; Stevens-Johnson syndrome; toxic epidural necrolysis. Hyperglycemia and insulin-dependent diabetes mellitus (often permanent) may occur even months after therapy.

NURSING IMPLICATIONS
Baseline Assessment:

Question history of anaphylactic reaction to pentamidine isethionate. Avoid concurrent use of nephrotoxic drugs. Establish baseline for B/P, blood glucose. Obtain specimens for diagnostic tests before giving first dose.

INTERVENTION/EVALUATION:

Monitor B/P during administration until stable for both IM and IV administration (pt should remain supine). Check glucose levels and clinical signs for hypoglycemia (sweating, nervousness, tremor, tachycardia, palpitation, lightheadedness, headache, numbness of lips, double vision, incoordination), hyperglycemia (polyuria, polyphagia, polydipsia, malaise, visual changes, abdominal pain, headache, nausea/vomiting). Evaluate IM sites for pain, redness, and induration; IV sites for phlebitis (heat, pain, red streaking over vein). Monitor renal, hepatic, and hematology test results. Assess skin for rash. Determine food tolerance. Evaluate equilibrium during ambulation. Be alert for respiratory difficulty when administering by inhalation route.

PATIENT/FAMILY TEACHING:

Remain flat in bed during administration of medication and get up slowly w/assistance when B/P stable. Notify nurse immediately of sweating, shakiness, lightheadedness, palpitations. Even several months after therapy stops, drowsiness, increased urination, thirst, anorexia may develop—notify nurse/physician immediately. Mouthwash, hard candy, or gum may help w/unpleasant taste that can occur.

pentazocine

pen-**tah**-zoe-seen
(Talwin [parenteral])

FIXED-COMBINATION(S):
W/naloxone, a narcotic antagonist (oral) (**Talwin NX**); w/aspirin (oral) (**Talwin Compound**); w/acetaminophen (oral) (**Talacen**).

CANADIAN AVAILABILITY:
Talwin

CLASSIFICATION

Opioid analgesic (**Schedule IV**)

AVAILABILITY (Rx)

Tablets: 12.5 mg and 325 mg aspirin; 25 mg and 650 mg acetaminophen; 50 mg. **Injection:** 30 mg

PHARMACOKINETICS

	ONSET	PEAK	DURATION
PO	15–30 min	1–3 hrs	>3 hrs
SubQ	15–20 min	—	—
IM	15–20 min	1 hr	2 hrs
IV	2–3 min	15 min	1 hr

Well absorbed from GI tract after IM, SubQ administration. Widely distributed. Metabolized in liver. Primarily excreted in urine. Half-life: 2–3 hrs.

ACTION/THERAPEUTIC EFFECT

Binds w/opioid receptors within CNS, *altering processes affecting pain perception, emotional response to pain.* May displace opioid agonists and competitively inhibit their action (may precipitate withdrawal symptoms).

USES

Relief of moderate to severe pain. Parenteral form used preop or preanesthetic or as supplement to surgical anesthesia.

STORAGE/HANDLING

Store oral, parenteral form at room temperature.

PO/SUBQ/IM/IV ADMINISTRATION

PO:

1. Scored tablets may be crushed; do not crush or break Talwin Compound caplets.

2. May give w/o regard to meals but give w/food or milk if GI distress is evident.

SubQ:

Give SubQ only if absolutely necessary (severe tissue damage possible at injection sites).

IM:

Give deep into upper outer quadrant of buttock, always rotating sites (severe sclerosing of skin, tissue and muscle damage may occur at repeated injection site).

IV:

1. Do not mix in same syringe w/soluble barbiturates (precipitation will occur).

2. May be given undiluted or diluted (each 5 mg w/1 ml sterile water for direct injection).

3. Administer each 5 mg or fraction thereof >1 min.

INDICATIONS/DOSAGE/ROUTES

Analgesia:
PO: Adults: 50 mg q3–4h. May increase to 100 mg q3–4h, if needed. **Maximum:** 600 mg/day.
SubQ/IM/IV: Adults: 30 mg q3–4h. Do not exceed 30 mg IV or 60 mg SubQ/IM per dose. **Maximum:** 360 mg/day.

Usual elderly dosage:
PO: 50 mg q4h p.r.n.
IM: 25 mg q4h p.r.n.

Obstetric labor:
IM: Adults: 30 mg.
IV: Adults: 20 mg when contractions are regular. May repeat 2–3 times q2–3h.

PRECAUTIONS

CONTRAINDICATIONS: Hypersensitivity to pentazocine. **CAUTIONS:** Impaired hepatic/renal function, elderly, debilitated, head injury, respiratory disease, prior to biliary tract surgery (produces spasm of sphincter of Oddi), MI w/nausea, vomiting. **PREGNANCY/LACTATION:** Readily crosses placenta; unknown whether distributed in breast milk. Prolonged use during pregnancy may produce withdrawal symptoms (irritability, excessive crying, tremors, hyperactive reflexes, fever, vomiting, diarrhea, yawning, sneezing, seizures) in neonate. **Pregnancy Category C.** (Category D if used for prolonged periods or in high doses at term.)

INTERACTIONS

DRUG INTERACTIONS: Alcohol, CNS depressants may increase CNS or respiratory depression, hypotension. MAO inhibitors may produce severe, fatal reaction (reduce dose to $1/4$ usual dose). Effects may be decreased w/buprenorphine. **ALTERED LAB VALUES:** May increase amylase, lipase.

SIDE EFFECTS

FREQUENT: Drowsiness, euphoria, nausea, vomiting. **OCCASIONAL:** Allergic reaction, shortness of breath, pounding heartbeat, histamine reaction (decreased B/P, increased sweating, flushing, wheezing), decreased urination, altered vision, constipation, dizziness, dry mouth, headache, hypotension, pain/burning at injection site.

RARE: Confusion, seizures, paralytic ileus, ringing in ears, trembling, stomach cramps, decreased appetite, insomnia.

ADVERSE REACTIONS/TOXIC EFFECTS

Overdosage results in severe respiratory depression, skeletal muscle flaccidity, cyanosis, extreme somnolence progressing to convulsions, stupor, coma. Abrupt withdrawal after prolonged use may produce symptoms of narcotic withdrawal (abdominal cramps, rhinorrhea, lacrimation, nausea, vomiting, restlessness, anxiety, increased temperature, piloerection [goose bumps]). Tolerance to analgesic effect and physical dependence may occur w/chronic use.

NURSING IMPLICATIONS
BASELINE ASSESSMENT:

Raise bed rails. Obtain vital signs before giving medication. If respirations are 12/min or lower, withhold medication, contact physician. Assess onset, type, location, and duration of pain. Effect of medication is reduced if full pain recurs before next dose.

INTERVENTION/EVALUATION:

Encourage deep breathing and coughing exercises. Check vital signs periodically (5–10 min after IV dose). Monitor for change in respirations, B/P, change in rate/quality of pulse. Initiate deep breathing and coughing exercises, particularly in those w/impaired pulmonary function. Change pt's position q2–4h. Assess for clinical improvement and record onset of relief of pain. Contact physician if pain is not adequately relieved.

PATIENT/FAMILY TEACHING:

Change positions slowly to avoid dizziness. Head-low position may help relieve lightheadedness, nausea. Explain need for assistance if ambulating. Avoid alcohol. Request pain medication before pain fully recurs.

---

pentobarbital
(Nembutal)
See Classification section under:
Sedative-Hypnotics

P

---

pentosan
(Elmiron)
See Supplement

---

pentostatin

pen-toe-**stat**-inn
(Nipent)

CLASSIFICATION

Antineoplastic

AVAILABILITY (Rx)

Powder for Injection: 10 mg vial

PHARMACOKINETICS

After IV administration, rapidly distributed to body tissues (poorly distributed to CSF). Excreted primarily in urine unchanged or as active metabolite. Half-life: 5.7 hrs (increased in decreased renal function).

ACTION / *THERAPEUTIC EFFECT*

Inhibits enzyme ADA (increases intracellular levels of adenine deoxynucleotide *leading to cell death*). Greatest activity in T cells of lymphoid system. Inhibits ADA and RNA synthesis. Produces DNA damage.

USES

Treatment of hairy cell leukemia refractory to, or poor response to, interferon alpha therapy.

STORAGE / HANDLING

Refrigerate vial. Contains no preservatives; after reconstitution or dilution, use within 8 hrs when given at room temperature, environmental light. Discard unused portion. Follow institutional procedures for handling antineoplastic medication. Use protective clothing/gloves when handling.

IV ADMINISTRATION

Note: Give by IV injection or IV infusion (*never* SubQ or IM). Gloves, gowns, eye goggles recommended during preparation and administration of medication. If powder or solution comes in contact w/skin, wash thoroughly. Avoid small veins, swollen/edematous extremities, and areas overlying joints, tendons.

1. Adequately hydrate pt before and immediately after (decreases risk of adverse renal effects).

2. Reconstitute each 10 mg vial w/5 ml 0.9% NaCl injection to provide a concentration of 2 mg/ml. Shake thoroughly to ensure dissolution.

3. For direct injection, give over 5 min.

4. For IV infusion, further dilute w/25–50 ml 5% dextrose or 0.9% NaCl and give over 20–30 min.

INDICATIONS / DOSAGE / ROUTES

Note: Dosage individualized based on clinical response, tolerance to adverse effects. When used in combination therapy, consult specific protocols for optimum dosage, sequence of drug administration.

Hairy cell leukemia:

IV: Adults, elderly: 4 mg/m^2 q2 wks until complete response attained (w/o any major toxicity). Discontinue if no response in 6 mos; partial response in 12 mos. **Note:** Withhold/discontinue in those w/severe reaction to pentostatin, nervous system toxicity, active underlying infections, increased serum creatinine, in pt w/neutrophil count <200/mm^3 w/baseline count >500/mm^3.

Dosage in renal impairment:

Only when benefits justify risks, give 2–3 mg/m^2 in pt w/Ccr 50–60 ml/min.

PRECAUTIONS

CONTRAINDICATIONS: None significant. **EXTREME CAUTION:** Preexisting myelosuppression, cardiac disease, impaired hepatic/renal function. Current or recent chickenpox, infection, herpes zoster, history of gout. **PREGNANCY/LACTATION:** If possible, avoid use during pregnancy (may be embryotoxic). Unknown whether drug is distributed in breast milk (advise to discontinue nursing before drug initiation). **Pregnancy Category D.**

INTERACTIONS

DRUG INTERACTIONS: May increase pulmonary toxicity w/fludarabine. May increase effects, toxicity of vidarabine. May decrease effect of antigout medications. Bone marrow depressants may increase bone marrow depression. Live virus vaccines may potentiate virus replication, increase vaccine side effects, decrease pt's antibody response to vaccine. **ALTERED LAB VALUES:** May increase SGOT (AST), SGPT (ALT), alkaline phosphatase, LDH, uric acid, creatinine.

SIDE EFFECTS

FREQUENT (>15%): Nausea, vomiting, unexplained fever, fatigue, rash (occasionally severe), cough, upper respiratory infection, anorexia, diarrhea. **OCCASIONAL (3-15%):** Hematuria, dysuria, headache, pharyngitis, sinusitis, myalgia, arthralgia, peripheral edema, anorexia, blurred vision, conjunctivitis, skin discoloration, sweating, easy bruising, anxiety, depression, dizziness, confusion.

ADVERSE REACTIONS/TOXIC EFFECTS

Bone marrow depression manifested as hematologic toxicity (principally leukopenia, anemia, thrombocytopenia). Doses higher than recommended (20–50 mg/m^2 in divided doses >5 days) may produce severe renal, hepatic, pulmonary, or CNS toxicity, death.

NURSING IMPLICATIONS

BASELINE ASSESSMENT:

Provide emotional support to pt and family. Obtain CBC, differential count (particularly platelets, neutrophils, lymphocytes), liver function studies (esp. SGOT [AST], SGPT [ALT], LDH, GGT, alkaline phosphatase), creatinine before initiating therapy. Antiemetics may be effective in preventing, treating nausea.

INTERVENTION/EVALUATION:

Obtain CBC, differential count,

liver function studies, creatinine at frequent intervals during therapy. Severe occurrence of rash, severe hematologic, blood chemistry values that have significantly changed from baseline or evidence of pulmonary or CNS toxicity may indicate need to terminate medication. Contact physician. Monitor closely for bone marrow suppression: evidence of infection (fever, sore throat), bleeding (easy bruising, unusual bleeding from any site), symptoms of anemia (excessive tiredness, weakness). Be alert for CNS toxicity (agitation, nervousness, confusion, anxiety, depression, insomnia). Avoid IM injections, rectal temperatures, or other trauma that may induce bleeding.

PATIENT/FAMILY TEACHING:

Bone marrow aspiration and biopsy may be a necessary part of program at 2–3 mo intervals to assess treatment response. Do not have immunizations w/o physician's approval (drug lowers body's resistance). Avoid crowds, those w/infection. Promptly report fever, sore throat, signs of local infection, easy bruising, or unusual bleeding from any site, emotional changes.

P

pentoxifylline

pen-tox-ih-**fill**-in
(Pentoxil, Trental)

CANADIAN AVAILABILITY:
Trental

CLASSIFICATION

Hemorheologic

AVAILABILITY (Rx)

Tablets (controlled-release): 400 mg

PHARMACOKINETICS

Completely absorbed from GI tract. Bound to erythrocyte membrane. Metabolized in erythrocytes, liver to active metabolite. Primarily excreted in urine. Half-life: 0.4–0.8 hrs; metabolite: 1–1.6 hrs.

ACTION / *THERAPEUTIC EFFECT*

Improves erythrocyte flexibility, microcirculatory flow, tissue oxygen concentration; *reduces blood viscosity.*

USES

Symptomatic treatment of intermittent claudication associated w/occlusive peripheral vascular disease, diabetic angiopathies.

PO ADMINISTRATION

1. Do not crush or break film-coated tablets.
2. Give w/meals to avoid GI upset.

INDICATIONS/DOSAGE/ROUTES

Intermittent claudication:
PO: Adults, elderly: 400 mg 3 times/day. Decrease to 400 mg 2 times/day if GI or CNS side effects occur. Continue for at least 8 wks.

PRECAUTIONS

CONTRAINDICATIONS: History of intolerance to xanthine derivatives (caffeine, theophylline, theobromine). CAUTIONS: Coronary artery disease, cerebrovascular disease, impaired renal function. PREGNANCY/LACTATION: Unknown whether drug crosses placenta; distributed in breast milk. Pregnancy Category C.

INTERACTIONS

DRUG INTERACTIONS: May increase effect of antihypertensives. ALTERED LAB VALUES: None significant.

SIDE EFFECTS

OCCASIONAL (2–5%): Dizziness, nausea, bad taste, dyspepsia (heartburn, gastric pain, indigestion). RARE (<2%): Rash, pruritus, anorexia, constipation, dry mouth, blurred vision, edema, nasal congestion, anxiety.

ADVERSE REACTIONS/TOXIC EFFECTS

Angina, chest pain occur rarely. May be accompanied by palpitations, tachycardia, arrhythmias. Overdosage (flushing, hypotension, nervousness, agitation, hand tremor, fever, somnolence) noted 4–5 hrs after ingestion, lasts 12 hrs.

NURSING IMPLICATIONS

INTERVENTION/EVALUATION:

Assist w/ambulation if dizziness occurs. Assess for hand tremor. Monitor for relief of symptoms of intermittent claudication (pain, aching, cramping in calf muscles, buttocks, thigh, feet). Symptoms generally occur while walking/exercising and not at rest or w/weight bearing in absence of walking/exercising. Monitor B/P, EKG.

PATIENT/FAMILY TEACHING:

Therapeutic effect generally noted in 2–4 wks. Avoid driving, tasks requiring alert response until response to drug known. Do not smoke (causes constriction and occlusion of peripheral blood vessels).

pergolide mesylate

purr-go-lied
(Permax)

CANADIAN AVAILABILITY:
Permax

CLASSIFICATION

Antiparkinson

AVAILABILITY (Rx)

Tablets: 0.05 mg, 0.25 mg, 1 mg

PHARMACOKINETICS

Well absorbed from GI tract. Metabolized in liver (undergoes extensive first-pass effect). Primarily excreted in urine.

ACTION / *THERAPEUTIC EFFECT*

Inhibits prolactin secretion; directly stimulates postsynaptic dopamine receptors, *assisting in reduction in tremor, improvement in akinesia (absence of movement), posture and equilibrium disorders, rigidity of parkinsonism.*

USES

Adjunctive treatment w/levodopa/carbidopa in those w/ Parkinson's disease.

PO ADMINISTRATION

1. Scored tablets may be crushed.
2. May be given w/o regard to meals.

INDICATIONS/DOSAGE/ROUTES

Note: Daily doses usually given in 3 divided doses.

Parkinsonism:
PO: Adults, elderly: Initially, 0.05 mg/day for 2 days. Increase by 0.1–0.15 mg/day q3 days over the following 12 days; then may increase by 0.25 mg/day q3 days. **Maximum:** 5 mg/day. **Range:** 3–4.6 mg/day.

PRECAUTIONS

CONTRAINDICATIONS: None significant. **CAUTIONS:** Cardiac dysrhythmias. **PREGNANCY/LACTATION:** Unknown whether drug crosses placenta or is distributed in breast milk. May interfere w/lactation. **Pregnancy Category B.**

INTERACTIONS

DRUG INTERACTIONS: Haloperidol, loxapine, methyldopa, metoclopramide, phenothiazines may decrease effect. Hypotension-producing medications may increase hypotensive effect. **ALTERED LAB VALUES:** May increase plasma growth hormone.

SIDE EFFECTS

Note: Dyskinesia (impaired voluntary movement) occurs in 62% of pts. **FREQUENT (10–24%):** Nausea, dizziness, hallucinations, constipation, rhinitis, dystonia (impaired muscle tone), confusion, somnolence. **OCCASIONAL (3–9%):** Postural hypotension, insomnia, dry mouth, peripheral edema, anxiety, diarrhea, dyspepsia, abdominal pain, headache, abnormal vision, anorexia, tremor, depression, rash. **RARE (<2%):** Urinary frequency, vivid dreams, neck pain, hypotension, vomiting.

ADVERSE REACTIONS/TOXIC EFFECTS

Overdosage may require supportive measures to maintain arterial B/P (monitor cardiac function, vital signs, blood gases, serum electrolytes). Activated charcoal may be more effective than emesis or lavage.

P

NURSING IMPLICATIONS
INTERVENTION/EVALUATION:

Be alert to neurologic effects: headache, lethargy, mental confusion, agitation. Monitor for evidence of dyskinesia (difficulty w/movement). Assess for clinical reversal of Parkinson symptoms (improvement of tremor of head/hands at rest, mask-like facial expression, shuffling gait, muscular rigidity).

PATIENT/FAMILY TEACHING:

Tolerance to feeling of light-headedness develops during therapy. To reduce hypotensive effect, rise slowly from lying to sitting position and permit legs to dangle momentarily before standing. Avoid tasks that require alertness, motor skills until response to drug is established. Dry mouth, drowsiness, dizziness may be expected responses of drug. Avoid alcoholic beverages during therapy. Coffee or tea may help reduce drowsiness.

---

perindopril
(Aceon)
See Supplement

---

perphenazine

per-**fen**-ah-zeen
(Trilafon)

FIXED-COMBINATION(S):
W/amitriptyline, a tricyclic antidepressant (**Etrafon, Triavil**)

CANADIAN AVAILABILITY:
Apo-Perphenazine, Trilafon

CLASSIFICATION

Antipsychotic

AVAILABILITY (Rx)

Tablets: 2 mg, 4 mg, 8 mg, 16 mg. **Oral Concentrate:** 16 mg/5 ml. **Injection:** 5 mg/ml.

PHARMACOKINETICS

Well absorbed from GI tract. Widely distributed. Metabolized in liver to active metabolite. Primarily excreted in urine.

ACTION/*THERAPEUTIC EFFECT*

Blocks postsynaptic dopamine receptor sites in brain. *Suppresses behavioral response in psychosis, produces antiemetic effect, terminates intractable hiccups.*

USES

Management of psychotic disorders; control of nausea, vomiting, intractable hiccups.

STORAGE/HANDLING

Store oral, parenteral form at room temperature. Yellow discoloration of solution does not affect potency, but discard if markedly discolored or if precipitate forms.

PO/IM/IV ADMINISTRATION

PO:

1. Do not mix oral concentrate w/caffeine (coffee, cola, tea), apple juice because of physical incompatibility.

2. Mix each 5 ml oral concentrate w/60 ml water, carbonated lemon-lime or orange drink, milk, vegetable, pineapple, apricot, prune, orange, tomato, grapefruit juice.

Parenteral Administration: Pt must remain recumbent for 30–60 min in head-low position w/legs raised, to minimize hypotensive effect.

IM:

1. Inject slow, deep IM into upper outer quadrant of gluteus

maximus. If irritation occurs, dilute further injections w/0.9% NaCl or 2% procaine hydrochloride.

2. Massage IM injection site to reduce discomfort.

IV:

Note: Give by fractional IV injection or IV infusion.

1. For fractional IV, dilute each 5 mg (1 ml) w/9 ml 0.9% NaCl, producing final concentration of 0.5 mg/ml.

2. Do not give more than 1 mg per injection at slow rate at not less than 1–2 min intervals.

3. For IV infusion, dilute further and give at rate of 0.5 mg or less/min.

INDICATIONS/DOSAGE/ROUTES

Note: Decrease dose gradually to optimum response. Decrease to lowest effective level for maintenance. Replace parenteral therapy w/oral therapy as soon as possible.

Hospitalized psychotic:
PO: Adults, children >12 yrs: 8–16 mg 2–4 times/day.
IM: Adults, children >12 yrs: 5 mg q6h, as needed.

Nonhospitalized:
PO: Adults, children >12 yrs: 4–8 mg 3 times/day.

Severe nausea, vomiting, intractable hiccups:
PO: Adults: 8–16 mg/day.
IM: Adults: 5 mg.
IV: Adults: Up to 5 mg.

Usual elderly dosage (nonpsychotic):
PO: Initially, 2–4 mg/day. May increase by 2–4 mg/day every 4–7 days. **Maximum:** 32 mg/day.

PRECAUTIONS

CONTRAINDICATIONS: Severe CNS depression, comatose states, severe cardiovascular disease, bone marrow depression, subcortical brain damage. **CAUTIONS:** Impaired respiratory/hepatic/renal/cardiac function, alcohol withdrawal, history of seizures, urinary retention, glaucoma, prostatic hypertrophy, hypocalcemia (increases susceptibility to dystonias). **PREGNANCY/LACTATION:** Crosses placenta; distributed in breast milk. **Pregnancy Category C.**

INTERACTIONS

DRUG INTERACTIONS: Alcohol, CNS depressants may increase CNS, respiratory depression, hypotensive effects. Tricyclic antidepressants, MAO inhibitors may increase sedative, anticholinergic effects. Antithyroid agents may increase risk of agranulocytosis. Extrapyramidal symptoms (EPS) may increase w/EPS-producing medications. Hypotensives may increase hypotension. May decrease levodopa effects. Lithium may decrease absorption, produce adverse neurologic effects. **ALTERED LAB VALUES:** May produce false-positive pregnancy test, phenylketonuria (PKU). EKG changes may occur, including Q and T wave disturbances.

SIDE EFFECTS

FREQUENT: Hypotension, dizziness, fainting occur frequently after parenteral form is given and occasionally thereafter but rarely w/oral dosage. **OCCASIONAL:** Marked photosensitivity. Drowsiness during early therapy, dry mouth, blurred vision, lethargy, constipation/diarrhea, nasal congestion, peripheral edema, urinary retention. **RARE:** Ocular changes, skin pigmentation (those on high doses for prolonged periods).

ADVERSE REACTIONS/TOXIC EFFECTS

Extrapyramidal symptoms appear dose related (particularly high dosage) and are divided into 3 categories: akathisia (inability to sit still, tapping of feet, urge to move around), parkinsonian symptoms (mask-like face, tremors, shuffling gait, hypersalivation), and acute dystonias: torticollis (neck muscle spasm), opisthotonos (rigidity of back muscles), and oculogyric crisis (rolling back of eyes). Dystonic reaction may also produce profuse sweating, pallor. Tardive dyskinesia (protrusion of tongue, puffing of cheeks, chewing/puckering of the mouth) occurs rarely (may be irreversible). Abrupt withdrawal following long-term therapy may precipitate nausea, vomiting, gastritis, dizziness, tremors. Blood dyscrasias, particularly agranulocytosis, mild leukopenia may occur. May lower seizure threshold.

NURSING IMPLICATIONS

BASELINE ASSESSMENT:

Avoid skin contact w/solutions (contact dermatitis). *Antiemetic:* Assess for dehydration (poor skin turgor, dry mucous membranes, longitudinal furrows in tongue). *Antipsychotic:* Assess behavior, appearance, emotional status, response to environment, speech pattern, thought content.

INTERVENTION/EVALUATION:

Monitor B/P for hypotension. Assess for extrapyramidal symptoms. Monitor WBC, differential count for blood dyscrasias. Monitor for fine tongue movement (may be early sign of tardive dyskinesia). Supervise suicidal risk pt closely during early therapy (as depression lessens, energy level improves increasing suicide potential). Assess for therapeutic response (interest in surroundings, improvement in self-care, increased ability to concentrate, relaxed facial expression). For antiemetic use: Monitor I&O and food tolerance.

PATIENT/FAMILY TEACHING:

Full therapeutic effect may take up to 6 wks. Urine may turn pink or reddish brown. Do not abruptly withdraw from long-term drug therapy. Report visual disturbances. Sugarless gum, sips of tepid water may relieve dry mouth. Drowsiness generally subsides during continued therapy. Avoid tasks that require alertness, motor skills until response to drug is established. Avoid alcohol and CNS depressants. Wear protective clothing, sunscreens in sunlight.

phenazopyridine hydrochloride

feen-ah-zoe-**peer**-ih-deen
(Pyridium, Urodine)

CANADIAN AVAILABILITY:
Phenazo, Pyridium

CLASSIFICATION

Urinary analgesic

AVAILABILITY (Rx)

Tablets: 100 mg, 200 mg

PHARMACOKINETICS

Well absorbed from GI tract. Partially metabolized in liver. Primarily excreted in urine.

ACTION/THERAPEUTIC EFFECT

Exact mechanism unknown. *Excreted in urine where it produces topical analgesic effect on urinary tract mucosa.*

USES

Symptomatic relief of pain, burning, urgency, frequency resulting from lower urinary tract mucosa irritation (may be caused by infection, trauma, surgery).

PO ADMINISTRATION

Give after meals.

INDICATIONS/DOSAGE/ROUTES

Analgesic:
PO: Adults: 200 mg 3 times/day. **Children >6 yrs:** 12 mg/kg/day in 3 divided doses for 3–15 days.

PRECAUTIONS

CONTRAINDICATIONS: Renal insufficiency. **CAUTIONS:** None significant. **PREGNANCY/LACTATION:** Unknown whether drug crosses placenta or is distributed in breast milk. **Pregnancy Category B.**

INTERACTIONS

DRUG INTERACTIONS: None significant. **ALTERED LAB VALUES:** May interfere w/urinalysis color reactions, e.g., urinary glucose, ketone tests, urinary protein, or determination of urinary steroids.

SIDE EFFECTS

OCCASIONAL: Headache, GI disturbance, rash, pruritus.

ADVERSE REACTIONS/TOXIC EFFECTS

Overdosage levels or those w/impaired renal function or severe hypersensitivity may develop renal toxicity, hemolytic anemia, hepatic toxicity. Methemoglobinemia generally occurs as result of massive, acute overdosage.

NURSING IMPLICATIONS
INTERVENTION/EVALUATION

Assess for therapeutic response: relief of pain, burning, urgency, frequency of urination.

PATIENT/FAMILY TEACHING:

A reddish-orange discoloration of urine should be expected. May stain fabric. Take after meals (reduces possibility of GI upset).

phenelzine sulfate

fen-ell-zeen
(Nardil)

CANADIAN AVAILABILITY:
Nardil

CLASSIFICATION

Antidepressant: MAO inhibitor

AVAILABILITY (Rx)

Tablets: 15 mg

PHARMACOKINETICS

Well absorbed from GI tract. Metabolized in liver. Primarily excreted in urine.

ACTION/THERAPEUTIC EFFECT

Inhibits monoamine oxidase (MAO) enzyme system at CNS storage sites. The reduced MAO activity causes an increased concentration in epinephrine, norepinephrine, serotonin, dopamine at neuron receptor sites, *producing antidepressant effect.*

USES/UNLABELED

Management of atypical, nonendogenous, neurotic depression associated w/anxiety, phobic, hypochondriacal features in those not responsive to other antidepressant therapy. *Treatment of panic disorder, vascular/tension headaches.*

PO ADMINISTRATION

Give w/food if GI distress occurs.

INDICATIONS/DOSAGE/ROUTES

Depression:
PO: Adults <60 yrs: 15 mg 3 times daily. Increase rapidly to 60 mg daily until therapeutic response noted (2–6 wks). Thereafter, reduce dose gradually to maintenance level. **Maintenance:** 15–60 mg/day in 3–4 divided doses.

PRECAUTIONS

CONTRAINDICATIONS: Pts >60 yrs, debilitated/hypertensive pts, cerebrovascular/cardiovascular disease, foods containing tryptophan/tyramine, within 10 days of elective surgery, pheochromocytoma, CHF, history of liver disease, abnormal liver function tests, severe renal impairment, history of severe/recurrent headache. **CAUTIONS:** Impaired renal function, history of seizures, parkinsonian syndrome, diabetic pts, hyperthyroidism. **PREGNANCY/LACTATION:** Crosses placenta; unknown whether distributed in breast milk. **Pregnancy Category C.**

INTERACTIONS

DRUG INTERACTIONS: Alcohol, CNS depressants may increase CNS depressant effects. Tricyclic antidepressants, fluoxetine, trazodone may cause serotonin syndrome. May increase effect of oral hypoglycemics, insulin. B/P may increase w/buspirone. Caffeine-containing medications may increase cardiac arrhythmias, hypertension. May precipitate hypertensive crises w/carbamazepine, cyclobenzaprine, maprotiline, other MAO inhibitors. Meperidine, other opioid analgesics may produce immediate excitation, diaphoresis, rigidity, severe hypertension or hypotension, severe respiratory distress, coma, convulsions, vascular collapse, death. May increase CNS stimulant effects of methylphenidate. Sympathomimetics may increase cardiac stimulant, vasopressor effects. Tyramine, foods w/pressor amines (e.g., aged cheese) may cause sudden, severe hypertension. **ALTERED LAB VALUES:** None significant.

SIDE EFFECTS

FREQUENT: Postural hypotension, restlessness, GI upset, insomnia, dizziness, headache, lethargy, weakness, dry mouth, peripheral edema. **OCCASIONAL:** Flushing, increased perspiration, rash, urinary frequency, increased appetite, transient impotence. **RARE:** Visual disturbances.

ADVERSE REACTIONS/TOXIC EFFECTS

Hypertensive crisis may be noted by hypertension, occipital headache radiating frontally, neck stiffness/soreness, nausea, vomit-

ing, sweating, fever/chilliness, clammy skin, dilated pupils, palpitations. Tachycardia or bradycardia, constricting chest pain may also be present. Antidote for hypertensive crisis: 5–10 mg phentolamine IV injection.

NURSING IMPLICATIONS
BASELINE ASSESSMENT:

Periodic liver function tests should be performed in those requiring high dosage undergoing prolonged therapy. MAO inhibitor therapy should be discontinued for 7–14 days prior to elective surgery.

INTERVENTION/EVALUATION:

Assess appearance, behavior, speech pattern, level of interest, mood. Monitor for occipital headache radiating frontally and/or neck stiffness/soreness (may be first signal of impending hypertensive crisis). Monitor blood pressure diligently for hypertension. Discontinue medication immediately if palpitations or frequent headaches occur.

PATIENT/FAMILY TEACHING:

Antidepressant relief may be noted during first week of therapy; maximum benefit noted in 2–6 wks. Report headache, neck stiffness/soreness immediately. To avoid orthostatic hypotension, change from lying to sitting position slowly and dangle legs momentarily before standing. Avoid tasks that require alertness, motor skills until response to drug is established. Avoid foods that require bacteria or molds for their preparation or preservation or those that contain tyramine, e.g., cheese, sour cream, beer, wine, pickled her-

ring, liver, figs, raisins, bananas, avocados, soy sauce, yeast extracts, yogurt, papaya, broad beans, meat tenderizers, or excessive amounts of caffeine (coffee, tea, chocolate), or OTC preparations for hay fever, colds, weight reduction. Avoid alcohol.

phenobarbital
feen-oh-**bar**-bih-tall
(Barbita, Sulfoton)

phenobarbital sodium
(Luminal)

FIXED-COMBINATION(S):
W/phenytoin sodium, an anticonvulsant (Dilantin w/Phenobarbital Kapseals); w/belladonna, an anticholinergic and ergotamine (Bellergal-S)

CLASSIFICATION
Anticonvulsant, hypnotic

AVAILABILITY (Rx)
Tablets: 15 mg, 30 mg, 60 mg, 100 mg. **Elixir:** 15 mg/5 ml, 20 mg/5 ml. **Injection:** 30 mg/ml, 60 mg/ml, 130 mg/ml.

PHARMACOKINETICS

	ONSET	PEAK	DURATION
PO	20–60 min	—	—
IM	10–15 min	—	4–6 hrs
IV	5 min	30 min	4–6 hrs

Well absorbed after oral, parenteral administration. Rapidly, widely distributed. Metabolized in liver. Primarily excreted in urine. Half-life: 53–118 hrs.

ACTION/*THERAPEUTIC EFFECT*

Decreases motor activity to electrical/chemical stimulation, *producing anticonvulsant effect.* CNS depressant effect produces all levels from mild sedation, hypnosis to deep coma.

USES/*UNLABELED*

Management of generalized tonic-clonic (grand mal) seizures, partial seizures, control of acute convulsive episodes (status epilepticus, eclampsia, febrile seizures). Relieves anxiety, provides preop sedation. *Prophylaxis/treatment of hyperbilirubinemia.*

STORAGE/HANDLING

Store oral, parenteral form at room temperature. Do not use oral liquid or parenteral form if solution is cloudy or contains precipitate.

PO/IM/IV ADMINISTRATION

PO:

1. Give w/o regard to meals. Tablets may be crushed.
2. Elixir may be mixed w/water, milk, fruit juice.

Parenteral Form: Do not mix w/acidic solutions (forms precipitate). May be diluted w/normal saline, 5% dextrose, lactated Ringer's.

IM:

1. Do not inject more than 5 ml in any one IM injection site (produces tissue irritation).

2. Inject IM deep into gluteus maximus or lateral aspect of thigh.

IV:

1. Administer at rate not greater than 60 mg/min (too rapid IV may produce severe hypotension, marked respiratory depression).
2. Monitor vital signs q3–5 min during and q15 min for 1–2 hrs after administration.
3. Inadvertent intra-arterial injection may result in arterial spasm w/severe pain, tissue necrosis. Extravasation in subcutaneous tissue may produce redness, tenderness, tissue necrosis. If either occurs, treat w/injection of 0.5% procaine solution into affected area, apply moist heat.

INDICATIONS/DOSAGE/ROUTES

Note: When replacement by another anticonvulsant is necessary, decrease phenobarbital over 1 wk as therapy begins w/low replacement dose.

Anticonvulsant:
PO: Adults, elderly: 60–250 mg/day as single or divided doses. **Children:** 1–6 mg/kg/day as single or divided doses.
IV: Adults, elderly: 100–320 mg. May repeat up to total daily dose of 600 mg/24 hrs. **Children:** Initially, 20 mg/kg as single dose, then 1–6 mg/kg/day.

Hypnotic:
IM/IV/PO: Adults, elderly: 100–320 mg at bedtime.

Sedative:
IM/IV/PO: Adults, elderly: 30–120 mg in 2–3 divided doses per day. **Children:** 2 mg/kg 3 times/day.

Status epilepticus:
IV: Adults, elderly: 10–20 mg/kg; may repeat. **Children:** 15–20 mg/kg, given over 10–15 min.

PRECAUTIONS

CONTRAINDICATIONS: History of porphyria, bronchopneumonia. **EXTREME CAUTION:** Nephritis, renal insufficiency. **CAUTIONS:** Uncontrolled pain (may produce paradoxical reaction), impaired liver function. **PREGNANCY/LACTATION:** Readily crosses placenta; distributed in breast milk. Produces respiratory depression in neonates during labor. May cause postpartum hemorrhage, hemorrhagic disease in newborn. Withdrawal symptoms may appear in neonates born to women receiving barbiturates during last trimester of pregnancy. Lowers serum bilirubin concentration in neonates. **Pregnancy Category D.**

INTERACTIONS

DRUG INTERACTIONS: May decrease effects of glucocorticoids, digoxin, metronidazole, oral anticoagulants, quinidine, tricyclic antidepressants. Alcohol, CNS depressants may increase effect. May increase metabolism of carbamazepine. Valproic acid decreases metabolism, increases concentration, toxicity. **ALTERED LAB VALUES:** May decrease bilirubin.

SIDE EFFECTS

OCCASIONAL (1–3%): Somnolence. **RARE (<1%):** Confusion, paradoxical CNS hyperactivity/nervousness in children, excitement/restlessness in elderly (generally noted during first 2 wks of therapy, particularly noted in presence of uncontrolled pain).

ADVERSE REACTIONS/TOXIC EFFECTS

Abrupt withdrawal after prolonged therapy may produce effects ranging from markedly increased dreaming, nightmares and/or insomnia, tremor, sweating, vomiting, to hallucinations, delirium, seizures, status epilepticus. Skin eruptions appear as hypersensitivity reaction. Blood dyscrasias, liver disease, hypocalcemia occur rarely. Overdosage produces cold, clammy skin, hypothermia, severe CNS depression, cyanosis, rapid pulse, Cheyne-Stokes respirations. Toxicity may result in severe renal impairment.

NURSING IMPLICATIONS

BASELINE ASSESSMENT:

Assess B/P, pulse, respirations immediately before administration. Liver function tests, blood counts should be performed before therapy begins and periodically during therapy. *Hypnotic:* Raise bed rails, provide environment conducive to sleep (back rub, quiet environment, low lighting). *Seizures:* Review history of seizure disorder (length, presence of auras, level of consciousness). Observe frequently for recurrence of seizure activity. Initiate seizure precautions.

INTERVENTION/EVALUATION:

Assess elderly, debilitated, children for evidence of paradoxical reaction, particularly during early therapy. Evaluate for therapeutic response: decrease in length, number of seizures. Monitor for therapeutic serum level (10–30 mcg/ml).

PATIENT/FAMILY TEACHING:

Drowsiness may gradually decrease/disappear w/continued use. Do not abruptly withdraw medication following long-term use (may precipitate seizures). Avoid tasks that require alertness, motor skills until response to drug is established. Tolerance/dependence may occur w/prolonged use of high doses. Strict maintenance of drug therapy is essential for seizure control. Avoid alcohol and other CNS depressants. Notify physician promptly of pregnancy.

phenoxybenzamine hydrochloride

fen-ox-ee-**bends**-ah-mean
(Dibenzyline)

CLASSIFICATION

Alpha-adrenergic blocking agent

AVAILABILITY (Rx)

Capsules: 10 mg

PHARMACOKINETICS

	ONSET	PEAK	DURATION
PO	Several hrs	—	3–4 days

Variably absorbed from GI tract. Metabolized in liver. Primarily excreted in urine. Half-life: 24 hrs.

ACTION/THERAPEUTIC EFFECT

Irreversibly combines w/postganglionic alpha-adrenergic receptors, prevents or reverses effects of catecholamines in exocrine glands, smooth muscle. *Increases blood flow to skin, mucosa, and abdominal viscera; lowers both supine and standing B/P.*

USES/UNLABELED

Controls/prevents hypertension and sweating in pts w/pheochromocytoma. *Treatment of benign prostatic hypertrophy.*

PO ADMINISTRATION

Do not crush or break capsules.

INDICATIONS/DOSAGE/ROUTES

Pheochromocytoma:
PO: Adults, elderly: Initially, 10 mg 2 times/day. **Maintenance:** 20–40 mg 2–3 times/day. May increase dose every other day. **Children:** Initially, 0.2 mg/kg once daily. **Maximum:** 10 mg. **Maintenance:** 0.4–1.2 mg/kg/day in divided doses.

PRECAUTIONS

CONTRAINDICATIONS: Conditions when decrease in B/P is unwarranted. CAUTIONS: Compounds that produce further fall in B/P, marked cerebral/coronary arteriosclerosis, renal impairment/damage. PREGNANCY/LACTATION: Unknown whether drug crosses placenta or is distributed in breast milk. Pregnancy Category C.

INTERACTIONS

DRUG INTERACTIONS: May decrease effects of sympathomimetics (e.g., dopamine, phenylephrine). ALTERED LAB VALUES: None significant.

SIDE EFFECTS

FREQUENT: Miosis, nasal stuffiness,

reflex tachycardia. **OCCASIONAL:** Confusion, drowsiness, dry mouth, headache, inhibition of ejaculation, drowsiness, lack of energy.

ADVERSE REACTIONS/TOXIC EFFECTS

Severe hypotension occurs rarely.

NURSING IMPLICATIONS
INTERVENTION/EVALUATION:

Assist w/ambulation if dizziness, drowsiness occurs. Monitor B/P.

PATIENT/FAMILY TEACHING:

Side effects tend to diminish as therapy continues. Avoid alcoholic beverages. Avoid OTC cough, cold medications. Change positions slowly to prevent postural hypotension. Avoid driving or tasks that require alert response until drug effects known.

phentolamine

fen-**toll**-ah-mean
(Regitine)

CANADIAN AVAILABILITY:
Rogitine

CLASSIFICATION

Alpha-adrenergic blocking agent

AVAILABILITY (Rx)

Injection: 5 mg vials

PHARMACOKINETICS

Excreted in urine. Half-life: 19 min.

ACTION/*THERAPEUTIC EFFECT*

Blocks presynaptic (alpha$_2$) and postsynaptic (alpha$_1$) adrenergic receptors, acting on both arterial tree and venous bed. *Decreases total peripheral resistance, diminishes venous return to heart.*

USES/*UNLABELED*

Diagnosis of pheochromocytoma. Controls/prevents hypertensive episodes immediately before, during surgical excision. Prevents/treats dermal necrosis and sloughing following IV administration of norepinephrine/dopamine. *Treatment of CHF.*

IM/IV ADMINISTRATION

Note: Maintain pt in supine position (preferably in quiet, darkened room) during pheochromocytoma testing. Decrease in B/P noted generally <2 min.

IV:

1. Reconstitute 5 mg vial w/1 ml sterile water to provide concentration of 5 mg/ml.
2. After reconstitution, stable for 48 hrs at room temperature or 1 wk refrigerated.
3. Inject rapidly. Monitor B/P immediately after injection, q30 sec for 3 min, then q60 sec for 7 min.

INDICATIONS/DOSAGE/ROUTES

Diagnosis of pheochromocytoma:
IV: Adults, elderly: 2.5–5 mg. **Children:** 1 mg.

Prevent/control hypertension in pheochromocytoma:
IV: Adults, elderly: 5 mg 1–2 hrs

before surgery. May repeat. **Children:** 1 mg.

Prevent/treat necrosis/sloughing:
IV: Adults, elderly: 5–10 mg in 10 ml saline infiltrated into affected area. **Children:** 0.1–0.2 mg/kg up to maximum of 10 mg.
Note: 10 mg may be added to each liter of solution containing norepinephrine.

PRECAUTIONS

CONTRAINDICATIONS: Epinephrine, myocardial infarction, coronary insufficiency, angina, coronary artery disease. **CAUTIONS:** Severe coronary insufficiency, recent MI, cerebrovascular disease, chronic renal failure, Raynaud's disease, thromboangitis obliterans. **PREGNANCY/LACTATION:** Unknown whether drug crosses placenta or is distributed in breast milk. **Pregnancy Category C**.

INTERACTIONS

DRUG INTERACTIONS: May decrease effects of sympathomimetics (e.g., dopamine, phenylephrine). **ALTERED LAB VALUES:** None significant.

SIDE EFFECTS

FREQUENT: Reflex tachycardia, diarrhea, nausea, vomiting, orthostatic hypotension, abdominal pain. **OCCASIONAL:** Fainting, weakness, flushed face, nasal stuffiness. **RARE:** Myocardial infarction, cerebrovascular spasm/occlusion (confusion, headache, loss of coordination, slurred speech).

ADVERSE REACTIONS/TOXIC EFFECTS

Tachycardia, arrhythmias, acute/prolonged hypotension may occur. Do not use epinephrine (will produce further drop in B/P).

NURSING IMPLICATIONS
BASELINE ASSESSMENT:

Positive pheochromocytoma test indicated by decrease in B/P >35 mm Hg systolic, >25 mm Hg diastolic pressure. Negative test indicated by no B/P change, elevated B/P, or B/P elevated 35 mm Hg systolic and 25 mm Hg diastolic. Preinjection B/P generally occurs within 15–30 min after administration.

INTERVENTION/EVALUATION:

Assist w/ambulation if dizziness occurs. Monitor B/P continuously during therapy/tests.

phenylephrine hydrochloride

fen-ill-**eh**-frin
(Alconefrin, Neo-Synephrine, Prefrin)

FIXED-COMBINATION(S):
W/zinc sulfate, an astringent **(Zincfrin);** w/pyrilamine maleate, an antihistamine **(Prefrin-A);** w/sulfacetamide, an anti-infective **(Vasosulf);** w/pheniramine maleate, an antihistamine **(Dristan);** w/naphazoline, a vasoconstrictor, and pyrilamine, an antihistamine **(4 Way Nasal Spray).**

CANADIAN AVAILABILITY:
Neo-Synephrine

CLASSIFICATION
Sympathomimetic

AVAILABILITY (OTC)

Injection (Rx): 1% (10 mg/ml).
Nasal Solution: 0.125%, 0.16%, 0.25%, 0.5%, 1%. **Ophthalmic Solution:** 0.12%, 2.5% **(Rx)**, 10% **(Rx)**.

PHARMACOKINETICS

	ONSET	PEAK	DURATION
Ophthalmic			
	Immediate	—	0.5–4 hrs
Nasal			
	Immediate	—	0.5–4 hrs
IV	Immediate	—	15–20 min
IM	10–15 min	—	0.5–2 hrs

Minimal absorption following intranasal, ophthalmic administration. Metabolized in liver, GI tract. Primarily excreted in urine. Half-life: 2.5 hrs.

ACTION / *THERAPEUTIC EFFECT*

Acts on alpha-adrenergic receptors of vascular smooth muscle. *Increases systolic/diastolic B/P, produces constriction of blood vessels, conjunctival arterioles, nasal arterioles.*

USES

Nasal: Topical application to nasal mucosa reduces nasal secretion, promoting drainage of sinus secretions. *Ophthalmic:* Topical application to conjunctiva relieves congestion, itching, minor irritation; whitens sclera of eye. *Parenteral:* Vascular failure in shock, drug-induced hypotension.

STORAGE / HANDLING

Store nasal, ophthalmic, parenteral forms at room temperature. Appears clear, colorless, slightly yellow. Do not use if discolored.

NASAL / OPHTHALMIC / IV ADMINISTRATION

NASAL:

1. Blow nose before medication is administered. W/head tilted back, apply drops in 1 nostril. Remain in same position and wait 5 min before applying drops in other nostril.

2. Sprays should be administered into each nostril w/head erect. Sniff briskly while squeezing container. Wait 3–5 min before blowing nose gently. Rinse tip of spray bottle.

OPHTHALMIC:

1. For topical ophthalmic use only.

2. Instruct pt to tilt head backward and look up.

3. Gently pull lower lid down to form pouch and instill medication.

4. Do not touch tip of applicator to lids or any surface.

5. When lower lid is released, have pt keep eye open w/o blinking for at least 30 secs.

6. Apply gentle finger pressure to lacrimal sac (bridge of the nose, inside corner of the eye) for 1–2 min.

7. Remove excess solution around eye w/tissue. Wash hands immediately to remove medication on hands.

PARENTERAL:

Dilute each 10 mg vial w/500 ml 5% dextrose to provide a concentration of 2 mcg/ml.

INDICATIONS / DOSAGE / ROUTES

Nasal decongestant:
PO: **Adults, children >12 yrs:** 2–3 drops, 1–2 sprays of 0.25–0.5% solution into each nostril. **Children 6–12 yrs:** 2–3 drops or 1–2 sprays of 0.25% solution in each nostril. **Children <6 yrs:** 2–3 drops of 0.125% solution in each nostril. Repeat q4h as needed. Do not use longer than 3 days.

P

Ophthalmic:
Ophthalmic: Adults, children >12 yrs: 1–2 drops of 0.125% solution q3–4h.

Usual elderly dosage:
Nasal: 2–3 drops or 1–2 sprays q4h for 3 days.
Ophthalmic: 1 drop (2.5%). May repeat in 1 hr.

Hypotension:
IV Infusion: Adults, elderly: Initially, 100–180 mcg/min. **Maintenance:** 40–60 mcg/min.

PRECAUTIONS

CONTRAINDICATIONS: Idiosyncrasy to sympathomimetics manifested by insomnia, dizziness, weakness, tremor, arrhythmias, MAO inhibitor therapy. *Ophthalmic:* Angle-closure glaucoma, those w/soft contact lenses, use of 10% solution in infants. *Nasal:* Those w/insomnia, tremor, asthenia, dizziness, arrhythmias due to previous drug doses. **CAUTIONS:** Marked hypertension, cardiac disorders, advanced arteriosclerotic disease, type I (insulin-dependent) diabetes mellitus, hyperthyroidism, children w/low body weight, elderly. **PREGNANCY/LACTATION:** Crosses placenta; is distributed in breast milk. **Pregnancy Category C.**

INTERACTIONS

DRUG INTERACTIONS: Tricyclic antidepressants, maprotiline may increase cardiovascular effects. May decrease effect of methyldopa. May have mutually inhibitory effects w/beta blockers. May increase risk of arrhythmias w/ digoxin. Ergonovine, oxytocin may increase vasoconstriction. MAO inhibitors may increase vasopressor effects. **ALTERED LAB VALUES:** None significant.

SIDE EFFECTS

FREQUENT: *Nasal:* Rebound nasal congestion due to overuse (longer than 3 days). **OCCASIONAL:** Mild CNS stimulation (restlessness, nervousness, tremors, headache, insomnia), particularly in those hypersensitive to sympathomimetics (generally, elderly patients). *Nasal:* Stinging, burning, drying of nasal mucosa. *Ophthalmic:* Transient burning/stinging, brow ache, blurred vision.

ADVERSE REACTIONS/TOXIC EFFECTS

Large doses may produce tachycardia, palpitations (particularly in those with cardiac disease), lightheadedness, nausea, vomiting. Overdosage in those >60 yrs may result in hallucinations, CNS depression, seizures. Prolonged nasal use may produce chronic swelling of nasal mucosa, rhinitis.

NURSING IMPLICATIONS
BASELINE ASSESSMENT:

If phenylephrine 10% ophthalmic is instilled into denuded or damaged corneal epithelium, corneal clouding may result.

PATIENT/FAMILY TEACHING:

Discontinue drug if adverse reactions occur. Do not use for nasal decongestion longer than 3–5 days (rebound congestion). Discontinue drug if insomnia, dizziness, weakness, tremor, or feeling of irregular heartbeat occurs. *Nasal:* Stinging/burning of inside nose may occur. *Ophthalmic:* Blurring of vision w/eye instillation generally subsides w/continued therapy. Discontinue medication if redness/swelling of eyelids, itching appears.

phenytoin

phen-ih-toyn
(Dilantin)

phenytoin sodium

(Dilantin)

FIXED-COMBINATION(S):
W/phenobarbital, a barbiturate
(Dilantin w/Phenobarbital)

CANADIAN AVAILABILITY:
Dilantin

CLASSIFICATION

Anticonvulsant

AVAILABILITY (Rx)

Capsules: 30 mg, 100 mg.
Tablets (chewable): 50 mg. **Oral
Suspension:** 30 mg/5 ml, 125
mg/5 ml. **Injection:** 50 mg/ml.

PHARMACOKINETICS

Slow, variably absorbed after
oral administration; slow but complete absorption following IM administration. Widely distributed.
Metabolized in liver. Primarily excreted in urine. Half-life: 22 hrs.

ACTION/THERAPEUTIC EFFECT

Anticonvulsant: Stabilizes neuronal membranes in motor cortex,
*limits spread of seizure activity. Sta-
bilizes threshhold against hyperexcitability. Decreases post-tetanic
potentiation and repetitive discharge.* **Antiarrhythmic:** Decreases abnormal ventricular automaticity *(shortens refractory
period, QT interval, action potential
duration).*

USES/UNLABELED

Management of generalized
tonic-clonic seizures (grand mal),
complex partial seizures (psychomotor), cortical focal seizures,
status epilepticus. Ineffective in
absence seizures, myoclonic
seizures, atonic epilepsy when
used alone. Treatment of cardiac
arrhythmias due to digitalis intoxication. *Treatment of digoxin-induced arrhythmias, trigeminal neuralgia; muscle relaxant in treatment
of muscle hyperirritability; adjunct
in treatment of tricyclic antidepressant toxicity.*

STORAGE/HANDLING

Store oral suspension, tablets,
capsules, parenteral form at room
temperature. Precipitate may form
if parenteral form is refrigerated
(will dissolve at room temperature). Slight yellow discoloration of
parenteral form does not affect
potency, but do not use if solution
is not clear or if precipitate is present.

PO/IV ADMINISTRATION

PO:

1. Give w/food if GI distress
occurs.
2. Do not chew/break cap-
sules. Tablets may be chewed.
3. Shake oral suspension well
before using.

IV:

Note: Give by direct IV injection.
Do not add to IV infusion (precipitate may form).
1. Severe hypotension, cardiovascular collapse occurs if rate of
IV injection exceeds 50 mg/min
for adults. Administer 50 mg >2–3
min for elderly. In neonates, administer at rate not exceeding 1–3
mg/kg/min.
2. IV injection very painful
(chemical irritation of vein due to
alkalinity of solution). To minimize

effect, flush vein w/sterile saline solution through same IV needle/catheter following each IV injection.

3. IV toxicity characterized by CNS depression, cardiovascular collapse.

INDICATIONS/DOSAGE/ROUTES

Note: Pts who are stabilized on 100 mg 3 times daily may receive 300 mg once daily w/extended-release medication. When replacement by another anticonvulsant is necessary, phenytoin should be decreased over 1 wk as therapy is begun w/low dose of replacement drug.

Seizure control:
PO: Adults, elderly: Initially, 100 mg 3 times daily. May be increased in 100 mg increments q2–4 wks until therapeutic response achieved. **Usual dose range:** 300–400 mg daily. **Maximum daily dose:** 600 mg daily (300 mg for extended-release). **Children:** Initially, 5 mg/kg daily in 2–3 equally divided doses. **Usual maintenance dose:** 4–8 mg/kg. **Maximum daily dose:** 300 mg daily.

Status epilepticus:
IV: Adults, elderly: 15–20 mg/kg. **Children:** 15–20 mg/kg in divided doses of 5–10 mg/kg.

Arrhythmias:
IV: Adults, elderly: 100 mg at 5 min intervals until arrhythmias disappear or undesirable effects occur. **Maximum:** 15 mg/kg total dose.

Management of arrhythmias:
PO: Adults, elderly: 100 mg 2–4 times daily.

PRECAUTIONS

CONTRAINDICATIONS: Seizures due to hypoglycemia, hydantoin hypersensitivity. *IV route only:* Sinus bradycardia, sinoatrial block, second- and third-degree heart block, Adam-Stokes syndrome. **EXTREME CAUTION:** *IV route only:* Respiratory depression, myocardial infarction, CHF, damaged myocardium. **CAUTIONS:** Impaired hepatic/renal function, severe myocardial insufficiency, hypotension, hyperglycemia. **PREGNANCY/LACTATION:** Crosses placenta; is distributed in small amount in breast milk. Fetal hydantoin syndrome (craniofacial abnormalities, nail/digital hypoplasia, prenatal growth deficiency) has been reported. There is increased frequency of seizures in pregnant women due to altered absorption of metabolism of phenytoin. May increase risk of hemorrhage in neonate, maternal bleeding during delivery. **Pregnancy Category D**.

INTERACTIONS

DRUG INTERACTIONS: May decrease effect of glucocorticoids. Alcohol, CNS depressants may increase CNS depression. Antacids may decrease absorption. Amiodarone, anticoagulants, cimetidine, disulfiram, fluoxetine, isoniazid, sulfonamides may increase phenytoin concentration, effects, toxicity. Fluconazole, ketoconazole, miconazole may increase concentration. Lidocaine, propranolol may increase cardiac depressant effects. Valproic acid may increase concentration, decrease metabolism. May increase xanthine metabolism. **ALTERED LAB VALUES:** May increase alkaline phosphatase, GGT, glucose.

SIDE EFFECTS

FREQUENT: Drowsiness, lethargy, confusion, slurred speech, irritability, gingival hyperplasia, hypersensitivity reaction (fever, rash, lymphadenopathy), constipation, dizziness, nausea. **OCCASIONAL:** Headache, hair growth, insomnia, muscle twitching.

ADVERSE REACTIONS/TOXIC EFFECTS

Abrupt withdrawal may precipitate status epilepticus. Blood dyscrasias, lymphadenopathy, osteomalacia (due to interference of vitamin D metabolism) may occur. Phenytoin blood concentration of 25 mcg/ml (toxic) may produce ataxia (muscular incoordination), nystagmus (rhythmic oscillation of eyes), double vision. As level increases, extreme lethargy to comatose states occur.

NURSING IMPLICATIONS
BASELINE ASSESSMENT:

Anticonvulsant: Review history of seizure disorder (intensity, frequency, duration, level of consciousness). Initiate seizure precautions. Liver function tests, CBC, platelet count should be performed before therapy begins and periodically during therapy. Repeat CBC, platelet count 2 wks after therapy begins and 2 wks after maintenance dose is given.

INTERVENTION/EVALUATION:

Observe frequently for recurrence of seizure activity. Assess for clinical improvement (decrease in intensity/frequency of seizures). Monitor EKG for cardiac arrhythmias. Assess B/P, EKG diligently w/IV administration. Assist w/ambulation if drowsiness, lethargy, vertigo occurs. Monitor for therapeutic serum level (10–20 mcg/ml).

PATIENT/FAMILY TEACHING:

Pain may occur w/IV injection. To prevent gingival hyperplasia (bleeding, tenderness, swelling of gums), encourage good oral hygiene care, gum massage, regular dental visits. CBC should be performed every month for 1 yr after maintenance dose is established and q3 mos thereafter. Urine may appear pink, red, or red brown. Report sore throat, fever, glandular swelling, skin reaction (hematologic toxicity). Drowsiness usually diminishes w/continued therapy. Do not abruptly withdraw medication following long-term use (may precipitate seizures). Strict maintenance of drug therapy is essential for seizure control, arrhythmias. Avoid tasks that require alertness, motor skills until response to drug is established. Avoid alcohol.

phosphates
potassium phosphate
(Neutra-phos K, K-Phosphate)
sodium phosphate
(Na-Phosphate)
potassium-sodium phosphate
(Neutraphos)

CANADIAN AVAILABILITY:
Potassium phosphate

CLASSIFICATION

Electrolyte

AVAILABILITY (Rx)

Injection: 3 mM/ml. **Tablets. Capsules. Powder.**

PHARMACOKINETICS

Well absorbed from GI tract. Primarily excreted in urine.

ACTION / THERAPEUTIC EFFECT

Modifies calcium concentration and buffer effect on acid-base equilibrium; influences renal excretion of hydrogen.

USES / UNLABELED

Prophylactic treatment of hypophosphatemia. *Prevents calcium renal calculi.*

PO ADMINISTRATION

1. Dissolve tablets in water.
2. Take after meals or w/food (decreases GI upset).
3. Maintain high fluid intake (prevents kidney stones).

INDICATIONS / DOSAGE / ROUTES

ELECTROLYTE REPLACEMENT:

Potassium phosphate:
IV: **Adults, elderly, adolescents:** 10 mmP (310 mg)/day. **Children:** 1.5–2 mmP (46.5–62 mg phosphate)/day.
PO: **Adults, elderly, adolescents:** 1.45 g (250 mg phosphate) in 75 ml water/juice 4 times/day.
Children: 200 mg phosphate in 60 ml water/juice 4 times/day.

Sodium phosphate:
IV: **Adults, elderly, adolescents:** 10–15 mmP (310–465 mg phosphate)/day. **Children:** 1.5–2 mmP/kg/day.

Potassium-sodium phosphate:
PO: **Adults, elderly, adolescents:** 1.25 g (250 mg phosphate) in 75 ml water/juice 4 times/day. **Children <4 yrs:** 1 g (200 mg phosphate) in 60 ml water/juice 4 times/day.

PRECAUTIONS

CONTRAINDICATIONS: Addison's disease, hyperkalemia, acidification of urine in urinary stone disease, those w/infected urolithiasis or struvite stone formation, severely impaired renal function (<30% of normal), hyperphosphatemia. **CAUTIONS:** Those on sodium/potassium-restricted diet, cardiac disease, dehydration, renal impairment, tissue breakdown, myotonia congenita (spasm/rigidity of muscle upon attempts at muscle movement), cardiac failure, cirrhosis/severe hepatic disease, peripheral and pulmonary edema, hypernatremia, hypertension, preeclampsia, hypoparathyroidism, osteomalacia, acute pancreatitis. **PREGNANCY/LACTATION:** Unknown whether drug crosses placenta or is distributed in breast milk. **Pregnancy Category C**.

INTERACTIONS

DRUG INTERACTIONS: Glucocorticoids w/sodium phosphate may cause edema. Antacids may decrease absorption. Calcium-containing medications may increase risk of calcium deposition in soft tissues, decrease phosphate absorption. NSAIDs, ACE inhibitors, potassium-sparing diuretics, potassium-containing medications, salt substitutes w/potassium phosphate may increase potassium concentration. Digoxin and potassium phosphate may increase risk of heart block (due to hyperkalemia). Phosphate-containing medications may increase risk of hyperphosphatemia. Sodium-containing medication w/sodium phosphate may increase risk of edema. **ALTERED LAB VALUES:** None significant.

SIDE EFFECTS

FREQUENT: Mild laxative effect first few days of therapy. **OCCASIONAL:** GI upset (diarrhea, nausea, abdominal pain, vomiting). **RARE:** Headache, dizziness, mental confusion, heaviness of legs, fatigue, muscle cramps, numbness/tingling of hands, feet, around lips, peripheral edema, irregular heartbeat, weight gain, thirst.

ADVERSE REACTIONS/TOXIC EFFECTS

High phosphate levels may produce extra skeletal calcification.

NURSING IMPLICATIONS
INTERVENTION/EVALUATION:

Monitor serum calcium, phosphorus, potassium, sodium levels routinely.

PATIENT/FAMILY TEACHING:

Report diarrhea, nausea, vomiting.

physostigmine salicylate

phy-sew-**stig**-meen
(Antilirium)

physostigmine sulfate

(Eserine Sulfate)

CLASSIFICATION

Anticholinesterase agent

AVAILABILITY (Rx)

Injection: 1 mg/ml. **Ophthalmic Ointment:** 0.25%.

PHARMACOKINETICS

	ONSET	PEAK	DURATION
IM	3–8 min	—	30 min–5 hrs
IV	<5 min	—	45–60 min
Ophthalmic	2 min	1–2 hrs	12–48 hrs

Readily absorbed after IM, SubQ, ophthalmic administration. Widely distributed. Penetrates blood-brain barrier. Hydrolyzed by cholinesterases. Primarily destroyed by hydrolysis. Half-life: 1–2 hrs.

ACTION/*THERAPEUTIC EFFECT*

Inhibits destruction of acetylcholine by enzyme acetylcholinesterase. *Improves skeletal muscle tone, stimulates salivary and sweat gland secretion.* Constricts iris sphincter and ciliary muscle, *producing miosis and increasing accommodation. Intraocular pressure (IOP) reduced by increasing aqueous humor outflow.*

USES/*UNLABELED*

Antidote for reversal of toxic CNS effects due to anticholinergic drugs, tricyclic antidepressants; reduces IOP in primary glaucoma. *Systemic: Treatment of hereditary ataxia. Ophthalmic: Treatment of secondary glaucoma, angle-closure glaucoma during/after iridectomy.*

STORAGE/HANDLING

Store ophthalmic solutions, parenteral form at room temperature. May produce a red tint after extended contact w/metals or long exposure to heat, light, or air. May further degrade to blue/brown color. Discard if discolored.

IM/IV/OPHTHALMIC ADMINISTRATION

IM/IV:

For IV injection, administer at rate no more than 1 mg/min for adults, 0.5 mg/min in children. A too rapid IV may produce bradycardia, hypersalivation, bronchospasm, seizures.

OPHTHALMIC:

1. Instruct pt to lie down or tilt head backward and look up.

2. Gently pull lower eyelid down until a pocket (pouch) is formed between eye and lower lid (conjunctival sac).

3. Hold applicator tube above pocket. Without touching the applicator tip to eyelid or conjunctival sac, place prescribed amount of ointment ($1/4$–$1/2$ inch) into the center pocket (placing ointment directly in eye may cause discomfort).

4. Instruct pt to close eye for 1–2 min, rolling eyeball in all directions (increases contact area of drug to eye).

5. Inform pt of temporary blurring of vision.

INDICATIONS/DOSAGE/ROUTES

Antidote:

IM/IV: Adults, elderly: Initially, 0.5–2 mg. If no response, repeat q20 min until response occurs or adverse cholinergic effects occur. If initial response occurs, may give additional doses of 1–4 mg at 30–60 min intervals as life-threatening signs recur (arrhythmias, seizures, deep coma). **Children:**

0.02 mg/kg. May give additional doses at 5–10 min intervals until response occurs, adverse cholinergic effects occur, or total dose of 2 mg given.

Glaucoma:

Ophthalmic: Adults, elderly: *Ointment:* Apply small quantity 1–3 times/day.

PRECAUTIONS

CONTRAINDICATIONS: Asthma, gangrene, diabetes, cardiovascular disease, mechanical obstruction of intestinal/urogenital tract, vagotonic state, those receiving ganglionic blocking agents. Hypersensitivity to cholinesterase inhibitors or any component of the preparation; active uveal inflammation; angle-closure (narrow-angle) glaucoma before iridectomy; glaucoma associated w/iridocyclitis. **CAUTIONS:** Bronchial asthma, gastrointestinal disturbances, peptic ulcer, bradycardia, hypotension, recent myocardial infarction, epilepsy, parkinsonism, and other disorders that may respond adversely to vagotonic effects. Safety and efficacy in children not established. Use ophthalmic physostigmine only when shorter acting miotics are not adequate, except in aphakics. Discontinue at least 3 wks before ophthalmic surgery. **PREGNANCY/LACTATION:** Probably crosses placenta. Unknown whether distributed in breast milk. May produce uterine irritability, induce premature labor if administered IV near term. **Pregnancy Category C**.

INTERACTIONS

DRUG INTERACTIONS: May increase effects of cholinesterases (e.g., bethanechol, carbachol). May prolong action of succinylcholine. **ALTERED LAB VALUES:** None significant.

SIDE EFFECTS

COMMON: Miosis, increased GI and skeletal muscle tone, reduced pulse rate, constriction of bronchi and ureters, salivary and sweat gland secretion. *Ophthalmic:* Stinging, burning, tearing, hypersensitivity reactions (including allergic conjunctivitis, dermatitis, or keratitis), painful ciliary/accommodative spasm, blurred vision/myopia, poor vision in dim light. **OCCASIONAL:** Slight, temporary decrease in diastolic B/P w/mild reflex tachycardia, short periods of atrial fibrillation in hyperthyroid pts. Hypertensive pts may react w/marked fall in B/P. *Ophthalmic:* Iris cysts (more frequent in children), increased visibility of floaters, headache, brow ache, photophobia, ocular pain. **RARE:** Allergic reaction. *Ophthalmic:* Lens opacities, paradoxical increase in intraocular pressure.

ADVERSE REACTIONS/TOXIC EFFECTS

Parenteral overdosage produces a cholinergic reaction manifested as abdominal discomfort/cramping, nausea, vomiting, diarrhea, flushing, feeling of warmth/heat about face, excessive salivation and sweating, lacrimation, pallor, bradycardia/tachycardia, hypotension, urinary urgency, blurred vision, bronchospasm, pupillary contraction, involuntary muscular contraction visible under the skin (fasciculation).

Overdosage may also produce a *cholinergic crisis,* manifested by increasingly severe muscle weakness (appears first in muscles involving chewing, swallowing, followed by muscular weakness of shoulder girdle and upper extremities), respiratory muscle paralysis, followed by pelvic girdle and leg muscle paralysis. Requires a withdrawal of all anticholinergic drugs and immediate use of 0.6–1.2 mg atropine sulfate IM/IV for adults, 0.01 mg/kg in infants and children under 12 yrs. *Ophthalmic:* Conjunctivitis occurs frequently with chronic use. Retinal detachment and vitreous hemorrhage have occurred occasionally. Systemic effects (nausea, vomiting, diarrhea, abdominal cramps, respiratory difficulty, excessive salivation, bradycardia, cardiac arrhythmias) occur infrequently, require parenteral administration of atropine sulfate.

NURSING IMPLICATIONS

BASELINE ASSESSMENT:

Have tissues readily available at pt's bedside.

INTERVENTION/EVALUATION:

Parenteral therapy: Assess vital signs immediately before and every 15–30 min following administration. Monitor diligently for cholinergic reaction (sweating, irregular heartbeat, muscle weakness, abdominal pain, dyspnea, hypotension). Reduce dosage if excessive sweating, nausea occurs; discontinue if excessive salivation, vomiting, urination, defecation occurs. *Ophthalmic:* Be alert for systemic toxicity: severe nausea, vomiting, diarrhea, frequent urination, excessive salivation, bradycardia (may trigger asthma attack in asthmatics). Assess vision acuity and provide assistance w/ambulation as needed.

PATIENT/FAMILY TEACHING:

Teach proper administration. Do not use more often than directed because of risk of overdosage. Adverse effects often subside after the first few days of therapy. Avoid night driving, activities requiring visual acuity in dim light. Avoid insecticides, pesticides; inhalation/absorption through skin may add to systemic effects of physostigmine. Report promptly any systemic effects (see above) or ocular problems.

---

pilocarpine
(Ocusert)

pilocarpine hydrochloride
(Pilocar, Isopto, Carpine, Ocu-Carpine, Piloptic, Adsorbocarpine, Akarpine, Pilopine, Pilostat, Salagen)

pilocarpine nitrate
(Pilagan Liquifilm)

FIXED COMBINATION(S):
W/epinephrine bitartrate, a vasco-constrictor (E-Pilo-1, 2, 3, 4 or 6); w/physostigmine salicylate, a miotic (Isopto P-ES)

See Classification section under: Antiglaucoma agents

---

pimozide

pim-oh-zied
(Orap)

CANADIAN AVAILABILITY:
Orap

CLASSIFICATION

Antipsychotic

AVAILABILITY (Rx)

Tablets: 2 mg

PHARMACOKINETICS

Poorly absorbed from GI tract. Undergoes first-pass effect. Widely distributed. Metabolized in liver to active metabolite. Primarily excreted in urine. Half-life: 55 hrs.

ACTION/*THERAPEUTIC EFFECT*

Inhibits dopamine receptors in CNS, *interrupting impulse movement.* Produces strong extrapyramidal, moderate anticholinergic, sedative effects.

USES/*UNLABELED*

Suppression of severely compromising motor and phonic tics in those w/Tourette's disorders who have failed to respond adequately to standard treatment. Sjogren's syndrome. *Treatment of psychotic disorders.*

PO ADMINISTRATION

May give w/o regard to meals.

INDICATIONS/DOSAGE/ROUTES

Tourette's disorder:
PO: Adults: Initially, 1–2 mg/day in divided doses. Increase every other day. **Maintenance:** <0.2 mg/kg/day or 10 mg/day, whichever is less. **Maximum:** 0.2 mg/kg/day or 10 mg/day.

Sjogren's syndrome:
PO: Adults: 5 mg 4 times/day.

PRECAUTIONS

CONTRAINDICATIONS: Congenital QT syndrome, history of cardiac arrhythmias, administration w/other drugs that prolong QT interval (azithromycin, clarithromycin, dirithromycin, erythromycin), severe toxic CNS depression, comatose states.

CAUTIONS: History of seizures, cardiovascular disease, impaired respiratory, hepatic/renal function, alcohol withdrawal, urinary retention, glaucoma, prostatic hypertrophy. **PREGNANCY/LACTATION:** Unknown whether drug crosses placenta or is distributed in breast milk. **Pregnancy Category C**.

INTERACTIONS

DRUG INTERACTIONS: Alcohol, CNS depressants may increase CNS depressant effect. Methylphenidate, pemoline may mask signs of tics. Anticholinergics may increase anticholinergic effects. Tricyclic antidepressants, phenothiazines, quinidine may increase risk of cardiac arrhythmias. Extrapyramidal symptom–producing medications (EPS) may increase anticholinergic, CNS depressant, and EPS effects. Clarithromycin may inhibit metabolism. **ALTERED LAB VALUES:** None significant.

SIDE EFFECTS

FREQUENT: Drowsiness, salivation, constipation, dizziness, tachycardia. **OCCASIONAL:** Nausea, sweating, dry mouth, headache, hypotension, GI upset, weight gain. **RARE:** Visual disturbances, diarrhea, rash, urinary abnormalities.

ADVERSE REACTIONS/TOXIC EFFECTS

Extrapyramidal reactions occur frequently but are usually mild and reversible (generally noted during first few days of therapy). Motor restlessness, dystonia, hyperreflexia occur much less frequently. Persistent tardive dyskinesia has occurred. Those on long-term maintenance may experience transient dyskinetic signs following abrupt withdrawal.

NURSING IMPLICATIONS
BASELINE ASSESSMENT:

Obtain baseline EKG. Potassium level should be checked and corrected if necessary.

INTERVENTION/EVALUATION:

EKG should be periodically monitored. Assess for extrapyramidal symptoms. Monitor WBC, differential count for blood dyscrasias. Monitor for fine tongue movement (may be early sign of tardive dyskinesia). Assess for therapeutic response (decreased tic activity).

PATIENT/FAMILY TEACHING:

Do not exceed prescribed dose. Do not abruptly withdraw from long-term drug therapy. Report visual disturbances. Drowsiness generally subsides during continued therapy. Avoid tasks that require alertness, motor skills until response to drug is established. Avoid alcohol and CNS depressants.

pindolol
pin-doe-lol
(Visken)

FIXED-COMBINATION(S):
W/hydrochlorothiazide, a diuretic
(Viskazide)

CANADIAN AVAILABILITY:
Apo-Pindol, Visken

CLASSIFICATION

Beta-adrenergic blocker

AVAILABILITY (Rx)

Tablets: 5 mg, 10 mg

PHARMACOKINETICS

	ONSET	PEAK	DURATION
PO	3 hrs	—	24 hrs

Completely absorbed from GI tract. Metabolized in liver. Primarily excreted in urine. Half-life: 3–4 hrs (increased in decreased renal function, elderly).

ACTION/ *THERAPEUTIC EFFECT*

Nonselective beta blocker. Blocks beta$_1$-adrenergic receptors, *slowing sinus heart rate, decreasing cardiac output, decreasing B/P.* Blocks beta$_2$-adrenergic receptors, *increasing airway resistance. Decreases myocardial ischemia severity* by decreasing oxygen requirements.

USES/ *UNLABELED*

Management of hypertension. May be used alone or in combination w/diuretic. *Treatment of chronic angina pectoris, hypertrophic cardiomyopathy, tremors, mitral valve prolapse syndrome. Increases antidepressant effect with fluoxetine, other SSRIs.*

PO ADMINISTRATION

1. May give w/o regard to food.
2. Tablets may be crushed.

INDICATIONS/DOSAGE/ROUTES

Hypertension:
PO: Adults: Initially, 5 mg 2 times/day. Gradually increase dose by 10 mg/day at 2–4 week intervals. **Maintenance:** 10–30 mg/day in 2–3 divided doses. **Maximum:** 60 mg/day.

Usual elderly dosage:
PO: Initially, 5 mg/day. May increase by 5 mg q3–4 wks.

PRECAUTIONS

CONTRAINDICATIONS: Bronchial asthma, COPD, uncontrolled cardiac failure, sinus bradycardia, heart block greater than first degree, cardiogenic shock, CHF, unless secondary to tachyarrhythmias. **CAUTIONS:** Inadequate cardiac function, impaired renal/hepatic function, diabetes mellitus, hyperthyroidism. **PREGNANCY/LACTATION:** Readily crosses placenta; is distributed in breast milk. May produce bradycardia, apnea, hypoglycemia, hypothermia during delivery, small birth weight infants. **Pregnancy Category B**. (Category D if used in 2nd or 3rd trimester.)

INTERACTIONS

DRUG INTERACTIONS: Diuretics, other hypotensives may increase hypotensive effect; sympathomimetics, xanthines may mutually inhibit effects; may mask symptoms of hypoglycemia, prolong hypoglycemic effect of insulin, oral hypoglycemics; NSAIDs may decrease antihypertensive effect; cimetidine may increase concentration. **ALTERED LAB VALUES:** May increase ANA titer, SGOT (AST), SGPT (ALT), alkaline phosphatase, LDH, bilirubin, BUN, creatinine, potassium, uric acid, lipoproteins, triglycerides.

SIDE EFFECTS

FREQUENT: Decreased sexual ability, drowsiness, trouble sleeping, unusual tiredness/weakness. **OCCASIONAL:** Bradycardia, difficulty breathing, depression, cold hands/feet, diarrhea, constipation, anxiety, nasal congestion, nausea, vomiting. **RARE:** Altered taste, dry eyes, itching, numbness of fingers, toes, scalp.

ADVERSE REACTIONS/TOXIC EFFECTS

Abrupt withdrawal (particularly

in those w/coronary artery disease) may produce angina, CHF or precipitate MI. May precipitate thyroid crisis in those w/thyrotoxicosis.

NURSING IMPLICATIONS
BASELINE ASSESSMENT:

Assess baseline renal/liver function tests. Assess B/P, apical pulse immediately before drug is administered (if pulse is 60/min or below or systolic B/P is below 90 mm Hg, withhold medication, contact physician).

INTERVENTION/EVALUATION:

Assess pulse for strength/weakness, irregular rate, bradycardia. Monitor EKG for cardiac changes. Assist w/ambulation if dizziness occurs. Assess for peripheral edema of hands, feet (usually, first area of low extremity swelling is behind medial malleolus in ambulatory, sacral area in bedridden). Monitor pattern of daily bowel activity, stool consistency. Assess skin for development of rash. Monitor any unusual changes in pt.

PATIENT/FAMILY TEACHING:

Do not abruptly discontinue medication. Compliance w/therapy regimen is essential to control hypertension. If dizziness occurs, sit or lie down immediately. Full therapeutic response may not occur for up to 2 wks. Avoid tasks that require alertness, motor skills until response to drug is established. Report excessive slow pulse rate (<60/min), peripheral numbness, dizziness. Do not use nasal decongestants, OTC cold preparations (stimulants) w/o physician approval. Outpatients should monitor B/P, pulse before taking medication. Restrict salt, alcohol intake.

pioglitazone
(Actos)
See Supplement
See Classification section under:
Antidiabetic

pipecuronium
(Arduan)
See Classification section under:
Neuromuscular blockers

piperacillin sodium
(Pipracil)
See Classification section under:
Antibiotic: Penicillins

piperacillin sodium/tazobactam sodium
pip-ur-ah-**sill**-in/tay-zoe-**back**-tam
(Zosyn)

CANADIAN AVAILABILITY:
Tazocin

CLASSIFICATION

Antibiotic: Penicillin

AVAILABILITY (Rx)

Powder for Injection: 2.25 g, 3.375 g, 4.5 g

PHARMACOKINETICS

Widely distributed. Primarily excreted unchanged in urine. Re-

moved by hemodialysis. Half-life:
0.7–1.2 hrs (increased in decreased
renal function, hepatic cirrhosis).

ACTION/*THERAPEUTIC EFFECT*

Piperacillin: Binds to bacterial
membranes, *inhibiting cell wall
synthesis. Bactericidal.* **Tazobac-
tam:** Inactivates bacterial beta-
lactamase enzymes. *Protects
piperacillin from inactivation by
beta-lactamase-producing organisms, extends spectrum of activity,
prevents bacterial overgrowth.*

USES

Treatment of appendicitis (complicated by rupture or abscess),
peritonitis, uncomplicated and
complicated skin and skin structure infections including cellulitis,
cutaneous abscesses, ischemic/
diabetic foot infections, postpartum endometritis, pelvic inflammatory disease, community-acquired pneumonia (moderate
severity only), moderate to severe
nosocomial pneumonia.

STORAGE/HANDLING

Reconstituted vials stable for 24
hrs at room temperature or 48 hrs
if refrigerated. After further dilution, stable for 24 hrs at room temperature or 7 days if refrigerated.

IV ADMINISTRATION

1. Reconstitute each 1 g w/5
ml diluent.
2. Further dilute w/at least 50
ml 5% dextrose, 0.9% NaCl, or
other compatible diluent.
3. Infuse over 30 min.
4. Alternating IV sites, use
large veins to prevent phlebitis.

INDICATIONS/DOSAGE/ROUTES

Usual parenteral dosage:
IV: Adults, elderly: 12 g/1.5 g/day
as 3.375 g every 6 hrs.

Dosage in renal impairment:
Dose and/or frequency based
on creatinine clearance.

CREATININE CLEARANCE	OSAGE
20–40 ml/min	8 g/1 g/day (2.25 g q6h)
<20 ml/min	6 g/0.75 g/day (2.25 g q8h)

PRECAUTIONS

CONTRAINDICATIONS: Hypersensitivity to any penicillin. **CAU-
TIONS:** History of allergies, esp.
cephalosporins, other drugs.
PREGNANCY/LACTATION: Readily crosses placenta; appears in cord
blood, amniotic fluid. Distributed in
breast milk in low concentrations.
May lead to allergic sensitization, diarrhea, candidiasis, skin rash in infant. **Pregnancy Category B**.

INTERACTIONS

DRUG INTERACTIONS: Probenecid may increase concentration,
risk of toxicity. Hepatotoxic medications may increase hepatotoxicity. **ALTERED LAB VALUES:** May
increase SGOT (AST), SGPT
(ALT), alkaline phosphatase,
bilirubin, LDH, sodium. May cause
positive Coombs' test. May decrease potassium.

SIDE EFFECTS

FREQUENT: Diarrhea, headache,
constipation, nausea, insomnia,
rash. **OCCASIONAL:** Vomiting,
dyspepsia, pruritus, fever, agitation, pain, moniliasis, dizziness,
abdominal pain, edema, anxiety,
dyspnea, rhinitis.

ADVERSE REACTIONS/TOXIC EFFECTS

Superinfections, potentially fatal
antibiotic-associated colitis may
result from bacterial imbalance.
Seizures, neurologic reactions

w/overdosage (more often w/renal impairment). Severe hypersensitivity reactions, including anaphylaxis, occur rarely.

NURSING IMPLICATIONS
BASELINE ASSESSMENT:

Question for history of allergies, esp. penicillins, cephalosporins, other drugs. Obtain specimen for culture and sensitivity before giving first dose (may begin therapy before results are known).

INTERVENTION/EVALUATION:

Hold medication and promptly report rash (hypersensitivity) or diarrhea (w/fever, abdominal pain, mucus and blood in stool may indicate antibiotic-associated colitis). Evaluate IV site for phlebitis (heat, pain, red streaking over vein). Monitor I&O, urinalysis, renal function tests. Monitor electrolytes, esp. potassium. Be alert for superinfection: increased fever, onset of sore throat, diarrhea, vomiting, ulceration, or other oral changes, anal/genital pruritus.

PATIENT/FAMILY TEACHING:

Continue antibiotic for full length of treatment. Space doses evenly. Notify physician in event of rash, diarrhea, bleeding, bruising, other new symptom.

piroxicam

purr-**ox**-i-kam
(Feldene)

CANADIAN AVAILABILITY:
Apo-Piroxicam, Feldene, Fexicam, Novopirocam

CLASSIFICATION

Nonsteroidal anti-inflammatory

AVAILABILITY (Rx)

Capsules: 10 mg, 20 mg

PHARMACOKINETICS

ONSET	PEAK	DURATION
PO (analgesic)		
1 hr	—	48–72 hrs
PO (antirheumatic)		
7–12 days	2–3 wks	—

Well absorbed from GI tract. Metabolized in liver. Primarily excreted in urine. Half-life: 30–86 hrs (increased in decreased renal function).

ACTION/*THERAPEUTIC EFFECT*

Produces analgesic and anti-inflammatory effect by inhibiting prostaglandin synthesis, *reducing inflammatory response and intensity of pain stimulus reaching sensory nerve endings.*

USES/*UNLABELED*

Symptomatic treatment of acute/chronic rheumatoid arthritis, osteoarthritis. *Treatment of ankylosing spondylitis, acute gouty arthritis, dysmenorrhea.*

PO ADMINISTRATION

1. Do not crush or break capsule form.
2. May give w/food, milk, or antacids if GI distress occurs.

INDICATIONS/DOSAGE/ROUTES

Acute/chronic rheumatoid arthritis, osteoarthritis:
PO: **Adults, elderly:** Initially, 20 mg/day as single/divided doses. Some pts may require up to 30–40 mg/day.

PRECAUTIONS

CONTRAINDICATIONS: Active peptic ulcer, GI ulceration, chronic inflammation of GI tract, GI bleeding disorders, history of hypersensitivity to aspirin/NSAIDs. **CAU-TIONS:** Impaired renal/hepatic function, history of GI tract disease, predisposition to fluid retention. **PREGNANCY/LACTATION:** Distributed in breast milk. Avoid use during third trimester (may adversely affect fetal cardiovascular system: premature closure of ductus arteriosus). **Pregnancy Category B**. (Category D if used in 3rd trimester or near delivery.)

INTERACTIONS

DRUG INTERACTIONS: May increase effects of oral anticoagulants, heparin, thrombolytics. May decrease effect of antihypertensives, diuretics. Salicylates, aspirin may increase risk of GI side effects, bleeding. Bone marrow depressants may increase risk of hematologic reactions. May increase concentration, toxicity of lithium. May increase methotrexate toxicity. Probenecid may increase concentration. **ALTERED LAB VALUES:** May increase serum transaminase activity. May decrease uric acid.

SIDE EFFECTS

FREQUENT (3–9%): Dyspepsia, nausea, dizziness. **OCCASIONAL (1–3%):** Diarrhea, constipation, abdominal cramping/pain, flatulence, stomatitis. **RARE (<1%):** Increased B/P, hives, painful/difficult urination, ecchymosis, blurred vision, insomnia.

ADVERSE REACTIONS/TOXIC EFFECTS

Peptic ulcer, GI bleeding, gastritis, severe hepatic reaction (cholestasis, jaundice) occur rarely. Nephrotoxicity (dysuria, hematuria, proteinuria, nephrotic syndrome), severe hypersensitivity reaction (fever, chills, bronchospasm), hematologic toxicity (anemia, leukopenia, eosinophilia, thrombocytopenia) may occur rarely w/long-term treatment.

NURSING IMPLICATIONS
BASELINE ASSESSMENT:

Assess onset, type, location, duration of pain/inflammation. Inspect appearance of affected joints for immobility, deformities, and skin condition.

INTERVENTION/EVALUATION:

Assist w/ambulation if dizziness occurs. Monitor pattern of daily bowel activity, stool consistency. Check behind medial malleolus for fluid retention (usually first area noted). Monitor for evidence of nausea, GI distress. Assess skin for evidence of rash. Evaluate for therapeutic response (relief of pain, stiffness, swelling, increase in joint mobility, reduced joint tenderness, improved grip strength).

PATIENT/FAMILY TEACHING:

Avoid aspirin, alcohol during therapy (increases risk of GI bleeding). If GI upset occurs, take w/food, milk, or antacids. Avoid tasks that require alertness until response to drug is established. Do not crush or chew capsule form.

plasma protein fraction
(Plasmanate, Plasma-Plex, Plasmatein)

CLASSIFICATION

Plasma volume expander

AVAILABILITY (Rx)

Injection: 5%

ACTION/*THERAPEUTIC EFFECT*

Regulates both the volume of circulating blood and tissue fluid balance. *Binds and functions as a carrier of intermediate metabolites (hormones, enzymes, drugs) in the transport and exchange of tissue products.*

USES

Plasma volume expansion in treatment of shock complicated by circulatory volume deficit. Management of protein deficiencies in pts with hypoproteinemia.

STORAGE/HANDLING

Store at room temperature. Liquid is typically transparent, slightly brown, and odorless. Do not use if solution has been frozen, if solution appears turbid or contains sediment, or if not used within 4 hrs of opening vial.

IV ADMINISTRATION

1. Give by IV infusion.
2. May be administered without regard to pt's blood group/Rh factor.
3. Do not administer near site of any trauma/infection.
4. Monitor blood pressure during infusion.

INDICATIONS/DOSAGE/ROUTES

Hypovolemic shock:
IV: **Adults, elderly:** Initially, 250–500 ml at a rate not exceeding 10 ml/min (minimizes hypotension). **Infants, children:** 20–30 ml/kg at a rate not to exceed 10 ml/min.

Hypoproteinemia:
IV: **Adults, elderly:** 1,000–1,500 ml/day at a rate not to exceed 5–8 ml/min (prevents hypervolemia).

PRECAUTIONS

CONTRAINDICATIONS: Severe anemia, cardiac failure, history of allergic reactions to albumin, renal insufficiency, no albumin deficiency. **CAUTIONS:** Low cardiac reserve, pulmonary disease, hepatic/renal failure. **PREGNANCY/LACTATION:** Unknown whether drug crosses placenta or is distributed in breast milk. **Pregnancy Category C**.

INTERACTIONS

DRUG INTERACTIONS: None significant. **ALTERED LAB VALUES:** None significant.

SIDE EFFECTS

OCCASIONAL: Hypotension. *High dosage, repeated therapy:* Allergy or protein overload (chills, fever, flushing, low back pain, nausea, urticaria, vital sign changes).

ADVERSE REACTIONS/TOXIC EFFECTS

Fluid overload (headache, weakness, blurred vision, behavioral changes, incoordination, isolated muscle twitching) and pulmonary edema (rapid breathing, rales, wheezing, coughing, increased B/P, distended neck veins) may occur.

NURSING IMPLICATIONS
BASELINE ASSESSMENT:

Obtain B/P, pulse, respirations immediately before administration. There should be adequate hydration before administration.

INTERVENTION/EVALUATION:

Monitor B/P for hypotension. Assess frequently for evidence of fluid overload, pulmonary edema (see Adverse Reactions/Toxic Effects). Check skin for flushing, urticaria. Monitor hemoglobin, hematocrit. Monitor I&O ratio (watch for decreased output). Assess for therapeutic response (increased B/P, decreased edema).

plicamycin

ply-kah-**my**-sin
(Mithracin)

CLASSIFICATION

Antineoplastic, antihypercalcemic

AVAILABILITY (Rx)

Powder for Injection: 2,500 mcg

PHARMACOKINETICS

Localized in liver, kidney, formed bone surfaces. Crosses blood-brain barrier, enters CSF. Primarily excreted in urine.

ACTION/ *THERAPEUTIC EFFECT*

Forms complexes w/DNA, inhibiting DNA-directed RNA synthesis. *Lowers serum calcium concentration. Blocks hypercalcemic action of vitamin D and blocks action of parathyroid hormone. Decreases serum phosphate levels.*

USES/ *UNLABELED*

Treatment of malignant testicular tumors, hypercalcemia, hypercalcuria associated w/advanced neoplasms. *Treatment of Paget's disease refractory to other therapy.*

STORAGE/HANDLING

Note: May be carcinogenic, mutagenic, or teratogenic. Handle w/extreme care during preparation/administration.

Refrigerate vials. Solutions must be freshly prepared before use; discard unused portions.

IV ADMINISTRATION

Note: Give by IV infusion.

1. Reconstitute 2,500 mcg (2.5 mg) vial w/4.9 ml sterile water for injection to provide concentration of 500 mcg/ml (0.5 mg/ml).

2. Dilute w/500–1,000 ml 5% dextrose or 0.9% NaCl fluid for injection. Infuse over 4–6 hrs.

3. Extravasation produces painful inflammation, induration. Sloughing may occur. Aspirate as much drug as possible. Apply warm compresses.

INDICATIONS/DOSAGE/ROUTES

Note: Dosage individualized based on clinical response, tolerance to adverse effects. Dose based on actual body weight. Use ideal body weight for obese or edematous pts. Do not exceed 30 mcg/kg/day or more than 10 daily doses (increases potential for hemorrhage).

Testicular tumors:
IV: Adults, elderly: 25–30 mcg/kg/day for 8–10 days. Repeat at monthly intervals.

Hypercalcemia/hyperuricemia:
IV: Adults, elderly: 15–25 mcg/kg/day for 3–4 days. Repeat at weekly or longer intervals until desired response achieved.

PRECAUTIONS

CONTRAINDICATIONS: Existing thrombocytopenia, thrombocytopathy, coagulation disorders, tendency to hemorrhage, impaired bone marrow function. **EXTREME CAUTION:** Renal/hepatic impairment. **CAUTIONS:** Electrolyte imbalance. **PREGNANCY/LACTATION:** Contraindicated during pregnancy. Breast-feeding not recommended. **Pregnancy Category D.**

INTERACTIONS

DRUG INTERACTIONS: May increase effect of oral anticoagulants, heparin, thrombolytics. May increase risk of hemorrhage w/NSAIDs, aspirin, dipyridamole, sulfinpyrazone, valproic acid. Bone marrow depressants, hepatotoxic, nephrotoxic medications may increase toxicity. Calcium-containing medications, vitamin D may decrease effect. Live virus vaccines may potentiate virus replication, increase vaccine side effects, decrease pt's antibody response to vaccine. **ALTERED LAB VALUES:** None significant.

SIDE EFFECTS

FREQUENT: Nausea, vomiting, anorexia, diarrhea, stomatitis. **OCCASIONAL:** Fever, drowsiness, weakness, lethargy, malaise, headache, mental depression, nervousness, dizziness, rash, acne.

ADVERSE REACTIONS/TOXIC EFFECTS

Hematologic toxicity noted by marked facial flushing, persistent nosebleeds, hemoptysis, purpura, ecchymoses, leukopenia, thrombocytopenia. Risk of bleeding tendencies increase w/higher doses and/or when more than 10 doses are given. May produce electrolyte imbalance.

NURSING IMPLICATIONS

BASELINE ASSESSMENT:

Question for possibility of pregnancy before initiating therapy (Pregnancy Category X). Antiemetics may be effective in preventing, treating nausea. Discontinue therapy if platelet count falls below 150,000/mm^3, if WBC falls below 4,000/mm^3, or if prothrombin time is 4 secs higher than control test. Renal/hepatic studies should be performed daily in those w/impairment.

INTERVENTION/EVALUATION:

Monitor hematologic, renal, hepatic function studies; platelet count; prothrombin, bleeding times; serum calcium, phosphorus, potassium levels. Assess pattern of daily bowel activity, stool consistency. Monitor for stomatitis (burning/erythema of oral mucosa at inner margin of lips, sore throat, difficulty swallowing, oral ulceration). Monitor for thrombocytopenia (bleeding from gums, tarry stool, petechiae, small subcutaneous hemorrhages). Avoid IM injections, rectal temperatures, any trauma that may induce bleeding.

PATIENT/FAMILY TEACHING:

Maintain fastidious oral hygiene. Do not have immunizations w/o physician's approval (drug lowers body's resistance). Avoid crowds, those w/infection. Promptly report fever, sore throat, signs of local infection, easy bruising, unusual bleeding from any site. Contact physician if nausea/vomiting continues at home. Use nonhormonal contraception.

podofilox
(Condylox)
See Supplement

polycarbophil

polly-**car**-bow-fill
(Fibercon, Mitrolan)

CANADIAN AVAILABILITY:
Replens

CLASSIFICATION

Laxative: Bulk-forming

AVAILABILITY (OTC)

Tablets: 500 mg, 1000 mg.
Tablets (chewable): 500 mg.

PHARMACOKINETICS

	ONSET	PEAK	DURATION
PO	12–72 hrs	—	—

Acts in small/large intestine.

ACTION/THERAPEUTIC EFFECT

Laxative: Retains water in intestine, opposes dehydrating forces of the bowel (promotes well-formed stools). **Antidiarrheal:** Absorbs free fecal water (forms gel, producing formed stool). *Restores normal moisture level, provides bulk.*

USES

Treatment of diarrhea associated w/irritable bowel syndrome, diverticulosis, acute nonspecific diarrhea. Relieves constipation associated w/irritable or spastic bowel.

INDICATIONS/DOSAGE/ROUTES

Note: For severe diarrhea, give every ½ hr up to maximum daily dosage; for laxative, give w/8 oz liquid.

Laxative, antidiarrheal:
PO: **Adults, elderly:** 1 g 4 times/day, or as needed. **Maximum:** 6 g/24 hrs. **Children 6–12 yrs:** 500 mg 1–3 times/day, or as needed. **Maximum:** 3 g/24 hrs. **Children 2–6 yrs:** 500 mg 1–2 times/day, or as needed. **Maximum:** 1.5 g/24 hrs.

PRECAUTIONS

CONTRAINDICATIONS: Abdominal pain, nausea, vomiting, symptoms of appendicitis, partial bowel obstruction, dysphagia. **CAUTIONS:** None significant. **PREGNANCY/LACTATION:** Safe for use in pregnancy. **Pregnancy Category C**.

INTERACTIONS

DRUG INTERACTIONS: May interfere w/effects of potassium-sparing diuretics, potassium supplements. May decrease effect of oral anticoagulants, digoxin, salicylates, tetracyclines by decreasing absorption. **ALTERED LAB VALUES:** May increase glucose. May decrease potassium.

SIDE EFFECTS

RARE: Some degree of abdominal discomfort, nausea, mild cramps, griping, faintness.

ADVERSE REACTIONS/TOXIC EFFECTS

Esophageal/bowel obstruction may occur if administered with insufficient liquid (less than 250 ml or 1 full glass).

NURSING IMPLICATIONS
INTERVENTION/EVALUATION:

Encourage adequate fluid intake. Assess bowel sounds for peristalsis. Monitor daily bowel activity, stool consistency (watery, loose, soft, semisolid, solid) and record time of evacuation. Monitor serum electrolytes in those exposed to prolonged, frequent, or excessive use of medication.

PATIENT/FAMILY TEACHING:

Institute measures to promote defecation (increase fluid intake, exercise, high-fiber diet). Drink 6–8 glasses of water/day when used as laxative (aids stool softening).

polyethylene glycol-electrolyte solution (PEG-ES)

poly-**eth**-ah-leen
(Colovage, CoLyte, GoLYTELY, MiraLax, NuLytely, OCL)

CANADIAN AVAILABILITY:
CoLyte, Golytely, Klean-Prep, Peglyte, Pro-Lax

CLASSIFICATION

Bowel evacuant

AVAILABILITY (Rx)

Powder for Oral Solution. Oral Solution

PHARMACOKINETICS

	ONSET	PEAK	DURATION
PO	30–60 min	—	Completed: 4 hrs

ACTION/THERAPEUTIC EFFECT

Osmotic effect. *Induces diarrhea, cleanses bowel* (electrolytes in solution prevent water/electrolyte imbalance).

USES

Bowel cleansing before GI examination and colon surgery. MiraLax: Treatment of occasional constipation.

STORAGE/HANDLING

Refrigerate reconstituted solutions; use within 48 hrs.

PO ADMINISTRATION

1. May use tap water to prepare solution. Shake vigorously several minutes to ensure complete dissolution of powder.
2. Fasting should occur at least 3 hrs before ingestion of solution (solid food should always be avoided <2 hrs before administration).
3. Only clear liquids permitted after administration.
4. May give via N-G tube.
5. Rapid drinking preferred.

INDICATIONS/DOSAGE/ROUTES

Bowel evacuant:
PO: Adults: 4 L prior to GI examination: 240 ml (8 oz) q10 min until 4 L consumed or rectal effluent clear. N-G tube: 20–30 ml/min.
Constipation:
PO: Adults (MiraLax): 17 g daily.

PRECAUTIONS

CONTRAINDICATIONS: GI obstruction, gastric retention, bowel perforation, toxic colitis, toxic megacolon, ileus. **CAUTIONS:** Ulcerative colitis. **PREGNANCY/LACTATION:** Unknown whether drug crosses placenta or is distributed in breast milk. **Pregnancy Category C.**

INTERACTIONS

DRUG INTERACTIONS: May decrease absorption of oral medications if given within 1 hr (may be flushed from GI tract). **ALTERED LAB VALUES:** None significant.

SIDE EFFECTS

FREQUENT (>10%): Some degree of abdominal fullness, nausea, bloating. **OCCASIONAL (1–10%):** Abdominal cramping, vomiting, anal irritation. **RARE (<1%):** Urticaria, rhinorrhea, dermatitis.

ADVERSE REACTIONS/TOXIC EFFECTS

None significant.

NURSING IMPLICATIONS
BASELINE ASSESSMENT:

Do not give oral medication within 1 hr of start of therapy (may not adequately be absorbed before GI cleansing).

INTERVENTION/EVALUATION:

Assess bowel sounds for peristalsis. Monitor bowel activity, stool consistency (watery, loose, soft, semisolid, solid) and record time of evacuation. Assess for abdominal disturbances.

---

polymyxin B sulfate

polly-**mix**-in
(Aerosporin)

FIXED-COMBINATION(S):
Ophthalmic: W/bacitracin, an anti-infective **(Ocumycin, Polysporin Ophthalmic, AK-Poly-Bac);** w/neomycin, an aminoglycoside **(Statrol);** w/neomycin and bacitracin, anti-infectives **(Neosporin, AK-Spore, Ocutricin);** w/neomycin and bacitracin, anti-infectives, and hydrocortisone, a corticosteroid **(Coracin);** w/dexamethasone, a corticosteroid, and neomycin, an aminoglycoside **(AK-Trol, Dexacidin, Dex-Ide, Maxitrol);** w/chloramphenicol, an antibiotic **(Ophthocort).** *Misc:*

W/neomycin, an aminoglycoside **(Neosporin GU irrigant).**

CLASSIFICATION

Antibiotic

AVAILABILITY (Rx)

Injection: 500,000 units. **Ophthalmic Powder for Solution.**

PHARMACOKINETICS

Widely distributed in tissues; excreted unchanged in urine. Serum concentration increased, half-life prolonged in those w/renal impairment. Half-life: 4–6 hrs (increased in decreased renal function).

ACTION/*THERAPEUTIC EFFECT*

Alters cell membrane permeability in susceptible microorganisms, *producing bactericidal activity.*

USES

Septicemia, infections of skin, urinary tract, meninges; treatment of superficial ocular infections, minor skin abrasions, external ear canal infections, mastoidectomy cavity infections. Prevents bacteriuria/bacteremia associated w/indwelling catheters (combination w/neomycin) as irrigating solution.

STORAGE/HANDLING

After reconstitution, solution stable for 72 hrs if refrigerated. Discard if precipitate forms.

IM/IV/OPHTHALMIC/ADMINISTRATION

Note: Pts must be hospitalized, closely supervised by physician for parenteral administration.

IM:

1. Reconstitute each 500,000 unit vial w/2 ml sterile water for in-

jection, 0.9% NaCl injection, or 1% procaine to provide concentration of 250,000 units/ml.

2. Administer deeply into upper outer quadrant of gluteus maximus.

3. Repeat IM injections at same site not recommended (produces tissue irritation, pain).

IV:

1. For IV infusion (piggyback), further dilute w/300–500 ml 5% dextrose. Infuse over 60–90 min.

2. Alternating IV sites, use large veins to reduce risk of phlebitis.

OPHTHALMIC:

1. Place finger on lower eyelid and pull out until a pocket is formed between eye and lower lid. Hold dropper above pocket and place correct number of drops ($1/4$–$1/2$ inch ointment) into pocket.

2. Have pt close eye gently; *w/solution,* apply digital pressure to lacrimal sac for 1–2 min (minimizes draining into nose and throat, reducing risk of systemic effects).

3. *W/ointment,* have pt close and roll eyes in all directions (increases contact area of drug to eye).

4. Remove excess solution or ointment around eye w/tissue.

INDICATIONS/DOSAGE/ROUTES

Note: Space doses evenly around the clock.

Mild to moderate infections:
IV: Adults, elderly, children >2 yrs: 15,000–25,000 units/kg/day in divided doses q12h. **Infants:** Up to 40,000 units/kg/day.
IM: Adults, elderly, children >2 yrs: 25,000–30,000 units/kg/day in divided doses q4–6h. **Infants:** Up to 40,000 units/kg/day.

Usual irrigation dosage:
Continuous Bladder Irrigation: Adults, elderly: 1 ml urogenital concentrate (contains 200,000 units polymyxin B, 57 mg neomycin) added to 1,000 ml 0.9% NaCl. Give each 1,000 ml >24 hrs for up to 10 days (may increase to 2,000 ml/day when urine output >2 L/day).

Usual ophthalmic dosage:
Ophthalmic: Adults, elderly, children: 1 drop q3–4h.

PRECAUTIONS

CONTRAINDICATIONS: Hypersensitivity to polymyxins or other components in fixed-combinations. **CAUTIONS:** Renal impairment, neuromuscular disorders. **PREGNANCY/LACTATION:** Does not cross placenta; unknown whether excreted in breast milk. **Pregnancy Category B.**

INTERACTIONS

DRUG INTERACTIONS: May produce muscle paralysis, prolonged or increased skeletal muscle relaxation w/neuromuscular blocking agents or anesthetics. Aminoglycosides, other nephrotoxic drugs may increase nephrotoxicity. **ALTERED LAB VALUES:** None significant.

SIDE EFFECTS

FREQUENT: Severe pain, irritation at IM injection sites, phlebitis, thrombophlebitis w/IV administration. **OCCASIONAL:** Fever, urticaria.

ADVERSE REACTIONS/TOXIC EFFECTS

Nephrotoxicity, esp. w/concurrent/sequential use of other nephrotoxic drugs, renal impairment, concurrent/sequential use of muscle relaxants. Neurotoxicity may occur, esp. w/other neurotoxic medications, following anesthesia. Superinfection, esp. w/fungi, may occur.

NURSING IMPLICATIONS
BASELINE ASSESSMENT:

Question pt for history of allergies to polymyxins, other ingredients when used in fixed-combinations. Avoid concurrent administration of other nephrotoxic, neurotoxic drugs if possible. Obtain specimens for culture, sensitivity before giving first dose (therapy may begin before results are known).

INTERVENTION/EVALUATION:

Evaluate IV sites for phlebitis (heat, pain, red streaking over vein). Assess pain, irritation from IM injections. Check I&O, renal function tests. Monitor level of consciousness. Assess for muscle weakness, steadiness on ambulation (support as needed). Obtain vital signs, be esp. alert to respiratory depression.

PATIENT/FAMILY TEACHING:

Therapy must be continued for full length of treatment. Doses are spaced evenly for full effectiveness. Discomfort may occur at IM injection sites. Notify physician in event of dizziness, drowsiness, difficulty breathing, or other new symptom; w/ophthalmic therapy, report any increased irritation, inflammation, itching, burning.

---

poractant
(Curosurf)
See Supplement

---

porfimer sodium
pour-fim-er
(Photofrin)

CANADIAN AVAILABILITY:
Photofrin

CLASSIFICATION

Antineoplastic; photosensitizing agent

AVAILABILITY (Rx)

Cake or Powder for Injection: 75 mg

PHARMACOKINETICS

Protein bound in serum. Accumulates primarily in abnormally active tissues. Light activates compound (absorbs light at wavelength of 630 nm clinically). Half-life: 250 hrs.

ACTION/*THERAPEUTIC EFFECT*

Photosensitizing agent (not cytotoxic until activated by light). Selective accumulation mainly in abnormally active tissues (e.g., cancer, organs of reticuloendothelial system). Tissues containing porfimer when activated by light cause a photochemical reaction *producing cell damage and death by oxidation.*

USES

Reduction of obstruction and palliation of symptoms in pts w/complete or partial obstructing endobronchial non–small cell lung cancer (NSCLC). Palliative tx w/complete or partial obstructing esophageal cancer in whom laser therapy is inadequate. Tx of micro-invasive endobronchial NSCLC when surgery or radiotherapy not indicated.

STORAGE/HANDLING

Store at room temperature. Protect reconstituted product from bright light; use immediately. Reconstituted solution appears opaque.

IV ADMINISTRATION

Note: Wipe spills of porfimer w/damp cloth. Avoid skin and eye contact (risk of photosensitivity reaction upon exposure to light). Use rubber gloves and eye protection. Dispose of all contaminated material in polyethylene bag.

1. Reconstitute each vial with 31.8 ml of either 5% dextrose injection or 0.9% NaCl resulting in concentration of 2.5 mg/ml and pH range of 7–8.

2. Shake well until dissolved.

3. Do not mix w/other drugs in same solution.

4. Give over 3–5 min.

5. If extravasation occurs, protect area from light.

INDICATIONS/DOSAGE/ROUTES

Esophageal cancer, lung cancer:
IV Injection: Adults, elderly: 2 mg/kg. Illuminate w/laser light (630 nm wavelength) 40–50 hrs following injection w/porfimer. A second laser light application may be given 96–120 hrs after initial light application. May be preceded by gentle debridement of tumor via endoscopy. A second course of PDT may be given no earlier than 30 days after initial therapy, up to three courses of PDT. Each course separated by 30 days rest period.

PRECAUTIONS

CONTRAINDICATIONS: *Porfimer:* Porphyria, known allergies to porphyrins. *PDT:* Existing tracheoesophageal or bronchoesophageal fistula; tumors eroding into major blood vessel. **CAUTIONS:** Extreme sensitivity to any light source. **PREGNANCY/LACTATION:** May produce fetal harm. Unknown whether distributed in breast milk. Avoid pregnancy. **Pregnancy Category C**.

INTERACTIONS

DRUG INTERACTIONS: Photosensitizing agents (tetracyclines, sulfonamides, phenothiazines, sulfonylureas, thiazide diuretics, griseofulvin) increase photosensitivity reaction. Alcohol, mannitol, beta-carotene, dimethyl sulfoxide decrease PDT activity. Allopurinol, calcium channel blockers, prostaglandin synthesis inhibitors interfere w/porfimer effect. Glucocorticoids decrease efficacy of treatment. Thromboxane A_2 inhibitors decrease PDT efficacy. **ALTERED LAB VALUES:** None significant.

SIDE EFFECTS

EXPECTED: Photosensitivity. **FREQUENT (>10%):** Photosensitivity reaction to sunlight, bright indoor light (mild erythema on face and hands), fever, nausea, constipation, chest pain, dyspnea, abdominal pain, vomiting, insomnia, back pain. **OCCASIONAL (5–10%):** Dysphagia, respiratory insufficiency, decrease in weight, anorexia, confusion, moniliasis, esophageal disturbances, urinary tract infection.

ADVERSE REACTIONS/TOXIC EFFECTS

Pleural effusion, pneumonia, anemia occurs commonly. Atrial fibrillation occurs occasionally. Esophageal perforation, peritonitis, angina pectoris, myocardial infarction, sick-sinus syndrome occur rarely.

NURSING IMPLICATIONS

INTERVENTION/EVALUATION:

Encourage pts to expose their skin to encircling indoor light (exposure of skin to indoor light inactivates the remaining drug gradually through a photobleaching reaction).

PATIENT/FAMILY TEACHING:

Observe precautions to avoid exposure of skin and eyes to direct sunlight or bright indoor light (examination lamps, dental lamps, operating room lamps, unshaded light bulbs at close proximity) for 30 days. When outdoors during 30 day period, cover all skin, wear sunglasses (eye pain may occur due to sun, bright light, or even car headlights). Encircling indoor light, however, is beneficial, so avoid a darkened room during the 30 day period, other than sleep. After 30 day period, test for photosensitivity by exposing small area of skin to sunlight for 10 min. If no reaction (redness, edema, blistering) occurs within 24 hrs, may gradually resume normal outdoor activity. Do not use face for testing for photosensitivity. If photosensitivity reaction occurs to limited skin test, retry in 2 wks. Sunscreens are of no value in protecting against photosensitivity reaction.

potassium acetate
(Potassium acetate)

potassium bicarbonate/citrate
(K-Lyte)

potassium chloride
(K-Lor, K-Lyte-Cl, Klotrix, K-Dur, Kaochlor, Micro-K, Slow-K)

potassium gluconate
(Kaon)

potassium phosphate
(Potassium phosphate)

CANADIAN AVAILABILITY:
Apo-K, Kaochlor, Kaon, K-Dur, K-Lor, Micro-K, Slow-K

CLASSIFICATION
Electrolyte

AVAILABILITY (Rx)
Acetate: Injection: 2 mEq/ml
Bicarbonate/Citrate: Effervescent Tablets: 25 mEq, 50 mEq
Chloride: Tablets: 6.7 mEq, 8 mEq, 10 mEq, 20 mEq. **Liquid:** 20 mEq/15 ml, 30 mEq/15 ml, 40 mEq/15 ml, 45 mEq/15 ml. **Oral Powder:** 15 mEq, 20 mEq, 25 mEq. **Injection:** 2 mEq/ml, 4 mEq/ml.
Gluconate: Liquid: 20 mEq/15 ml
Phosphate: Injection: 3 mM/ml (mM = millimoles)

PHARMACOKINETICS
Well absorbed from GI tract. Enters cells via active transport from extracellular fluid. Primarily excreted in urine.

ACTION/ *THERAPEUTIC EFFECT*
Necessary for multiple cellular metabolic processes. Primary action intracellular. Necessary *for nerve impulse conduction, contraction of cardiac, skeletal, smooth muscle; maintains normal renal function, acid-base balance.*

USES
Treatment of potassium deficiency found in severe vomiting, diarrhea, loss of GI fluid, malnutrition, prolonged diuresis, debilitated, poor GI absorption, metabolic alkalosis, prolonged parenteral ali-

mentation; prevents hypokalemia in risk pts.

STORAGE/HANDLING

Store oral, parenteral forms at room temperature.

PO/IV ADMINISTRATION

PO:

1. Take w/or after meals and w/full glass of water (decreases GI upset).

2. Liquids, powder, or effervescent tablets: Mix, dissolve w/juice, water before administering.

3. Do not chew, crush tablets; swallow whole.

IV:

1. For IV infusion only, must dilute before administration/mixed well/infused slowly.

2. Generally, no more than 40 mEq/L; no faster than 20 mEq/hr. (Higher concentrations/faster rates may sometimes be necessary.)

3. Use largest peripheral vein/small-bore needle.

4. Avoid adding potassium to hanging IV.

5. Check IV site closely during infusion for evidence of phlebitis (heat, pain, red streaking of skin over vein, hardness to vein), extravasation (swelling, pain, cool skin, little or no blood return).

INDICATIONS/DOSAGE/ROUTES

Treatment/prevention of hypokalemia:
Note: Dosage is individualized.
PO: Adults, elderly: *Prevention:* 20 mEq/day. *Treatment:* 40–100 mEq/day. **Children:** No more than 3 mEq/kg/day. **Infants:** 2–3 mEq/kg/day. Give in 2–4 divided doses.

IV: Adults, elderly, children: Individualize based on EKG, serum potassium concentrations.

PRECAUTIONS

CONTRAINDICATIONS: Severe renal impairment, untreated Addison's disease, postop oliguria, shock w/hemolytic reaction and/or dehydration, hyperkalemia, those receiving potassium-sparing diuretics, digitalis toxicity, heat cramps, severe burns. **CAUTIONS:** Cardiac disease, tartrazine sensitivity (mostly noted in those w/aspirin hypersensitivity). **PREGNANCY/LACTATION:** Unknown whether drug crosses placenta or is distributed in breast milk. **Pregnancy Category A**.

INTERACTIONS

DRUG INTERACTIONS: Angiotensin-converting enzyme (ACE) inhibitors, NSAIDs, beta-adrenergic blockers, potassium-sparing diuretics, heparin, potassium-containing medications, salt substitutes may increase potassium concentration. Anticholinergics may increase risk of GI lesions. **ALTERED LAB VALUES:** None significant.

SIDE EFFECTS

OCCASIONAL: Nausea, vomiting, diarrhea, flatulence, abdominal discomfort w/distention, phlebitis w/IV administration (particularly when potassium concentration of more than 40 mEq/L is infused). **RARE:** Rash.

ADVERSE REACTIONS/TOXIC EFFECTS

Hyperkalemia (observed particularly in elderly or in those w/impaired renal function) manifested as paresthesia of extremities, heaviness of legs, cold skin, grayish pallor, hypotension, mental confusion, irritability, flaccid paralysis, cardiac arrhythmias.

NURSING IMPLICATIONS
BASELINE ASSESSMENT:

Oral dose should be given w/food or after meals w/full glass of water or fruit juice (minimizes GI irritation).

INTERVENTION/EVALUATION:

Monitor serum potassium level (particularly in renal function impairment). If GI disturbance is noted, dilute preparation further or give w/meals. Be alert to decrease in urinary output (may be indication of renal insufficiency). Monitor daily bowel activity, stool consistency. Assess I&O diligently during diuresis, IV site for extravasation, phlebitis. Be alert to evidence of hyperkalemia (skin pallor/coldness, complaints of paresthesia of extremities, feeling of heaviness of legs).

PATIENT/FAMILY TEACHING:

Foods rich in potassium include beef, veal, ham, chicken, turkey, fish, milk, bananas, dates, prunes, raisins, avocado, watermelon, cantaloupe, apricots, molasses, beans, yams, broccoli, brussel sprouts, lentils, potatoes, spinach. Report paresthesia of extremities, feeling of heaviness of legs.

---

pramipexole
(Mirapex)
See Supplement

---

pravastatin

pra-vah-sta-tin
(Pravachol)

CLASSIFICATION

Antihyperlipoproteinemic

AVAILABILITY (Rx)

Tablets: 10 mg, 20 mg, 40 mg

PHARMACOKINETICS

Poorly absorbed from GI tract. Metabolized in liver (minimal active metabolites). Primarily excreted in feces via biliary system. Half-life: 2.7 hrs.

ACTION/*THERAPEUTIC EFFECT*

Interferes w/cholesterol biosynthesis by preventing the conversion of HMG-CoA reductase to mevalonate, a precursor to cholesterol. *Lowers LDL cholesterol, VLDL, plasma triglycerides; increases HDL concentration.*

USES

Preventive therapy to reduce risks of the following in pts w/previous myocardial infarction (MI) and normal cholesterol levels: recurrent MI, undergoing myocardial revascularization procedures; stroke or transient ischemic attack. Prevents CV events in pts w/elevated cholesterol levels.

PO ADMINISTRATION

1. Give w/o regard to meals.
2. Administer in evening.

INDICATIONS/DOSAGE/ROUTES

Note: Before initiating therapy, pt should be on standard cholesterol-lowering diet for minimum of 3–6 mos. Continue diet throughout pravastatin therapy.

Usual dosage:
PO: Adults: Initially, 10–20 mg/day at bedtime. **Elderly:** Initially, 10

mg/day at bedtime. **Range:** 10–40 mg/day at bedtime.

PRECAUTIONS

CONTRAINDICATIONS: Hypersensitivity to pravastatin or any component of the preparation, active liver disease or unexplained, persistent elevations of liver function tests. Safety and efficacy in individuals less than 18 yrs of age has not been established. **CAUTIONS:** History of liver disease, substantial alcohol consumption. Withholding/discontinuing pravastatin may be necessary when pt at risk for renal failure secondary to rhabdomyolysis. Severe metabolic, endocrine, or electrolyte disorders. **PREGNANCY/LACTATION:** Contraindicated in pregnancy (suppression of cholesterol biosynthesis may cause fetal toxicity) and lactation. Unknown whether drug is distributed in breast milk, but there is risk of serious adverse reactions in nursing infants. **Pregnancy Category X**.

INTERACTIONS

DRUG INTERACTIONS: Increased risk of rhabdomyolysis, acute renal failure w/cyclosporine, erythromycin, gemfibrozil, niacin, other immunosuppressants. **ALTERED LAB VALUES:** May increase creatinine kinase, serum transaminase concentrations.

SIDE EFFECTS

Generally well tolerated. Side effects usually mild and transient. **OCCASIONAL (4–7%):** Nausea, vomiting, diarrhea, constipation, abdominal pain, headache, rhinitis, rash, pruritus. **RARE (2–3%):** Heartburn, myalgia, dizziness, cough, fatigue, flu-like symptoms.

ADVERSE REACTIONS/TOXIC EFFECTS

Potential for malignancy, cataracts. Hypersensitivity syndrome has been reported rarely.

NURSING IMPLICATIONS

BASELINE ASSESSMENT:

Question for possibility of pregnancy before initiating therapy (Pregnancy Category X). Question history of hypersensitivity to pravastatin. Assess baseline lab results: cholesterol, triglycerides, liver function tests.

INTERVENTION/EVALUATION:

Monitor cholesterol and triglyceride lab results for therapeutic response. Monitor liver function tests. Evaluate food tolerance. Determine pattern of bowel activity. Check for headache, dizziness (provide assistance as needed). Assess for rash, pruritus. Be alert for malaise, muscle cramping/weakness; if accompanied by fever, may require discontinuation of medication.

PATIENT/FAMILY TEACHING:

Take w/o regard to meals. Follow special diet (important part of treatment). Periodic lab tests are essential part of therapy. Do not take other medications w/o physician's knowledge. Do not stop medication w/o consulting physician. Report promptly any muscle pain/weakness, esp. if accompanied by fever or malaise. Do not drive/perform activities that require alert response if dizziness occurs. Use nonhormonal contraception.

praziquantel

pray-zih-**kwon**-tel
(Biltricide)

CANADIAN AVAILABILITY:
Biltricide

CLASSIFICATION

Anthelmintic

AVAILABILITY (Rx)

Tablets: 600 mg

PHARMACOKINETICS

Rapidly absorbed from GI tract (undergoes extensive first-pass metabolism). Distributed in serum, CSF. Metabolized in liver. Primarily excreted in urine. Half-life: 0.8–1.5 hrs (metabolite: 4–6 hrs).

ACTION/*THERAPEUTIC EFFECT*

Vermicidal. Increases cell permeability in susceptible helminths resulting in loss of intracellular calcium, massive contractions and paralysis of their musculature, followed by attachment of phagocytes to the parasites, *dislodging the dead and dying worms.*

USES

Treatment of all stages of schistosomiasis (bilharziasis or fluke infections), infections due to liver flukes, clonorchiasis and opisthorchiasis.

PO ADMINISTRATION

1. Tablets must not be chewed, but can be halved or quartered.
2. Give w/meals, w/sufficient fluid to swallow w/o gagging.

INDICATIONS/DOSAGE/ROUTES

Schistosomiasis:
PO: Adults, elderly: 3 doses of 20 mg/kg as 1 day treatment. Do not give doses <4 hrs or >6 hrs apart.

Clonorchiasis/opisthorchiasis:
PO: Adults, elderly: 3 doses of 25 mg/kg as 1 day treatment.

PRECAUTIONS

CONTRAINDICATIONS: Ocular cysticercosis, hypersensitivity to praziquantel. **CAUTIONS:** None significant. **PREGNANCY/LACTATION:** Distributed in breast milk; nursing should be discontinued until 72 hrs after last dose (milk should be expressed, thrown away during this period). **Pregnancy Category B.**

INTERACTIONS

DRUG INTERACTIONS: None significant. **ALTERED LAB VALUES:** None significant.

SIDE EFFECTS

FREQUENT: Headache, dizziness, malaise, abdominal pain occur in 90% of pts. **OCCASIONAL:** Anorexia, vomiting, diarrhea. Severe cramping abdominal pain may occur within 1 hr of administration w/fever, sweating, bloody stools. **RARE:** Giddiness, urticaria.

ADVERSE REACTIONS/TOXIC EFFECTS

Overdose should be treated w/fast-acting laxative.

NURSING IMPLICATIONS

BASELINE ASSESSMENT:

Question for history of hypersensitivity to praziquantel. Obtain stool, urine specimens to confirm diagnosis.

INTERVENTION/EVALUATION:

Collect stool, urine specimens as required to monitor effectiveness of therapy. Assess food tolerance, encourage adequate nutrition. Monitor CNS reactions, provide safety measures for ambulation. Check hematology results for anemia. Assess for urticaria.

PATIENT/FAMILY TEACHING:

Complete full course of therapy. If iron supplements are ordered, continue as directed (may be up to 6 mos post therapy). Notify physician if symptoms do not improve in a few days, or if they become worse. Follow-up office visits (several months after therapy is complete) are essential to assure cure. Don't drive, use machinery if dizzy or drowsy.

prazosin hydrochloride

pray-zoe-sin
(Minipress)

FIXED-COMBINATION(S):
W/polythiazide, a diuretic
(Minizide)

CANADIAN AVAILABILITY:
Minipress

CLASSIFICATION

Antihypertensive

AVAILABILITY (Rx)

Capsules: 1 mg, 2 mg, 5 mg

PHARMACOKINETICS

	ONSET	PEAK	DURATION
PO	2 hrs	2–4 hrs	24 hrs

Well absorbed from GI tract. Widely distributed. Metabolized in liver. Primarily eliminated in feces and bile. Not removed by hemodialysis. Half-life: 2–3 hrs.

ACTION/*THERAPEUTIC EFFECT*

Blocks alpha-adrenergic receptors. *Produces vasodilation, decreases peripheral resistance.*

USES/*UNLABELED*

Treatment of mild to moderate hypertension. Used alone or in combination w/other antihypertensives. *Treatment of CHF, ergot alkaloid toxicity, pheochromocytoma, Raynaud's phenomena, benign prostate hypertrophy.*

PO ADMINISTRATION

1. May give w/o regard to food.
2. Administer first dose at bedtime (minimizes risk of fainting due to "first-dose syncope").

INDICATIONS/DOSAGE/ROUTES

Hypertension (alone):
PO: Adults: Initially, 0.5–1 mg 2–3 times/day. Increase gradually up to 20–40 mg/day in divided doses. **Maintenance:** 6–15 mg/day in divided doses.

Hypertension (in combinations w/antihypertensives):
PO: Adults: 1–2 mg 3 times/day and retitrate.

Usual elderly dosage:
PO: Initially, 1 mg 1–2 times/day.

PRECAUTIONS

CONTRAINDICATIONS: None significant. **CAUTIONS:** Chronic renal failure, impaired hepatic function. **PREGNANCY/LACTATION:** Unknown whether drug crosses placenta; distributed in small amount in breast milk. **Pregnancy Category C.**

INTERACTIONS

DRUG INTERACTIONS: Estrogen, NSAIDs, sympathomimetics may decrease effect. Hypotension-producing medications may increase antihypertensive effect. **ALTERED LAB VALUES:** None significant.

SIDE EFFECTS

FREQUENT (7–10%): Dizziness, drowsiness, headache, asthenia (loss of strength, energy). **OCCASIONAL (4–5%):** Palpitations, nausea, dry mouth, nervousness. **RARE (<1%):** Angina, urinary urgency.

ADVERSE REACTIONS/TOXIC EFFECTS

"First-dose syncope" (hypotension w/sudden loss of consciousness) generally occurs 30–90 min after giving initial dose of 2 mg or greater, a too rapid increase in dose, or addition of another hypotensive agent to therapy. May be preceded by tachycardia (120–160 beats/min).

NURSING IMPLICATIONS
BASELINE ASSESSMENT:

Give first dose at bedtime. If initial dose is given during daytime, pt must remain recumbent for 3–4 hrs. Assess B/P, pulse immediately before each dose and q15–30 min until stabilized (be alert to B/P fluctuations).

INTERVENTION/EVALUATION:

Monitor pulse diligently (first-dose syncope may be preceded by tachycardia). Monitor pattern of daily bowel activity and stool consistency. Assist w/ambulation if dizziness, lightheadedness occurs.

PATIENT/FAMILY TEACHING:

May cuase syncope (fainting). Avoid driving for 12–24 hrs after first dose or increase in dosage. Use caution driving or operating machinery and when rising from sitting or lying position. Report dizziness or palpitations if bothersome.

prednicarbate
(Dermatop)
See Supplement
See Classification section under:
Corticosteroids: topical

prednisolone
pred-**niss**-oh-lone
(Prelone, Delta-Cortef)

prednisolone acetate
(Econopred, Inflamase, Pred Mild, Pred Forte, Predolone)

prednisolone sodium phosphate
(Hydeltrasol, Pediapred)

prednisolone tebutate
(Hydeltra TBA, Predalone TBA)

FIXED-COMBINATION(S): Prednisolone acetate w/sulfacetamide sodium, a sulfonamide (Blephamide Liquifilm, Isopto Cetopred); w/atropine sulfate, a mydriatic (Mydrapred); w/neomycin and polymyxin B, anti-infectives (Poly-Pred Liquifilm).

Prednisolone sodium phosphate w/sulfacetamide, a sulfonamide **(Vasocidin, Optimyd).**

CANADIAN AVAILABILITY:
Inflamase, Pediapred

CLASSIFICATION

Corticosteroid

AVAILABILITY (Rx)

Tablets: 5 mg. **Syrup:** 15 mg/5 ml. **Ophthalmic Suspension:** 0.125%, 1%. **Ophthalmic Solution:** 1%.

Acetate: Injection: 25 mg/ml, 50 mg/ml

Phosphate: Injection: 20 mg/ml. **Oral Liquid:** 5 mg/5 ml.

Tebutate: Injection: 20 mg/ml

PHARMACOKINETICS

Well absorbed from GI tract, after IM administration. Widely distributed. Metabolized in liver, tissues. Primarily excreted in urine. Half-life: 3–6 hrs.

ACTION/ *THERAPEUTIC EFFECT*

Inhibits accumulation of inflammatory cells at inflammation sites, phagocytosis, lysosomal enzyme release and synthesis, and/or release of mediators of inflammation. *Prevents/suppresses cell-mediated immune reactions. Decreases/prevents tissue response to inflammatory process.*

USES

Substitution therapy in deficiency states: Acute/chronic adrenal insufficiency, congenital adrenal hyperplasia, adrenal insufficiency secondary to pituitary insufficiency. *Nonendocrine disorders:* Arthritis, rheumatic carditis; allergic, collagen, intestinal tract, liver, ocular, renal, skin diseases; bronchial asthma, cerebral edema, malignancies.

PO/IM/IV/OPHTHALMIC ADMINISTRATION

PO:

1. Give w/food or milk.
2. Single doses given before 9 AM; multiple doses at evenly spaced intervals.

IM:

Give deep IM in gluteus maximus.

IV:

1. May add to 5% dextrose in water or 0.9% NaCl; use within 24 hrs.
2. Prednisolone tebutate not for IV use.

OPHTHALMIC:

1. Place finger on lower eyelid and pull out until a pocket is formed between eye and lower lid. Hold dropper above pocket and place correct number of drops ($1/4$–$1/2$ inch ointment) into pocket. Close eye gently. *Solution:* Apply digital pressure to lacrimal sac for 1–2 min (minimizes drainage into nose and throat, reducing risk of systemic effects). Remove excess solution around eye w/tissue.
2. As w/other corticosteroids, taper dosage slowly when discontinuing.

INDICATIONS/DOSAGE/ROUTES

Note: Individualize dose based on disease, pt, and response.

USUAL ORAL DOSAGE:

PO: Adults, elderly: 5–60 mg/day.

Multiple sclerosis:
PO: Adults, elderly: 200 mg/day

for 1 wk; then 80 mg every other day for 1 mo.

PREDNISOLONE ACETATE:

IM: Adults, elderly: 4–60 mg/day. **Intralesional, Intra-articular, Soft Tissue: Adults, elderly:** 5 mg up to 100 mg/day.

Multiple sclerosis:
IM: Adults, elderly: 200 mg/day for 7 days; then 80 mg every other day for 30 days.

PREDNISOLONE TEBUTATE:

Intralesional, Intra-articular, Soft Tissue: Adults, elderly: 4–30 mg.

PREDNISOLONE SODIUM PHOSPHATE:

IM/IV Adults, elderly: 4–60 mg/day. **Intralesional, Intra-articular, Soft Tissue: Adults, elderly:** 2–30 mg.

Multiple sclerosis:
IM: Adults, elderly: 200 mg/day for 7 days; then 80 mg every other day for 30 days.

USUAL OPHTHALMIC DOSAGE:

Ophthalmic: Adults, elderly: *Solution:* 1–2 drops q1h during day; q2h during night; after response, decrease dose to 1 drop q4h, then 1 drop 3–4 times/day. *Ointment:* thin coat 3–4 times/day; after response, decrease to 2 times/day; then once daily.

PRECAUTIONS

CONTRAINDICATIONS: Hypersensitivity to any corticosteroid or tartrazine, systemic fungal infection, peptic ulcers (except life-threatening situations). Avoid live virus vaccine such as smallpox. **CAUTIONS:** Thromboembolic disorders, history of tuberculosis (may reactivate disease), hypothyroidism, cirrhosis, nonspe-cific ulcerative colitis, CHF, hypertension, psychosis, renal insufficiency, seizure disorders. Prolonged therapy should be discontinued slowly. **PREGNANCY/LACTATION:** Drug crosses placenta, distributed in breast milk. May cause cleft palate (chronic use first trimester). Nursing contraindicated. **Pregnancy Category D.** *Ophthalmic:* Unknown if topical steroids could have sufficient absorption to be distributed in breast milk. **Pregnancy Category B.**

INTERACTIONS

DRUG INTERACTIONS: Amphotericin may increase hypokalemia. May decrease effect of oral hypoglycemics, insulin, diuretics, potassium supplements. May increase digoxin toxicity (due to hypokalemia). Hepatic enzyme inducers may decrease effect. Live virus vaccines may potentiate virus replication, increase vaccine side effects, decrease pt's antibody response to vaccine. **ALTERED LAB VALUES:** May decrease calcium, potassium, thyroxine. May increase cholesterol, lipids, glucose, sodium, amylase.

SIDE EFFECTS

FREQUENT: Insomnia, heartburn, nervousness, abdominal distention, increased sweating, acne, mood swings, increased appetite, facial flushing, delayed wound healing, increased susceptibility to infection, diarrhea/constipation. **OCCASIONAL:** Headache, edema, change in skin color, frequent urination. **RARE:** Tachycardia, allergic reaction (rash, hives), psychic changes, hallucinations, depression. *Ophthalmic:* Stinging or burning, posterior subcapsular cataracts.

ADVERSE REACTIONS/TOXIC EFFECTS

Long-term therapy: Hypocalcemia, hypokalemia, muscle wasting (esp. arms, legs), osteoporosis, spontaneous fractures, amenorrhea, cataracts, glaucoma, peptic ulcer, CHF. *Abrupt withdrawal following long-term therapy:* Anorexia, nausea, fever, headache, sudden, severe joint pain, rebound inflammation, fatigue, weakness, lethargy, dizziness, orthostatic hypotension. Sudden discontinuance may be fatal.

NURSING IMPLICATIONS

BASELINE ASSESSMENT:

Question for hypersensitivity to any corticosteroids. Obtain baselines for height, weight, B/P, glucose, electrolytes. Check results of initial tests, e.g., TB skin test, x-rays, EKG. Never give live virus vaccine (i.e., smallpox).

INTERVENTION/EVALUATION:

Evaluate food tolerance and bowel activity; report hyperacidity promptly. Check B/P, temperature, pulse, respiration at least 2 times/day. Be alert to infection (sore throat, fever, or vague symptoms); assess mouth daily for signs of candida infection (white patches, painful tongue and mucous membranes). Monitor electrolytes. Monitor I&O, daily weight; assess for edema. Watch for hypokalemia (weakness and muscle cramps, numbness/tingling esp. lower extremities, nausea and vomiting, irritability, EKG changes) or hypocalcemia (muscle twitching, cramps, positive Trousseau's or Chvostek's signs). Assess emotional status, ability to sleep.

PATIENT/FAMILY TEACHING:

Carry identification of drug and dose, physician's name and phone number. Do not change dose/schedule or stop taking drug; must taper off gradually under medical supervision. Notify physician of fever, sore throat, muscle aches, sudden weight gain/swelling. W/dietician give instructions for prescribed diet (may be sodium restricted, high protein and potassium). Maintain careful personal hygiene, avoid exposure to disease or trauma. Severe stress (serious infection, surgery, or trauma) may require increased dosage. Do not take any other medication w/o consulting physician. Follow-up visits, lab tests are necessary; children must be assessed for growth retardation. Inform dentist or other physicians of prednisolone therapy now or within past 12 mos. Caution against overuse of joints injected for symptomatic relief. *Ophthalmic:* Teach proper administration.

prednisone
pred-nih-sewn
(Orasone, Deltasone, Meticorten)

CANADIAN AVAILABILITY:
Apo-Prednisone, Deltasone, Winpred

CLASSIFICATION
Corticosteroid

AVAILABILITY (Rx)
Tablets: 1 mg, 2.5 mg, 5 mg, 10

mg, 20 mg, 50 mg. **Oral Solution:** 5 mg/5 ml, 5 mg/ml. **Syrup:** 5 mg/5 ml.

PHARMACOKINETICS

Well absorbed from GI tract. Widely distributed. Metabolized in liver (converted to prednisolone). Primarily excreted in urine. Half-life: 3.4–3.8 hrs.

ACTION / THERAPEUTIC EFFECT

Inhibits accumulation of inflammatory cells at inflammation sites, phagocytosis, lysosomal enzyme release and synthesis, and/or release of mediators of inflammation. *Prevents/suppresses cell-mediated immune reactions. Decreases/prevents tissue response to inflammatory process.*

USES

Substitution therapy in deficiency states: Acute/chronic adrenal insufficiency, congenital adrenal hyperplasia, adrenal insufficiency secondary to pituitary insufficiency. *Nonendocrine disorders:* Arthritis, rheumatic carditis; allergic, collagen, intestinal tract, liver, ocular, renal, skin diseases; bronchial asthma, cerebral edema, malignancies.

PO ADMINISTRATION

1. Give w/o regard to meals (give w/food if GI upset occurs).

2. Give single doses before 9 AM, multiple doses at evenly spaced intervals.

INDICATIONS / DOSAGE / ROUTES

Usual oral dosage:
PO: Adults, elderly: 5–60 mg/day. **Children:** 0.14–2 mg/kg/day.

PRECAUTIONS

CONTRAINDICATIONS: Hypersensitivity to any corticosteroid, systemic fungal infection, peptic ulcer (except life-threatening situations), breast-feeding. **CAUTIONS:** Thromboembolic disorders, history of tuberculosis (may reactivate disease), hypothyroidism, cirrhosis, nonspecific ulcerative colitis, CHF, hypertension, psychosis, renal insufficiency, seizure disorders. **PREGNANCY/LACTATION:** Crosses placenta; is distributed in breast milk. Cleft palate generally occurs w/chronic use, first trimester. **Pregnancy Category B**.

INTERACTIONS

DRUG INTERACTIONS: Amphotericin may increase hypokalemia. May decrease effect of oral hypoglycemics, insulin, diuretics, potassium supplements. May increase digoxin toxicity (due to hypokalemia). Hepatic enzyme inducers may decrease effect. Live virus vaccines may potentiate virus replication, increase vaccine side effects, decrease pt's antibody response to vaccine. **ALTERED LAB VALUES:** May decrease calcium, potassium, thyroxine. May increase cholesterol, lipids, glucose, sodium, amylase.

SIDE EFFECTS

FREQUENT: Insomnia, heartburn, nervousness, abdominal distention, increased sweating, acne, mood swings, increased appetite, facial flushing, delayed wound healing, increased susceptibility to infection, diarrhea/constipation. **OCCASIONAL:** Headache, edema, change in skin color, frequent urination. **RARE:** Tachycardia, allergic reaction (rash, hives), psychic changes, hallucinations, depression.

ADVERSE REACTIONS/TOXIC EFFECTS

Long-term therapy: Muscle wasting (esp. arms, legs), osteoporosis, spontaneous fractures, amenorrhea, cataracts, glaucoma, peptic ulcer, CHF. *Abrupt withdrawal following long-term therapy:* Anorexia, nausea, fever, headache, sudden or severe joint pain, rebound inflammation, fatigue, weakness, lethargy, dizziness, orthostatic hypotension. Sudden discontinuance may be fatal.

NURSING IMPLICATIONS
BASELINE ASSESSMENT:

Question for hypersensitivity to any corticosteroids. Obtain baselines for height, weight, B/P, glucose, electrolytes. Check results of initial tests, e.g., TB skin test, x-rays, EKG. Never give live virus vaccine.

INTERVENTION/EVALUATION:

Monitor I&O, daily weight; assess for edema. Check lab results for blood coagulability, clinical evidence of thromboembolism. Evaluate food tolerance, bowel activity; report hyperacidity promptly. Check B/P, temperature, pulse, respiration, at least 2 times/day. Be alert to infection: sore throat, fever/vague symptoms. Assess mouth daily for signs of candida infection (white patches, painful tongue and mucous membranes). Monitor electrolytes. Watch for hypocalcemia (muscle twitching, cramps, positive Trousseau's or Chvostek's signs) or hypokalemia (weakness and muscle cramps, numbness/tingling, esp. lower extremities, nausea and vomiting, irritability, EKG changes). As-

sess emotional status, ability to sleep.

PATIENT/FAMILY TEACHING:

Carry identification of drug and dose, physician's name and phone number. Do not change dose/schedule or stop taking drug (must taper off gradually under medical supervision). Notify physician of fever, sore throat, muscle aches, sudden weight gain/swelling. Give instructions for prescribed diet (may be sodium restricted, high protein and potassium). Maintain careful personal hygiene, avoid exposure to disease/trauma. Severe stress (serious infection, surgery, or trauma) may require increased dosage. Do not take any other medication w/o consulting physician. Follow-up visits, lab tests are necessary; children must be assessed for growth retardation. Inform dentist or other physicians of prednisone therapy now or within past 12 mos. Caution against overuse of joints injected for symptomatic relief.

primidone
prih-mih-doan
(Mysoline)

CANADIAN AVAILABILITY:
Apo-Primidone, Mysoline

CLASSIFICATION
Anticonvulsant

AVAILABILITY (Rx)
Tablets: 50 mg, 250 mg. **Oral Suspension:** 250 mg/5 ml.

PHARMACOKINETICS

Rapidly, completely absorbed from GI tract. Widely distributed. Metabolized in liver to active metabolite (phenobarbital). Primarily excreted in urine. Half-life: 3–23 hrs; metabolite: 75–126 hrs.

ACTION/ *THERAPEUTIC EFFECT*

Decreases motor activity to electrical/chemical stimulation, stabilizes threshhold against hyperexcitability, *producing anticonvulsant effect.*

USES/ *UNLABELED*

Management of partial seizures w/complex symptomatology (psychomotor seizures), generalized tonic-clonic (grand mal) seizures. *Treatment of essential tremor.*

PO ADMINISTRATION

1. Give w/o regard to meals.

2. Shake oral suspension well before administering (may be mixed w/food).

3. Tablets may be crushed.

INDICATIONS/DOSAGE/ROUTES

Note: When replacement by another anticonvulsant is necessary, decrease primidone gradually as therapy begins w/low replacement dose.

Anticonvulsant:
PO: Adults, elderly, children >8 yrs: 100–125 mg daily for 3 days at bedtime, then 100–125 mg 2 times/day for days 4–6, then 100–125 mg 3 times/day for days 7–9, then maintenance of 250 mg 3 times/day. **Children <8 yrs:** 50 mg at bedtime for 3 days, then 50 mg 2 times/day for days 4–6, then 100 mg 2 times/day for days 7–9, then maintenance of 125–250 mg 3 times/day.

PRECAUTIONS

CONTRAINDICATIONS: History of porphyria, bronchopneumonia. **EXTREME CAUTION:** Nephritis, renal insufficiency. **CAUTIONS:** Uncontrolled pain (may produce paradoxical reaction), impaired liver function. **PREGNANCY/LACTATION:** Readily crosses placenta; is distributed in breast milk in substantial quantities. Produces respiratory depression in the neonate during labor. May cause postpartum hemorrhage, hemorrhagic disease in newborn. Withdrawal symptoms may occur in neonates born to women who receive barbiturates during last trimester of pregnancy. Lowers serum bilirubin concentrations in neonates. **Pregnancy Category D**.

INTERACTIONS

DRUG INTERACTIONS: May decrease effects of glucocorticoids, digoxin, metronidazole, oral anticoagulants, quinidine, tricyclic antidepressants. Alcohol, CNS depressants may increase effect. May increase metabolism of carbamazepine. Valproic acid decreases metabolism, increases concentration, toxicity. **ALTERED LAB VALUES:** May decrease bilirubin.

SIDE EFFECTS

FREQUENT: Ataxia, dizziness. **OCCASIONAL:** Loss of appetite, drowsiness, mental changes, nausea, vomiting, paradoxical excitement. **RARE:** Skin rash.

ADVERSE REACTIONS/TOXIC EFFECTS

Abrupt withdrawal after prolonged therapy may produce effects ranging from markedly increased dreaming, nightmares and/or insomnia, tremor, sweating, vomiting, to hallucinations, delirium, seizures, status epilepticus. Skin eruptions may appear as hypersensitivity reaction. Blood dyscrasias, liver disease, hypocalcemia occur rarely. Overdosage produces cold clammy skin, hypothermia, severe CNS depression followed by high fever, coma.

NURSING IMPLICATIONS

BASELINE ASSESSMENT:

Review history of seizure disorder (intensity, frequency, duration, level of consciousness). Observe frequently for recurrence of seizure activity. Initiate seizure precautions.

INTERVENTION/EVALUATION:

For those on long-term therapy, liver/renal function tests, blood counts should be performed periodically. Assist w/ambulation if dizziness, ataxia occurs. Assess children, elderly for paradoxical reaction (particularly during early therapy). Assess for clinical improvement (decrease in intensity/frequency of seizures). Monitor for therapeutic serum level (5–12 mcg/ml).

PATIENT/FAMILY TEACHING:

Do not abruptly withdraw medication following long-term use (may precipitate seizures). Strict maintenance of drug therapy is essential for seizure control. Drowsiness usually disappears during continued therapy. If dizziness occurs, change positions slowly from recumbent to sitting position before standing. Avoid tasks that require alertness, motor skills until response to drug is established. Avoid alcohol.

probenecid

pro-**ben**-ah-sid
(Benemid, Probalan)

FIXED-COMBINATION(S):
W/colchicine, antigout agent (Col-Benemid, Proben-C)

CANADIAN AVAILABILITY:
Benemid, Benuryl

CLASSIFICATION

Uricosuric

AVAILABILITY (Rx)

Tablets: 500 mg

PHARMACOKINETICS

Rapidly, completely absorbed from GI tract. Widely distributed. Metabolized in liver to active metabolite. Primarily excreted in urine. Half-life: 3–12 hrs.

ACTION/*THERAPEUTIC EFFECT*

Inhibits tubular reabsorption of urate at proximal renal tubule, *increasing urinary excretion of uric acid.*

USES

Treatment of hyperuricemia associated w/gout or gouty arthritis. Adjunctive therapy w/penicillins or cephalosporins to elevate and prolong antibiotic plasma levels.

PO ADMINISTRATION

1. May give w/or immediately after meals or milk.
2. Instruct pt to drink at least 6–8 glasses (8 oz) of water/day

(prevents kidney stone development).

INDICATIONS/DOSAGE/ROUTES

Gout:
Note: Do not start until acute gout attack subsides; continue if acute attack occurs during therapy.
PO: Adults, elderly: Initially, 250 mg 2 times/day for 1 wk; then 500 mg 2 times/day. May increase by 500 mg q4 wks. **Maximum:** 2–3 g/day. **Maintenance:** Dosage that maintains normal uric acid levels.

Penicillin/cephalosporin therapy:
Note: Do not use in presence of renal impairment.
PO: Adults, elderly: 2 g/day in divided doses. **Children (2–14 yrs):** Initially, 25 mg/kg. **Maintenance:** 40 mg/kg/day in 4 divided doses. **Children >50 kg:** Receive adult dosage.

PRECAUTIONS

CONTRAINDICATIONS: Blood dyscrasias, uric acid kidney stones, concurrent use w/penicillin in presence of renal impairment. **CAUTIONS:** Impaired renal function, history of peptic ulcer. **PREGNANCY/LACTATION:** Crosses placenta, appears in cord blood. Unknown whether distributed in breast milk. **Pregnancy Category B**.

INTERACTIONS

DRUG INTERACTIONS: May increase concentrations of cephalosporins, methotrexate, NSAIDs, nitrofurantoin, penicillins, zidovudine. Antineoplastics may increase risk of uric acid nephropathy. Salicylates may decrease uricosuric effect. May increase, prolong effects of heparin. **ALTERED LAB VALUES:** May inhibit renal excretion of PSP (phenolsulfonphthalein), 17-ketosteroids, BSP (sulfobromophthalein) tests.

SIDE EFFECTS

FREQUENT (5–10%): Headache, anorexia, nausea, vomiting. **OCCASIONAL (1–5%):** Lower back/side pain, rash, hives, itching, dizziness, flushed face, frequent urge to urinate, gingivitis.

ADVERSE REACTIONS/TOXIC EFFECTS

Severe hypersensitivity reactions (including anaphylaxis) occur rarely (usually within a few hours after readministration following previous use). Discontinue immediately, contact physician. Pruritic maculopapular rash should be considered a toxic reaction. May be accompanied by malaise, fever, chills, joint pain, nausea, vomiting, leukopenia, aplastic anemia.

NURSING IMPLICATIONS
BASELINE ASSESSMENT:

Do not initiate therapy until acute gouty attack has subsided. Question pt for hypersensitivity to probenecid or if taking penicillin or cephalosporin antibiotics. Instruct pt to drink 6–8 glasses (8 oz) of fluid daily while on medication.

INTERVENTION/EVALUATION:

If exacerbation of gout recurs following therapy, use other agents for gout. Discontinue medication immediately if rash or other evidence of allergic reaction appears. Encourage high fluid intake (3,000 ml/day). Monitor I&O (output should be at least 2,000 ml/day). Assess CBC, serum uric acid levels. Assess urine for cloudiness, unusual color, odor. Assess for therapeutic response (reduced joint tenderness, swelling, redness, limitation of motion).

PATIENT/FAMILY TEACHING:

Encourage low-purine food intake (reduce/omit meat, fowl, fish; use eggs, cheese, vegetables). Foods high in purine: kidneys, liver, sweetbreads, sardines, anchovies, meat extracts. May take 1 or more wks for full therapeutic effect. Drink 6–8 glasses (8 oz) of fluid daily while on medication. Avoid tasks that require alertness, motor skills until response to drug is established. Contact physician, nurse if rash, irritation of eyes, swelling of lips/mouth occurs.

procainamide hydrochloride

pro-**cane**-ah-myd
(ProcanBid, Procan-SR, Pronestyl, Rhythmin)

CANADIAN AVAILABILITY:
Pronestyl, Procan SR

CLASSIFICATION

Antiarrhythmic

AVAILABILITY (Rx)

Capsules: 250 mg, 375 mg, 500 mg. **Tablets:** 250 mg, 375 mg, 500 mg. **Tablets (sustained-release):** 250 mg, 500 mg, 750 mg, 1,000 mg. **Injection:** 100 mg/ml, 500 mg/ml.

PHARMACOKINETICS

Rapidly, completely absorbed from GI tract. Widely distributed. Metabolized in liver to active metabolite. Primarily excreted in urine. Removed by hemodialysis. Half-life: 2.5–4.5 hrs; metabolite: 6 hrs.

ACTION/*THERAPEUTIC EFFECT*

Prolongs refractory period by direct effect, decreasing myocardial excitability and conduction velocity. *Depresses myocardial contractility.*

USES/*UNLABELED*

Prophylactic therapy to maintain normal sinus rhythm after conversion of atrial fibrillation and/or flutter. Treatment of premature ventricular contractions, paroxysmal atrial tachycardia, atrial fibrillation, ventricular tachycardia. *Conversion/management of atrial fibrillation and PAT.*

STORAGE/HANDLING

Solution appears clear, colorless to light yellow. Discard if solution darkens/appears discolored or if precipitate forms. When diluted w/5% dextrose, solution is stable for 24 hrs at room temperature or for 7 days if refrigerated.

PO/IM/IV ADMINISTRATION

PO:

Do not crush or break sustained-release tablets.

IM/IV:

Note: May give by IM, IV injection, or IV infusion.
1. B/P, EKG should be monitored continuously during IV administration and rate of infusion adjusted to eliminate arrhythmias.
2. For direct IV injection, dilute w/5% dextrose and, w/pt in supine position, administer at rate not exceeding 25–50 mg/min.
3. For initial loading infusion,

add 1 g to 50 ml 5% dextrose to provide a concentration of 20 mg/ml. Infuse 1 ml/min for up to 25–30 min.

4. For IV infusion, add 1 g to 250–500 ml 5% dextrose to provide concentration of 2–4 mg/ml. Infuse at 1–3 ml/min.

5. Check B/P q5–10 min during infusion. If fall in B/P exceeds 15 mm Hg, discontinue drug, contact physician.

6. Monitor EKG for cardiac changes, particularly widening of QRS, prolongation of PR and QT interval. Notify physician of any significant interval changes.

INDICATIONS/DOSAGE/ROUTES

Note: Dose, interval of administration individualized based on underlying myocardial disease, pt's age, renal function, clinical response. Extended-release capsules used for maintenance therapy.

Usual oral dosage (to provide 50 mg/kg/day):
PO: Adults, elderly (40–50 kg): 250 mg q3h up to 500 mg q6h. **(60–70 kg):** 375 mg q3h up to 750 mg q6h. **(80–90 kg):** 500 mg q3h up to 1 g q6h. **(>100 kg):** 625 mg q3h up to 1.25 g q6h.
PO (extended-release): Adults, elderly (40–50 kg): 500 mg q6h. **(60–70 kg):** 750 mg q6h. **(80–90 kg):** 1 g q6h. **(>100 kg):** 1.25 g q6h. ProCanbid: 500–1,000 mg q12 h.

Usual parenteral dosage:
IM: Adults, elderly: 50 mg/kg/day in divided doses q3–6h.
IV: Adults, elderly: 100 mg q5 min until arrhythmias suppressed or 500 mg administered.
IV Infusion: Adults, elderly: Initially, loading infusion of 20 mg/ml at 1 ml/min for 25–30 min to deliver 500–600 mg procainamide. **Maintenance:** Infusion of 2 mg/ml at 1–3 ml/min to deliver 2–6 mg/min.

PRECAUTIONS

CONTRAINDICATIONS: Complete AV block, second- and third-degree AV block w/o pacemaker, abnormal impulses/rhythms because of escape mechanism. **CAUTIONS:** Ventricular tachycardia during coronary occlusion, renal/hepatic disease, incomplete AV nodal block, digitalis intoxication, CHF, preexisting hypotension. **PREGNANCY/LACTATION:** Crosses placenta; unknown whether distributed in breast milk. **Pregnancy Category C.**

INTERACTIONS

DRUG INTERACTIONS: Pimozide, other antiarrhythmics may increase cardiac effects. May increase effects of antihypertensives (IV procainamide), neuromuscular blockers. May decrease antimyasthenic effect on skeletal muscle. **ALTERED LAB VALUES:** May cause positive ANA, Coombs' test, EKG changes. May increase SGOT (AST), SGPT (ALT), alkaline phosphatase, bilirubin, LDH.

SIDE EFFECTS

FREQUENT: *Oral:* Abdominal pain/cramping, nausea, diarrhea, vomiting. **OCCASIONAL:** Dizziness, giddiness, weakness, hypersensitivity reaction (rash, urticaria, pruritus, flushing). **INFREQUENT:** *IV:* Transient, but at times, marked hypotension. **RARE:** Confusion, mental depression, psychosis.

ADVERSE REACTIONS/TOXIC EFFECTS

Paradoxical, extremely rapid ventricular rate may occur during treatment of atrial fibrillation/flutter. Systemic lupus erythematosus–like syndrome (fever, joint pain, pleuritic chest pain) w/prolonged therapy. Cardiotoxic effects occur most commonly w/IV administration, observed as conduction changes (50% widening of QRS complex, frequent ventricular premature contractions, ventricular tachycardia, complete AV block). Prolonged PR and QT intervals, flattened T waves occur less frequently (discontinue drug immediately).

NURSING IMPLICATIONS

BASELINE ASSESSMENT:

Check B/P and pulse for 1 full min (unless pt is on continuous monitor) before giving medication.

INTERVENTION/EVALUATION:

Monitor EKG for cardiac changes, particularly widening of QRS, prolongation of PR and QT interval. Assess pulse for strength/weakness, irregular rate. Monitor I&O, electrolyte serum level (potassium, chloride, sodium). Assess for complaints of GI upset, headache, dizziness, joint pain. Monitor pattern of daily bowel activity, stool consistency. Assess for dizziness. Monitor B/P for hypotension. Assess skin for evidence of hypersensitivity reaction (esp. in those on high-dose therapy). Monitor for therapeutic serum level (3–10 mcg/ml).

PATIENT/FAMILY TEACHING:

Take medication at evenly spaced doses around the clock. Contact physician if fever, joint pain/stiffness, signs of upper respiratory infection occur. Do not abruptly discontinue medication. Compliance w/therapy regimen is essential to control arrhythmias. **Do not use nasal decongestants, OTC cold preparations (stimulants) w/o physician approval. Restrict salt, alcohol intake. Report any arthralgia, myalgia, fever, chills, rash, easy bruising, sore throat, dark urine, nausea, vomiting, diarrhea, palpitations.**

procaine hydrochloride
(Novocain)
See Classification section under: Anesthetics: local

procarbazine hydrochloride
pro-**car**-bah-zeen
(Matulane)

CLASSIFICATION

Antineoplastic

AVAILABILITY (Rx)

Capsules: 50 mg

PHARMACOKINETICS

Completely absorbed from GI tract. Widely distributed (crosses blood-brain barrier). Metabolized in liver to active metabolite. Primarily excreted in urine. Half-life: 10 min.

ACTION/*THERAPEUTIC EFFECT*

Inhibits DNA, RNA, protein synthesis. *Cytotoxic effects occur in tissue w/high rate of cellular proliferation.* Cell cycle-specific for S phase of cell division.

USES/*UNLABELED*

Treatment of advanced Hodgkin's disease. *Treatment of non-Hodgkin's lymphoma, primary brain tumors, lung carcinoma, malignant melanoma, multiple myeloma, polycythemia vera.*

INDICATIONS/DOSAGE/ROUTES

Note: May be carcinogenic, mutagenic, or teratogenic. Handle w/extreme care during administration. Dosage individualized based on clinical response, tolerance to adverse effects. When used in combination therapy, consult specific protocols for optimum dosage, sequence of drug administration. Dosage based on actual weight. Use ideal body weight for obese and edematous pts.

Hodgkin's disease:
PO: Adults, elderly: Initially, 2–4 mg/kg daily as single or divided dose for 1 wk, then 4–6 mg/kg day. **Children:** 50 mg/m^2 daily for 1 wk, then 100 mg/m^2 daily. Continue until maximum response, leukocyte count falls below 4,000/mm^3, or platelets fall below 100,000/mm^3.

Maintenance:
PO: Adults, elderly: 1–2 mg/kg/ day. **Children:** 50 mg/m^2 daily.

Component of MOPP:
PO: Adults, elderly: 100 mg/m^2 daily on days 1–14 of 28 day cycle.

PRECAUTIONS

CONTRAINDICATIONS: Inadequate bone marrow reserve. **CAUTIONS:** Impaired renal/hepatic function. **PREGNANCY/ LACTATION:** If possible, avoid use during pregnancy, esp. first trimester. Breast-feeding not recommended. **Pregnancy Category D**.

INTERACTIONS

DRUG INTERACTIONS: Alcohol may cause disulfiram reaction. Anticholinergics, antihistamines may increase anticholinergic effects. Tricyclic antidepressants may increase anticholinergic effects, cause hyperpyretic crisis, convulsions. May increase effects of oral hypoglycemics, insulin. Bone marrow depressants may increase bone marrow depression. May increase B/P w/buspirone, caffeine-containing medications. May cause hyperpyretic crisis, seizures, death w/carbamazepine, cyclobenzaprine, maprotiline, MAO inhibitors. CNS depressants may increase CNS depression. Meperidine may produce immediate excitation, sweating, rigidity, severe hypertension or hypotension, severe respiratory distress, coma, convulsions, vascular collapse, death. Sympathomimetics may increase cardiac stimulant, vasopressor effects. **ALTERED LAB VALUES:** None significant.

SIDE EFFECTS

FREQUENT: Severe nausea, vomiting, respiratory disorders (cough, effusion), myalgia, arthralgia, drowsiness, nervousness, insomnia, nightmares, sweating, hallucinations, seizures. **OCCASIONAL:** Hoarseness, tachycardia, nystagmus, retinal hemorrhage, photophobia, photosensitivity, urinary frequency, nocturia, hypotension, diarrhea, stomatitis, paresthesia, unsteadiness, confusion, decreased reflexes, foot drop. **RARE:** Hypersensitivity reaction (dermatitis, pruritus, rash, urticaria), hyperpigmentation, alopecia.

ADVERSE REACTIONS/TOXIC EFFECTS

Major toxic effects are bone marrow depression manifested as hematologic toxicity (principally leukopenia, thrombocytopenia, anemia) and hepatotoxicity manifested by jaundice, ascites. Urinary tract infection secondary to leukopenia may occur. Therapy should be discontinued if stomatitis, diarrhea, paresthesia, neuropathies, confusion, hypersensitivity reaction occurs.

NURSING IMPLICATIONS
BASELINE ASSESSMENT:

Obtain bone marrow tests, Hgb, Hct, leukocyte, differential, reticulocyte, platelet, urinalysis, serum transaminase, serum alkaline phosphatase, BUN results before therapy and periodically thereafter. Therapy should be interrupted if WBC falls below 4,000/mm³ or platelet count falls below 100,000/mm³.

INTERVENTION/EVALUATION:

Monitor hematologic status, renal, hepatic function studies. Assess for stomatitis (burning/erythema of oral mucosa at inner margin of lips, sore throat, difficulty swallowing, oral ulceration). Monitor for hematologic toxicity (fever, sore throat, signs of local infection, easy bruising, unusual bleeding from any site), symptoms of anemia (excessive tiredness, weakness). Avoid IM injections, rectal temperatures, trauma that may induce bleeding.

PATIENT/FAMILY TEACHING:

Do not drink alcoholic beverages during or for 2 wks after therapy (Antabuse-like reaction: severe headache, tachycardia, chest pain, stiff neck). Avoid foods with high tyramine content (e.g., yogurt, ripe cheese, smoked meat, overripe fruit). Avoid OTC medications. Do not have immunizations w/o physician's approval (drug lowers body's resistance). Avoid crowds, those w/infection. Promptly report fever, sore throat, signs of local infection, easy bruising, or unusual bleeding from any site. Contact physician if nausea/vomiting continues at home. Wear protective clothing, sunscreens to protect from sun/ultraviolet light.

prochlorperazine
pro-klor-**pear**-ah-zeen
(Compazine suppositories)
prochlorperazine edisylate
(Compazine syrup, injection)
prochlorperazine maleate
(Compazine spansule, tablets)

CANADIAN AVAILABILITY: Stemetil

CLASSIFICATION

Antiemetic, antipsychotic

AVAILABILITY (Rx)

Tablets: 5 mg, 10 mg, 25 mg. **Capsules (sustained-release):** 10 mg, 15 mg, 30 mg. **Syrup:** 5 mg/5 ml. **Suppository:** 2.5 mg, 5 mg, 25 mg. **Injection:** 5 mg/ml.

PHARMACOKINETICS

	ONSET	PEAK	DURATION
Tablets, syrup (antiemetic)	30–40 min	—	3–4 hrs
Extended-Release (antiemetic)	30–40 min	—	10–12 hrs
IM (antiemetic)	10–20 min	—	3–4 hrs
Rectal (antiemetic)	60 min	—	3–4 hrs

Variably absorbed after oral administration, well absorbed after IM administration. Widely distributed. Metabolized in liver, GI mucosa. Primarily excreted in urine. Half-life: 23 hrs.

ACTION/THERAPEUTIC EFFECT

Antiemetic: Acts centrally to inhibit/block dopamine receptors in chemoreceptor trigger zone and peripherally to block vagus nerve in GI tract. *Relieves nausea and vomiting.* **Antipsychotic:** Antagonizes dopamine neurotransmission at synapses by blocking postsynaptic dopaminergic receptors in brain. *Suppresses behavioral response in psychosis.*

USES

Control of severe nausea and vomiting, management of psychotic disorders, moderate to severe anxiety and tension in psychoneurotic pts.

STORAGE/HANDLING

Store at room temperature (including suppositories), protect from light (darkens on exposure). Slight yellow discoloration of solution does not affect potency, but discard if markedly discolored or precipitate forms.

PO/IM/IV/RECTAL ADMINISTRATION

PO:

Give w/o regard to meals.
Parenteral Administration: Pt must remain recumbent for 30–60 min in head-low position w/legs raised to minimize hypotensive effect.

IM:

1. Inject slow, deep IM into upper outer quadrant of gluteus maximus. If irritation occurs, further injections may be diluted w/0.9% NaCl or 2% procaine hydrochloride.
2. Massage IM injection site to reduce discomfort.

IV:

Note: Give by direct IV injection or IV infusion.
1. For direct IV, administer each 5 mg >1 min.
2. For IV infusion, dilute 20 mg (4 ml) prochlorperazine w/0.9% NaCl and administer 5 mg/min rate of infusion.
3. Monitor B/P diligently for hypotension during IV administration.

RECTAL:

Moisten suppository w/cold water before inserting well up into rectum.

INDICATIONS/DOSAGE/ROUTES

Severe nausea, vomiting:
PO: Adults, elderly: 5–10 mg 3–4 times/day. **PO/Rectal Children >2 yrs, 20–29 lbs:** 2.5 mg q12–24h. Do not exceed 7.5 mg/day. **Children 30–39 lbs:** 2.5 mg 2–3 times/day. Do not exceed 10 mg/day. **Children 40–85 lbs:** 2.5 mg 3 times/day or 5 mg 2

times/day. Do not exceed 15 mg/day.
IM: Adults, elderly: 5–10 mg q3–4h. Do not exceed 40 mg/day.
Children >20 lbs, >2 yrs: 0.13 mg/kg.
Rectal: Adults, elderly: 25 mg 2 times/day. .

Severe nausea, vomiting after surgery:
IM: Adults, elderly: 5–10 mg. Repeat once in 30 min, if needed.
IV: Adults, elderly: 5–10 mg. Repeat once, if needed.

Psychotic disorders, outpatient:
PO: Adults, elderly: 5–10 mg 3–4 times/day. Increase dosage gradually every 2–3 days until therapeutic response noted.
PO/Rectal: Children 2–12 yrs: 2.5 mg 2–3 times/day. Increase gradually to therapeutic response.
Maximum: Children 2–5 yrs: 20 mg/day. **6–12 yrs:** 25 mg/day.

Psychotic disorders, inpatient:
PO: Adults, elderly: 10 mg 3–4 times/day.
IM: Adults, elderly: 10–20 mg q1–4h to control symptoms.

PRECAUTIONS

CONTRAINDICATIONS: Suspected Reye's syndrome, severe CNS depression, comatose states, severe cardiovascular disease, bone marrow depression, subcortical brain damage. **CAUTIONS:** Impaired respiratory/hepatic/renal/cardiac function, alcohol withdrawal, history of seizures, urinary retention, glaucoma, prostatic hypertrophy, hypocalcemia (increases susceptibility to dystonias).
PREGNANCY/LACTATION: Crosses placenta; is distributed in breast milk. **Pregnancy Category C.**

INTERACTIONS

DRUG INTERACTIONS: Alcohol, CNS depressants may increase CNS, respiratory depression, hypotensive effects. Tricyclic antidepressants, MAO inhibitors may increase sedative, anticholinergic effects. Antithyroid agents may increase risk of agranulocytosis. Extrapyramidal symptoms (EPS) may increase w/EPS-producing medications. Hypotensives may increase hypotension. May decrease levodopa effects. Lithium may decrease absorption, produce adverse neurologic effects.
ALTERED LAB VALUES: None significant.

P

SIDE EFFECTS

FREQUENT: Drowsiness, hypotension, dizziness, fainting occur frequently after first dose, occasionally after subsequent dosing, and rarely w/oral dosage.
OCCASIONAL: Dry mouth, blurred vision, lethargy, constipation/diarrhea, muscular aches, nasal congestion, peripheral edema, urinary retention.

ADVERSE REACTIONS/TOXIC EFFECTS

Extrapyramidal symptoms appear dose related (particularly w/high dosage) and are divided into 3 categories: akathisia (inability to sit still, tapping of feet, urge to move around), parkinsonian symptoms (mask-like face, tremors, shuffling gait, hypersalivation), and acute dystonias: torticollis (neck muscle spasm), opisthotonos (rigidity of back muscles) and oculogyric crisis (rolling back of eyes). Dystonic reaction may also produce profuse sweating, pallor. Tardive dyskinesia (protrusion of tongue, puffing of cheeks, chewing/puckering of the mouth) occurs rarely (may be irreversible). Abrupt withdrawal following long-term therapy may precipitate nausea, vomiting, gastritis, dizziness, tremors. Blood dyscrasias, particularly agranulocytosis, mild leukopenia (sore mouth/gums/throat) may occur. May lower seizure threshold.

NURSING IMPLICATIONS
BASELINE ASSESSMENT:

Avoid skin contact w/solution (contact dermatitis). *Antiemetic:* Assess for dehydration (poor skin turgor, dry mucous membranes, longitudinal furrows in tongue). *Antipsychotic:* Assess behavior, appearance, emotional status, response to environment, speech pattern, thought content.

INTERVENTION/EVALUATION:

Monitor B/P for hypotension. Assess for extrapyramidal symptoms. Monitor WBC, differential count for blood dyscrasias. Monitor for fine tongue movement (may be early sign of tardive dyskinesia). Supervise suicidal risk pt closely during early therapy (as depression lessens, energy level improves, increasing suicide potential). Assess for therapeutic response (interest in surroundings, improvement in self-care, increased ability to concentrate, relaxed facial expression).

PATIENT/FAMILY TEACHING:

Urine may turn pink or reddish brown. Do not abruptly withdraw from long-term drug therapy. Report visual disturbances. Sugarless gum, sips of tepid water may relieve dry mouth. Drowsiness generally subsides during continued therapy. Avoid tasks that require alertness, motor skills until response to drug is established. Avoid alcohol, CNS depressants. Use sunscreen, protective clothing in sun or ultraviolet light. Use caution in hot weather (possibility of heat stroke).

progesterone

proe-**jess**-ter-one
(Crinone, Gesterol, Prometrium)

CANADIAN AVAILABILITY:
Prometrium

CLASSIFICATION

Progestin

AVAILABILITY (Rx)

Injection: 50 mg/ml. Intrauterine System. Soft Gel Capsule: 200 mg, 400 mg. Vaginal Gel: 4%, 8%.

PHARMACOKINETICS

Slow absorption after IM administration. Metabolized in liver. Primarily excreted in urine.

ACTION/ THERAPEUTIC EFFECT

Transforms endometrium from proliferative to secretory (in an estrogen-primed endometrium); inhibits secretion of pituitary gonadotropins, preventing follicular maturation and ovulation. Stimulates the growth of mammary alveolar tissue; relaxes uterine smooth muscle. *Restores hormonal balance.*

USES/ UNLABELED

Treatment of primary or secondary amenorrhea, abnormal uterine bleeding due to hormonal imbalance, endometriosis. Prevention of endometrial hyperplasia in estrogen recipients. Vaginal Gel

(8%): Treatment of infertility. *Treatment of corpus luteum dysfunction.*

IM ADMINISTRATION

1. For IM use only.
2. Administer deep IM in large muscle.

INDICATIONS/DOSAGE/ROUTES

Amenorrhea:

IM: Adults: 5–10 mg for 6–8 days. Withdrawal bleeding expected in 48–72 hrs if ovarian activity produced proliferative endometrium.
Vaginal: Adults: Apply every other day for up to 6 doses.
PO: Adults: 400 mg daily in evening for 10 days.

Abnormal uterine bleeding:

IM: Adults: 5–10 mg for 6 days. (When estrogen given concomitantly, begin progesterone after 2 wks of estrogen therapy; discontinue when menstrual flow begins.)

Prevention of endometrial hyperplasia:

PO: Adults: 200 mg in evening for 12 days per 28-day cycle in combination w/daily conjugated estrogen.

PRECAUTIONS

CONTRAINDICATIONS: Hypersensitivity to progestins; thrombophlebitis, thromboembolic disorders, cerebral apoplexy or history of these conditions; severe liver dysfunction; breast cancer; undiagnosed vaginal bleeding; missed abortion; use as a diagnostic test for pregnancy. **CAUTIONS:** Diabetes, conditions aggravated by fluid retention (e.g., asthma, epilepsy, migraine, cardiac/renal dysfunction), history of mental depression. **PREGNANCY/LACTATION:** Not recommended during pregnancy, esp. first 4 mos (congenital heart, limb reduction defects). Distributed in breast milk. **Pregnancy Category D**.

INTERACTIONS

DRUG INTERACTIONS: May interfere w/effects of bromocriptine. **ALTERED LAB VALUES:** May increase alkaline phosphatase, LDL. May decrease HDL. May cause abnormal thyroid, metapyrone, liver, endocrine function tests, decrease glucose tolerance.

SIDE EFFECTS

FREQUENT: Breakthrough bleeding or spotting at beginning of therapy. Amenorrhea, change in menstrual flow, breast tenderness. **OCCASIONAL:** Edema, weight gain or loss, rash, pruritus, photosensitivity, skin pigmentation. **RARE:** Pain/swelling at injection site, acne, mental depression, alopecia, hirsutism.

ADVERSE REACTIONS/TOXIC EFFECTS

Thrombophlebitis, cerebrovascular disorders, retinal thrombosis, pulmonary embolism occurs rarely.

NURSING IMPLICATIONS

BASELINE ASSESSMENT:

Question for possibility of pregnancy or hypersensitivity to progestins before initiating therapy. Obtain baseline weight, blood glucose level, B/P.

INTERVENTION/EVALUATION:

Check weight daily; report weekly gain of 5 lbs or more. Assess skin for rash, hives. Immediately report the development of chest pain, sudden shortness of breath, sudden decrease in vision, migraine headache, pain (esp. w/swelling, warmth, and redness) in calves, numbness of an arm/leg (thrombotic disorders). Check B/P periodically. Note progesterone therapy on pathology specimens.

PATIENT/FAMILY TEACHING:

Importance of medical supervision. Do not take other medications w/o physician's approval. Use sunscreens, protective clothing to protect from sunlight/ultraviolet light until tolerance determined. Notify physician of abnormal vaginal bleeding or other symptoms. Teach how to perform Homans' test, signs and symptoms of blood clots (report these to physician immediately). Teach breast self-exam. Stop taking medication and contact physician at once if pregnancy suspected. Give labeling from drug package.

promethazine hydrochloride

pro-**meth**-ah-zeen
(Phenergan)

FIXED-COMBINATION(S):

W/codeine, a narcotic analgesic **(Phenergan w/Codeine)**; w/dextromethorphan, an antitussive **(Phenergan w/Dextromethorphan)**; w/meperidine, a narcotic analgesic **(Mepergan)**; w/phenylephrine, a nasal vasoconstrictor **(Phenergan VC)**; w/phenylephrine and codeine **(Phenergan VC w/Codeine)**.

CANADIAN AVAILABILITY:
Phenergan

CLASSIFICATION

Antihistamine

AVAILABILITY (Rx)

Tablets: 12.5 mg, 25 mg, 50 mg. **Syrup:** 6.25 mg/5 ml, 25 mg/5 ml.

Suppository: 12.5 mg, 25 mg, 50 mg. **Injection:** 25 mg/ml, 50 mg/ml.

PHARMACOKINETICS

	ONSET	PEAK	DURATION
PO	20 min	—	2–8 hrs
IM	20 min	—	2–8 hrs
Rectal			
	20 min	—	2–8 hrs
IV	3–5 min	—	2–8 hrs

Well absorbed from GI tract, after IM administration. Widely distributed. Metabolized in liver. Primarily excreted in urine.

ACTION/*THERAPEUTIC EFFECT*

Antihistamine: Inhibits histamine at histamine receptor sites, *preventing, antagonizing most allergic effects (e.g., urticaria, pruritus)*. **Antiemetic:** Diminishes vestibular stimulation, depresses labyrinthine function, acts on chemoreceptor trigger zone, *producing antiemetic effect.* **Sedative-hypnotic:** Decreases stimulation to brain stem reticular formation, *producing CNS depression.*

USES

Provides symptomatic relief of allergic symptoms; sedative/antiemetic in surgery/labor; decreases postop nausea/vomiting; adjunct to analgesics in control of pain; management of motion sickness.

STORAGE/HANDLING

Store oral, parenteral forms at room temperature. Refrigerate suppositories.

PO/IM/IV/RECTAL ADMINISTRATION

PO:

Give w/o regard to meals. Scored tablets may be crushed.

IM:

Note: Significant tissue necrosis may occur if given SubQ. Inadvertent intra-arterial injection may produce severe arteriospasm, resulting in severe circulation impairment.

    1. May be given undiluted.

    2. Inject deep IM.

IV:

    1. Final dilution should not exceed 25 mg/ml.

    2. Administer at 25 mg/min rate thru IV infusion tube.

    3. A too rapid rate of infusion may result in transient fall in blood pressure, producing orthostatic hypotension, reflex tachycardia.

    4. If pt complains of pain at IV site, stop injection immediately (possibility of intra-arterial needle placement/perivascular extravasation).

RECTAL:

    Moisten suppository w/cold water before inserting well up into rectum.

INDICATIONS/DOSAGE/ROUTES

Allergic symptoms:
PO: Adults, elderly: 25 mg at bedtime or 12.5 mg 4 times/day. **Children:** Up to 25 mg at bedtime or up to 12.5 mg 3 times/day.
Rectal/IM/IV: Adults, elderly: 25 mg, may repeat in 2 hrs.

Motion sickness:
PO: Adults, elderly: 25 mg 30–60 min before departure; may repeat in 8–12 hrs, then every morning on arising and before evening meal. **Children:** 12.5–25 mg (same regimen).

Prevention of nausea, vomiting:
PO/IM/IV/Rectal: Adults, elderly: 12.5–25 mg q4–6h as needed.

Children: 0.25–0.5 mg/kg q4–6h as needed.

Pre- and postop sedation; adjunct to analgesics:
IM/IV: Adults, elderly: 25–50 mg. **Children:** 12.5–25 mg.

PRECAUTIONS

CONTRAINDICATIONS: Comatose, those receiving large doses of other CNS depressants, acutely ill/dehydrated children, acute asthmatic attack, vomiting of unknown etiology in children, Reye's syndrome, those receiving MAO inhibitors. **EXTREME CAUTION:** History of sleep apnea, young children, family history of sudden infant death syndrome (SIDS), those difficult to arouse from sleep. **CAUTIONS:** Narrow-angle glaucoma, peptic ulcer, prostatic hypertrophy, pyloroduodenal/bladder neck obstruction, asthma, COPD, increased intraocular pressure, cardiovascular disease, hyperthyroidism, hypertension, seizure disorders. **PREGNANCY/LACTATION:** Readily crosses placenta; unknown whether drug is excreted in breast milk. May inhibit platelet aggregation in neonates if taken within 2 wks of birth. May produce jaundice, extrapyramidal symptoms in neonates if taken during pregnancy. **Pregnancy Category C**.

INTERACTIONS

DRUG INTERACTIONS: Alcohol, CNS depressants may increase CNS depressant effects. Anticholinergics may increase anticholinergic effects. MAO inhibitors may prolong, intensify anticholinergic, CNS depressant effects. **ALTERED LAB VALUES:** May suppress wheal and flare reactions to antigen skin testing, unless discontinued 4 days before testing.

P

SIDE EFFECTS

HIGH INCIDENCE: Drowsiness, disorientation. Hypotension, confusion, syncope more likely noted in elderly. **FREQUENT:** Dry mouth, urinary retention, thickening of bronchial secretions. **OCCASIONAL:** Epigastric distress, flushing, visual disturbances, hearing disturbances, wheezing, paresthesia, sweating, chills. **RARE:** Dizziness, urticaria, photosensitivity, nightmares. Fixed-combination form with pseudoephedrine may produce mild CNS stimulation.

ADVERSE REACTIONS/TOXIC EFFECTS

Paradoxical reaction (particularly in children) manifested as excitation, nervousness, tremor, hyperactive reflexes, convulsions. CNS depression has occurred in infants and young children (respiratory depression, sleep apnea, SIDS). Long-term therapy may produce extrapyramidal symptoms noted as dystonia (abnormal movements), pronounced motor restlessness (most frequently occurs in children), and parkinsonian symptoms (esp. noted in elderly). Blood dyscrasias, particularly agranulocytosis, have occurred.

NURSING IMPLICATIONS
BASELINE ASSESSMENT:

Assess B/P and pulse for bradycardia/tachycardia if pt is given parenteral form. If used as an antiemetic, assess for dehydration (poor skin turgor, dry mucous membranes, longitudinal furrows in tongue).

INTERVENTION/EVALUATION:

Monitor serum electrolytes in pts w/severe vomiting. Assist w/ambulation if drowsiness, lightheadedness occurs.

PATIENT/FAMILY TEACHING:

Drowsiness, dry mouth may be an expected response to drug. Sugarless gum, sips of tepid water may relieve dry mouth. Coffee/tea may help reduce drowsiness. Report visual disturbances. Avoid tasks that require alertness, motor skills until response to drug is established. Avoid alcohol and other CNS depressants. Use caution in sun; wear-protective clothing and use sunscreens.

propafenone hydrochloride

pro-**pah**-phen-own
(Rythmol)

CANADIAN AVAILABILITY:
Rythmol

CLASSIFICATION

Antiarrhythmic

AVAILABILITY (Rx)

Tablets: 150 mg, 300 mg

PHARMACOKINETICS

Well absorbed from GI tract (undergoes first-pass effect). Distributed primarily to heart, liver, lung. Metabolized in liver to active metabolite. Primarily eliminated in feces. Half-life: 2–10 hrs.

ACTION/THERAPEUTIC EFFECT

Decreases the fast sodium current in Purkinje/myocardial cells. *Decreases excitability, automaticity; prolongs conduction velocity, refractory period.* Greatest effects on Purkinje system.

USES / *UNLABELED*

Treatment of documented, life-threatening ventricular arrhythmias (e.g., sustained ventricular tachycardias). Prolongs time to recurrence of paroxysmal supraventricular tachycardia (PSVT) and paroxysmal atrial fibrillation/flutter (PAF) associated w/disabling symptoms. *Treatment of supraventricular arrhythmias.*

PO ADMINISTRATION

1. Scored tablets may be crushed.

2. Give w/o regard to meals (food may increase serum concentrations).

INDICATIONS / DOSAGE / ROUTES

Usual dosage:
PO: **Adults, elderly:** Initially, 150 mg q8h, may increase at 3–4 day intervals to 225 mg q8h, then to 300 mg q8h. **Maximum:** 900 mg/day.

PRECAUTIONS

CONTRAINDICATIONS: Uncontrolled CHF, cardiogenic shock, sinoatrial, AV and intraventricular disorders of impulse/conduction (sick-sinus syndrome [bradycardia-tachycardia], AV block) w/o presence of pacemaker, bradycardia, marked hypotension, bronchospastic disorders, manifest electrolyte imbalance. **CAUTIONS:** Impaired renal/hepatic function, recent myocardial infarction, CHF, conduction disturbances. **PREGNANCY/LACTATION:** Unknown whether drug crosses placenta or is distributed in breast milk. **Pregnancy Category C**.

INTERACTIONS

DRUG INTERACTIONS: May increase concentrations of digoxin, propranolol. May increase effects of warfarin. **ALTERED LAB VAL-UES:** May cause EKG changes (e.g., QRS widening, PR prolongation), positive ANA titers.

SIDE EFFECTS

FREQUENT (>5%): Dizziness, unusual taste, nausea, vomiting, constipation, blurred vision. **OCCASIONAL (1–5%):** Headache, dyspepsia, weakness. **RARE (<1%):** Dry mouth, diarrhea, rash, edema, hot flashes.

ADVERSE REACTIONS / TOXIC EFFECTS

May produce/worsen existing arrhythmias. Overdosage may produce hypotension, somnolence, bradycardia, intra-atrial and intraventricular conduction disturbances.

NURSING IMPLICATIONS

BASELINE ASSESSMENT:

Correct electrolyte imbalance before administering medication.

INTERVENTION / EVALUATION:

Assess pulse for strength/weakness, irregular rate. Monitor EKG for cardiac performance/changes, particularly widening of QRS, prolongation of PR interval. Question for visual disturbances, headache, GI upset. Monitor fluid, electrolyte serum levels. Monitor pattern of daily bowel activity, stool consistency. Assess for dizziness, unsteadiness. Monitor liver enzymes results. Monitor for therapeutic serum level (0.06–1 μ/ml).

PATIENT / FAMILY TEACHING:

Compliance w/therapy regimen is essential to control arrhythmias. Unusual taste sensation may occur. Report headache, blurred vision, fever.

proparacaine
(Ophthaine, AK-Taine, Alcaine, I-Paracaine, Kainair, Ophthetic)

FIXED-COMBINATION(S):
W/fluorescein, a water-soluble dye **(Fluoracaine, Parascein, Ocu-Flurcaine)**

See Classification section under: Anesthetics: local

propofol
pro-**poe**-foal
(Diprivan)

CANADIAN AVAILABILITY:
Diprivan

CLASSIFICATION

Anesthetic: General

AVAILABILITY (Rx)

Injection: 10 mg/ml

PHARMACOKINETICS

	ONSET	PEAK	DURATION
IV	40 sec	—	—

Rapidly, extensively distributed. Metabolized in liver. Primarily excreted in urine. Half-life: 3–12 hrs.

ACTION / THERAPEUTIC EFFECT

Unknown. *Produces hypnosis rapidly.*

USES

Induction and maintenance of anesthesia. Continuous sedation in intubated/respiratory controlled adult pts in ICU.

STORAGE / HANDLING

Store at room temperature. Discard unused portions. Do not use if emulsion separates. Shake well before using.

IV ADMINISTRATION

Note: Do not give through same IV line w/blood or plasma.
 1. Dilute only w/5% dextrose.
 2. Do not dilute to concentration <2 mg/ml.
 3. Use larger veins of forearm or antecubital fossa to minimize IV pain.
 4. Transient, local pain at IV site may be reduced w/1 ml of 1% IV lidocaine solution.
 5. A too rapid IV may produce marked severe hypotension, respiratory depression, irregular muscular movements.
 6. Observe for signs of intra-arterial injection (pain, discolored skin patches, white/blue color to hand, delayed onset of drug action).
 7. Inadvertent intra-arterial injection may result in arterial spasm w/severe pain, thrombosis, gangrene.

INDICATIONS / DOSAGE / ROUTES

ICU sedation:
IV: Adults, elderly: Initially, 5 mcg/kg/min for at least 5 min until onset of peak effect. May increase by increments of 5–10 mcg/kg/min over 5–10 min intervals. **Maintenance:** 5–50 mcg/kg/min (some pts may require higher dosage).

Anesthesia:
IV: Adults ASA I & II: 2–2.5 mg/kg (about 40 mg q10 secs until onset of anesthesia). **IV: Elderly, debilitated, hypovolemic, or ASA III or IV:** 1–1.5 mg/kg q10 secs until onset of anesthesia.

Maintenance:
IV: Adults ASA I & II: 0.1–0.2 mg/kg/min. **IV: Elderly, debilitated, hypovolemic, or ASA III or IV:** 0.05–0.1 mg/kg/min.

PRECAUTIONS

CONTRAINDICATIONS: Increased intracranial pressure, impaired cerebral circulation. **CAUTIONS:** Debilitated, impaired respiratory, circulatory, renal, hepatic, lipid metabolism disorders. **PREGNANCY/LACTATION:** Unknown whether drug crosses placenta. Distributed in breast milk. Not recommended for obstetrics, nursing mothers. **Pregnancy Category B.**

INTERACTIONS

DRUG INTERACTIONS: Alcohol, CNS depressants may increase CNS, respiratory, depression, hypotensive effect. **ALTERED LAB VALUES:** None significant.

SIDE EFFECTS

FREQUENT: Involuntary muscular movement, apnea (common during induction; lasts >60 secs), hypotension, nausea, vomiting, burning/stinging at IV site. **OCCASIONAL:** Twitching, bucking, jerking, thrashing, headache, dizziness, bradycardia, hypertension, fever, abdominal cramping, tingling, numbness, coldness, cough, hiccups, facial flushing. **RARE:** Rash, dry mouth, agitation, confusion, myalgia, thrombophlebitis.

ADVERSE REACTIONS/TOXIC EFFECTS

Continuous/repeated intermittent infusion may result in extreme somnolence, respiratory/circulatory depression. A too rapid IV may produce marked severe hypotension, respiratory depression, irregular muscular movements. Acute allergic reaction (erythema, pruritus, urticaria, rhinitis, dyspnea, hypotension, restlessness, anxiety, abdominal pain) may occur.

NURSING IMPLICATIONS
BASELINE ASSESSMENT:

Resuscitative equipment, endotracheal tube, suction, oxygen must be available. Obtain vital signs before administration.

INTERVENTION/EVALUATION:

Monitor for hypotension, bradycardia q3–5 min during and after administration until recovery is achieved. Assess diligently for apnea during administration. Monitor for involuntary skeletal muscle movement.

PATIENT/FAMILY TEACHING:

Discomfort along IV route may occur.

propoxyphene hydrochloride

pro-**pox**-ih-feen
(Darvon)

FIXED-COMBINATION(S):
W/aspirin, caffeine **(Darvon Compound-65);** w/acetaminophen **(Wygesic)**

propoxyphene napsylate

(Darvon-N)

FIXED-COMBINATION(S):
W/acetaminophen **(Darvocet-N)**

CLASSIFICATION

Opioid analgesic

AVAILABILITY (Rx)

Hydrochloride: Capsules: 32 mg, 65 mg
Napsylate: Tablets: 100 mg.
Suspension: 10 mg/ml.

PHARMACOKINETICS

	ONSET	PEAK	DURATION
PO	15–60 min	—	4–6 hrs

Well absorbed from GI tract. Widely distributed. Metabolized in liver. Primarily excreted in urine. Half-life: 6–12 hrs; metabolite: 30–36 hrs.

ACTION/THERAPEUTIC EFFECT

Binds w/opioid receptors within CNS, *altering processes affecting pain perception, emotional response to pain.*

USES

Relief of mild to moderate pain.

PO ADMINISTRATION

1. Give w/o regard to meals.
2. Capsules may be emptied and mixed w/food.
3. Shake oral suspension well.
4. Do not crush or break film-coated tablets.

INDICATIONS/DOSAGE/ROUTES

Note: Reduce initial dosage in those w/hypothyroidism, concurrent CNS depressants, Addison's disease, renal insufficiency, elderly/debilitated.

Propoxyphene hydrochloride:
PO: Adults, elderly: 65 mg q4h, as needed. **Maximum:** 390 mg/day.

Propoxyphene napsylate:
PO: Adults, elderly: 100 mg q4h, as needed. **Maximum:** 600 mg/day.

PRECAUTIONS

CONTRAINDICATIONS: None significant. **EXTREME CAUTION:** Severe CNS depression, anoxia, hypercapnia, respiratory depression, seizures, acute alcoholism, shock, untreated myxedema, respiratory dysfunction. **CAUTIONS:** Increased intracranial pressure, impaired hepatic function, acute abdominal conditions, hypothyroidism, prostatic hypertrophy, Addison's disease, urethral stricture, COPD. **PREGNANCY/LACTATION:** Crosses placenta; minimal amount distributed in breast milk. Respiratory depression may occur in neonate if mother received opiates during labor. Regular use of opiates during pregnancy may produce withdrawal symptoms in neonate (irritability, excessive crying, tremors, hyperactive reflexes, fever, vomiting, diarrhea, yawning, sneezing, seizures). **Pregnancy Category C**. (Category D if used for prolonged periods.)

INTERACTIONS

DRUG INTERACTIONS: Alcohol, CNS depressants may increase CNS or respiratory depression, risk of hypotension. May increase concentration, toxicity of carbamazepine. Effects may be decreased w/buprenorphine. MAO inhibitors may produce severe, fatal reaction (reduce dose to $1/4$ usual dose). **ALTERED LAB VALUES:** May increase amylase, lipase, SGOT (AST), SGPT (ALT), LDH, alkaline phosphatase, bilirubin.

SIDE EFFECTS

Note: Effects dependent on dosage amount. Ambulatory pts and those not in moderate pain may experience dizziness, nausea, vomiting, hypotension more frequently than those in supine position or having moderate pain.

FREQUENT: Dizziness, drowsiness, dry mouth, euphoria, hypotension, nausea, vomiting, unusual tiredness. **OCCASIONAL:** Histamine reaction (decreased B/P, increased sweating, flushing, wheezing), trembling, decreased urination, altered vision, constipation, headache. **RARE:** Confusion, increased B/P, depression, stomach cramps, anorexia.

ADVERSE REACTIONS/TOXIC EFFECTS

Overdosage results in respiratory depression, skeletal muscle flaccidity, cold clammy skin, cyanosis, extreme somnolence progressing to convulsions, stupor, coma. Hepatotoxicity may occur w/overdosage of acetaminophen component. Tolerance to analgesic effect, physical dependence may occur w/repeated use.

NURSING IMPLICATIONS
BASELINE ASSESSMENT:

Obtain vital signs before giving medication. If respirations are 12/min or lower (20/min or lower in children), withhold medication, contact physician. Assess onset, type, location, and duration of pain. Effect of medication is reduced if full pain recurs before next dose.

INTERVENTION/EVALUATION:

Palpate bladder for urinary retention. Monitor pattern of daily bowel activity, stool consistency. Initiate deep breathing and coughing exercises, particularly in those w/impaired pulmonary

function. Assess for clinical improvement, record onset of relief of pain. Contact physician if pain is not adequately relieved.

PATIENT/FAMILY TEACHING:

Change positions slowly to avoid orthostatic hypotension. Avoid tasks that require alertness, motor skills until response to drug is established. Tolerance/dependence may occur w/prolonged use of high doses.

propranolol hydrochloride
pro-**pran**-oh-lol
(Inderal)

FIXED-COMBINATION(S): W/hydrochlorothiazide, a diuretic (Inderide)

CANADIAN AVAILABILITY: Apo-Propranolol, Inderal

CLASSIFICATION
Beta-adrenergic blocker

AVAILABILITY (Rx)
Tablets: 10 mg, 20 mg, 40 mg, 60 mg, 80 mg, 90 mg. **Capsules (sustained-release):** 60 mg, 80 mg, 120 mg, 160 mg. **Oral Solution:** 4 mg/ml, 8 mg/ml. **Solution (concentrate):** 80 mg/ml. **Injection:** 1 mg/ml.

PHARMACOKINETICS

	ONSET	PEAK	DURATION
PO	—	60–90 min	—
PO (long-acting)	—	6 hrs	—
IV	Immediate	1 min	—

Almost completely absorbed from GI tract. Widely distributed. Metabolized in liver. Primarily excreted in urine. Not removed by hemodialysis. Half-life: 3–5 hrs.

ACTION / THERAPEUTIC EFFECT

Nonselective beta blocker. Blocks beta$_1$-adrenergic receptors, *slowing sinus heart rate, decreasing cardiac output, decreasing B/P.* Blocks beta$_2$-adrenergic receptors, *increasing airway resistance. Decreases myocardial ischemia severity* by decreasing oxygen requirements. Slows AV conduction, increases refractory period in AV node; *exhibits antiarrhythmic activity.*

USES / UNLABELED

Treatment of hypertension, angina, various cardiac arrhythmias, hypertrophic subaortic stenosis, migraine headache, essential tremor, and as an adjunct to alpha-blocking agents in the treatment of pheochromocytoma. Used to reduce risk of cardiovascular mortality and reinfarction in pts who have previously suffered a myocardial infarction (MI). *Treatment of adjunct anxiety, thyrotoxicosis, mitral valve prolapse syndrome, essential tremor.*

PO / IV ADMINISTRATION

PO:

1. May crush scored tablets.
2. Give at same time each day.

IV:

1. Give undiluted for direct injection.
2. Do not exceed 1 mg/min injection rate.
3. For IV infusion, may dilute each 1 mg in 10 ml 5% dextrose in water.
4. Give 1 mg over 10–15 min.

INDICATIONS / DOSAGE / ROUTES

Hypertension:
PO: Adults, elderly: Initially, 40 mg 2 times/day or 80 mg daily as extended-release capsule. Increase at 3–7 day intervals. **Maintenance:** 120–240 mg/day as tablets or oral solution, 120–160 mg/day as extended-release capsules. **Maximum:** 640 mg/day. **Children:** Initially, 1 mg/kg/day in 2 equally divided doses. Increase at 3–5 day intervals up to 2 mg/kg/day.

Angina pectoris:
PO: Adults, elderly: Initially, 80–320 mg/day in 2–4 divided doses or 80 mg/day (sustained-release). **Maximum:** 320 mg/day. **Maintenance:** 160 mg/day.

Cardiac arrhythmias:
PO: Adults, elderly: 10–30 mg 3–4 times/day.

Life-threatening arrhythmias:
IV: Adults, elderly: 0.5–3 mg. Repeat once in 2 min. Give additional doses at intervals of at least 4 hrs.

Hypertrophic subaortic stenosis:
PO: Adults, elderly: 20–40 mg in 3–4 divided doses or 80–160 mg/day as extended-release capsule.

Pheochromocytoma:
PO: Adults, elderly: 60 mg/day in divided doses w/alpha blocker for 3 days before surgery. **Maintenance (inoperable tumor):** 30 mg/day w/alpha blocker.

Migraine headache:
PO: Adults, elderly: 80 mg/day in divided doses or 80 mg once daily as extended-release capsule. Increase up to 160–240 mg/day in divided doses.

Myocardial infarction:
PO: Adults, elderly: 180–240 mg/day in divided doses beginning 5–21 days after MI.

Essential tremor:
PO: Adults, elderly: Initially, 40 mg 2 times/day increased up to 120–320 mg/day in 3 divided doses.

Usual pediatric dosage:
PO: 2–4 mg/kg/day in 2 equally divided doses up to 16 mg/kg/day in divided doses.

PRECAUTIONS

CONTRAINDICATIONS: Bronchial asthma, COPD, uncontrolled cardiac failure, sinus bradycardia, heart block greater than first degree, cardiogenic shock, CHF, unless secondary to tachyarrhythmias, those on MAO inhibitors. **CAUTIONS:** Inadequate cardiac function, impaired renal/hepatic function, those w/Wolff-Parkinson-White syndrome, diabetes mellitus, hyperthyroidism. **PREGNANCY/LACTATION:** Crosses placenta; is distributed in breast milk. Avoid use during first trimester. May produce bradycardia, apnea, hypoglycemia, hypothermia during delivery, small birth weight infants. **Pregnancy Category C**. (Category D if used in 2nd or 3rd trimester.)

INTERACTIONS

DRUG INTERACTIONS: Diuretics, other hypotensives may increase hypotensive effect. Sympathomimetics, xanthines may mutually inhibit effects. May mask symptoms of hypoglycemia, prolong hypoglycemic effect of insulin, oral hypoglycemics. NSAIDs may decrease antihypertensive effect. May increase cardiac depressant effect w/IV phenytoin. **ALTERED**

LAB VALUES: May increase ANA titer, SGOT (AST), SGPT (ALT), alkaline phosphatase, LDH, bilirubin, BUN, creatinine, potassium, uric acid, lipoproteins, triglycerides.

SIDE EFFECTS

FREQUENT: Decreased sexual ability, drowsiness, difficulty sleeping, unusual tiredness/weakness. **OCCASIONAL:** Bradycardia, depression, cold hands/feet, diarrhea, constipation, anxiety, nasal congestion, nausea, vomiting. **RARE:** Altered taste, dry eyes, itching, numbness of fingers, toes, scalp.

ADVERSE REACTIONS/TOXIC EFFECTS

May produce profound bradycardia, hypotension. Abrupt withdrawal may result in sweating, palpitations, headache, tremulousness. May precipitate CHF, MI in those w/cardiac disease, thyroid storm in those w/thyrotoxicosis, peripheral ischemia in those w/existing peripheral vascular disease. Hypoglycemia may occur in previously controlled diabetics.

NURSING IMPLICATIONS
BASELINE ASSESSMENT:

Assess baseline renal/liver function tests. Assess B/P, apical pulse immediately before drug is administered (if pulse is 60/min or below or systolic B/P is below 90 mm Hg, withhold medication, contact physician). *Anginal:* Record onset, type (sharp, dull, squeezing), radiation, location, intensity, and duration of anginal pain and precipitating factors (exertion, emotional stress).

INTERVENTION/EVALUATION:

Assess pulse for strength/

weakness, irregular rate, brady-cardia. Monitor EKG for cardiac arrhythmias. Assess fingers for color, numbness (Raynaud's). Assist w/ambulation if dizziness occurs. Assess for evidence of CHF (dyspnea [particularly on exertion or lying down], night cough, peripheral edema, distended neck veins). Monitor I&O (increase in weight, decrease in urine output may indicate CHF). Assess for rash, fatigue, behavioral changes. Therapeutic response ranges from a few days to several weeks. Measure B/P near end of dosing interval (determines if B/P is controlled throughout day).

PATIENT/FAMILY TEACHING:

Do not abruptly discontinue medication. Compliance w/therapy regimen is essential to control hypertension, arrhythmia, anginal pain. To avoid hypotensive effect, rise slowly from lying to sitting position, wait momentarily before standing. Avoid tasks that require alertness, motor skills until response to drug is established. Report excessively slow pulse rate (<60 beats/min), peripheral numbness, dizziness. Do not use nasal decongestants, OTC cold preparations (stimulants) w/o physician approval. Outpatients should monitor B/P, pulse before taking medication. Restrict salt, alcohol intake.

propylthiouracil

pro-pill-thye-oh-**your**-ah-sill
(Propylthiouracil)

CANADIAN AVAILABILITY:
Propyl-Thyracil

CLASSIFICATION

Antithyroid

AVAILABILITY (Rx)

Tablets: 50 mg

PHARMACOKINETICS

Readily absorbed from GI tract. Concentrated in thyroid. Metabolized in liver. Primarily excreted in urine. Minimally removed by hemodialysis. Half-life: 1–2 hrs.

ACTION/ *THERAPEUTIC EFFECT*

In hyperthyroidism, *inhibits synthesis of thyroid hormone.* Diverts iodine from thyroid hormone synthesis.

USES

Palliative treatment of hyperthyroidism; adjunct to ameliorate hyperthyroidism in preparation for surgical treatment or radioactive iodine therapy.

PO ADMINISTRATION

Space doses evenly.

INDICATIONS/DOSAGE/ROUTES

Hyperthyroidism:
PO: Adults, elderly: Initially: 300–400 mg/day. **Maintenance:** 100–150 mg/day. **Children (6–10 yrs):** Initially: 50–150 mg/day; **(>10 yrs):** 150–300 mg/day. **Maintenance:** Determined by pt response.

PRECAUTIONS

CONTRAINDICATIONS: Hypersensitivity to the drug. **CAUTIONS:** Pts over 40 years of age or in combination w/other agranulocytosis-inducing drugs. **PREGNANCY/LACTATION:** Do not give to nursing mothers. **Pregnancy Category D.**

INTERACTIONS

DRUG INTERACTIONS: Amiodarone, iodinated glycerol, iodine, potassium iodide may decrease response. May decrease effect of oral anticoagulants. May increase concentration of digoxin (as pt becomes euthyroid). May decrease thyroid uptake of I^{131}. **ALTERED LAB VALUES:** May increase SGOT (AST), SGPT (ALT), alkaline phosphatase, LDH, bilirubin, prothrombin time.

SIDE EFFECTS

FREQUENT: Urticaria, rash, pruritus, nausea, skin pigmentation, hair loss, headache, paresthesia. **OCCASIONAL:** Drowsiness, lymphadenopathy, vertigo. **RARE:** Drug fever, lupus-like syndrome.

ADVERSE REACTIONS/TOXIC EFFECTS

Agranulocytosis (which may occur as long as 4 mos after therapy), pancytopenia, fatal hepatitis have occurred.

NURSING IMPLICATIONS

BASELINE ASSESSMENT:

Question for hypersensitivity. Obtain baseline weight, pulse.

INTERVENTION/EVALUATION:

Monitor pulse, weight daily. Assess food tolerance. Check for skin eruptions, itching, swollen lymph glands. Be alert to hepatitis (nausea, vomiting, drowsiness, jaundice). Monitor hematology results for bone marrow suppression; check for signs of infection/bleeding.

PATIENT/FAMILY TEACHING:

Do not exceed ordered dose; follow-up w/physician is essential. Space evenly around the clock. Take resting pulse daily (teach pt/family), report as directed. Do not take other medications w/o approval of physician. Seafood, iodine products may be restricted. Report illness, unusual bleeding/bruising immediately. Inform physician of sudden/continuous weight gain, cold intolerance, or depression.

protamine sulfate

pro-tah-meen
(Protamine sulfate)

CANADIAN AVAILABILITY:
Protamine

CLASSIFICATION

Heparin antagonist

AVAILABILITY (Rx)

Injection: 10 mg/ml

PHARMACOKINETICS

	ONSET	PEAK	DURATION
IV	5 min	—	2 hrs

After IV administration, protamine neutralizes heparin within 5 min (forms complex).

ACTION/*THERAPEUTIC EFFECT*

Complexes w/heparin to form a stable salt, *resulting in reduction of anticoagulant activity of heparin.*

USES/*UNLABELED*

Treatment of severe heparin overdose (causing hemorrhage). Neutralizes effects of heparin administered during extracorporeal circulation. *Treatment of enoxaparin toxicity.*

STORAGE/HANDLING

Keep at room temperature. Use only colorless solutions. Discard unused portions.

IV ADMINISTRATION

IV:

1. Administer *slowly,* over 1–3 min (less than 50 mg over any 10 min period).
2. Give by IV injection only.
3. May be administered undiluted or diluted w/5% dextrose/0.9% NaCl fluid for injection.

INDICATIONS/DOSAGE/ROUTES

Antidote:
IV: **Adults, elderly:** 1 mg protamine sulfate neutralizes 90–115 units of heparin. Heparin disappears rapidly from circulation, reducing the dosage demand for protamine as time elapses.

PRECAUTIONS

CONTRAINDICATIONS: None significant. **CAUTIONS:** History of allergy to fish, vasectomized/infertile men, those on isophane (NPH) insulin or previous protamine therapy (propensity to hypersensitivity reaction). **PREGNANCY/LACTATION:** Unknown whether drug crosses placenta or is distributed in breast milk. **Pregnancy Category C**.

INTERACTIONS

DRUG INTERACTIONS: None significant. **ALTERED LAB VALUES:** None significant.

SIDE EFFECTS

FREQUENT: Decreased B/P, dyspnea. **OCCASIONAL:** Hypersensitivity reaction: urticaria, angioedema; nausea, vomiting (generally occurs in those sensitive to fish, vasectomized or infertile men, those on isophane [NPH], insulin, or previous protamine therapy). **RARE:** Back pain.

ADVERSE REACTIONS/TOXIC EFFECTS

A too rapid IV administration may produce acute hypotension, bradycardia, pulmonary hypertension, dyspnea, transient flushing, feeling of warmth. Heparin rebound may occur several hours after heparin has been neutralized by protamine (usually evident 8–9 hrs after protamine administration). Occurs most often following arterial/cardiac surgery.

NURSING IMPLICATIONS

BASELINE ASSESSMENT:

Check prothrombin time, activated partial thromboplastin time (APTT), hematocrit; assess for bleeding.

INTERVENTION/EVALUATION:

Monitor pts closely after cardiac surgery for evidence of hyperheparinemia/bleeding. Monitor APTT or activated coagulation time (ACT) 5–15 min after protamine administration. Because of possibility of heparin rebound, repeat tests in 2–8 hrs. Assess hematocrit, platelet count, urine/stool culture for occult blood. Assess for decrease in B/P, increase in pulse rate, complaint of abdominal/back pain, severe headache (may be evidence of hemorrhage). Question for increase in amount of discharge during menses. Assess peripheral pulses; skin for bruises, petechiae. Check for excessive bleeding from minor cuts, scratches. Assess gums for erythema, gingival bleeding. Assess urine output for hematuria.

protriptyline hydrochloride

pro-**trip**-teh-leen
(Vivactil)

CANADIAN AVAILABILITY:
Triptil

CLASSIFICATION

Antidepressant: Tricyclic

AVAILABILITY (Rx)

Tablets: 5 mg, 10 mg

PHARMACOKINETICS

Well absorbed from GI tract. Widely distributed. Metabolized in liver (undergoes first-pass effect). Primarily excreted in urine. Half-life: 67–89 hrs.

ACTION/*THERAPEUTIC EFFECT*

Blocks reuptake of neurotransmitters (norepinephrine, serotonin) at neuronal presynaptic membranes, increasing availability at postsynaptic receptor sites. *Resulting enhancements of synaptic activity produce antidepressant effect.*

USES

Treatment of various forms of depression, often in conjunction w/psychotherapy.

PO ADMINISTRATION

1. Give w/food or milk if GI distress occurs.
2. Do not break or chew tablets.

INDICATIONS/DOSAGE/ROUTES

Depression:
PO: Adults: Initially, 15–40 mg daily, given in 1–4 divided doses. Increase dosage gradually to 60 mg daily, then reduce dosage to lowest effective maintenance level. **Adolescents:** Initially, 5 mg 3 times daily.

Usual elderly dosage:
PO: Initially, 5–10 mg/day. May increase by 5–10 mg/day q3–7 days. **Maintenance:** 10–20 mg/day.

PRECAUTIONS

CONTRAINDICATIONS: Acute recovery period following MI, within 14 days of MAO inhibitor therapy. **CAUTIONS:** Prostatic hypertrophy, history of urinary retention/obstruction, glaucoma, diabetes mellitus, history of seizures, hyperthyroidism, cardiac/hepatic/renal disease, schizophrenia, increased intraocular pressure, hiatal hernia. **PREGNANCY/LACTATION:** Crosses placenta; is distributed in breast milk. **Pregnancy Category C**.

INTERACTIONS

DRUG INTERACTIONS: Alcohol, CNS depressants may increase CNS, respiratory depression, hypotensive effects. Antithyroid agents may increase risk of agranulocytosis. Phenothiazines may increase sedative, anticholinergic effects. Cimetidine may increase concentration, toxicity. May decrease effects of clonidine, guanadrel. May increase cardiac effects w/sympathomimetics. May increase risk of hypertensive crisis, hyperpyretic convulsions w/MAO inhibitors. **ALTERED LAB VALUES:** May alter EKG readings, glucose.

SIDE EFFECTS

FREQUENT: Drowsiness, fatigue,

dry mouth, blurred vision, constipation, delayed micturition, postural hypotension, excessive sweating, disturbed concentration, increased appetite, urinary retention. **OCCASIONAL:** GI disturbances (nausea, GI distress, metallic taste sensation). **RARE:** Paradoxical reaction (agitation, restlessness, nightmares, insomnia), extrapyramidal symptoms (particularly fine hand tremor).

ADVERSE REACTIONS/TOXIC EFFECTS

High dosage may produce cardiovascular effects (severe postural hypotension, dizziness, tachycardia, palpitations, arrhythmias) and seizures. May also result in altered temperature regulation (hyperpyrexia/hypothermia). Abrupt withdrawal from prolonged therapy may produce headache, malaise, nausea, vomiting, vivid dreams.

NURSING IMPLICATIONS
BASELINE ASSESSMENT:

For those on long-term therapy, liver/renal function tests, blood counts should be performed periodically.

INTERVENTION/EVALUATION:

Supervise suicidal risk patient closely during early therapy (as depression lessens, energy level improves, increasing suicide potential). Assess appearance, behavior, speech pattern, level of interest, mood. Monitor stools; avoid constipation. Monitor B/P, pulse for hypotension, arrhythmias. Closely monitor for cardiac disturbances in elderly pts receiving more than 20 mg daily. Assess for urinary retention by bladder palpation.

PATIENT/FAMILY TEACHING:

Change positions slowly to avoid hypotensive effect. Tolerance to postural hypotension, sedative and anticholinergic effects usually develops during early therapy. Therapeutic effect may be noted within 2–5 days, maximum effect within 2–3 wks. Photosensitivity to sun may occur; use sunscreens, wear protective clothing. Dry mouth may be relieved by sugarless gum, sips of tepid water. Report visual disturbances. Do not abruptly discontinue medication. Avoid tasks that require alertness, motor skills until response to drug is established. Avoid alcohol and other CNS depressants.

pseudoephedrine hydrochloride
su-do-eh-**fed**-rin
(Novafed, Sudafed)
pseudoephedrine sulfate
(Afrinol Repetabs)

FIXED-COMBINATION(S):
W/acrivastine, an antihistamine (Semprex-D); w/loratidine, an antihistamine (Claritin-D); w/fexofenidine, an antihistamine (Allegra-D).

CANADIAN AVAILABILITY:
Eltor, Sudafed

CLASSIFICATION
Sympathomimetic

AVAILABILITY (OTC)
Tablets: 30 mg, 60 mg. **Tablets**

(extended-release): 120 mg. **Capsules:** 60 mg. **Capsules (extended-release):** 120 mg. **Liquid:** 15 mg/5 ml, 30 mg/5 ml. **Drops:** 7.5 mg/0.8 ml.

PHARMACOKINETICS

	ONSET	PEAK	DURATION
Tablets, syrup	15–30 min	—	4–6 hrs
Extended-release	—	—	8–12 hrs

Well absorbed from GI tract. Partially metabolized in liver. Primarily excreted in urine. Half-life: 9–16 hrs.

ACTION/*THERAPEUTIC EFFECT*

Acts directly on alpha-adrenergic receptors and, to lesser extent, on beta-adrenergic receptors, *producing vasoconstriction of respiratory tract mucosa, resulting in shrinkage of nasal mucous membranes, edema, nasal congestion.* Produces little, if any, rebound nasal congestion.

USES

For nasal congestion, treatment of obstructed eustachian ostia in those w/otic inflammation, infection.

PO ADMINISTRATION

Do not crush, chew extended-release tablets; swallow whole.

INDICATIONS/DOSAGE/ROUTES

Decongestant:
PO: Adults, children >12 yrs: 60 mg q4–6h. **Maximum:** 240 mg/day. **Children 6–12 yrs:** 30 mg q6h. **Maximum:** 120 mg/day. **Children 2–5 yrs:** 15 mg q6h. **Maximum:** 60 mg/day.

Usual elderly dose:
PO: 30–60 mg q6h as needed.

Extended-release:
PO: Adults, children >12 yrs: 120 mg q12h.

PRECAUTIONS

CONTRAINDICATIONS: Severe hypertension, coronary artery disease, lactating women, MAO inhibitor therapy. **CAUTIONS:** Elderly, hyperthyroidism, diabetes, ischemic heart disease, prostatic hypertrophy. **PREGNANCY/LACTATION:** Crosses placenta; is distributed in breast milk. **Pregnancy Category C**.

INTERACTIONS

DRUG INTERACTIONS: May decrease effects of antihypertensive, diuretics, beta-adrenergic blockers. MAO inhibitors may increase cardiac stimulant, vasopressor effects. **ALTERED LAB VALUES:** None significant.

SIDE EFFECTS

OCCASIONAL (5–10%): Nervousness, restlessnss, insomnia, trembling, headache. **RARE (1–4%):** Increased sweating, weakness.

ADVERSE REACTIONS/TOXIC EFFECTS

Large doses may produce tachycardia, palpitations (particularly in those with cardiac disease), lightheadedness, nausea, vomiting. Overdosage in those >60 yrs may result in hallucinations, CNS depression, seizures.

NURSING IMPLICATIONS
PATIENT/FAMILY TEACHING

Discontinue drug if adverse reactions occur. Report insomnia, dizziness, tremors, rapid or irregular heartbeat.

psyllium

sill-ee-um
(Fiberall, Hydrocil, Konsyl, Metamucil, Perdiem)

CANADIAN AVAILABILITY:
Metamucil, Prodiem Plain

CLASSIFICATION

Laxative: Bulk forming

AVAILABILITY (OTC)

Powder. Wafer.

PHARMACOKINETICS

	ONSET	PEAK	DURATION
PO	12–72 hrs	—	—

Acts in small/large intestine.

ACTION/*THERAPEUTIC EFFECT*

Powder, wafer dissolves and swells in water (provides increased bulk, moisture content in stool). *Increased bulk promotes peristalsis, bowel motility.*

USES

Prophylaxis in those who should not strain during defecation. Facilitates defecation in those w/diminished colonic motor response.

PO ADMINISTRATION

1. Drink 6–8 glasses of water/day (aids stool softening).
2. Do not swallow in dry form; mix w/at least 1 full glass (8 oz) liquid.

INDICATIONS/DOSAGE/ROUTES

Laxative:
PO: Adults, elderly: 1 rounded tsp, packet, or wafer in water 1–3 times/day.

PRECAUTIONS

CONTRAINDICATIONS: Abdominal pain, nausea, vomiting, symptoms of appendicitis, partial bowel obstruction, dysphagia. **CAUTIONS:** None significant. **PREGNANCY/LACTATION:** Safe for use in pregnancy. **Pregnancy Category C**.

INTERACTIONS

DRUG INTERACTIONS: May interfere w/effects of potassium-sparing diuretics, potassium supplements. May decrease effect of oral anticoagulants, digoxin, salicylates by decreasing absorption. **ALTERED LAB VALUES:** May increase glucose. May decrease potassium.

SIDE EFFECTS

RARE: Some degree of abdominal discomfort, nausea, mild cramps, griping, faintness.

ADVERSE REACTIONS/TOXIC EFFECTS

Esophageal/bowel obstruction may occur if administered with insufficient liquid (less than 250 ml or 1 full glass).

NURSING IMPLICATIONS

INTERVENTION/EVALUATION:

Encourage adequate fluid intake. Assess bowel sounds for peristalsis. Monitor daily bowel activity, stool consistency (watery, loose, soft, semisolid, solid). Monitor serum electrolytes in those exposed to prolonged, frequent, or excessive use of medication.

PATIENT/FAMILY TEACHING:

Institute measures to promote defecation (increase fluid intake, exercise, high-fiber diet).

pyrazinamide

peer-a-**zin**-a-mide
(Pyrazinamide)

FIXED-COMBINATION(S):
W/ioniazid and rifampin, antituberculars (**Rifater**)

CANADIAN AVAILABILITY:
Tebrazid

CLASSIFICATION

Antitubercular

AVAILABILITY (Rx)

Tablets: 500 mg

PHARMACOKINETICS

Rapidly, completely absorbed from GI tract. Widely distributed. Metabolized in liver to active metabolite. Removed by hemodialysis. Half-life: 9.5 hrs (increased in decreased renal function).

ACTION/ *THERAPEUTIC EFFECT*

Exact mechanism unknown. *Either bacteriostatic or bactericidal, depending on its concentration at infection site and susceptibility of infecting bacteria.*

USES

In conjunction w/at least one other antitubercular agent in treatment of clinical tuberculosis after failure of primary agents (isoniazid, rifampin).

INDICATIONS/DOSAGE/ROUTES

Tuberculosis:
PO: Adults: 20–35 mg/kg/day as single dose. **Maximum:** 3 g/day. **Children:** 15–30 mg/kg/day in 1 or 2 doses. **Maximum:** 1.5 g/day.

PRECAUTIONS

CONTRAINDICATIONS: Hypersensitivity to pyrazinamide, severe hepatic dysfunction. **CAUTIONS:** Diabetes mellitus, renal impairment, history of gout, children (safety not established). Possible cross-sensitivity w/isoniazid, ethionamide, niacin. **PREGNANCY/LACTATION:** Excreted in breast milk. **Pregnancy Category C**.

INTERACTIONS

DRUG INTERACTIONS: May decrease effects of allopurinol, colchicine, probenecid, sulfinpyrazone. **ALTERED LAB VALUES:** May increase SGOT (AST), SGPT (ALT), uric acid concentrations.

SIDE EFFECTS

FREQUENT: Arthralgia, myalgia (usually mild and self-limiting). **RARE:** Hypersensitivity (rash, urticaria, pruritus), photosensitivity.

ADVERSE REACTIONS/TOXIC EFFECTS

Hepatoxicity, thrombocytopenia, anemia occurs rarely.

NURSING IMPLICATIONS

BASELINE ASSESSMENT:

Question for hypersensitivity to pyrazinamide, isoniazid, ethionamide, niacin. Assure collection of specimens for culture, sensitivity. Evaluate results of initial CBC, hepatic function tests, uric acid levels.

INTERVENTION/EVALUATION:

Monitor hepatic function results and be alert for hepatic reactions: jaundice, malaise, fever, liver tenderness, anorexia/nausea/vomiting (stop drug, notify physician promptly). Check serum uric acid levels and assess for hot, painful, swollen joints, esp. big toe, ankle, or knee (gout). Evaluate blood sugars, diabetic status carefully (pyrazinamide makes management difficult). Assess for rash, skin eruptions. Monitor CBC results for thrombocytopenia, anemia.

PATIENT/FAMILY TEACHING:

Do not skip doses; complete full length of therapy (may be months, years). Office visits, lab tests are essential part of treatment. Take w/food to reduce GI upset. Do not take any other medications w/o consulting physician. Avoid too much sun or ultraviolet light until photosensitivity is determined. Notify physician of any new symptom, immediately for yellow eyes or skin; unusual tiredness; fever; loss of appetite; hot, painful, or swollen joints.

pyridostigmine bromide

pier-id-oh-**stig**-meen
(Mestinon, Regonol)

CANADIAN AVAILABILITY:
Mestinon

CLASSIFICATION

Anticholinesterase agent

AVAILABILITY (Rx)

Tablets: 60 mg. **Tablets (sustained-release):** 180 mg. **Syrup:** 60 mg/5 ml. **Injection:** 5 mg/ml.

PHARMACOKINETICS

	ONSET	PEAK	DURATION
PO	30–45 min	—	3–6 hrs
IM	<15 min	—	2–4 hrs
IV	2–5 min	—	2–3 hrs

Minimally absorbed from GI tract. Metabolized in liver, by plasma cholinesterases. Primarily excreted in urine. Half-life: 63–112 min.

ACTION/*THERAPEUTIC EFFECT*

Prevents destruction of acetylcholine by enzyme, anticholinesterase. *Produces miosis, increases tone of intestinal and skeletal muscles, stimulates salivary, sweat gland secretions.*

USES

Improvement of muscle strength in control of myasthenia gravis, reversal of effects of nondepolarizing neuromuscular blocking agents after surgery.

STORAGE/HANDLING

Store oral, parenteral forms at room temperature.

PO/IM/IV ADMINISTRATION

PO:

1. Give w/food or milk.
2. Tablets may be crushed; do not chew, crush extended-release tablets (may be broken).
3. Give larger dose at times of increased fatigue (e.g., for those w/difficulty in chewing, 30–45 min before meals).

IM/IV:

Give large parenteral doses concurrently w/0.6–1.2 mg atropine sulfate IV to minimize side effects.

INDICATIONS/DOSAGE/ROUTES

Note: Dosage, frequency of administration dependent on daily clinical pt response (remissions, exacerbations, physical and emotional stress).

Myasthenia gravis:
PO: Adults, elderly: Initially, 60 mg 3 times/day. Increase dose at intervals of 48 hrs or more until therapeutic response is achieved. When increased dosage does not produce further increase in muscle strength, reduce dose to previous dosage level. **Maintenance:** 60–1,500 mg/day. **Children:** Initially, 7 mg/kg/day in 5–6 divided doses.
Extended-Release: Adults, elderly: 180–540 mg 1–2 times/day (must maintain at least 6 hrs between doses).
IM/IV: Adults, elderly: 2 mg q2–3h.
PO: Neonate: 5 mg q4–6h.
IM: Neonate: 0.05–0.15 mg/kg q4–6h.

Reversal of nondepolarizing muscle relaxants:
IV: Adults, elderly: 10–20 mg with, or shortly after, 0.6–1.2 mg atropine sulfate or 0.2–0.6 mg glycopyrrolate.

PRECAUTIONS

CONTRAINDICATIONS: Mechanical GI, urinary obstruction. **CAUTIONS:** Bronchial asthma, bradycardia, epilepsy, recent coronary occlusion, vagotonia, hyperthyroidism, cardiac arrhythmias, peptic ulcer. **PREGNANCY/LACTATION:** Transient muscular weakness occurs in 10–20% of neonates born to mothers treated with drug therapy for myasthenia gravis during pregnancy. Myasthenic mothers may be given 1/30 of their usual oral dose by IM or slow IV injection 1 hr before completion of second stage of labor. **Pregnancy Category C**.

INTERACTIONS

DRUG INTERACTIONS: Anticholinergics reverse/prevent effects. Cholinesterase inhibitors may increase toxicity. Antagonizes neuromuscular blocking agents. Quinidine, procainamide may antagonize action. **ALTERED LAB VALUES:** None significant.

SIDE EFFECTS

COMMON: Miosis, increased GI and skeletal muscle tone, reduced pulse rate, constriction of bronchi and ureters, salivary and sweat gland secretion. **OCCASIONAL:** Headache, slight temporary decrease in diastolic B/P w/mild reflex tachycardia, short periods of atrial fibrillation in hyperthyroid pts. Hypertensive pts may react w/marked fall in B/P. **RARE:** Rash.

ADVERSE REACTIONS/TOXIC EFFECTS

Overdosage produces cholinergic reaction manifested as abdominal discomfort/cramping, nausea, vomiting, diarrhea, flushing, feeling of warmth/heat about face, excessive salivation and sweating, lacrimation, pallor, bradycardia/tachycardia, hypotension, urinary urgency, blurred vision, bronchospasm, pupillary contraction, involuntary muscular contraction visible under the skin (fasciculation).

Overdosage may also produce a *cholinergic crisis,* manifested by increasingly severe muscle weakness (appears first in muscles involving chewing, swallowing, followed by muscular weakness of shoulder girdle and upper extremities), respiratory muscle paralysis followed by pelvis girdle and leg muscle paralysis. Requires withdrawal of all cholinergic drugs and immediate use of 1–4 mg atropine sulfate IV for adults, 0.01 mg/kg in infants and children under 12 yrs.

Myasthenic crisis (due to underdosage) also produces extreme muscle weakness but requires a *more* intensive drug therapy program (differentiation between the two crises is imperative for accurate treatment). Weakness beginning 1 hr after drug administration suggests overdosage; weakness occurring 3 hrs or more after administration suggests underdosage/resistance to anticholinesterase drugs. Extremely high doses may produce CNS stimulation followed by CNS depression. Resistance to pyridostigmine therapy may occur following prolonged treatment in myasthenic pts. Responsiveness may be restored by decreasing dose/temporarily discontinuing therapy for several days.

NURSING IMPLICATIONS
BASELINE ASSESSMENT:

Larger doses should be given at time of greatest fatigue. Assess muscle strength before testing for diagnosis of myasthenia gravis and after drug administration. Avoid large doses in those w/megacolon or reduced GI motility. Have tissues readily available at pt's bedside.

INTERVENTION/EVALUATION:

Monitor respirations closely during myasthenia gravis testing or if dosage is increased. Assess diligently for cholinergic reaction, as well as bradycardia in the myasthenic pt in crisis. Coordinate dosage time vs. periods of fatigue and increased/decreased muscle strength. Monitor for therapeutic response to medication (increased muscle strength, decreased fatigue, improved chewing, swallowing functions).

PATIENT/FAMILY TEACHING:

Report nausea, vomiting, diarrhea, sweating, increased salivary secretions, irregular heartbeat, muscle weakness, severe abdominal pain, or difficulty in breathing.

---

pyridoxine hydrochloride (vitamin B$_6$)

(Pyridoxine)
pie-rih-**docks**-in

CANADIAN AVAILABILITY:
Hexa-Betalin

CLASSIFICATION

Vitamin (B$_6$), coenzyme

AVAILABILITY (OTC)

Tablets: 25 mg, 50 mg, 100 mg.
Tablets (time-release): 100 mg.
Injection (Rx): 100 mg/ml.

PHARMACOKINETICS

Readily absorbed primarily in jejunum. Stored in liver, muscle, brain. Metabolized in liver. Primarily excreted in urine. Removed by hemodialysis. Half-life: 15–20 days.

ACTION/THERAPEUTIC EFFECT

Coenzyme for various metabolic functions *affecting protein, carbohydrate, lipid utilization.*

USES

Prevention, treatment of pyridoxine deficiency caused by inadequate diet, drug-induced (e.g., INH, penicillamine, cyclosporine) or inborn error of metabolism. Treatment of INH poisoning. Treatment of seizures in neonate unresponsive to conventional therapy. Treatment of sideroblastic anemia associated w/increased serum iron concentrations.

PO/SUBQ/IM/IV ADMINISTRATION

Note: Give orally unless nausea, vomiting, or malabsorption occurs. Avoid IV use in cardiac pts.

IV:

Give undiluted or add to IV solutions and give as infusion.

INDICATIONS/DOSAGE/ROUTES

Pyridoxine deficiency:
PO: Adults, elderly: *(Diet):* 2.5–10 mg/day; after signs of deficiency decrease, 2.5–5 mg/day for several wks. *(Drug-Induced):* 10–50 mg/day (INH, penicillamine); 100–300 mg/day (cyclosporine). *(Error metabolism):* 100–500 mg/day.

INH toxicity (>10 g); with other anticonvulsants:
IV: Adults, elderly: 4 g, then 1 g IM q30 min until entire dose given. *Total dose:* Equal to amount INH ingested.

Seizures in neonates:
IM/IV: Neonates: 10–100 mg/day; then oral therapy of 2–100 mg/day for life.

Sideroblastic anemia:
PO: Adults, elderly: 200–600 mg/day. After adequate response, 30–50 mg/day for life.

PRECAUTIONS

CONTRAINDICATIONS: IV therapy in cardiac pts. **CAUTIONS:** Megadosage in pregnancy. **PREGNANCY/LACTATION:** Crosses placenta; is excreted in breast milk. High doses in utero may produce seizures in neonates. **Pregnancy Category A.** (Category C if doses above RDA.)

INTERACTIONS

DRUG INTERACTIONS: Immunosuppressants, isoniazid, penicillamine may antagonize pyridoxine (may cause anemia/peripheral neuritis). Reverses effects of levodopa. **ALTERED LAB VALUES:** None significant.

SIDE EFFECTS

OCCASIONAL: Stinging at IM injection site. **RARE:** Headache, nausea, somnolence; high doses cause sensory neuropathy (paresthesia, unstable gait, clumsiness of hands).

ADVERSE REACTIONS/TOXIC EFFECTS

Long-term megadoses (2–6 g more than 2 mos) may produce sensory neuropathy (reduced deep tendon reflex, profound impairment of sense of position in distal limbs, gradual sensory ataxia). Toxic symptoms reverse w/drug discontinuance. Seizures have occurred following IV megadoses.

NURSING IMPLICATIONS

INTERVENTION/EVALUATION:

Observe for improvement of deficiency symptoms, including nervous system abnormalities (anxiety, depression, insomnia, motor difficulty, peripheral numbness and tremors), skin lesions (glossitis, seborrhealike lesions around mouth, nose, eyes). Evaluate for nutritional adequacy.

PATIENT/FAMILY TEACHING:

Discomfort may occur w/IM injection. Foods rich in pyridoxine include legumes, soybeans, eggs, sunflower seeds, hazelnuts, organ meats, tuna, shrimp, carrots, avocado, banana, wheat germ, bran.

quazepam
(Doral)
See Classification section under:
Sedative-hypnotics

quetiapine
(Seroquel)
See Supplement
See Classification section under:
Antipsychotics

quinapril hydrochloride
quin-ah-prill
(Accupril)

CANADIAN AVAILABILITY:
Accupril

CLASSIFICATION

Antihypertensive

AVAILABILITY (Rx)

Tablets: 5 mg, 10 mg, 20 mg, 40 mg

PHARMACOKINETICS

	ONSET	PEAK	DURATION
PO	1 hr	2–4 hrs	—

Readily absorbed from GI tract. Metabolized in liver, GI tract, extra-vascular tissue to active metabolite. Primarily excreted in urine. Minimal removal by hemodialysis. Half-life: 1–2 hrs; metabolite: 3 hrs (increased in decreased renal function).

ACTION/THERAPEUTIC EFFECT

Suppresses renin-angiotensin-aldosterone system (prevents conversion of angiotensin I to angiotensin II, a potent vasoconstrictor; may also inhibit angiotensin II at local vascular and renal sites). *Reduces peripheral arterial resistance, B/P, pulmonary capillary wedge pressure; improves cardiac output.*

USES/UNLABELED

Treatment of hypertension. Used alone or in combination w/other antihypertensives. Adjunctive therapy in management of heart failure. *Treatment of hypertension/renal crisis in scleroderma.*

PO ADMINISTRATION

1. May give w/o regard to food.
2. Tablets may be crushed.

INDICATIONS/DOSAGE/ROUTES

Hypertension (used alone):
PO: Adults: Initially, 10–20 mg/day. May adjust dose after at least 2 wk intervals. **Maintenance:** 20–80 mg/day as single or 2 divided doses. **Maximum:** 80 mg/day.

Hypertension (combination therapy):
Note: Discontinue diuretic 2–3 days before initiating quinapril therapy.
PO: Adults: Initially, 5 mg/day titrated to pt's needs.

Usual elderly dose:
PO: Initially, 2.5–5 mg/day. May increase by 2.5–5 mg q1–2 wks.

Heart failure:
PO: Adults, elderly: Initially, 5 mg 2 times/day. **Range:** 20–40 mg/day.

Dosage in renal impairment:

Titrate to pt need after following initial doses:

CREATININE CLEARANCE	INITIAL DOSE
>60 ml/min	10 mg
30–60 ml/min	5 mg
10–30 ml/min	2.5 mg

PRECAUTIONS

CONTRAINDICATIONS: MI, coronary insufficiency, angina, evidence of coronary artery disease, hypersensitivity to phentolamine, history of angioedema w/previous treatment w/ACE inhibitors. **CAUTIONS:** Renal impairment, those w/sodium depletion or on diuretic therapy, dialysis, hypovolemia, coronary/cerebrovascular insufficiency. **PREGNANCY/LACTATION:** Crosses placenta; unknown whether distributed in breast milk. May cause fetal-neonatal mortality/morbidity. **Pregnancy Category D.**

INTERACTIONS

DRUG INTERACTIONS: Alcohol, diuretics, hypotensive agents may increase effects. NSAIDs may decrease effect. Potassium-sparing diuretics, potassium supplements may cause hyperkalemia. May increase lithium concentration, toxicity. **ALTERED LAB VALUES:** May increase potassium, SGOT (AST), SGPT (ALT), alkaline phosphatase, bilirubin, BUN, creatinine. May decrease sodium. May cause positive ANA titer.

SIDE EFFECTS

FREQUENT (5–7%): Headache, dizziness. **OCCASIONAL (2–4%):** Fatigue, vomiting, nausea, hypotension, chest pain, cough, syncope. **RARE (<2%):** Diarrhea, cough, dyspnea, rash, palpitations, impotence, insomnia, drowsiness, malaise.

ADVERSE REACTIONS/TOXIC EFFECTS

Excessive hypotension ("first-dose syncope") may occur in those w/CHF, severely salt/volume depleted. Angioedema (swelling of face/lips), hyperkalemia occur rarely. Agranulocytosis, neutropenia may be noted in those w/impaired renal function or collagen vascular disease (systemic lupus erythematosus, scleroderma). Nephrotic syndrome may be noted in those w/history of renal disease.

NURSING IMPLICATIONS

BASELINE ASSESSMENT:

Obtain B/P immediately before each dose in addition to regular monitoring (be alert to fluctuations). If excessive reduction in B/P occurs, place pt in supine position w/legs slightly elevated. Renal function tests should be performed before therapy begins. In those w/prior renal disease, urine test for protein by dipstick method should be made w/first urine of day before therapy begins and periodically thereafter. In those w/renal impairment, autoimmune disease or those taking drugs that affect leukocytes/immune response, CBC and differential count should be performed before therapy begins and q2 wks for 3 mos, then periodically thereafter.

INTERVENTION/EVALUATION:

Assist w/ambulation if dizziness occurs. Question for evidence of headache.

PATIENT/FAMILY TEACHING:

To reduce hypotensive effect, rise slowly from lying to sitting position and permit legs to dangle from bed momentarily before standing. Noncola carbonated beverage, unsalted crackers, dry toast may relieve nausea. Full therapeutic effect may take 1–2 wks. Report any sign of infection (sore throat, fever). Skipping doses or voluntarily discontinuing drug may produce severe rebound hypertension. Avoid driving and other tasks that require alert responses until reaction to drug is known. Do not use salt substitutes w/o consulting physician.

quinidine gluconate
kwin-ih-deen
(Duraquin, Quinaglute)
quinidine polygalacturonate
(Cardioquin)
quinidine sulfate
(Cin-quin, Quinidex)

CANADIAN AVAILABILITY:
Apo-Quinidine, Cardioquin, Quinate, Quinidex

CLASSIFICATION
Antiarrhythmic

AVAILABILITY (Rx)
Gluconate: Tablets (sustained-release): 324 mg. **Injection:** 80 mg/ml (50 mg/ml quinidine).
Polygalacturonate: Tablets: 275 mg (200 mg quinidine)
Sulfate: Tablets: 200 mg, 300 mg. **Tablets (sustained-release):** 300 mg.

PHARMACOKINETICS

	ONSET	PEAK	DURATION
PO	1–3 hrs	—	6–8 hrs

Completely absorbed from GI tract. Widely distributed. Metabolized in liver. Primarily excreted in urine. Small amounts removed by hemodialysis. Half-life: 6 hrs (increased in CHF, cirrhosis, elderly).

ACTION/THERAPEUTIC EFFECT
Direct cardiac effects *(decreases excitability, conduction velocity, automaticity, membrane responsiveness; prolongs refractory period).*

USES/UNLABELED
Prophylactic therapy to maintain normal sinus rhythm after conversion of atrial fibrillation and/or flutter. Prevention of premature atrial, AV and ventricular contractions, paroxysmal atrial tachycardia, paroxysmal AV junctional rhythm, atrial fibrillation, atrial flutter, paroxysmal ventricular tachycardia not associated w/complete heart block. *Treatment of malaria (IV only).*

STORAGE/HANDLING
For parenteral form, use only clear, colorless solution. Solution is stable for 24 hrs at room temperature when diluted w/5% dextrose.

PO/IM/IV ADMINISTRATION
PO:
1. Do not crush or chew sustained-release tablets.
2. GI upset can be reduced if given w/food.

IV:
Note: B/P, EKG should be monitored continuously during IV administration and rate of infusion adjusted to eliminate arrhythmias.
1. For IV infusion, dilute 800 mg w/40 ml 5% dextrose to provide concentration of 16 mg/ml.
2. Administer w/pt in supine position.

3. For IV injection, give at rate of 1 ml (16 mg)/min (too rapid IV rate may markedly decrease arterial pressure).

4. Monitor EKG for cardiac changes, particularly prolongation of PR, QT interval, widening of QRS complex. Notify physician of any significant interval changes.

INDICATIONS/DOSAGE/ROUTES

Note: Extended-release tablets used only for maintenance therapy; 267 mg quinidine gluconate = 275 mg quinidine polygalacturonate or 200 mg quinidine sulfate.

Conversion of atrial fibrillation:
PO: Adults, elderly: 200 mg q2–3h for 5–8 doses. Increase dose until sinus rhythm achieved/toxicity occurs. **Maximum:** 4 g/day. Control ventricular rate w/digoxin before quinidine administration.

Atrial flutter:
PO: Adults, elderly: Individualize, give after digitalization.

Paroxysmal supraventricular tachycardia:
PO: Adults, elderly: 400–600 mg q2–3h.

Premature atrial/ventricular contractions:
PO: Adults, elderly: 200–300 mg 3–4 times/day.

Maintenance therapy:
PO: Adults, elderly: 200–400 mg 3–4 times/day or 300–600 mg (as extended-release tablets) q8–12h.

Usual parenteral dosage:
IM: Adults, elderly: Initially, 600 mg, then 400 mg q2h adjusting each subsequent dose according to effect achieved by previous dose.
IV: Adults, elderly: 300 mg (may give 500–750 mg) infused at initial rate of 16 mg/min (1 ml/min).

PRECAUTIONS

CONTRAINDICATIONS: Complete AV block, intraventricular conduction defects, abnormal impulses and rhythms due to escape mechanism, myasthenia gravis. **EXTREME CAUTION:** Incomplete AV block, digitalis intoxication, CHF, preexisting hypotension. **CAUTIONS:** Preexisting asthma, muscle weakness, infection w/fever, hepatic/renal insufficiency. **PREGNANCY/LACTATION:** Crosses placenta; is distributed in breast milk. **Pregnancy Category C**.

INTERACTIONS

DRUG INTERACTIONS: May increase concentration of digoxin. Pimozide, other antiarrhythmics may increase cardiac effects. Urinary alkalizers (e.g., antacids) may decrease excretion. May increase effects of oral anticoagulants, neuromuscular blockers. May decrease effects of antimyasthenics on skeletal muscle. **ALTERED LAB VALUES:** None significant.

SIDE EFFECTS

FREQUENT: Abdominal pain/cramps, nausea, diarrhea, vomiting (can be immediate, intense). **OCCASIONAL:** Mild cinchonism (ringing in ears, blurred vision, hearing loss) or severe cinchonism (headache, vertigo, sweating, lightheadedness, photophobia, confusion, delirium). **RARE:** Hypotension (particularly w/IV administration), hypersensitivity reaction (fever, anaphylaxis, thrombocytopenia).

ADVERSE REACTIONS/TOXIC EFFECTS

Cardiotoxic effects occur most commonly w/IV administration, particularly at high concentration, observed as conduction changes

(50% widening of QRS complex, prolonged QT interval, flattened T waves, disappearance of P wave), ventricular tachycardia/flutter, frequent PVCs, complete AV block. Quinidine-induced syncope may occur w/usual dosage (discontinue drug). Severe hypotension may result from high doses. Atrial flutter/fibrillation pts may experience a paradoxical, extremely rapid ventricular rate (may be prevented by prior digitalization). Hepatotoxicity w/jaundice due to drug hypersensitivity.

NURSING IMPLICATIONS

BASELINE ASSESSMENT:

Check B/P and pulse for 1 full min (unless pt is on continuous monitor) before giving medication. For those on long-term therapy, CBC and liver/renal function tests should be performed periodically.

INTERVENTION/EVALUATION:

Monitor EKG for cardiac changes, particularly prolongation of PR, QT interval, widening of QRS complex. Monitor I&O, CBC, serum potassium, hepatic/renal function tests. Monitor pattern of daily bowel activity, stool consistency. Assess for dizziness, syncope. Monitor B/P for hypotension (esp. in those on high-dose therapy). If cardiotoxic effect occurs (see Adverse Reactions/Toxic Effects), notify physician immediately. Monitor for therapeutic serum level (2–6 mcg/ml).

PATIENT/FAMILY TEACHING:

Report rash, fever, unusual bleeding or bruising, visual disturbances, ringing in ears. Teach pt/family to take pulse properly. Photophobia may occur—sunglasses will provide some relief.

quinine sulfate

kwye-nine
(Quinine)

FIXED-COMBINATION(S):
W/vitamin E for nocturnal leg cramps **(M-KYA, Q-vel)**

CANADIAN AVAILABILITY:
Quinine

CLASSIFICATION

Antimalarial, antimyotonic

AVAILABILITY (Rx)

Capsules: 65 mg, 200 mg, 300 mg, 325 mg. **Tablets:** 162.5 mg, 260 mg.

PHARMACOKINETICS

Rapidly, completely absorbed from GI tract. Widely distributed. Metabolized in liver. Primarily excreted in urine. Minimal removal by hemodialysis. Half-life: 11 hrs.

ACTION/*THERAPEUTIC EFFECT*

Myotonia: *Relaxes skeletal muscle* by increasing the refractory period, decreasing excitability of motor end plates (curarelike), and affecting distribution of calcium w/muscle fiber. **Antimalaria:** Elevates pH in intracellular organelles of parasites, *producing parasitic death.*

USES

Prevention, treatment of nocturnal recumbency leg cramps. Generally replaced by more effective, less toxic antimalarials. Used alone, w/pyrimethamine and sulfonamide (or w/oral tetracycline) for treatment of chloraquine-resistant falciparum malaria.

PO ADMINISTRATION

1. Do *not* crush tablets (irritating to gastric mucosa, bitter).

2. Give w/or after meals to reduce GI distress.

3. Bedtime dose should be given w/milk or snack.

INDICATIONS/DOSAGE/ROUTES

Nocturnal leg cramps:
PO: Adults, elderly: 260–300 mg at bedtime as needed.

Treatment of malaria:
PO: Adults, elderly: 260–650 mg 3 times a day for 6–12 days. **Children:** 10 mg/kg q8h for 5–7 days.

PRECAUTIONS

CONTRAINDICATIONS: Hypersensitivity to quinine (possible cross-sensitivity to quinidine), G-6-PD deficiency, tinnitus, optic neuritis, history of thrombocytopenia during previous quinine therapy, blackwater fever. **CAUTIONS:** Cardiovascular disease (as w/ quinidine), myasthenia gravis, asthma. **PREGNANCY/LACTATION:** Contraindicated in pregnancy. Crosses placenta; is distributed in breast milk. Do not breast-feed. May cause congenital malformations (i.e., deafness, limb anomalies, visceral defects, visual changes, stillbirths). **Pregnancy Category D.**

INTERACTIONS

DRUG INTERACTIONS: May increase concentration of digoxin. Mefloquine may increase seizures, EKG abnormalities. **ALTERED LAB VALUES:** May interfere w/17-OH steroid determinations.

SIDE EFFECTS

FREQUENT: Nausea, headache, tinnitus, slight visual disturbances (mild cinchonism). **OCCASIONAL:** Extreme flushing of skin w/intense generalized pruritus is most typical hypersensitivity reaction; also rash, wheezing, dyspnea, angioedema. Prolonged therapy: cardiac conduction disturbances, decreased hearing.

ADVERSE REACTIONS/TOXIC EFFECTS

Overdosage (severe cinchonism): cardiovascular effects, severe headache, intestinal cramps w/vomiting and diarrhea, apprehension, confusion, seizures, blindness, respiratory depression. Hypoprothrombinemia, thrombocytopenic purpura, hemoglobinuria, asthma, agranulocytosis, hypoglycemia, deafness, optic atrophy occur rarely.

NURSING IMPLICATIONS
BASELINE ASSESSMENT:

Question for possibility of pregnancy before initiating therapy (Pregnancy Category X). Question for hypersensitivity to quinine, quinidine. Evaluate initial EKG, CBC results.

INTERVENTION/EVALUATION:

Check for hypersensitivity: flushing, rash/urticaria, itching, dyspnea, wheezing (hold drug, inform physician at once). Assess level of hearing, visual acuity, presence of headache/tinnitus, nausea and report adverse effects promptly (possible cinchonism). Monitor CBC results for blood dyscrasias; be alert to infection (fever, sore throat) and bleeding/bruising or unusual tiredness/weakness. Assess pulse, EKG for arrhythmias. Check FBS levels and watch for hypoglycemia (cold sweating, tremors, tachycardia, hunger, anxiety).

PATIENT/FAMILY TEACHING:

Use appropriate contraceptive measures (Pregnancy Category

X). Use nonhormonal contraception. Take w/food; do not crush tablets. Do not take any other medication w/o consulting physician. Report *any* new symptom immediately, esp. visual/hearing difficulties, shortness of breath, rash/itching, nausea. Periodic lab tests are part of therapy.

quinupristin-dalfopristin

quin-you-pris-tin/**dal**-foh-pris-tin
(Synercid)

CLASSIFICATION

Antimicrobial

AVAILABILITY (Rx)

Injection: 500 mg vial (350 mg dalfopristin/150 mg quinupristin)

PHARMACOKINETICS

After IV administration, both are extensively metabolized in the liver, with dalfopristin to active metabolite. Primarily eliminated in feces. Half-life: 1–2 hrs.

ACTION/ *THERAPEUTIC EFFECT*

Bactericidal (in combination). Two chemically distinct compounds that, when given together, bind to different sites on bacterial ribosomes forming a drug-ribosome complex. Protein synthesis is interrupted, *resulting in bacterial cell death.*

USES

Treatment of intra-abdominal, skin/skin structure, urinary tract, central catheter, bone and joint, respiratory infections, endocarditis, bacteremia.

STORAGE/HANDLING

Refrigerate vials. Reconstitute w/5% dextrose (compatibility w/0.9% NaCl unknown). After reconstitution, stable for 6 hrs at room temperature, 72 hrs refrigerated.

IV ADMINISTRATION

Note: Space doses evenly around the clock for full effectiveness.

IV:

1. For intermittent IV infusion (piggyback), infuse over 1 hr.
2. Alternating IV sites, use large veins to reduce risk of phlebitis.

INDICATIONS/DOSAGE/ROUTES

Usual adult dosage:
IV Infusion: Adults, elderly: 7.5 mg/kg q8–12h.

PRECAUTIONS

CONTRAINDICATIONS. Hypersensitivity to quinupristin-dalfopristin. **CAUTIONS:** Liver/renal dysfunction. **PREGNANCY/LACTATION:** Unknown if drug crosses placenta or is distributed in breast milk. **Pregnancy Category B**.

INTERACTIONS

DRUG INTERACTIONS: None significant. **ALTERED LAB VALUES:** May increase SGOT (AST), SGPT (ALT), LDH, serum creatinine, bilirubin.

SIDE EFFECTS

Generally well tolerated. **FREQUENT:** Mild erythema, itching, pain, or burning at infusion site for doses of 7 mg/kg or higher. **OCCASIONAL:** Headache, diarrhea. **RARE:** Vomiting, arthralgia, myalgia.

ADVERSE REACTIONS/TOXIC EFFECTS

Superinfection, including antibiotic-associated colitis, may result from bacterial imbalance. Liver function abnormalities, peripheral venous intolerability may occur.

NURSING IMPLICATIONS

BASELINE ASSESSMENT:

Question history of allergies, esp. penicillins, cephalosporins. Obtain specimen for culture and sensitivity before giving first dose (therapy may begin before results are known). Assess temperature, B/P, respiratory rate, pulse. Obtain baseline liver function tests, BUN, CBC w/differential, urinalysis.

INTERVENTION/EVALUATION:

Hold medication and promptly inform physician of diarrhea (w/fever, abdominal pain, mucous and blood in stool may indicate antibiotic-associated colitis). Evaluate IV site for mild erythema, itching, pain, or burning. Be alert for superinfection: increased fever, onset sore throat, nausea, vomiting, diarrhea, ulceration or changes of oral mucosa, anal/genital pruritus. Check liver function studies. Assess cultures of infection site. Monitor temperature for sign of infection.

---

rabeprazole

(Aciphex)
See Supplement

---

raloxifene

(Evista)
See Supplement

---

ramipril

ram-ih-prill
(Altace)

CANADIAN AVAILABILITY:
Altace

CLASSIFICATION

Antihypertensive

AVAILABILITY (Rx)

Capsules: 1.25 mg, 2.5 mg, 5 mg, 10 mg

PHARMACOKINETICS

	ONSET	PEAK	DURATION
PO	1–2 hrs	3–6 hrs	24 hrs

Well absorbed from GI tract. Metabolized in liver to active metabolite. Primarily excreted in urine. Half-life: 5.1 hrs.

ACTION/*THERAPEUTIC EFFECT*

Suppresses renin-angiotensin-aldosterone system. Decreases plasma angiotensin II, increases plasma renin activity, decreases aldosterone secretion. *Reduces peripheral arterial resistance.*

USES/*UNLABELED*

Treatment of hypertension. Used alone or in combination w/other antihypertensives. Treatment of CHF. *Treatment of hypertension/renal crisis in scleroderma. Prevention of heart attacks, stroke.*

PO ADMINISTRATION

1. May give w/o regard to food.
2. Do not chew or break capsules.
3. May mix w/water, apple juice/sauce.

INDICATIONS/DOSAGE/ROUTES

Hypertension (used alone):
PO: **Adults, elderly:** Initially, 2.5

mg/day. **Maintenance:** 2.5–20 mg/day as single or in 2 divided doses.

Hypertension (combination therapy):
Note: Discontinue diuretic 2–3 days before initiating ramipril therapy.
PO: Adults, elderly: Initially, 1.25 mg/day titrated to pt's needs.

CHF:
PO: Adults, elderly: Initially, 1.25–2.5 mg 2 times/day. **Maximum:** 5 mg 2 times/day.

Dosage in renal impairment (Ccr <40 ml/min; serum creatinine >2.5 mg/dl):
Initially, 1.25 mg/day titrated up to maximum of 5 mg/day.

PRECAUTIONS

CONTRAINDICATIONS: History of angioedema w/previous treatment w/ACE inhibitors. **CAUTIONS:** Renal impairment, those w/sodium depletion or on diuretic therapy, dialysis, hypovolemia, coronary/cerebrovascular insufficiency. **PREGNANCY/LACTATION:** Crosses placenta; is distributed in breast milk. May cause fetal/neonatal mortality/morbidity. **Pregnancy Category D**.

INTERACTIONS

DRUG INTERACTIONS: Alcohol, diuretics, hypotensive agents may increase effects. NSAIDs may decrease effect. Potassium-sparing diuretics, potassium supplements may cause hyperkalemia. May increase lithium concentration, toxicity. **ALTERED LAB VALUES:** May increase potassium, SGOT (AST), SGPT (ALT), alkaline phosphatase, bilirubin, BUN, creatinine. May decrease sodium. May cause positive ANA titer.

SIDE EFFECTS

FREQUENT (5–12%): Cough, headache. **OCCASIONAL (2–4%):** Dizziness, fatigue, nausea, asthenia (loss of strength). **RARE (<2%):** Palpitations, insomnia, nervousness, malaise, abdominal pain, myalgia.

ADVERSE REACTIONS/TOXIC EFFECTS

Excessive hypotension ("first-dose syncope") may occur in those w/CHF, severely salt/volume depleted. Angioedema (swelling of face/lips), hyperkalemia occur rarely. Agranulocytosis, neutropenia may be noted in those w/impaired renal function or collagen vascular disease (systemic lupus erythematosus, scleroderma). Nephrotic syndrome may be noted in those w/history of renal disease.

NURSING IMPLICATIONS
BASELINE ASSESSMENT:

Obtain B/P immediately before each dose, in addition to regular monitoring (be alert to fluctuations). If excessive reduction in B/P occurs, place pt in supine position w/legs elevated. Renal function tests should be performed before therapy begins. In those w/prior renal disease, urine test for protein by dipstick method should be made w/first urine of day before therapy begins and periodically thereafter. In those w/renal impairment, autoimmune disease, or taking drugs that affect leukocytes/immune response, CBC and differential count should be performed before therapy begins and q2 wks for 3 mos, then periodically thereafter.

INTERVENTION/EVALUATION:

Assess for cough (common effect). Assist w/ambulation if

dizziness occurs. Assess lung sounds for rales, wheezing in those w/CHF. Monitor urinalysis for proteinuria. Monitor serum potassium levels in those on concurrent diuretic therapy. Monitor pattern of daily bowel activity, stool consistency.

PATIENT/FAMILY TEACHING:

Report any sign of infection (sore throat, fever). Several weeks may be needed for full therapeutic effect of B/P reduction. Skipping doses or voluntarily discontinuing drug may produce severe, rebound hypertension. To reduce hypotensive effect, rise slowly from lying to sitting position and permit legs to dangle from bed momentarily before standing.

ranitidine
rah-**nih**-tih-deen
(Zantac)
ranitidine bismuth citrate
(Tritec)

CANADIAN AVAILABILITY:
Apo-Ranitidine, Novo-Ranidine, Zantac

CLASSIFICATION

Histamine H_2 receptor antagonist

AVAILABILITY (Rx)

Tablets: 75 mg **(OTC),** 150 mg, 300 mg. **Tablets (effervescent):** 150 mg. **Capsules:** 150 mg, 300 mg. **Syrup:** 15 mg/ml. **Granules (effervescent):** 150 mg. **Injection:** 25 mg/ml, 0.5 mg/ml, 100 ml infusion.

Bismuth citrate: Tablets: 400 mg.

PHARMACOKINETICS

Rapidly absorbed from GI tract. Widely distributed. Metabolized in liver. Primarily excreted in urine. Half-life: *Oral:* 2.5 hrs; *IV:* 2–2.5 hrs (increased in decreased renal function).

ACTION/*THERAPEUTIC EFFECT*

Inhibits histamine action at H_2 receptors of parietal cells, *inhibiting basal and nocturnal gastric acid secretion.*

USES/*UNLABELED*

Short-term treatment of active duodenal ulcer. Prevention of duodenal ulcer recurrence. Treatment of active benign gastric ulcer, pathologic GI hypersecretory conditions, acute gastroesophageal reflux disease (GERD) including erosive esophagitis. Maintenance of healed erosive esophagitis. *Bismuth citrate:* Treatment of duodenal ulcers associated w/*H. Pylori.* Prophylaxis of aspiration pneumonia.

STORAGE/HANDLING

Store tablets, syrup at room temperature. IV solutions appear clear, colorless to yellow (slight darkening does not affect potency). IV infusion (piggyback) is stable for 48 hrs at room temperature (discard if discolored or precipitate forms).

PO/IM/IV ADMINISTRATION
PO:

1. Give w/o regard to meals. Best given after meals or at bedtime.

2. Do not administer within 1 hr of magnesium- or aluminum-containing antacids (decreases absorption by 33%).

IM:

1. May be given undiluted.

R

2. Give deep IM into large muscle mass.

IV:

1. For direct IV, dilute w/20 ml NaCl or other compatible IV fluid. Administer over minimum of 5 min (prevents arrhythmias, hypotension).

2. For intermittent IV infusion (piggyback), dilute w/50 ml 0.9% NaCl, 5% dextrose, or other compatible IV fluid. Infuse over 15–20 min.

3. For IV infusion, dilute w/100–1,000 ml 0.9% NaCl, 5% dextrose solution. Infuse over 24 hrs.

INDICATIONS/DOSAGE/ROUTES

Active duodenal ulcer:
PO: Adults, elderly: 150 mg 2 times/day or 300 mg at bedtime. **Maintenance:** 150 mg at bedtime.

Pathologic hypersecretory conditions:
PO: Adults, elderly: 150 mg 2 times/day up to 6 g/day.

Benign gastric ulcer, GERD:
PO: Adults, elderly: 150 mg 2 times/day.

Erosive esophagitis:
PO: Adults, elderly: 150 mg 4 times/day. **Maintenance:** 150 mg 2 times/day.

H. Pylori *duodenal ulcer:*
PO: Adults, elderly: 400 mg 2 times/day for 28 days (days 1–14 w/clarithromycin).

Usual parenteral dosage:
IM/IV: Adults, elderly: 50 mg q6–8h. **Maximum:** 400 mg/day.
IV Infusion: Adults, elderly: 150 mg/day up to 2.5 mg/kg/hr (Zollinger-Ellison).

Dosage in renal impairment (creatinine clearance <50 ml/min):
PO: 150 mg q24h.
IM/IV: 50 mg q18–24h.

PRECAUTIONS

CONTRAINDICATIONS: None significant. **CAUTIONS:** Impaired renal/hepatic function, elderly. **PREGNANCY/LACTATION:** Unknown whether drug crosses placenta or is distributed in breast milk. **Pregnancy Category B**.

INTERACTIONS

DRUG INTERACTIONS: Antacids may decrease absorption (do not give within 1 hr). May decrease absorption of ketoconazole (give at least 2 hrs after). **ALTERED LAB VALUES:** Interferes w/skin tests using allergen extracts. May increase liver function tests, creatinine, gamma-glutamyl transpeptidase.

SIDE EFFECTS

OCCASIONAL (2%): Diarrhea. **RARE (1%):** Constipation, headache (may be severe).

ADVERSE REACTIONS/TOXIC EFFECTS

Reversible hepatitis, blood dyscrasias occur rarely.

NURSING IMPLICATIONS

BASELINE ASSESSMENT:

Do not confuse medication w/Xanax (alprazolam).

INTERVENTION/EVALUATION:

Monitor serum SGOT (AST), SGPT (ALT) levels. Assess mental status in elderly.

PATIENT/FAMILY TEACHING:

Smoking decreases effectiveness of medication. Do not take medicine within 1 hr of magnesium- or aluminum-containing antacids. Transient burning/itching may occur w/IV administration. Report headache. Avoid alcohol, aspirin.

rapacuronium
(Raplon)
See Classification section under:
Neuromuscular blockers

remifentanil hydrochloride
(Ultiva)
See Classification section under:
Opioid analgesics

repaglinide
(Prandin
See Supplement
See Classification section under:
Antidiabetics

respiratory syncytial virus immune globulin
(Respigam)
See Supplement

reteplase
(Retavase)
See Supplement
See Classification section under:
Anticoagulants, antiplatelets, thrombolytics

Rho (D) immune globulin IV
(WinRho SD)
See Supplement

ribavirin
rye-bah-**vi**-rin
(Virazole)

FIXED-COMBINATION(S):
W/interferon, alfa 2b (Rebetron)

CANADIAN AVAILABILITY:
Virazole

CLASSIFICATION
Antiviral

AVAILABILITY (Rx)
Powder for Reconstitution (Aerosol): 6 g/100 ml

PHARMACOKINETICS
Small amount systemically absorbed after inhalation. Rapidly absorbed from GI tract. Primarily distributed to plasma, respiratory tract secretions, RBCs. Metabolized in liver to active metabolite. Primarily excreted in urine. Half-life: 9.5 hrs.

ACTION / *THERAPEUTIC EFFECT*
Appears to be virustatic through disruption of RNA and DNA synthesis, *interfering with viral replication, protein synthesis.*

USES / *UNLABELED*
Severe lower respiratory tract infections due to respiratory syncytial viruses in select infants, children. *Treatment of influenza A or B.*

STORAGE / HANDLING
Solutions appear clear and colorless, are stable for 24 hrs at room temperature. Discard solutions for nebulization after 24 hrs. Discard if discolored or cloudy.

INHALATION ADMINISTRATION
Note: May be given via nasal or oral inhalation.
1. Add 50–100 ml sterile water for injection or inhalation to 6 g vial.
2. Transfer to a flask, serving as reservoir for aerosol generator.
3. Further dilute to final volume of 300 ml, giving a solution concentration of 20 mg/ml.
4. Use only aerosol generator available from manufacturer of drug.
5. Do not give concomitantly w/other drug solutions for nebulization.

R

6. Discard reservoir solution when fluid levels are low and at least q24h.

7. Controversy over safety in ventilator-dependent pts; only experienced personnel should administer.

INDICATIONS/DOSAGE/ROUTES

Severe lower respiratory tract infection caused by RSV.
Inhalation: Children, infants: Deliver mist containing 190 mcg/L at rate of 12.5 L of mist/min continuously for 12–18 hrs/day for 3–7 days.

PRECAUTIONS

CONTRAINDICATIONS: Hypersensitivity to drug, potential for pregnancy. CAUTIONS: Use care in assisted ventilation because of mechanical problems associated w/precipitate and "rainout" when fluid accumulates in tubing.

INTERACTIONS

DRUG INTERACTIONS: May have antagonistic effect w/zidovudine. ALTERED LAB VALUES: None significant.

SIDE EFFECTS

OCCASIONAL: Rash, conjunctivitis, reticulocytosis. RARE: Hypotension, digitalis toxicity.

ADVERSE REACTIONS/TOXIC EFFECTS

Cardiac arrest, apnea and ventilator dependence, bacterial pneumonia, pneumonia, pneumothorax occur rarely. If therapy exceeds 7 days, anemia may occur.

NURSING IMPLICATIONS
BASELINE ASSESSMENT:

Obtain respiratory tract secretions before giving first dose or at least during first 24 hrs of therapy. Assess respiratory status for baseline.

INTERVENTION/EVALUATION:

Monitor I&O, fluid balance carefully. Check hematology reports for anemia due to reticulocytosis when therapy exceeds 7 days. For ventilator-assisted pts watch for "rainout" in tubing and empty frequently; be alert to impaired ventilation and gas exchange due to drug precipitate. Assess skin for rash. Monitor B/P, respirations; assess lung sounds.

PATIENT/FAMILY TEACHING:

Therapy must be continued for full length of treatment. Report immediately any difficulty breathing, chest discomfort or itching/swelling/redness of eyes.

rifabutin
rye-fah-**byew**-tin
(Mycobutin)

CANADIAN AVAILABILITY:
Mycobutin

CLASSIFICATION

Antibacterial (antimycobacterial)

AVAILABILITY (Rx)

Capsules: 150 mg

PHARMACOKINETICS

Readily absorbed from GI tract (high-fat meals slow absorption). Widely distributed. Crosses blood-brain barrier. Extensive intracellular tissue uptake. Metabolized in liver to active metabolite. Excreted in urine; eliminated in feces. Half-life: 16–69 hrs.

ACTION/ *THERAPEUTIC EFFECT*

Inhibits DNA-dependent RNA polymerase, an enzyme in susceptible strains of *E. coli* and *Bacil-*

lus subtilis, preventing *M avium complex (MAC) disease*.

USES

Prevention of disseminated *Mycobacterium avium* complex (MAC) disease in those w/advanced HIV infection.

PO ADMINISTRATION

1. May take w/o regard to food. Give w/food to decrease GI irritation.

2. May mix w/applesauce if pt is unable to swallow capsules whole.

INDICATIONS/DOSAGE/ROUTES

MAC:
PO: Adults, elderly, adolescents: 300 mg/day as single dose or in two divided doses.

PRECAUTIONS

CONTRAINDICATIONS: Hypersensitivity to rifabutin, other rifamycins (e.g., rifampin). Active tuberculosis. **CAUTIONS:** Safety in children not established. **PREGNANCY/LACTATION:** Unknown whether drug crosses placenta or is excreted in breast milk. **Pregnancy Category B**.

INTERACTIONS

DRUG INTERACTIONS: May decrease effects of oral contraceptives. May decrease concentration of zidovudine (does not affect inhibition of HIV by zidovudine). **ALTERED LAB VALUES:** May increase SGOT (AST), SGPT (ALT), alkaline phosphatase. May cause anemia, neutropenia, leukopenia, thrombocytopenia.

SIDE EFFECTS

FREQUENT (>10%): Skin rash, red-orange/red-brown discoloration of urine, feces, saliva, skin, sputum, sweat, or tears. **OCCASIONAL (2–10%):** Arthralgia, altered taste, muscle pain, uveitis (eye pain, loss of vision), nausea, diarrhea, decreased appetite. **RARE (<2%):** Vomiting, insomnia.

ADVERSE REACTIONS/TOXIC EFFECTS

Hepatitis, thrombocytopenia occur rarely.

NURSING IMPLICATIONS
BASELINE ASSESSMENT:

Chest x-ray, sputum or blood cultures, biopsy of suspicious node must be done to rule out active tuberculosis (given in active tuberculosis may cause resistance to both rifabutin and rifampin). Obtain baseline CBC, platelets, differential count, hepatic function tests.

INTERVENTION/EVALUATION:

Monitor CBC, platelets, differential count. Avoid IM injections, rectal temperatures, other trauma that may induce bleeding. Check temperature and notify physician of flulike syndrome, rash, or GI intolerance. If jaundice occurs w/nausea, vomiting, and fatigue, may indicate hepatitis.

PATIENT/FAMILY TEACHING:

Urine, feces, saliva, sputum, perspiration, tears, skin may be discolored brown orange. Soft contact lenses may be permanently discolored. Rifabutin may decrease efficacy of oral contraceptives; nonhormonal methods should be considered. Avoid crowds, those w/infections. Notify physician immediately of signs and symptoms of MAC and tuberculosis: night sweats, fatigue, fever, weight loss, abdom-

R

inal pain. **Report any yellowing of skin or eyes.**

rifampin

rif-**am**-pin
(Rifadin, Rimactane)

FIXED-COMBINATION(S):
W/isoniazid, an antitubercular **(Rifamate);** w/isoniazid and pyrazinamide, antituberculars **(Rifater)**

CANADIAN AVAILABILITY:
Rifadin, Rimactane, Rofact

CLASSIFICATION

Antitubercular

AVAILABILITY (Rx)

Capsules: 150 mg, 300 mg. **Powder for Injection:** 600 mg.

PHARMACOKINETICS

Well absorbed from GI tract (food delays absorption). Widely distributed. Metabolized in liver to active metabolite. Primarily eliminated via biliary system. Not removed by hemodialysis. Half-life: 3–5 hrs.

ACTION/THERAPEUTIC EFFECT

Interferes bacterial RNA synthesis by binding to DNA-dependent RNA polymerase, preventing attachment of the enzyme to DNA, thereby blocking RNA transcription. *Bactericidal activity occurs in susceptible microorganisms.*

USES/UNLABELED

In conjunction w/at least one other antitubercular agent for initial treatment and retreatment of clinical tuberculosis. Eliminates *Neisseria* meningococci from the nasopharynx of asymptomatic carriers in situations w/high risk of meningococcal meningitis (prophylaxis, not cure). Recommended by WHO as adjunctive therapy w/dapsone for leprosy. *Prophylaxis of H. Influenza type b infection, treatment of atypical mycobacterial infection, serious infections caused by Staphylococcus species.*

STORAGE/HANDLING

Store capsules at room temperature. Reconstituted vial stable for 24 hrs. Use diluted solution within 4 hrs.

PO/IV ADMINISTRATION

PO:

1. Preferably give 1 hr before or 2 hrs after meals w/8 oz water (may give w/food to decrease GI upset; will delay absorption).
2. For those unable to swallow capsules, contents may be mixed w/applesauce, jelly.
3. Administer at least 1 hr before antacids, esp. those containing aluminum.

IV:

1. For IV infusion only. Avoid IM, SubQ administration.
2. Avoid extravasation (local irritation, inflammation).
3. Reconstitute 600 mg vial w/10 ml sterile water to provide concentration of 60 mg/ml.
4. Withdraw desired dose and further dilute w/500 ml 5% dextrose; infuse over 3 hrs (may dilute w/100 ml D_5W and infuse over 30 min).

INDICATIONS/DOSAGE/ROUTES

Tuberculosis:
IV/PO: Adults, elderly: 600 mg/day. **Children:** 10–20 mg/kg/day. **Maximum:** 600 mg/day.

Meningococcal carrier:
PO: Adults, elderly: 600 mg/day.
Children: 10–20 mg/kg/day. **Maximum:** 600 mg for 4 consecutive days.

PRECAUTIONS

CONTRAINDICATIONS: Hypersensitivity to rifampin or any rifamycin, intermittent therapy. **CAUTIONS:** Hepatic dysfunction, active/treated alcoholism. Dosage not established in children under 5 yrs of age. **PREGNANCY/LACTATION:** Crosses placenta; is distributed in breast milk. **Pregnancy Category C**.

INTERACTIONS

DRUG INTERACTIONS: Alcohol, hepatotoxic medications may increase risk of hepatotoxicity. May increase clearance of aminophylline, theophylline. May decrease effects of oral anticoagulants, oral hypoglycemics, chloramphenicol, digoxin, disopyramide, mexiletine, quinidine, tocainide, fluconazole, methadone, phenytoin, verapamil. **ALTERED LAB VALUES:** May increase SGOT (AST), SGPT (ALT), alkaline phosphatase, bilirubin, BUN, uric acid.

SIDE EFFECTS

EXPECTED: Red-orange/red-brown discoloration of urine, feces, saliva, skin, sputum, sweat, or tears. **OCCASIONAL (2–5%):** Hypersensitivity reaction (pruritus, flushing, rash). **RARE (1–2%):** Diarrhea, dyspepsia, nausea, fungal overgrowth (sore mouth/tongue).

ADVERSE REACTIONS/TOXIC EFFECTS

Hepatotoxicity (risk increased w/isoniazid combination), hepatitis, blood dyscrasias, Stevens-Johnson syndrome, antibiotic-associated colitis occur rarely.

NURSING IMPLICATIONS
BASELINE ASSESSMENT:

Question for hypersensitivity to rifampin, rifamycins. Assure collection of diagnostic specimens. Evaluate initial hepatic function and CBC results.

INTERVENTION/EVALUATION:

Assess IV site at least hourly during infusion; restart at another site at the first sign of irritation/inflammation. Monitor hepatic function tests and assess for hepatitis: jaundice, anorexia/nausea/vomiting, fatigue, weakness (hold rifampin and inform physician at once). Report hypersensitivity reactions promptly: any type skin eruption, pruritus, flulike syndrome w/high dosage. Monitor frequency, consistency of stools esp. w/potential for antibiotic-associated colitis. Evaluate mental status. Check for visual difficulties. Assess for dizziness, assist w/ambulation as needed. Monitor CBC results for blood dyscrasias and be alert for infection (fever, sore throat), bleeding/bruising, or unusual tiredness/weakness.

PATIENT/FAMILY TEACHING:

Do not skip doses, take full length of treatment (may take for months, years). Office visits, vision and lab tests are important part of treatment. Preferably take on empty stomach w/8 oz water 1 hr before or 2 hrs after meal (w/food if GI upset). Avoid alcohol during treatment. Do not take *any* other medications w/o consulting physician, including antacids; must take rifampin at least 1 hr before antacid. Urine, feces, sputum, sweat, tears may become red orange; soft contact lenses may be permanently stained. Notify physician of *any* new symptom, immediately for yellow eyes/skin, fatigue, weakness, nausea/vomiting, sore throat, fever, "flu," unusual bruising/bleeding. Be certain no vision difficulty, dizziness, or other impairment exists before driving, using machinery. If taking oral contraceptives check w/physician (reliability may be affected).

---

rifapentine
(Priftin)
See Supplement

---

rimantadine
rye-**man**-tah-deen
(Flumadine)

CLASSIFICATION

Antiviral

AVAILABILITY (Rx)

Tablets: 100 mg. **Syrup:** 50 mg/5 ml.

PHARMACOKINETICS

Readily absorbed from GI tract. Metabolized in liver. Primarily excreted in urine. Half-life: 20–65 hrs (increased in severe liver and/or renal impairment).

ACTION / *THERAPEUTIC EFFECT*

Exact mechanism unknown. Appears to exert inhibitory effect early in viral replication cycle. May inhibit uncoating of virus, *preventing replication of influenza A virus.*

USES

Adults: Prophylaxis and treatment of illness due to influenza A virus. *Children:* Prophylaxis against influenza A virus.

PO ADMINISTRATION:

May give w/o regard to food.

INDICATIONS/DOSAGE/ROUTES

Prophylaxis against influenza A virus:
PO: Adults, elderly, children >10 yrs: 100 mg 2 times/day. **Severe hepatic/renal impairment, elderly nursing home pts:** 100 mg/day. **Children <10 yrs:** 5 mg/kg once daily. **Maximum:** 150 mg.

Treatment of influenza virus A:
PO: Adults, elderly: 100 mg 2 times/day for 7 days. **Severe hepatic/renal impairment, elderly nursing home pts:** 100 mg/day for 7 days.

PRECAUTIONS

CONTRAINDICATIONS: Hypersensitivity to amantadine, rimantadine. **CAUTIONS:** Pts w/renal, liver impairment; history of seizures (increased incidence of seizures). **PREGNANCY/LACTATION:** Avoid use in nursing mothers. Potentially carcinogenic. Unknown whether drug crosses placenta or is excreted in breast milk. **Pregnancy Category C**.

INTERACTIONS

DRUG INTERACTIONS: Acetaminophen, aspirin may decrease concentrations. Cimetidine may increase concentrations. **ALTERED LAB VALUES:** None significant.

SIDE EFFECTS

OCCASIONAL (1–3%): Insomnia, dizziness, headache, nervousness, fatigue, asthenia. Nausea, vomiting, anorexia, dry mouth, abdominal pain. **RARE (<1%):** Diarrhea, dyspepsia, agitation, impaired concentration, ringing in ears, dyspnea.

ADVERSE REACTIONS/TOXIC EFFECTS

None significant.

NURSING IMPLICATIONS

INTERVENTION/EVALUATION:

Assess for nervousness and evaluate sleep pattern for insomnia. Provide assistance if dizziness occurs. Check food tolerance. When administering for illness, monitor temperature.

PATIENT/FAMILY TEACHING:

Avoid contact w/those who are at high risk for influenza A (rimantadine-resistant virus may be shed during therapy). Do not drive or perform tasks that require alert response if dizziness or decreased concentration occurs. Do not take aspirin, acetaminophen, or compounds containing these drugs.

---

risedronate
(Actonel)
See Supplement

---

risperidone
ris-**pear**-ih-doan
(**Risperdal**)

CANADIAN AVAILABILITY:
Risperdal

CLASSIFICATION

Antipsychotic

AVAILABILITY (Rx)

Tablets: 0.25 mg, 0.5 mg, 1 mg, 2 mg, 3 mg, 4 mg. **Oral Solution:** 1 mg/ml.

PHARMACOKINETICS

Well absorbed from GI tract (unaffected by food). Extensively metabolized in liver to active metabolite. Primarily excreted in urine. Half-life: 3–20 hrs; metabolite: 21–30 hrs (increased in elderly).

ACTION/*THERAPEUTIC EFFECT*

Exact mechanism unknown. Action may be due to dopamine and serotonin receptor antagonism. *Suppresses behavioral response in psychosis.*

USES

Management of manifestations of psychotic disorders.

PO ADMINISTRATION

May take w/o regard to food.

INDICATIONS/DOSAGE/ROUTES

Antipsychotic:
PO: Adults: Initially, 1 mg 2 times/day for 1 day; then, 2 mg 2 times/day for 1 day; then, 3 mg 2 times/day for 1 day. Further adjustments of 1 mg 2 times/day made at at least 1 wk intervals. Maximum effect in range of 4–6 mg/day. **Elderly, debilitated, pts w/severe liver/renal impairment, risk of hypotension:** Initially, 0.5 mg 2 times/day for 1 day; then, 1 mg 2 times/day for 1 day; then, 1.5 mg 2 times/day for 1 day. Further adjustments made at at least 1 wk intervals.

PRECAUTIONS

CONTRAINDICATIONS: Hypersensitivity to risperidone. **CAUTIONS:** Cardiac pts (e.g., history of MI, ischemia, CHF, conduction abnormality); pts w/cerebrovascular disease, dehydration, hypovolemia, use of antihypertensives. History of seizures. Safety in children unknown. May mask signs of drug overdose, intestinal obstruction. **PREGNANCY/LACTATION:** Unknown whether drug crosses placenta or is excreted in breast milk. Recommend against breastfeeding. **Pregnancy Category C**.

INTERACTIONS

DRUG INTERACTIONS: May decrease effects of levodopa, dopamine agonists. Carbamazepine may decrease concentration. Clozapine may increase concentration. Alcohol, CNS depressants may increase CNS depression. **ALTERED LAB VALUES:** May increase creatine phosphokinase, uric acid, triglycerides, SGOT (AST), SGPT (ALT), prolactin. May decrease potassium, sodium, protein, glucose. May cause EKG changes.

SIDE EFFECTS

FREQUENT (13–26%): Agitation, anxiety, insomnia, headache, constipation. **OCCASIONAL (4–10%):** Dyspepsia, rhinitis, drowsiness, dizziness, nausea, vomiting, rash, abdominal pain, dry skin, tachycardia. **RARE (2–3%):** Visual disturbances, fever, back pain, pharyngitis, cough, arthralgia, angina, aggressive reaction.

ADVERSE REACTIONS/TOXIC EFFECTS

Neuroleptic malignant syndrome (NMS): hyperpyrexia, muscle rigidity, change in mental status, irregular pulse or B/P, tachycardia, diaphoresis, cardiac dysrhythmias, elevated creatine phosphokinase, rhabdomyolysis, acute renal failure. Tardive dyskinesia: irreversible, involuntary, dyskinetic movements. Extension of action: drowsiness, sedation, tachycardia, hypotension, EPS.

NURSING IMPLICATIONS

BASELINE ASSESSMENT:

Renal and liver function tests should be done before therapy. Assess behavior, appearance, emotional status, response to environment, speech pattern, thought content.

INTERVENTION/EVALUATION:

Monitor for fine tongue movement (may be first sign of tardive dyskinesia, which may be irreversible: protrusion of tongue, puffing of cheeks, chewing/puckering of the mouth). Supervise suicidal risk pt closely during early therapy (as depression lessens, energy level improves, increasing suicide potential). Smallest prescription possible reduces risk of overdose. Assess for therapeutic response (greater interest in surroundings, improved self-care, increased ability to concentrate, relaxed facial expression). Monitor for potential NMS: fever, muscle rigidity, irregular B/P or pulse, altered mental status. Possible antiemetic effect may mask signs and symptoms of other conditions.

PATIENT/FAMILY TEACHING:

Change positions slowly to prevent hypotensive effect. Wear protective clothing, use sunscreens to protect from sunlight, ultraviolet light. Do not drive or perform tasks requiring alert response until assured that drug does not cause impairment. Consult physician before taking any other medications. Inform physician if become or plan to become pregnant; do not breast-feed.

ritodrine

rih-toe-dreen
(Yutopar)

CANADIAN AVAILABILITY:
Yutopar

CLASSIFICATION

Uterine relaxant

AVAILABILITY (Rx)

Injection: 10 mg/ml, 15 mg/ml

PHARMACOKINETICS

Undergoes first-pass metabolism. Metabolized in liver. Primarily excreted in urine. Removed by hemodialysis. Half-life: 15–17 hrs.

ACTION/ *THERAPEUTIC EFFECT*

Beta$_2$-adrenergic stimulant that relaxes uterine muscle, *suppresses uterine contractions.*

USES

To prolong gestation by inhibiting uterine contractions in preterm labor.

STORAGE/HANDLING

Stable for 48 hrs at room temperature after dilutions of 150 mg in 500 ml 0.9% NaCl or 5% dextrose in water. Do not use if discolored or if precipitate forms.

PO/IV ADMINISTRATION

IV:

    1. Hospitalization advised.
    2. Place pt in left lateral position to prevent hypotension.
    3. Dilute 15 ml of concentrate for injection (150 mg) in 500 ml of 5% dextrose injection (provides solution of 0.3 mg/ml). Because of potential for pulmonary edema, NaCl-containing solutions are used only when dextrose medically undesirable (e.g., diabetes mellitus).
    4. Use infusion device to carefully control rate of flow.

INDICATIONS/DOSAGE/ROUTES

Usual parenteral dosage:
IV Infusion: Adults: Initially, 0.05 mg/min (10 ml/hr); gradually increase by 0.05 mg/min (10 ml/hr) q10 min until desired result reached. **Range:** 0.15–0.35 mg/min (30–70 ml/hr). Continue for 12 hrs after uterine contractions cease.

PRECAUTIONS

CONTRAINDICATIONS: Before 20th week of pregnancy. Preexisting medical conditions for mother that would be adversely affected by the effects of ritodrine: cardiac arrhythmias, uncontrolled hypertension, bronchial asthma treated w/betamimetics or steroids, hypovolemia. When continuation of pregnancy is hazardous to mother or fetus: eclampsia, severe preeclampsia, antepartum hemorrhage, intrauterine fetal death, pulmonary hypertension, pheochromocytoma, hyperthyroidism, cardiac disease, chorioamnionitis, uncontrolled diabetes mellitus. W/injection, sulfite sensitivity (often w/aspirin sensitivity). **CAUTIONS:** Migraine headache, diabetes mellitus, concomitant use of potassium-depleting diuretics. **PREGNANCY/LACTATION:** Drug crosses placenta; unknown whether distributed in breast milk. **Pregnancy Category B.**

INTERACTIONS

DRUG INTERACTIONS: Beta-adrenergic blockers antagonize effects. Glucocorticoids enhance fetal lung maturity; may increase risk of pulmonary edema in

R

mother. **ALTERED LAB VALUES:**
May increase SGOT (AST), SGPT
(ALT), FFA, blood glucose, serum
insulin. May decrease potassium.

SIDE EFFECTS

FREQUENT: Increased maternal
and fetal heart rates widening maternal pulse pressure (80–100%);
palpitations (33%); nausea, vomiting, headache, erythema (10–15%).
OCCASIONAL (3–10%): Tremors,
jitteriness, chest pain/tightness, constipation, diarrhea, bloating, sweating, chills, weakness. *Neonate:*
Hypo/hyperglycemia, ileus, hypocalcemia, hypotension. **RARE:** Impaired liver function.

ADVERSE REACTIONS/TOXIC EFFECTS

Ketoacidosis occurs infrequently.
Pulmonary edema (may be fatal,
esp. w/preexisting cardiopulmonary disease or concomitant
use of corticosteroids), anaphylactic shock, hepatitis occur rarely.

NURSING IMPLICATIONS
BASELINE ASSESSMENT:

Question for hypersensitivity
to ritodrine, sulfite, or aspirin.
Assess baselines for temperature, pulse, respiration, B/P, glucose and potassium levels, EKG,
fetal heart rate. Check lungs, determine hydration status. Determine frequency, duration, and
strength of contractions.

INTERVENTION/EVALUATION:

Take temperature at start and
conclusion of IV infusion. B/P,
pulse, respirations, and fetal
heart rate are monitored every
15 min until stable, then hourly
until infusion complete. Check
uterine contractions frequently
throughout the infusion. Assess
lungs for rales; pay particular attention to evidence of impending pulmonary edema (persistent tachycardia, fluid retention
[I&O], increased respiratory
rate/shortness of breath). Monitor potassium and glucose levels. Evaluate for palpitations,
chest pain/tightness, nausea/
vomiting, headache, jitteriness.

PATIENT/FAMILY TEACHING:

Keep pt, family informed of
therapeutic response during infusion. Explain importance of left
lateral position during IV infusion.

ritonavir
rih-**tone**-ah-vir
(Norvir)

CANADIAN AVAILABILITY:
Norvir

CLASSIFICATION
Antiviral

AVAILABILITY (Rx)
Soft Gelatin Capsules: 100 mg.
Oral Solution: 80 mg/ml.

PHARMACOKINETICS

Slowly absorbed following oral
administration (extent of absorption
increased with food). Extensively
metabolized by liver to active
metabolite. Primarily eliminated in
feces. Half-life: 2.7–5 hrs.

ACTION/ THERAPEUTIC EFFECT

Inhibits HIV-1 and HIV-2 proteas-
es, rendering the enzymes incapable of processing the polypep-
tide precursor that leads to
production of immature HIV particles, *slowing HIV replication, reducing progression of HIV infection.*

USES

Used in combination w/nucleoside analogues or as monotherapy for treatment of HIV infection.

STORAGE/HANDLING

Store capsules, solution in refrigerator. Protect from light. Refrigeration of oral solution by pt is recommended but not necessary if used within 30 days and stored below 77°F.

PO ADMINISTRATION

1. May give w/o regard to meals (preferably give w/food).

2. May improve taste of oral solution by mixing w/chocolate milk, Ensure, or Advera within 1 hr of dosing.

INDICATIONS/DOSAGE/ROUTES

HIV infection:
PO: Adults: 600 mg 2 times/day. If nausea becomes apparent upon initiation of 600 mg twice daily, give 300 mg twice daily for 1 day, 400 mg twice daily for 2 days, 500 mg twice daily for 1 day, then 600 mg twice daily thereafter.
Children: 400 mg/m^2 twice daily.
Maximum: 600 mg twice daily.

PRECAUTIONS

CONTRAINDICATIONS: Hypersensitivity to drug; amiodarone, astemizole, bepridil, bupropion, cisapride, clozapine, encainide, flecainide, meperidine, piroxicam, propafenone, propoxyphene, quinidine, rifabutin, and terfenadine increase risk of arrhythmias, hematologic abnormalities, seizures. Alprazolam, clorazepate, diazepam, estrazolam, flurazepam, midazolam, triazolam and zolpidem may produce extreme sedation and respiratory depression. **CAUTIONS:** Impaired hepatic function. **PREGNANCY/LACTATION:** Breast-feeding not recommended (possibility of HIV transmission). **Pregnancy Category B.**

INTERACTIONS

DRUG INTERACTIONS: May produce disulfiramlike reaction if taken w/disulfiram or drugs causing disulfiramlike reaction (e.g., metronidazole). Enzyme inducers (e.g., nevirapine, phenobarbital, carbamazepine, dexamethasone, phenytoin, rifampin, rifabutin) may increase metabolism, decrease efficacy. May decrease effectiveness of theophylline, oral contraceptives. May increase concentration of desipramine, other antidepressants. Cisapride may cause serious arrhythmias. **ALTERED LAB VALUES:** May alter SGPT (ALT), SGOT (AST), creatinine clearance, GGT, CPK, uric acid, triglycerides.

SIDE EFFECTS

FREQUENT: GI disturbances (nausea, diarrhea, vomiting, anorexia, abdominal pain), neurologic disturbances (taste perversion, circumoral and peripheral paresthesias), headache, dizziness, paresthesia (esp. around lips, hands, or feet), fatigue, weakness. **OCCASIONAL:** Allergic reaction, flu syndrome, hypotension.

ADVERSE REACTIONS/TOXIC EFFECTS

Numerous body system effects may occur (<2%).

NURSING IMPLICATIONS

BASELINE ASSESSMENT:

Pts beginning combination therapy w/ritonavir and nucleosides may promote GI tolerance by beginning ritonavir alone and subsequently adding nucleosides before completing 2 wks of ritonavir monotherapy. Obtain baseline laboratory testing, esp. liver function tests, triglycerides before beginning ritonavir thera-

R

py and at periodic intervals during therapy. Offer emotional support. Obtain medication history.

INTERVENTION/EVALUATION:

Closely monitor for evidence of GI disturbances or neurologic abnormalities (particularly paresthesias). Monitor clinical chemistry tests for marked laboratory abnormalities.

PATIENT/FAMILY TEACHING:

Continue therapy for full length of treatment. Doses should be evenly spaced. Do not take any medications, including OTC drugs, w/o consulting physician (many interacting medications). Ritonavir is not a cure for HIV infection, nor does it reduce risk of transmission to others. Pts may continue to acquire illnesses associated w/advanced HIV infection. If possible, take ritonavir w/food. Taste of solution may be mixed w/chocolate, Ensure, or Advera.

rituximab
(Rituxan)
See Supplement

rizatriptan
(Maxalt)
See Supplement

rocuronium bromide
(Zemuron)
See Classification section under: Neuromuscular blockers

rofecoxib
(Vioxx)
See Supplement

ropinirole
(Requip)
See Supplement

rizatriptan
(Maxalt)
See Supplement

rosiglitazone
(Avandia)
See Supplement
See Classification section under: Antidiabetic

sacrosidase
(Sucraid)
See Supplement

salicylate salts
sal-**ih**-sah-late

choline salicylate
(Arthropan)

magnesium salicylate
(Magan, Mobidin)

sodium salicylate
(Trilisate combination)

CLASSIFICATION

Nonsteroidal anti-inflammatory

AVAILABILITY (OTC)

Choline: Liquid: 870 mg/5 ml
Magnesium: Caplets: 325 mg, 500 mg. **Tablets (Rx):** 545 mg, 600 mg.
Sodium: Tablets: 325 mg, 650 mg

PHARMACOKINETICS

Rapidly, completely absorbed from GI tract. Hydrolyzed in GI tract, liver, blood; further metabolized in liver. Primarily excreted in urine. Removed by hemodialysis. Half-life: dose dependent (*low dose:* 2–3 hrs; *high dose:* 20 hrs).

ACTION/*THERAPEUTIC EFFECT*

Produces analgesic and anti-inflammatory effect by inhibiting prostaglandin synthesis, *reducing inflammatory response and intensity of pain stimulus reaching sensory nerve endings.* Antipyresis produced by drug's effect on hypothalamus, producing vasodilation, *decreasing elevated body temperature.*

USES

Relieves mild to moderate musculoskeletal, arthritic pain of low to moderate intensity; reduces fever.

PO ADMINISTRATION

1. May give w/food, milk, or antacids if GI distress occurs.

2. Choline salicylate may be mixed w/water, fruit juice, carbonated beverage to mask taste (do not mix w/antacid).

INDICATIONS/DOSAGE/ROUTES
ANALGESIC, ANTIPYRETIC:

Choline salicylate:
PO: Adults, elderly, children >11 yrs: 2.5–5 ml q4h as needed. **Children, 2–11 yrs:** 11.5 ml/m^2/day in 4–6 divided doses.

Magnesium salicylate:
PO: Adults, elderly, children >11 yrs: 300–600 mg q4h as needed. **Children, 2–11 yrs:** 150–450 mg q4h as needed.

Sodium salicylate:
PO: Adults, elderly, children >11 yrs: 325–650 mg q4h as needed.

Children, 2–11 yrs: 25–50 mg/kg/day in 4–6 divided doses.

RHEUMATOID ARTHRITIS, OSTEOARTHRITIS, INFLAMMATORY CONDITIONS:

Choline salicylate:
PO: Adults, elderly: 5–10 ml up to 20–40 ml/day in divided doses. **Children:** 0.6–0.8 ml/kg/day in divided doses.

Magnesium salicylate:
PO: Adults, elderly: 545–1,200 mg 3–4 times/day.

Sodium salicylate:
PO: Adults, elderly: 3.6–5.4 g/day in divided doses. **Children:** 80–100 mg/kg/day up to 130 mg/kg/day in divided doses.

PRECAUTIONS

CONTRAINDICATIONS: Chicken pox or flu in children/teenagers, GI bleeding/ulceration, bleeding disorders, history of hypersensitivity to aspirin/NSAIDs, impaired hepatic function. **CAUTIONS:** Vitamin K deficiency, chronic renal insufficiency, those w/"aspirin triad" (rhinitis, nasal polyps, asthma). **PREGNANCY/LACTATION:** Readily crosses placenta, is distributed in breast milk. Avoid use during last trimester (may adversely affect fetal cardiovascular system: premature closure of ductus arteriosus). **Pregnancy Category C**.

INTERACTIONS

DRUG INTERACTIONS: Alcohol, NSAIDs may increase risk of GI effects (e.g., ulceration). Urinary alkalinizer, antacids increase excretion. Anticoagulants, heparin, thrombolytics increase risk of bleeding. Large dose may increase effect of insulin, oral hypoglycemics. Valproic acid, platelet aggregation inhibitors may increase risk of bleeding. May increase toxicity of methotrexate, zidovudine. Ototoxic medications, vancomycin may increase ototoxicity. May decrease effect of probenecid, sulfinpyrazone. **ALTERED LAB VALUES:** May alter SGOT (AST), SGPT (ALT), alkaline phosphatase, uric acid; prolong prothrombin time, bleeding time. May decrease cholesterol, potassium, T_3, T_4.

SIDE EFFECTS

FREQUENT (5–25%): Nausea, dyspepsia. **OCCASIONAL (1–5%):** Heartburn, loss of appetite, epigastric distress, thirst.

ADVERSE REACTIONS/TOXIC EFFECTS

High doses may produce GI bleeding and/or gastric mucosal lesions. Low-grade toxicity characterized by ringing in ears, generalized pruritus (may be severe), decreased hearing ability, headache, dizziness, flushing, tachycardia, hyperventilation, sweating, thirst. Febrile, dehydrated children can reach toxic levels quickly. Marked intoxication may be manifested by hyperthermia, restlessness, abnormal breathing pattern, convulsions, respiratory failure, coma.

NURSING IMPLICATIONS
BASELINE ASSESSMENT:

Do not give to children/teenagers who have flu/chicken pox (increases risk of Reye's syndrome). Assess onset, type, location, and duration of pain, fever, or inflammation. Inspect appearance of affected joints for immobility, deformities, and skin condition.

INTERVENTION/EVALUATION:

In long-term therapy, monitor plasma salicylic acid concentration. Monitor urinary pH (sudden acidification [pH from 6.5 to 5.5] may result in toxicity). Assess skin for evidence of bruising. If given as an antipyretic, assess temperature directly before and 1 hr after giving medication. Evaluate for therapeutic response: relief of pain/stiffness/swelling, increase in joint mobility, reduced joint tenderness, improved grip strength.

PATIENT/FAMILY TEACHING:

Take w/food if GI distress is noted. Minimize or avoid other NSAIDs, alcohol during therapy (increases possibility of GI irritation). Report ringing in ears, persistent GI pain.

salmeterol

sal-**met**-er-all
(Serevent, Serevent Diskus)

CANADIAN AVAILABILITY:
Serevent

CLASSIFICATION

Bronchodilator

AVAILABILITY (Rx)

Aerosol. Aerosol Powder: 50 mcg.

PHARMACOKINETICS

ONSET	PEAK	DURATION
Inhalation		
10–20 min	3 hrs	12 hrs

Primarily acts in lung; low systemic absorption. Metabolized by hydroxylation. Primarily eliminated in feces. Half-life: 5.5 hrs.

ACTION/*THERAPEUTIC EFFECT*

Stimulates beta$_2$-adrenergic receptors resulting in relaxation of bronchial smooth muscle, *relieving bronchospasm; reduces airway resistance.*

USES

Maintenance treatment for asthma, bronchospasm associated w/COPD. Prevention of exercise-induced bronchospasm, bronchospasm in pts w/reversible obstructive airway disease.

INHALATION ADMINISTRATION

1. Shake container well, then remove cap from mouthpiece.
2. Position mouthpiece to bottom, tilt head back.
3. Breathe out through mouth to functional volume.
4. Place mouthpiece in mouth or hold 1–2 inches away from open mouth.
5. Activate inhaler while breathing in slowly and deeply.
6. Hold breath 5–10 secs (or as long as possible).
7. Remove inhaler from mouth and breathe out slowly.
8. Wait 1–10 min before second inhalation.

INDICATIONS/DOSAGE/ROUTES

Maintenance of bronchodilation, prevention of asthma symptoms:
Inhalation: Adults, elderly, children >4 yrs: 1 50 mcg inhalation 2 times/day, morning and evening about 12 hrs apart.

Prevention of exercise-induced bronchospasm:
Inhalation: Adults, elderly, children >4 yrs: 1 50 mcg inhalation at least 30–60 min before exercise.

Long-term maintenance tx of COPD-induced bronchospasm:
Inhalation: Adults: 2 inhalations q12hrs.

PRECAUTIONS

CONTRAINDICATIONS: History of hypersensitivity to salmeterol. **CAUTIONS:** Not for acute symptoms. May cause paradoxical bronchospasm. Pts w/cardiovascular disorders (e.g., coronary insufficiency, arrhythmias, hypertension), seizure disorder, thyrotoxicosis. Safety in children <12 yrs not known. **PREGNANCY/LACTATION:** Unknown whether excreted in breast milk. **Pregnancy Category C.**

INTERACTIONS

DRUG INTERACTIONS: May decrease effects of beta-adrenergic blockers. **ALTERED LAB VALUES:** May decrease serum potassium levels.

SIDE EFFECTS

FREQUENT (28%): Headache. **OCCASIONAL (≤3–7%):** Cough, tremor, dizziness, vertigo, throat dryness/irritation, pharyngitis. **RARE (<3%):** Palpitations, tachycardia, shakiness, nausea, heartburn, GI distress.

ADVERSE REACTIONS/TOXIC EFFECTS

Tachycardia, arrhythmias, tremor, headache, muscle cramps. May prolong QT interval (may lead to ventricular arrhythmias). May cause hypokalemia, hyperglycemia.

NURSING IMPLICATIONS

INTERVENTION/EVALUATION:

Monitor rate, depth, rhythm, tape of respiration; quality and rate of pulse, B/P. Assess lungs for wheezing, rales, rhonchi. Periodically evaluate potassium levels.

PATIENT/FAMILY TEACHING:

Not for relief of acute episodes. Keep canister at room temperature (cold decreases effects). Teach pt correct use of aerosol. Do not stop medication or exceed recommended dosage. Notify physician promptly of chest pain, dizziness, or failure to respond to medication. Wait at least one full minute before second inhalation. Administer dose 30 to 60 min before exercise when used to prevent exercise-induced bronchospasm. Avoid excessive use of caffeine derivatives: coffee, tea, colas, chocolate.

salsalate

sal-sah-late
(Disalcid, Mono-Gesic)

CANADIAN AVAILABILITY: Disalcid

CLASSIFICATION

Nonsteroidal anti-inflammatory

AVAILABILITY (Rx)

Capsules: 500 mg. **Tablets:** 500 mg, 750 mg.

PHARMACOKINETICS

Rapidly, completely absorbed from GI tract. Hydrolyzed in GI tract, liver, blood; further metabolized in liver. Primarily excreted in urine. Removed by hemodialysis. Half-life: dose dependent (*low dose:* 7–8 hrs; *high dose:* 15–30 hrs).

ACTION/ *THERAPEUTIC EFFECT*

Produces analgesic, anti-inflammatory effect by inhibiting prostaglandin synthesis, reducing inflammatory response and intensity of pain stimulus reaching sensory nerve endings.

USES

Symptomatic treatment of acute and/or chronic rheumatoid arthritis and osteoarthritis, related inflammatory conditions.

PO ADMINISTRATION

Give w/food/large amount of water.

INDICATIONS/DOSAGE/ROUTES

Rheumatoid arthritis, osteoarthritis:
PO: Adults, elderly: Initially: 3 g/day in 2–3 divided doses. **Maintenance:** 2–4 g/day.

PRECAUTIONS

CONTRAINDICATIONS: History of hypersensitivity to salicylates; chicken pox/flu in children/teenagers. **CAUTIONS:** None significant. **PREGNANCY/LACTATION:** Avoid use during last trimester (may adversely affect fetal cardiovascular system: premature closure of ductus arteriosus). **Pregnancy Category C.**

INTERACTIONS

DRUG INTERACTIONS: Alcohol, NSAIDs may increase risk of GI effects (e.g., ulceration). Urinary alkalinizers, antacids increase excretion. Anticoagulants, heparin, thrombolytics increase risk of bleeding. Large dose may increase effect of insulin, oral hypoglycemics. Valproic acid, platelet aggregation inhibitors may increase risk of bleeding. May increase toxicity of methotrexate, zidovudine. Ototoxic medications, vancomycin may increase ototoxicity. May decrease effect of probenecid, sulfinpyrazone. **ALTERED LAB VALUES:** May alter SGOT (AST), SGPT (ALT), alkaline phosphatase, uric acid; prolong prothrombin time, bleeding time. May decrease cholesterol, potassium, T_3, T_4.

SIDE EFFECTS

OCCASIONAL: Nausea, dyspepsia (heartburn, indigestion, epigastric pain).

ADVERSE REACTIONS/TOXIC EFFECTS

Tinnitus may be first sign that blood salicylic acid concentration is reaching/exceeding upper therapeutic range. May also produce vertigo, headache, confusion, drowsiness, sweating, hyperventilation, vomiting, diarrhea. Severe overdosage may result in electrolyte imbalance, hyperthermia, dehydration, blood pH imbalance. Low incidence of GI bleeding, peptic ulcer.

NURSING IMPLICATIONS

BASELINE ASSESSMENT:

Do not give to children/teenagers who have flu/chicken pox (increases risk of Reye's syndrome). Assess type, location, duration of pain, inflammation. Inspect appearance of affected joints for immobility, deformities, and skin condition.

INTERVENTION/EVALUATION:

Monitor pattern of daily bowel activity, stool consistency. Assess skin for evidence of bruising. Check behind medial malleolus for evidence of fluid retention. Assess for evidence of nausea, dyspepsia. Evaluate for therapeutic response: relief of pain/stiffness/swelling, increase in joint mobility, reduced joint tenderness, improved grip strength.

PATIENT/FAMILY TEACHING:

Do not crush/chew capsules or film-coated tablets. Avoid antacids (decreases drug effectiveness). Report ringing in ears, persistent GI pain. Avoid alcohol.

saquinavir mesylate

sah-**quin**-ah-vir
(Fortovase, Invirase)

CANADIAN AVAILABILTY:
Invirase

CLASSIFICATION

Antiviral

AVAILABILITY (Rx)

Capsules, Soft Gelatin Capsules: 200 mg

PHARMACOKINETICS

Poorly absorbed following oral administration (high-caloric/high-fat meal increases absorption). Metabolized in liver to inactive metabolite. Primarily eliminated in feces.

ACTION/*THERAPEUTIC EFFECT*

Inhibits HIV protease, rendering the enzyme incapable of processing the polyprotein precursor to generate functional proteins in HIV-infected cells, *slowing HIV replication, reducing progression of HIV infection.*

USES

Used in combination w/nucleoside analogues for treatment of advanced HIV infection in selected pts.

PO ADMINISTRATION

Give within 2 hrs after a full meal (if taken w/o food in stomach, may result in no antiviral activity).

INDICATIONS/DOSAGE/ROUTES

Note: Complete prescribing information for saquinavir should be consulted before concurrent therapy w/zidovudine (AZT), zalcitabine (ddC).

HIV infection (combination therapy):

PO: Adults, elderly: Fortovase: 1,200 mg 3 times/day. Saquinavir: Three 200 mg capsules given 3 times daily within 2 hrs after a full meal. Do not give <600 mg/day (does not produce antiviral activity). Recommended daily doses of ddC or AZT: ddC 0.75 mg 3 times daily; AZT 200 mg 3 times daily.

PRECAUTIONS

CONTRAINDICATIONS: Clinically significant hypersensitivity to drug. **CAUTIONS:** Impaired hepatic function. **PREGNANCY/LACTATION:** Breast-feeding not recommended (possibility of HIV transmission). **Pregnancy Category B.**

INTERACTIONS

DRUG INTERACTIONS: Ketoconazole increases saquinavir concentration. Rifampin, phenobarbital, phenytoin, dexamethasone, carbamazepine may reduce saquinavir plasma concentration. May increase terfenadine, astemizole, calcium channel blockers, clindamycin, dapsone, quinidine, triazolam plasma concentrations. **ALTERED LAB VALUES:** May elevate serum transaminase, lower glucose level, alter CPK. **FOOD:** Grapefruit juice may increase saquinavir concentrations.

SIDE EFFECTS

OCCASIONAL: Diarrhea, abdominal discomfort or pain, nausea, photosensitivity, buccal mucosa ulceration. **RARE:** Confusion, ataxia, weakness, headache, rash.

ADVERSE REACTIONS/TOXIC EFFECTS

None significant.

NURSING IMPLICATIONS

BASELINE ASSESSMENT:

Obtain baseline laboratory testing, esp. liver function tests, before beginning saquinavir therapy and at periodic intervals during therapy. Offer emotional support. Obtain medication history.

INTERVENTION/EVALUATION:

Closely monitor for evidence of GI discomfort. Monitor stool frequency and consistency (watery, loose, soft). Inspect mouth for signs of mucosal ulceration. Monitor clinical chemistry tests for marked laboratory abnormalities. If serious or severe toxicities occur, interrupt therapy, contact physician.

PATIENT/FAMILY TEACHING:

Continue therapy for full length of treatment. Doses should be evenly spaced. Do not take any medications, including OTC drugs, w/o consulting physician. Saquinavir is not a cure for HIV infection, nor does it reduce risk of transmission to others. Pts may continue to acquire illnesses associated w/advanced HIV infection. Take within 2 hrs after a full meal. Take protective measures against exposure to ultraviolet or sunlight (i.e., sunscreens, protective clothing) until tolerance is established. Avoid coadministration w/grapefruit products.

---

sargramostim

sar-gra-**moh**-stim
(Leukine, Prokine)

CLASSIFICATION

Colony-stimulating factor

AVAILABILITY (Rx)

Powder for Injection: 250 mcg, 500 mcg. **Liquid for Injection:** 500 mcg/ml.

PHARMACOKINETICS

Half-life: *IV:* 2 hrs; *SubQ:* 3 hrs.

ACTION / THERAPEUTIC EFFECT

Stimulates proliferation/differentiation of hematopoietic cells to activate mature granulocytes and macrophages, *assisting bone marrow in making new WBCs.* Chemotactic, antifungal, and antiparasite activities increase. Increases cytotoxicity of monocytes to certain neoplastic cells; *activates neutrophils to inhibit tumor cell growth.*

USES / UNLABELED

Accelerates myeloid recovery in pt w/non-Hodgkin's lymphoma, acute lymphoblastic leukemia, and Hodgkin's disease undergoing autologous bone marrow transplantation. Used in pts w/allogenic or autologous bone marrow transplantation where engraftment is delayed or has failed. Shortens time of neutrophil recovery following induction chemotherapy in pts w/AML. Mobilizes autologous peripheral blood progenitor cells (PBPC) following induction of chemotherapy in pt >55 yrs w/acute myelogenous leukemia; used in myeloid reconstitution after allogenic bone marrow transplantation. *Treatment of AIDS-related neutropenia; chronic, severe neutropenia, drug-induced neutropenia; myelodysplastic syndrome.*

STORAGE / HANDLING

Refrigerate powder, reconstituted solution, diluted solution for injection. Do not shake. Do not use past expiration date. Reconstituted solutions are clear, colorless. Use within 6 hrs; discard unused portions. Use 1 dose/vial; do not reenter vial.

IV ADMINISTRATION

1. To 250 mcg/500 mcg vial, add 1 ml sterile water for injection (preservative free).

2. Direct sterile water to side of vial, gently swirl contents to avoid foaming; do not shake/vigorously agitate.

3. After reconstitution, further dilute w/0.9% NaCl. If final concentration <10 mcg/ml, add 1 mg albumin/ml 0.9% NaCl to provide a final albumin concentration of 0.1%. **Note:** Albumin is added before addition of sargramostim (prevents drug adsorption to components of drug delivery system).

4. Administer within 6 hrs of preparation/dilution.

5. Monitor for supraventricular arrhythmias during administration (particularly in those w/history of cardiac arrhythmias).

6. Assess closely for dyspnea during and immediately following infusion (particularly in those w/history of lung disease). If dyspnea occurs during infusion, cut infusion rate by half. If dyspnea continues, stop infusion immediately.

7. If neutrophil count exceeds 20,000 cells/mm^3 or platelet count exceeds 500,000/mm^3, stop infusion or reduce dose by half, based on clinical condition of pt.

INDICATIONS / DOSAGE / ROUTES

Note: Administer by IV infusion.

Usual parenteral dosage:
IV Infusion: Adults, elderly: 250 mcg/m^2/day for 21 days (as a 2 hr infusion). Begin 2–4 hrs after autologous bone marrow infusion and not less than 24 hrs after last dose

of chemotherapy or not less than 12 hrs after last radiation treatment. Discontinue if blast cells appear or underlying disease progresses.

Bone marrow transplantation failure/engraftment delay:
IV Infusion: Adults, elderly: 250 mcg/m²/day for 14 days. Infuse over 2 hrs. May repeat after 7 days of therapy if engraftment not occurred w/500 mcg/m²/day for 14 days.

Mobilization or post PBPC transplant:
IV/SubQ: Adults: 250 mcg/m²/day.

Allogeneic transplantation:
IV Infusion: Adults: 250 mcg/m²/day × 21 days starting 2–4 hrs after bone marrow infusion and not less than 24 hrs after last chemotherapy dose or 12 hrs after last radiation dose.

PRECAUTIONS

CONTRAINDICATIONS: Excessive leukemic myeloid blasts in bone marrow/peripheral blood (greater than/equal to 10%), known hypersensitivity to GM-CSF, yeast-derived products, any component of drug, 24 hrs before/after chemotherapy, 12 hrs before/after radiation therapy. **CAUTIONS:** Preexisting cardiac disease, hypoxia, preexisting fluid retention, pulmonary infiltrates, CHF, impaired renal/hepatic function. **PREGNANCY/LACTATION:** Unknown whether drug crosses placenta or is distributed in breast milk. **Pregnancy Category C.**

INTERACTIONS

DRUG INTERACTIONS: Lithium, steroids may increase effect. **ALTERED LAB VALUES:** May decrease albumin. May increase bilirubin, creatinine, liver enzymes.

SIDE EFFECTS

FREQUENT: GI disturbances, (nausea, diarrhea, vomiting, stomatitis, anorexia, abdominal pain), arthralgia/myalgia, headache, malaise, rash, pruritus. **OCCASIONAL:** Peripheral edema, weight gain, dyspnea, asthenia (loss of strength), fever, leukocytosis, capillary leak syndrome (e.g., fluid retention, irritation at local injection site, peripheral edema). **RARE:** Rapid/irregular heartbeat, thrombophlebitis.

ADVERSE REACTIONS/TOXIC EFFECTS

Pleural/pericardial effusion occurs rarely following infusion.

NURSING IMPLICATIONS
BASELINE ASSESSMENT:

Assess renal, hepatic function tests before initial therapy and biweekly. Note that excessive blood counts return to normal or baseline 3–7 days after discontinuation of therapy. Obtain baseline weight.

INTERVENTION/EVALUATION:

Monitor urinalysis reports, alkaline phosphatase, serum creatinine, bilirubin, SGOT (AST), SGPT (ALT) levels, CBC w/differential diligently. Monitor body weight. Assess for peripheral edema, particularly behind medial malleolus (usually first area showing peripheral edema), skin turgor, mucous membranes for hydration status. Note skin temperature, moisture. Assess muscle strength. Monitor daily bowel activity, stool consistency (watery, loose, soft, semi-solid, solid). **Assess injection site for redness, irritation.**

scopolamine
(Scopolamine, Transderm Scop)
See Supplement

scopolamine bromide
(Isopto Hyoscine)
See Classification section under: Anticholinergics

secobarbital sodium
(Seconal)
See Classification section under: Sedative-hypnotics

selegiline hydrochloride

sell-**eh**-geh-leen
(Eldepryl)

CANADIAN AVAILABILITY:
Eldepryl, Novo-Selegiline

CLASSIFICATION
Antiparkinson

AVAILABILITY (Rx)
Capsules: 5 mg. **Tablets:** 5 mg.

PHARMACOKINETICS
Rapidly absorbed from GI tract. Crosses blood-brain barrier. Metabolized in liver to active metabolites. Primarily excreted in urine. Half-life: 16–69 hrs.

ACTION / *THERAPEUTIC EFFECT*
Irreversibly inhibits monoamine oxidase type B activity. Increases dopaminergic action, *assisting in reduction in tremor, akinesia (absence of sense of movement), posture and equilibrium disorders, rigidity of parkinsonism.*

USES
Adjunctive to levodopa/carbidopa in treatment of Parkinson's disease.

PO ADMINISTRATION
May be given w/meals.

INDICATIONS/DOSAGE/ROUTES
Note: Therapy should begin w/lowest dosage, then be increased in gradual increments over 3–4 wks.

Parkinsonism:
PO: **Adults:** 10 mg/day in divided doses (5 mg at breakfast and lunch). **Elderly:** Initially, 5 mg in morning. May increase up to 10 mg/day.

PRECAUTIONS
CONTRAINDICATIONS: None significant. **CAUTIONS:** History of peptic ulcer disease, dementia, psychosis, tardive dyskinesia, profound tremor. Cardiac dysrhythmias. **PREGNANCY/LACTATION:** Unknown whether drug crosses placenta or is distributed in breast milk. **Pregnancy Category C.**

INTERACTIONS
DRUG INTERACTIONS: Fluoxetine may cause mania, serotonin syndrome (mental changes, restlessness, diaphoresis, diarrhea, fever). Meperidine may cause a potentially fatal reaction (e.g., excitation, sweating, rigidity, hypertension or hypotension, coma, and death). Tyramine-rich foods may produce hypertensive reactions. **ALTERED LAB VALUES:** None significant.

SIDE EFFECTS
FREQUENT (>3%): Nausea, dizziness, lightheadedness, faintness,

abdominal discomfort. **OCCA-SIONAL (2–3%):** Confusion, hallucinations, dry mouth, vivid dreams, dyskinesia (impairment of voluntary movement). **RARE (1%):** Headache, generalized aches.

ADVERSE REACTIONS/TOXIC EFFECTS

Overdosage may vary from CNS depression (sedation, apnea, cardiovascular collapse, death) to severe paradoxical reaction (hallucinations, tremor, seizures). Impaired motor coordination (loss of balance, blepharospasm [blinking], facial grimace, feeling of heavy leg/stiff neck, involuntary movements), hallucinations, confusion, depression, nightmares, delusions, overstimulation, sleep disturbance, anger occurs in some pts.

NURSING IMPLICATIONS
INTERVENTION/EVALUATION:

Be alert to neurologic effects (headache, lethargy, mental confusion, agitation). Monitor for evidence of dyskinesia (difficulty w/movement). Assess for clinical reversal of symptoms (improvement of tremor of head/hands at rest, mask-like facial expression, shuffling gait, muscular rigidity).

PATIENT/FAMILY TEACHING:

Tolerance to feeling of lightheadedness develops during therapy. To reduce hypotensive effect, rise slowly from lying to sitting position and permit legs to dangle momentarily before standing. Avoid tasks that require alertness, motor skills until response to drug is established. Dry mouth, drowsiness, dizziness may be an expected response of drug. Avoid alcoholic beverages during therapy. Coffee/tea may help reduce drowsiness. Inform other physicians, dentist of Eldepryl therapy.

senna
sen-ah
(Senokot, Senolax)

FIXED-COMBINATION(S): W/docusate, a stool softener (**Gentlax-S, Senokap DSS, Senokot-S**)

CANADIAN AVAILABILITY: Senokot

CLASSIFICATION
Laxative: Stimulant

AVAILABILITY (OTC)
Tablets: 187 mg, 217 mg, 374 mg, 600 mg. **Granules:** 326 mg/tsp. **Suppository:** 652 mg. **Syrup:** 218 mg/5 ml. **Liquid:** 33.3 mg/ml.

PHARMACOKINETICS

	ONSET	PEAK	DURATION
PO	6–12 hrs	—	—
Rectal	0.5–2 hrs	—	—

Minimal absorption after oral administration. Hydrolyzed to active form by enzymes of colonic flora. Absorbed drug metabolized in liver; eliminated in feces via biliary system.

ACTION/THERAPEUTIC EFFECT
Increases peristalsis by direct effect on intestinal smooth musculature (stimulates intramural nerve plexi). Builds fluid and ion accumulation in colon, *promoting laxative effect.*

USES

Facilitates defecation in those w/diminished colonic motor response, for evacuation of colon for rectal, bowel examination, elective colon surgery.

PO/RECTAL ADMINISTRATION

PO:

1. Give on an empty stomach (faster results).
2. Offer at least 6–8 glasses of water/day (aids stool softening).
3. Avoid giving within 1 hr of other oral medication (decreases drug absorption).

RECTAL:

1. If suppository is too soft, chill for 30 min in refrigerator or run cold water over foil wrapper.
2. Moisten suppository w/cold water before inserting well up into rectum.

INDICATIONS/DOSAGE/ROUTES

Laxative:
PO: Adults, elderly: 2 tablets (or 1 tsp granules) at bedtime. **Maximum:** 4 tablets (2 tsp) 2 times/day. **Children:** 1 tablet (1/2 tsp granules) at bedtime.
PO: Adults, elderly: (Syrup): 10–15 ml at bedtime. **Children 5–15 yrs:** 5–10 ml at bedtime. **Children 1–5 yrs:** 2.5–5 ml at bedtime. **Children 1 mo–1 yr:** 1.25–2.5 ml at bedtime.
Rectal: Adults, elderly: 1 suppository at bedtime, may repeat in 2 hrs. **Children:** 1/2 suppository at bedtime.

PRECAUTIONS

CONTRAINDICATIONS: Abdominal pain, nausea, vomiting, appendicitis, intestinal obstruction. **CAUTIONS:** None significant. **PREGNANCY/LACTATION:** Unknown whether distributed in breast milk. **Pregnancy Category C.**

INTERACTIONS

DRUG INTERACTIONS: May decrease transit time of concurrently administered oral medication, decreasing absorption. **ALTERED LAB VALUES:** May increase glucose, may decrease potassium.

SIDE EFFECTS

FREQUENT: Pink red, red violet, red brown, or yellow brown discoloration of urine. **OCCASIONAL:** Some degree of abdominal discomfort, nausea, mild cramps, griping, faintness.

ADVERSE REACTIONS/TOXIC EFFECTS

Long-term use may result in laxative dependence, chronic constipation, loss of normal bowel function. Chronic use/overdosage may result in electrolyte disturbances (hypokalemia, hypocalcemia, metabolic acidosis/alkalosis), persistent diarrhea, malabsorption, weight loss. Electrolyte disturbance may produce vomiting, muscle weakness.

NURSING IMPLICATIONS

INTERVENTION/EVALUATION:

Encourage adequate fluid intake. Assess bowel sounds for peristalsis. Monitor stool frequency, consistency (watery, loose, soft, semisolid, solid). Assess for abdominal disturbances. Monitor serum electrolytes in those exposed to prolonged, frequent, or excessive use of medication.

PATIENT/FAMILY TEACHING:

Urine may turn pink red, red violet, red brown, or yellow brown (only temporary and not harmful). Institute measures to promote defecation (increase

S

fluid intake, exercise, high-fiber diet). Laxative effect generally occurs in 6–12 hrs, but may take 24 hrs. Suppository produces evacuation in 30 min to 2 hrs. Do not take other oral medication within 1 hr of taking this medicine (decreased effectiveness).

---

sermorelin
(Geref)
See Supplement

---

sertraline hydrochloride

sir-trah-leen
(Zoloft)

CANADIAN AVAILABILITY:
Zoloft

CLASSIFICATION

Antidepressant

AVAILABILITY (Rx)

Tablets: 50 mg, 100 mg

PHARMACOKINETICS

Incompletely, slowly absorbed from GI tract (food increases absorption). Widely distributed. Undergoes extensive first-pass metabolism in liver to active compound. Excreted in urine, eliminated in feces. Half-life: 26 hrs.

ACTION / THERAPEUTIC EFFECT

Blocks reuptake of the neurotransmitter serotonin at CNS neuronal presynaptic membranes, increasing availability at postsynaptic receptor sites, *producing antidepressant, anxiolytic effect.*

USES

Treatment of major depressive disorders, panic disorder, obsessive compulsive disorder (OCD). Post traumatic-stress disorder.

PO ADMINISTRATION

Give w/food or milk if GI distress occurs.

INDICATIONS/DOSAGE/ROUTES

Antidepressant:
PO: Adults: Initially, 50 mg/day w/morning or evening meal. May increase at intervals no sooner than 1 wk. **Elderly:** Initially, 25 mg/day. May increase by 25 mg q2–3 days. **Maximum:** 200 mg/day.

Panic disorder:
PO: Adults: Initially, 25 mg/day titrated individually.

OCD:
PO: Adults: Initially, 50 mg/day titrated individually. **Children 13–17 yrs:** Initially, 50 mg/day. **Children 6–12 yrs:** Initially, 25 mg/day.

PRECAUTIONS

CONTRAINDICATIONS: During or within 14 days of MAO inhibitor antidepressant therapy. **CAUTIONS:** Severe hepatic/renal impairment. **PREGNANCY/LACTATION:** Unknown whether drug crosses placenta or is distributed in breast milk. **Pregnancy Category B.**

INTERACTIONS

DRUG INTERACTIONS: May increase concentration, toxicity of highly protein-bound medications (e.g., digoxin, warfarin). MAO inhibitors may cause serotonin syndrome (mental changes, restlessness, diaphoresis, shivering, diarrhea, fever), confusion, agitation, hyperpyretic convulsions. **ALTERED LAB VALUES:** May increase SGOT (AST), SGPT (ALT), total cholesterol, triglycerides. May decrease uric acid.

SIDE EFFECTS

FREQUENT (12–26%): Headache, nausea, diarrhea, insomnia, drowsiness, dizziness, fatigue, rash, dry mouth. **OCCASIONAL (4–6%):** Anxiety, nervousness, agitation, tremor, dyspepsia, excessive sweating, vomiting, constipation, abnormal ejaculation, change in vision, change in taste. **RARE (<3%):** Flatulence, urinary frequency, paresthesia, hot flashes, chills.

ADVERSE REACTIONS/TOXIC EFFECTS

None significant.

NURSING IMPLICATIONS

BASELINE ASSESSMENT:

For those on long-term therapy, liver/renal function tests, blood counts should be performed periodically.

INTERVENTION/EVALUATION:

Supervise suicidal risk pt closely during early therapy (as depression lessens, energy level improves, increasing suicide potential). Assess appearance, behavior, speech pattern, level of interest, mood. Monitor pattern of daily bowel activity, stool consistency. Assist w/ambulation if dizziness occurs.

PATIENT/FAMILY TEACHING:

Dry mouth may be relieved by sugarless gum, sips of tepid water. Report headache, fatigue, tremor, sexual dysfunction. Avoid tasks that require alertness, motor skills until response to drug is established. Take w/food if nausea occurs. Inform physician if become pregnant. Avoid alcohol. Do not take OTC medications w/o consulting physician.

sevelamer
(Renagel)
See Supplement

sibutramine
(Meridia)
See Supplement

sildenafil
(Viagra)
See Supplement

silver sulfadiazine
sul-fah-**dye**-ah-zeen
(Silvadene, Flint SSD)

CANADIAN AVAILABILITY:
Flamazine

CLASSIFICATION

Burn preparation

AVAILABILITY (Rx)

Cream

PHARMACOKINETICS

Variably absorbed. Significant systemic absorption may occur if applied to extensive burns. Absorbed medication excreted unchanged in urine. Half-life: 10 hrs (increased in decreased renal function).

ACTION/ *THERAPEUTIC EFFECT*

Acts upon cell wall and cell membrane to *produce bactericidal effect.* Silver is released slowly in concentrations selectively toxic to bacteria.

USES/ *UNLABELED*

Prevention, treatment of infection in second- and third-degree burns, protection against conversion from partial- to full-thickness wounds (infection causes extended tissue destruction). *Treatment of minor bacterial skin infection, dermal ulcer.*

TOPICAL ADMINISTRATION

1. Apply to cleansed, debrided burns using sterile glove.

2. Keep burn areas covered w/silver sulfadiazine cream at all times; reapply to areas where removed by pt activity.

3. Dressings may be ordered on individual basis.

INDICATIONS/DOSAGE/ROUTES

Usual topical dosage:
Topical: Adults, elderly: Apply 1–2 times/day.

PRECAUTIONS

CONTRAINDICATIONS: Hypersensitivity to silver sulfadiazine, components of preparation. **CAUTIONS:** Impaired renal/hepatic function, G-6-PD deficiency, premature neonates, infants <2 mos. Cross-sensitivity w/other sulfonamides unknown. **PREGNANCY/LACTATION:** Not recommended during pregnancy unless burn area is greater than 20% of body surface. Unknown whether distributed in breast milk. Risk of kernicterus in neonates. **Pregnancy Category B**.

INTERACTIONS

DRUG INTERACTIONS: Collagenase, papain, sutilains may be inactivated. **ALTERED LAB VALUES:** None significant.

SIDE EFFECTS

Side effects characteristic of all sulfonamides may occur when systemically absorbed, e.g., extensive burn areas (over 20% of body surface): anorexia, nausea, vomiting, headache, diarrhea, dizziness, photosensitivity, joint pain. **FREQUENT:** Burning feeling at treatment site. **OCCASIONAL:** Brown-gray skin discoloration, rash, itching. **RARE:** Increased sensitivity of skin to sunlight.

ADVERSE REACTIONS/TOXIC EFFECTS

If significant systemic absorption occurs, less often but serious are hemolytic anemia, hypoglycemia, diuresis, peripheral neuropathy, Stevens-Johnson syndrome, agranulocytosis, disseminated lupus erythematosus, anaphylaxis, hepatitis, toxic nephrosis. Fungal superinfections may occur. Interstitial nephritis occurs rarely.

NURSING IMPLICATIONS
BASELINE ASSESSMENT:

Question for hypersensitivity to silver sulfadiazine/components, other sulfonamides. Determine initial CBC, renal/hepatic function test results.

INTERVENTION/EVALUATION:

Evaluate fluid balance, renal function: Check I&O, renal function tests and report changes promptly. Monitor vital signs. Check serum sulfonamide concentrations carefully. Assess burns, surrounding areas for pain, burning, itching, rash (antihistamines may provide relief, silver sulfadiazine therapy continued unless reactions severe). Check CBC results.

PATIENT/FAMILY TEACHING:

Therapy must be continued until healing is satisfactory or the site is ready for grafting.

simethicone
sye-**meth**-ih-cone
(**Mylicon, Phazyme, Silain**)

FIXED-COMBINATION(S):
W/aluminum and magnesium hy-

droxide, antacids **(Digel, Gelusil, Maalox Plus, Mylanta)**; w/loperamide, an antidiarrheal **(Imodium Advanced)**; w/magaldrate, an antacid **(Riopan)**

CANADIAN AVAILABILITY:
Ovol, Phazyme

CLASSIFICATION

Antiflatulent

AVAILABILITY (OTC)

Tablets: 60 mg, 95 mg. **Tablets (chewable):** 40 mg, 80 mg, 125 mg. **Capsules:** 125 mg. **Drops:** 40 mg/0.6 ml.

PHARMACOKINETICS

Does not appear to be absorbed from GI tract. Excreted unchanged in feces.

ACTION/*THERAPEUTIC EFFECT*

Changes surface tension of gas bubbles allowing for easier elimination of gas. *Disperses, prevents formation of gas pockets in GI tract.*

USES/*UNLABELED*

Treatment of flatulence, gastric bloating, postop gas pain or when gas retention may be problem (i.e., peptic ulcer, spastic colon, air swallowing). *Adjunct to gastroscopy, bowel radiography.*

PO ADMINISTRATION

1. Give after meals and at bedtime as needed. Chewable tablets are to be chewed thoroughly before swallowing. Enteric-coated tablets are swallowed whole; do not crush.

2. Shake suspension well before using.

INDICATIONS/DOSAGE/ROUTES

Antiflatulent:
PO: Adults, elderly: (capsules): 125 mg 4 times/day; (tablets): 50–125 mg 4 times/day; (suspension): 40 mg (0.6 ml) 4 times/day; (chewable tablets): 40–80 mg 4 times/day.

PRECAUTIONS

CONTRAINDICATIONS: None significant. **CAUTIONS:** None significant. **PREGNANCY/LACTATION:** Unknown whether drug crosses placenta or is distributed in breast milk. **Pregnancy Category C**.

INTERACTIONS

DRUG INTERACTIONS: None significant. **ALTERED LAB VALUES:** None significant.

SIDE EFFECTS

None significant.

ADVERSE REACTIONS/TOXIC EFFECTS

None significant.

NURSING IMPLICATIONS
INTERVENTION/EVALUATION:

Evaluate for therapeutic response: relief of flatulence, abdominal bloating.

simvastatin
sim-vah-**stay**-tin
(Zocor)

CANADIAN AVAILABILITY:
Zocor

CLASSIFICATION

Antihyperlipoproteinemic

AVAILABILITY (Rx)

Tablets: 5 mg, 10 mg, 20 mg, 40 mg, 80 mg

PHARMACOKINETICS

Well absorbed from GI tract. Undergoes extensive first-pass metabolism. Hydrolyzed to active metabolite. Primarily eliminated in feces.

ACTION/THERAPEUTIC EFFECT

Interferes w/cholesterol biosynthesis by inhibiting the conversion of the enzyme HMG-CoA to mevalonate. *Decreases LDL, cholesterol, VLDL, plasma triglycerides, slight increase in HDL concentration.*

USES

Adjunct to diet therapy to decrease elevated total and LDL cholesterol concentrations in those w/primary hypercholesterolemia (types IIa and IIb), lowers triglyceride levels, increases HDL. Reduces deaths, prevents heart attacks in pts w/heart disease, high cholesterol. Decreases risk of mortality by decreasing coronary death, risk of nonfatal myocardial infarction, need for myocardial revascularization procedures. Decreases risk for stroke/TIA.

PO ADMINISTRATION

1. Give w/o regard to meals.
2. Administer in evening.

INDICATIONS/DOSAGE/ROUTES

Note: Before initiating therapy, pt should be on standard cholesterol-lowering diet for minimum of 3–6 mos. Continue diet throughout simvastatin therapy.

Hyperlipidemia/decreased mortality:

PO: Adults: Initially, 10–20 mg/day in evening. Dosage adjustment at 4 wk intervals. **Elderly:** Initially, 10 mg/day. May increase by 5–10 mg/day q4 wks. **Range:** 5–80 mg/day. **Maximum:** 80 mg/day.

PRECAUTIONS

CONTRAINDICATIONS: Pregnancy, hypersensitivity to simvastatin/any component of the preparation, active liver disease or unexplained, persistent elevations of liver function tests, <18 yrs. **CAUTIONS:** History of liver disease, substantial alcohol consumption. Withholding/discontinuing simvastatin may be necessary when pt at risk for renal failure secondary to rhabdomyolysis. Severe metabolic, endocrine, or electrolyte disorders. **PREGNANCY/LACTATION:** Contraindicated in pregnancy (suppression of cholesterol biosynthesis may cause fetal toxicity) and lactation. Risk of serious adverse reactions in nursing infants. **Pregnancy Category X.**

INTERACTIONS

DRUG INTERACTIONS: Increased risk of rhabdomyolysis, acute renal failure w/cyclosporine, erythromycin, gemfibrozil, niacin, other immunosuppressants. Erythromycin, itraconazole, ketoconazole may increase concentration, cause muscle pain, inflammation or weakness. **ALTERED LAB VALUES:** May increase creatinine kinase, serum transaminase concentrations.

SIDE EFFECTS

Generally well tolerated. Side effects usually mild and transient. **OCCASIONAL:** Abdominal pain, headache, constipation, upper respiratory infection. **RARE:** Diarrhea, flatulence, asthenia (loss of strength and energy), nausea/vomiting.

ADVERSE REACTIONS/TOXIC EFFECTS

Potential for lens opacities. Hypersensitivity reaction, hepatitis occurs rarely.

NURSING IMPLICATIONS
BASELINE ASSESSMENT:

Question for possibility of pregnancy before initiating therapy (Pregnancy Category X). Question history of hypersensitivity to simvastatin. Assess baseline lab results: cholesterol, triglycerides, liver function tests.

INTERVENTION/EVALUATION:

Monitor cholesterol and triglyceride lab results for therapeutic response. Monitor liver function tests. Evaluate food tolerance. Determine pattern of bowel activity. Check for headache, dizziness (provide assistance as needed). Assess for rash, pruritus. Be alert for malaise, muscle cramping/ weakness; if accompanied by fever, may require discontinuation of medication.

PATIENT/FAMILY TEACHING:

Take w/o regard to meals. Use appropriate contraceptive measures (Pregnancy Category X). Follow special diet (important part of treatment). Periodic lab tests are essential part of therapy. Do not take other medications w/o physician knowledge. Do not stop medication w/o consulting physician. Report promptly any muscle pain/weakness, esp. if accompanied by fever/malaise. Do not drive or perform activities that require alert response if dizziness occurs.

sirolimus
(Rapamune)
See Supplement

sodium bicarbonate
(Sodium bicarbonate)

CANADIAN AVAILABILITY:
Sodium bicarbonate

CLASSIFICATION
Antacid, alkalinizing agent

AVAILABILITY (OTC)
Tablets: 325 mg, 520 mg, 650 mg. **Injection (Rx):** 0.5 mEq/ml (4.2%), 0.6 mEq/ml (5%), 0.9 mEq/ml (7.5%), 1 mEq/ml (8.4%).

PHARMACOKINETICS
After administration, sodium bicarbonate dissociates to sodium and bicarbonate ions. Forms/excretes CO_2 (w/increased hydrogen ions combines to form carbonic acid, then dissociates to carbon dioxide, which is excreted by lungs). Plasma concentration regulated by kidney (ability to excrete/make bicarbonate).

ACTION/*THERAPEUTIC EFFECT*
Systemic alkalizer. Increases plasma bicarbonate, buffers excess hydrogen ion concentration, *increases pH, reverses acidosis.* **Urinary alkalizer:** Increases excretion of free bicarbonate in urine, *increases urinary pH.* **Antacid:** Neutralizes existing quantities of stomach acid, *increases pH of stomach contents.*

USES
Corrects metabolic acidosis occurring in severe renal disease and for advanced cardiac life support during cardiopulmonary resuscitation. Used in treatment of drug intoxicants and hyperacidity, associated stomach upset. Treat-

ment of symptoms of peptic ulcer disease; reduces uric acid crystallization (prophylactic).

PO/IV ADMINISTRATION

PO:

1. Individualize dose (based on neutralizing capacity of antacids).

2. *Chewable tablets:* Thoroughly chew tablets before swallowing (follow w/glass of water or milk).

IV:

1. The 4.2%, 7.5%, and 8.4% solutions can be used for direct IV administration.

2. For IV injection, give up to 1 mEq/kg over 1–3 min for cardiac arrest.

3. The 5% solution is administered by IV piggyback.

4. For IV infusion, do not exceed rate of infusion of 50 mEq/hr. For children <2 yrs, premature infants, neonates, administer by slow infusion, up to 8 mEq/daily.

INDICATIONS/DOSAGE/ROUTES

Note: May give by direct IV, IV infusion, or orally. Dose individualized (based on severity of acidosis, laboratory values, pt age, weight, clinical conditions). Do not fully correct bicarbonate deficit during first 24 hrs (may cause metabolic alkalosis).

Cardiac arrest:
IV: Adults, elderly: Initially, 1 mEq/kg (as 7.5–8.4% solution). May repeat w/0.5 mEq/kg q10 min during continued arrest. Postresuscitation phase based on arterial blood pH, $PaCO_2$ base deficit. **Children, infants:** Initially, 1 mEq/kg.

Metabolic acidosis (less severe):
IV Infusion: Adults, elderly, older children: 2–5 mEq/kg over 4–8 hrs. May repeat based on laboratory values.

Acidosis (associated w/chronic renal failure):
Note: Give when plasma bicarbonate <15 mEq/L.
PO: Adults, elderly: Initially, 20–36 mEq/day in divided doses.

Renal tubular acidosis (prevents renal failure, osteomalacia):
PO: Adults, elderly: 4–6 g/day in divided doses or 0.5–10 mEq/kg/day in divided doses (higher doses for proximal renal tubular acidosis).

Alkalinization of urine:
PO: Adults, elderly: Initially, 4 g, then 1–2 g q4h. **Maximum:** 16 g/day. **Children:** 84–840 mg/kg/day in divided doses.

Antacid:
PO: Adults, elderly: 300 mg to 2 g 1–4 times/day.

PRECAUTIONS

CONTRAINDICATIONS: Metabolic/respiratory alkalosis, hypocalcemia, excessive chloride loss due to vomiting/diarrhea/GI suction. **CAUTIONS:** CHF, edematous states, renal insufficiency, those on corticosteroid therapy. **PREGNANCY/LACTATION:** May produce hypernatremia, increase tendon reflexes in neonate/fetus whose mother is a chronic, high-dose user. May be distributed in breast milk. **Pregnancy Category C**.

INTERACTIONS

DRUG INTERACTIONS: May decrease excretion of quinidine, ketoconazole, tetracyclines. Calcium-containing products, milk, milk products may result in milk-alkali syndrome. May increase excretion of salicylates, lithium. May decrease effect of methenamine. **ALTERED LAB VALUES:** May increase serum, urinary pH.

SIDE EFFECTS

FREQUENT: Abdominal distention, flatulence, belching.

ADVERSE REACTIONS/TOXIC EFFECTS

Excessive/chronic use may produce metabolic alkalosis (irritability, twitching, numbness/tingling of extremities, cyanosis, slow/shallow respiration, headache, thirst, nausea). Fluid overload results in headache, weakness, blurred vision, behavioral changes, incoordination, muscle twitching, rise in B/P, decrease in pulse rate, rapid respirations, wheezing, coughing, distended neck veins. Extravasation may occur at IV site, resulting in necrosis, ulceration.

NURSING IMPLICATIONS
BASELINE ASSESSMENT:

Do not give other oral medication within 1–2 hrs of antacid administration.

INTERVENTION/EVALUATION:

Monitor blood and urine pH, CO_2 level, serum electrolytes, plasma bicarbonate, and $PaCO_2$ levels. Watch for signs of metabolic alkalosis, fluid overload. Assess for clinical improvement of metabolic acidosis (relief from hyperventilation, weakness, disorientation). Assess pattern of daily bowel activity, stool consistency. Monitor serum phosphate, calcium, uric acid levels. Assess for relief of gastric distress.

PATIENT/FAMILY TEACHING:

Chewable tablets: Chew tablets thoroughly before swallowing (may be followed by water or milk). Tablets may discolor stool. Maintain adequate fluid intake.

---

sodium chloride
(Salinex, Ocean Mist)

CANADIAN AVAILABILITY:
Salinex, Sodium chloride

CLASSIFICATION

Electrolyte

AVAILABILITY (OTC)

Tablets: 650 mg, 1 g, 2.25 g.
Tablets (slow-release): 600 mg.
Nasal Solution: 0.4%, 0.6%, 0.75%. **Ophthalmic Solution:** 2%, 5%. **Ophthalmic Ointment:** 5%.
Injection (concentrate) (Rx): 14.6%, 23.4%. **Injection (Infusion) (Rx):** 0.45%, 0.9%, 3%, 5%. **Irrigation (Rx):** 0.45%, 0.9%.

PHARMACOKINETICS

Well absorbed from GI tract. Widely distributed. Primarily excreted in urine.

ACTION/THERAPEUTIC EFFECT

Sodium (a major cation of extracellular fluid) primarily *controls water distribution, fluid/electrolyte balance, osmotic pressure of body fluids.* Associated w/chloride and bicarbonate, *maintains acid-base balance.*

USES

Parenteral: Source of hydration; prevent/treats sodium and chloride

S

deficiencies (hypertonic for severe deficiencies). Prevents muscle cramps/heat prostration occurring w/excessive perspiration. *Hypotonic:* Hydrating solution, used to assess renal function status and manage hyperosmolar diabetes. Diluent for reconstitution. *Nasal:* Restores moisture, relieves dry and inflamed nasal membranes. *Ophthalmic:* Therapy in reduction of corneal edema, diagnostic aid in ophthalmoscopic exam.

STORAGE/HANDLING

Store nasal, ophthalmic, parenteral forms at room temperature.

PO/NASAL/OPHTHALMIC/ IV ADMINISTRATION

PO:

Do not crush or break enteric-coated or extended-release tablets.

NASAL:

1. Instruct pt to begin inhaling slowly just before releasing medication into nose.
2. Inhale slowly, then release air gently through mouth.
3. Continue technique for 20–30 secs.

OPHTHALMIC:

1. Position pt w/head tilted back, looking up.
2. Gently pull lower lid down to form pouch and instill drops (or apply thin strip of ointment).
3. Do not touch tip of applicator to lids or any surface.
4. When lower lid is released, have pt keep eye open w/o blinking for at least 30 secs for solution; for ointment have pt close eye and roll eyeball around to distribute medication.
5. Apply gentle finger pressure to lacrimal sac (bridge of the nose, inside corner of the eye) for 1–2 min after administration of solution.
6. Remove excess solution around eye w/tissue.

IV:

1. Hypertonic solutions (3 or 5%) administered via large vein; avoid infiltration; do not exceed 100 ml/hr.
2. Vials containing 2.5–4 mEq/ml (concentrated NaCl) must be diluted before administration.

INDICATIONS/DOSAGE/ROUTES

Usual parenteral dosage:
Note: Dosage based on age, weight, clinical condition, fluid, electrolyte, acid-base status.
IV Infusion: Adults, elderly: (0.9 or 0.45%): 1–2 L/day. (3 or 5%): 100 ml over 1 hr; assess serum electrolyte concentration before additional fluid given.

Usual oral dosage:
PO: Adults, elderly: 1–2 g 3 times/ day.

Usual nasal dosage:
Intranasal: Adults, elderly: Take as needed.

Usual ophthalmic dosage:
Ophthalmic: Adults, elderly: (Solution): 1–2 drops q3–4h. (Ointment): Once/day or as directed.

PRECAUTIONS

CONTRAINDICATIONS: Hypernatremia, fluid retention. **CAUTIONS:** CHF, circulatory insufficiency, kidney dysfunction, hypoproteinemia. Do not use NaCl preserved w/benzyl alcohol in neonates. **PREGNANCY/LACTATION: Pregnancy Category C.**

INTERACTIONS

DRUG INTERACTIONS: Hypertonic saline and oxytocics may cause uterine hypertonus, possible uterine ruptures or lacerations. **ALTERED LAB VALUES:** None significant.

SIDE EFFECTS

FREQUENT: Flushed face. **OCCASIONAL:** Fever, irritation/phlebitis/extravasation at injection site. *Ophthalmic:* Temporary burning/irritation.

ADVERSE REACTIONS/TOXIC EFFECTS

Too rapid administration may produce peripheral edema, CHF, pulmonary edema. Excessive dosage produces hypokalemia, hypervolemia, hypernatremia.

NURSING IMPLICATIONS

BASELINE ASSESSMENT:

Assess fluid balance (I&O, edema).

INTERVENTION/EVALUATION:

Monitor fluid balance (e.g., I&O, daily weight, edema, lung sounds), IV site for extravasation. Monitor serum electrolytes, acid-base balance, B/P. Hypernatremia associated w/edema, weight gain, elevated B/P; hyponatremia associated w/muscle cramps, nausea, vomiting, dry mucous membranes.

PATIENT/FAMILY TEACHING:

Temporary burning, irritation may occur upon instillation of eye medication. Discontinue eye medication if severe pain, headache, rapid change in vision (side and straight ahead), sudden appearance of floating spots, acute redness of eyes, pain on exposure to light, or double vision occurs and contact physician.

---

sodium ferric gluconate
(Ferrlecit)
See Supplement

---

sodium polystyrene sulfonate

sew-dee-um pah-lee-**sty**-reen **sul**-foe-nate
(SPS, Kayexalate)

CANADIAN AVAILABILITY:
Kayexalate

CLASSIFICATION

Cation exchange resin

AVAILABILITY (Rx)

Suspension: 15 g/60 ml. **Powder.**

ACTION/*THERAPEUTIC EFFECT*

Resin either passes through intestine or is retained in colon; *releases sodium ions in exchange for primarily potassium ions.* Occurs from 2–12 hrs after oral administration, longer after rectal administration.

USES

Treatment of hyperkalemia.

STORAGE/HANDLING

After preparation, suspension stable for 24 hrs.

PO/RECTAL ADMINISTRATION

PO:

1. Give w/20–100 ml sorbitol (facilitates passage of resin through intestinal tract, prevents constipation, aids in potassium removal, increases palatability).
2. Do not mix w/foods, liquids containing potassium.

RECTAL:

1. Initial cleansing enema, then insert large rubber tube into

rectum well into sigmoid colon, tape in place.

2. Introduce suspension (w/100 ml sorbitol) via gravity.

3. Flush w/50–100 ml fluid and clamp.

4. Retain for several hours if possible.

5. Irrigate colon w/nonsodium-containing solution to remove resin.

INDICATIONS/DOSAGE/ROUTES

Hyperkalemia:
PO: Adults, elderly: 60 ml (15 g) 1–4 times/day.
Rectal: Adults, elderly: 30–50 g as needed q6h.

Usual pediatric dosage:
PO/Rectal: Based on 1 g resin binding approx. 1 mEq potassium: 1 g/kg q6h.

PRECAUTIONS

CONTRAINDICATIONS: None significant. **CAUTIONS:** Those who cannot tolerate increase in sodium (CHF, severe hypertension, marked edema). **PREGNANCY/LACTATION:** Unknown whether drug crosses placenta or is distributed in breast milk. **Pregnancy Category N/A.**

INTERACTIONS

DRUG INTERACTIONS: Cation-donating antacids, laxatives (e.g., magnesium hydroxide) may decrease effect, cause systemic alkalosis (pts w/renal impairment). **ALTERED LAB VALUES:** May decrease magnesium, calcium.

SIDE EFFECTS

High dosage: Anorexia, nausea, vomiting, constipation. High dosage in elderly: Fecal impaction (severe stomach pain w/nausea/vomiting). **OCCASIONAL:** Diarrhea, sodium retention (decreased urination, swelling hands/feet, increased weight), hypocalcemia (abdominal/muscle cramps).

ADVERSE REACTIONS/TOXIC EFFECTS

Serious potassium deficiency may occur. Early signs of hypokalemia: irritable confusion, delayed thought processes, often associated w/lengthened QT interval and widening, flattening, or conversion of T wave and prominent U waves. Arrhythmias, severe muscle weakness may be noted.

NURSING IMPLICATIONS
BASELINE ASSESSMENT:

Does not rapidly correct severe hyperkalemia (may take hours to days). Consider other measures in medical emergency (IV calcium, IV sodium bicarbonate, glucose, insulin, dialysis).

INTERVENTION/EVALUATION:

Frequent potassium levels within each 24 hrs should be maintained, monitored. Assess pt's clinical condition, EKG (valuable in determining when treatment should be discontinued). In addition to checking serum potassium, monitor magnesium, calcium levels. Monitor daily bowel activity, stool consistency (fecal impaction may occur in those on high doses, particularly in elderly).

somatrem
soe-ma-trem
(Protropin)

CANADIAN AVAILABILITY:
Protropin

CLASSIFICATION

Growth stimulator

AVAILABILITY (Rx)

Powder for Injection: 5 mg, 10 mg

PHARMACOKINETICS

Well absorbed following SubQ, IM administration. Metabolized in liver. Eliminated in feces via biliary system, excreted in urine. Half-life: *IM/SubQ:* 3–5 hrs.

ACTION/ THERAPEUTIC EFFECT

Stimulates linear growth. Increases number, size of muscle cells, increases red cell mass. Affects carbohydrate metabolism (antagonizes action of insulin), fats (increases mobilization of fats), and proteins (increases cellular protein synthesis).

USES

Long-term treatment of children who have growth failure due to endogenous growth hormone deficiency.

STORAGE/HANDLING

Refrigerate vials. After reconstitution, use within 7 days. Avoid freezing.

IM ADMINISTRATION

1. Reconstitute each 5 mg vial w/1–5 ml of bacteriostatic water for injection (benzyl alcohol preserved only). For newborns (because of toxicity w/benzyl alcohol), reconstitute w/water for injection.

2. To prepare solution, inject diluent into vial aiming the stream of liquid against the glass wall. Swirl gently until dissolved. DO NOT SHAKE.

3. Use one dose per vial; discard unused portion.

4. Do not administer if solution is cloudy/contains particulate matter.

5. To prevent contamination, use disposable needle/syringe for each entry into vial.

INDICATIONS/DOSAGE/ROUTES

Usual parenteral dosage:
IM/SubQ: Up to 0.1 mg/kg (0.26 IU/kg) 3 times/wk.

PRECAUTIONS

CONTRAINDICATIONS: Pts w/ closed epiphyses, known sensitivity to benzyl alcohol, active neoplasia (intracranial tumors must be inactive and antitumor therapy complete before somatrem therapy; discontinue if tumor growth recurs). **CAUTIONS:** Diabetes mellitus, hypothyroidism, pts whose growth hormone deficiency is secondary to an intracranial lesion.

INTERACTIONS

DRUG INTERACTIONS: Glucocorticoids (chronic use) may decrease effects. **ALTERED LAB VALUES:** May increase fatty acid, phosphate concentration. May decrease glucose tolerance, thyroid function tests.

SIDE EFFECTS

FREQUENT: 30% of pts develop persistent antibodies to growth hormone (generally does not cause failure to respond to somatrem). **OCCASIONAL:** Headache, muscle pain, weakness, mild hyperglycemia, allergic reaction (rash, itching), pain/swelling at injection site, pain in hip/knee.

ADVERSE REACTIONS/TOXIC EFFECTS

Hypothyroidism (must be treated or will interfere w/response to somatrem).

NURSING IMPLICATIONS

BASELINE ASSESSMENT:

Question sensitivity to benzyl alcohol. Baseline blood glucose, thyroid function, and bone age determinations should be established.

INTERVENTION/EVALUATION:

Monitor blood glucose levels and check for hyperglycemia (polyuria, polydipsia, polyphagia). Assess for developing hypothyroidism: forgetfulness, dry skin and hair, feeling cold, apathy, lethargy, weight gain, bradycardia.

PATIENT/FAMILY TEACHING:

Somatrem therapy may continue for years, as long as pt is responsive, until mature adult height is reached or epiphyses close. Importance of regular visits to the physician, tests during therapy. Record height, weight as directed by physician. Signs and symptoms of hypothyroidism, hyperglycemia: Report promptly.

---

somatropin

soe-mah-**troe**-pin
(Humatrope, Norditropin, Nutropin, Nutropin AQ, Saizen)

CANADIAN AVAILABILITY:
Humatrope, Nutropin, Saizen

CLASSIFICATION

Growth stimulator

AVAILABILITY (Rx)

Powder for Injection: 5 mg, 10 mg

PHARMACOKINETICS

Well absorbed following SubQ, IM administration. Metabolized in liver. Eliminated in feces via biliary system, excreted in urine. Half-life: *IM/SubQ:* 3–5 hrs.

ACTION/*THERAPEUTIC EFFECT*

Stimulates linear growth. Increases number, size of muscle cells, increases red cell mass. Affects carbohydrate metabolism (antagonizes action of insulin), fats (increases mobilization of fats), and proteins (increases cellular protein synthesis).

USES

Long-term treatment of children who have growth failure due to endogenous growth hormone deficiency or associated w/chronic renal insufficiency (Nutropin only). Long-term therapy in adults w/growth hormone deficiency. Long-term treatment of short stature associated w/Turner's syndrome, treatment of AIDS-wasting syndrome.

STORAGE/HANDLING

Refrigerate vials. After reconstitution, stable for 14 days refrigerated. Avoid freezing.

SUBQ/IM ADMINISTRATION

1a. *Humatrope:* Reconstitute each 5 mg vial w/1.5–5 ml diluent or sterile water for injection. (If sterile water used, use 1 dose/vial, refrigerate solution if not used immediately, use within 24 hrs, discard unused portion.)

1b. *Nutropin:* Reconstitute 5 mg vial w/1–5 mg (10 mg w/1–10 ml) bacteriostatic water for injection.

2. Do not shake.

3. Do not inject if solution is cloudy or contains particulate matter.

INDICATIONS/DOSAGE/ROUTES

Growth hormone deficiency:
IM/SubQ: *(Humatrope):* Up to 0.06 mg/kg 3 times/wk.
SubQ: *(Nutropin):* 0.3 mg/kg/wk.
Adults: SubQ: 0.04 mg/kg/wk in 6–7 injections/wk. **Maximum:** 0.08 mg/kg/wk.

Chronic renal insufficiency:

SubQ: *(Nutropin):* 0.35 mg/kg/wk.

Turner's syndrome:
SubQ: 0.375 mg/kg/wk divided into 3–7 equal doses/wk.

AIDS-wasting syndrome:
SubQ: 4–6 mg at bedtime.

PRECAUTIONS

CONTRAINDICATIONS: Pts w/ closed epiphyses, active neoplasia (intracranial tumors must be inactive and antitumor therapy complete before somatropin therapy; discontinue if tumor growth recurs). Do not use supplied diluent when sensitivity to m-cresol or glycerin is known. **CAUTIONS:** Diabetes mellitus, hypothyroidism, pts whose growth hormone deficiency is secondary to an intracranial lesion.

INTERACTIONS

DRUG INTERACTIONS: Glucocorticoids (chronic use) may decrease effects. **ALTERED LAB VALUES:** May increase fatty acid, phosphate concentration. May decrease glucose tolerance, thyroid function tests.

SIDE EFFECTS

FREQUENT: Development of persistent antibodies to growth hormone (generally does not cause failure to respond to somatropin); hypercalciuria during first 2–3 mos of therapy. **OCCASIONAL:** Headache, muscle pain, weakness, mild hyperglycemia, allergic reaction (rash, itching), pain/swelling at injection site, pain in hip/knee.

ADVERSE REACTIONS/TOXIC EFFECTS

Hypothyroidism (must be treated or will interfere w/response to somatropin).

NURSING IMPLICATIONS
BASELINE ASSESSMENT:

Question sensitivity to m-cresol, glycerin. Establish baseline blood glucose, thyroid function, and bone age determinations.

INTERVENTION/EVALUATION:

Monitor blood glucose levels and check for hyperglycemia (polyuria, polydipsia, polyphagia). Assess for developing hypothyroidism: forgetfulness, dry skin and hair, feeling cold, apathy, lethargy, weight gain, bradycardia. During early therapy, be alert to renal calculi associated w/hypercalciuria (flank pain and colic, chills, fever, urinary frequency, hematuria).

PATIENT/FAMILY TEACHING:

Somatropin therapy may continue for years, as long as pt is responsive, until mature adult height is reached or epiphyses close. Importance of regular visits to the physician, tests during therapy. Record height, weight as directed by physician. Signs and symptoms of hypothyroidism, hyperglycemia, renal calculi: Report promptly.

sotalol
sew-tah-lol
(Betapace)

CANADIAN AVAILABILITY: Sotacor

CLASSIFICATION

Beta-adrenergic blocking agent

AVAILABILITY (Rx)

Tablets: 80 mg, 120 mg, 160 mg, 240 mg

PHARMACOKINETICS

Well absorbed from GI tract. Widely distributed. Primarily excreted unchanged in urine. Half-life: 12 hrs (increased in elderly, pts w/decreased renal function).

ACTION/ *THERAPEUTIC EFFECT*

Prolongs action potential and effective refractory period, QT interval. Decreases heart rate, AV nodal conduction; increases AV nodal refractoriness, *producing antiarrhythmic activity.*

USES/ *UNLABELED*

Treatment of documented, life-threatening ventricular arrhythmias. *Treatment of chronic angina pectoris, hypertension, hypertrophic cardiomyopathy, myocardial infarction, pheochromocytoma, tremors, anxiety, thyrotoxicosis, mitral valve prolapse syndrome. Maintenance of normal heart rhythm in chronic or recurring atrial fibrillation or flutter.*

PO ADMINISTRATION

May give w/o regard to food.

INDICATIONS/DOSAGE/ROUTES

Antiarrhythmic:
PO: Adults, elderly: Initially, 80 mg 2 times/day. May increase gradually at 2–3 day intervals. **Range:** 240–320 mg/day.
Note: Some patients may require 480–640 mg/day. Dosing more than 2 times/day usually not necessary due to long half-life.

Dosage in renal impairment:

CREATININE CLEARANCE	DOSAGE INTERVAL
30–60 ml/min	24 hrs
10–30 ml/min	36–48 hrs
<10 ml/min	Individualized

PRECAUTIONS

CONTRAINDICATIONS: Bronchial asthma, uncontrolled cardiac failure, sinus bradycardia, second- and third-degree heart block, cardiogenic shock, long QT syndrome (unless functioning pacemaker present). **CAUTIONS:** Pts w/history of ventricular tachycardia, ventricular fibrillation, cardiomegaly, CHF, diabetes mellitus, excessive prolongation of QT interval, hypokalemia, and hypomagnesium. Severe, prolonged diarrhea. Pts w/sick-sinus syndrome; pts at risk of developing thyrotoxicosis. Avoid abrupt withdrawal. **PREGNANCY/LACTATION:** Crosses placenta; excreted in breast milk. **Pregnancy Category B.** (Category D if used in 2nd or 3rd trimester.)

INTERACTIONS

DRUG INTERACTIONS: Antiarrhythmics, phenothiazine, tricyclic antidepressants, terfenadine, astemizole may increase prolonged QT interval. May increase proarrhythmia w/digoxin. Calcium channel blockers may increase effect on AV conduction, B/P. May mask signs of hypoglycemia, prolong effect of insulin, oral hypoglycemics. May inhibit effects of sympathomimetics. May potentiate rebound hypertension seen after discontinuing clonidine. **ALTERED LAB VALUES:** May increase glucose, alkaline phosphatase, LDH, SGOT (AST), SGPT (ALT), lipoproteins, triglycerides.

SIDE EFFECTS

FREQUENT: Decreased sexual ability, drowsiness, difficulty sleeping, unusual tiredness/weakness. **OCCASIONAL:** Depression, cold hands/feet, diarrhea, constipation, anxiety, nasal congestion, nausea, vomiting. **RARE:** Altered taste, dry eyes, itching, numbness of fingers, toes, scalp.

ADVERSE REACTIONS/TOXIC EFFECTS

Bradycardia, CHF, hypotension,

bronchospasm, hypoglycemia, prolonged QT interval, torsade de pointes, ventricular tachycardia, premature ventricular complexes.

NURSING IMPLICATIONS
BASELINE ASSESSMENT:

Pt must be on continuous cardiac monitoring upon initiation of therapy. Establish baseline B/P and pulse. Do not administer w/o consulting physician if pulse is below 60 beats/min.

INTERVENTION/EVALUATION:

Monitor B/P for hypotension, pulse for bradycardia. Assess for CHF: dyspnea, peripheral edema, jugular vein distention, increased weight, rales in lungs, decreased urine output.

PATIENT/FAMILY TEACHING:

May have lightheadedness; do not drive or perform tasks that require alert response if this occurs. Carry identification bracelet/card. Teach pt/family to correctly take B/P, pulse before dosing; contact physician if below parameters, usually systolic B/P of 90 mm Hg, pulse of 60 beats/min. Change positions slowly to prevent orthostatic hypotension. Do not take OTC cold medications, nasal decongestants. Restrict sodium and alcohol as ordered. Do not stop taking drug suddenly. Report chest pain, fatigue, shortness of breath.

sparfloxacin

(Zagam)
See Supplement
See Classification section under:
Antibiotics: fluoroquinolones

spectinomycin hydrochloride

speck-tin-oh-**my**-sin
(Trobicin)

CLASSIFICATION

Antibiotic

AVAILABILITY (Rx)

Powder for Injection: 400 mg/ml (2 g, 4 g vials)

PHARMACOKINETICS

Rapidly, completely absorbed after IM administration. Primarily concentrated in urine. Excreted in urine. Removed by hemodialysis. Half-life: 1–3 hrs (increased in decreased renal function).

ACTION/*THERAPEUTIC EFFECT*

Inhibits protein synthesis of bacterial cells, *producing bacterial cell death.*

USES/*UNLABELED*

Treatment of acute gonococcal urethritis, proctitis in males, acute gonococcal cervicitis and proctitis in females. *Treatment of disseminated gonorrhea.*

STORAGE/HANDLING

Following reconstitution, stable for 24 hrs at room temperature. Use within 24 hrs.

IM ADMINISTRATION

1. For IM injection, reconstitute each 2 g vial w/3.2 ml bacteriostatic water for injection containing 0.9% benzyl alcohol (6.2 ml to 4 g vial) to provide concentration of 400 mg/ml.
2. Shake vigorously.

S

3. Inject deep IM into upper outer quadrant of gluteal muscle (use 20 gauge needle).

4. Do not inject more than 5 ml in one site.

5. Observe pt for 1 hr after injection for potential anaphylaxis.

INDICATIONS/DOSAGE/ROUTES

Usual adult dosage:
IM: 2 g once. In areas where antibiotic resistance is known to be prevalent, 4 g (10 ml) divided between 2 injection sites is preferred.

PRECAUTIONS

CONTRAINDICATIONS: None significant. **CAUTIONS:** History of allergies. **PREGNANCY/LACTATION:** Unknown whether drug crosses placenta or is distributed in breast milk. **Pregnancy Category B**.

INTERACTIONS

DRUG INTERACTIONS: None significant. **ALTERED LAB VALUES:** None significant.

SIDE EFFECTS

FREQUENT: Pain at injection site. **OCCASIONAL:** Dizziness, insomnia. **RARE:** Decreased urine output.

ADVERSE REACTIONS/TOXIC EFFECTS

Hypersensitivity reaction characterized as chills, fever, nausea, vomiting, urticaria.

NURSING IMPLICATIONS
BASELINE ASSESSMENT:

Question pt for history of allergies, particularly to spectinomycin. Obtain culture and sensitivity test before giving first dose (therapy may begin before results are known). Serologic test for syphilis should be completed before therapy.

INTERVENTION/EVALUATION:

Observe pt for 1 hr after injection because of potential for anaphylaxis.

PATIENT/FAMILY TEACHING:

May have discomfort at injection site.

spironolactone

spear-own-oh-**lak**-tone
(Aldactone)

FIXED-COMBINATION(S):
W/hydrochlorothiazide, a thiazide diuretic **(Aldactazide, Spironazide)**

CANADIAN AVAILABILITY:
Aldactone, Novospiroton

CLASSIFICATION

Diuretic: Potassium sparing

AVAILABILITY (Rx)

Tablets: 25 mg, 50 mg, 100 mg

PHARMACOKINETICS

	ONSET	PEAK	DURATION
PO	24–48 hrs	48–72 hrs	48–72 hrs

Well absorbed from GI tract (increased w/food). Metabolized in liver to active metabolite. Primarily excreted in urine. Half-life: 9–24 hrs.

ACTION/*THERAPEUTIC EFFECT*

Competitively inhibits action of aldosterone. Interferes w/sodium reabsorption in distal tubule, *increasing potassium retention while promoting sodium and water excretion.*

USES/*UNLABELED*

Treatment of excessive aldosterone production, essential hypertension, edema due to CHF, CHF, cirrhosis of liver/nephrotic syndrome. Adjunct to potassium-losing diuretics or to potentiate action of other diuretics. Diagnosis of hyperaldosteronism. *Treatment of polycystic ovary syndrome, female hirsutism.*

STORAGE/HANDLING

Oral suspension containing crushed tablets in cherry syrup is stable for up to 30 days if refrigerated.

PO ADMINISTRATION

1. Cherry suspension available for pediatric administration.
2. Drug absorption enhanced if taken w/food.
3. Scored tablets may be crushed.
4. Do not crush or break film-coated tablets.

INDICATIONS/DOSAGE/ROUTES

Note: Use loading dose to prevent delay in therapeutic effect (may take up to 3 days).

CHF:
PO: Adults, elderly: 25 mg/day.

Edema:
PO: Adults: 25–200 mg daily. Give in single or equally divided doses. **Children:** 3.3 mg/kg daily.

Hypokalemia:
PO: Adults: 25–100 mg daily.

Hypertension:
PO: Adults: 50–100 mg daily.

Usual elderly dosage:
PO: Initially, 25–50 mg/day. May increase by 25–50 mg/day every 5 days.

Diagnosis of primary aldosteronism:
PO: Adults: 400 mg daily for 3–4 wks. Increase in potassium and reduction in hypertension point to primary aldosteronism. This dosage may be tried for 4 days w/increase in potassium levels during use as the diagnostic indicator. **Children:** 125–375 mg/m^2 over 24 hrs.

Preop or maintenance therapy for hyperaldosteronism:
PO: Adults: 100–400 mg daily for preop therapy; 400 mg initial dose followed by lowest therapeutic dose at 100–300 mg/day for maintenance if surgery cannot be done.

PRECAUTIONS

CONTRAINDICATIONS: Acute renal insufficiency/impairment, anuria, BUN/creatinine over twice normal values levels, hyperkalemia. **CAUTIONS:** Hepatic/renal impairment. **PREGNANCY/LACTATION:** Active metabolite excreted in breast milk—nursing not advised. **Pregnancy Category D.**

INTERACTIONS

DRUG INTERACTIONS: May decrease effect of anticoagulants, heparin. NSAIDs may decrease antihypertensive effect. ACE inhibitors (e.g., captopril), potassium-containing medications, potassium supplements may increase potassium. May decrease lithium clearance, increase toxicity. May increase digoxin half-life. **ALTERED LAB VALUES:** May increase BUN, calcium excretion, creatinine, glucose, magnesium, potassium, uric acid. May decrease sodium.

SIDE EFFECTS

FREQUENT: Hyperkalemia for those on potassium supplements or those w/renal insufficiency; dehydration, hyponatremia, lethargy. **OCCASIONAL:** Nausea, vomiting, anorexia, cramping, diarrhea, headache, ataxia, drowsiness, confusion, fever. *Male:* Gynecomastia, impotence, decreased libido. *Female:* Menstrual irregularities/amenorrhea, postmenopausal bleeding, breast tenderness. **RARE:** Rash, urticaria, hirsutism.

ADVERSE REACTIONS/TOXIC EFFECTS

Severe hyperkalemia may produce arrhythmias, bradycardia, tented T waves, widening QRS, ST depression. These can proceed to cardiac standstill or ventricular fibrillation. Cirrhosis pts at risk for hepatic decompensation if dehydration/hyponatremia occurs. Those w/primary aldosteronism may experience rapid weight loss, severe fatigue during high-dose therapy.

NURSING IMPLICATIONS
BASELINE ASSESSMENT:

Weigh pt; initiate strict I&O. Evaluate hydration status by assessing mucous membranes, skin turgor. Obtain baseline electrolytes, renal/hepatic functions, urinalysis. EKG may be ordered. Assess for edema; note location and extent. Check baseline vital signs, note pulse rate/regularity.

INTERVENTION/EVALUATION:

Monitor electrolyte values, esp. for increased potassium. Monitor B/P levels. Monitor for hyponatremia: mental confusion, thirst, cold/clammy skin, drowsiness, dry mouth. Monitor for hyperkalemia: colic, diarrhea, muscle twitching followed by weakness/paralysis, arrhythmias. Obtain daily weight. Note changes in edema, skin turgor.

PATIENT/FAMILY TEACHING:

Expect increase in volume, frequency of urination. Therapeutic effect takes several days to begin and can last for several days when drug is discontinued. This may not apply if pt is on a potassium-losing drug concomitantly (diet and use of supplements should be established by physician). Notify physician for irregular/slow pulse, electrolyte imbalance (signs noted above). Avoid foods high in potassium such as whole grains (cereals), legumes, meat, bananas, apricots, orange juice, potatoes (white, sweet), raisins.

stavudine (d4T)

stah-view-deen
(Zerit)

CANADIAN AVAILABILITY:
Zerit

CLASSIFICATION

Antiviral

AVAILABILITY (Rx)

Capsules: 15 mg, 20 mg, 30 mg, 40 mg. **Oral Solution:** 1 mg/ml.

PHARMACOKINETICS

Rapidly, completely absorbed following oral administration. Equally distributed into extravascular spaces. Undergoes minimal metabolism. Excreted in urine. Half-life: 1.5 hrs (increased in decreased renal function).

ACTION/*THERAPEUTIC EFFECT*

Inhibits HIV reverse transcriptase via viral DNA chain termination. Also inhibits RNA- and DNA-dependent DNA polymerase, an enzyme necessary for viral HIV replication, *slowing HIV replication, reducing progression of HIV infection.*

USES

Treatment of adults w/advanced HIV infection who are intolerant or have experienced deterioration w/other drug therapy. First line component in tx of HIV.

PO ADMINISTRATION

May give w/o regard to meals.

INDICATIONS/DOSAGE/ROUTES

HIV infection:
PO: Adults ≥60 kg: 40 mg twice daily. **Adults ≤60 kg:** 30 mg twice daily. If peripheral neuropathy or elevated hepatic transaminases present, stop therapy. If symptoms resolve completely, resume treatment using following schedule: **Adults ≥60 kg:** 20 mg twice daily. **Adults <60 kg:** 15 mg twice daily. **Children >30 kg:** Same as adults; **<30 kg:** 2 mg/kg/day.

Dosage in renal impairment:
Dose and/or frequency is modified based on creatinine clearance, pt weight.

CREATININE CLEARANCE	≥ 60 KG	≤ 60 KG
> 50	40 mg q12h	30 mg q12h
26–50	20 mg q12h	15 mg q12h
10–25	20 mg q24h	15 mg q24h

PRECAUTIONS

CONTRAINDICATIONS: None significant. **CAUTIONS:** History of peripheral neuropathy. **PREGNANCY/LACTATION:** Breast-feeding not recommended (possibility of HIV transmission). **Pregnancy Category C.**

INTERACTIONS

DRUG INTERACTIONS: None significant. **ALTERED LAB VALUES:** Commonly increases SGOT (AST), SGPT (ALT). May decrease neutrophil count.

SIDE EFFECTS

FREQUENT: Headache (55%), diarrhea (50%), chills/fever (38%), nausea/vomiting, myalgia (35%), rash (33%), asthenia [loss of strength, energy] (28%), insomnia, abdominal pain (26%), anxiety (22%), arthralgia (18%), back pain (20%), sweating (19%), malaise (17%), depression (14%). **OCCASIONAL:** Anorexia, weight loss, nervousness, dizziness, conjunctivitis, dyspepsia, dyspnea. **RARE:** Constipation, vasodilation, confusion, migraine, urticaria, abnormal vision.

ADVERSE REACTIONS/TOXIC EFFECTS

Peripheral neuropathy, characterized by numbness, tingling, or pain in hands or feet, occurs frequently (15%–21%). Ulcerative stomatitis (erythema/ulcers of oral mucosa, glossitis, gingivitis), pneumonia, benign skin neoplasms occur occasionally. Pancreatitis occurs rarely.

NURSING IMPLICATIONS

BASELINE ASSESSMENT:

Obtain baseline laboratory testing, esp. liver function tests, before beginning stavudine therapy and at periodic intervals during therapy. Offer emotional support. Obtain medication history. Question pt for previous history of peripheral neuropathy.

INTERVENTION/EVALUATION:

Monitor for peripheral neuropathy (characterized by numbness, tingling, or pain in hands or feet). Symptoms resolve promptly if therapy is discontinued (symptoms may worsen temporarily after drug is withdrawn). If symptoms resolve completely, reduced dosage may be resumed. Assess for headache, nausea, skin rash. Monitor skin for evidence of rash, signs of chills/fever. Determine pattern of bowel activity and stool consistency. Assess for muscle or joint aches, dizziness, sleep pattern. Assess eating pattern; monitor for weight loss. Check eyes for signs of conjunctivitis.

PATIENT/FAMILY TEACHING:

Continue therapy for full length of treatment. Doses should be evenly spaced. Do not take any medications, including OTC drugs, w/o consulting physician. Stavudine is not a cure for HIV infection, nor does it reduce risk of transmission to others. Pt may continue to experience illnesses, including opportunistic infections. Do not drive, use machinery, or engage in other activities that require mental acuity if experiencing dizziness.

streptokinase

strep-toe-**kine**-ace
(Kabikinase, Streptase)

CANADIAN AVAILABILITY:
Kabikinase, Streptase

CLASSIFICATION

Thrombolytic

AVAILABILITY (Rx)

Powder for Injection: 250,000 IU, 600,000 IU, 750,000 IU, 1.5 million IU

PHARMACOKINETICS

Rapidly cleared from plasma by antibodies, reticuloendothelial system. Route of elimination unknown. Duration of action continues for several hours after discontinuing medication. Half-life: 23 min.

ACTION/ *THERAPEUTIC EFFECT*

Activates fibrinolytic system by converting plasminogen to plasmin (enzyme that degrades fibrin clots). Acts indirectly by forming complex w/plasminogen, which converts plasminogen to plasmin. *Resultant effect destroys thrombi.* Action occurs within thrombus, on its surface, and in circulating blood.

USES

Management of acute myocardial infarction (lyses thrombi obstructing coronary arteries, decreases infarct size, improves ventricular function after MI, decreases CHF, mortality associated w/AMI). Lysis of diagnosed pulmonary emboli, acute/extensive thrombi of deep veins, and acute arterial thrombi/emboli. Clears totally/partially occluded arteriovenous cannulae.

STORAGE/HANDLING

Store vials at room temperature. Reconstitute vials immediately before use. Solution for direct IV administration may be used within 8 hrs of reconstitution. Discard unused portion.

IV/INTRACORONARY ADMINISTRATION

Note: Must be administered within 12–14 hrs of clot formation (little effect on older, organized clots).

IV:

1. Give by direct IV/IV infusion (via infusion pump). Infuse into se-

lected thrombosed coronary artery, intra-arterially, or by cannula.

2. Reconstitute vial w/5 ml 5% dextrose or 0.9% NaCl solution. (Add diluent slowly to side of vial, roll and tilt to avoid foaming. Do not shake vial.)

3. Slight flocculation may occur; does not affect safe use of the drug.

4. Further dilute w/50–500 ml 5% dextrose or 0.9% NaCl.

5. If minor bleeding occurs at puncture sites, apply pressure for 30 min, then apply pressure dressing.

6. Monitor B/P during infusion (hypotension may be severe, occurs in 1–10%). Decrease of infusion rate may be necessary.

7. If uncontrolled hemorrhage occurs, discontinue infusion immediately (slowing rate of infusion may produce worsening hemorrhage). Do not use dextran to control hemorrhage.

INTRACORONARY:

Monitor for arrhythmias during and immediately after infusion (atrial/ventricular).

INDICATIONS/DOSAGE/ROUTES

Note: Do not use from 5 days to 6 mos of previous streptokinase treatment of streptococcal infection (pharyngitis, rheumatic fever, acute glomerulonephritis secondary to streptococcal infection).

Acute evolving transmural myocardial infarction (give as soon as possible after symptoms occur):
IV Infusion: Adults, elderly: (1.5 million units diluted to 45 ml): 1.5 million IU infused over 60 min. **Intracoronary Infusion: Adults, elderly: 250,000 units diluted to 125 ml):** Initially, 20,000 IU (10 ml)

bolus; then, 2,000 IU/min for 60 min. **Total dose:** 140,000 IU.

Pulmonary embolism, deep vein thrombosis, arterial thrombosis/embolism (give within 7 days after onset):
IV Infusion: Adults, elderly: (1.5 million units diluted to 90 ml): Initially, 250,000 IU infused over 30 min; then, 100,000 IU/hr for 24–72 hrs for arterial thrombosis/embolism, 24–72 hrs for pulmonary embolism, 72 hrs for deep vein thrombosis.
Intracoronary Infusion: Adults, elderly: (1.5 million units diluted to 45 ml): Initially, 250,000 IU infused over 30 min; then, 100,000 IU/hr for maintenance.

Arteriovenous cannulae occlusion:
Instill 100,000–250,000 IU into each occluded cannula limb; clamp for 2 hrs. Aspirate contents of infused cannula limb; flush w/saline, reconnect cannula.

PRECAUTIONS

CONTRAINDICATIONS: Active internal bleeding, recent (within 2 mos) cerebrovascular accident, intracranial/intraspinal surgery, intracranial neoplasm, severe uncontrolled hypertension. **CAUTIONS:** Recent (10 days) major surgery/GI bleeding, obstetrical delivery, organ biopsy, trauma (cardiopulmonary resuscitation); uncontrolled arterial hypertension, left heart thrombus, endocarditis, severe hepatic/renal disease, pregnancy, elderly, cerebrovascular disease, diabetic retinopathy, thrombophlebitis, occluded AV cannula at infected site. **PREGNANCY/LACTATION:** Use only when benefit outweighs potential risk to fetus. Unknown whether drug crosses placenta or is distributed in breast milk. **Pregnancy Category C**.

INTERACTIONS

DRUG INTERACTIONS: Anticoagulants, heparin may increase risk of hemorrhage. Platelet aggregation inhibitors (e.g., aspirin) may increase risk of bleeding. **ALTERED LAB VALUES:** Decreases plasminogen and fibrinogen level during infusion, decreasing clotting time (confirms presence of lysis).

SIDE EFFECTS

FREQUENT: Fever, superficial bleeding at puncture sites, decreased B/P. **OCCASIONAL:** Allergic reaction (rash, wheezing), bruising. **RARE:** Skin lesions.

ADVERSE REACTIONS/TOXIC EFFECTS

Severe internal hemorrhage may occur. Lysis of coronary thrombi may produce atrial/ventricular arrhythmias.

NURSING IMPLICATIONS
BASELINE ASSESSMENT:

Assess Hct, platelet count, thrombin (TT), activated thromboplastin (APTT), prothrombin (PT) time, fibrinogen level, before therapy is instituted. If heparin is component of treatment, discontinue before streptokinase is instituted (TT/APTT should be less than twice normal value before institution of therapy).

INTERVENTION/EVALUATION:

Monitor EKG continuously. Assess clinical response, vital signs (pulse, temperature, respiratory rate, B/P) q4h or per protocol. Handle pt carefully and as infrequently as possible to prevent bleeding. Do not obtain B/P in lower extremities (possible deep vein thrombi). Monitor TT, PT, APTT, fibrinogen level q4h after initiation of therapy. Check stool for occult blood. Assess for decrease in B/P, increase in pulse rate, complaint of abdominal/back pain, severe headache (may be evidence of hemorrhage). Question for increase in amount of discharge during menses. Assess area of thromboembolus for color, temperature. Assess peripheral pulses, skin for bruises and petechiae. Check for excessive bleeding from minor cuts, scratches. Assess urine output for hematuria.

streptomycin sulfate
(Streptomycin)
See Classification section under:
Antibiotics: Aminoglycosides

streptozocin

strep-to-**zoe**-sin
(Zanosar)

CANADIAN AVAILABILITY:
Zanosar

CLASSIFICATION

Antineoplastic

AVAILABILITY (Rx)

Powder for Injection: 1 g

PHARMACOKINETICS

Rapidly distributed primarily in liver, kidneys, intestine, pancreas. Metabolized in liver. Primarily excreted in urine. Half-life: 35 min; metabolite: 40 min.

ACTION/THERAPEUTIC EFFECT

Cross-links strands of DNA, inhibiting DNA synthesis, *promoting cell death.* Cell cycle-phase nonspecific.

USES/UNLABELED

Treatment of metastatic islet cell carcinoma of pancreas. *Treatment of carcinoid tumors.*

STORAGE/HANDLING

Note: May be carcinogenic, mutagenic, or teratogenic. Handle w/extreme care during preparation/administration.

Refrigerate unopened vials. Solutions are clear to pale gold. Discard if color changes to dark brown (indicates decomposition). Discard solution within 12 hrs after reconstitution.

IV ADMINISTRATION

Note: May give by IV injection or infusion. Wear gloves when preparing solution (topical contact may be carcinogenic hazard). If powder or solution comes in contact w/skin, wash immediately, thoroughly w/soap, water.

1. Reconstitute 1 g vial w/9.5 ml 5% dextrose or 0.9% NaCl injection to provide concentration of 100 mg/ml.

2. For IV injection, administer over 10–15 min.

3. For IV infusion, further dilute w/10–200 ml 5% dextrose or 0.9% NaCl solution and infuse over 15 min–6 hrs.

4. Extravasation may produce severe tissue necrosis. Apply warm compresses to reduce severity of irritation at IV site.

INDICATIONS/DOSAGE/ROUTES

Note: Dosage individualized based on clinical response, tolerance to adverse effects. When used in combination therapy, consult specific protocols for optimum dosage, sequence of drug administration. Dosage based on body surface area (BSA).

Daily:
IV: Adults, elderly: 500 mg/m^2 of BSA for 5 consecutive days q6 wks.

Weekly:
IV: Adults, elderly: Initially, 1 g/m^2 BSA weekly for 2 wks. May increase up to 1.5 g/m^2 BSA.

PRECAUTIONS

CONTRAINDICATIONS: None significant. **EXTREME CAUTION:** Impaired renal function. **CAUTION:** Impaired hepatic function. **PREGNANCY/LACTATION:** If possible, avoid use during pregnancy, esp. first trimester. Unknown whether distributed in breast milk. Breast-feeding not recommended. **Pregnancy Category C**.

INTERACTIONS

DRUG INTERACTIONS: Nephrotoxic medications may increase nephrotoxicity. May decrease effects of phenytoin. Live virus vaccines may potentiate virus replication, increase vaccine side effects, decrease pt's antibody response to vaccine. **ALTERED LAB VALUES:** May increase SGOT (AST), SGPT (ALT), alkaline phosphatase, bilirubin, LDH, BUN, creatinine, urinary protein. May decrease albumin, phosphate concentrations.

SIDE EFFECTS

FREQUENT (>90%): Severe nausea, vomiting (usually begins 1–4 hrs after administration; may persist over 24 hrs). **OCCASIONAL:** A burning sensation originating at IV site and moving up arm (occurs particularly w/rapid IV injection), diarrhea, confusion, lethargy, depression, particularly in those receiving continuous IV infusion over 5 days.

ADVERSE REACTIONS/TOXIC EFFECTS

High incidence of nephrotoxicity manifested by azotemia, anuria, proteinuria, hyperchloremia, hypophosphatemia. Proximal renal tubular acidosis evidenced by glycosuria, acetonuria, aminoaciduria. Mild to moderate bone marrow depression manifested as hematologic toxicity (leukopenia, thrombocytopenia, anemia). Severe myelosuppression, hepatotoxicity occur rarely.

NURSING IMPLICATIONS

BASELINE ASSESSMENT:

Phenothiazine antiemetics only minimally effective in preventing/reducing nausea, vomiting; droperidol, metoclopramide appear to be more effective. Obtain renal function tests, electrolytes, CBC before and weekly during therapy. Obtain hepatic function tests before therapy.

INTERVENTION/EVALUATION:

Monitor urinalysis, creatinine clearance, BUN, serum creatinine, electrolyte, CBC. (Earliest sign of renal toxicity is mild proteinuria, glycosuria.) Inform physician if urine is positive for proteinuria or if vomiting exceeds 600–800 ml/8 hrs. Monitor for hematologic toxicity (fever, sore throat, signs of local infection, easy bruising, unusual bleeding from any site), symptoms of anemia (excessive tiredness, weakness).

PATIENT/FAMILY TEACHING:

Do not have immunizations w/o physician's approval (drug lowers body's resistance). Avoid contact w/those who have recently received live virus vaccine. Promptly report fever, sore throat, signs of local infection, easy bruising/unusual bleeding from any site. Increase fluid intake (decreases risk of nephrotoxicity). A burning sensation may be noted w/IV administration. Contact physician if nausea/vomiting continues at home.

---

succinylcholine chloride
(Anectine, Quelicin)
See Classification section under: Neuromuscular blockers

---

sucralfate
sue-**kral**-fate
(Carafate)

CANADIAN AVAILABILITY:
Novo-Sucralate, Sulcrate

CLASSIFICATION

Antiulcer

AVAILABILITY (Rx)

Tablets: 1 g. **Oral Suspension:** 500 mg/5 ml.

PHARMACOKINETICS

Minimally absorbed from GI tract. Eliminated in feces w/small amount excreted in urine.

ACTION/*THERAPEUTIC EFFECT*

Forms adhesive gel that adheres to ulcer site. *Gel protects* damaged mucosa from further destruction by absorbing gastric acid, pepsin, bile salts and reacting w/exudation of proteins.

USES / *UNLABELED*

Short-term treatment (up to 8 wks) of duodenal ulcer. Maintenance therapy of duodenal ulcer after healing of acute ulcers. *Treatment of gastric ulcer, rheumatoid arthritis (relieves GI symptoms associated w/NSAIDs), prevents/treatment of stress-related mucosal damage especially ICU pts, treatment of gastroesophageal reflux.*

PO ADMINISTRATION

1. Administer 1 hr before meals and at bedtime.
2. Tablets may be crushed/dissolved in water.
3. Avoid antacids $\frac{1}{2}$ hr before or after giving sucralfate.

INDICATIONS / DOSAGE / ROUTES

Note: 1 g = 10 ml suspension.

Duodenal ulcers, active:
PO: Adults, elderly: 1 g 4 times/day (before meals and at bedtime) for up to 8 wks.

Duodenal ulcers, maintenance:
PO: Adults, elderly: 1 g 2 times/day.

PRECAUTIONS

CONTRAINDICATIONS: None significant. **CAUTIONS:** None significant. **PREGNANCY/LACTATION:** Unknown whether drug crosses placenta or is distributed in breast milk. **Pregnancy Category B.**

INTERACTIONS

DRUG INTERACTIONS: Antacids may interfere w/binding (do not give within $\frac{1}{2}$ hr). May decrease absorption of digoxin, phenytoin, quinolones (e.g., ciprofloxacin), theophylline (do not give within 2–3 hrs of sucralfate). **ALTERED LAB VALUES:** None significant.

SIDE EFFECTS

FREQUENT (2%): Constipation. **OCCASIONAL (<2%):** Dry mouth, backache, diarrhea, dizziness, drowsiness, nausea, indigestion, skin rash/hives/itching, stomach discomfort.

ADVERSE REACTIONS / TOXIC EFFECTS

None significant.

NURSING IMPLICATIONS

INTERVENTION / EVALUATION:

Monitor stool consistency and frequency.

PATIENT / FAMILY TEACHING:

Take medication on an empty stomach. Antacids may be given as an adjunct but should not be taken for 30 min before or after sucralfate (formation of sucralfate gel is activated by stomach acid). Dry mouth may be relieved by sour hard candy or sips of tepid water.

sufentanil citrate
(Sufenta)
See Classification section under:
Opioid analgesics

sulconazole nitrate
(Exelderm)
See Classification section under:
Antifungals: topical

sulfacetamide sodium

sul-fah-**see**-tah-mide
(AK-Sulf, Bleph-10, Isopto
Cetamide, Ophthacet, Sodium
Sulamyd, Sulfair)

FIXED-COMBINATION(S):
W/phenylephrine hydrochloride, a
sympathomimetic (**Vasosulf**);
w/prednisolone, a steroid (**Blephamide, Cetapred, Metimyd,
Optimyd, Sulphrin, Vasocidin**)

CANADIAN AVAILABILITY:
Cetamide, Diosulf, Sodium Sulamyd

CLASSIFICATION

Sulfonamide

AVAILABILITY (Rx)

Ophthalmic Solution: 10%,
15%, 30%. **Ophthalmic Ointment:**
10%. **Topical Lotion:** 10%.

PHARMACOKINETICS

Minimal absorption after ophthalmic administration.

ACTION/*THERAPEUTIC EFFECT*

Interferes w/synthesis of folic
acid that bacteria require for
growth, *preventing further bacterial growth.* Bacteriostatic.

USES/*UNLABELED*

Treatment of corneal ulcers,
conjunctivitis and other superficial
infections of the eye, prophylaxis
after injuries to the eye/removal of
foreign bodies, adjunctive therapy
for trachoma and inclusion conjunctivitis. **Topical lotion:** Seborrheic dermatitis, seborrheic sicca
(dandruff), secondary bacterial
skin infections. **Ophthalmic:** *Treatment of bacterial blepharitis, ble-*
pharoconjunctivitis, bacterial kerati-
tis, keratoconjunctivitis.

STORAGE/HANDLING

Protect from light. May develop
a yellow-brown or reddish-brown
color. Do not use if color change
occurs/precipitate forms.

OPHTHALMIC ADMINISTRATION

1. Place finger on lower eyelid
and pull out until a pocket is
formed between eye and lower lid.

2. Hold dropper above pocket
and place correct number of
drops ($1/4$–$1/2$ inch ointment) into
pocket. Close eye gently.

3. For solution: Apply digital
pressure to lacrimal sac for 1–2 min
(minimizes drainage into nose and
throat, reducing risk of systemic effects). For ointment: Close eye for
1–2 min, rolling eyeball (increases
contact area of drug to eye).

4. Remove excess solution/
ointment around eye w/tissue.

INDICATIONS/DOSAGE/ROUTES

Usual ophthalmic dosage:
Ophthalmic: Adults, elderly:
Ointment: Apply small amount in
lower conjunctival sac 1–4
times/day and at bedtime. Solution: 1–3 drops to lower conjunctival sac q2–3h.

Usual topical dosage:
Topical: Adults, elderly: Apply
1–4 times/day.

PRECAUTIONS

CONTRAINDICATIONS: Hypersensitivity to sulfonamides or any
component of preparation (some
products contain sulfite). **CAU-
TIONS:** Extremely dry eye. Application of lotion to large infected,
denuded, or debrided areas.
PREGNANCY/LACTATION: Un-

known whether excreted in breast milk. **Pregnancy Category C**.

INTERACTIONS

DRUG INTERACTIONS: Silver-containing preparations are incompatible. **ALTERED LAB VALUES:** None significant.

SIDE EFFECTS

FREQUENT: Transient burning, stinging w/ophthalmic application. **OCCASIONAL:** Headache, local irritation. **RARE:** Hypersensitivity: erythema, rash, itching, swelling. Retarded corneal healing, photosensitivity.

ADVERSE REACTIONS/TOXIC EFFECTS

Superinfection, drug-induced lupus erythematosus, Stevens-Johnson syndrome occur rarely; nephrotoxicity w/high dermatologic concentrations.

NURSING IMPLICATIONS
BASELINE ASSESSMENT:

Question for hypersensitivity to sulfonamides, any ingredients of preparation (e.g., sulfite).

INTERVENTION/EVALUATION:

Withhold medication and notify physician at once of hypersensitivity reaction (redness, itching, urticaria, rash). Assess for fever, joint pain, or sores in mouth—discontinue drug and inform physician immediately.

PATIENT/FAMILY TEACHING:

Continue therapy as directed. May have transient burning, stinging upon ophthalmic application; may cause sensitivity to light—wear sunglasses, avoid bright light. Notify physician of

any new symptom, esp. swelling, itching, rash, joint pain, fever. For topical skin/scalp treatment, cleanse (shampoo) area before application to ensure direct contact w/affected areas.

sulfasalazine
sul-fah-**sal**-ah-zeen
(Azulfidine, Azulfidine EN-tabs)

CANADIAN AVAILABILITY: Salazopyrin, SAS-500

CLASSIFICATION

Sulfonamide, anti-inflammatory

AVAILABILITY (Rx)

Tablets: 500 mg. **Oral Suspension:** 250 mg/5 ml.

PHARMACOKINETICS

Poorly absorbed from GI tract. Cleaved in colon by intestinal bacterial forming sulfapyridine and mesalamine (5-ASA). Absorbed in colon. Widely distributed. Metabolized in liver. Primarily excreted in urine. Half-life: sulfapyridine: 6–14 hrs; 5-ASA: 0.6–1.4 hrs.

ACTION/*THERAPEUTIC EFFECT*

Blocks prostaglandin synthesis, *producing anti-inflammatory and antibacterial effect.*

USES/*UNLABELED*

Treatment of ulcerative colitis, inflammatory bowel disease, rheumatoid arthritis. *Treatment of ankylosing spondylitis.*

PO ADMINISTRATION

1. Space doses evenly (intervals not to exceed 8 hrs).

2. Administer after meals if possible (prolong intestinal passage).

3. Swallow enteric-coated tablets whole; do not chew.

4. Give w/8 oz water; encourage several glasses of water between meals.

INDICATIONS/DOSAGE/ROUTES

Ulcerative colitis:
PO: **Adults, elderly:** Initially, 1–4 g/day in divided doses. **Maintenance:** 2 g/day in 4 divided doses. **Children >2 yrs:** Initially, 40–60 mg/kg/day in 4–6 divided doses. **Maintenance:** 20–30 mg/kg in 4 divided doses. **Maximum:** 2 g/day.

Rheumatoid arthritis:
PO: **Adults, elderly:** Initially, 0.5–1 g/day for 1 wk. Increase by 0.5 g/wk, up to 3 g/day.

PRECAUTIONS

CONTRAINDICATIONS: Hypersensitivity to salicylates, sulfonamides, sulfonylureas, thiazide or loop diuretics, carbonic anhydrase inhibitors, sunscreens containing PABA, local anesthetics, pregnancy at term, severe hepatic/renal dysfunction, porphyria, intestinal/urinary tract obstruction, children <2 yrs. **CAUTIONS:** Severe allergies, bronchial asthma, impaired hepatic/renal function, G-6-PD deficiency. **PREGNANCY/LACTATION:** May produce infertility, oligospermia in men while on medication. Readily crosses placenta; if given near term, may produce jaundice, hemolytic anemia, kernicterus. Excreted in breast milk. Do not nurse premature infant or those w/hyperbilirubinemia or G-6-PD deficiency. **Pregnancy Category B**. (Category D if given near term.)

INTERACTIONS

DRUG INTERACTIONS: May increase effects of oral anticoagulants, anticonvulsants, oral hypoglycemics, methotrexate. Hemolytics may increase toxicity. Hepatotoxic medications may increase hepatotoxicity. **ALTERED LAB VALUES:** None significant.

SIDE EFFECTS

FREQUENT (33%): Anorexia, nausea, vomiting, headache, oligospermia (generally reversed by withdrawal of drug). **OCCASIONAL (3%):** Hypersensitivity reaction: rash, urticaria, pruritus, fever, anemia. **RARE (<1%):** Tinnitus, hypoglycemia, diuresis, photosensitivity.

ADVERSE REACTIONS/TOXIC EFFECTS

Anaphylaxis, Stevens-Johnson syndrome, hematologic toxicity (leukopenia, agranulocytosis); hepatotoxicity, nephrotoxicity occur rarely.

NURSING IMPLICATIONS
BASELINE ASSESSMENT:

Question for hypersensitivity to medications (see Contraindications). Check initial urinalysis, CBC, hepatic and renal function tests.

INTERVENTION/EVALUATION:

Check I&O, urinalysis, renal function tests; assure adequate hydration (minimum output 1,500 ml/24 hr) to prevent nephrotoxicity. Evaluate food tolerance (distribute doses more evenly or consult physician regarding enteric-coated tablets, reduction of dose). Assess skin for rash (discontinue drug/notify physician at first sign). Check pattern of bowel activity, stool consistency (dosage may need to be increased if diarrhea continues/recurs). Monitor CBC closely; assess for/report immediately hematologic effects: bleeding, bruising, fever, sore throat, pallor, weakness, purpura, jaundice.

PATIENT/FAMILY TEACHING:

May cause orange-yellow discoloration of urine, skin. Space doses evenly around the clock. Take after food w/8 oz water; drink several glasses of water between meals. Continue for full length of treatment; may be necessary to take drug even after symptoms relieved. Do not take any other medications (including vitamins) w/o consulting physician. Follow-up, lab tests are essential. In event of dental/other surgery inform dentist/surgeon of sulfasalazine therapy. Notify physician of any new symptom, immediately for fever, sore throat, shortness of breath, rash, any bleeding, ringing in ears. Avoid exposure to sun/ultraviolet light until photosensitivity determined (may last for months after last dose).

sulindac
suel-**in**-dak
(Clinoril)

CANADIAN AVAILABILITY:
Apo-Sulin, Novo Sundac

CLASSIFICATION

Nonsteroidal anti-inflammatory

AVAILABILITY (Rx)

Tablets: 150 mg, 200 mg

PHARMACOKINETICS

ONSET	PEAK	DURATION
PO (antirheumatic):		
7 days	2–3wks	—

Well absorbed from GI tract. Me-tabolized in liver to active metabolite. Primarily excreted in urine. Half-life: 7.8 hrs; metabolite: 16.4 hrs.

ACTION/*THERAPEUTIC EFFECT*

Produces analgesic and anti-inflammatory effect by inhibiting prostaglandin synthesis, *reducing inflammatory response and intensity of pain stimulus reaching sensory nerve endings.*

USES

Treatment of pain of rheumatoid arthritis, osteoarthritis, ankylosing spondylitis, acute painful shoulder, bursitis/tendinitis, acute gouty arthritis.

PO ADMINISTRATION

May give w/food, milk, or antacids if GI distress occurs.

INDICATIONS/DOSAGE/ROUTES

Rheumatoid arthritis, osteoarthritis, ankylosing spondylitis:
PO: Adults, elderly: Initially, 150 mg 2 times/day, up to 400 mg/day.

Acute painful shoulder, gouty arthritis, bursitis, tendinitis:
PO: Adults, elderly: 200 mg 2 times/day.

PRECAUTIONS

CONTRAINDICATIONS: Active peptic ulcer, GI ulceration, chronic inflammation of GI tract, GI bleeding disorders, history of hypersensitivity to aspirin/NSAIDs. **CAUTIONS:** Impaired renal/hepatic function, history of GI tract disease, predisposition to fluid retention. **PREGNANCY/LACTATION:** Unknown whether drug is excreted in breast milk. Avoid use during third trimester (may adversely affect fetal cardiovascular system: premature closure of ductus arteriosus). **Pregnancy Category B**. (Category D if used in 3rd trimester or near delivery.)

INTERACTIONS

DRUG INTERACTIONS: May increase effects of oral anticoagulants, heparin, thrombolytics. May decrease effect of antihypertensives, diuretics. Salicylates, aspirin may increase risk of GI side effects, bleeding. Bone marrow depressants may increase risk of hematologic reactions. May increase concentration, toxicity of lithium. May increase methotrexate toxicity. Probenecid may increase concentration. Antacids may decrease concentration. **ALTERED LAB VALUES:** May increase alkaline phosphatase, liver function tests.

SIDE EFFECTS

Note: Age increases possibility of side effects.
FREQUENT (3–9%): Diarrhea/constipation, indigestion, nausea, maculopapular rash, dermatitis, dizziness, headache. **OCCASIONAL (1–3%):** Anorexia, GI cramps, flatulence.

ADVERSE REACTIONS/TOXIC EFFECTS

GI bleeding, peptic ulcer occur infrequently. Nephrotoxicity (glomerular nephritis, interstitial nephritis, and nephrotic syndrome) may occur in those w/preexisting impaired renal function. Acute hypersensitivity reaction (fever, chills, joint pain) occurs rarely.

NURSING IMPLICATIONS

BASELINE ASSESSMENT:

Assess onset, type, location, and duration of pain, fever, or inflammation. Inspect appearance of affected joints for immobility, deformities, and skin condition.

INTERVENTION/EVALUATION:

Assist w/ambulation if dizziness occurs. Monitor pattern of daily bowel activity, stool consistency. Assess for evidence of rash. Evaluate for therapeutic response: relief of pain, stiffness, swelling, increase in joint mobility, reduced joint tenderness, improved grip strength.

PATIENT/FAMILY TEACHING:

Therapeutic antiarthritic effect noted 1–3 wks after therapy begins. Avoid aspirin, alcohol during therapy (increases risk of GI bleeding). If GI upset occurs, take w/food, milk.

sumatriptan succinate injection

sue-mah-**trip**-tan
(Imitrex)

CANADIAN AVAILABILITY:
Imitrex

CLASSIFICATION

Antimigraine

AVAILABILITY (Rx)

Tablets: 25 mg, 50 mg. **Injection:** 12 mg/ml. **Nasal Spray:** 5 mg, 20 mg.

PHARMACOKINETICS

	ONSET	PEAK	DURATION
SubQ	<10 min	<2 hrs	—

Rapidly absorbed after SubQ administration. Widely distributed, protein binding (10–21%). Undergoes first-pass hepatic metabolism; excreted in urine. Half-life: 2 hrs.

ACTION/THERAPEUTIC EFFECT

Binds selectively to vascular receptors producing a vasoconstrictive effect on cranial blood vessels, *producing relief of migraine headache.* Efficiency of relief unaffected by aura, duration of attack, concurrent use of other antimigraine medications (e.g., beta blockers).

USES:

Acute treatment of migraine headache with or without aura; treatment of cluster headaches.

STORAGE/HANDLING

Store at room temperature.

INDICATIONS/DOSAGE/ROUTES

Vascular headache:
SubQ: Adults, elderly: 6 mg. **Maximum:** No more than two 6 mg injections within a 24 hr period separated by at least 1 hr between injections.
PO: Adults, elderly: 50 mg. **Maximum single dose:** 100 mg. May repeat no sooner than 2 hrs. **Maximum:** 300 mg/24 hrs.
Nasal: Adults, elderly: 5–20 mg; may repeat in 2 hrs. **Maximum:** 40 mg/24 hrs.

PRECAUTIONS

CONTRAINDICATIONS: IV use, those w/ischemic heart disease (angina pectoris, history of myocardial infarction), silent ischemia, Prinzmetal's angina, uncontrolled hypertension, concurrent ergotamine-containing preparations, hemiplegic or basilar migraine. **CAUTIONS:** Hepatic, renal impairment. Pt profile suggesting cardiovascular risks. **PREGNANCY/LACTATION:** Unknown whether distributed in breast milk. **Pregnancy Category C.**

INTERACTIONS

DRUG INTERACTIONS: Ergotamine-containing drugs may produce vasospastic reaction. Monoamine oxidase inhibitors may increase concentration, half-life. **ALTERED LAB VALUES:** None significant.

SIDE EFFECTS

FREQUENT: *Oral (5–10%):* Tingling, nasal discomfort. *Subcutaneous (>10%):* Injection site reactions, tingling, warm, hot sensation, dizziness, vertigo. *Nasal (>10%):* Bad, unusual taste, nausea, vomiting. **OCCASIONAL:** *Oral (1–5%):* Flushing, weakness, visual disturbances. *Subcutaneous (2–10%):* Burning sensation, numbness, chest discomfort, drowsiness, weakness. *Nasal (1–5%):* Discomfort of nasal cavity/throat, dizziness. **RARE:** *Oral (<1%):* Agitation, eye irritation, dysuria. *Subcutaneous (<2%):* Anxiety, fatigue, sweating, muscle cramps, muscle pain. *Nasal (<1%):* Burning sensation.

ADVERSE REACTIONS/TOXIC EFFECTS

Excessive dosage may produce tremor, redness of extremities, reduced respirations, cyanosis, convulsions, paralysis. Serious arrhythmias occur rarely, but particularly in those w/hypertension, obesity, smokers, diabetics, and those w/strong family history of coronary artery disease.

NURSING IMPLICATIONS

BASELINE ASSESSMENT:

Question pt regarding history of peripheral vascular disease, renal/hepatic impairment, or possibility of pregnancy. Question pt regarding onset, location, and duration of migraine and possible precipitating symptoms.

INTERVENTION/EVALUATION:

Evaluate for relief of migraine headache and resulting photophobia, phonophobia (sound sensitivity), nausea and vomiting.

PATIENT/FAMILY TEACHING:

Teach pt proper loading of autoinjector, injection technique, and discarding of syringe. Do not use more than 2 injections during any 24 hr period and allow at least 1 hr between injections. If experience wheezing, heart throbbing, skin rash, swelling of eyelids/face/lips, pain/tightness in chest or throat, contact physician immediately.

---

tacrine

tay-crin
(Cognex)

CLASSIFICATION

Antidementia

AVAILABILITY (Rx)

Capsules: 10 mg, 20 mg, 30 mg, 40 mg

PHARMACOKINETICS

Rapidly absorbed from GI tract. Undergoes first-pass metabolism in liver. Half-life: 2–4 hrs.

ACTION/ *THERAPEUTIC EFFECT*

Elevates acetylcholine concentrations in cerebral cortex by slowing degeneration of acetylcholine released by still intact cholinergic neurons (Alzheimer's disease involves degeneration of cholinergic neuronal pathways). *Resultant effect slows Alzheimer's disease process.*

USES

Symptomatic treatment of pts w/Alzheimer's disease.

PO ADMINISTRATION

May give w/o regard to food.

INDICATIONS/DOSAGE/ROUTES

Alzheimer's disease:
PO: Adults, elderly: Initially, 10 mg 4 times/day for 6 wks; then 20 mg 4 times/day for 6 wks; then 30 mg 4 times/day for 12 wks; then to maximum of 40 mg 4 times/day if needed.
Note: If medication is stopped for >14 days, must retitrate as noted above.

PRECAUTIONS

CONTRAINDICATIONS: Known hypersensitivity to cholinergics; current treatment w/other cholinesterase inhibitors; severe, active liver disease; active, untreated gastric/duodenal ulcers; mechanical obstruction of intestine/urinary tract; pregnancy, nursing, or childbearing potential. **CAUTIONS:** Known liver dysfunction, asthma, COPD, seizure disorders, bradycardia, hyperthyroidism, cardiac arrhythmias, history of gastric/intestinal ulcers, alcohol abuse. **PREGNANCY/LACTATION:** May cause fetal harm; unknown whether secreted in breast milk. **Pregnancy Category C**.

INTERACTIONS

DRUG INTERACTIONS: May increase theophylline concentration; cimetidine may increase tacrine concentrations; may interfere w/anticholinergics; may increase adverse effects of NSAIDs. **ALTERED LAB VALUES:** Increases SGOT (AST), SGPT (ALT); alters hematocrit, hemoglobin, electrolytes.

SIDE EFFECTS

FREQUENT (11–28%): Headache, nausea, vomiting, diarrhea, dizziness. **OCCASIONAL (4–9%):** Fatigue, chest pain, dyspepsia, anorexia, abdominal pain, flatulence, constipation, confusion, agitation, rash, depression, ataxia (muscular incoordination), insomnia, rhinitis, myalgia. **RARE (<3%):** Weight loss, anxiety, cough, facial flushing, urinary frequency, back pain, tremor.

ADVERSE REACTIONS/TOXIC EFFECTS

Overdose can cause cholinergic crises (increased salivation, lacrimation, urination, defecation, bradycardia, hypotension, increased muscle weakness). Treatment aimed at general supportive measures, use of anticholinergics (e.g., atropine).

NURSING IMPLICATIONS

BASELINE ASSESSMENT:

Assess cognitive, behavioral, and functional deficits of pt. Assess liver function.

INTERVENTION/EVALUATION:

Monitor cognitive, behavioral, and functional status of pt. Monitor SGOT (AST), SGPT (ALT). EKG evaluation, periodic rhythm strips in pts w/underlying arrhythmias. Monitor for symptoms of ulcer, GI bleeding.

PATIENT/FAMILY TEACHING:

Take at regular intervals, between meals (may take w/meals if GI upset occurs). Do not reduce or stop medication; do not increase dosage w/o physician direction. Report increasing or new symptoms. Do not smoke (reduces plasma concentration of tacrine). Periodic lab tests are essential. Inform family of local chapter of Alzheimer's Disease Association (provides a guide to services for these pts).

tacrolimus

tack-row-**lee**-mus
(Prograf)

CANADIAN AVAILABILITY:
Prograf

CLASSIFICATION

Immunosuppressant

AVAILABILITY (Rx)

Capsules: 1 mg, 5 mg. **Injection:** 5 mg/ml.

PHARMACOKINETICS

Variably absorbed following oral administration (food reduces absorption). Extensively metabolized in the liver. Excreted in urine. Half-life: 11.7 hrs.

ACTION/*THERAPEUTIC EFFECT*

Binds to intracellular protein, forming a complex, inhibiting phosphatase activity. This effect results in inhibition of T-lymphocyte activation, suppressing immunologically mediated inflammatory response. *Assists in prevention of liver transplant rejection.*

USES/*UNLABELED*

Prophylaxis of organ rejection in pts receiving allogeneic liver transplants, kidney transplants. Should be used concurrently w/adrenal corticosteroids. *Bone marrow, cardiac, pancreas, pancreatic island cell, and small-bowel transplantation. Treatment of autoimmune disease, severe recalcitrant psoriasis.*

STORAGE/HANDLING

Store diluted infusion solution in glass or polyethylene containers and discard after 24 hrs. Do not store in a PVC container (decreased stability, potential for extraction).

IV ADMINISTRATION

1. Dilute w/0.9% NaCl injection or 5% dextrose injection to concentration between 0.004 and 0.02 mg/ml.
2. Give as continuous IV infusion.
3. Continuously monitor pt for anaphylaxis for at least 30 min fol-

T

lowing start of infusion. Stop infusion immediately at first sign of hypersensitivity reaction.

INDICATIONS/DOSAGE/ROUTES

Note: In pts unable to take capsules, initiate therapy with IV infusion. Give oral dose 8–12 hrs after discontinuing IV infusion. Titrate dosing based on clinical assessments of rejection and tolerability. In pts w/hepatic/renal function impairment, give lowest IV and oral dosing range (delay dosing up to 48 hrs or longer in pts w/postop oliguria).

Liver transplantation:
IV Infusion: Adults, elderly: 0.05–0.1 mg/kg/day with initial dose given no sooner than 6 hrs after transplant. Titrate dosing based. Give adult pts doses at lower end of dosing range. Give in combination w/adrenal corticosteroids. Transfer to oral therapy when oral tolerance is apparent (usually occurs within 2–3 days).
PO: Adults: 0.15–0.3 mg/kg/day given in 2 divided daily doses q12h. Give initial dose no sooner than 6 hrs after transplant. Give in combination w/adrenal corticosteroids.

Pediatric dosage
(w/o preexisting renal or hepatic dysfunction):
IV Infusion: 0.1 mg/kg/day.
PO: 0.3 mg/kg/day

PRECAUTIONS

CONTRAINDICATIONS: Hypersensitivity to tacrolimus, hypersensitivity to HCO-60 polyoxyl 60 hydrogenated castor oil (used in vehicle for injection), cyclosporine (increased risk of ototoxicity). **CAUTIONS:** Immunosuppressed pts, renal/hepatic function impairment. **PREGNANCY/LACTA-**

TION: Crosses placenta. Neonatal hyperkalemia, renal dysfunction noted in neonates. Excreted in breast milk. Avoid nursing. **Pregnancy Category C.**

INTERACTIONS

DRUG INTERACTIONS: Aminoglycosides, amphotericin B, cisplatin increase risk of renal dysfunction. Cyclosporine increases risk of nephrotoxicity. Antifungals, bromocriptine, calcium channel blockers, cimetidine, clarithromycin, cyclosporine, danazol, diltiazem, erythromycin, methylprednisolone, metoclopramide increase tacrolimus blood levels. Carbamazepine, phenobarbital, phenytoin, rifamycins decrease tacrolimus blood levels. Other immunosuppressants may increase risk of infection or development of lymphomas. Live virus vaccines may potentiate virus replication, increase vaccine side effects, decrease pt's antibody response to vaccine. **ALTERED LAB VALUES:** May increase creatinine, BUN, WBCs, glucose. May decrease thrombocytes, RBCs, magnesium. Alters potassium level.

SIDE EFFECTS

FREQUENT (>30%): Headache, tremor, insomnia, paresthesia, diarrhea, nausea, constipation, vomiting, abdominal pain, hypertension. **OCCASIONAL (10–30%):** Rash, pruritus, anorexia, asthenia, peripheral edema.

ADVERSE REACTIONS/TOXIC EFFECTS

Nephrotoxicity, pleural effusion occur frequently. Overt nephrotoxicity characterized by increasing serum creatinine, decrease in urine output. Thrombocytopenia, leukocytosis, anemia, atelectasis occur occasionally. Neurotoxicity, including tremor, headache, mental status changes, occur commonly. Sepsis, infection occur occasionally. Significant anemia, thrombocytopenia, leukocytosis may occur.

NURSING IMPLICATIONS
BASELINE ASSESSMENT:

Assess medical history, esp. renal function, drug history, esp. other immunosuppressants. Have aqueous solution of epinephrine 1:1,000 available at bedside as well as O_2 before beginning IV infusion. Assess pt continuously for first 30 min following start of infusion and at frequent intervals thereafter.

INTERVENTION/EVALUATION:

Closely monitor pts w/impaired renal function. Monitor lab values, esp. serum creatinine, serum potassium levels. CBC w/differential, hepatic function tests. Monitor I&O closely. CBC should be performed weekly during first month of therapy, twice monthly during second and third months of treatment, then monthly throughout the first year. Report any major change in assessment of pt. Routinely watch for any change from normal.

PATIENT/FAMILY TEACHING:

Contact physician if unusual bleeding or bruising, sore throat, mouth sores, abdominal pain, or fever occurs. Inform pts of need for laboratory tests while taking medication, increased risk of neoplasia.

---

talc
(Sclerosol)
See Supplement

---

tamoxifen citrate
tam-**ox**-ih-fen
(Nolvadex)

CANADIAN AVAILABILITY:
Apo-Tamox, Nolvaldex-D, Novo-Tamoxifen, Tamofen, Tamone

CLASSIFICATION
Antineoplastic

AVAILABILITY (Rx)
Tablets: 10 mg, 20 mg

PHARMACOKINETICS
Well absorbed from GI tract. Metabolized in liver. Primarily eliminated in feces via biliary system. Half-life: 7 days.

ACTION/*THERAPEUTIC EFFECT*
Competes w/estradiol for binding to estrogen in tissues containing high concentration of receptors (e.g., breasts, uterus, vagina). *Reduces DNA synthesis, estrogen response.*

USES
Treatment of metastatic breast carcinoma in women/men. Effective in delaying recurrence following total mastectomy and axillary dissection or segmental mastectomy, axillary dissection and breast irradiation in women w/axillary node–negative breast carcinoma. Prevention of breast cancer in high-risk women.

INDICATIONS/DOSAGE/ROUTES
Usual dosage:
PO: Adults, elderly: 10–20 mg 2 times/day in morning and evening. (20 mg a single daily dose = 10 mg 2 times/day).

PRECAUTIONS
CONTRAINDICATIONS: None significant. **CAUTIONS:** Leukopenia, thrombocytopenia, increased risk of uterine cancer. **PREGNAN-**

T

CY/LACTATION: If possible, avoid use during pregnancy, esp. first trimester. May cause fetal harm. Breast-feeding not recommended. **Pregnancy Category D.**

INTERACTIONS

DRUG INTERACTIONS: Estrogens may decrease effect. **ALTERED LAB VALUES:** May increase calcium, cholesterol, triglycerides.

SIDE EFFECTS

FREQUENT: *Women (>10%):* Hot flashes, nausea, vomiting. **OCCASIONAL:** *Women (1–10%):* Changes in menstrual period, gential itching, vaginal discharge, endometrial hyperplasia/polyps. *Males:* Impotence, decreased sexual interest. *Men/Women:* Headache, nausea, vomiting, rash, bone pain, confusion, weakness, sleepiness.

ADVERSE REACTIONS/TOXIC EFFECTS

Retinopathy, corneal opacity, decreased visual acuity noted in those receiving extremely high doses (240–320 mg/day) for >17 mos.

NURSING IMPLICATIONS
BASELINE ASSESSMENT:

An estrogen receptor assay should be done before therapy is begun. CBC, platelet count, serum calcium levels should be checked before and periodically during therapy.

INTERVENTION/EVALUATION:

Be alert to increased bone pain and assure adequate pain relief. Monitor I&O, weight; check for edema, esp. of dependent areas. Assess for hypercalcemia (increased urine volume, excessive thirst, nausea, vomiting, constipation, hypotonicity of muscles, deep bone or flank pain, renal stones).

PATIENT/FAMILY TEACHING:

Report vaginal bleeding/discharge/itching, leg cramps, weight gain, shortness of breath, weakness. May initially experience increase in bone, tumor pain (appears to indicate good tumor response). Contact physician if nausea/vomiting continues at home. Nonhormone contraceptives are recommended during treatment. Have regular gynecologic exams. Report menstrual irregularities, pelvic pain, pressure.

tamsulosin
(Flomax)
See Supplement

tazarotene
(Tazorac)
See Supplement

telmisartan
(Micardis)
See Supplement

temazepam
tem-**az**-eh-pam
(Restoril)

CANADIAN AVAILABILITY: Restoril

CLASSIFICATION
Sedative-hypnotic **(Schedule IV)**

AVAILABILITY (Rx)
Capsules: 7.5 mg, 15 mg, 30 mg

PHARMACOKINETICS
Well absorbed from GI tract. Widely distributed. Crosses blood-brain barrier. Metabolized

in liver. Primarily excreted in urine. Half-life: 8–15 hrs.

ACTION/*THERAPEUTIC EFFECT*

Enhances action of inhibitory neurotransmitter gamma-aminobutyric acid (GABA), *producing hypnotic effect due to CNS depression.*

USES

Short-term treatment of insomnia (up to 5 wks). Reduces sleep-induction time, number of nocturnal awakenings; increases length of sleep.

PO ADMINISTRATION

1. Give w/o regard to meals.
2. Capsules may be emptied and mixed w/food.

INDICATIONS/DOSAGE/ROUTES

Hypnotic:
PO: Adults >18 yrs: 15–30 mg at bedtime. **Elderly/debilitated:** 7.5–15 mg at bedtime.

PRECAUTIONS

CONTRAINDICATIONS: Acute narrow-angle glaucoma, acute alcohol intoxication. **CAUTIONS:** Impaired renal/hepatic function. **PREGNANCY/LACTATION:** Crosses placenta; may be distributed in breast milk. Chronic ingestion during pregnancy may produce withdrawal symptoms, CNS depression in neonates. **Pregnancy Category X.**

INTERACTIONS

DRUG INTERACTIONS: Alcohol, CNS depressants may increase CNS depressant effect. **ALTERED LAB VALUES:** None significant.

SIDE EFFECTS

FREQUENT: Drowsiness, sedation, rebound insomnia (may occur for 1–2 nights after drug is discontinued), dizziness, confusion, euphoria. **OCCASIONAL:** Weakness, anorexia, diarrhea. **RARE:** Paradoxical CNS excitement, restlessness (particularly noted in elderly/debilitated).

ADVERSE REACTION/TOXIC EFFECTS

Abrupt or too rapid withdrawal may result in pronounced restlessness, irritability, insomnia, hand tremors, abdominal/muscle cramps, sweating, vomiting, seizures. Overdosage results in somnolence, confusion, diminished reflexes, coma.

NURSING IMPLICATIONS

BASELINE ASSESSMENT:

Question for possibility of pregnancy before initiating therapy (Pregnancy Category X). Assess B/P, pulse, respirations immediately before administration. Raise bed rails. Provide environment conducive to sleep (back rub, quiet environment, low lighting).

INTERVENTION/EVALUATION:

Assess sleep pattern of pt. Assess elderly/debilitated for paradoxical reaction, particularly during early therapy. Evaluate for therapeutic response: decrease in number of nocturnal awakenings, increase in length of sleep.

PATIENT/FAMILY TEACHING:

Do not exceed prescribed dosage. Smoking reduces drug effectiveness. Rebound insomnia may occur when drug is discontinued after short-term therapy. Avoid alcohol and other CNS depressants. Inform physician if you are or are planning to become pregnant.

temozolomide
(Temodar)
See Supplement
See Classification section under:
Antineoplastics

teniposide

ten-**ih**-poe-side
(Vumon)

CANADIAN AVAILABILITY:
Vumon

CLASSIFICATION

Antineoplastic

AVAILABILITY (Rx)

Injection: 50 mg

PHARMACOKINETICS

Does not efficiently cross blood-brain barrier. Metabolized extensively in liver. Primarily excreted in urine. Half-life: 5 hrs.

**ACTION/ *THERAPEUTIC EFFECT* **

Induces single- and double-stranded breaks in DNA, inhibiting or altering DNA synthesis, *preventing cells from entering mitosis.* Phase specific acting in late S and early G_2 phases of cell cycle.

USES

In combination w/other antineoplastic agents, induction therapy in pts w/refractory childhood acute lymphoblastic leukemia.

STORAGE/HANDLING

Refrigerate unopened ampules. Protect from light. Reconstituted solutions stable for 24 hrs at room temperature. Discard if precipitation occurs. Use 1 mg/ml solutions within 4 hrs of preparation (reduces potential for precipitation). Do not refrigerate reconstituted solutions.

IV ADMINISTRATION

Note: Administer by slow IV infusion. Wear gloves when preparing solution. If powder or solution comes in contact w/skin, wash immediately and thoroughly w/soap, water.
    1. Dilute teniposide w/5% dextrose, 0.9% NaCl injection to provide final concentration of 0.1, 0.2, 0.4, or 1 mg/ml.
    2. Avoid contact of undiluted teniposide w/plastic (may cause softening/cracking and possible drug leakage).
    3. Prepare/administer in non-DEHP-containing LVP containers such as glass or polyolefin plastic bags/containers. Avoid use of PVC containers.
    4. Give over at least 30–60 min (decreases hypotension). Do not give by rapid IV injection.
    5. Avoid contact w/other drugs/fluids.
    6. Monitor for anaphylactic reaction during infusion (chills, fever, dyspnea, sweating, lacrimation, sneezing, throat/back/chest pain).

INDICATIONS/DOSAGE/ROUTES

Dosage individualized based on clinical response, tolerance to adverse effects. When used in combination therapy, consult specific protocols for optimum dosage, sequence of drug administration.

PRECAUTIONS

CONTRAINDICATIONS: Hypersensitivity to etoposide, teniposide, or Cremophor EL (polyoxyethylated castor oil); platelet count <50,000 mm³; absolute neutrophil count <500/mm³. **CAUTIONS:** Pts w/brain tumors/neuroblastoma (increased risk of anaphylaxis). Retreating pts w/hypersensitivity reaction to teniposide. Pts w/Down syndrome, decreased liver function. **PREGNANCY/LACTATION:**

If possible, avoid use during pregnancy, esp. during first trimester. May cause fetal harm. Breast-feeding not recommended. Unknown whether excreted in breast milk. **Pregnancy Category D**.

INTERACTIONS

DRUG INTERACTIONS: May increase intracellular accumulation of methotrexate. May increase severity of peripheral neuropathy w/vincristine. Bone marrow depressants may increase bone marrow depression. Live virus vaccines may potentiate virus replication, increase vaccine side effects, decrease pt's antibody response to vaccine. **ALTERED LAB VALUES:** None significant.

SIDE EFFECTS

FREQUENT (>30%): Mucositis, nausea, vomiting, diarrhea, anemia. **OCCASIONAL (3–5%):** Alopecia, rash. **RARE (<3%):** Liver dysfunction, fever, renal dysfunction, peripheral neurotoxicity.

ADVERSE REACTIONS/TOXIC EFFECTS

Bone marrow depression manifested as hematologic toxicity (principally leukopenia, neutropenia, thrombocytopenia) w/increased risk of infection or bleeding. Hypersensitivity reaction, including anaphylaxis (chills, fever, tachycardia, bronchospasm, dyspnea, facial flushing).

NURSING IMPLICATIONS

BASELINE ASSESSMENT:

Assess hematology (platelet count, Hgb, WBC, differential), renal and hepatic function tests before and frequently during therapy.

INTERVENTION/EVALUATION:

Have antihistamines, corticosteroids, epinephrine, IV fluids, and other supportive measures readily available for first dose (possible life-threatening anaphylaxis as evidenced by chills, fever, tachycardia, bronchospasm, dyspnea, hyper/hypotension, facial flushing). Monitor for myelosuppression: infection (fever, sore throat, signs of local infection); unusual bleeding or bruising; anemia (excessive tiredness, weakness). Pretreat w/antiemetics for nausea, vomiting but be alert to hypotension and CNS depression that may occur w/these drug combinations (because of benzyl alcohol in teniposide, esp. w/high doses).

PATIENT/FAMILY TEACHING:

Avoid crowds, those w/infection. Do not have immunizations w/o physician's approval. Promptly report fever, signs of infection, easy bruising, unusual bleeding from any site, difficulty breathing. Avoid pregnancy. Alopecia is reversible, but new hair growth may have different color or texture.

terazosin hydrochloride

tear-**aye**-zoe-sin
(Hytrin)

CANADIAN AVAILABILITY:
Apo-Terazosin, Hytrin

CLASSIFICATION

Antihypertensive

AVAILABILITY (Rx)

Capsules: 1 mg, 2 mg, 5 mg, 10 mg

PHARMACOKINETICS

	ONSET	PEAK	DURATION
PO	15 min	1–2 hrs	12–24 hrs

Rapid, complete absorption from GI tract. Metabolized in liver to active metabolite. Primarily eliminated in feces via biliary system; excreted in urine. Half-life: 12 hrs.

ACTION/ THERAPEUTIC EFFECT

Blocks alpha-adrenergic receptors. **Hypertension:** *Produces vasodilation, decreases peripheral resistance.* **Benign prostatic hypertrophy:** *Relaxes smooth muscle in bladder neck and prostate.*

USES

Treatment of mild to moderate hypertension. Used alone or in combination w/other antihypertensives. Treatment of benign prostatic hypertrophy.

PO ADMINISTRATION

1. May give w/o regard to food.

2. Tablets may be crushed.

3. Administer first dose at bedtime (minimizes risk of fainting due to "first-dose syncope").

INDICATIONS/DOSAGE/ROUTES

Note: If medication is discontinued for several days, retitrate initially using 1 mg dose at bedtime.

Hypertension:
PO: Adults, elderly: Initially, 1 mg at bedtime. Slowly increase dose to desired levels. **Range:** 1–5 mg/day as single or 2 divided doses. **Maximum:** 20 mg.

Benign prostatic hypertrophy:
PO: Adults, elderly: Initially, 1 mg at bedtime. May increase up to 10 mg/day. **Maximum:** 20 mg/day.

PRECAUTIONS

CONTRAINDICATIONS: None significant. **CAUTIONS:** Chronic renal failure, impaired hepatic function. **PREGNANCY/LACTATION:** Unknown whether drug crosses placenta or is distributed in breast milk. **Pregnancy Category C.**

INTERACTIONS

DRUG INTERACTIONS: Estrogen, NSAIDs, sympathomimetics may decrease effect. Hypotension-producing medications may increase antihypertensive effect. **ALTERED LAB VALUES:** May decrease albumin, total protein, Hgb, Hct, WBC.

SIDE EFFECTS

FREQUENT (5–9%): Dizziness, headache, unusual tiredness. **RARE (<2%):** Peripheral edema, orthostatic hypotension, back/joint pain, blurred vision, nausea, vomiting, nasal congestion, drowsiness.

ADVERSE REACTIONS/TOXIC EFFECTS

"First-dose syncope" (hypotension w/sudden loss of consciousness) generally occurs 30–90 min after giving initial dose of ≥2 mg, a too rapid increase in dose, or addition of another hypotensive agent to therapy. May be preceded by tachycardia (120–160 beats/min).

NURSING IMPLICATIONS

BASELINE ASSESSMENT:

Give first dose at bedtime. If initial dose is given during daytime, pt must remain recumbent for 3–4 hrs. Assess B/P, pulse immediately before each dose, and q15–30 min until stabilized (be alert to B/P fluctuations).

INTERVENTION/EVALUATION:

Monitor pulse diligently ("first-dose syncope" may be preceded by tachycardia). Assist w/ambulation if dizziness occurs. Assess for peripheral edema of hands, feet (usually, first area of low extremity swelling is behind medial malleolus in ambulatory, sacral area in bedridden).

PATIENT/FAMILY TEACHING:

Noncola carbonated beverage, unsalted crackers, dry toast may relieve nausea. Nasal congestion may occur. Full therapeutic effect may not occur for 3–4 wks. Use caution driving, performing tasks requiring mental alertness. Use caution rising from sitting position. Report dizziness, palpitations.

---

terbinafine hydrochloride

tur-**bin**-ah-feen
(Lamisil, Lamisil Derma Gel)

CANADIAN AVAILABILITY:
Lamisil

CLASSIFICATION

Antifungal

AVAILABILITY (Rx)

Tablets: 250 mg. **Gel. Cream:** 1% (OTC). **Solution:** 1%.

PHARMACOKINETICS

Oral: Well absorbed following oral administration (unaffected by food). Distributed to sebum and skin. Extensively metabolized.

Eliminated in urine. Half-life: 200–400 hrs. *Topical:* Minimal systemic absorption.

ACTION/THERAPEUTIC EFFECT

Fungicidal. Inhibits the enzyme, squalene epoxidase, interfering w/biosynthesis in fungi, *resulting in fungal cell death.*

USES

Systemic: Treatment of onychomycosis (fungal disease of nails due to dermatophytes). *Topical:* Treatment of *Tinea cruris* (jock itch), *T. pedis* (athlete's foot), *T. corporis* (ringworm). *Derma Gel:* Treatment of *Tinea corporis, T. pedis,* and *T. versicolor.*

PO ADMINISTRATION

May give w/o regard to food.

INDICATIONS/DOSAGE/ROUTES

Note: Topical therapy for minimum 1 wk, not to exceed 4 wks.

Tinea pedis:
Topical: Adults, elderly, adolescents: Apply 2 times/day until signs/symptoms significantly improved.

Tinea cruris, T. corporis:
Topical: Adults, elderly, adolescents: Apply 1–2 times/day until signs/symptoms significantly improved.

Onychomycosis:
PO: Adults, elderly, adolescents: 250 mg/day for 6 wks (fingernails), 12 wks (toenails).

PRECAUTIONS

CONTRAINDICATIONS: Hypersensitivity to terbinafine or any component in formulation. *Oral:* Preexisting liver disease or renal impairment (creatinine clearance ≤ 50 ml/min). Safety in children

<12 yrs not established. **CAUTIONS:** None significant. **PREGNANCY/LACTATION:** Both topical and oral medication are excreted in breast milk. Oral treatment not recommended in nursing mothers. **Pregnancy Category B**.

INTERACTIONS

DRUG INTERACTIONS: Alcohol, other hepatotoxic medications may increase risk hepatotoxicity. Liver enzyme inhibitors may decrease clearance (e.g., cimetidine). Liver enzyme inducers may increase clearance (e.g., rifampin). **ALTERED LAB VALUES:** May increase SGPT (ALT), SGOT (AST).

SIDE EFFECTS

FREQUENT: *Oral:* Headache (13%). **OCCASIONAL:** *Oral:* Diarrhea, rash (6%), dyspepsia (4%), pruritus, taste disturbance, nausea (3%). **RARE:** *Oral:* Abdominal pain, flatulence, urticaria, visual disturbance. *Topical:* Irritation, burning, itching, dryness.

ADVERSE REACTIONS/TOXIC EFFECTS

Hepatobiliary dysfunction (including cholestatic hepatitis), serious skin reactions, severe neutropenia occur rarely. Ocular lens and retina changes have been noted.

NURSING IMPLICATIONS

BASELINE ASSESSMENT:

Assure that diagnostic tests have been completed, e.g., culture or direct microscopic examination of scrapings from infected tissue. Liver function tests should be obtained in pts receiving treatment for >6 wks. Assess medication history. Obtain medical history, esp. alcoholism, liver/renal impairment.

INTERVENTION/EVALUATION:

Check for therapeutic response. Discontinue medication, notify physician if local reaction occurs (irritation, redness, swelling, itching, oozing, blistering, burning). Monitor CBC, liver function tests in pts receiving treatment for >6 wks.

PATIENT/FAMILY TEACHING:

Complete full course of treatment. Use only as directed for the time indicated. Do not use topical cream for oral or intravaginal use; use externally only. Keep areas clean and dry; wear light clothing to promote ventilation. Separate personal items. Avoid topical cream contact w/eyes, nose, mouth, or other mucous membranes. Rub well into affected, surrounding area. Do not cover w/occlusive dressing or use other preparations w/o consulting physician. Notify physician if skin irritation, diarrhea occurs.

terbutaline sulfate

tur-**byew**-ta-leen
(Brethaire, Brethine, Bricanyl)

CANADIAN AVAILABILITY:
Bricanyl

CLASSIFICATION

Sympathomimetic

AVAILABILITY (Rx)

Tablets: 2.5 mg, 5 mg. **Aerosol:** 0.2 mg/activation. **Injection:** 1 mg/ml.

PHARMACOKINETICS

	ONSET	PEAK	DURATION
PO	30 min	1–3 hrs	4–8 hrs
SubQ	15 min	30–60 min	1.5–4 hrs
Inhalation			
	5–30 min	1–2 hrs	3–4 hrs

Moderately absorbed from GI tract; well absorbed after SubQ administration. Metabolized in liver. Primarily excreted in urine. Half-life: 11–16 hrs.

ACTION/THERAPEUTIC EFFECT

Bronchospasm: Stimulates beta$_2$-adrenergic receptors, *relaxes bronchial smooth muscle, relieves bronchospasm, reduces airway resistance.* **Labor:** *Relaxes uterine muscle, inhibiting uterine contractions.*

USES

Symptomatic relief of reversible bronchospasm due to bronchial asthma, bronchitis, emphysema. Delays premature labor in pregnancies between 20 and 34 wks.

STORAGE/HANDLING

Store oral, parenteral forms at room temperature. Do not use if solution appears discolored.

PO/INHALATION/SUBQ ADMINISTRATION

PO:

1. May give w/o regard to food (take w/food if GI upset occurs).
2. Tablets may be crushed.

INHALATION:

1. Shake container well, exhale completely. Holding mouthpiece 1 inch away from lips, inhale and hold breath as long as possible before exhaling.
2. Wait 1–10 min before inhaling second dose (allows for deeper bronchial penetration).

3. Rinse mouth w/water immediately after inhalation (prevents mouth/throat dryness).

SubQ:

Inject SubQ into lateral deltoid region.

INDICATIONS/DOSAGE/ROUTES

Bronchospasm:
PO: Adults, elderly, children >15 yrs: Initially, 2.5 mg 3–4 times/day. **Maintenance:** 2.5–5 mg 3 times/day q6h while awake. **Maximum:** 15 mg/day. **Children 12–15 yrs:** 2.5 mg 3 times/day. **Maximum:** 7.5 mg/day.

Inhalation: Adults, elderly, children >12 yrs: 2 inhalations q4–6h. Allow at least 1 min between inhalations.

SubQ: Adults: Initially, 0.25 mg. Repeat in 15–30 min if substantial improvement does not occur. **Maximum:** No more than 0.5 mg/4 hrs.

Premature labor:
PO: Adults: 2.5 mg q4–6h until term.

IV Infusion: Adults: Initially, 10 mcg/min, increase by 5 mcg/min q10 min up to maximum of 80 mcg/min or until contractions cease. (After contractions cease for ½–1 hr, decrease by 5 mcg/min to lowest effective dose).

SubQ: Adults: 0.25 mg q1h until contractions cease.

PRECAUTIONS

CONTRAINDICATIONS: History of hypersensitivity to sympathomimetics. **CAUTIONS:** Impaired cardiac function, diabetes mellitus, hypertension, hyperthyroidism, history of seizures. **PREGNANCY/LACTATION:** Transient hypokalemia, pulmonary edema, hypoglycemia may occur if given during labor. Hypoglycemia may be found in neonate. Distributed in breast milk. **Pregnancy Category B**.

INTERACTIONS

DRUG INTERACTIONS: Tricyclic antidepressants may increase cardiovascular effects. MAO inhibitors may increase risk of hypertensive crises. May decrease effects of beta blockers. Digoxin, sympathomimetics may increase risk of arrhythmias. **ALTERED LAB VALUES:** May decrease serum potassium levels.

SIDE EFFECTS

FREQUENT (23–38%): Tremor, shakiness, nervousness. **OCCASIONAL (10–11%):** Drowsiness, headache, nausea, heartburn, dizziness. **RARE (1–3%):** Flushing, weakness, drying or irritation of oropharynx noted with inhalation therapy.

ADVERSE REACTIONS/TOXIC EFFECTS

Too frequent or excessive use may lead to loss of bronchodilating effectiveness and/or severe, paradoxical bronchoconstriction. Excessive sympathomimetic stimulation may cause palpitations, extrasystoles, tachycardia, chest pain, slight increase in B/P followed by a substantial decrease, chills, sweating, and blanching of skin.

NURSING IMPLICATIONS

BASELINE ASSESSMENT:

Bronchospasm: Offer emotional support (high incidence of anxiety due to difficulty in breathing and sympathomimetic response to drug). *Preterm labor:* Assess uterine contractions (intensity, frequency, duration).

INTERVENTION/EVALUATION:

Bronchospasm: Monitor rate, depth, rhythm, type of respiration; quality and rate of pulse. Assess lung sounds for rhonchi, wheezing, rales. Monitor arterial blood gases. Observe lips, fingernails for blue or dusky color in light-skinned patients; gray in dark-skinned pts. Observe for clavicular retractions, hand tremor. Evaluate for clinical improvement (quieter, slower respirations, relaxed facial expression, cessation of clavicular retractions). *Preterm labor:* Assess maternal heart rate, B/P, blood glucose, fluid status. Determine fetal heart rate.

PATIENT/FAMILY TEACHING:

Bronchospasm: Increase fluid intake (decreases lung secretion viscosity). Do not take more than 2 inhalations at any one time (excessive use may produce paradoxical bronchoconstriction, or a decreased bronchodilating effect). Rinsing mouth w/water immediately after inhalation may prevent mouth/throat dryness. Avoid excessive use of caffeine derivatives (chocolate, coffee, tea, cola, cocoa). *Preterm labor:* Contractions may resume while on oral therapy. Contact physician if 4–6 contractions per hour occur.

terconazole

ter-**con**-ah-zole
(Terazol)

CANADIAN AVAILABILITY:
Terazol

CLASSIFICATION

Antifungal

AVAILABILITY (Rx)

Vaginal Cream: 0.4%, 0.8%.
Vaginal Suppository: 80 mg.

PHARMACOKINETICS

Systemic absorption minimal following intravaginal administration.

ACTION / *THERAPEUTIC EFFECT*

Disrupts fungal cell membrane permeability, *producing antifungal activity.*

USES

Treatment of vulvovaginal candidiasis (moniliasis).

INTRAVAGINAL ADMINISTRATION

1. Use disposable gloves; always wash hands thoroughly after application.
2. Follow manufacturer's directions for use of applicator.
3. Insert suppository, applicator high in vagina.
4. Administration at bedtime is preferred.

INDICATIONS / DOSAGE / ROUTES

Vulvovaginal candidiasis:
Intravaginal: Adults, elderly:
Tablet: 1 suppository vaginally at bedtime for 3 days. *Cream* (0.4%): 1 applicatorful at bedtime for 7 days; 0.8% for 3 days.

PRECAUTIONS

CONTRAINDICATIONS: Hypersensitivity to terconazole or any component of the cream or suppository. **CAUTIONS:** Safety and efficacy in children not established. **PREGNANCY/LACTATION:** Unknown whether excreted in breast milk. **Pregnancy Category C**.

INTERACTIONS

DRUG INTERACTIONS: None significant. **ALTERED LAB VALUES:** None significant.

SIDE EFFECTS

FREQUENT (>10%): Headache, vulvovaginal burning. **OCCASIONAL (1–10%):** Dysmenorrhea, pain in female genitalia, abdominal pain, fever, itching. **RARE (<1%):** Chills.

ADVERSE REACTIONS / TOXIC EFFECTS

None significant.

NURSING IMPLICATIONS
BASELINE ASSESSMENT:

Question for hypersensitivity to terconazole or components of preparation. Confirm that a potassium hydroxide (KOH) culture and/or smear were done for accurate diagnosis; therapy may begin before results known. For suppository, inquire about use of vaginal contraceptives (such as diaphragm), since base of suppository interacts w/rubber latex.

INTERVENTION / EVALUATION:

Monitor temperature at least daily. Assess for therapeutic response or burning, itching, pain, or irritation.

PATIENT / FAMILY TEACHING:

Do not interrupt or stop regimen, even during menses. Teach pt proper insertion. Not affected by oral contraception. Notify physician of increased itching, irritation, burning. Consult physician about sexual intercourse, douching, or the use of other vaginal products. Do not use vaginal contraceptive di-

T

aphragms, condoms within 72 hrs after treatment. Avoid contact w/eyes. Wash hands thoroughly after application.

terfenadine

turr-**phen**-ah-deen
(Seldane)

FIXED-COMBINATION(S):
W/pseudoephedrine, a sympathomimetic **(Seldane-D)**

CLASSIFICATION

Antihistamine

AVAILABILITY (Rx)

Tablets: 60 mg

PHARMACOKINETICS

	ONSET	PEAK	DURATION
PO	1–2 hrs	3–6 hrs	>12 hrs

Well absorbed from GI tract. Undergoes first-pass metabolism. Primarily distributed in liver, lungs, GI tract. Metabolized in liver to active metabolite. Primarily eliminated in feces. Half-life: 20.3 hrs.

ACTION / *THERAPEUTIC EFFECT*

Competes w/histamine for receptor site *to prevent allergic responses mediated by histamine (urticaria, pruritus).*

USES / *UNLABELED*

Relief of seasonal allergic rhinitis (hay fever). Provides symptomatic relief of rhinorrhea, sneezing, oronasopharyngeal irritation, itching, lacrimation, red/irritated/itching eyes. *Adjunct in treatment of bronchial asthma.*

PO ADMINISTRATION

1. May give w/food (decreases GI distress).
2. Do not crush, chew extended-release tablets.

INDICATIONS / DOSAGE / ROUTES

Allergic rhinitis:
PO: Adults, children >12 yrs: 60 mg 2 times/day. **Children 7–12 yrs:** 30 mg 2 times/day. **Children 3–6 yrs:** 15 mg 2 times/day.

Usual elderly dosage:
PO: 60 mg 1–2 times/day.

PRECAUTIONS

CONTRAINDICATIONS: Acute asthmatic attack, those receiving MAO inhibitors. **CAUTIONS:** Narrow-angle glaucoma, peptic ulcer, prostatic hypertrophy, pyloroduodenal or bladder neck obstruction, asthma, COPD, increased intraocular pressure, cardiovascular disease, hyperthyroidism, hypertension, seizure disorders. **PREGNANCY/LACTATION:** Unknown whether drug crosses placenta or is detected in breast milk. Increased risk of seizures in neonates, premature infants if used during third trimester of pregnancy. May prohibit lactation. **Pregnancy Category C.**

INTERACTIONS

DRUG INTERACTIONS: Alcohol, CNS depressants may increase CNS depressant effects. Anticholinergics may increase anticholinergic effects. MAO inhibitors may increase anticholinergic, CNS depressant effects. Clarithromycin, erythromycin, itraconazole, ketoconazole, nafazodone may increase risk of cardiotoxic effects. Medications that prolong QT interval may increase risk of arrhythmias (e.g., procainamide, quinidine). **ALTERED LAB VALUES:** May suppress wheal and flare reactions to antigen skin testing. Discontinue at least 4 days before testing.

SIDE EFFECTS

OCCASIONAL: Headache, nausea, vomiting, constipation/diarrhea, increased appetite, insomnia, paresthesia, tremor, reduced concentration, nightmares, mental depression, confusion. **RARE:** Irritability, incoordination, vertigo, dizziness, muscular weakness, hypersensitivity reaction (rash, urticaria, bronchospasm), skin dryness, photosensitivity reaction, sweating.

ADVERSE REACTIONS/TOXIC EFFECTS

Children may experience dominant paradoxical reaction (restlessness, insomnia, euphoria, nervousness, tremors). Hypersensitivity reaction (eczema, pruritus, rash, photosensitivity) may occur.

NURSING IMPLICATIONS
BASELINE ASSESSMENT:

If pt is undergoing allergic reaction, obtain history of recently ingested foods, drugs, environmental exposure, recent emotional stress. Monitor rate, depth, rhythm, type of respiration; quality and rate of pulse. Assess lung sounds for rhonchi, wheezing, rales.

INTE'RVENTION/EVALUATION:

Monitor B/P, esp. in elderly (increased risk of hypotension). Monitor children closely for paradoxical reaction.

PATIENT/FAMILY TEACHING:

Tolerance to antihistaminic effect generally does not occur; tolerance to sedative effect may occur. Avoid tasks that require alertness, motor skills until response to drug is established. Dry mouth, drowsiness, dizziness may be an expected response of drug. Avoid alcoholic beverages during antihistamine therapy. Sugarless gum, sips of tepid water may relieve dry mouth. Coffee/tea may help reduce drowsiness.

testolactone
tes-toe-**lack**-tone
(Teslac)

CLASSIFICATION

Antineoplastic

AVAILABILITY (Rx)

Tablets: 50 mg

PHARMACOKINETICS

Well absorbed from GI tract. Metabolized in liver; excreted in urine.

ACTION

Inhibits steroid aromatase activity, an enzyme that reduces estrone synthesis (estrone is major source of estrogen in postmenopausal women).

USES

Adjunctive therapy in treatment of advanced disseminated breast carcinoma in postmenopausal women when hormonal therapy is indicated, and in premenopausal women where ovarian function has been terminated.

INDICATIONS/DOSAGE/ROUTES

Breast carcinoma:
PO: **Adults, elderly:** 250 mg 4 times/day.

PRECAUTIONS

CONTRAINDICATIONS: Breast cancer in men. **CAUTIONS:** Renal, liver, cardiac disease. **PREGNANCY/LACTATION:** If possible, avoid use during pregnancy, esp. first trimester. Breast-feeding not recommended. **Pregnancy Category C.**

INTERACTIONS

DRUG INTERACTIONS: May increase effects of oral anticoagulants. **ALTERED LAB VALUES:** May increase calcium, creatinine, 17-ketosteroids. May decrease estradiol.

SIDE EFFECTS

RARE: Maculopapular erythema, increase in B/P, alopecia, nail growth disturbances, paresthesia, aches, edema of extremities, glossitis, anorexia, hot flashes, nausea, vomiting, diarrhea.

ADVERSE REACTIONS/TOXIC EFFECTS

None significant.

NURSING IMPLICATIONS
INTERVENTION/EVALUATION:

Monitor plasma calcium levels (hypercalcemia is evidence of active remission of bone metastasis). Assess for signs of hypercalcemia (decreased muscle tone, bone/flank pain, thirst, excessive urination). Assess skin for maculopapular erythema.

PATIENT/FAMILY TEACHING:

Therapeutic effects usually noted in 6–12 wks. Therapy should continue for at least 3 mos. If alopecia occurs, it is reversible, but new hair growth may have different color or texture. Contact physician if nausea/vomiting continues at home.

testosterone
tess-**toss**-ter-own
(Andronaq, Histerone)

testosterone cypionate
(Depotest, Depo-Testosterone)

testosterone enanthate
(Delatest)

testosterone propionate
(Testex)

testosterone transdermal
(Androderm, Testoderm, Testoderm TTS)

FIXED-COMBINATION(S):
Testosterone cypionate w/estradiol cypionate, an estrogen (**depAndrogyn, Duratestrin, De-Comberol**); testosterone enanthate w/estradiol cypionate (**Deladumone**)

CANADIAN AVAILABILITY:
Delatestryl

CLASSIFICATION
Androgen

AVAILABILITY (Rx)

Injection: 25 mg/ml, 50 mg/ml, 100 mg/ml. **Transdermal Patch:** 2.5 mg/24 hr, 4 mg/24 hr, 6 mg/24 hr.

Cypionate: Injection: 100 mg/ml, 200 mg/ml

Enanthate: Injection: 100 mg/ml, 200 mg/ml

Propionate: Injection: 100 mg/ml

PHARMACOKINETICS

Well absorbed after IM administration. Metabolized in liver (undergoes first-pass metabolism). Primarily excreted in urine. Half-life: 10–20 min.

ACTION/*THERAPEUTIC EFFECT*

Stimulates spermatogenesis, development of male secondary sex characteristics, sexual maturation at puberty. Stimulates production of RBCs. *Initiates male puberty, corrects hormonal deficiency, suppresses tumor growth in breast cancer.*

USES

Treatment of delayed puberty; testicular failure due to cryptorchidism, bilateral orchism, orchitis, vanishing testis syndrome, or orchidectomy; hypogonadotropic hypogonadism due to pituitary/hypothalamic injury (tumors, trauma, or radiation), idiopathic gonadotropin or luteinizing hormone releasing hormone deficiency. Palliative therapy in women 1–5 yrs postmenopausal w/advancing, inoperable metastatic breast cancer or premenopausal women who have benefited from oophorectomy and have a hormone-responsive tumor. Prevention of postpartum breast pain and engorgement. In combination w/estrogens for management of moderate to severe vasomotor symptoms associated w/menopause when estrogens alone are not effective.

IM/TRANSDERMAL ADMINISTRATION

IM:

1. Give deep in gluteal muscle.
2. Do *not* give IV.
3. Warming and shaking redissolves crystals that may form in long-acting preparations.
4. Wet needle of syringe may cause solution to become cloudy; this does not affect potency.

TRANSDERMAl:

Testoderm:
Apply to clean, dry scrotal skin that has been dry-shaved (optimal skin contact). Testoderm TTS may be applied to arm, back, or upper buttock.

Androderm:
1. Apply to clean, dry area on skin on back, abdomen, upper arms, or thighs.
2. Do not apply to bony prominences (e.g., shoulder) or oily, damaged, irritated skin. Do not apply to scrotum.
3. Rotate application site with 7-day interval to same site.

INDICATIONS/DOSAGE/ROUTES

Testosterone, Testosterone Propionate:

Androgen replacement therapy:
IM: Adults: 25–50 mg 2–3 times/wk.

Palliation of mammary cancer:
IM: Adults, elderly: 50–100 mg 3 times/wk.

Postpartum breast engorgement (propionate):
IM: Adults: 25–50 mg/day for 3–4 days (begin at time of delivery).

TESTOSTERONE CYPIONATE, TESTOSTERONE ENANTHATE:

Male hypogonadism (replacement therapy):
IM: **Adults:** 50–400 mg q2–4 wks.

Males (delayed puberty):
IM: **Adults:** 50–200 mg q2–4 wks.

Females: (palliation of inoperable breast cancer):
IM: **Adults, elderly:** 200–400 mg q2–4 wks.

TESTOSTERONE TRANSDERMAL:

Males (replacement therapy):
Topical: **Adults:** 6 mg/day system.

PRECAUTIONS

CONTRAINDICATIONS: Hypersensitivity to drug or components of preparation; serious cardiac, renal, or hepatic dysfunction. Do not use for men w/carcinomas of the breast or prostate. **EXTREME CAUTION:** In children because of bone maturation effects. **CAUTIONS:** Epilepsy, migraine, or other conditions aggravated by fluid retention; metastatic breast cancer or immobility increases risk of hypercalcemia. **PREGNANCY/LACTATION:** Contraindicated during lactation. **Pregnancy Category X.**

INTERACTIONS

DRUG INTERACTIONS: May increase effect of oral anticoagulants. Hepatotoxic medications may increase hepatotoxicity. **ALTERED LAB VALUES:** May increase SGOT (AST), alkaline phosphatase, bilirubin, calcium, potassium, sodium, Hgb, Hct, LDL. May decrease HDL.

SIDE EFFECTS

FREQUENT: Gynecomastia, acne, amenorrhea or other menstrual irregularities. *Females:* hirsutism, deepening of voice, clitoral enlargement (may not be reversible when drug discontinued). **OCCASIONAL:** Edema, nausea, insomnia, oligospermia, priapism, male pattern of baldness, bladder irritability, hypercalcemia in immobilized pts or those w/breast cancer, hypercholesterolemia, inflammation and pain at IM injection site. *Transdermal:* Itching, erythema, skin irritation. **RARE:** Polycythemia w/high dosage, hypersensitivity.

ADVERSE REACTIONS/TOXIC EFFECTS

Peliosis hepatitis (liver, spleen replaced w/blood-filled cysts), hepatic neoplasms and hepatocellular carcinoma have been associated w/prolonged high-dosage, anaphylactoid reactions.

NURSING IMPLICATIONS
BASELINE ASSESSMENT:

Question for hypersensitivity to testosterone. Establish baseline weight, B/P, Hgb, and Hct. Check liver function test results, electrolytes, and cholesterol if ordered. Wrist x-rays may be ordered to determine bone maturation in children.

INTERVENTION/EVALUATION:

Weigh daily and report weekly gain of more than 5 lbs; evaluate for edema. Monitor I&O. Check B/P at least 2 times/day. Assess electrolytes, cholesterol, Hgb, and Hct (periodically for high dosage), liver function test results. W/breast cancer or immobility, check for hypercalcemia (lethargy, muscle weakness, confusion, irritability). Assure adequate intake of protein, calories. Assess for virilization. Monitor sleep patterns.

Check injection site for redness, swelling, or pain.

PATIENT/FAMILY TEACHING:

Regular visits to physician and monitoring tests are necessary. Do not take any other medications w/o consulting physician. Teach diet high in protein, calories. Food may be tolerated better in small, frequent feedings. Weigh daily, report 5 lbs/gain/week. Notify physician if nausea, vomiting, acne, or ankle swelling occurs. *Females:* Promptly report menstrual irregularities, hoarseness, deepening of voice. *Males:* Report frequent erections, difficulty urinating, gynecomastia.

---

tetracaine
(Pontocaine)
*See Classification section under:
Anesthetics: local*

---

tetracycline hydrochloride

tet-rah-**sigh**-clean
(**Achromycin, Actisite, Panmycin, Robitet, Sumycin, Topicycline**)

CANADIAN AVAILABILITY:
Apo-Tetra, Novotetra

CLASSIFICATION

Antibiotic: Tetracycline

AVAILABILITY (Rx)

Capsules: 250 mg, 500 mg. **Tablets:** 250 mg, 500 mg. **Topical Solution. Topical Ointment:** 3%.

PHARMACOKINETICS

Readily absorbed from GI tract. Widely distributed. Excreted in urine; eliminated in feces via biliary system. Slowly removed by hemodialysis. Half-life: 6–11 hrs (increased in decreased renal function).

ACTION/*THERAPEUTIC EFFECT*

Inhibits protein synthesis by binding to ribosomes, *preventing bacterial cell growth.* Bacteriostatic.

USES/*UNLABELED*

Treatment of uncomplicated gonorrhea, syphilis (when allergic to penicillin), adjunctive therapy for acne, urinary tract infection, Rocky Mountain spotted fever, typhus, Q fever, cholera, psittacosis, brucellosis, yaws, bejel, pinta, anthrax, actinomycosis, Whipple's disease, rat bite fever. Treatment of H. Pylori–associated peptic ulcer disease (w/bismuth subsalicylate/metronidazole). *Topical:* Inflammatory acne vulgaris, superficial infections. *Treatment of gonorrhea, malaria.*

STORAGE/HANDLING

Store capsules, oral suspension at room temperature.

PO/TOPICAL ADMINISTRATION

PO:

Give capsules, tablets w/full glass of water 1 hr before or 2 hrs after meals, milk.

TOPICAL:

1. Cleanse area gently before application.
2. Apply only to affected area.

INDICATIONS/DOSAGE/ROUTES

Note: Space doses evenly around the clock.

Usual dosage:
PO: Adults, elderly: 1–3 g/day in 2–4 divided doses. **Children >8 yrs:** 25–50 mg/kg/day in 2–4 divided doses.

H. Pylori peptic ulcer:
PO: Adults: 500 mg 4 times/day for 14 days (w/bismuth subsalicylate, metronidazole).

Usual topical dosage:
Topical: Adults, elderly: Apply 2 times/day in morning, evening.

PRECAUTIONS

CONTRAINDICATIONS: Hypersensitivity to tetracyclines, sulfite, children ≤ age 8 yrs. **CAUTIONS:** Sun/ultraviolet light exposure (severe photosensitivity reaction). **PREGNANCY/LACTATION:** Readily crosses placenta, is distributed in breast milk. Avoid use in women during last half of pregnancy. May produce permanent teeth discoloration/enamel hypoplasia, inhibit fetal skeletal growth in children ≤ 8 yrs. **Pregnancy Category D**.

INTERACTIONS

DRUG INTERACTIONS: Cholestyramine, colestipol may decrease absorption. May decrease effect of oral contraceptives. Carbamazepine, phenytoin may decrease concentrations. **ALTERED LAB VALUES:** May increase BUN, SGOT (AST), SGPT (ALT), alkaline phosphatase, amylase, bilirubin concentrations.

SIDE EFFECTS

FREQUENT: Dizziness, lightheadedness, diarrhea, nausea, vomiting, stomach cramps, increased sensitivity of skin to sunlight. *Topical:* Dry scaly skin, stinging, burning feeling. **OCCASIONAL:** Pigmentation of skin, mucus membranes, itching in rectal/genital area, sore mouth/tongue. *Topical:* Pain, redness, swelling, other skin irritation.

ADVERSE REACTIONS/TOXIC EFFECTS

Superinfection (esp. fungal), anaphylaxis, increased intracranial pressure, bulging fontanelles occur rarely in infants.

NURSING IMPLICATIONS
BASELINE ASSESSMENT:

Question for history of allergies, esp. tetracyclines, sulfite. Obtain specimens for culture and sensitivity before giving first dose (therapy may begin before results are known).

INTERVENTION/EVALUATION:

Assess skin for rash. Determine pattern of bowel activity and stool consistency. Monitor food intake, tolerance. Be alert for superinfection: diarrhea, ulceration, or changes of oral mucosa, anal/genital pruritus. Monitor B/P and level of consciousness because of potential for increased intracranial pressure.

PATIENT/FAMILY TEACHING:

Continue antibiotic for full length of treatment. Space doses evenly. Take oral doses on empty stomach (1 hr before or 2 hrs after food/beverages). Drink full glass of water w/capsules and avoid bedtime doses. Notify physician in event of diarrhea, rash, other new symptom. Protect skin from sun exposure. Consult physician before taking any other medication. *Topical:* Skin may turn yellow w/Topicycline application (washing removes solution); fabrics may be stained by heavy application. Do not apply to deep/open wounds.

tetrahydrozyline hydrochloride

tet-rah-high-**droz**-ah-leen
(Visine, Tyzine)

FIXED-COMBINATION(S):

W/benzalkonium chloride, a wetting agent, and edetate disodium, a chelating agent (**Murine Plus, Visine A.C.**)

CLASSIFICATION

Sympathomimetic

AVAILABILITY (OTC)

Nasal Solution: 0.05%, 0.1%.
Ophthalmic Solution: 0.05%.

PHARMACOKINETICS

	ONSET	PEAK	DURATION
Ophthalmic			
	Several min	—	4–8 hrs
Intranasal			
	Several min	—	4–8 hrs

May be systemically absorbed. Metabolic, elimination rates unknown.

ACTION/ *THERAPEUTIC EFFECT*

Stimulates alpha-adrenergic receptors in sympathetic nervous system. **Ophthalmic:** Constricts arterioles, *reduces redness, irritation.* **Intranasal:** Constricts arterioles, *reduces congestion.*

USES

Ophthalmic: Relief of itching, minor irritation and to control hyperemia in pts w/superficial corneal vascularity. Combination solutions relieve discomfort due to minor eye irritations and symptoms related to dry eyes. *Intranasal:* Relief of nasal congestion of rhinitis, the common cold, sinusitis, hay fever, or other allergies; reduces swelling and improves visualization for surgery or diagnostic procedures; opens obstructed eustachian ostia in pts w/ear inflammation.

OPHTHALMIC/INTRANASAL ADMINISTRATION

OPHTHALMIC:

1. Instruct pt to tilt head backward and look up.
2. Gently pull lower lid down to form pouch and instill medication.
3. Do not touch tip of applicator to lids or any surface.
4. After releasing lower lid, have pt close eyes w/o squeezing.
5. Apply gentle finger pressure to lacrimal sac (bridge of the nose, inside corner of the eye) for 1–2 min.
6. Remove excess solution around eye w/tissue. Wash hands immediately to remove medication on hands.

INTRANASAL:

1. Drops should be administered w/pt in lateral, head-low position or reclining w/head tilted back as far as possible.
2. Pt should maintain same position for 5 min, then drops applied to other nostril.
3. Dropper containers should be used by only one person; tips of dispensers or droppers should be rinsed well w/hot water after use.

INDICATIONS/DOSAGE/ROUTES

Usual nasal dosage:
Adults, elderly, children >6 yrs: 2–4 drops (0.1% solution) to each nostril q4–6h (no sooner than q3h). **Children, 2–6 yrs:** 2–3 drops

(0.05% solution) to each nostril q4–6h (no sooner than q3h).

Usual ophthalmic dosage:
Adults, elderly, children: 1–2 drops (0.05%) 2–4 times/day.

PRECAUTIONS

CONTRAINDICATIONS: Known hypersensitivity to tetrahydrozyline or components of preparation; children <2 yrs of age (the 0.1% nasal solution is contraindicated in children <6 yrs of age); pts w/angle closure glaucoma or other serious eye diseases. **CAUTIONS:** Some caution should be taken when using w/cardiac disease, hyperthyroidism, hypertension, diabetes mellitus, cerebral arteriosclerosis, bronchial asthma, monoamine oxidase inhibitors. **PREGNANCY/LACTATION:** Safety in pregnancy and lactation has not been established. **Pregnancy Category C**.

INTERACTIONS

DRUG INTERACTIONS: Maprotiline, tricyclic antidepressants may increase pressor effects. MAO inhibitors may cause severe hypertensive reaction. **ALTERED LAB VALUES:** None significant.

SIDE EFFECTS

OCCASIONAL: *Intranasal:* Transient burning, stinging, sneezing, dryness of mucosa. *Ophthalmic:* Irritation, blurred vision, mydriasis. Systemic sympathomimetic effects may occur w/either route: headache, hypertension, weakness, sweating, palpitations, tremors. Prolonged use may result in rebound congestion.

ADVERSE REACTIONS/TOXIC EFFECTS

Overdosage may result in CNS depression w/drowsiness, decreased body temperature, bradycardia, hypotension, coma, apnea.

NURSING IMPLICATIONS

PATIENT/FAMILY TEACHING:

Discard if solution becomes cloudy or discolored. Overuse of vasoconstrictors may produce rebound congestion, hyperemia. Avoid excessive dosage, prolonged or too frequent use. *Ophthalmic:* Do not use w/glaucoma unless under advice and direction of physician. Remove contact lenses before administration. Do not use w/wetting agents for contact lenses. Discontinue and consult physician immediately if ocular pain or visual changes occur, if condition worsens or continues for more than 72 hrs. *Intranasal:* Discontinue and consult physician if rebound congestion occurs.

thalidomide
(Sinovir)
See Supplement

thiamine hydrochloride (vitamin B₁)
thigh-ah-min
(Betalin)

CANADIAN AVAILABILITY:
Betaxin

CLASSIFICATION

Vitamin: B-complex

AVAILABILITY (OTC)

Tablets: 5 mg, 10 mg, 25 mg, 50

mg, 100 mg, 250 mg, 500 mg. **Injection (Rx):** 100 mg/ml.

PHARMACOKINETICS

Readily absorbed from GI tract primarily in duodenum, after IM administration. Widely distributed. Metabolized in liver. Primarily excreted in urine.

ACTION/*THERAPEUTIC EFFECT*

Combines w/adenosine triphosphate (ATP) in liver, kidney, leukocytes to form thiamine diphosphate, which is *necessary for carbohydrate metabolism*.

USES

Prevention/treatment of thiamine deficiency (e.g., beriberi, alcoholic w/altered sensorium).

STORAGE/HANDLING

Store oral, parenteral forms at room temperature.

PO/IM/IV ADMINISTRATION

Note: IM/IV administration used only in acutely ill or those unresponsive to oral route (GI malabsorption syndrome). IM route preferred to IV use. Give by direct IV, or add to most IV solutions and give as infusion.

INDICATIONS/DOSAGE/ROUTES

Dietary supplement:
PO: Adults, elderly: 1–2 mg/day. **Children:** 0.5–1 mg/day. **Infants:** 0.3–0.5 mg/day.

Thiamine deficiency:
PO: Adults, elderly: 5–30 mg/day, in single or 3 divided doses, for 1 mo. **Children:** 10–50 mg/day in 3 divided doses.

Critically ill/malabsorption syndrome:
IM/IV: Adults, elderly: 5–100 mg,
3 times/day. **Children:** 10–25 mg/day.

Metabolic disorders:
PO: Adults, elderly, children: 10–20 mg/day; up to 4 g in divided doses/day.

PRECAUTIONS

CONTRAINDICATIONS: None significant. **CAUTIONS:** None significant. **PREGNANCY/LACTATION:** Crosses placenta; unknown whether excreted in breast milk. **Pregnancy Category A.** (Category C if used in doses above RDA.)

INTERACTIONS

DRUG INTERACTIONS: None significant. **ALTERED LAB VALUES:** None significant.

SIDE EFFECTS

FREQUENT: Pain, induration, tenderness at IM injection site.

ADVERSE REACTIONS/TOXIC EFFECTS

Rare, severe hypersensitivity reaction w/IV administration may result in feeling of warmth, pruritus, urticaria, weakness, sweating, nausea, restlessness, tightness of throat, angioedema (swelling of face/lips), cyanosis, pulmonary edema, GI tract bleeding, cardiovascular collapse.

NURSING IMPLICATIONS
INTERVENTION/EVALUATION:

Monitor lab values for erythrocyte activity, EKG readings. Assess for clinical improvement (improved sense of well-being, weight gain). Observe for reversal of deficiency symptoms (*neurologic:* peripheral neuropathy, hyporeflexia, nystagmus, ophthalmoplegia, ataxia, muscle weakness; *cardiac:* ve-

T

nous hypertension, bounding arterial pulse, tachycardia, edema; *mental:* confused state).

PATIENT/FAMILY TEACHING:

Discomfort may occur w/IM injection. Foods rich in thiamine include pork, organ meats, whole grain and enriched cereals, legumes, nuts, seeds, yeast, wheat germ, rice bran.

thiethylperazine maleate

thigh-eth-ill-**pear**-ah-zeen
(Torecan)

CLASSIFICATION

Antiemetic

AVAILABILITY (Rx)

Tablets: 10 mg. **Suppository:** 10 mg. **Injection:** 5 mg/ml.

PHARMACOKINETICS

	ONSET	PEAK	DURATION
PO	30–60 min	—	4 hrs
IM	30 min	—	4 hrs
Rectal			
	30–60 min	—	4 hrs

Well absorbed after oral, rectal, IM administration. Widely distributed, primarily in CNS. Metabolized in liver. Excreted in urine.

ACTION/*THERAPEUTIC EFFECT*

Acts centrally to block dopamine receptors in chemoreceptor trigger zone (CTZ) in CNS, *relieving nausea and vomiting.*

USES

Control of nausea and vomiting.

STORAGE/HANDLING

Store oral, rectal, parenteral forms at room temperature.

PO/IM/RECTAL ADMINISTRATION

PO:

Give w/o regard to meals.

IM:

Give deep IM into large muscle mass, preferably upper outer gluteus maximus.

RECTAL:

1. If suppository is too soft, chill for 30 min in refrigerator or run cold water over foil wrapper.
2. Moisten suppository w/cold water before inserting well into rectum.

INDICATIONS/DOSAGE/ROUTES

Note: Do not use IV route (produces severe hypotension).

Nausea, vomiting:
PO, Rectal, IM: Adults, elderly: 10 mg, 1–3 times/day.

PRECAUTIONS

CONTRAINDICATIONS: Severe CNS depression, comatose states, hypersensitivity to phenothiazines, pregnancy. **CAUTIONS:** Elderly, debilitated, dehydration, electrolyte imbalance, high fever. **PREGNANCY/LACTATION:** Unknown whether drug crosses placenta or is distributed in breast milk. Contraindicated during pregnancy. **Pregnancy Category unknown.**

INTERACTIONS

DRUG INTERACTIONS: Alcohol,

CNS depressants may increase CNS, respiratory depression, increase hypotension. May block alpha-adrenergic effects of epinephrine (causing hypotension, tachycardia). Extrapyramidal symptom (EPS)–producing medications may increase risk of EPS. May inhibit effects of levodopa. May increase cardiac effects w/quinidine. **ALTERED LAB VALUES:** None significant.

SIDE EFFECTS

FREQUENT: Drowsiness, dizziness. **OCCASIONAL:** Blurred vision, decreased color/night vision, fever, headache, orthostatic hypotension, rash, ringing in ears, constipation, dry mouth, decreased sweating.

ADVERSE REACTIONS/TOXIC EFFECTS

Extrapyramidal symptoms manifested as torticollis (neck muscle spasm), oculogyric crisis (rolling back of eyes), akathisia (motor restlessness, anxiety) occur rarely.

NURSING IMPLICATIONS
BASELINE ASSESSMENT:

Assess for dehydration if excessive vomiting occurs (poor skin turgor, dry mucous membranes, longitudinal furrows in tongue).

INTERVENTION EVALUATION:

Monitor B/P esp. before dosing. Assist w/ambulation if dizziness or hypotension occurs. Assess for improvement of dehydration status. Monitor I&O. Monitor for evidence of fever. Assess any vomitus. Be alert for extrapyramidal symptoms.

PATIENT/FAMILY TEACHING:

Report visual disturbances, headache. Dry mouth is expected response to medication. Relief from nausea/vomiting generally occurs within 30 min of drug administration. Avoid alcohol and other CNS depressants. Change positions slowly to prevent postural hypotension. Avoid tasks requiring alert response until assured drug does not cause impairment.

thioguanine
thigh-oh-**guan**-een
(Thioguanine)

CANADIAN AVAILABILITY:
Lanvis

CLASSIFICATION

Antineoplastic

AVAILABILITY (Rx)

Tablets: 40 mg

PHARMACOKINETICS

Incompletely, variably absorbed from GI tract. Metabolized in liver. Primarily excreted in urine. Half-life: 25–240 min.

ACTION/ *THERAPEUTIC EFFECT*

Converted intracellularly to active nucleotide, inhibiting DNA, RNA synthesis, *producing malignant cell death.* Cell cycle-specific for S phase of cell division.

USES/ *UNLABELED*

Treatment of acute myelogenous leukemia, chronic myelogenous leukemia. *Treatment of acute lymphocytic leukemia.*

INDICATIONS/DOSAGE/ROUTES

Note: May be carcinogenic, mutagenic, or teratogenic. Handle w/extreme care during administration.

Dosage individualized based on clinical response, tolerance to adverse effects. When used in combination therapy, consult specific protocols for optimum dosage, sequence of drug administration.

Initial treatment:
PO: Adults, elderly, children: 2 mg/kg/day as single dose. Increase to 3 mg/kg/day after 4 wks if no leukocyte, platelet depression appears and no clinical improvement obvious.

Maintenance:
PO: Adults, elderly, children: 2–3 mg/kg/day.

PRECAUTIONS

CONTRAINDICATIONS: Disease resistance to prior therapy w/drug. **EXTREME CAUTION:** Preexisting liver disease, pts receiving other hepatotoxic drugs. **PREGNANCY/LACTATION:** If possible, avoid use during pregnancy, esp. first trimester. May cause fetal harm. Unknown whether distributed in breast milk. Breast-feeding not recommended. **Pregnancy Category D**.

INTERACTIONS

DRUG INTERACTIONS: May decrease effect of antigout medications. Bone marrow depressants may increase bone marrow depression. Live virus vaccines may potentiate virus replication, increase vaccine side effects, decrease pt's antibody response to vaccine. **ALTERED LAB VALUES:** May increase uric acid.

SIDE EFFECTS

FREQUENT: Hyperuricemia. **OCCASIONAL:** Nausea, vomiting, anorexia, stomatitis, diarrhea (particularly w/excessive dosage), rash, dermatitis, unsteady gait, loss of vibration sensitivity, jaundice.

ADVERSE REACTIONS/TOXIC EFFECTS

Major effects are bone marrow depression manifested as leukopenia, thrombocytopenia, anemia, pancytopenia, hepatotoxicity manifested as jaundice, hepatomegaly, veno-occlusive liver disease.

NURSING IMPLICATIONS

BASELINE ASSESSMENT:

Obtain liver function tests weekly during initial therapy, monthly intervals thereafter. Obtain hematology tests at least weekly during therapy. Discontinue therapy if abnormally large/rapid decrease (over few days) of WBC, platelet, Hgb level occurs or at first sign of clinical jaundice.

INTERVENTION/EVALUATION:

Monitor serum transaminase, alkaline phosphatase, bilirubin, blood uric acid, Hgb, Hct, WBC, differential, platelet count. Assess skin, sclera for evidence of jaundice. Encourage fluid intake. Monitor for stomatitis (burning/erythema of oral mucosa at inner margin of lips, sore throat, difficulty swallowing, oral ulceration). Monitor for hematologic toxicity; infection (fever, sore throat, signs of local infection), easy bruising, unusual bleeding from any site, symptoms of anemia (excessive tiredness, weakness). Assess pattern of daily bowel activity and stool consistency.

PATIENT/FAMILY TEACHING:

Drink plenty of fluid. Maintain fastidious oral hygiene. Do not have immunizations w/o physician's approval (drug lowers body's resistance). Avoid crowds, those w/infection. Use nonhormonal contraceptive during therapy; notify physician at once if pregnancy is suspected. Promptly report fever, sore throat, signs of local infection, easy bruising, unusual bleeding from any site, yellowing of skin or eyes, flank pain. Contact physician if nausea/vomiting continues at home.

---

thiopental sodium
(Pentothal)
See Classification section under: Anesthetics: general

---

thioridazine
thigh-oh-**rid**-ah-zeen
(Mellaril-S)

thioridazine hydrochloride
(Mellaril)

CANADIAN AVAILABILITY:
Apo-Thioridazine, Melaril

CLASSIFICATION

Antipsychotic

AVAILABILITY (Rx)

Tablets: 10 mg, 15 mg, 25 mg, 50 mg, 100 mg, 150 mg, 200 mg. **Oral Concentrate:** 30 mg/ml, 100 mg/ml. **Oral Suspension:** 25 mg/5 ml, 100 mg/5 ml.

PHARMACOKINETICS

Variably absorbed from GI tract. Widely distributed. Metabolized in liver to some active metabolites. Excreted in urine, eliminated in feces.

ACTION/*THERAPEUTIC EFFECT*

Blocks dopamine at postsynaptic receptor sites, *suppressing behavioral response in psychosis, reducing locomotor activity, aggressiveness, suppressing conditioned responses.* Possesses strong anticholinergic, sedative effects.

USES

Management of psychotic disorders, severe behavioral disturbances in children, including those w/excessive motor activity, conduct disorders. Used in short-term treatment of moderate to marked depression w/variable degrees of anxiety.

PO ADMINISTRATION

1. Dilute oral concentrate solution in water or fruit juice just before administration.
2. Do not crush, chew, or break tablets.

INDICATIONS/DOSAGE/ROUTES

Psychotic disorders:
PO: Adults: 50–100 mg 3 times/day in hospitalized pts. May gradually increase to 800 mg/day maximum. Dosage from 200–800 mg/day

should be divided into 2–3 doses. Reduce dose gradually when therapeutic response is achieved.

Depression w/anxiety:
PO: Adults: 25 mg 3 times/day. **Total dose range/day:** 10 mg 2 times/day to 50 mg 3–4 times/day.

Usual elderly dosage (nonpsychotic):
PO: Initially, 10–25 mg 12 times/day. May increase by 10–25 mg q4–7 days. **Maximum:** 400 mg/day.

Usual pediatric dosage:
PO: Children 2–12 yrs: 0.5–3 mg/kg/day.

PRECAUTIONS

CONTRAINDICATIONS: Severe CNS depression, comatose states, severe cardiovascular disease, bone marrow depression, subcortical brain damage. **CAUTIONS:** Impaired respiratory/hepatic/renal/cardiac function, alcohol withdrawal, history of seizures, urinary retention, glaucoma, prostatic hypertrophy, hypocalcemia (increases susceptibility to dystonias). **PREGNANCY/LACTATION:** Crosses placenta; distributed in breast milk. **Pregnancy Category C.**

INTERACTIONS

DRUG INTERACTIONS: Alcohol, CNS depressants may increase CNS, respiratory depression, hypotensive effects. Tricyclic antidepressants, MAO inhibitors may increase sedative, anticholinergic effects. Antithyroid agents may increase risk of agranulocytosis. Extrapyramidal symptoms (EPS) may increase w/EPS–producing medications. Hypotensives may increase hypotension. May decrease levodopa effects. Lithium may decrease absorption, pro-

duce adverse neurologic effects. **ALTERED LAB VALUES:** May cause EKG changes.

SIDE EFFECTS

Generally well tolerated w/only mild and transient effects. **OCCASIONAL:** Drowsiness during early therapy, dry mouth, blurred vision, lethargy, constipation or diarrhea, nasal congestion, peripheral edema, urinary retention. **RARE:** Ocular changes, skin pigmentation (those on high doses for prolonged periods).

ADVERSE REACTIONS/TOXIC EFFECTS

Extrapyramidal symptoms appear dose related (particularly high dosage) and are divided into 3 categories: akathisia (inability to sit still, tapping of feet, urge to move around); parkinsonian symptoms (mask-like face, tremors, shuffling gait, hypersalivation); and acute dystonias: torticollis (neck muscle spasm), opisthotonos (rigidity of back muscles), and oculogyric crisis (rolling back of eyes). Dystonic reaction may also produce profuse sweating, pallor. Tardive dyskinesia (protrusion of tongue, puffing of cheeks, chewing/puckering of the mouth) occurs rarely (may be irreversible). Abrupt withdrawal following long-term therapy may precipitate nausea, vomiting, gastritis, dizziness, tremors. Blood dyscrasias, particularly agranulocytosis, mild leukopenia (sore mouth/gums/throat) may occur. May lower seizure threshold.

NURSING IMPLICATIONS
BASELINE ASSESSMENT:

Avoid skin contact w/solution (contact dermatitis). Assess behavior, appearance, emotion-

al status, response to environment, speech pattern, thought content.

INTERVENTION EVALUATION:

Monitor B/P for hypotension. Assess for extrapyramidal symptoms. Monitor WBC, differential count for blood dyscrasias. Monitor for fine tongue movement (may be early sign of tardive dyskinesia). Supervise suicidal risk pt closely during early therapy (as depression lessens, energy level improves, but suicide potential increases). Assess for therapeutic response (interest in surroundings, improvement in self-care, increased ability to concentrate, relaxed facial expression).

PATIENT/FAMILY TEACHING:

Full therapeutic effect may take up to 6 wks. Urine may darken. Do not abruptly withdraw from long-term drug therapy. Report visual disturbances. Sugarless gum, sips of tepid water may relieve dry mouth. Drowsiness generally subsides during continued therapy. Avoid tasks that require alertness, motor skills until response to drug is established.

thiotepa

thigh-oh-**teh**-pah
(Thioplex, Thiotepa)

CANADIAN AVAILABILITY:
Thiotepa

CLASSIFICATION

Antineoplastic

AVAILABILITY (Rx)

Powder for Injection: 15 mg

PHARMACOKINETICS

Variable systemic absorption occurs following local administration. Primarily excreted in urine as metabolites.

ACTION/ THERAPEUTIC EFFECT

Binds w/many intracellular structures. Cross-links strands of DNA, RNA, disrupting protein synthesis, *producing malignant cell death.* Cell cycle-phase nonspecific.

USES/ UNLABELED

Treatment of superficial papillary carcinoma of urinary bladder, adenocarcinoma of breast and ovary, Hodgkin's disease, lymphosarcoma. Intracavitary injection to control pleural, pericardial, or peritoneal effusions due to metastatic tumors. *Treatment of lung carcinoma.*

STORAGE/HANDLING

Note: May be carcinogenic, mutagenic, or teratogenic. Handle w/extreme care during preparation/administration.

Refrigerate unopened vials. Reconstituted solutions appear clear to slightly opaque; stable for 5 days if refrigerated. Discard if solution appears grossly opaque or precipitate forms.

PARENTERAL ADMINISTRATION

Note: Give by IV, intrapleural, intraperitoneal, intrapericardial, or intratumor injection; intravesical instillation.

1. Reconstitute 15 mg vial w/1.5 ml sterile water for injection to provide concentration of 10 mg/ml.

2. For IV injection, administer over 1 min.

3. Further dilute w/5% dextrose, 0.9% NaCl injection for intracavitary use, IV infusion, perfusion therapy.

INDICATIONS/DOSAGE/ROUTES

Note: Dosage individualized based on clinical response, tolerance to adverse effects. When used in combination therapy, consult specific protocols for optimum dosage, sequence of drug administration.

Initial treatment:
IV: Adults, elderly: 0.3–0.4 mg/kg q1–4 wks. Maintenance dose adjusted weekly on basis of blood counts.
Intracavitary: Adults, elderly: 0.6–0.8 mg/kg q1–4 wks.
Intratumor: Adults, elderly: Initially, 0.6–0.8 mg/kg given directly into tumor. **Maintenance:** 0.7–0.8 mg/kg q1–4 wks.
Intravesical: Adults, elderly: 30–60 mg in 30–60 ml sterile water instilled by catheter into bladder of pt who has been dehydrated for 8–12 hrs. Retain in bladder for 2 hrs. Reposition pt q15 min for maximum area contact. Repeat once weekly for 4 wks.

PRECAUTIONS

CONTRAINDICATIONS: Existing hepatic, renal, bone marrow damage unless drug administered in low doses, concurrent use w/alkylating agents or radiation therapy until pt recovers from myelosuppression. **CAUTIONS:** None significant. **PREGNANCY/LACTATION:** If possible, avoid use during pregnancy, esp. first trimester. Breastfeeding not recommended. **Pregnancy Category D**.

INTERACTIONS

DRUG INTERACTIONS: May decrease effect of antigout medications. Bone marrow depressants may increase bone marrow depression. Live virus vaccines may potentiate virus replication, increase vaccine side effects, decrease pt's antibody response to vaccine. **ALTERED LAB VALUES:** May increase uric acid.

SIDE EFFECTS

OCCASIONAL: Pain at injection site, headache, dizziness, tightness of throat, amenorrhea, decreased spermatogenesis, hives, skin rash, nausea, vomiting, anorexia. **RARE:** Alopecia, cystitis, hematuria following intravesical dosing.

ADVERSE REACTIONS/TOXIC EFFECTS

Hematologic toxicity manifested as leukopenia, anemia, thrombocytopenia, pancytopenia due to bone marrow depression. Although WBC falls to lowest point at 10–14 days after initial therapy, bone marrow effects not evident for 30 days. Stomatitis, ulceration of intestinal mucosa may be noted.

NURSING IMPLICATIONS

BASELINE ASSESSMENT:

Interrupt therapy if WBC falls below 3,000/mm^3, platelet count below 150,000/mm^3, WBC or platelet count declines rapidly. Obtain hematologic status at least weekly during therapy and for 3 wks after therapy discontinued.

INTERVENTION/EVALUATION:

Monitor uric acid serum levels, hematology tests. Assess for stomatitis (burning/erythema of oral mucosa at inner margin of lips, sore throat, difficulty swallowing, oral ulceration). Monitor for hematologic toxicity: infection (fever, sore throat, signs of local infection), easy bruising, unusual bleeding from any site, symptoms of anemia (excessive tiredness, weakness). Assess skin for rash, hives.

PATIENT/FAMILY TEACHING:

Discomfort may occur w/IV administration. Maintain fastidious oral hygiene. Do not have immunizations w/o physician's approval (drug lowers body's resistance). Avoid crowds, those w/infection. Promptly report fever, sore throat, signs of local infection, easy bruising, unusual bleeding from any site. Contact physician if nausea/vomiting continues at home.

thiothixene

thigh-oh-**thicks**-een
(Navane caps)

thiothixene hydrochloride

(Navane solution, injection)

CANADIAN AVAILABILITY: Navane

CLASSIFICATION

Antipsychotic

AVAILABILITY (Rx)

Capsules: 1 mg, 2 mg, 5 mg, 10 mg, 20 mg. **Oral Concentrate:** 5 mg/ml. **Injection:** 2 mg/ml, 5 mg/ml.

PHARMACOKINETICS

	ONSET	PEAK	DURATION
IM	—	1–6 hrs	—

Well absorbed from GI tract, after IM administration. Widely distrib-

uted. Metabolized in liver. Primarily excreted in urine. Half-life: 34 hrs.

ACTION/*THERAPEUTIC EFFECT*

Blocks postsynaptic dopamine receptor sites in brain. Has alpha-adrenergic blocking effects; depresses release of hypothalamic, hypophyseal hormones. *Suppresses behavioral response in psychosis.*

USES

Symptomatic management of psychotic disorders.

STORAGE/HANDLING

Reconstituted solutions stable for 48 hrs at room temperature.

PO/IM ADMINISTRATION

PO:

1. Give w/o regard to meals.
2. Avoid skin contact w/oral solution (contact dermatitis).

IM:

1. Following parenteral form, pt must remain recumbent for 30–60 min in head-low position w/legs raised, to minimize hypotensive effect.
2. For IM injection, reconstitute 10 mg thiothixene hydrochloride w/2.2 ml sterile water for injection, yielding final solution of 5 mg/ml.
3. Inject slow, deep IM into upper outer quadrant of gluteus maximus or midlateral thigh.

INDICATIONS/DOSAGE/ROUTES

Note: Reduce dosage gradually to optimum response, then decrease to lowest effective level for maintenance. Replace parenteral therapy w/oral therapy as soon as possible.

Mild to moderate symptoms:
PO: Adults: 2 mg 3 times/day. May

be increased gradually to 15 mg/day.

Severe symptoms:
PO: Adults: 5 mg 2 times/day. Increase gradually to 60 mg if needed. **Usual dose range:** 20–30 mg/day.
IM: Adults: 4 mg 2–4 times/day. May increase to maximum 30 mg/day. **Usual dose range:** 16–20 mg/day.

Usual elderly dosage:
PO: Initially, 1–2 mg 1–2 times/day. May increase by 1–2 mg q4–7 days. **Maximum:** 30 mg/day.

PRECAUTIONS

CONTRAINDICATIONS: Comatose states, circulatory collapse, CNS depression, blood dyscrasias. **EXTREME CAUTION:** History of seizures. **CAUTIONS:** Severe cardiovascular disorders, alcoholic withdrawal, pt exposure to extreme heat, glaucoma, prostatic hypertrophy. **PREGNANCY/LACTATION:** Crosses placenta; distributed in breast milk. **Pregnancy Category C.**

INTERACTIONS

DRUG INTERACTIONS: Alcohol, CNS depressants may increase CNS, respiratory depression, increase hypotension. Extrapyramidal symptom (EPS)–producing medications may increase risk of EPS. May inhibit effects of levodopa. May increase cardiac effects w/quinidine. **ALTERED LAB VALUES:** May decrease uric acid.

SIDE EFFECTS

Hypotension, dizziness, fainting occur frequently after first injection, occasionally after subsequent injections, rarely w/oral dosage. **FREQUENT:** Transient drowsiness, dry mouth, constipation, blurred vision, nasal congestion. **OCCASIONAL:** Diarrhea, peripheral edema, urinary retention, nausea. **RARE:** Ocular changes, skin pigmentation (those on high dosage for prolonged periods).

ADVERSE REACTIONS/TOXIC EFFECTS

Frequently noted extrapyramidal symptom is akathisia (motor restlessness, anxiety). Occurring less frequently is akinesia (rigidity, tremor, salivation, mask-like facial expression, reduced voluntary movements). Infrequently noted are dystonias: torticollis (neck muscle spasm), opisthotonos (rigidity of back muscles), and oculogyric crisis (rolling back of eyes). Tardive dyskinesia (protrusion of tongue, puffing of cheeks, chewing/puckering of mouth) occurs rarely but may be irreversible. Risk is greater in female geriatric pts. Grand mal seizures may occur in epileptic pts (risk higher w/IM administration).

NURSING IMPLICATIONS

BASELINE ASSESSMENT:

Assess behavior, appearance, emotional status, response to environment, speech pattern, thought content.

INTERVENTION/EVALUATION:

Supervise suicidal risk pt closely during early therapy (as depression lessens, energy level improves, increasing suicide potential). Monitor B/P for hypotension. Assess for peripheral edema behind medial malleolus (sacral area in bedridden pts). Assess stools; prevent constipation. Monitor for EPS, tardive dyskinesia (see Adverse Reactions/Toxic Effects) and potentially fatal, rare neuroleptic malignant syndrome: fever, irregular pulse or B/P, muscle rigidity, altered mental status. Assess for therapeutic response (interest in surroundings, improvement in self-care, increased ability to concentrate, relaxed facial expression).

PATIENT/FAMILY TEACHING:

Full therapeutic effect may take up to 6 wks. Report visual disturbances. Sugarless gum, sips of tepid water may relieve dry mouth. Drowsiness generally subsides during continued therapy. Avoid tasks that require alertness, motor skills until response to drug is established. Avoid alcohol and other CNS depressants.

thyroid
(S-P-T, Thyrar, Armour Thyroid)
See Classification section under: Thyroid

tiagabine
(Gabitril)
See Supplement
See Classifination section under: Anticonvulsants

ticarcillin disodium
(Ticar)
See Classification section under: Antibiotics: penicillins

ticarcillin disodium/ clavulanate potassium

tie-car-**sill**-in/klah-view-**lan**-ate
(Timentin)

CANADIAN AVAILABILITY:
Timentin

CLASSIFICATION
Antibiotic: Penicillin

AVAILABILITY (Rx)
Powder for Injection: 3.1 g. **Solution for Infusion:** 3.1 g/100 ml.

PHARMACOKINETICS
Widely distributed. Minimal metabolism in liver. Primarily excreted unchanged in urine. Moderately removed by hemodialysis. Half-life: 1–1.2 hrs (increased in decreased renal function).

ACTION/*THERAPEUTIC EFFECT*
Ticarcillin: Binds to bacterial cell wall inhibiting bacterial cell wall synthesis, *causing cell lysis, death.* **Clavulanate:** Inhibits bacterial beta-lactamase *protecting ticarcillin from enzymatic degradation.* Bactericidal.

USES
Treatment of septicemia, skin/skin structure, bone and joint, lower respiratory, urinary tract infections, endometritis.

STORAGE/HANDLING
Solution appears colorless to pale yellow (if solution darkens, indicates loss of potency). IV infusion (piggyback) stable for 24 hrs at room temperature, 3 days if refrigerated. Discard if precipitate forms.

IV ADMINISTRATION
Note: Space doses evenly around the clock.
1. For IV infusion (piggyback), reconstitute each 3.1 g vial w/13 ml sterile water for injection or 0.9% NaCl injection to provide concentration of 200 mg ticarcillin and 6.7 mg clavulanic acid per ml.
2. Shake vial to assist reconstitution.
3. Further dilute w/50–100 ml

5% dextrose or 0.9% NaCl. Infuse over 30 min.

4. Because of potential for hypersensitivity/anaphylaxis, start initial dose at few drops/min, increase slowly to ordered rate; stay w/pt first 10–15 min, then check q10 min.

5. Alternating IV sites, use large veins to reduce risk of phlebitis.

INDICATIONS/DOSAGE/ROUTES

Systemic and urinary tract infections:
IV: Adults >60 kg: 3.1 g q4–6h. **Adults <60 kg, children >12 yrs:** 200–300 mg/kg/day in divided doses q4–6h.

Gynecologic infections:
IV: Adults >60 kg: 200 mg/kg/day in divided doses q6h up to 300 mg/kg/day in divided doses q4h.

Usual pediatric dose:
IV: Children <60 kg: 200–300 mg/kg/day **>60 kg:** 3.1 g q4–6h.

Dosage in renal/hepatic impairment:
Hepatic impairment alone usually requires no change. Renal impairment alone, administer 3.1 g initially, then modify dose and/or frequency based on creatinine clearance and/or severity of infection.

CREATININE CLEARANCE	DOSAGE
30–60 ml/min	2 g IV q4h
10–30 ml/min	2 g q8h
<10 ml/min	2 g q12h
10 ml/min w/liver impairment	2 g q24h

PRECAUTIONS

CONTRAINDICATIONS: Hypersensitivity to any penicillin. **CAUTIONS:** History of allergies, esp. cephalosporins. **PREGNANCY/LACTATION:** Readily crosses placenta, appears in cord blood, am-

niotic fluid. Distributed in breast milk in low concentrations. May lead to allergic sensitization, diarrhea, candidiasis, skin rash in infant. **Pregnancy Category B**.

INTERACTIONS

DRUG INTERACTIONS: Anticoagulants, heparin, thrombolytics, NSAIDs may increase risk of hemorrhage w/high doses of ticarcillin. Probenecid may increase concentration, risk of toxicity. **ALTERED LAB VALUES:** May cause positive Coombs' test. May increase SGOT (AST), SGPT (ALT), alkaline phosphatase, bilirubin, creatinine, LDH, bleeding time. May decrease potassium, sodium, uric acid.

SIDE EFFECTS

FREQUENT: Phlebitis, thrombophlebitis w/IV dose, rash, urticaria, pruritus, taste/smell disturbances. **OCCASIONAL:** Nausea, diarrhea, vomiting. **RARE:** Headache, fatigue, hallucinations, bruising/bleeding.

ADVERSE REACTIONS/TOXIC EFFECTS

Overdosage may produce seizures, neurologic reactions. Superinfections, potentially fatal antibiotic-associated colitis may result from bacterial imbalance. Severe hypersensitivity reactions, including anaphylaxis, occur rarely.

NURSING IMPLICATIONS

BASELINE ASSESSMENT:

Question for history of allergies, esp. penicillins, cephalosporins. Obtain specimen for culture and sensitivity before giving first dose (therapy may begin before results are known).

INTERVENTION/EVALUATION:

Hold medication and promptly report rash (hypersensitivity) or diarrhea (w/fever, abdominal pain, mucus and blood in stool may indicate antibiotic-associated colitis). Assess food tolerance. Provide mouth care, sugarless gum or hard candy to offset taste, smell effects. Evaluate IV site for phlebitis (heat, pain, red streaking over vein). Monitor I&O, urinalysis, renal function tests. Assess for bleeding: overt bleeding, bruising or tissue swelling; check hematology reports. Monitor electrolytes, particularly potassium. Be alert for superinfection: increased fever, onset of sore throat, diarrhea, vomiting, ulceration or other oral changes, anal/genital pruritus.

PATIENT/FAMILY TEACHING:

Continue antibiotic for full length of treatment. Space doses evenly. Notify physician in event of rash, diarrhea, bleeding, bruising, or other new symptom.

ticlopidine hydrochloride

tie-**clow**-pih-deen
(Ticlid)

CANADIAN AVAILABILITY:
Apo-Ticlopidine, Ticlid

CLASSIFICATION

Platelet aggregation inhibitor

AVAILABILITY (Rx)

Tablets: 250 mg

PHARMACOKINETICS

Rapidly, well absorbed from GI tract (absorption increases after meals). Metabolized in liver to active metabolite. Primarily excreted in urine. Half-life: single dose: 7.9–12.6 hrs; repeated doses: 4–5 days.

ACTION/ *THERAPEUTIC EFFECT*

Inhibits release of platelet granule constituents, platelet-platelet interactions, and adhesion to endothelium and atheromatous plaque, *preventing platelet aggregation.*

USES/ *UNLABELED*

To reduce risk of stroke in those who have experienced strokelike warnings or those w/history of thrombotic stroke. *Treatment of intermittent claudication, subarachnoid hemorrhage, sickle cell disease.*

PO ADMINISTRATION

Give w/food or just after meals (bioavailability increased, GI discomfort decreased).

INDICATIONS/DOSAGE/ROUTES

Prevention of stroke:
PO: **Adults, elderly:** 250 mg 2 times/day.

PRECAUTIONS

CONTRAINDICATIONS: Hematopoietic disorders (neutropenia, thrombocytopenia), presence of hemostatic disorder, active pathologic bleeding (bleeding peptic ulcer, intracranial bleeding), severe liver impairment. **CAUTIONS:** Those at risk of increased bleeding from trauma, surgery, pathologic conditions. **PREGNANCY/LACTATION:** Unknown whether drug crosses placenta or is distributed in breast milk. **Pregnancy Category B.**

T

INTERACTIONS

DRUG INTERACTIONS: May increase risk of bleeding w/oral anticoagulants, heparin, thrombolytics, aspirin. **ALTERED LAB VALUES:** May increase alkaline phosphatase, bilirubin, liver function tests, cholesterol, triglycerides. May prolong bleeding time. May decrease neutrophil, platelet count.

SIDE EFFECTS

FREQUENT (5–13%): Diarrhea, nausea, dyspepsia (heartburn, indigestion, GI discomfort, bloating). **RARE (1–2%):** Vomiting, flatulence, pruritus, dizziness.

ADVERSE REACTIONS/TOXIC EFFECTS

Thrombotic thrombocytopenia purpura (TTD).

NURSING IMPLICATIONS

BASELINE ASSESSMENT:

Drug should be discontinued 10–14 days before surgery if antiplatelet effect is not desired.

INTERVENTION/EVALUATION:

Assist w/ambulation if dizziness occurs. Monitor heart sounds by auscultation. Assess B/P for hypotension. Assess skin for flushing, rash.

PATIENT/FAMILY TEACHING:

If nausea occurs, cola, unsalted crackers, or dry toast may relieve effect. Therapeutic response may not be achieved before 2–3 mos of continuous therapy. Report any unusual bleeding/bruising or rash.

---

tiludronate

(Skelid)
See Supplement

---

timolol maleate

tim-oh-lol
(Betimol, Blocadren, Timoptic, Timoptic XE)

FIXED-COMBINATION(S):
W/hydrochlorothiazide, a diuretic **(Timolide)**; w/dorzolamide, a carbonic anhydrase inhibitor **(Cosopt)**

CANADIAN AVAILABILITY:
Apo-Timol, Blocadren, Timoptic

CLASSIFICATION

Beta-adrenergic blocker

AVAILABILITY (Rx)

Tablets: 5 mg, 10 mg, 20 mg. **Ophthalmic Solution:** 0.25%, 0.5%. **Ophthalmic Gel:** 0.25%, 0.5%.

PHARMACOKINETICS

	ONSET	PEAK	DURATION
Eye drops	30 min	1–2 hrs	12–24 hrs

Well absorbed from GI tract. Minimal absorption following ophthalmic administration. Metabolized in liver. Primarily excreted in urine. Not removed by hemodialysis. Half-life: 4 hrs. *Ophthalmic:* Systemic absorption may occur.

ACTION/ *THERAPEUTIC EFFECT*

Nonselective beta-adrenergic blocking agent. Blocks beta$_1$-adrenergic receptors, *slowing sinus heart rate, decreasing cardiac output, decreasing B/P*. Blocks beta$_2$-adrenergic receptors, *increasing airway resistance*. Decreases myocardial ischemia severity by decreasing oxygen requirements. *Reduces intraocular pressure (IOP)*.

USES/ *UNLABELED*

Management of mild to moderate hypertension. Used alone or in combination w/diuretics, esp. thiazide type. Reduces cardiovascular mortality in those w/definite/suspected acute MI. Prophylaxis of migraine headache. *Ophthalmic: Reduces IOP in management of open-angle glaucoma, aphakic glaucoma, ocular hypertension, secondary glaucoma. Systemic: Treatment of chronic angina pectoris, cardiac arrhythmias, hypertrophic cardiomyopathy, pheochromocytoma, tremors, anxiety, thyrotoxicosis. Ophthalmic: W/miotics decreases IOP in acute/chronic angle closure glaucoma, treatment of secondary glaucoma, malignant glaucoma, angle closure glaucoma during/after iridectomy.*

STORAGE/HANDLING

Store oral form, ophthalmic solution, gel at room temperature.

PO/OPHTHALMIC ADMINISTRATION

PO:

1. May be given w/o regard to meals.
2. Tablets may be crushed.

OPHTHALMIC:

Note: When using gel, invert container, shake once prior to each use.
1. Place finger on lower eyelid and pull out until pocket is formed between eye and lower lid.
2. Hold dropper above pocket and place prescribed number of drops into pocket. Instruct pt to close eyes gently so medication will not be squeezed out of sac.
3. Apply gentle finger pressure to the lacrimal sac at inner canthus for 1 min following installation (lessens risk of systemic absorption).

INDICATIONS/DOSAGE/ROUTES

Hypertension:
PO: Adults, elderly: Initially, 10

mg 2 times/day, alone or in combination w/other therapy. Gradually increase at intervals of not less than 1 wk. **Maintenance:** 20–60 mg/day in 2 divided doses.

Myocardial infarction:
PO: Adults, elderly: 10 mg 2 times/day, beginning within 1–4 wks after infarction.

Migraine prophylaxis:
PO: Adults, elderly: Initially, 10 mg 2 times/day. **Range:** 10–30 mg/day.

Glaucoma:
Ophthalmic: Adults, elderly: 1 drop of 0.25% solution in affected eye(s) 2 times/day. May be increased to 1 drop of 0.5% solution in affected eye(s) 2 times/day. When IOP is controlled, dosage may be reduced to 1 drop 1 time/day. If pt is transferred to timolol from another antiglaucoma agent, administer concurrently for 1 day. Discontinue other agent on following day. *Timoptic XE:* 1 drop/day.

PRECAUTIONS

Precautions apply to oral and ophthalmic administration (because of systemic absorption of ophthalmic). **CONTRAINDICATIONS:** Bronchial asthma, COPD, uncontrolled cardiac failure, sinus bradycardia, heart block greater than first degree, cardiogenic shock, CHF unless secondary to tachyarrhythmias, those on MAO inhibitors. **CAUTIONS:** Inadequate cardiac function, impaired renal/hepatic function, hyperthyroidism. **PREGNANCY/LACTATION:** Distributed in breast milk; not for use in nursing women because of potential for serious adverse effect on nursing infant. Avoid use during first trimester. May produce bradycardia, apnea, hypoglycemia, hypothermia during delivery, small birth weight infants. **Pregnancy Category C**. (Category D if used in 2nd or 3rd trimester.)

INTERACTIONS

DRUG INTERACTIONS: Diuretics, other hypotensives may increase hypotensive effect. Sympathomimetics, xanthines may mutually inhibit effects. May mask symptoms of hypoglycemia, prolong hypoglycemic effect of insulin, oral hypoglycemics. NSAIDs may decrease antihypertensive effect. **ALTERED LAB VALUES:** May increase ANA titer, SGOT (AST), SGPT (ALT), alkaline phosphatase, LDH, bilirubin, BUN, creatinine, potassium, uric acid, lipoproteins, triglycerides.

SIDE EFFECTS

FREQUENT: Decreased sexual ability, drowsiness, difficulty sleeping, unusual tiredness/weakness. *Ophthalmic:* Eye irritation, visual disturbances. **OCCASIONAL:** Depression, cold hands/feet, diarrhea, constipation, anxiety, nasal congestion, nausea, vomiting. **RARE:** Altered taste, dry eyes, itching, numbness of fingers, toes, scalp.

ADVERSE REACTIONS/TOXIC EFFECTS

Oral form may produce profound bradycardia, hypotension, bronchospasm. Abrupt withdrawal may result in sweating, palpitations, headache, tremulousness. May precipitate CHF, myocardial infarction in those w/cardiac disease, thyroid storm in those w/thyrotoxicosis, peripheral ischemia in those w/existing peripheral vascular disease. Hypoglycemia may occur in previously controlled diabetics. Ophthalmic overdosage may produce bradycardia, hy-

potension, bronchospasm, acute cardiac failure.

NURSING IMPLICATIONS
BASELINE ASSESSMENT:

Assess B/P, apical pulse immediately before drug is administered (if pulse is 60/min or below, or systolic B/P is below 90 mm Hg, withhold medication, contact physician).

INTERVENTION/EVALUATION:

Monitor B/P for hypotension, respiration for shortness of breath. Assess pulse for strength/weakness, irregular rate, bradycardia. Monitor EKG for cardiac arrhythmias, particularly PVCs. Monitor stool frequency and consistency. Assist w/ambulation if dizziness occurs. Assess for evidence of CHF: dyspnea (particularly on exertion or lying down), night cough, peripheral edema, distended neck veins. Monitor I&O (increase in weight, decrease in urine output may indicate CHF). Assess for nausea, diaphoresis, headache, fatigue. *Ophthalmic:* Monitor B/P and pulse regularly.

PATIENT/FAMILY TEACHING:

Do not abruptly discontinue medication. Compliance w/therapy regimen is essential to control glaucoma, hypertension, angina, arrhythmias. To avoid hypotensive effect, rise slowly from lying to sitting position, wait momentarily before standing. Avoid tasks that require alertness, motor skills until response to drug is established. Report shortness of breath, excessive fatigue, prolonged dizziness/headache. Do not use nasal decongestants, OTC cold preparations (stimulants) w/o physician approval. Monitor B/P, pulse before taking medication. Restrict salt, alcohol intake. *Ophthalmic:* Teach pt how to instill drops correctly, how to take pulse. Importance of maintaining regimen, of keeping office visits to check IOP. Transient stinging, discomfort may occur upon instillation. Report difficulty breathing immediately.

tioconazole

tie-oh-**con**-ah-zole
(Vagistat, Monostat-1)

CANADIAN AVAILABILITY: Gynecure, Trosyd

CLASSIFICATION

Antifungal

AVAILABILITY (OTC)

Vaginal Ointment: 6.5%

PHARMACOKINETICS

Systemic absorption minimal.

ACTION/*THERAPEUTIC EFFECT*

Inhibits synthesis of ergosterol (vital component of fungal cell formation), *damaging fungal cell membrane. Fungistatic.*

USES

Treatment of vulvovaginal candidiasis (moniliasis).

INTRAVAGINAL ADMINISTRATION

1. Use disposable gloves; always wash hands thoroughly after application.
2. Follow manufacturer's directions for use of applicator.
3. Insert applicator high in vagina.

4. Administer preferably at bedtime.

INDICATIONS/DOSAGE/ROUTES

Vulvovaginal candidiasis:
Intravaginal: Adults, elderly: 1 applicatorful just before bedtime as a single dose.

PRECAUTIONS

CONTRAINDICATIONS: Hypersensitivity to tioconazole, other imidazole antifungal agents, or any component of the cream/suppository. **CAUTIONS:** Safety and efficacy in children and diabetic pts not established. **PREGNANCY/LACTATION:** Unknown whether excreted in breast milk. **Pregnancy Category C.**

INTERACTIONS

DRUG INTERACTIONS: None significant. **ALTERED LAB VALUES:** None significant.

SIDE EFFECTS

FREQUENT: Headache (26% of pts). **OCCASIONAL (1–6%):** Burning, itching. **RARE (<1%):** Irritation, vaginal pain, dysuria, dryness of vaginal secretions, vulvar edema/swelling.

ADVERSE REACTIONS/TOXIC EFFECTS

None significant.

NURSING IMPLICATIONS

BASELINE ASSESSMENT:

Question for hypersensitivity to tioconazole, other imidazole antifungal agents, or components of preparation. Confirm that potassium hydroxide culture and/or smears were done for accurate diagnosis; therapy may begin before results known. Inquire about use of rubber/latex

T

contraceptives, since there is interaction between such products and the medication.

INTERVENTION/EVALUATION:

Assess for therapeutic response or burning, itching, pain, or irritation.

PATIENT/FAMILY TEACHING:

Do not interrupt/stop regimen, even during menses. Teach pt proper insertion. Not affected by oral contraception. Notify physician of increased itching, irritation, burning. Consult physician about sexual intercourse, douching, or the use of other vaginal products. Do not use vaginal contraceptive diaphragms, condoms within 72 hrs after treatment. Avoid contact w/eyes. Wash hands thoroughly after application.

---

tirobifan
(Aggrastat)
See Supplement

---

tizanidine
(Zanaflex)
See Supplement

---

tobramycin sulfate

tow-bra-**my**-sin
(Nebcin, Tobi, Tobrex)

FIXED-COMBINATION(S):
W/dexamethasone, a steroid (**To-braDex**)

CANADIAN AVAILABILITY:
Nebcin, Tobrex

CLASSIFICATION

Antibiotic: Aminoglycoside

AVAILABILITY (Rx)

Injection: 10 mg/ml, 40 mg/ml. **Powder for Injection:** 1.2 g. **Ophthalmic Solution:** 0.3%. **Ophthalmic Ointment:** 3 mg/g. **Inhalation Solution:** 300 mg/5 ml.

PHARMACOKINETICS

Rapid, complete absorption after IM administration. Widely distributed (does not cross blood-brain barrier, low concentrations in CSF). Excreted unchanged in urine. Removed by hemodialysis. Half-life: 2–4 hrs (increased in decreased renal function, neonates; decreased in cystic fibrosis, burn or febrile pts).

ACTION/*THERAPEUTIC EFFECT*

Irreversibly binds to protein on bacterial ribosome, *interfering in protein synthesis of susceptible microorganisms.*

USES

Skin/skin structure, bone, joint, respiratory tract infections; postop, burn, intra-abdominal infections, complicated urinary tract infections, septicemia, meningitis. *Ophthalmic:* Superficial eye infections: blepharitis, conjunctivitis, keratitis, corneal ulcers. *Inhalation:* Bronchopulmonary infections in pts w/cystic fibrosis.

STORAGE/HANDLING

Store vials, ophthalmic ointment, solution at room temperature. Solutions may be discolored by light/air (does not affect potency). Intermittent IV infusion (piggyback) stable for 24 hrs at room temperature. Discard if precipitate forms.

IM/IV/OPHTHALMIC ADMINISTRATION

Note: Coordinate peak and trough lab draws w/administration times.

IM:

To minimize discomfort, give deep IM slowly. Less painful if injected into gluteus maximus rather than lateral aspect of thigh.

IV:

1. Dilute w/50–200 ml 5% dextrose, 0.9% NaCl, or other compatible fluid. Amount of diluent for infants, children depends upon individual need.

2. Infuse over 20–60 min.

3. Alternating IV sites, use large veins to reduce risk of phlebitis.

OPHTHALMIC:

1. Place finger on lower eyelid and pull out until a pocket is formed between eye and lower lid.

2. Hold dropper above pocket and place correct number of drops ($1/4$–$1/2$ inch ointment) into pocket. Have pt close eye gently.

3. *Solution:* Apply digital pressure to lacrimal sac for 1–2 min (minimizes drainage into nose and throat, reducing risk of systemic effects.) *Ointment:* Close eye for 1–2 min, rolling eyeball (increases contact area of drug to eye).

4. Remove excess solution or ointment around eye w/tissue.

INDICATIONS/DOSAGE/ROUTES

Note: Space parenteral doses evenly around the clock. Dosage based on ideal body weight. Peak, trough level is determined periodically to maintain desired serum concentrations (minimizes risk of toxicity). *Recommended peak level:* 4–10 mcg/ml; *trough level:* 1–2 mcg/ml.

Moderate to severe infections:
IM/IV: Adults, elderly: 3 mg/kg/day in divided doses q8h.

Life-threatening infections:
IM/IV: Adults, elderly: Up to 5 mg/kg/day in divided doses q6–8h.

Usual dosage for children, infants:
IM/IV: Children, infants: 6–7.5 mg/kg/day in 3–4 divided doses.

Dosage in renal impairment:
Dose and/or frequency is modified based on degree of renal impairment, serum concentration of drug. After loading dose of 1–2 mg/kg, maintenance dose/frequency based on serum creatinine/creatinine clearance.

Usual ophthalmic dosage:
Ophthalmic Ointment: Adults, elderly: Thin strip to conjunctiva q8–12h (q3–4h for severe infections). **Ophthalmic Solution: Adults, elderly:** 1–2 drops q4h (2 drops every hour for severe infections).

Usual inhalation dosage:
Adults: Twice daily for 28 days, then off for 28 days.

PRECAUTIONS

CONTRAINDICATIONS: Hypersensitivity to tobramycin, other aminoglycosides (cross-sensitivity). **CAUTIONS:** Elderly, neonates because of renal insufficiency/immaturity; neuromuscular disorders (potential for respiratory depression), prior hearing loss, vertigo, renal impairment. Cumulative effects may occur w/concurrent ophthalmic and systemic administration. **PREGNANCY/LACTATION:** Readily crosses placenta; is distributed in breast milk. May cause fetal nephrotoxicity. **Pregnancy Category D**. Ophthalmic form should not be used in nursing mothers and only when specifically indicated in pregnancy. **Pregnancy Category B**.

INTERACTIONS

DRUG INTERACTIONS: Other

aminoglycosides, nephrotoxic, ototoxic-producing medications may increase toxicity. May increase effects of neuromuscular blocking agents. **ALTERED LAB VALUES:** May increase BUN, SGPT (ALT), SGOT (AST), bilirubin, creatinine, LDH concentrations; may decrease serum calcium, magnesium, potassium, sodium concentrations.

SIDE EFFECTS

OCCASIONAL: Pain, induration at IM injection site; phlebitis, thrombophlebitis w/IV administration; hypersensitivity reaction (rash, fever, urticaria, pruritus). *Ophthalmic:* Tearing, itching, redness, swelling of eyelid. **RARE:** Hypotension, nausea, vomiting.

ADVERSE REACTIONS/TOXIC EFFECTS

Nephrotoxicity (evidenced by increased BUN and serum creatinine, decreased creatinine clearance) may be reversible if drug stopped at first sign of symptoms; irreversible ototoxicity (tinnitus, dizziness, ringing/roaring in ears, reduced hearing) and neurotoxicity (headache, dizziness, lethargy, tremors, visual disturbances) occur occasionally. Risk is greater w/higher dosages, prolonged therapy, or if solution is applied directly to mucosa. Superinfections, particularly w/fungi, may result from bacterial imbalance via any route of administration; anaphylaxis.

NURSING IMPLICATIONS
BASELINE ASSESSMENT:

Dehydration must be treated before parenteral therapy is begun. Question for history of allergies, esp. to aminoglycosides and sulfite (and parabens for topical/ophthalmic routes). Establish baseline for hearing acuity. Obtain specimens for culture, sensitivity before giving first dose (therapy may begin before results are known).

INTERVENTION/EVALUATION:

Monitor I&O (maintain hydration), urinalysis (casts, RBCs, WBCs, decrease in specific gravity). Monitor results of peak/trough blood tests. Be alert to ototoxic and neurotoxic symptoms (see Adverse Reactions/Toxic Effects). Check IM injection site for pain, induration. Evaluate IV site for phlebitis (heat, pain, red streaking over vein). Assess for rash (*ophthalmic*—assess for redness, swelling, itching, tearing). Be alert for superinfection particularly genital/anal pruritus, changes of oral mucosa, diarrhea. When treating pts w/neuromuscular disorders, assess respiratory response carefully.

PATIENT/FAMILY TEACHING:

Continue antibiotic for full length of treatment. Space doses evenly. Discomfort may occur w/IM injection. Notify physician in event of any hearing, visual, balance, urinary problems even after therapy is completed. Do not take other medication w/o consulting physician. Lab tests are an essential part of therapy. *Ophthalmic:* Blurred vision/tearing may occur briefly after application. Contact physician if tearing, redness, or irritation continues.

tocainide hydrochloride

toe-**kay**-nied
(Tonocard)

CANADIAN AVAILABILITY:
Tonocard

CLASSIFICATION

Antiarrhythmic

AVAILABILITY (Rx)

Tablets: 400 mg, 600 mg

PHARMACOKINETICS

Completely absorbed from GI tract. Widely distributed. Metabolized in liver. Primarily excreted in urine. Removed by hemodialysis. Half-life: 15 hrs (increased in decreased renal function).

ACTION / *THERAPEUTIC EFFECT*

Shortens action potential duration, decreases effective refractory period, automaticity in His-Purkinje system of myocardium by blocking sodium transport across myocardial cell membranes, *suppressing ventricular arrhythmias.*

USES

Suppression, prevention of ventricular arrhythmias including frequent unifocal/multifocal coupled premature ventricular contractions and paroxysmal ventricular tachycardia.

PO ADMINISTRATION

1. Do not crush or break film-coated tablets.
2. May give w/food (decreases GI upset).
3. Monitor EKG for cardiac changes, particularly shortening of QT interval. Notify physician of any significant interval changes.

INDICATIONS/DOSAGE/ROUTES

Note: When giving tocainide in those receiving IV lidocaine, give single 600 mg dose 6 hrs before cessation of lidocaine and repeat in 6 hrs. Then give standard tocainide maintenance doses.

Ventricular arrhythmias:
PO: Adults, elderly: Initially, 400 mg q8h. **Maintenance:** 1.2–1.8 g/day in divided doses q8h. **Maximum:** 2,400 mg/day.

PRECAUTIONS

CONTRAINDICATIONS: Hypersensitivity to local anesthetics, second- or third-degree AV block. **CAUTIONS:** CHF, elderly, severe respiratory depression, bradycardia, incomplete heart block. **PREGNANCY/LACTATION:** Unknown whether drug crosses placenta or is distributed in breast milk. **Pregnancy Category C.**

INTERACTIONS

DRUG INTERACTIONS: Other antiarrhythmics may increase risk of adverse cardiac effects. Beta-adrenergic blockers may increase pulmonary wedge pressure, decrease cardiac index. **ALTERED LAB VALUES:** None significant.

SIDE EFFECTS

Generally well tolerated. **FREQUENT (3–10%):** Minor, transient lightheadedness, dizziness, nausea, paresthesia, rash, tremor. **OCCASIONAL (1–3%):** Clammy skin, night sweats, joint pain. **RARE (<1%):** Restlessness, nervousness, disorientation, mood changes, ataxia (muscular incoordination), visual disturbances.

ADVERSE REACTIONS/TOXIC EFFECTS

High dosage may produce bradycardia/tachycardia, hypotension, palpitations, increased ventricular arrhythmias, PVCs, chest pain, exacerbation of CHF.

NURSING IMPLICATIONS

BASELINE ASSESSMENT:

Assess pulse for strength/weakness, irregular rate. Monitor EKG for cardiac changes, particularly shortening of QT interval. Notify physician of any significant interval changes. Monitor fluid and electrolyte serum levels. Assess hand movement for sign of tremor (usually first clinical sign that maximum dose is being reached). Assess sleeping pt for night sweats. Question for tingling/numbness in hands/feet. Assess skin for rash, clamminess. Observe for CNS disturbances (restlessness, disorientation, mood changes, incoordination). Assist w/ambulation if lightheadedness, dizziness occur. Assess for evidence of CHF: dyspnea (particularly on exertion or lying down), night cough, peripheral edema, distended neck veins. Monitor I&O (increase in weight, decrease in urine output may indicate CHF). Monitor for therapeutic serum level (3–10 mcg/ml).

PATIENT/FAMILY TEACHING:

Avoid tasks that require alertness, motor skills until response to drug is established. Side effects generally disappear w/continued therapy. Unsalted crackers, dry toast may relieve nausea.

tolazamide

(Tolinase, Tolamide)
See Classification section under: Antidiabetic agents

tolazoline hydrochloride

toe-**laze**-oh-lean
(Priscoline)

CLASSIFICATION

Antihypertensive

AVAILABILITY (Rx)

Injection: 25 mg/ml

PHARMACOKINETICS

Rapidly, completely absorbed. Concentrated primarily in liver, kidney. Excreted unchanged in urine. Half-life: 3–10 hrs.

ACTION/*THERAPEUTIC EFFECT*

Directly relaxes vascular smooth muscle, *causes vasodilation, decreases peripheral resistance.* Has moderate alpha-adrenergic blocking activity.

USES

Treatment of persistent pulmonary vasoconstriction and hypertension of newborn (persistent fetal circulation). Improves oxygenation.

PARENTERAL ADMINISTRATION

Monitor B/P diligently for systemic hypotension. If hypotension occurs, place in supine position w/feet elevated, give IV fluids. Do not administer epinephrine. Tolazoline may cause "epinephrine reversal" (further B/P decrease followed by rebound hypertension).

INDICATIONS/DOSAGE/ROUTES

Persistent fetal circulation:
IV: Newborn: Initially, 1–2 mg/kg via scalp vein over 10 min; then, IV infusion of 1–2 mg/kg/hr.

PRECAUTIONS

CONTRAINDICATIONS: None significant. **CAUTIONS:** Known/suspected mitral stenosis.

INTERACTIONS

DRUG INTERACTIONS: Antagonizes vasoconstriction caused by dopamine. Decreases effects of metaraminol, ephedrine, phenylephrine. **ALTERED LAB VALUES:** None significant.

SIDE EFFECTS

OCCASIONAL: Nausea, diarrhea, vomiting, increased pilomotor activity (goose bumps), peripheral vasodilation (flushing), tachycardia. **RARE:** Mydriasis.

ADVERSE REACTIONS/TOXIC EFFECTS

GI hemorrhage, hypochloremic alkalosis, cardiac arrhythmias, hypotension, oliguria, hepatitis, thrombocytopenia, leukopenia may occur.

NURSING IMPLICATIONS

BASELINE ASSESSMENT:

Obtain B/P immediately before each dose, in addition to regular monitoring (be alert to fluctuations). If excessive reduction in B/P occurs, place pt in supine position w/feet elevated, give IV fluids.

INTERVENTION/EVALUATION:

Monitor vital signs, oxygenation, acid-base balance, fluid and electrolytes.

tolbutamide
(Orinase, Oramide)
See Classification section under: Antidiabetic agents

tolcapone
(Tasmar)
See Supplement

tolmetin sodium

toll-meh-tin
(Tolectin)

CANADIAN AVAILABILITY:
Tolectin

CLASSIFICATION

Nonsteroidal anti-inflammatory

AVAILABILITY (Rx)

Tablets: 200 mg, 600 mg. **Capsules:** 400 mg.

PHARMACOKINETICS

	ONSET	PEAK	DURATION
PO (antirheumatic):			
	7 days	1–2 wks	—

Rapidly, completely absorbed from GI tract. Metabolized in liver. Excreted in urine. Half-life: 5 hrs.

ACTION/THERAPEUTIC EFFECT

Produces analgesic and anti-inflammatory effect by inhibiting prostaglandin synthesis, *reducing inflammatory response and intensity of pain stimulus reaching sensory nerve endings.*

USES/UNLABELED

Relief of pain, disability associated w/rheumatoid arthritis, juvenile rheumatoid arthritis, osteoarthritis. *Treatment of ankylosing spondylitis, psoriatic arthritis.*

PO ADMINISTRATION

May give w/food, milk, or antacids if GI distress occurs.

INDICATIONS/DOSAGE/ROUTES

Rheumatoid arthritis, osteoarthritis:
PO: **Adults, elderly:** Initially, 400 mg 3 times/day (including 1 dose upon arising, 1 dose at bedtime). Adjust dose at 1–2 wk intervals. **Maintenance:** 600–1,800 mg/day in 3–4 divided doses.

Juvenile rheumatoid arthritis:
PO: **Children >2 yrs:** Initially, 20 mg/kg/day in 3–4 divided doses. **Maintenance:** 15–30 mg/kg/day in 3–4 divided doses.

PRECAUTIONS

CONTRAINDICATIONS: History of hypersensitivity to aspirin or other NSAIDs, those severely incapacitated, bedridden, wheelchair bound. **CAUTIONS:** Impaired renal function, impaired cardiac function, coagulation disorders, history of upper GI disease. **PREGNANCY/LACTATION:** Distributed in breast milk. Avoid use during third trimester (may adversely affect fetal cardiovascular system: premature closure of ductus arteriosus). **Pregnancy Category C**. (Category D if used in 3rd trimester or near delivery.)

INTERACTIONS

DRUG INTERACTIONS: May increase effects of oral anticoagulants, heparin, thrombolytics. May decrease effect of antihypertensives, diuretics. Salicylates, aspirin may increase risk of GI side effects, bleeding. Bone marrow depressants may increase risk of hematologic reactions. May increase concentration, toxicity of lithium. May increase methotrexate toxicity. Probenecid may increase concentration. Antacids may decrease concentration. **ALTERED LAB VALUES:** May increase BUN, potassium, liver function tests. May decrease Hgb, Hct. May prolong bleeding time.

SIDE EFFECTS

OCCASIONAL (3–11%): Nausea, vomiting, diarrhea, abdominal cramping, dyspepsia (heartburn, indigestion, epigastric pain), flatulence, dizziness, headache, weight decrease or increase. **RARE (1–3%):** Constipation, anorexia, rash, pruritus.

ADVERSE REACTIONS/TOXIC EFFECTS

Peptic ulcer, GI bleeding, gastritis, severe hepatic reaction (cholestasis, jaundice) occur rarely. Nephrotoxicity (dysuria, hematuria, proteinuria, nephrotic syndrome) and severe hypersensitivity reaction (fever, chills, bronchospasm) occur rarely.

NURSING IMPLICATIONS

BASELINE ASSESSMENT:

Assess onset, type, location, and duration of pain/inflammation. Inspect appearance of affected joints for immobility, deformities, and skin condition.

INTERVENTION/EVALUATION:

Monitor pattern of daily bowel activity, stool consistency. Assist w/ambulation if dizziness occurs. Monitor for evidence of GI distress. Evaluate for therapeutic response (relief of pain, stiffness, swelling; increase in joint mobility, reduced joint tenderness, improved grip strength).

PATIENT/FAMILY TEACHING:

Therapeutic effect noted in 1–3 wks. Avoid tasks that require alertness, motor skills until response to drug is established. If GI upset occurs, take w/food, milk. Avoid aspirin, alcohol during therapy (increases risk of GI bleeding). Report headache, GI distress.

tolnaftate
(Tinactin, Aftate)
See Classification section under: Antifungals: topical

tolterodine
(Detrol)
See Supplement

topiramate
(Topamax)
See Supplement
See Classification section under: Anticonvulsants

topotecan
toe-**poh**-teh-can
(Hycamtin)

CANADIAN AVAILABILITY:
Hycamtin

CLASSIFICATION

Antineoplastic

AVAILABILITY (Rx)

Powder for Injection: 4 mg (single-dose vial)

PHARMACOKINETICS

Following IV administration, hydrolyzed to active form. Excreted in urine. Half-life: 2–3 hrs (half-life increased in renal impairment).

ACTION/THERAPEUTIC EFFECT

Interacts w/topoisomerase I, an enzyme, which relieves torsional strain in DNA by inducing reversible

single-strand breaks. Binds to topoisomerase-DNA complex preventing relegation of these single-strand breaks. Double-strand DNA damage occurring during DNA synthesis *produces cytoxic effect.*

USES

Treatment of metastatic carcinoma of ovary after failure of initial or recurrent chemotherapy. Treatment of sensitive, relapsed small cell lung cancer.

STORAGE/HANDLING

Store vials at room temperature in original cartons. Reconstituted vials diluted for infusion stable at room temperature, ambient lighting for 24 hrs.

IV ADMINISTRATION

1. Reconstitute each 4 mg vial with 4 ml sterile water for injection.
2. Dilute appropriate volume of reconstituted solution either with 0.9% NaCl or 5% dextrose.
3. Administer all doses as IV solution over 30 min.
4. Extravasation associated w/only mild local reactions (erythema, bruising).

INDICATIONS/DOSAGE/ROUTES

Note: Do not give topotecan if baseline neutrophil count <1,500 cells/mm^3 and platelet count <100,000/mm^3.

Carcinoma of ovary; small-cell lung cancer:
IV Infusion: Adults, elderly: 1.5 mg/m^2 over 30 min daily for 5 consecutive days, beginning on day 1 of a 21 day course. Minimum of four courses recommended. If severe neutropenia occurs during treatment, reduce dose by 0.25 mg/m^2 for subsequent courses or as an alternative, give G-CSF fol-

lowing the subsequent course beginning day 6 of the course (24 hrs after completion of topotecan administration).

Note: No dosage adjustment necessary in pts w/mild renal impairment (creatinine clearance 40–60 ml/min).

Moderate renal impairment (creatinine clearance 20–39 ml/min): **IV Infusion: Adults, elderly:** 0.75 mg/m^2.

PRECAUTIONS

CONTRAINDICATIONS: Hypersensitivity to topotecan, baseline neutrophil count <1,500 cells/mm^3, pregnancy, breast feeding, severe bone marrow depression. **CAUTIONS:** Mild bone marrow depression, liver or renal impairment. **PREGNANCY/LACTATION:** May cause fetal harm. Avoid pregnancy; discontinue nursing. **Pregnancy Category D**.

INTERACTIONS

DRUG INTERACTIONS: Other myelosuppressants may increase risk of myelosuppression. Concurrent use of cisplatin may increase severity of myelosuppression. Live virus vaccines may potentiate virus replication, increase vaccine side effects, decrease antibody response to vaccine. **ALTERED LAB VALUES:** May decrease neutrophil, leukocyte, thrombocyte, RBC levels. May increase SGOT (AST), SGPT (ALT), bilirubin.

SIDE EFFECTS

FREQUENT: Nausea (77%), vomiting (58%), diarrhea, total alopecia (42%), headache (21%), dyspnea (21%). **OCCASIONAL:** Paresthesia (9%), constipation, abdominal pain (3%). **RARE:** Anorexia, malaise, arthralgia, asthenia, myalgia.

ADVERSE REACTIONS/TOXIC EFFECTS

Severe neutropenia (<500 cells/mm^3) occurs in 60% of pts (develops at median of 11 days after day 1 of initial therapy). Thrombocytopenia (<25,000/mm^3) occurs in 26% of pts and severe anemia (< 8 g/dl) occurs in 40% of pts (develops at median of 15 days after day 1 of initial therapy).

NURSING IMPLICATIONS

BASELINE ASSESSMENT:

Offer emotional support to pt and family. Assess CBC w/differential, hemoglobin, and platelet count before each dose. Myelosuppression may precipitate life-threatening hemorrhage, infection, anemia. If platelet count drops, avoid even slightest trauma to body (injection site, assisting movement). Premedicate w/antiemetics on day of treatment, starting at least 30 min prior to administration.

INTERVENTION/EVALUATION:

Monitor frequently for CBC w/differential during treatment. Assess for bleeding, signs of infection, anemia. Monitor hydration status, I/O, electrolytes (diarrhea, vomiting are common side effects). Monitor CBC w/differential, Hgb, platelets for evidence of myelosuppression. Assess response to medication; provide interventions, e.g., small, frequent meals/antiemetics for nausea and vomiting. Question for complaints of headache. Assess breathing pattern for evidence of dyspnea.

PATIENT/FAMILY TEACHING:

Explain that alopecia is reversible, but new hair may have different color, texture. Inform pt of possible late diarrhea causing dehydration, electrolyte depletion. Provide antiemetic/antidiarrheal regimen for subsequent use. Notify physician if diarrhea, vomiting continues at home. Do not have immunizations without physician's approval (drug lowers body's resistance). Avoid contact with those who have recently received live virus vaccine.

___

toremifene
(Fareston)
See Supplement
See Classification section under:
Antineoplastics

___

torsemide
tore-seh-mide
(Demadex)

CANADIAN AVAILABILITY:
Demadex

CLASSIFICATION
Diuretic: Loop

AVAILABILITY (Rx)
Tablets: 5 mg, 10 mg, 20 mg, 100 mg. **Injection:** 10 mg/ml.

PHARMACOKINETICS

	ONSET	PEAK	DURATION
PO	1 hr	1–2 hrs	6–8 hrs
IV	20 min	1 hr	6–8 hrs

Rapidly, well absorbed from GI tract. Metabolized in liver. Primarily excreted in urine. Half-life: 3.3 hrs.

ACTION/*THERAPEUTIC EFFECT*
Diuretic: Enhances excretion of sodium, chloride, potassium, water at ascending limb of loop of Henle, *producing diuretic effect.*
Antihypertensive: Reduces plasma, extracellular fluid volume, *lowering B/P.*

USES
Treatment of hypertension either alone or in combination w/other antihypertensives. Edema associated w/CHF, renal disease, hepatic cirrhosis, chronic renal failure.

STORAGE/HANDLING
Store oral, parenteral forms at room temperature.

PO/IV ADMINISTRATION
PO:
May take w/o regard to food. Give w/food to avoid GI upset, preferably w/breakfast (prevents nocturia).

IV:
1. Give slowly over 2 min or as continuous IV infusion.
2. Give high doses slowly (minimizes risk of ototoxicity).

INDICATIONS/DOSAGE/ROUTES

Hypertension:
PO: Adults, elderly: Initially, 5 mg/day. May increase to 10 mg/day if no response in 4–6 wks. If no response, additional antihypertensive added.

Congestive heart failure:
IV/PO: Adults, elderly: Initially, 10–20 mg/day. May increase by approximately doubling dose until desired diuretic dose attained. (Dose >200 mg not adequately studied.)

Chronic renal failure:
IV/PO: Adults, elderly: Initially, 20 mg/day. May increase by approximately doubling dose until desired diuretic dose attained. (Dose >200 mg not adequately studied.)

Hepatic cirrhosis:
IV/PO: Adults, elderly: Initially, 5

mg/day (w/aldosterone antagonist or potassium-sparing diuretic). May increase by approximately doubling dose until desired diuretic dose attained. (Dose >40 mg not adequately studied.)

PRECAUTIONS

CONTRAINDICATIONS: Anuria, hepatic coma, severe electrolyte depletion. **EXTREME CAUTION:** Hypersensitivity to sulfonamides. **CAUTIONS:** Elderly, cardiac pts, pts w/history of ventricular arrhythmias, pts w/hepatic cirrhosis, ascites. Renal impairment, systemic lupus erythematosus. Safety in children not known. **PREGNANCY/ LACTATION:** Unknown whether drug is excreted in breast milk. Pregnancy Category B.

INTERACTIONS

DRUG INTERACTIONS: May increase antihypertensive effect of other antihypertensives. NSAIDs, probenecid may decrease effect. May increase risk of digoxin-induced arrhythmias (due to hypokalemia). Amphotericin may increase risk nephrotoxicity. Effects of anticoagulants, heparin, thrombolytics may be decreased, hypokalemia-causing medications may increase risk of hypokalemia; may increase risk of lithium toxicity. Nephrotoxic/ototoxic medications may increase nephrotoxicity/ototoxicity. **ALTERED LAB VALUES:** May increase uric acid, BUN, creatinine. May decrease calcium, chloride, magnesium, potassium, sodium.

SIDE EFFECTS

FREQUENT (3–10%): Headache, dizziness, rhinitis. **OCCASIONAL (1–3%):** Asthenia, insomnia, nervousness, diarrhea, constipation, nausea, dyspepsia, edema, EKG changes, sore throat, cough, arthral-gia, myalgia. **RARE (<1%):** Syncope, hypotension, arrhythmias.

ADVERSE REACTIONS/TOXIC EFFECTS

Overdosage produces acute, profound water loss, volume and electrolyte depletion, dehydration, decreased blood volume, circulatory collapse. Ototoxicity may occur: High IV doses must be given slowly to minimize ototoxicity.

NURSING IMPLICATIONS
BASELINE ASSESSMENT:

Assess B/P for hypotension. Check electrolyte levels, esp. potassium. Obtain baseline weight; check for edema, rales in lungs.

INTERVENTION/EVALUATION:

Monitor B/P, electrolytes (esp. potassium), I&O, weight. Notify physician of any hearing abnormality. Note extent of diuresis. Assess lungs for rales. Check for signs of edema, particularly of dependent areas. Although less potassium is lost w/torsemide than furosemide, assess for signs of hypokalemia (change of muscle strength, tremor, muscle cramps, change in mental status, cardiac arrhythmias).

PATIENT/FAMILY TEACHING:

Take medication in morning to prevent nocturia. Expect increased frequency and volume of urination. Report irregular heartbeats, signs of hypokalemia (see above), muscle weakness, cramps, nausea, or dizziness. Change positions slowly to prevent orthostatic hypotension. Do not take other medications (including OTC drugs) w/o consulting physician. Eat foods high in potassium such as whole grains (cereals), legumes, meat, bananas, apricots, orange juice, potatoes (white, sweet), raisins.

tramadol hydrochloride

tray-mah-doal
(Ultram)

CLASSIFICATION

Analgesic

AVAILABILITY (Rx)

Tablets: 50 mg

PHARMACOKINETICS

	ONSET	PEAK	DURATION
PO	<1 hr	2–3 hrs	4–6 hrs

Rapidly, almost completely absorbed following oral administration. Extensively metabolized in liver to active metabolite (reduced in pts w/advanced cirrhosis). Primarily excreted in urine. Minimally removed by hemodialysis. Half-life: 6–7 hrs.

ACTION / THERAPEUTIC EFFECT

Binds to μ-opiate receptors and inhibits reuptake of norepinephrine and serotonin. *Reduces intensity of pain stimuli incoming from sensory nerve endings, altering pain perception and emotional response to pain.*

USES

Management of moderate to moderately severe pain.

PO ADMINISTRATION

Give w/o regard to meals.

INDICATIONS / DOSAGE / ROUTES

Moderate to moderately severe pain:

PO: Adults, elderly: 50–100 mg q4–6h. **Maximum <75 yrs:** 400 mg/day. **Maximum >75 yrs:** 300 mg/day.

Renal function impairment (creatinine clearance <30 ml/min):
Note: Dialysis pts can receive their regular dose on day of dialysis.
PO: Adults, elderly: Increase dosing interval to 12 hrs. **Maximum daily dose:** 200 mg.

Hepatic function impairment:
PO: Adults, elderly: 50 mg q12h.

PRECAUTIONS

CONTRAINDICATIONS: Hypersensitivity to tramadol, acute intoxication w/alcohol, hypnotics, centrally acting analgesics, opioids or psychotropic drugs. **EXTREME CAUTION:** CNS depression, anoxia, advanced liver cirrhosis, epilepsy, respiratory depression, acute alcoholism, shock. **CAUTIONS:** Sensitivity to opioids, increased intracranial pressure, impaired hepatic/renal function, acute abdominal conditions, opioid-dependent pts. **PREGNANCY/LACTATION:** Crosses placenta; distributed in breast milk. May prolong labor if administered in latent phase of first stage of labor, or before cervical dilation of 4–5 cm has occurred. Respiratory depression may occur in neonate if mother received opiates during labor. Regular use of opiates during pregnancy may produce withdrawal symptoms (irritability, excessive crying, tremors, hyperactive reflexes, fever, vomiting, diarrhea, yawning, sneezing, seizures) in the neonate. **Pregnancy Category C**.

INTERACTIONS

DRUG INTERACTIONS: Alcohol, CNS depressants may increase

CNS effects or respiratory depression, hypotension. MAO inhibitors increase tramadol concentration. Carbamazepine increases tramadol metabolism, decreases concentration. **ALTERED LAB VALUES:** May increase creatinine, liver enzymes. May decrease hemoglobin, proteinuria.

SIDE EFFECTS

FREQUENT (15–25%): Dizziness/vertigo, nausea, constipation, headache, somnolence. **OCCASIONAL (5–10%):** Vomiting, pruritus, CNS stimulation (nervousness, anxiety, agitation, tremor, euphoria, mood swings, hallucinations), asthenia, sweating, dyspepsia, dry mouth, diarrhea. **RARE (<5%):** Malaise, vasodilation, anorexia, flatulence, rash, visual disturbance, urinary retention/frequency, menopausal symptoms.

ADVERSE REACTIONS/TOXIC EFFECTS

Overdosage results in respiratory depression, skeletal muscle flaccidity, cold clammy skin, cyanosis, extreme somnolence progressing to seizures, stupor, coma. Tolerance to analgesic effect, physical dependence may occur w/repeated use. Prolonged duration of action, cumulative effect may occur in those w/impaired hepatic, renal function.

NURSING IMPLICATIONS
BASELINE ASSESSMENT:

Assess onset, type, location, and duration of pain. Effect of medication is reduced if full pain recurs before next dose. Assess drug history, esp. carbamazepine, CNS depressant medication, MAO inhibitors. Review past medical history, esp. epilepsy/seizures. Assess renal/liver function lab values.

INTERVENTION/EVALUATION:

Assist w/ambulation if dizziness, vertigo occurs. Dry crackers, cola may relieve nausea. Question bowel activity, frequency. Palpate bladder for urinary retention. Monitor pattern of daily bowel activity and stool consistency. Sips of tepid water may relieve dry mouth. Assess for clinical improvement and record onset of relief of pain. Assess skin for evidence of rash, pruritus.

PATIENT/FAMILY TEACHING:

Avoid tasks that require alertness, motor skills until response to drug is established. Tolerance/dependence may occur w/prolonged use of high doses.

trandolapril
tran-**doal**-ah-prill
(Mavik)

FIXED-COMBINATION(S):
W/verapamil, a calcium channel blocker **(Tarka)**

CANADIAN AVAILABILITY:
Mavik

CLASSIFICATION

Angiotensin-converting enzyme (ACE) inhibitor, antihypertensive

AVAILABILITY (Rx)

Tablets: 1 mg, 2 mg, 4 mg

PHARMACOKINETICS

Slowly absorbed from GI tract. Metabolized in liver, GI mucosa to active metabolite. Primarily excreted in urine. Minimal removal by hemodialysis. Half-life: 6–10 hrs.

ACTION/ *THERAPEUTIC EFFECT*

Suppresses renin-angiotensin-aldosterone system (prevents conversion of angiotensin I to angiotensin II, a potent vasoconstrictor; may also inhibit angiotensin II at local vascular and renal sites). Decreases plasma angiotensin II, increases plasma renin activity, decreases aldosterone secretion. *Reduces peripheral arterial resistance, pulmonary capillary wedge pressure; improves cardiac output, exercise tolerance.*

USES

Treatment of hypertension. Used alone or in combination w/other antihypertensives. Treatment of congestive heart failure (CHF)

PO ADMINISTRATION

1. May give w/o regard to meals.

2. Tablets may be crushed.

INDICATIONS/DOSAGE/ROUTES

Hypertension (w/o diuretic):
PO: Adults, elderly: Initially, 1 mg once daily in nonblack pts, 2 mg once daily in black pts. Adjust dose at least at 7 day intervals. **Maintenance:** 2–4 mg/day. **Maximum:** 8 mg/day.

CHF:
PO: Adults, elderly: Initially, 0.5–1 mg, titrated to target dose of 4 mg/day.

PRECAUTIONS

CONTRAINDICATIONS: History of angioedema w/previous treatment w/ACE inhibitors. **CAUTIONS:** Renal impairment, those w/sodium depletion or on diuretic therapy, dialysis, hypovolemia, coronary or cerebrovascular insufficiency. **PREGNANCY/LACTATION:** Crosses placenta; distributed in breast milk. May cause fetal/neonatal mortality/morbidity. **Pregnancy Category C** (first trimester); **Pregnancy Category D** (second and third trimesters).

INTERACTIONS

DRUG INTERACTIONS: Alcohol, diuretics, hypotensive agents may increase effects. NSAIDs may decrease effect. Potassium-sparing diuretics, potassium supplements may cause hyperkalemia. May increase lithium concentration, toxicity. **ALTERED LAB VALUES:** May increase potassium, SGOT (AST), SGPT (ALT), alkaline phosphatase, bilirubin, BUN, creatinine. May decrease sodium. May cause positive ANA titer.

SIDE EFFECTS

FREQUENT (23–35%): Dizziness, cough. **OCCASIONAL (3–11%):** Hypotension, dyspepsia (heartburn, epigastric pain, indigestion), syncope, asthenia (loss of strength), tinnitus. **RARE (<1%):** Palpitations, insomnia, drowsiness, nausea, vomiting, constipation, flushed skin.

ADVERSE REACTIONS/TOXIC EFFECTS

Excessive hypotension ("first-dose syncope") may occur in those w/CHF, severely salt/volume depleted. Angioedema (swelling of face/lips), hyperkalemia occur rarely. Agranulocytosis, neutropenia may be noted in those w/impaired renal function or collagen vascular disease (systemic lupus erythematosus, scleroderma). Nephrotic syndrome may be noted in those w/history of renal disease.

NURSING IMPLICATIONS

BASELINE ASSESSMENT:

Obtain B/P immediately before each dose, in addition to regular monitoring (be alert to fluctuations). Renal function tests should be performed before therapy begins. In those w/renal impairment, autoimmune disease, or taking drugs that affect leukocytes or immune response, CBC and differential count should be performed before therapy begins and q2 wks for 3 mos, then periodically thereafter.

INTERVENTION/EVALUATION:

If excessive reduction in B/P occurs, place pt in supine position w/legs elevated. Assist w/ambulation if dizziness occurs. Assess for urinary frequency. Auscultate lung sounds for rales, wheezing in those w/CHF. Monitor urinalysis for proteinuria. Monitor serum potassium levels in those on concurrent diuretic therapy. Monitor pattern of daily bowel activity and stool consistency.

PATIENT/FAMILY TEACHING:

Report any sign of infection (sore throat, fever). Several weeks may be needed for full therapeutic effect of B/P reduction. Skipping doses or voluntarily discontinuing drug may produce severe, rebound hypertension. To reduce hypotensive effect, rise slowly from lying to sitting position and permit legs to dangle from bed momentarily before standing. Report facial swelling, difficulty swallowing. Avoid potassium supplements/salt substitutes.

tranylcypromine sulfate

tran-ill-**sip**-roe-meen
(Parnate)

CANADIAN AVAILABILITY:
Parnate

CLASSIFICATION

Antidepressant: MAO inhibitor

AVAILABILITY (Rx)

Tablets: 10 mg

PHARMACOKINETICS

Well absorbed from GI tract. Metabolized in liver. Primarily excreted in urine. Half-life: 1.5–3 hrs.

ACTION/*THERAPEUTIC EFFECT*

Inhibits MAO enzyme (assists in metabolism of sympathomimetic amines) at CNS storage sites. Levels of epinephrine, norepinephrine, serotonin, dopamine increased at neuron receptor sites, *producing antidepressant effect.*

USES

Symptomatic treatment of severe depression in hospitalized or closely supervised pts who have not responded to other antidepressant therapy, including electroconvulsive therapy.

PO ADMINISTRATION

Give w/food if GI distress occurs.

INDICATIONS/DOSAGE/ROUTES

PO: Adults, elderly: 30 mg/day in divided doses. May increase dose by 10 mg/day at intervals of 1–3 wks. **Maximum:** 60 mg/day.

PRECAUTIONS

CONTRAINDICATIONS: Pts >60 yrs, debilitated/hypertensive pts, cerebrovascular/cardiovascular disease, foods containing tryptophan/tyramine, within 10 days of elective surgery, pheochromocytoma, congestive heart failure, history of liver disease, abnormal liver function tests, severe renal impairment, history of severe/

recurrent headache. **CAUTIONS:** Impaired renal function, history of seizures, parkinsonian syndrome, diabetic pts, hyperthyroidism. **PREGNANCY/LACTATION:** Crosses placenta; unknown whether distributed in breast milk. **Pregnancy Category C**.

INTERACTIONS

DRUG INTERACTIONS: Alcohol, CNS depressants may increase CNS depressant effects. Tricyclic antidepressants, fluoxetine, trazodone may cause serotonin syndrome. May increase effect of oral hypoglycemics, insulin. B/P may increase w/buspirone. Caffeine-containing medications may increase cardiac arrhythmias, hypertension. May precipitate hypertensive crises w/carbamazepine, cyclobenzaprine, maprotiline, other MAO inhibitors. Meperidine, other opioid analgesics may produce immediate excitation, sweating, rigidity, severe hypertension or hypotension, severe respiratory distress, coma, convulsions, vascular collapse, death. May increase CNS stimulant, vasopressor effects. Tyramine, foods w/pressor amines (e.g., aged cheese) may cause sudden, severe hypertension. **ALTERED LAB VALUES:** None significant.

SIDE EFFECTS

FREQUENT: Postural hypotension, restlessness, GI upset, insomnia, dizziness, lethargy, weakness, dry mouth, peripheral edema. **OCCASIONAL:** Flushing, increased perspiration, rash, urinary frequency, increased appetite, transient impotence. **RARE:** Visual disturbances.

ADVERSE REACTIONS/TOXIC EFFECTS

Hypertensive crisis may be noted by hypertension, occipital headache radiating frontally, neck stiffness/soreness, nausea, vomiting, sweating, fever/chilliness, clammy skin, dilated pupils, palpitations. Tachycardia/bradycardia, constricting chest pain may also be present. Antidote for hypertensive crisis: 5–10 mg phentolamine IV injection.

NURSING IMPLICATIONS

BASELINE ASSESSMENT:

Periodic liver function tests should be performed in those requiring high dosage and/or undergoing prolonged therapy. MAO inhibitor therapy should be discontinued for 7–14 days before elective surgery.

INTERVENTION/EVALUATION:

Assess appearance, behavior, speech pattern, level of interest, mood. Monitor for occipital headache radiating frontally, and/or neck stiffness or soreness (may be first signal of impending hypertensive crisis). Monitor blood pressure diligently for hypertension. Assess skin temperature for fever. Discontinue medication immediately if palpitations or frequent headaches occur.

PATIENT/FAMILY TEACHING:

Antidepressant relief may be noted during first week of therapy; maximum benefit noted within 3 wks. Report headache, neck stiffness/soreness immediately. To avoid orthostatic hypotension, change from lying to sitting position slowly and dangle legs momentarily before standing. Avoid tasks that require alertness, motor skills until response to drug is established. Avoid foods that require bacteria/molds for their prepara-

T

tion/preservation or those that contain tyramine, e.g., cheese, sour cream, beer, wine, pickled herring, liver, figs, raisins, bananas, avocados, soy sauce, yeast extracts, yogurt, papaya, broad beans, meat tenderizers, or excessive amounts of caffeine (coffee, tea, chocolate), or OTC preparations for hay fever, colds, weight reduction.

---

trastuzumab
(Herceptin)
See Supplement

---

trazodone hydrochloride

tra-zoh-doan
(Desyrel)

CANADIAN AVAILABILITY:
Desyrel

CLASSIFICATION

Antidepressant

AVAILABILITY (Rx)

Tablets: 50 mg, 100 mg, 150 mg, 300 mg

PHARMACOKINETICS

Well absorbed from GI tract. Metabolized in liver. Primarily excreted in urine. Half-life: 5–9 hrs.

ACTION/ *THERAPEUTIC EFFECT*

Blocks reuptake of serotonin by CNS presynaptic neuronal membranes, increasing availability at postsynaptic neuronal receptor sites. Resulting enhancement of synaptic activity *produces antidepressant effect.*

USES/ *UNLABELED*

Treatment of depression exhibited as persistent, prominent dysphoria (occurring nearly every day for at least 2 wks) manifested by 4 of 8 symptoms: appetite change, sleep pattern change, increased fatigue, impaired concentration, feelings of guilt or worthlessness, loss of interest in usual activities, psychomotor agitation or retardation, suicidal tendencies. *Treatment of neurogenic pain.*

PO ADMINISTRATION

1. Give shortly after snack, meal (reduces risk of dizziness, lightheadedness).
2. Tablets may be crushed.

INDICATIONS/DOSAGE/ROUTES

Antidepressant:
PO: Adults: Initially, 150 mg daily in equally divided doses. Increase by 50 mg/day at 3–4 day intervals until therapeutic response is achieved. Do not exceed 400 mg/day for outpatients, 600 mg/day for hospitalized pts.

Usual elderly dosage:
PO: Initially, 25–50 mg at bedtime. May increase by 25–50 mg q3–7 days. **Range:** 75–150 mg/day.

PRECAUTIONS

CONTRAINDICATIONS: Recovery phase of MI, surgical pts, electroconvulsive therapy. **CAUTIONS:** Cardiovascular disease, MAO inhibitor therapy. **PREGNANCY/ LACTATION:** Crosses placenta; minimally distributed in breast milk. **Pregnancy Category C.**

INTERACTIONS

DRUG INTERACTIONS: Alcohol,

CNS depression–producing medications may increase CNS depression. May increase effects of antihypertensives. May increase concentration of digoxin, phenytoin. **ALTERED LAB VALUES:** May decrease neutrophil, leukocyte counts.

SIDE EFFECTS

FREQUENT (3–9%): Drowsiness, dry mouth, lightheadedness/dizziness, headache, blurred vision, nausea/vomiting. **OCCASIONAL (1–3%):** Nervousness, fatigue, constipation, generalized aches and pains, mild hypotension.

ADVERSE REACTIONS/TOXIC EFFECTS

Priapism (painful, prolonged penile erection), decreased/increased libido, retrograde ejaculation, impotence have been noted rarely. Appears to be less cardiotoxic than other antidepressants, although arrhythmias may occur in pts w/preexisting cardiac disease.

NURSING IMPLICATIONS

BASELINE ASSESSMENT:

For those on long-term therapy, liver/renal function tests, blood counts should be performed periodically.

INTERVENTION/EVALUATION:

Supervise suicidal risk pt closely during early therapy (as depression lessens, energy level improves, increasing suicide potential). Assess appearance, behavior, speech pattern, level of interest, mood. Monitor WBC and neutrophil count (drug should be stopped if levels fall below normal). Assist w/ambulation if dizziness or lightheadedness occurs.

PATIENT/FAMILY TEACHING:

Immediately discontinue medication and consult physician if priapism occurs. Change positions slowly to avoid hypotensive effect. Tolerance to sedative and anticholinergic effects usually develops during early therapy. Photosensitivity to sun may occur. Dry mouth may be relieved by sugarless gum, sips of tepid water. Report visual disturbances. Do not abruptly discontinue medication. Avoid tasks that require alertness, motor skills until response to drug is established. Avoid alcohol.

tretinoin

tret-ih-noyn
(Avita, Renova, Retin-A, Retin-A Micro, Vesanoid)

FIXED-COMBINATION(S):
W/octyl methoxycinnamate and oxybenzone, moistures, and SPF-12, a sunscreen **(Retin-A Regimen Kit)**

CANADIAN AVAILABILITY:
Retin-A, Stieva-A, Vesanoid, Vitamin A Acid

CLASSIFICATION

Antiacne, transdermal, antineoplastic

AVAILABILITY (Rx)

Capsules: 10 mg. **Cream:** 0.025%, 0.05%, 0.1%. **Cream (Avita):** 0.025%. **(Renova):** 0.05%. **Gel:** 0.025%, 0.01%. **(Retin-A Micro):** 0.1%. **Liquid:** 0.05%.

PHARMACOKINETICS

Topical: Minimally absorbed. *Oral:* Well absorbed following oral administration. Primarily excreted in urine. Half-life: 0.5–2 hrs.

ACTION/*THERAPEUTIC EFFECT*

Antiacne: Decreases cohesiveness of follicular epithelial cells. Increases turnover of follicular epithelial cells, *causing expulsion of blackheads*. Bacterial skin counts are not altered. **Transdermal:** Exerts its effects on growth and differentiation of epithelial cells, *alleviating fine wrinkles, hyperpigmentation.* **Antineoplastic:** Induces maturation, decreases proliferation of acute promyelocytic leukemia (APL) cells, *followed by repopulation of bone marrow and blood by normal hematopoietic cells.*

USES/*UNLABELED*

Topical: Treatment of acne vulgaris, esp. grades I–III in which blackheads, papules, pustules predominate. **Transdermal:** Treatment of fine wrinkles, hyperpigmentation. **Antineoplastic:** Induction of remission in pts with acute promyelocytic leukemia (APL). *Treatment of disorders of keratinization, including photo-aged skin, liver spots.*

ORAL/TOPICAL ADMINISTRATION

PO:

Do not crush or break capsule.

TOPICAL:

1. Thoroughly cleanse area before applying tretinoin.

2. Lightly cover only the affected area. Liquid may be applied w/fingertip, gauze, or cotton, taking care to avoid running onto unaffected skin.

3. Keep medication away from eyes, mouth, angles of nose, mucous membranes.

4. Wash hands immediately after application.

INDICATIONS/DOSAGE/ROUTES

Acne:
Topical: Adults: Apply once daily at bedtime.

Transdermal:
Topical: Adults: Apply to face once daily at bedtime.

Acute promyelocytic leukemia:
PO: Adults: 45 mg/m^2/day given as two evenly divided doses until complete remission is documented. Discontinue therapy 30 days after complete remission or after 90 days of treatment, whichever comes first.

PRECAUTIONS

CONTRAINDICATIONS: Hypersensitivity to any component of the preparation, sensitivity to parabens (used as preservative in gelatin capsule). **EXTREME CAUTION:** *Topical:* Eczema, sun exposure. **CAUTIONS:** *Topical:* Those w/considerable sun exposure in their occupation or hypersensitivity to sun. *Oral:* Elevated cholesterol/triglycerides. **PREGNANCY/LACTATION:** *Topical:* Use during pregnancy only if clearly needed. Unknown whether excreted in breast milk; exercise caution in nursing mother. **Pregnancy Category C**. *(Topical).* *Oral:* Teratogenic, embryotoxic effect. **Pregnancy Category D**.

INTERACTIONS

DRUG INTERACTIONS: *Topical:* Keratolytic agents (e.g., sulfur, benzoyl peroxide, salicylic acid), medicated soaps, shampoos, astringents, spice or lime cologne, permanent wave solutions, hair depilatories may increase skin irritation. Photosensitive medication (thiazides, tetracyclines, fluoroquinolones, phenothiazines, sulfonamides) augments phototoxicity. *Oral:* Ketoconazole may increase tretinoin concentration. **AL-**

TERED LAB VALUES: *Oral:* Leukocytosis occurs commonly (40%). May elevate liver function tests, cholesterol, triglycerides.

SIDE EFFECTS

Topical: Local inflammatory reactions are to be expected and are reversible w/discontinuation of tretinoin. **FREQUENT (>10%):** Headache, dry skin/oral mucosa, cheilitis (crusting, swelling of lips), nausea, vomiting, bone pain, arthralgia, myalgia, rash, fever, weakness, fatigue. *Topical:* Transient feeling of warmth or stinging, erythema, peeling. **OCCASIONAL (1–10%):** *Oral:* Pruritus, increased sweating visual disturbances, alopecia, skin changes, dizziness, flushing, abdominal pain. *Topical:* Temporary hyperpigmentation, severe erythema, crusting, blistering, edema. **RARE (<1%):** *Topical:* Contact allergy.

ADVERSE REACTIONS/TOXIC EFFECTS

Oral: Retinoic acid syndrome (fever, dyspnea, weight gain, abnormal chest auscultatory findings [pulmonary infiltrates, pleural or pericardial effusions], episodic hypotension) occurs commonly (25%) as does leukocytosis (40%). Syndrome generally occurs during first month of therapy (sometimes occurs following first dose). High-dose steroids (dexamethasone 10 mg IV) at first suspicion of syndrome reduces morbidity, mortality. Pseudo tumor cerebri may be noted, esp. in children (headache, nausea, vomiting, visual disturbances). *Topical:* Possible tumorigenic potential when combined w/ultraviolet radiation.

NURSING IMPLICATIONS
BASELINE ASSESSMENT:

Oral: Inform women of childbearing potential of risk to fetus if pregnancy occurs. Instruct in need for use of two reliable forms of contraceptives concurrently during therapy and for 1 mo after discontinuation of therapy, even in infertile, premenopausal women. Pregnancy test should be obtained within 1 wk prior to institution of therapy. Obtain initial liver function tests, cholesterol, triglyceride levels.

INTERVENTION/EVALUATION:

Oral: Monitor liver function tests, hematologic, coagulation profiles, cholesterol, triglycerides. Monitor signs/symptoms of pseudo tumor cerebri in children.

PATIENT/FAMILY TEACHING:

Topical: Avoid exposure to sunlight or sunbeds; use sunscreens and protective clothing. Affected areas should also be protected from wind, cold. If skin is already sunburned, do not use until fully recovered. Do not use more often than instructed or use larger amount of medication (does not lead to more rapid or better results). Keep tretinoin away from eyes, mouth, angles of nose and mucous membranes. Do not use medicated, drying, or abrasive soaps; wash face no more than 2–3 times/day with bland soap. Avoid use of preparations containing alcohol, menthol, spice, or lime such as shaving lotions, astringents, perfume. Application may cause temporary warmth or stinging feeling. Mild redness, peeling are expected; decrease frequency or discontinue medication if excessive reaction occurs. Nonmedicated cosmetics may be used; however, cosmetics must be removed before tretinoin application. Improvement noted during first 24 wks of therapy. *Antiacne:* Therapeutic results noted in 2–3 wks; optimal results in 6 wks. *Oral:* Explain purpose of medication, adverse effects. Report adverse effects to physician.

triamcinolone
try-am-**sin**-oh-lone
(Aristocort, Kenacort)

triamcinolone diacetate
(Amcort, Aristocort Intralesional, Trilone)

triamcinolone acetonide
(Aristocort, Azmacort, Kenalog, Nasacort AQ)

triamcinolone hexacetonide
(Aristospan)

FIXED-COMBINATION(S):
Triamcinolone acetonide w/nystatin, an antifungal **(Myco-Aricin, Myco II, Myco-Biotic, Mycogen II, Nystolone)**

CANADIAN AVAILABILITY:
Aristocort, Azmacort, Kenalog, Triaderm

CLASSIFICATION

Corticosteroid

AVAILABILITY (Rx)

Tablets: 1 mg, 2 mg, 4 mg, 8 mg. **Syrup:** 4 mg/5 ml. **Aerosol (respiratory inhalant), Nasal Spray, Ointment:** 0.025%, 0.1%, 0.5%. **Cream:** 0.025%, 0.1%, 0.5%. **Lotion:** 0.025%, 0.1%.
   Acetonide: Injection: 3 mg/ml, 10 mg/ml, 40 mg/ml
   Diacetate: Injection: 25 mg/ml, 40 mg/ml
   Hexacetone: Injection: 5 mg/ml, 20 mg/ml

PHARMACOKINETICS

Rapidly absorbed after inhalation. Completely absorbed after oral administration; well absorbed after IM administration. Widely distributed. Metabolized in liver. Primarily excreted in urine. Half-life: 2–5 hrs.

ACTION/ *THERAPEUTIC EFFECT*

Inhibits accumulation of inflammatory cells at inflammation sites, phagocytosis, lysosomal enzyme release and synthesis and/or release of mediators of inflammation. *Prevents/suppresses cell-mediated immune reactions. Decreases/ prevents tissue response to inflammatory process.*

USES

Substitution therapy in deficiency states: Acute/chronic adrenal insufficiency, congenital adrenal hyperplasia, adrenal insufficiency secondary to pituitary insufficiency. *Nonendocrine disorders:* Arthritis, rheumatic carditis, allergic, collagen, intestinal tract, liver, ocular, renal, and skin diseases, bronchial asthma, cerebral edema, malignancies. Allergic rhinitis. *Inhalation:* Maintenance prophylaxis of asthma.

PO/IM/INHALATION/ TOPICAL ADMINISTRATION

PO:

   1. Give w/food or milk.

2. Single doses given before 9 AM; multiple doses at evenly spaced intervals.

IM:

1. Do *not* give IV.
2. Give deep IM in gluteus maximus.

INHALATION:

1. Shake and inhale immediately before use.
2. Pt should exhale completely; place mouthpiece 2 fingers' width away from mouth.
3. Tilt head back; while activating inhaler, take slow, deep breath for 3–5 secs.
4. Pt should hold breath as long as possible (5–10 secs) then exhale slowly.
5. Wait 1 min between inhalations when multiple inhalations ordered.
6. Following treatment, pt should thoroughly rinse mouth w/water or mouthwash.

TOPICAL:

1. Gently cleanse area before application.
2. Use occlusive dressings only as ordered.
3. Apply sparingly and rub into area thoroughly.

INDICATIONS/DOSAGE/ROUTES

Usual oral dosage:
PO: Adults, elderly: 4–60 mg/day.

Triamcinolone diacetate:
IM: Adults, elderly: 40 mg/wk.
Intra-articular, Intralesional: Adults, elderly: 5–40 mg.

Triamcinolone acetonide:
IM: Adults, elderly: Initially, 2.5–60 mg/day.
Intra-articular: Adults, elderly: Initially, 2.5–40 mg up to 100 mg.

Triamcinolone hexacetonide:
Intra-articular: Adults, elderly: 2–20 mg.

Control of bronchial asthma:
Inhalation: Adults, elderly: 2 inhalations 3–4 times/day. **Children 6–12 yrs:** 1–2 inhalations 3–4 times/day. **Maximum:** 12 inhalations/day.

Rhinitis:
Intranasal: Adults, children >6 yrs: 2 sprays each nostril daily.

Usual topical dosage:
Topical: Adults, elderly: Sparingly 2–4 times/day. May give 1–2 times/day or intermittent therapy.

PRECAUTIONS

CONTRAINDICATIONS: Hypersensitivity to any corticosteroid or tartrazine, systemic fungal infection, peptic ulcers (except life-threatening situations). IM injection, oral inhalation not for children <6 yrs of age. Avoid immunizations, smallpox vaccination. *Topical:* Marked circulation impairment. **CAUTIONS:** History of tuberculosis (may reactivate disease), hypothyroidism, cirrhosis, nonspecific ulcerative colitis, CHF, hypertension, psychosis, renal insufficiency. Prolonged therapy should be discontinued slowly. **PREGNANCY/LACTATION:** Drug crosses placenta, is distributed in breast milk. May cause cleft palate (chronic use during first trimester). Nursing contraindicated. **Pregnancy Category C.**

INTERACTIONS

DRUG INTERACTIONS: Amphotericin may increase hypokalemia. May decrease effect of oral hypoglycemics, insulin, diuretics, potassium supplements. May increase digoxin toxicity (due to hypokalemia). Hepatic enzyme inducers may decrease effect. Live virus vaccines may potentiate virus replication, increase vaccine side effects, decrease pt's antibody response to vaccine. **ALTERED LAB VALUES:** May decrease calcium, potassium, thyroxine. May increase cholesterol, lipids, glucose, sodium, amylase.

SIDE EFFECTS

FREQUENT: Insomnia, heartburn, nervousness, abdominal distention, increased sweating, acne, mood swings, increased appetite, facial flushing, delayed wound healing, increased susceptibility to infection, diarrhea/constipation. **OCCASIONAL:** Headache, edema, change in skin color, frequent urination. **RARE:** Tachycardia, allergic reaction (rash, hives), psychic changes, hallucinations, depression. *Topical:* Allergic contact dermatitis.

ADVERSE REACTIONS/TOXIC EFFECTS

Long-term therapy: muscle wasting (esp. arms, legs), osteoporosis, spontaneous fractures, amenorrhea, cataracts, glaucoma, peptic ulcer, CHF. *Abrupt withdrawal following long-term therapy:* anorexia, nausea, fever, headache, joint pain, rebound inflammation, fatigue, weakness, lethargy, dizziness, orthostatic hypotension. Anaphylaxis w/parenteral administration. Sudden discontinuance may be fatal. Blindness has occurred rarely after intralesional injection around face, head.

NURSING IMPLICATIONS
BASELINE ASSESSMENT:

Question for hypersensitivity to any of the corticosteroids or tartrazine (Kenacort). Obtain baselines for height, weight, B/P, glucose, electrolytes. Check results of initial tests, e.g., TB skin test, x-rays, EKG.

INTERVENTION/EVALUATION:

Monitor I&O, daily weight; assess for edema. Evaluate food tolerance and bowel activity; promptly report hyperacidity. Check B/P, temperature, pulse, respiration at least 2 times/day. Be alert to infection: sore throat, fever, or vague symptoms. Monitor electrolytes. Watch for hypocalcemia (muscle twitching, cramps, positive Trousseau's or Chvostek's signs) or hypokalemia (weakness and muscle cramps, numbness/tingling, esp. in lower extremities, nausea and vomiting, irritability, EKG changes). Assess emotional status, ability to sleep. Check lab results for blood coagulability and clinical evidence of thromboembolism. Provide assistance w/ambulation.

PATIENT/FAMILY TEACHING:

Take w/food or milk. Carry identification of drug and dose, physician name and phone number. Do not change dose/schedule or stop taking drug, must taper off gradually under medical supervision. Notify physician of fever, sore throat, muscle aches, sudden weight gain/swelling. W/dietician give instructions for prescribed diet (usually sodium restricted w/high vitamin D, protein, and potassium). Maintain careful personal hygiene, avoid exposure to disease or trauma. Severe stress (serious infection, surgery, or trauma) may require increased dosage. Do not take any other medication w/o consulting physician. Follow-up visits, lab tests are necessary; children must be assessed for growth retardation. Inform dentist or other physicians of triamcinolone therapy now or within past 12 mos. Caution against overuse of joints injected for symptomatic relief. Teach proper oral inhalation technique. *Topical:* Apply after shower/bath for best absorption. Do not cover unless physician orders; do not use tight diapers, plastic pants or coverings. Avoid contact w/eyes. Do not expose treated area to sunlight.

triamterene

try-**am**-tur-een
(Dyrenium)

FIXED-COMBINATION(S): W/hydrochlorothiazide, a thiazide diuretic (Dyazide, Maxzide)

CANADIAN AVAILABILITY: Dyrenium

CLASSIFICATION

Diuretic: Potassium sparing

AVAILABILITY (Rx)

Capsules: 50 mg, 100 mg

PHARMACOKINETICS

	ONSET	PEAK	DURATION
PO	2–4 hrs	6–8 hrs	12–16 hrs

Incompletely absorbed from GI tract. Widely distributed. Metabolized in liver. Primarily eliminated in feces via biliary route. Half-life: 1.5–2 hrs (increased in decreased renal function).

ACTION/ THERAPEUTIC EFFECT

Competitively inhibits action of aldosterone. Interferes w/sodium reabsorption in distal tubule, *increasing potassium retention while promoting sodium and water excretion.*

USES/ UNLABELED

Treatment of edema associated w/CHF, hepatic cirrhosis, nephrotic syndrome, steroid-induced edema, idiopathic edema, edema due to secondary hyperaldosteronism. May be used alone or w/other diuretics. *Treatment adjunct for hypertension, prophylaxis/treatment of hypokalemia.*

PO ADMINISTRATION

1. May give w/food if GI disturbances occur.

2. Do not crush or break capsules.

INDICATIONS/DOSAGE/ROUTES

Note: Fixed-combination medication should not be used for initial therapy but rather for maintenance therapy.

Dyrenium:
PO: Adults: Initially, 100 mg twice daily after meals. **Maintenance:** 100 mg/day or every other day. **Maximum:** 300 mg/day. When used concurrently w/other diuretics, decrease dosage of each drug initially; adjust to pt's needs.

Usual elderly dosage:
PO: Initially, 50 mg/day. **Maximum:** 100 mg/day in 1–2 doses.

Dyazide, Maxzide:
PO: Adults: 1–2 capsules/tablets per day.

PRECAUTIONS

CONTRAINDICATIONS: Severe or progressive renal disease, severe hepatic disease, preexisting or drug-induced hyperkalemia. **CAUTIONS:** Impaired hepatic or kidney function, history of renal calculi, diabetes mellitus. **PREGNANCY/LACTATION:** Crosses placenta; is distributed in breast milk. Nursing is not advised. **Pregnancy Category D**.

INTERACTIONS

DRUG INTERACTIONS: May decrease effect of anticoagulants, heparin. NSAIDs may decrease antihypertensive effect. ACE inhibitors (e.g., captopril), potassium-containing medications, potassium supplements may increase potassium. May decrease lithium clearance, increase toxicity. **ALTERED LAB VALUES:** May increase BUN, calcium excretion, creatinine, glucose, magnesium, potassium, uric acid. May decrease sodium.

SIDE EFFECTS

OCCASIONAL: Tiredness, nausea, diarrhea, abdominal distress, leg aches, headache. **RARE:** Anorexia, weakness, rash, dizziness.

ADVERSE REACTIONS/TOXIC EFFECTS

May produce hyponatremia (drowsiness, dry mouth, increased thirst, lack of energy) or severe hyperkalemia (irritability, anxiety, heaviness of legs, paresthesia, hypotension, bradycardia, tented T waves, widening QRS, ST depression). Agranulocytosis, nephrolithiasis, thrombocytopenia occur rarely.

NURSING IMPLICATIONS

BASELINE ASSESSMENT:

Assess baseline electrolytes, particularly check for low potassium. Assess renal/hepatic functions. Assess edema (note location, extent), skin turgor, mucous membranes for hydration status. Assess muscle strength, mental status. Note skin temperature, moisture. Obtain baseline weight. Initiate strict I&O. Note pulse rate/regularity.

INTERVENTION/EVALUATION:

Monitor B/P, vital signs, electrolytes (particularly potassium), I&O, weight. Note extent of diuresis. Watch for changes from initial assessment (hyperkalemia may result in muscle strength changes, tremor, muscle cramps), change in mental status (orientation, alertness, confusion), cardiac arrhythmias. Monitor potassium level, particularly during initial therapy. Weigh daily. Assess lung sounds for rhonchi, wheezing.

PATIENT/FAMILY TEACHING:

Expect increase in volume and frequency of urination. Therapeutic effect takes several days to begin and can last for several days when drug is discontinued. High-potassium diet/potassium supplements can be dangerous, esp. if pt has renal/hepatic problems. Avoid prolonged exposure to sunlight. Report severe or persistent weakness, headache, dry mouth, nausea, vomiting, fever, sore throat, unusual bleeding/bruising.

triazolam

try-**aye**-zoe-lam
(Halcion)

CANADIAN AVAILABILITY:
Apo-Triazo, Halcion

CLASSIFICATION

Sedative-hypnotic (**Schedule IV**)

AVAILABILITY (Rx)

Tablets: 0.125 mg, 0.25 mg

PHARMACOKINETICS

Well absorbed from GI tract. Widely distributed (crosses blood-brain barrier). Metabolized in liver (undergoes first-pass liver extraction). Primarily excreted in urine. Half-life: 1.5–5.5 hrs.

ACTION / THERAPEUTIC EFFECT

Enhances action of inhibitory neurotransmitter gamma-aminobutyric acid (GABA), *producing hypnotic effect due to CNS depression.*

USES

Short-term treatment of insomnia (up to 6 wks). Reduces sleep-induction time, number of nocturnal awakenings; increases length of sleep.

PO ADMINISTRATION

1. Give w/o regard to meals.
2. Tablets may be crushed.
3. Grapefruit juice may alter absorption.

INDICATIONS / DOSAGE / ROUTES

Hypnotic:
PO: Adults >18 yrs: 0.125–0.5 mg at bedtime. **Elderly:** 0.0625–0.125 mg at bedtime.

PRECAUTIONS

CONTRAINDICATIONS: Acute narrow-angle glaucoma, acute alcohol intoxication. **CAUTIONS:** Impaired renal/hepatic function. **PREGNANCY/LACTATION:** Crosses placenta; may be distributed in breast milk. Chronic ingestion during pregnancy may produce withdrawal symptoms, CNS depression in neonates. **Pregnancy Category X.**

INTERACTIONS

DRUG INTERACTIONS: Alcohol, CNS depressants may increase CNS depressant effect. **ALTERED LAB VALUES:** None significant.

SIDE EFFECTS

FREQUENT: Drowsiness, sedation, headache, dizziness, nervousness, lightheadedness, incoordination, nausea. **OCCASIONAL:** Euphoria, tachycardia, abdominal cramps, visual disturbances. **RARE:** Paradoxical CNS excitement, restlessness, particularly noted in elderly, debilitated.

ADVERSE REACTIONS / TOXIC EFFECTS

Abrupt or too rapid withdrawal may result in pronounced restlessness, irritability, insomnia, hand tremors, abdominal/muscle cramps, sweating, vomiting, seizures. Overdosage results in somnolence, confusion, diminished reflexes, coma.

NURSING IMPLICATIONS

BASELINE ASSESSMENT:

Question for possibility of pregnancy before initiating therapy (Pregnancy Category X). Assess B/P, pulse, respirations immediately before administration. Raise bed rails. Provide

T

environment conducive to sleep (backrub, quiet environment, low lighting).

INTERVENTION/EVALUATION:

Assess sleep pattern of pt. Assess elderly/debilitated for paradoxical reaction, particularly during early therapy. Evaluate for therapeutic response to insomnia: decrease in number of nocturnal awakenings, increase in length of sleep.

PATIENT/FAMILY TEACHING:

Smoking reduces drug effectiveness. Rebound insomnia may occur when drug is discontinued after short-term therapy. Avoid alcohol and other CNS depressants. Inform physician if you are or are planning to become pregnant. May experience disturbed sleep for 1–2 nights after discontinuing triazolam. Avoid concomitant grapefruit juice.

trifluoperazine hydrochloride

try-floo-oh-**pear**-ah-zeen
(Stelazine)

CANADIAN AVAILABILITY:
Apo-Trifluoperazine, Stelazine

CLASSIFICATION

Antipsychotic

AVAILABILITY (Rx)

Tablets: 1 mg, 2 mg, 5 mg, 10 mg. **Oral Concentrate:** 10 mg/ml. **Injection:** 2 mg/ml.

PHARMACOKINETICS

Variably absorbed after oral administration, well absorbed after IM administration. Widely distributed. Metabolized in liver to some active metabolites. Primarily excreted in urine.

ACTION/*THERAPEUTIC EFFECT*

Blocks dopamine at postsynaptic receptor sites, *suppressing behavioral response in psychosis, reducing locomotor activity/aggressiveness, suppressing conditioned responses.* Has strong extrapyramidal, antiemetic action; weak anticholinergic, sedative effects.

USES

Management of psychotic disorders, nonpsychotic anxiety.

STORAGE/HANDLING

Store oral solutions, parenteral form at room temperature. Slight yellow discoloration of solutions does not affect potency, but discard if markedly discolored or if precipitate forms.

PO/IM ADMINISTRATION

PO:

Add oral concentrate to 60 ml tomato or fruit juice, milk, carbonated beverages, coffee, tea, water. May also add to semisolid food.

IM:

1. Pt must remain recumbent for 30–60 min in head-low position w/legs raised, to minimize hypotensive effect.
2. Inject slow, deep IM into upper outer quadrant of gluteus maximus. If irritation occurs, further injections may be diluted w/0.9% NaCl or 2% procaine hydrochloride.

INDICATIONS/DOSAGE/ROUTES

Note: Decrease dosage gradually to optimum response, then decrease to lowest effective level for maintenance. Replace parenteral therapy w/oral therapy as soon as possible.

Psychotic disorders (hospitalized):
PO: Adults: 2–5 mg twice daily. Gradually increase to average daily dose of 15–20 mg (up to 40 mg may be required in severe cases). **Children 6–12 yrs:** 1 mg 1–2 times/day. Gradually increase to maximum daily dose of 15 mg.
IM: Adults: 1–2 mg q4–6h. Do not exceed 6 mg/24 hrs. **Children 6–12 yrs:** 1 mg 1–2 times/day.

Psychotic disorders (outpatient):
PO: Adults: 1–2 mg 2 times/day.

Nonpsychotic anxiety:
PO/IM: Adults: 1–2 mg 2 times/day.

Usual elderly dosage:
PO: Initially, 1–5 mg 2 times/day. **Range:** 15–20 mg/day. **Maximum:** 40 mg/day.
IM: Initially, 1 mg q4–6h as needed. **Maximum:** 6 mg/day.

PRECAUTIONS

CONTRAINDICATIONS: Severe CNS depression, comatose states, severe cardiovascular disease, bone marrow depression, subcortical brain damage. **CAUTIONS:** Impaired respiratory/hepatic/renal/cardiac function, alcohol withdrawal, history of seizures, urinary retention, glaucoma, prostatic hypertrophy, hypocalcemia (increases susceptibility to dystonias). **PREGNANCY/LACTATION:** Crosses placenta; distributed in breast milk. **Pregnancy Category C.**

INTERACTIONS

DRUG INTERACTIONS: Alcohol, CNS depressants may increase CNS, respiratory depression, hypotensive effects. Tricyclic antidepressants, MAO inhibitors may increase sedative, anticholinergic effects. Antithyroid agents may increase risk of agranulocytosis. Extrapyramidal symptoms (EPS) may increase w/EPS-producing medications. Hypotensives may increase hypotension. May decrease levodopa effects. Lithium may decrease absorption, produce adverse neurologic effects. **ALTERED LAB VALUES:** May cause EKG changes.

SIDE EFFECTS

FREQUENT: Hypotension, dizziness, and fainting occur frequently after first injection, occasionally after subsequent injections, and rarely w/oral dosage. **OCCASIONAL:** Drowsiness during early therapy, dry mouth, blurred vision, lethargy, constipation or diarrhea, nasal congestion, peripheral edema, urinary retention. **RARE:** Ocular changes, skin pigmentation (those on high doses for prolonged periods).

ADVERSE REACTIONS/TOXIC EFFECTS

Extrapyramidal symptoms appear dose related (particularly high dosage) and are divided into 3 categories: akathisia (inability to sit still, tapping of feet, urge to move around); parkinsonian symptoms (mask-like face, tremors, shuffling gait, hypersalivation); and acute dystonias: torticollis (neck muscle spasm), opisthotonos (rigidity of back muscles), and oculogyric crisis (rolling back of eyes). Dystonic reaction may also produce profuse sweating, pallor. Tardive dyskinesia (protrusion of tongue, puffing of cheeks, chewing/puckering of the mouth) occurs rarely (may be irreversible). Abrupt withdrawal following long-term therapy may precipitate nausea, vomiting, gastritis, dizziness, tremors. Blood dyscrasias, particularly agranulocytosis, mild leukopenia (sore mouth/gums/throat) may occur. May lower seizure threshold.

NURSING IMPLICATIONS

BASELINE ASSESSMENT:

Avoid skin contact w/solution (contact dermatitis). Assess behavior, appearance, emotional status, response to environment, speech pattern, thought content.

INTERVENTION/EVALUATION:

Monitor B/P for hypotension. Assess for extrapyramidal symptoms. Monitor WBC, differential count for blood dyscrasias. Monitor for fine tongue movement (may be early sign of tardive dyskinesia). Supervise suicidal risk pt closely during early therapy (as depression lessens, energy level improves, increasing suicide potential). Assess for therapeutic response (interest in surroundings, improvement in self-care, increased ability to concentrate, relaxed facial expression).

PATIENT/FAMILY TEACHING:

Maximum therapeutic response occurs in 2–3 wks. Urine may darken. Do not abruptly withdraw from long-term drug therapy. Report visual disturbances. Sugarless gum, sips of tepid water may relieve dry mouth. Drowsiness generally subsides during continued therapy. Avoid tasks that require alertness, motor skills until response to drug is established. Avoid alcohol.

trifluridine

try-**fleur**-ih-deen
(Viroptic)

CANADIAN AVAILABILITY:
Viroptic

CLASSIFICATION

Antiviral

AVAILABILITY (Rx)

Ophthalmic Solution: 1%

PHARMACOKINETICS

Intraocular penetration occurs after instillation. Half-life: 12–18 min.

ACTION/*THERAPEUTIC EFFECT*

Incorporated into DNA causing increased rate of mutation and errors in protein formation, *preventing viral replication.*

USES

Recurrent epithelial keratitis and primary keratoconjunctivitis caused by herpes simplex types I and II. Treatment of epithelial keratitis not responding to idoxuridine or resistant to vidarabine.

STORAGE/HANDLING

Refrigerate ophthalmic solution.

OPHTHALMIC ADMINISTRATION

1. Instruct pt to lie down or tilt head backward and look up.

2. Gently pull lower eyelid down to form pocket between eye and lower lid. Hold dropper above pocket and place prescribed

number of drops in pocket (do not touch tip of applicator to any surface).

3. Close eye gently. Apply gentle finger pressure to lacrimal sac (bridge of nose, inside corner of eye) for 1–2 min (minimized drainage into nose and throat, reducing risk of systemic effects).

4. Remove excess solution around eye w/tissue.

5. Tell pt not to close eyes tightly or blink more often than necessary.

6. Never rinse dropper.

INDICATIONS/DOSAGE/ROUTES

Usual ophthalmic dosage:
Adults, elderly: 1 drop onto cornea q2h while awake. **Maximum:** 9 drops/day. Continue until corneal ulcer has completely reepithelialized; then, 1 drop q4h while awake (minimum: 5 drops/day) for an additional 7 days.

PRECAUTIONS

CONTRAINDICATIONS: Hypersensitivity to trifluridine or any component of the preparation. **PREGNANCY/LACTATION:** Not recommended during pregnancy or lactation due to mutagenic effects in vitro. **Pregnancy Category C**.

INTERACTIONS

DRUG INTERACTIONS: None significant. **ALTERED LAB VALUES:** None significant.

SIDE EFFECTS

FREQUENT: Transient stinging or burning w/instillation. **OCCASIONAL:** Edema of eyelid. **RARE:** Hypersensitivity reaction: itching, redness, swelling, increased irritation; superficial punctate ker-

atopathy, increased intraocular pressure, keratitis sicca.

ADVERSE REACTIONS/TOXIC EFFECTS

Ocular toxicity may occur if used longer than 21 days.

NURSING IMPLICATIONS

BASELINE ASSESSMENT:

Question for hypersensitivity to trifluridine or components of preparation.

INTERVENTION/EVALUATION:

Evaluate for therapeutic response or burning/stinging, edema of eyelid, hypersensitivity reaction.

PATIENT/FAMILY TEACHING:

Use only as directed by physician (assure proper administration); do not stop or increase frequency of doses. Contact physician if no improvement after 7 days or complete healing after 14. Do not continue longer than 21 days. Refrigerate; avoid freezing. Mild, transient burning, stinging may occur when instilled. Promptly report itching, swelling, redness, or any increased irritation. Medication and personal items in contact w/eye should not be shared. Do not use any other products, including makeup, around the eye w/o advice of physician.

trihexyphenidyl hydrochloride

try-hex-eh-**fen**-ih-dill
(Artane)

CANADIAN AVAILABILITY:
Apo-Trihex

CLASSIFICATION

Anticholinergic, antiparkinson

AVAILABILITY (Rx)

Tablets: 2 mg, 5 mg. **Capsules (sustained-release):** 5 mg. **Elixir:** 2 mg/5 ml.

PHARMACOKINETICS

	ONSET	PEAK	DURATION
PO	1 hr	2–3 hrs	6–12 hrs

Well absorbed from GI tract. Primarily excreted in urine. Half-life: 5.6–10.2 hrs.

ACTION / THERAPEUTIC EFFECT

Blocks central cholinergic receptors (aids in balancing cholinergic and dopaminergic activity). *Decreases salivation, relaxes smooth muscle.*

USES

Adjunctive treatment for all forms of Parkinson's disease, including postencephalitic, arteriosclerotic, idiopathic types. Controls symptoms of drug-induced extrapyramidal symptoms.

PO ADMINISTRATION

1. May take w/o regard to food; give w/food if GI distress occurs.
2. Scored tablets may be crushed; do not crush or break sustained-release capsules.

INDICATIONS / DOSAGE / ROUTES

Parkinsonism:
Note: Do not use sustained-release capsules for initial therapy. Once stabilized, may switch, on mg-for-mg basis, giving a single daily dose after breakfast or 2 divided doses 12 hrs apart.
PO: Adults, elderly: Initially, 1 mg on first day. May increase by 2 mg/day at 3–5 day intervals up to 6–10 mg/day (12–15 mg/day in pts w/postencephalitic parkinsonism).

Drug-induced extrapyramidal symptoms:
PO: Adults, elderly: Initially, 1 mg/day. **Range:** 5–15 mg/day.

PRECAUTIONS

CONTRAINDICATIONS: Angle closure glaucoma, GI obstruction, paralytic ileus, intestinal atony, severe ulcerative colitis, prostatic hypertrophy, myasthenia gravis, megacolon. **CAUTIONS:** Treated open-angle glaucoma, autonomic neuropathy, pulmonary disease, esophageal reflux, hiatal hernia, heart disease, hyperthyroidism, hypertension. **PREGNANCY/ LACTATION:** Unknown whether drug crosses placenta; is distributed in breast milk. **Pregnancy Category C.**

INTERACTIONS

DRUG INTERACTIONS: Alcohol, CNS depressants may increase sedative effect. Amantadine, anticholinergics, MAO inhibitors may increase anticholinergic effects. Antacids, antidiarrheals may decrease absorption, effects. **ALTERED LAB VALUES:** None significant.

SIDE EFFECTS

Note: Elderly (>60 yrs) tend to develop mental confusion, disorientation, agitation, psychotic-like symptoms.
FREQUENT: Drowsiness, dry mouth. **OCCASIONAL:** Blurred vi-

sion, urinary retention, constipation, dizziness, headache, muscle cramps. **RARE:** Skin rash, seizures, depression.

ADVERSE REACTIONS/TOXIC EFFECTS

Children may experience dominant paradoxical reaction (restlessness, insomnia, euphoria, nervousness, tremors). Overdosage in children may result in hallucinations, convulsions, death. Hypersensitivity reaction (eczema, pruritus, rash, cardiac disturbances, photosensitivity) may occur. Overdosage may vary from CNS depression (sedation, apnea, cardiovascular collapse, death) to severe paradoxical reaction (hallucinations, tremor, seizures).

NURSING IMPLICATIONS
BASELINE ASSESSMENT:

If pt is undergoing allergic reaction, obtain history of recently ingested foods, drugs, environmental exposure, recent emotional stress. Monitor rate, depth, rhythm, type of respiration; quality and rate of pulse. Assess lung sounds for rhonchi, wheezing, rales.

INTERVENTION/EVALUATION:

Be alert to neurologic effects: headache, lethargy, mental confusion, agitation. Monitor children closely for paradoxical reaction. Assess for clinical reversal of symptoms (improvement of tremor of head/hands at rest, masklike facial expression, shuffling gait, muscular rigidity).

PATIENT/FAMILY TEACHING:

Avoid tasks that require alertness, motor skills until response to drug is established. Dry mouth, drowsiness, dizziness may be an expected response of drug. Avoid alcoholic beverages during therapy. Sugarless gum, sips of tepid water may relieve dry mouth. Coffee/tea may help reduce drowsiness.

trimethobenzamide hydrochloride
try-meth-oh-**benz**-ah-mide
(Tigan)

CLASSIFICATION
Antiemetic

AVAILABILITY (Rx)
Capsules: 100 mg, 250 mg.
Suppositories: 100 mg, 200 mg.
Injection: 100 mg/ml.

PHARMACOKINETICS

	ONSET	PEAK	DURATION
PO	10–40 min	—	3–4 hrs
IM	15–30 min	—	2–3 hrs

Partially absorbed from GI tract. Distributed primarily to liver. Metabolic fate unknown. Excreted in urine.

ACTION/THERAPEUTIC EFFECT
Acts at the chemoreceptor trigger zone in CNS (medulla oblongata), *relieving nausea and vomiting.*

USES
Control of nausea and vomiting.

STORAGE/HANDLING

Store oral, rectal, parenteral form at room temperature.

PO/IM/RECTAL ADMINISTRATION

PO:

1. Give w/o regard to meals.
2. Do not crush or break capsule form.

IM:

Give deep IM into large muscle mass, preferably upper outer gluteus maximus.

RECTAL:

1. If suppository is too soft, chill for 30 min in refrigerator or run cold water over foil wrapper.
2. Moisten suppository w/cold water before inserting well up into rectum.

INDICATIONS/DOSAGE/ROUTES

Note: Do not use IV route (produces severe hypotension).

Nausea, vomiting:
PO: Adults, elderly: 250 mg 3–4 times/day. **Children 30–100 lbs:** 100–200 mg 3–4 times/day.
IM: Adults, elderly: 200 mg 3–4 times/day.
Rectal: Adults, elderly: 200 mg 3–4 times/day. **Children 30–100 lbs:** 100–200 mg 3–4 times/day. **Children <30 lbs:** 100 mg 3–4 times/day. Do not use in premature or newborn infants.

PRECAUTIONS

CONTRAINDICATIONS: Hypersensitivity to benzocaine or similar local anesthetics; parenteral form in children, suppositories in premature infants or neonates. **CAUTIONS:** Elderly, debilitated, dehydration, electrolyte imbalance, high fever. **PREGNANCY/LACTATION:** Unknown whether drug crosses placenta or is distributed in breast milk. **Pregnancy Category C**.

INTERACTIONS

DRUG INTERACTIONS: CNS depression–producing medications may increase CNS depression. **ALTERED LAB VALUES:** None significant.

SIDE EFFECTS

Note: Elderly (>60 yrs) tend to develop mental confusion, disorientation, agitation, psychotic-like symptoms.
FREQUENT: Drowsiness. **OCCASIONAL:** Blurred vision, diarrhea, dizziness, headache, muscle cramps. **RARE:** Skin rash, seizures, depression, opisthotonus, Parkinson's syndrome, Reye's syndrome (vomiting, seizures).

ADVERSE REACTIONS/TOXIC EFFECTS

Hypersensitivity reaction manifested as extrapyramidal symptoms (muscle rigidity, allergic skin reactions) occurs rarely. Children may experience dominant paradoxical reaction (restlessness, insomnia, euphoria, nervousness, tremors). Overdosage may vary from CNS depression (sedation, apnea, cardiovascular collapse, death) to severe paradoxical reaction (hallucinations, tremor, seizures).

NURSING IMPLICATIONS
BASELINE ASSESSMENT:

Assess for dehydration if excessive vomiting occurs (poor skin turgor, dry mucous membranes, longitudinal furrows in tongue).

INTERVENTION/EVALUATION:

Check B/P, esp. in elderly (increased risk of hypotension). Assess children closely for paradoxical reaction. Monitor serum electrolytes in those with severe vomiting. Assess skin turgor, mucous membranes to evaluate hydration status. Assess for extrapyramidal symptoms (hypersensitivity). Measure I&O and assess any vomitus.

PATIENT/FAMILY TEACHING:

Report visual disturbances, headache. Dry mouth is expected response to medication. Relief from nausea/vomiting generally occurs within 30 min of drug administration.

trimethoprim

try-**meth**-oh-prim
(Primsol, Proloprim, Trimpex)

FIXED-COMBINATION(S):
W/sulfamethoxazole, a sulfonamide (Bactrim, Septra)

CANADIAN AVAILABILITY:
Proloprim

CLASSIFICATION

Anti-infective

AVAILABILITY (Rx)

Tablets: 100 mg, 200 mg

PHARMACOKINETICS

Rapidly, completely absorbed from GI tract. Widely distributed including CSF. Metabolized in liver. Primarily excreted in urine. Moderately removed by hemodialysis. Half-life: 8–10 hrs (increased in decreased renal function, newborns; decreased in children).

ACTION/*THERAPEUTIC EFFECT*

Blocks bacterial biosynthesis of nucleic acids and proteins by interfering with metabolism of folinic acid, *producing antibacterial activity.*

USES/*UNLABELED*

Treatment of initial acute uncomplicated urinary tract infections (UTIs). *Prophylaxis of bacterial UTI, treatment of pneumonia caused by Pneumocystis carinii.*

PO ADMINISTRATION

1. Space doses evenly to maintain constant level in urine.
2. Give w/o regard to meals (if stomach upset occurs, give w/food).

INDICATIONS/DOSAGE/ROUTES

Acute, uncomplicated UTIs:
PO: Adults, elderly: 100 mg q12h or 200 mg once daily for 10 days.

Dosage in renal impairment:
The dose and/or frequency is modified in response to degree of renal impairment, severity of infection, and serum concentration of drug.

CREATININE CLEARANCE	DOSAGE
>30 ml/min	No change
15–30 ml/min	50 mg q12h

PRECAUTIONS

CONTRAINDICATIONS: Hypersensitivity to trimethoprim, infants <2 mos, megaloblastic anemia due to folic acid deficiency. **CAUTIONS:** Impaired renal or hepatic function, children who have X chromosome w/mental retardation, pts who have possible folic acid deficiency. **PREGNANCY/LACTATION:** Readily crosses placenta; is distributed in breast milk. **Pregnancy Category C.**

INTERACTIONS

DRUG INTERACTIONS: Folate antagonists (e.g., methotrexate) may increase risk of myeloblastic anemia. **ALTERED LAB VALUES:** May increase BUN, SGOT (AST), SGPT (ALT), serum bilirubin, creatinine concentration.

SIDE EFFECTS

OCCASIONAL: Nausea, vomiting, diarrhea, decreased appetite, stomach cramps, headache. **RARE:** Hypersensitivity reaction (rash, itching), methemoglobinemia (blue color on fingernails, lips, or skin, pale skin, sore throat, fever, unusual tiredness).

ADVERSE REACTIONS/TOXIC EFFECTS

Stevens-Johnson syndrome, erythema multiforme, exfoliative dermatitis, anaphylaxis occur rarely. Hematologic toxicity (thrombocytopenia, neutropenia, leukopenia, megaloblastic anemia) more likely to occur in elderly, debilitated, alcoholics, those w/impaired renal function or receiving prolonged high dosage.

NURSING IMPLICATIONS

BASELINE ASSESSMENT:

Question for history of hypersensitivity to trimethoprim. Obtain specimens for diagnostic tests before giving first dose (therapy may begin before results are known). Identify hematology baseline reports.

INTERVENTION/EVALUATION:

Assess skin for rash. Evaluate food tolerance. Monitor hematology reports, renal, hepatic test results if ordered. Check for developing signs of hematologic toxicity: pallor, fever, sore throat, malaise, bleeding, or bruising.

PATIENT/FAMILY TEACHING:

Space doses evenly. Complete full length of therapy (may be 10–14 days). May take on empty stomach or w/food if stomach upset occurs. Avoid sun/ultraviolet light; use sunscreen, wear protective clothing. Immediately report pallor, tiredness, sore throat, bleeding, bruising or discoloration of skin, fever to physician.

trimetrexate glucuronate

try-meh-**trex**-ate
(Neutrexin)

CANADIAN AVAILABILITY: Neutrexin

CLASSIFICATION

Antiprotozoal

AVAILABILITY (Rx)

Powder for Injection: 25 mg

PHARMACOKINETICS

Following IV administration, distributed readily into ascitic fluid. Metabolized in liver. Eliminated in urine. Half-life: 11–20 hrs.

ACTION/*THERAPEUTIC EFFECT*

Inhibits the enzyme dihydrofolate reductase (DHFR), *disrupting purine, DNA, RNA, protein synthesis, with consequent cell death.*

USES/*UNLABELED*

Alternative therapy w/concurrent leucovorin administration for treatment of moderate to severe *Pneumocystis carinii* pneumonia (PCP) in immunocompromised pts, including pts w/acquired immunodeficiency syndrome (AIDS), who are intolerant of, or are refractory to, trimethoprim-sulfamethoxazole (TMP/SMZ) therapy or for whom TMP/SMZ is contraindicated. *Treatment of non-small cell lung, prostate, and colorectal cancer.*

STORAGE/HANDLING

Store vials for parenteral use at room temperature. After reconstitution, solution is stable under refrigeration or at room temperature for up to 24 hrs. Reconstituted solution appears as pale greenish yellow. Inspect for particulate matter. Discard if cloudiness or precipitate is present. Do not freeze reconstituted solution. Discard unused portion after 24 hrs.

IV ADMINISTRATION

Note: If solution comes in contact w/skin or mucosa, wash w/soap and water immediately. Use proper cytoxic disposal technique. Do not reconstitute w/solution containing either chloride ion or leucovorin, since precipitate occurs instantly.

1. Reconstitute each 25 mg vial w/2 ml 5% dextrose injection or sterile water for injection to provide concentration of 12.5 mg/ml. Complete dissolution should occur within 30 secs.

2. Filter the reconstituted solution prior to further dilution.

3. Further dilute w/5% dextrose to yield a final concentration of 0.25–2 mg/ml.

4. Give diluted solution by IV infusion over 60–90 min.

5. Flush IV line thoroughly with at least 10 ml 5% dextrose before and after administering trimetrexate.

INDICATIONS/DOSAGE/ROUTES

Note: Even though trimetrexate and leucovorin are given concurrently, they must be administered separately or precipitate will occur instantly; flush IV line thoroughly with 10 ml 5% dextrose between infusions. Dilute leukovorin according to leukovorin instructions and give over 5–10 min q6h.

PCP:

IV Infusion: Adults: *Trimetrexate:* 45 mg/m² once daily over 60–90 min. *Leukovorin:* 20 mg/m² over 5–10 min q6h for total daily dose of 80 mg/m², or orally as 4 doses of 20 mg/m² spaced equally throughout the day. Round up the oral dose to the next higher 25 mg increment. **Recommended course of therapy:** 21 days trimetrexate, 24 days leucovorin.

Note: In event of hematologic, renal, hepatic toxicities, doses of trimetrexate and leukovorin should be modified.

PRECAUTIONS

CONTRAINDICATIONS: Clinically significant hypersensitivity to trimetrexate, leucovorin, or methotrexate. **CAUTIONS:** Fertility impairment, pts w/hematologic, renal, hepatic impairment. **PREGNANCY/LACTATION:** May cause fetal harm. Unknown if drug crosses placenta or is distributed in breast milk. **Pregnancy Category D.**

INTERACTIONS

DRUG INTERACTIONS: Erythromycin, rifampin, rifabutin, ketoconazole, fluconazole, acetaminophen may alter timetrexate plasma concentration. Cimetidine reduces trimetrexate metabolism. Clotrimazole, ketoconazole, miconazole may inhibit trimetrexate metabolism. **ALTERED LAB VAL-**

T

UES: May increase SGOT (AST), SGPT (ALT), alkaline phosphatase, bilirubin, BUN, serum creatinine. May decrease Hgb, Hct, leukocytes, platelet counts.

SIDE EFFECTS

OCCASIONAL: Fever, rash, pruritus, nausea, vomiting, confusion. **RARE:** Fatigue.

ADVERSE REACTIONS/TOXIC EFFECTS

Trimetrexate given without concurrent leucovorin may result in serious or fatal hematologic, hepatic, and/or renal complications, including bone marrow suppression, oral and GI mucosal ulceration, and renal and hepatic dysfunction. In event of overdose, stop trimetrexate and give leucovorin 40 mg/m^2 q6h for 3 days. Anaphylaxis occurs rarely.

NURSING IMPLICATIONS

BASELINE ASSESSMENT:

Offer emotional support to pt and family. Leucovorin therapy must extend for 72 hrs past the last dose of trimetrexate. Advise women of childbearing potential to avoid pregnancy. Blood tests should be performed twice weekly during therapy. Question for sensitivity to trimetrexate, methotrexate, leucovorin, medication history, particularly bone marrow depressants, hepato/nephrotoxic medication. To allow for full therapeutic effect of trimetrexate to occur, zidovudine treatment should be discontinued during trimetrexate therapy.

INTERVENTION/EVALUATION:

Closely monitor neutrophil count, platelet count, liver function tests (SGOT, SGPT, alkaline phosphatase), renal values (serum creatinine, BUN) for development of serious toxicities. Carefully assess and treat pts w/nephrotoxic, myelosuppressive, or hepatotoxic drugs given during trimetrexate therapy.

PATIENT/FAMILY TEACHING:

Failure to take the recommended dose and duration of leucovorin can lead to fatal toxicity. Use two forms of contraception during therapy. Avoid persons w/bacterial infections. Immediately contact physician if fever, chills, cough or hoarseness, lower back or side pain, or painful urination occurs. Report any unusual bleeding or bruising, black tarry stools, blood in urine or stools, pinpoint red spots on skin.

trovafloxacin
(Trovan)
See Supplement
See Classification section under:
Antibiotic: fluoroquinolones

tubocurarine chloride
(Tubarine)
See Classification section under:
Neuromuscular blockers

urokinase
your-oh-**kine**-ace
(Abbokinase)

CANADIAN AVAILABILITY:
Abbokinase

CLASSIFICATION

Thrombolytic

AVAILABILITY (Rx)

Powder for Injection: 250,000 IU/vial; 5,000 IU/ml

PHARMACOKINETICS

Rapidly cleared from circulation by liver. Small amounts eliminated in urine and via bile. Half-life: 20 min.

ACTION/ *THERAPEUTIC EFFECT*

Acts directly on the fibrinolytic system to convert plasminogen to plasmin, an enzyme *that degrades fibrin clots, fibrinogen, and other plasma proteins.*

USES

Lysis of acute pulmonary emboli, pulmonary emboli accompanied by unstable hemodynamics, acute thrombi obstructing coronary arteries associated with evolving transmural myocardial infarction. Restores patency to IV catheters obstructed by clotted blood or fibrin.

STORAGE/HANDLING

Refrigerate vials. Reconstitute immediately before use. After reconstitution, solution is stable for 24 hours at room temperature or if refrigerated. Solutions are clear, colorless to light straw. Do not use if solution is highly colored; discard unused portions.

IV ADMINISTRATION

Note: Must be administered within 12–14 hrs of clot formation (little effect on older, organized clots).

IV:

1. Give by IV infusion via pump; via coronary catheter into thrombosed coronary artery; or via syringe into occluded IV catheter.

2. For IV infusion, reconstitute each 250,000 IU vial with 5 ml sterile water for injection to provide a concentration of 50,000 IU/ml. Further dilute up to 200 ml with 5% dextrose or 0.9% NaCl.

3. For intracoronary administration, reconstitute three 250,000 IU vials with 5 ml sterile water for injection for each vial. Further dilute with 500 ml 5% dextrose or 0.9% NaCl to provide a concentration of 1,500 IU/ml.

4. Gently roll and tilt vial (minimizes formation of filaments). Do not shake vial.

5. Solutions may be filtered through 0.45 micron or smaller filter.

6. If minor bleeding occurs at puncture sites, apply pressure for 30 min, then apply pressure dressing.

7. If uncontrolled hemorrhage occurs, discontinue infusion immediately (slowing rate of infusion may produce worsening hemorrhage). Do not use dextran to control hemorrhage.

8. Avoid undue pressure when drug is injected into catheter (can rupture catheter or expel clot into circulation).

INDICATIONS/DOSAGE/ROUTES

Pulmonary embolism:
IV: Adults, elderly: Initially, 4,400 IU/kg at rate of 90 ml/hr over 10 min; then, 4,400 IU/kg at rate of 15 ml/hr for 12 hrs. Flush tubing. Follow with anticoagulant therapy.

Coronary artery thrombi:
Intracoronary: Adults, elderly: 6,000 IU/min for up to 2 hrs.
Note: Before therapy, give 2,500–10,000 U heparin by IV injection; continue heparin after artery is opened.

Occluded IV catheter:

Disconnect IV tubing from catheter; attach a 1 ml TB syringe with 5,000 U urokinase to catheter; inject urokinase slowly (equal to volume of catheter). Wait 5 min. Connect empty 5 ml syringe; aspirate residual clot. When patency is restored, aspirate 4–5 ml blood. Irrigate with 0.9% NaCl; reconnect IV tubing to catheter.

PRECAUTIONS

CONTRAINDICATIONS: Active internal bleeding, recent (within 2 mos) cerebrovascular accident, intracranial/intraspinal surgery, intracranial neoplasm. **CAUTIONS:** Recent (within 10 days) major surgery/GI bleeding, OB delivery, organ biopsy, recent trauma (cardiopulmonary resuscitation, uncontrolled arterial hypertension, left ventricular thrombus, endocarditis, severe hepatic/renal disease, pregnancy, elderly, cerebrovascular disease, diabetic retinopathy, thrombophlebitis, occluded AV cannula at infected site. **PREGNANCY/LACTATION:** Use only when benefit outweighs potential risk to fetus. Unknown whether drug crosses placenta or is distributed in breast milk. **Pregnancy Category B**.

INTERACTIONS

DRUG INTERACTIONS: Anticoagulants, heparin may increase risk of hemorrhage. NSAIDs, platelet aggregate inhibitors may increase risk of bleeding. Antifibrinolytics (e.g., aminocaproic acid) may antagonize effects. **ALTERED LAB VALUES:** Decreases plasminogen and fibrinogen level during infusion, decreasing clotting time (confirms presence of lysis). Increases APTT, PT, TT.

SIDE EFFECTS

FREQUENT: Superficial or surface bleeding at puncture sites (venous cutdowns, arterial punctures, surgical sites, IM sites, retroperitoneal/intracerebral sites); internal bleeding (GI/GU tract, vaginal). **RARE:** Mild allergic reaction (rash, wheezing).

ADVERSE REACTIONS/TOXIC EFFECTS

Severe internal hemorrhage may occur. Lysis of coronary thrombi may produce atrial/ventricular arrhythmias.

NURSING IMPLICATIONS

BASELINE ASSESSMENT:

Avoid arterial invasive technique before and during treatment. If arterial puncture is necessary, use upper extremity vessels. Assess Hct, platelet count, thrombin (TT), activated thromboplastin (APTT), prothrombin time (PT), fibrinogen level before therapy is instituted.

INTERVENTION/EVALUATION:

Handle pt as carefully and infrequently as possible to prevent bleeding. Never give urokinase via IM injection route. Monitor clinical response, vital signs (pulse, temperature, respiratory rate, B/P) q4h. Do not obtain B/P in lower extremities (possible deep vein thrombi). Monitor TT, PT, APTT, fibrinogen level q4h or per protocol after initiation of therapy, stool culture for occult blood. Assess for decrease in B/P, increase in pulse rate, complaint of abdominal/back pain, severe headache (may be evidence of hemorrhage). Question for increase in amount of discharge during menses. Assess peripheral pulses; assess skin for bruises, petechiae. Check for excessive bleeding from minor cuts, scratches. Assess urine for hematuria.

ursodiol (ursodeoxycholic acid)

er-**sew**-dee-ol
(Actigall, Urso)

CANADIAN AVAILABILITY:
Ursofalk

CLASSIFICATION

Gallstone solubilizing agent

AVAILABILITY (Rx)

Capsules: 300 mg

PHARMACOKINETICS

Readily absorbed from small bowel. Undergoes first-pass hepatic extraction. Distributed primarily in liver, bile, intestinal lumen. Protein binding: high. Metabolized in liver. Excreted into bile and eliminated in feces.

ACTION/*THERAPEUTIC EFFECT*

Suppresses hepatic synthesis, secretion of cholesterol and inhibits intestinal absorption of cholesterol. *Changes the bile of pts with gallstones from cholesterol precipitating (capable of forming crystals) to cholesterol solubilizing (capable of being dissolved).*

USES/*UNLABELED*

Dissolution of radiolucent, non-calcified gallstones when cholecystectomy is an unacceptable method of treatment. Treatment of biliary cirrhosis. Prevention of gallstones. *Treatment of biliary atresia, sclerosing cholangitis, alcoholic cirrhosis, chronic hepatitis; prophylaxis of liver transplant rejection, gallstone formation.*

INDICATIONS/DOSAGE/ROUTES

Usual dosage:
PO: Adults, elderly: 8–10 mg/kg/day in 2–3 divided doses. Treatment may require months of therapy. Obtain ultrasound image of gallbladder at 6 mo intervals for first year. If dissolved, continue therapy and repeat ultrasound within 1–3 mos.

Prevention of gallstones:
PO: Adults, elderly: 300 mg 2 times/day.

PRECAUTIONS

CONTRAINDICATIONS: Calcified cholesterol stones, radiopaque stones, radiolucent bile pigment stones, allergy to bile acids, chronic liver disease. **CAUTIONS:** None significant. **PREGNANCY/LACTATION:** Unknown whether drug crosses placenta or is distributed in breast milk. **Pregnancy Category B.**

INTERACTIONS

DRUG INTERACTIONS: Aluminum-containing antacids, cholestyramine, colestipol may decrease absorption, effects. Estrogens, oral contraceptives may decrease effect. **ALTERED LAB VALUES:** May alter liver function tests.

SIDE EFFECTS

OCCASIONAL: Diarrhea.

ADVERSE REACTIONS/TOXIC EFFECTS

None significant.

NURSING IMPLICATIONS

Baseline Assessment:

SGOT (AST) and SGPT (ALT) liver function tests should be obtained before therapy begins, after 1 and 3 mos of therapy, and q6 mos thereafter. Those w/significant liver test abnormalities should be monitored more frequently.

U

INTERVENTION/EVALUATION:

Monitor liver function tests in those w/impaired liver function (metabolic acidosis may occur during infusion).

PATIENT/FAMILY TEACHING:

Treatment requires months of therapy.

---

valacyclovir

val-ah-**sigh**-klo-veer
(Valtrex)

CANADIAN AVAILABILITY:
Valtrex

CLASSIFICATION

Antiviral

AVAILABILITY (Rx)

Tablets: 500 mg

PHARMACOKINETICS

Rapidly absorbed following oral administration. Rapidly converted by hydrolysis to active compound, acyclovir. Widely distributed to tissues/body fluids (including CSF). Primarily eliminated in urine. Half-life: 2.5–3.3 hrs (increased in reduced renal function).

ACTION/*THERAPEUTIC EFFECT*

Converted to acyclovir triphosphate, becoming part of DNA chain, *interfering w/DNA synthesis and viral replication of herpes simplex and varicella zoster virus.* Virustatic.

USES

Treatment of herpes zoster (shingles) in immunocompetent adults. Episodic treatment of recurrent genital herpes in immunocompetent adults. Prevention of recurrent genital herpes. Treatment of initial genital herpes.

PO ADMINISTRATION

1. Give w/o regard to meals.
2. Do not crush or break tablets.

INDICATIONS/DOSAGE/ROUTES

Note: Therapy should be initiated at first sign of shingles (most effective within 48 hrs of onset of zoster rash).

Herpes zoster (shingles):
PO: Adults, elderly: 1 g 3 times daily for 7 days.

Recurrent genital herpes:
PO: Adults, elderly: 500 mg twice daily for 5 days.

Prevention of herpes:
PO: Adults, elderly: 500–1,000 mg/day.

Initial treatment of genital herpes:
PO: Adults, elderly: 1 g twice daily for 10 days.

Dosage in renal impairment:

CREATININE CLEARANCE	HERPES ZOSTER	GENITAL HERPES
≥ 50	1 g q8h	500 mg q12h
30–49	1 g q12 h	500 mg q12h
10–29	1 g q24h	500 mg q24h
<10	500 mg q24h	500 mg q24h

PRECAUTIONS

CONTRAINDICATIONS: Hypersensitivity or intolerance to valacyclovir, acyclovir, or components of formulation. **CAUTIONS:** Bone marrow or renal transplantation, advanced HIV infections, renal or hepatic impairment, dehydration, fluid/electrolyte imbalance, concurrent use of nephrotoxic agents, neurologic abnormalities. **PREGNANCY/LACTATION:** May cross placenta; may be distributed in breast milk. **Pregnancy Category B.**

INTERACTIONS

DRUG INTERACTION: Probenecid, cimetidine may increase acyclovir concentration. **ALTERED LAB VALUES:** None significant.

SIDE EFFECTS

Herpes zoster: **FREQUENT (10–17%):** Nausea, headache. **OCCASIONAL (3–7%):** Vomiting, diarrhea, constipation (≥ 50 yrs), asthenia, dizziness (≥ 50 yrs). **RARE (1–3%):** Abdominal pain, anorexia. *Genital herpes:* **FREQUENT (17%):** Headache. **OCCASIONAL (3–8%):** Nausea, diarrhea, dizziness. **RARE (1–3%):** Asthenia, abdominal pain.

ADVERSE REACTION/TOXIC EFFECTS

None significant.

NURSING IMPLICATIONS

BASELINE ASSESSMENT:

Question history of allergies, particularly to valacyclovir, acyclovir. Tissue cultures for herpes zoster and herpes simplex should be done before giving first dose (therapy may proceed before results are known). Assess medical history, esp. advanced HIV infection, bone marrow/renal transplantation, hepatic/renal function.

INTERVENTION/EVALUATION:

Evaluate cutaneous lesions. Manage herpes zoster with strict isolation. Provide analgesics and comfort measures for herpes zoster; esp. exhausting to elderly. Encourage fluids. Keep pt's fingernails short, hands clean.

PATIENT/FAMILY TEACHING:

Drink adequate fluids. Do not touch lesions with fingers to avoid spreading infection to new site. *Genital herpes:* Continue therapy for full length of treatment. Space doses evenly. Avoid sexual intercourse during duration of lesions to prevent infecting partner. Valacyclovir does not cure herpes. Notify physician if lesions do not improve or recur.

Pap smears should be done at least annually due to increased risk of cancer of cervix in women w/genital herpes. Initiate treatment at first sign of a recurrent episode of genital herpes or herpes zoster (early treatment, that is, within first 24–48 hrs, is imperative for therapeutic results).

valproic acid

val-**pro**-ick
(Depakene)

valproate sodium

(Depakene syrup)

divalproex sodium

(Depacon, Depakote)

CANADIAN AVAILABILITY: Divalproex sodium (Epival), valproic acid (Depakene)

CLASSIFICATION

Anticonvulsant

AVAILABILITY (Rx)

Capsules: 250 mg (valproic acid). **Syrup:** 250 mg/5 ml (valproic acid). **Tablets (delayed-release):** 125 mg, 250 mg, 500 mg (divalproex). **Capsules (sprinkle):** 125 mg (divalproex). **Injection.**

PHARMACOKINETICS

Well absorbed from GI tract. Metabolized in liver. Primarily excreted in urine. Half-life: 6–16 hrs (may be increased in decreased liver function, elderly, children <18 mos).

ACTION/*THERAPEUTIC EFFECT*

Directly increases concentration of the inhibitory neurotransmitter gamma-aminobutyric acid (GABA), *producing anticonvulsant effect.*

USES / *UNLABELED*

Prophylaxis of absence seizures (petit mal), myoclonic, tonic-clonic seizure control. Used principally as adjunct w/other anticonvulsant agents. Treatment of manic episodes w/bipolar disorders, complex partial seizures. Prophylaxis of migraine headaches. *Treatment of myoclonic, simple partial, tonic-clonic seizures.*

PO ADMINISTRATION

1. Give w/food if GI distress occurs.

2. Do not crush, chew, or break enteric-coated tablets.

3. Do not mix solution w/carbonated drinks (may produce local mouth irritation, unpleasant taste).

INDICATIONS / DOSAGE / ROUTES

Anticonvulsant:

PO: **Adults, elderly, children:** Initially, 15 mg/kg daily (if dosage exceeds 250 mg daily, give in two or more equally divided doses). Increase at 1 wk intervals by 5–10 mg/kg daily until seizures are controlled or unacceptable effects occur. **Maximum daily dose:** 60 mg/kg.

Manic episodes:

PO: **Adults, elderly:** Initially, 750 mg/day in divided doses. **Maximum:** 60 mg/kg/day.

Migraines:

PO: **Adults:** 250 mg 2 times/day.

PRECAUTIONS

CONTRAINDICATIONS: Hepatic disease. **CAUTIONS:** History of hepatic disease, bleeding abnormalities. **PREGNANCY/LACTATION:** Crosses placenta; is distributed in breast milk. **Pregnancy Category D.**

INTERACTIONS

DRUG INTERACTIONS: Alcohol, CNS depressants may increase CNS depressant effects. May increase risk of bleeding w/anticoagulants, heparin, thrombolytics, platelet aggregation inhibitors. May increase concentration of amitriptyline, primidone. Carbamazepine may decrease concentration. Hepatotoxic medications may increase risk of hepatotoxicity. May alter phenytoin protein binding, increasing toxicity. Phenytoin may decrease effect. **ALTERED LAB VALUES:** May increase SGOT (AST), SGPT (ALT), LDH, bilirubin.

SIDE EFFECTS

FREQUENT: *Epilepsy:* Abdominal pain, irregular menses, diarrhea, transient alopecia, indigestion, nausea, vomiting, trembling, weight change. **OCCASIONAL:** Constipation, dizziness, drowsiness, headache, skin rash, unusual excitement, restlessness. **RARE:** Mood changes, double vision, nystagmus, spots before eyes, unusual bleeding/bruising. *Mania:* **FREQUENT (19–22%):** Nausea, somnolence. **OCCASIONAL (6–12%):** Asthenia, abdominal pain, dyspepsia, rash.

ADVERSE REACTIONS / TOXIC EFFECTS

Hepatotoxicity may occur, particularly in the first 6 mos of therapy. May not be preceded by abnormal liver function tests, but may be noted as loss of seizure control, malaise, weakness, lethargy, anorexia, and vomiting. Blood dyscrasias may occur.

NURSING IMPLICATIONS

BASELINE ASSESSMENT:

Review history of seizure disorder (intensity, frequency, duration, level of consciousness). Initiate safety measures, quiet dark environment. CBC, platelet count should be performed before and 2 wks after therapy begins, then 2 wks after maintenance dose is given.

INTERVENTION/EVALUATION:

Observe frequently for recurrence of seizure activity. Monitor liver function, CBC, platelet count. Assess skin for bruising, petechiae. Monitor for clinical improvement (decrease in intensity or frequency of seizures).

PATIENT/FAMILY TEACHING:

Do not abruptly withdraw medication following long-term use (may precipitate seizures). Strict maintenance of drug therapy is essential for seizure control. Drowsiness usually disappears during continued therapy. Avoid tasks that require alertness, motor skills until response to drug is established. Avoid alcohol. Carry identification card/bracelet to note anticonvulsant therapy. Teach pts about their seizure condition and role in its management. If noncompliance is an issue in causing acute seizures, discuss reasons for noncompliance and address them.

---

valrubicin
(Valstar)
See Supplement

---

valsartan
(Diovan)
See Supplement

---

vancomycin hydrochloride

van-koe-**my**-sin
(Vancocin, Vancoled)

CANADIAN AVAILABILITY:
Vancocin

CLASSIFICATION

Antibiotic

AVAILABILITY (Rx)

Capsules: 125 mg, 250 mg. **Powder for Oral Solution:** 1 g, 10 g. **Powder for Injection:** 500 mg, 1 g.

PHARMACOKINETICS

Oral: Poorly absorbed from GI tract. Primarily eliminated in feces. *Parenteral:* Widely distributed. Primarily excreted unchanged in urine. Not removed by hemodialysis. Half-life: 4–11 hrs (increased in decreased renal function).

ACTION/*THERAPEUTIC EFFECT*

Inhibits cell wall synthesis by binding to bacterial cell wall, altering cell membrane permeability, inhibiting RNA synthesis, *producing bacterial cell death.* Bactericidal.

USES/*UNLABELED*

Systemic: Treatment of respiratory tract, bone, skin/soft tissue infections, endocarditis, peritonitis, septicemia. Given prophylactically to those at risk for bacterial endocarditis (if penicillin contraindicated) when undergoing dental, respiratory, GI, GU, biliary surgery/invasive procedures. *Oral:* Treatment of antibiotic colitis, pseudomembranous colitis, antibiotic-associated diarrhea, staphylococcal enterocolitis. *Treatment of brain abscess, staphylococcal/streptococcal meningitis, perioperative infections.*

STORAGE/HANDLING

Store capsules at room temperature. Oral solutions stable for 2 wks if refrigerated. IV infusion (piggyback) stable for 24 hrs at room temperature, 96 hrs if refrigerated. Discard if precipitate forms.

PO/IV ADMINISTRATION

Note: Space doses evenly around the clock.

PO:

1. Generally not given for systemic infections because of poor absorption from GI tract; however, some pts w/colitis may have effective absorption.

2. Powder for oral solution may be reconstituted, given by mouth or nasogastric tube.

3. Do not use powder for oral solution for IV administration.

IV:

Note: Give by intermittent IV infusion (piggyback), continuous IV infusion. Do not give IV push (may result in exaggerated hypotension).

1. For intermittent IV infusion (piggyback), reconstitute each 500 mg vial w/10 ml sterile water for injection (20 ml for 1 g vial) to provide concentration of 50 mg/ml.

2. Further dilute each 500 mg w/at least 100 ml 5% dextrose, 0.9% NaCl, or other compatible IV fluid. Infuse over at least 1 hr.

3. For IV infusion, add 1–2 g reconstituted vancomycin to sufficient amount 5% dextrose or 0.9% NaCl to infuse over 24 hrs.

4. Monitor B/P closely during IV infusion.

5. ADD-Vantage vials should not be used in neonates, infants, children requiring less than 500 mg dose.

6. Alternating IV sites, use large veins every 2–3 days to reduce risk of phlebitis.

INDICATIONS/DOSAGE/ROUTES

Usual parenteral dosage:
IV: Adults, elderly: 500 mg q6h or 1 g q12h. **Children >1 mo:** 40 mg/kg/day in divided doses. **Max-imum:** 2 g/day. **Neonates:** 15 mg/kg initially, then 10 mg/kg q8–12h.

Dosage in renal impairment:
After a loading dose, subsequent dose and/or frequency is modified based on degree of renal impairment, severity of infection, serum concentration of drug.

Staphylococcal enterocolitis, antibiotic-associated pseudomembranous colitis caused by Clostridium difficile:
PO: Adults, elderly: 0.5–2 g/day in 3–4 divided doses for 7–10 days. **Children:** 40 mg/kg/day in 3–4 divided doses for 7–10 days. **Maximum:** 2 g/day.

PRECAUTIONS

CONTRAINDICATIONS: None significant. **CAUTIONS:** Renal dysfunction, preexisting hearing impairment, concurrent therapy w/other ototoxic/nephrotoxic medications. **PREGNANCY/LACTATION:** Drug crosses placenta; unknown whether distributed in breast milk. **Pregnancy Category C.**

INTERACTIONS

DRUG INTERACTIONS: *Oral:* Cholestyramine, colestipol may decrease effect. *Parenteral:* Aminoglycosides, amphotericin, aspirin, bumetanide, carmustine, cisplatin, cyclosporine, ethacrynic acid, furosemide, streptozocin may increase ototoxicity and/or nephrotoxicity. **ALTERED LAB VALUES:** May increase BUN.

SIDE EFFECTS

FREQUENT: *Oral:* Bitter/unpleasant taste, nausea, vomiting, mouth irritation (oral solution). **RARE:** *Systemic:* Phlebitis, thrombophlebitis, pain at IV site. Necrosis may occur w/extravasation.

Dizziness, vertigo, tinnitus, chills, fever, rash. *Oral:* Skin rash.

ADVERSE REACTIONS/TOXIC EFFECTS

Nephrotoxicity (change in amount/frequency of urination, nausea, vomiting, increased thirst, anorexia); ototoxicity (deafness due to damage to auditory branch of eighth cranial nerve); red-neck syndrome (too rapid injection): chills, fever, fast heartbeat, nausea, vomiting, itching, rash, redness on face/neck/arms/back; unpleasant taste.

NURSING IMPLICATIONS
BASELINE ASSESSMENT:

Question pt for history of allergy to vancomycin. Avoid other ototoxic and nephrotoxic medications if possible. Obtain culture and sensitivity test before giving first dose (therapy may begin before results are known).

INTERVENTION/EVALUATION:

Evaluate IV site for phlebitis (heat, pain, red streaking over vein). Monitor renal function tests, I&O. Assess skin for rash. Check hearing acuity, balance. Monitor B/P carefully during infusion.

PATIENT/FAMILY TEACHING:

Continue therapy for full length of treatment. Doses should be evenly spaced. Notify physician in event of tinnitus, rash, other new symptom. Lab tests are important part of total therapy.

vasopressin
vay-sew-**press**-in
(Pitressin)

CANADIAN AVAILABILITY:
Pressyn

CLASSIFICATION

Vasopressor, antidiuretic

AVAILABILITY (Rx)

Injection: 20 units/ml

PHARMACOKINETICS

	ONSET	PEAK	DURATION
IM/SubQ	—	—	2–8 hrs
IV	—	—	0.5–1 hr

Distributed throughout extracellular fluid. Metabolized in liver, kidney. Primarily excreted in urine. Half-life: 10–20 min.

ACTION/*THERAPEUTIC EFFECT*

Increases reabsorption of water by the renal tubules *resulting in decreased urinary flow rate,* increased urine osmolality. Urea is also reabsorbed by the collecting ducts. Directly stimulates contraction of smooth muscle, *preventing abdominal distension, intestinal paresis.* Causes vasoconstriction w/reduced blood flow in coronary, peripheral, cerebral, and pulmonary vessels, but particularly in portal and splanchnic vessels. In large doses, may cause mild uterine contractions.

USES/*UNLABELED*

Prevents/controls polydipsia, polyuria, dehydration in pts w/neurogenic diabetes insipidus. Stimulates peristalsis in the prevention or treatment of postop abdominal distention, intestinal paresis. *Adjunct in treatment of acute, massive hemorrhage.*

IV ADMINISTRATION
SubQ/IM:

Note: May give IM or Subq.

Give 1–2 glasses of water at time of administration to reduce side effects.

IV INFUSION:

Dilute w/5% dextrose in water or 0.9% NaCl to concentration of 0.1–1 units/ml.

INDICATIONS/DOSAGE/ROUTES

Diabetes insipidus:
Note: May administer intranasally on cotton pledgets, by nasal spray; individualize dosage.
IM/SubQ: Adults, elderly: 5–10 units, 2–4 times/day. **Range:** 5–60 units/day. **Children:** 2.5–10 units, 2–4 times/day.

Abdominal distention:
IM: Adults, elderly: Initially, 5 units. Subsequent doses of 10 units q3–4h.

GI hemorrhage:
IV Infusion: Adults, elderly: Initially, 0.2–0.4 units/min progressively increased to 0.9 units/min.

PRECAUTIONS

CONTRAINDICATIONS: Anaphylaxis or hypersensitivity to vasopressin or components, chronic nephritis w/nitrogen retention. **CAUTIONS:** Migraine, epilepsy, heart failure, asthma, or any condition in which rapid addition of extracellular water may be a risk. Extreme caution in pts w/vascular disease, esp. coronary artery disease. **PREGNANCY/LACTATION:** Caution in giving to nursing woman. **Pregnancy Category B.**

INTERACTIONS

DRUG INTERACTIONS: Carbamazepine, chlorpropamide, clofibrate may increase effects. Demeclocycline, lithium, norepinephrine may decrease effect. **ALTERED LAB VALUES:** None significant.

SIDE EFFECTS

FREQUENT: Pain at injection site w/vasopressin tannate. **OCCASIONAL:** Stomach cramps, nausea, vomiting, diarrhea, dizziness, diaphoresis, paleness, circumoral pallor, trembling, "pounding" in head, eructation, and flatulence. **RARE:** Chest pain, confusion. *Allergic reactions:* Rash or hives, pruritus, wheezing or difficulty breathing, swelling of mouth, face, feet, hands. Sterile abscess w/vasopressin tannate.

ADVERSE REACTIONS/TOXIC EFFECTS

Anaphylaxis, myocardial infarction, and water intoxication have occurred. Elderly and very young at higher risk for water intoxication.

NURSING IMPLICATIONS

BASELINE ASSESSMENT:

Question for hypersensitivity to vasopressin, components. Establish baselines for weight, B/P, pulse, electrolytes, urine specific gravity.

INTERVENTION/EVALUATION:

Monitor I&O closely, restrict intake as necessary to prevent water intoxication. Weigh daily if indicated. Check B/P and pulse 2 times/day. Monitor electrolytes, urine specific gravity. Evaluate injection site for erythema, pain, abscess. Report side effects to physician for dose reduction. Be alert for early signs of water intoxication (drowsiness, listlessness, headache). Hold medication and report immediately any chest pain/allergic symptoms.

PATIENT/FAMILY TEACHING:

Promptly report headache, chest pain, shortness of breath, or other symptom. Stress importance of I&O.

---

varicella vaccine
(Varivax)
See Classification section under: Immunizations

---

vecuronium bromide
(Norcuron)
See Classification section under: Neuromuscular blockers

---

venlafaxine
ven-lah-**facks**-een
(Effexor, Effexor XR)

CANADIAN AVAILABILITY:
Effexor

CLASSIFICATION

Antidepressant

AVAILABILITY (Rx)

Tablets: 25 mg, 37.5 mg, 50 mg, 75 mg, 100 mg. **Effexor XR:** 37.5 mg, 75 mg, 150 mg.

PHARMACOKINETICS

Well absorbed from GI tract. Metabolized in liver to active metabolite. Primarily excreted in urine. Half-life: 3–7 hrs; metabolite: 9–13 hrs (increased in pts w/liver and/or renal disease).

ACTION/*THERAPEUTIC EFFECT*

Potentiates CNS neurotransmitter activity. Inhibits reuptake of serotonin, norepinephrine (weakly inhibits dopamine reuptake), *producing antidepressant activity.*

USES

Treatment of depression exhibited as persistent, prominent dysphoria (occurring nearly every day for at least 2 wks) manifested by 4 of 8 symptoms: change in appetite, change in sleep pattern, increased fatigue, impaired concentration, feelings of guilt or worthlessness, loss of interest in usual activities, psychomotor agitation or retardation, or suicidal tendencies. Psychotherapy augments therapeutic result. *Venlafaxine XR:* Treatment of generalized anxiety disorder.

PO ADMINISTRATION

1. May give w/o regard to food. Give w/food or milk if GI distress occurs.
2. Scored tablet may be crushed.
3. Do not crush extended-release capsules

INDICATIONS/DOSAGE/ROUTES

Note: Decrease dose by 50% in pts w/moderate liver impairment; 25% in mild to moderate renal impairment (50% in pts on dialysis, withholding dose until completion of dialysis). When discontinuing the medication, taper slowly over 2 wks.

Depression:
PO: Adults, elderly: Initially, 75 mg/day in 2–3 divided doses w/food. May increase by 75 mg/day no sooner than 4 day intervals. **Maximum:** 375 mg/day in 3 divided doses. **Extended release:** 75 mg/day as single dose. May increase by 75 mg/day at in-

tervals of at least 4 days. **Maximum:** 225 mg/day.

Anxiety disorder:
PO: Adults: 37.5–225 mg/day.

PRECAUTIONS

CONTRAINDICATIONS: Hypersensitivity to venlafaxine. Children <18 yrs of age (safety unknown). Pts currently receiving MAO inhibitors (see Drug Interactions). **CAUTIONS:** Renal, hepatic impairment. History of mania, seizures, those w/metabolic or hemodynamic disease, hypertension, history of drug abuse. **PREGNANCY/LACTATION:** Unknown whether excreted in breast milk. **Pregnancy Category C**.

INTERACTIONS

DRUG INTERACTIONS: MAO inhibitors (MAOIs) may cause hyperthermia, rigidity, myoclonus, autonomic instability (including rapid fluctuations of vital signs), mental status changes, coma, extreme agitation. May cause neuroleptic malignant syndrome (wait 14 days after discontinuing MAOIs to start or wait 7 days after discontinuing venlafaxine before starting MAOIs). **ALTERED LAB VALUES:** May increase serum cholesterol, uric acid, alkaline phosphatase, SGOT (AST), SGPT (ALT), bilirubin, BUN. May decrease sodium, phosphate. May alter glucose, potassium.

SIDE EFFECTS

FREQUENT (>20%): Nausea, somnolence, headache, dry mouth. **OCCASIONAL (10–20%):** Dizziness, insomnia, constipation, sweating, nervousness, asthenia (loss of strength, energy), ejaculatory disturbance, anorexia. **RARE (<10%):** Anxiety, blurred vision, diarrhea, vomiting, tremor, abnormal dreams, impotence.

ADVERSE REACTIONS/TOXIC EFFECTS

Sustained increase in diastolic B/P (10–15 mm Hg) occurs occasionally.

NURSING IMPLICATIONS
BASELINE ASSESSMENT:

Obtain initial weight and B/P. Assess appearance, behavior, speech pattern, level of interest, mood.

INTERVENTION/EVALUATION:

Check B/P regularly for hypertension. Monitor weight and encourage small, frequent meals of favorite foods to prevent weight loss, esp. in underweight pts. Assess sleep pattern for insomnia. Check during waking hours for somnolence or dizziness and anxiety; provide assistance as necessary. Supervise suicidal risk pt closely during early therapy (as depression lessens, energy level improves, increasing suicide potential). Assess appearance, behavior, speech pattern, level of interest, mood for therapeutic response.

PATIENT/FAMILY TEACHING:

Take w/food. Do not increase, decrease, or suddenly stop medication. Venlafaxine may decrease appetite and cause weight loss. Do not drive or perform tasks that require alert response until certain drug does not cause impairment. Inform physician if breast-feeding, pregnant or planning to become pregnant. Avoid alcohol. Do not take any other medication including OTC preparations w/o consulting physician. Report rash, hives, or other allergic responses promptly.

verapamil hydrochloride

ver-**ap**-ah-mill
(Calan, Covera-HS, Isoptin, Verelan, Verelan PM)

FIXED COMBINATION(S):
W/trandolapril, an angiotensin inhibitor (Tarka)

CANADIAN AVAILABILITY:
Apo-Verap, Chronovera, Isoptin, Novoveramil, Verelan

CLASSIFICATION
Calcium channel blocker

AVAILABILITY (Rx)
Tablets: 40 mg, 80 mg, 120 mg. **Tablets (sustained-release):** 120 mg, 180 mg, 240 mg. **Capsules (sustained-release):** 120 mg, 180 mg, 240 mg, 360 mg. **Verelan PM:** 100 mg, 200 mg, 300 mg. **Injection:** 5 mg/2 ml.

PHARMACOKINETICS

	ONSET	PEAK	DURATION
PO	30 min	1–2 hrs	6–8 hrs
Extended-release			
	30 min	—	—
IV	1–2 min	3–5 min	10–60 min

Well absorbed from GI tract. Undergoes first-pass metabolism in liver. Metabolized in liver to active metabolite. Primarily excreted in urine. Not removed by hemodialysis. Half-life: *oral:* 2.8–7.4 hrs; *IV:* 2–5 hrs.

ACTION/*THERAPEUTIC EFFECT*

Inhibits calcium ion entry across cell membranes of cardiac and vascular smooth muscle (dilates coronary arteries, peripheral arteries, arterioles). *Decreases heart rate, myocardial contractility, slows SA and AV conduction. Decreases total peripheral vascular resistance by vasodilation.*

USES/*UNLABELED*

Parenteral: Management of supraventricular tachyarrhythmias, temporary control of rapid ventricular rate in atrial flutter/fibrillation. *Oral:* Management of spastic (Prinzmetal's variant) angina, unstable (crescendo, preinfarction) angina, chronic stable angina (effort-associated angina), hypertension, prevention of recurrent PSVT, and (w/digoxin) control of ventricular resting rate in those w/atrial flutter and/or fibrillation. *Treatment of hypertrophic cardiomyopathy, vascular headaches.*

PO/IV ADMINISTRATION
PO:

1. Give sustained-release tablets w/food. Verelan may be taken w/o regard to food.
2. Do not crush or break sustained-released tablets. Do not break capsules.
3. Verelan may be opened and sprinkled on food.
4. Grapefruit juice can increase concentration.

IV:

1. Administer direct IV >2 min for adults, children (administer >3 min for elderly).
2. Continuous EKG monitoring during IV injection is required

for children, recommended for adults.

3. Monitor EKG for rapid ventricular rates, extreme bradycardia, heart block, asystole, prolongation of PR interval. Notify physician of any significant changes.

4. Monitor B/P q5–10 min.

5. Pt should remain recumbent for at least 1 hr following IV administration.

INDICATIONS/DOSAGE/ROUTES

Supraventricular tachyarrhythmias:
IV: Adults, elderly: Initially, 5–10 mg, repeat in 30 min w/10 mg dose. **Children 1–15 yrs:** 2–5 mg, repeat in 30 min up to 10 mg. **Children <1 yr:** 0.75–2 mg, repeat after 30 min. **Maximum single dose:** 10 mg.

Arrhythmias:
PO: Adults, elderly: 240–480 mg/day in 3–4 divided doses.

Angina:
PO: Adults, elderly: Initially, 80–120 mg 3 times/day (40 mg in elderly, pts w/liver dysfunction). Titrate to optimal dose. **Maintenance:** 240–480 mg/day in 3–4 divided doses. *Covera-HS:* 180–480 mg/day at bedtime.

Hypertension:
PO: Adults, elderly: Initially, 40–80 mg 3 times/day. **Maintenance:** Up to 480 mg/day. *Covera-HS:* 180–480 mg/day at bedtime.
Extended-release tablets: 120–240 mg/day up to 480 mg/day in 2 divided doses. **Verelan PM:** 100–300 mg/day.

PRECAUTIONS

CONTRAINDICATIONS: Sicksinus syndrome/second- or third-degree AV block (except in presence of pacemaker), cardiogenic shock, severe hypotension (<90 mm Hg, systolic), severe CHF (unless secondary to supraventricular tachycardia). **CAUTIONS:** Impaired renal, hepatic function. **PREGNANCY/LACTATION:** Crosses placenta; is distributed in breast milk. Breast-feeding not recommended. **Pregnancy Category C.**

INTERACTIONS

DRUG INTERACTIONS: Beta blockers may have additive effect. May increase digoxin concentration. Procainamide, quinidine may increase risk of QT interval prolongation. Carbamazepine, quinidine, theophylline may increase concentration, toxicity. Disopyramide may increase negative inotropic effect. **ALTERED LAB VALUES:** PR interval may be increased.

SIDE EFFECTS

FREQUENT (7%): Constipation. **OCCASIONAL (2–4%):** Dizziness, lightheadedness, headache, asthenia (loss of strength, energy), nausea, peripheral edema, hypotension. **RARE (<1%):** Bradycardia, dermatitis/rash.

ADVERSE REACTIONS/TOXIC EFFECTS

Rapid ventricular rate in atrial flutter/fibrillation, marked hypotension, extreme bradycardia, CHF, asystole, and second- and third-degree AV block occur rarely.

NURSING IMPLICATIONS

BASELINE ASSESSMENT:

Concurrent therapy of sublingual nitroglycerin may be used for relief of anginal pain. Record onset, type (sharp, dull, squeezing), radiation, location, intensity, and duration of anginal pain and precipitating factors (exertion, emotional stress). Check B/P for hypotension, pulse for bradycardia immediately before giving medication.

INTERVENTION/EVALUATION:

Assess pulse for strength/weakness, irregular rate. Monitor EKG for cardiac changes, particularly prolongation of PR interval. Notify physician of any significant interval changes. Assist w/ambulation if dizziness occurs. Assess for peripheral edema behind medial malleolus (sacral area in bedridden pts). For those taking oral form, check stool consistency, frequency. Monitor for therapeutic serum level (0.1–0.3 mcg/ml).

PATIENT/FAMILY TEACHING:

Do not abruptly discontinue medication. Compliance w/therapy regimen is essential to control anginal pain. To avoid hypotensive effect, rise slowly from lying to sitting position, wait momentarily before standing. Avoid tasks that require alertness, motor skills until response to drug is established. Contact physician/nurse if irregular heartbeat, shortness of breath, pronounced dizziness, nausea, or constipation occurs. Avoid concomitant grapefruit juice.

vidarabine
vy-**dare**-ah-been
(Ara-A, Vira-A)

CLASSIFICATION
Antiviral

AVAILABILITY (Rx)
Ophthalmic ointment: 3%

PHARMACOKINETICS
Trace amounts in aqueous humor only if there is an epithelial defect in cornea.

ACTION/*THERAPEUTIC EFFECT*
Appears to interfere w/viral DNA synthesis, *regenerating corneal epithelium.*

USES
Treatment of keratitis, keratoconjunctivitis caused by herpes simplex virus, types 1 and 2.

STORAGE/HANDLING
Store at room temperature.

OPHTHALMIC ADMINISTRATION
1. Place finger on lower eyelid and pull out until a pocket is formed between eye and lower lid.
2. Place $1/4$–$1/2$ inch ointment into pocket.
3. Have pt close eye for 1–2 min, rolling eyeball (increases contact area of drug to eye).
4. Remove excess ointment around eye w/tissue.

INDICATIONS/DOSAGE/ROUTES
Usual ophthalmic dosage:
Ophthalmic: Adults, elderly: 0.5 inch into lower conjunctival sac 5 times/day at 3 hr intervals. After reepithelialization, treat additional 7 days at dosage of 2 times/day.

PRECAUTIONS
CONTRAINDICATIONS: Hyper-

sensitivity to vidarabine, components of preparation. **PREGNANCY/ LACTATION:** Unknown whether distributed in breast milk. **Pregnancy Category C**.

INTERACTIONS

DRUG INTERACTIONS: None significant. **ALTERED LAB VALUES:** None significant.

SIDE EFFECTS

FREQUENT: Burning, itching, irritation. **OCCASIONAL:** Foreign body sensation, tearing, sensitivity, pain, photophobia.

ADVERSE REACTIONS/TOXIC EFFECTS

None significant.

NURSING IMPLICATIONS
BASELINE ASSESSMENT:

Question history of allergy to vidarabine, components of preparation.

INTERVENTION/EVALUATION:

Assess for irritation, itching, burning.

PATIENT/FAMILY TEACHING:

Assure proper administration. Notify physician if there is no improvement in 7 days or if burning, irritation, pain develops. Do not stop or increase doses. Ointment should be continued for 5–7 days after infection is gone to prevent recurrence of infection. A temporary haze may occur after application to eye; sunglasses will decrease sensitivity to light. Use other eye products, including makeup, only w/advice of physician. Refrigerate, avoid freezing; if using another eye ointment, wait at least 10 min between dosing.

vigabatrin
(Sabril)
See Supplement
See Classifiction section under:
Anticonvulsants

vinblastine sulfate
vin-**blass**-teen
(Velban, Velsar)

CANADIAN AVAILABILITY:
Velbe

CLASSIFICATION
Antineoplastic

AVAILABILITY (Rx)
Powder for Injection: 10 mg.
Injection: 1 mg/ml.

PHARMACOKINETICS
Does not cross blood-brain barrier. Metabolized in liver to active metabolite. Primarily eliminated in feces via biliary system. Half-life: 24.8 hrs.

ACTION/ *THERAPEUTIC EFFECT*
Blocks mitosis by arresting cells in metaphase of cell division, *inhibiting cellular division*. Interferes w/amino acid metabolism, synthesis of nucleic acids, protein. Cell cycle-specific for M phase of cell division. Has some immunosuppressive activity.

USES/ *UNLABELED*
Treatment of disseminated Hodgkin's disease, non-Hodgkin's lymphoma, advanced stage of mycosis fungoides, advanced carcinoma of testis, Kaposi's sarcoma, Letterer-Siwe disease, breast carcinoma, choriocarcinoma. *Treatment of neuroblastoma, carcinoma*

of bladder, lung, head/neck, renal; germ cell ovarian tumors, chronic myelocytic leukemia.

STORAGE/HANDLING

Note: May be carcinogenic, mutagenic, or teratogenic. Handle w/extreme care during preparation/administration. Refrigerate unopened vials. Solutions are clear, colorless. Following reconstitution w/bacteriostatic 0.9% NaCl, solution stable for 30 days if refrigerated. Discard if precipitate forms, discoloration occurs.

IV ADMINISTRATION

Note: Give by IV injection. Leakage from IV site into surrounding tissue may produce extreme irritation. Avoid eye contact w/solution (severe eye irritation, possible corneal ulceration may result). If eye contact occurs, immediately irrigate eye w/water.

1. Reconstitute 10 mg vial w/10 ml 0.9% NaCl injection preserved w/phenol or benzyl alcohol to provide concentration of 1 mg/ml.

2. Inject into tubing of running IV infusion or directly into vein over 1 min.

3. Do not inject into extremity w/impaired or potentially impaired circulation caused by compression or invading neoplasm, phlebitis, varicosity.

4. Rinse syringe, needle w/venous blood before withdrawing needle (minimizes possibility of extravasation).

5. Extravasation may result in cellulitis, phlebitis. Large amount of extravasation may result in tissue sloughing. If extravasation occurs, give local injection of hyaluronidase and apply warm compresses.

INDICATIONS/DOSAGE/ROUTES

Note: Dosage individualized based on clinical response, tolerance to adverse effects. When used in combination therapy, consult specific protocols for optimum dosage, sequence of drug administration. Reduce dose if serum bilirubin >3 mg/dl. Repeat dosage at intervals of no less than 7 days and if the WBC count is at least 4,000/mm^3.

Induction remission:
IV: Adults, elderly: Initially, 3.7 mg/m^2 as single dose. Increase dose at weekly intervals of about 1.8 mg/m^2 until desired response is attained, WBC count falls below 3,000/mm^3, or maximum weekly dose of 18.5 mg/m^2 is reached. **Children:** Initially, 2.5 mg/m^2 as single dose. Increase dose at weekly intervals of about 1.25 mg/m^2 until desired response is attained, WBC count falls below 3,000/mm^3, or maximum weekly dose of 7.5–12.5 mg/m^2 is reached.

Maintenance dose:
IV: Adults, elderly, children: Use one increment less than dose required to produce leukocyte count of 3,000/mm^3. Each subsequent dose given when leukocyte count returns to 4,000/mm^3 and at least 7 days has elapsed since previous dose.

PRECAUTIONS

CONTRAINDICATIONS: Severe leukopenia, bacterial infection, significant granulocytopenia unless a result of disease being treated. **EXTREME CAUTION:** Debilitated, elderly (high susceptibility to leukopenia). **PREGNANCY/ LACTATION:** If possible, avoid use during pregnancy, esp. first trimester. Breast-feeding not recommended. **Pregnancy Category D**.

INTERACTIONS

DRUG INTERACTIONS: May decrease effect of antigout medications. Bone marrow depressants may increase bone marrow depression. Live virus vaccines may potentiate virus replication, increase vaccine side effects, decrease pt's antibody response to vaccine. **ALTERED LAB VALUES:** May increase uric acid.

SIDE EFFECTS

FREQUENT: Nausea, vomiting, alopecia. **OCCASIONAL:** Constipation/diarrhea, rectal bleeding, paresthesia, headache, malaise, weakness, dizziness, pain at tumor site, jaw/face pain, mental depression, dry mouth. GI distress, headache, paresthesia occurs 4–6 hrs after administration, persists for 2–10 hrs. **RARE:** Dermatitis, stomatitis, phototoxicity, hyperuricemia.

ADVERSE REACTIONS/TOXIC EFFECTS

Hematologic toxicity manifested most commonly as leukopenia, less frequently as anemia. WBC falls to lowest point 4–10 days after initial therapy w/recovery within another 7–14 days (high doses may require 21 day recovery period). Thrombocytopenia usually slight, transient, w/rapid recovery within few days. Hepatic insufficiency may increase risk of toxicity. Acute shortness of breath, bronchospasm may occur, particularly when administered concurrently with mitomycin.

NURSING IMPLICATIONS
BASELINE ASSESSMENT:

Nausea, vomiting easily controlled by antiemetics. Discontinue therapy if WBC, thrombocyte counts fall abruptly (unless drug is clearly destroying tumor cells in bone marrow). Obtain CBC weekly or before each dosing.

INTERVENTION/EVALUATION:

If WBC falls below 2,000/mm³, assess diligently for signs of infection. Assess for stomatitis (burning erythema of oral mucosa at inner margin of lips, sore throat, difficulty swallowing, oral ulceration). Monitor for hematologic toxicity: infection (fever, sore throat, signs of local infection); easy bruising, unusual bleeding from any site; symptoms of anemia (excessive tiredness, weakness). Assess frequency and consistency of stools; avoid constipation.

PATIENT/FAMILY TEACHING:

Immediately report any pain or burning at injection site during administration. Pain at tumor site may occur during or shortly after injection. Do not have immunizations w/o physician approval (drug lowers body's resistance). Avoid crowds, those w/infection. Promptly report fever, sore throat, signs of local infection, easy bruising, unusual bleeding from any site. Alopecia is reversible, but new hair growth may have different color or texture. Contact physician if nausea/vomiting continues at home. Avoid constipation by increasing fluids, bulk in diet, exercise as tolerated.

vincristine sulfate

vin-**cris**-teen
(Oncovin, Vincasar PFS)

CLASSIFICATION

Antineoplastic

AVAILABILITY (Rx)

Injection: 1 mg/ml

PHARMACOKINETICS

Does not cross blood-brain barrier. Metabolized in liver. Primarily eliminated in feces via biliary system. Half-life: 10–37 hrs.

ACTION / *THERAPEUTIC EFFECT*

Blocks mitosis by arresting cells in metaphase stage, *inhibiting cellular division.* Interferes w/amino acid metabolism, nucleic acid synthesis. Cell cycle-specific for M phase of cell division. Has some immunosuppressive effect.

USES / *UNLABELED*

Treatment of acute leukemia, disseminated Hodgkin's disease, advanced non-Hodgkin's lymphomas, neuroblastoma, rhabdomyosarcoma, Wilm's tumor. *Treatment of chronic lymphocytic, myelocytic leukemia, carcinoma of breast, lung, ovarian, cervical, colorectal, malignant melanoma, multiple myeloma, germ cell ovarian tumors, mycosis fungoides, idiopathic thrombocytopenia purpura.*

STORAGE / HANDLING

Note: May be carcinogenic, mutagenic, or teratogenic. Handle w/extreme care during preparation/administration. Refrigerate unopened vials. Solutions appear clear, colorless. Discard if precipitate forms or discoloration occurs.

IV ADMINISTRATION

Note: Give by IV injection. Use extreme caution in calculating, administering vincristine. Overdose may result in serious or fatal outcome.

1. Inject dose into tubing of running IV infusion or directly into vein >1 min.

2. Do not inject into extremity w/impaired or potentially impaired circulation caused by compression or invading neoplasm, phlebitis, varicosity.

3. Extravasation produces stinging, burning, edema at injection site. Terminate immediately, locally inject hyaluronidase and apply heat (disperses drug, minimizes discomfort, cellulitis).

INDICATIONS / DOSAGE / ROUTES

Note: Dosage individualized based on clinical response, tolerance to adverse effects. When used in combination therapy, consult specific protocols for optimum dosage, sequence of drug administration.

Usual dosage (administer at weekly intervals):
IV: Adults, elderly: 0.4–1.4 mg/m^2. **Maximum:** 2 mg. **Children:** 1.5–2 mg/m^2. **Children <10 kg or body surface area <1 m^2:** 0.05 mg/kg.

Hepatic function impairment:
Reduce dose by 50% in those w/ direct serum bilirubin concentration <3 mg/dl.

PRECAUTIONS

CONTRAINDICATIONS: Those receiving radiation therapy through ports that include liver.

EXTREME CAUTION: Hepatic impairment. **PREGNANCY/LACTATION:** If possible, avoid use during pregnancy, esp. first trimester. May cause fetal harm. Breast feeding not recommended. **Pregnancy Category D**.

INTERACTIONS

DRUG INTERACTIONS: May decrease effect of antigout medications. Live virus vaccines may potentiate virus replication, increase vaccine side effects, decrease pt's antibody response to vaccine. Asparaginase, neurotoxic medications may increase neurotoxicity. Doxorubicin may increase myelosuppression. **ALTERED LAB VALUES:** May increase uric acid.

SIDE EFFECTS

Peripheral neuropathy occurs in nearly every pt (first clinical sign: depression of Achilles tendon reflex). **FREQUENT:** Peripheral paresthesia, alopecia, constipation or obstipation (upper colon impaction w/empty rectum), abdominal cramps, headache, jaw pain, hoarseness, double vision, ptosis (drooping of eyelid), urinary tract disturbances. **OCCASIONAL:** Nausea, vomiting, diarrhea, abdominal distention, stomatitis, fever. **RARE:** Mild leukopenia, mild anemia, thrombocytopenia.

ADVERSE REACTIONS/TOXIC EFFECTS

Acute shortness of breath, bronchospasm may occur (esp. when used in combination w/mitomycin). Prolonged or high-dose therapy may produce foot/wrist drop, difficulty walking, slapping gait, ataxia, muscle wasting. Acute uric acid nephropathy may be noted.

NURSING IMPLICATIONS

BASELINE ASSESSMENT:

Monitor serum uric acid levels, renal, hepatic function studies, hematologic status. Assess Achilles tendon reflex. Assess stools for consistency, frequency. Monitor for ptosis, blurred vision. Question pt regarding urinary changes.

PATIENT/FAMILY TEACHING:

Immediately report any pain or burning at injection site during administration. Alopecia is reversible, but new hair growth may have different color/texture. Contact physician if nausea/vomiting continues at home. Teach signs of peripheral neuropathy.

---

vinorelbine

vin-oh-**rell**-bean
(Navelbine)

CANADIAN AVAILABILITY:
Navelbine

CLASSIFICATION

Antineoplastic

AVAILABILITY (Rx)

Injection: 10 mg/ml (1 ml, 5 ml vials)

PHARMACOKINETICS

Following IV administration, widely distributed. Metabolized in liver. Primarily eliminated via biliary/fecal route. Half-life: 28–43 hrs.

ACTION/*THERAPEUTIC EFFECT*

Interferes with mitotic microtubule assembly, *preventing cellular division*.

USES / *UNLABELED*

Single agent or in combination w/cisplatin for treatment w/unresectable, advanced, non small cell lung cancer (NSCLC). *Treatment of breast cancer, cisplatin-resistant ovarian carcinoma, Hodgkin's disease.*

STORAGE / HANDLING

Refrigerate unopened vials. Protect from light. Unopened vials are stable at room temperature for 72 hrs. Do not administer if particulate matter is noted. Diluted vinorelbine may be used for up to 24 hrs under normal room light when stored in polypropylene syringes or polyvinyl chloride bags at room temperature.

IV ADMINISTRATION

Note: Extremely important that IV needle or catheter is correctly positioned before administration. Leaking into surrounding tissue produces extreme irritation, local tissue necrosis, or thrombophlebitis. Wear gloves when preparing solution. If solution comes in contact w/skin or mucosa, wash immediately and thoroughly w/soap, water.

1. Must be diluted and administered via a syringe or IV bag.

2. *Syringe dilution:* Dilute calculated vinorelbine dose w/5% dextrose or 0.9% NaCl to a concentration between 1.5 and 3 mg/ml.

3. *IV bag dilution:* Dilute calculated vinorelbine dose w/5% dextrose, 0.45% or 0.9% NaCl, 5% dextrose and 0.45% NaCl, Ringer's or lactated Ringer's to a concentration between 0.5–2 mg/ml.

4. Administer diluted vinorelbine over 6–10 min into side port of free-flowing IV closest to IV bag followed by flushing with 75–125 ml of one of the solutions.

5. If extravasation occurs, stop injection immediately; give remaining portion of the dose into another vein.

INDICATIONS / DOSAGE / ROUTES

Note: Granulocyte count should be ≥ 1,000 cells/mm³ before vinorelbine administration. Dosage adjustments should be based on granulocyte count obtained on day of treatment, as follows:

GRANULOCYTES (CELLS/MM³) ON DAYS OF TREATMENT	DOSE (MG/M²)
≥ 1,500	30
1,000–1,499	15
< 1,000	Do not administer.

Non small cell lung cancer:
IV Injection: Adults, elderly: 30 mg/m², given over 6–10 min, administered weekly.

PRECAUTIONS

CONTRAINDICATIONS: Pretreatment granulocyte count <1,000 cells/mm³. **EXTREME CAUTION:** Immunocompromised pts. **CAUTIONS:** Existing or recent chicken pox, herpes zoster, infection, leukopenia, impaired pulmonary function, severe hepatic injury or impairment. **PREGNANCY/LACTATION:** If possible, avoid use during pregnancy, esp. during first trimester. May cause fetal harm. Breast-feeding not recommended. Unknown whether excreted in breast milk. **Pregnancy Category D.**

INTERACTIONS

DRUG INTERACTIONS: Significantly increased risk of granulocytopenia when cisplatin is used concurrently w/vinorelbine. Mitomycin may produce acute pulmonary reaction. Bone marrow depressants may increase risk of bone marrow depression. Live virus vaccines may potentiate virus replication, increase vaccine side effects, decrease pt's antibody response to vaccine. **ALTERED LAB VALUES:** Decreases granulocytes, leukocytes, thrombocytes, RBCs. May increase total bilirubin, SGOT (AST), liver function tests.

SIDE EFFECTS

FREQUENT: Asthenia (35%), mild or moderate nausea (34%), constipation (29%), injection site reaction manifested as erythema, pain, vein discoloration (28%), fatigue (27%), peripheral neuropathy manifested as paresthesia, hypesthesia (25%), diarrhea (17%), alopecia (12%). **OCCASIONAL:** Phlebitis (10%), dyspnea (7%), loss of deep tendon reflexes (5%). **RARE:** Chest pain, jaw pain, myalgia, arthralgia, rash.

ADVERSE REACTIONS/TOXIC EFFECTS

Bone marrow depression is manifested mainly as granulocytopenia (may be severe); other hematologic toxicity (neutropenia, thrombocytopenia, leukopenia, anemia) increases risk of infection, bleeding. Acute shortness of breath, severe bronchospasm occurs infrequently, particularly when there is preexisting pulmonary dysfunction.

NURSING IMPLICATIONS

BASELINE ASSESSMENT:

Review medication history. Assess hematology (CBC, platelet count, Hgb, differential) values before giving each dose. Granulocyte count should be ≥ 1,000 cells/mm^3 before vinorelbine administration. Granulocyte nadirs occur between 7 and 10 days after dosing. Do not give hematologic growth factors within 24 hrs before administration of chemotherapy or no earlier than 24 hrs after cytotoxic chemotherapy. Advise women of childbearing potential to avoid pregnancy during drug therapy.

INTERVENTION/EVALUATION:

Diligently monitor injection site for swelling, redness, pain at injection site. Frequently monitor for myelosuppression both during and after therapy: infection (fever, sore throat, signs of local infection); unusual bleeding or bruising; anemia (excessive tiredness, weakness). Monitor pts developing severe granulocytopenia for evidence of infection or fever. Crackers, dry toast, sips of cola may help relieve nausea. Assess bowel activity and frequency. Check injection site for reaction. Question for tingling, burning, numbness of hands/feet (peripheral neuropathy). Pt complaint of "walking on glass" is sign of hyperesthesia.

PATIENT/FAMILY TEACHING:

Notify nurse immediately if redness, swelling, pain occur at injection site. Avoid crowds, those w/infection. Do not have immunizations w/o physician's approval. Promptly report fever, signs of infection, easy bruising, unusual bleeding from any site, difficulty breathing. Avoid pregnancy. Alopecia is reversible, but new hair growth may have different color or texture.

vitamin A
(Aquasol A)

CLASSIFICATION

Fat-soluble vitamin

AVAILABILITY (OTC)

Tablets: 5,000 IU. **Capsules:** 10,000 IU, 25,000 IU **(Rx),** 50,000 IU **(Rx). Drops:** 5,000 IU/0.1 ml. **Injection:** 50,000 IU/ml **(Rx).**

PHARMACOKINETICS

Absorption dependent on bile salts, pancreatic lipase, dietary fat. Transported in blood to liver, stored in parenchymal liver cells, then transported in plasma as retinol, as needed. Metabolized in liver. Excreted in bile and to a lesser amount in urine.

ACTION/THERAPEUTIC EFFECT

May be a cofactor in biochemical reactions. *Essential for normal function of retina. Necessary for visual adaptation to darkness, bone growth, testicular and ovarian function, embryonic development.*

USES

Treatment of vitamin A deficiency (biliary tract or pancreatic disease, sprue, colitis, hepatic cirrhosis, celiac disease, regional enteritis, extreme dietary inadequacy, partial gastrectomy, cystic fibrosis).

STORAGE/HANDLING

Store oral forms at room temperature. Refrigerate vials.

PO/IM ADMINISTRATION

Note: IM administration used only in acutely ill or those unresponsive to oral route (GI malabsorption syndrome).

PO:

1. Do not crush or break capsule form.
2. May take w/o regard to food.

INDICATIONS/DOSAGE/ROUTES

Severe deficiency (Xerophthalmia):
PO: Adults, elderly: 25–50,000 IU/day. **Children >1 yr:** 200,000 IU as single dose; repeat following day and 4 wks later. **6 mos–1 yr:** 100,000 IU as single dose; repeat following day and 4 wks later.
IM: Adults, elderly, children >8 yrs: 50–100,000 IU/day for 3 days, then 50,000 IU daily for 2 wks. **Children 1–8 yrs:** 5–15,000 IU/day for 10 days. **<1 yr:** 5–10,000 IU/day for 10 days.

Dietary supplement:
PO: Adults, elderly: 4,000–5,000 IU/day. **Children 7–10 yrs:** 3,300–3,500 IU/day. **Children 4–6 yrs:** 2,500 IU/day. **Children 6 mos–3 yrs:** 1,500–2,000 IU/day. **Neonates to 6 mos:** 1,500 IU/day.

PRECAUTIONS

CONTRAINDICATIONS: Hypervitaminosis A, oral use in malabsorption syndrome. **CAUTIONS:** Renal impairment. **PREGNANCY/LACTATION:** Crosses placenta; is distributed in breast milk. **Pregnancy Category A**. (Category X if doses above RDA.)

INTERACTIONS

DRUG INTERACTIONS: Cholestyramine, colestipol, mineral oil may decrease absorption. Isotretinoin may increase toxicity. **ALTERED LAB VALUES:** May increase BUN, calcium, cholesterol, triglycerides. May decrease erythrocyte, leukocyte counts.

SIDE EFFECTS

None significant.

ADVERSE REACTIONS/TOXIC EFFECTS

Chronic overdosage produces malaise, nausea, vomiting, drying/cracking of skin/lips, inflammation of tongue/gums, irritability, loss of hair, night sweats. Bulging fontanelles in infants noted.

NURSING IMPLICATIONS

INTERVENTION/EVALUATION:

Closely supervise for overdosage symptoms during prolonged daily administration over 25,000 IU. Monitor for therapeutic serum vitamin A levels (80–300 IU/ml).

PATIENT/FAMILY TEACHING:

Foods rich in vitamin A include cod, halibut, tuna, shark (naturally occurring vitamin A found only in animal sources). Avoid taking mineral oil, cholestyramine (Questran) while taking vitamin A.

vitamin D calcifediol
(Calderol)
calcitriol
(Calcijex, Rocaltrol)
dihydrotachysterol
(DHT, Hytakerol)
ergocalciferol
(Calciferol, Deltalin, Drisdol)

CANADIAN AVAILABILITY:
Calciferol, Calcijex, Drisdol, Hytakerol, Rocaltrol

CLASSIFICATION

Fat-soluble vitamin

AVAILABILITY (Rx)

Calcifediol: Capsules: 20 mcg, 50 mcg

Calcitriol: Capsules: 0.25 mcg, 0.5 mcg. **Injection:** 1 mcg/ml, 2 mcg/ml.

Dihydrotachysterol: Tablets: 0.125 mg, 0.2 mg, 0.4 mg. **Capsules:** 0.125 mg. **Oral Solution:** 0.2 mg/ml, 0.25 mg/ml.

Ergocalciferol: Liquid (OTC): 8,000 IU/ml. **Capsules:** 50,000 IU. **Tablets:** 50,000 IU. **Injection:** 500,000 IU/ml.

PHARMACOKINETICS

Readily absorbed from small intestine. Concentrated primarily in liver, fat depots. Activated in liver, kidney. Eliminated via biliary system; excreted in urine. Half-life: calcifediol: 10–22 days; calcitrol: 3–6 hrs; ergocalciferol: 19–48 hrs.

ACTION/*THERAPEUTIC EFFECT*

Essential for absorption and utilization of calcium and phosphate, normal calcification of bone, regulation of serum calcium concentration (w/parathyroid, calcitonin).

USES

Prevention/treatment of rickets or osteomalacia; management of hypocalcemia associated w/hypoparathyroidism.

PO ADMINISTRATION

1. May take w/o regard to food.

2. Swallow whole; do not crush/chew.

INDICATIONS/DOSAGE/ROUTES

CALCIFEDIOL:

*Metabolic bone disease, hypocal-
cemia (dialysis pts):*
PO: Adults, elderly: Initially,
300–350 mcg/wk given daily or
every other day. May increase at 4
wk intervals. **Maintenance:**
50–100 mcg/day or 100 and 200
mcg on alternate days.

CALCITRIOL:

Hypocalcemia (dialysis pts):
PO: Adults, elderly: Initially, 0.25
mcg/day. May increase by 0.25
mcg/day q4–8 wks. **Range:** 0.25–1
mcg/day.

Hypoparathyroidism:
PO: Adults, elderly, children: Initially, 0.25 mcg/day. May increase
at 2–4 wk intervals. **Maintenance:**
Adults, children ≥6 yrs: 0.5–2
mcg/day. **Children 1–5 yrs:**
0.25–0.75 mcg/day.

CHOLECALCIFEROL:

Dietary supplement, deficiency:
PO: Adults, elderly: 400–1,000
IU/day.

DIHYDROTACHYSTEROL:

*Postop tetany, idiopathic tetany,
hypoparathyroidism:*
PO: Adults, elderly: Initially,
0.8–2.4 mg/day for several days.
Maintenance: 0.2–1 mg/day.

ERGOCALCIFEROL:

Familial hypophosphatemia:
PO: Adults, elderly: 10,000–
80,000 IU/day plus 1–2 g/day elemental phosphorus.

Hypoparathyroidism:
PO: Adults, elderly: 50,000–
200,000 IU/day plus 500 mg elemental calcium 6 times/day.

Refractory rickets:
PO: Adults, elderly: 12,000–
500,000 IU/day.

PRECAUTIONS

CONTRAINDICATIONS: Hypercalcemia, vitamin D toxicity, malabsorption syndrome, hypervitaminosis D, decreased renal
function, abnormal sensitivity to vitamin D effects (those w/idiopathic
hypercalcemia). **CAUTIONS:** Those
w/kidney stones, coronary disease,
renal function impairment, arteriosclerosis, hypoparathyroidism,
those w/tartrazine sensitivity. **PREG-
NANCY/LACTATION:** Unknown
whether drug crosses placenta; is
distributed in breast milk. **Pregnancy Category A.** (Category D if
used in doses above RDA.)

INTERACTIONS

DRUG INTERACTIONS: Aluminum-containing antacid (long-
term use) may increase aluminum
concentration, aluminum bone toxicity. Magnesium-containing
antacids may increase magnesium
concentration. Calcium-containing
preparations, thiazide diuretics
may increase risk of hypercalcemia. **ALTERED LAB VALUES:**
May increase calcium, cholesterol,
phosphate, magnesium. May decrease alkaline phosphatase.

SIDE EFFECTS

None significant.

ADVERSE REACTIONS/TOXIC
EFFECTS

Early signs of overdosage manifested as weakness, headache,
somnolence, nausea, vomiting,
dry mouth, constipation, muscle
and bone pain, metallic taste sensation. Later signs of overdosage
evidenced by polyuria, polydip-

sia, anorexia, weight loss, nocturia, photophobia, rhinorrhea, pruritus, disorientation, hallucinations, hyperthermia, hypertension, cardiac arrhythmias.

NURSING IMPLICATIONS
BASELINE ASSESSMENT:

Therapy should begin at lowest possible dose.

INTERVENTION/EVALUATION:

Monitor serum calcium and urinary calcium levels, serum phosphate, magnesium, creatinine, alkaline phosphatases and BUN determinations (therapeutic serum calcium level: 9–10 mg/dl). Estimate daily dietary calcium intake. Encourage adequate fluid intake.

PATIENT/FAMILY TEACHING:

Foods rich in vitamin D include vegetable oils, vegetable shortening, margarine, leafy vegetables, milk, eggs, meats. Do not take mineral oil while on vitamin D therapy. If on chronic renal dialysis, do not take magnesium-containing antacids during vitamin D therapy. Drink plenty of liquids.

vitamin E
(Aquasol E)

CANADIAN AVAILABILITY:
Aquasol E

CLASSIFICATION:

Fat-soluble vitamin

AVAILABILITY (OTC)
Tablets: 200 IU, 400 IU. **Cap-**sules: 100 IU, 200 IU, 400 IU, 500 IU, 600 IU, 1,000 IU. **Drops:** 50 mg/ml.

PHARMACOKINETICS

Variably absorbed from GI tract (requires bile salts, dietary fat, normal pancreatic function). Primarily concentrated in adipose tissue. Metabolized in liver. Primarily eliminated via biliary system.

ACTION/THERAPEUTIC EFFECT

Essential nutritional element. An antioxidant, *protects cells from oxidation. Protects red blood cells against hemolysis.* May act as cofactor in enzyme systems.

USES/UNLABELED

Treatment of vitamin E deficiency. *Decreases severity of tardive dyskinesia.*

PO ADMINISTRATION

1. Do not crush or break tablets/capsules.
2. May take w/o regard to food.

INDICATIONS/DOSAGE/ROUTES

Vitamin E deficiency:
PO: **Adults, elderly, children:** Individualized.

PRECAUTIONS

CONTRAINDICATIONS: None significant. **CAUTIONS:** None significant. **PREGNANCY/LACTATION:** Unknown whether drug crosses placenta or is distributed in breast milk. **Pregnancy Category A.** (Category C if used in doses above RDA.)

INTERACTIONS

DRUG INTERACTIONS: May impair hematologic response in pts w/iron deficiency anemia. Iron (large doses) may increase vitamin E requirements. Cholestyramine, colestipol, mineral oil may decrease absorption. **ALTERED LAB VALUES:** None significant.

SIDE EFFECTS

None significant.

ADVERSE/TOXIC EFFECTS

Chronic overdosage produces fatigue, weakness, nausea, headache, blurred vision, flatulence, diarrhea.

NURSING IMPLICATIONS

PATIENT/FAMILY TEACHING:

Foods rich in vitamin E include vegetable oils, vegetable shortening, margarine, leafy vegetables, milk, eggs, meats.

---

vitamin K

phytonadione (vitamin K₁)
fy-toe-na-**dye**-own
(AquaMEPHYTON, Konakion, Mephyton)

CLASSIFICATION

Nutritional supplement, antidote (drug-induced hypoprothrombinemia), antihemorrhagic

AVAILABILITY (Rx)

Tablets: 5 mg. **Injection:** 2 mg/ml, 10 mg/ml.

PHARMACOKINETICS

Readily absorbed from GI tract (duodenum), after IM, SubQ administration. Metabolized in liver. Excreted in urine, eliminated via biliary system. *Parenteral:* Controls hemorrhage within 3–6 hrs, normal prothrombin time in 12–14 hrs. *Oral:* Effect in 6–10 hrs.

ACTION/THERAPEUTIC EFFECT

Necessary for hepatic formation of coagulation factors II, VII, IX, and X, *which are essential for normal clotting of blood.*

USES

Prevention, treatment of hemorrhagic states in neonates; antidote for hemorrhage induced by oral anticoagulants, hypoprothombinemic states due to vitamin K deficiency. Will not counteract anticoagulation effect of heparin.

PO/SUBQ/IM/IV ADMINISTRATION

PO:

Scored tablets may be crushed.

SubQ/IM:

Inject into anterolateral aspect of thigh/deltoid region.

IV:

Note: Restrict to emergency use only.

1. May dilute w/preservative-free NaCl or 5% dextrose immediately before use. Do not use other diluents. Discard unused portions.

2. Administer slow IV at rate of 1 mg/min.

3. Monitor continuously for hypersensitivity, anaphylactic reaction during and immediately following IV administration.

INDICATIONS/DOSAGE/ROUTES

Anticoagulant-induced hypoprothrombinemia:
PO/IM/SubQ/IV: **Adults, elderly:** 2.5–10 mg up to 25 mg. Subsequent dosage based on pt condition, prothrombin time.

Hemorrhagic disease of newborn:
IM: **Infants:** 0.5–1 mg in first hour of birth.

PRECAUTIONS

CONTRAINDICATIONS: Last few weeks of pregnancy or neonates. **CAUTIONS:** Those w/asthma, impaired hepatic function. **PREGNANCY/LACTATION:** Crosses placenta; distributed in breast milk. **Pregnancy Category C**.

INTERACTIONS

DRUG INTERACTIONS: Broad-spectrum antibiotics, high-dose salicylates may increase vitamin K requirements. May decrease effect of oral anticoagulants. Cholestyramine, colestipol, mineral oil, sucralfate may decrease absorption. **ALTERED LAB VALUES:** None significant.

SIDE EFFECTS

Note: Oral or SubQ administration less likely to produce side effects than IM or IV route. **OCCASIONAL:** Pain, soreness, swelling at IM injection site; repeated injections: pruritic erythema; flushed face, unusual taste.

ADVERSE REACTIONS/TOXIC EFFECTS

May produce hyperbilirubinemia in newborn (esp. premature infants). Rarely, severe reaction occurs immediately following IV administration (cramp-like pain, chest pain, dyspnea, facial flushing, dizziness, rapid/weak pulse, rash, profuse sweating, hypotension; may progress to shock, cardiac arrest).

NURSING IMPLICATIONS

INTERVENTION/EVALUATION:

Monitor prothrombin time routinely in those taking anticoagulants. Assess skin for bruises, petechiae. Assess gums for gingival bleeding, erythema. Monitor urine output for hema-turia. Assess hematocrit, platelet count, urine/stool culture for occult blood. Assess for decrease in B/P, increase in pulse rate, complaint of abdominal or back pain, severe headache (may be evidence of hemorrhage). Question for increase in amount of discharge during menses. Assess peripheral pulses, skin for bruises, petechiae. Check for excessive bleeding from minor cuts, scratches. Assess urine output for hematuria.

PATIENT/FAMILY TEACHING:

Discomfort may occur w/parenteral administration. *Adults:* Use electric razor, soft toothbrush to prevent bleeding. Report any sign of red or dark urine, black or red stool, coffee-ground vomitus, red-speckled mucus from cough. Do not use any OTC medication w/o physician approval (may interfere w/platelet aggregation). Foods rich in vitamin K_1 include leafy green vegetables, meat, cow's milk, vegetable oil, egg yolks, tomatoes.

warfarin sodium
war-fair-in
(Coumadin, Panwarfin, Sofarin)

CANADIAN AVAILABILITY: Coumadin, Warfilone

CLASSIFICATION

Anticoagulant

AVAILABILITY (Rx)

Tablets: 1 mg, 2 mg, 2.5 mg, 3 mg, 5 mg, 6 mg, 7.5 mg, 10 mg. **Injection:** 5 mg vials.

PHARMACOKINETICS

	ONSET	PEAK	DURATION
PO	—	1.5–3 days	2–5 days

Well absorbed from GI tract. Metabolized in liver. Primarily excreted in urine. Half-life: 1.5–2.5 days.

ACTION/*THERAPEUTIC EFFECT*

Interferes w/hepatic synthesis of vitamin K–dependent clotting factors, resulting in depletion of coagulation factors II, VII, IX, X. *Prevents further extension of formed existing clot; prevents new clot formation or secondary thromboembolic complications.*

USES/*UNLABELED*

Prophylaxis, treatment of venous thrombosis, pulmonary embolism. Treatment of thromboembolism associated w/chronic atrial fibrillation. Adjunct in treatment of coronary occlusion. Prophylaxis/treatment of thromboembolic complications associated w/cardiac valve replacement. Reduces risk of death, recurrent MI, stroke, embolization after myocardial infarction. *Prophylaxis vs. recurrence cerebral embolism, myocardial reinfarction, treatment adjunct in transient ischemic attacks.*

PO ADMINISTRATION

1. Scored tablets may be crushed.
2. May give w/o regard to food. If GI upset occurs, give w/food.

INDICATIONS/DOSAGE/ROUTES

Note: Dosage highly individualized, based on prothrombin time (PT), INR.
PO/IV: Adults: Initially, 10–15 mg, then adjust dose. **Maintenance:** 2–10 mg/day based on prothrombin determinations.

Usual elderly dosage:
PO/IV: 2–5 mg/day (maintenance).

PRECAUTIONS

CONTRAINDICATIONS: Bleeding abnormalities, hemophilia, thrombocytopenia, brain/spinal cord surgery, spinal anesthesia, eye surgery; bleeding from GI, respiratory, or GU tract; threatened abortion, aneurysm, ascorbic acid deficiency, acute nephritis, cerebrovascular hemorrhage, eclampsia, pre-eclampsia, blood dyscrasias, hypertension, severe hepatic disease, pericardial effusion, bacterial endocarditis, visceral carcinoma, following spinal puncture, IUD insertion, or any potential for bleeding abnormalities. **CAUTIONS:** Factors increasing risk of hemorrhage, active tuberculosis, severe diabetes, GI tract ulcer disease, during menstruation, postpartum period. Long-term use may increase bone fractures. **PREGNANCY/LACTATION:** Contraindicated in pregnancy (fetal/neonatal hemorrhage, intrauterine death). Crosses placenta; is distributed in breast milk. **Pregnancy Category D.**

INTERACTIONS

DRUG INTERACTIONS: *Increased effect with:* Acetaminophen (regular use), allopurinol, amiodarone, anabolic steroids, androgens, aspirin, cefamandole, cefoperazone, chloral hydrate, chloramphenicol, cimetidine, clofibrate, danazol, dextrothyroxine, disulfiram, erythromycin, fenoprofen, gemfibrozil, indomethacin, methimazole, metronidazole, oral hypoglycemics, phenytoin, plicamycin, PTU, quinidine, salicylates, sulfinpyrazone, sulfonamides, sulindac, troplitazone. *Decreased effect with:* Barbiturates,

W

carbamazepine, cholestyramine, colestipol, estramustine, estrogens, griseofulvin, primidone, rifampin, vitamin K. **ALTERED LAB VALUES:** None significant.

SIDE EFFECTS

OCCASIONAL: GI distress (nausea, anorexia, abdominal cramps, diarrhea). **RARE:** Hypersensitivity reaction (dermatitis, urticaria, esp. in those sensitive to aspirin).

ADVERSE REACTIONS/TOXIC EFFECTS

Bleeding complications ranging from local ecchymoses to major hemorrhage. Drug should be discontinued immediately and vitamin K (phytonadione) administered. Mild hemorrhage: 2.5–10 mg PO/IM/IV. Severe hemorrhage: 10–15 mg IV and repeated q4h, as necessary. Hepatotoxicity, blood dyscrasias, necrosis, vasculitis, local thrombosis occur rarely.

NURSING IMPLICATIONS

BASELINE ASSESSMENT:

Cross-check dose w/co-worker. Determine INR before administration and daily after therapy initiation. When stabilized, follow w/INR determination q4–6 wks.

INTERVENTION/EVALUATION:

Monitor INR reports diligently. Assess Hct, platelet count, urine/stool culture for occult blood, SGOT (AST), SGPT (ALT), regardless of route of administration. Be alert to complaints of abdominal back pain, severe headache (may be signs of hemorrhage). Decrease in B/P, increase in pulse rate may also be sign of hemorrhage. Question for increase in amount of discharge during menses. Assess area of thromboembolus for color, temperature.

Assess peripheral pulses, skin for bruises, petechiae. Check for excessive bleeding from minor cuts, scratches. Assess gums for erythema, gingival bleeding. Assess urine output for hematuria.

PATIENT/FAMILY TEACHING:

Take medication exactly as prescribed. Do not take or discontinue any other medication except on advice of physician. Avoid alcohol, salicylates, or drastic dietary changes. Do not change from one brand to another. Consult w/physician before surgery or dental work. Urine may become red orange. Notify physician if bleeding, bruising, red or brown urine, black stools occur. Use electric razor, soft toothbrush to prevent bleeding. Report any sign of red or dark urine, black or red stool, coffee-ground vomitus, red-speckled mucus from cough. Do not use any OTC medication w/o physician approval (may interfere w/platelet aggregation).

zafirlukast

zay-**fur**-leu-cast
(Accolate)

CANADIAN AVAILABILITY: Accolate

CLASSIFICATION

Leukotriene receptor antagonist

AVAILABILITY (Rx)

Tablets: 10 mg, 20 mg

PHARMACOKINETICS

Rapidly absorbed following oral administration (food reduces absorption). Extensively metabolized in liver. Primarily excreted in feces. Half-life: 10 hrs.

ACTION/*THERAPEUTIC EFFECT*

Binds to leukotriene receptors. Inhibits bronchoconstriction due to sulfur dioxide, cold air, specific antigens (grass, cat dander, ragweed) *reducing airway edema, smooth muscle constriction, altered cellular activity associated w/inflammatory process.*

USES

Prophylaxis, chronic treatment of bronchial asthma.

PO ADMINISTRATION

1. Give 1 hr before or 2 hrs after meals.
2. Do not crush or break tablets.

INDICATIONS/DOSAGE/ROUTES

Bronchial asthma:
PO: Adults, elderly, children >12 yrs: 20 mg twice daily. **Children 7–12 yrs:** 10 mg twice daily.

PRECAUTIONS

CONTRAINDICATIONS: Hypersensitivity to zafirlukast. **CAUTIONS:** Impaired hepatic function. **PREGNANCY/LACTATION:** Distributed in breast milk. Do not administer to breast-feeding women. **Pregnancy Category B**.

INTERACTIONS

DRUG INTERACTIONS: Aspirin increases concentration. Coadministration of warfarin increases prothrombin time (PT). Erythromycin, terfenadine, theophylline decreases concentration. **ALTERED LAB VALUES:** May increase SGPT (ALT).

SIDE EFFECTS

FREQUENT (13%): Headache. **OCCASIONAL (3%):** Nausea, diarrhea. **RARE (<3%):** Generalized pain, asthenia, myalgia, fever, dyspepsia, vomiting, dizziness.

ADVERSE REACTIONS/TOXIC EFFECTS

Coadministration of inhaled corticosteroids increase risks of upper respiratory infection.

NURSING IMPLICATIONS
BASELINE ASSESSMENT:

Obtain medication history. Assess liver function lab values.

INTERVENTION/EVALUATION:

Monitor rate, depth, rhythm, type of respiration; quality and rate of pulse. Assess lung sounds for rhonchi, wheezing, rales. Observe lips, fingernails for blue or dusky color in light-skinned pts; gray in dark-skinned pts. Monitor liver function tests.

PATIENT/FAMILY TEACHING:

Increase fluid intake (decreases lung secretion viscosity). Take as prescribed, even during symptom-free periods. Do not use for acute asthma episodes. Do not alter/stop other asthma medications. Nursing mothers should not breast-feed. Report nausea, jaundice, abdominal pain, flu-like symptoms, or worsening of asthma.

zalcitabine
zal-**site**-ah-bean
(Hivid)

CANADIAN AVAILABILITY:
Hivid

CLASSIFICATION

Antiviral

AVAILABILITY (Rx)

Tablets: 0.375 mg, 0.75 mg

PHARMACOKINETICS

Readily absorbed from GI tract (food decreases absorption). Undergoes phosphorylation intracellularly to the active metabolite. Primarily excreted in urine. Unknown whether removed by hemodialysis. Half-life: 1–3 hrs; metabolite: 2.6–10 hrs (increased in decreased renal function).

ACTION/*THERAPEUTIC EFFECT*

Intracellularly converted to active metabolite. Inhibits viral DNA synthesis, *preventing replication of human immunodeficiency virus (HIV-1)*.

USES

Management of adult pts w/advanced HIV disease who are either intolerant to zidovudine or have disease progression while receiving zidovudine.

PO ADMINISTRATION

1. Best taken on empty stomach (food decreases absorption).
2. May take w/food to decrease GI distress.
3. Space doses evenly around the clock.

INDICATIONS/DOSAGE/ROUTES

HIV infection:
PO: Adults: 0.75 mg q8h (may be given w/zidovudine).

Dosage in renal impairment:
Based on creatinine clearance.

CREATININE CLEARANCE	DOSE
10–40 ml/min	0.75 mg q12h
<10 ml/min	0.75 mg q24h

PRECAUTIONS

CONTRAINDICATIONS: Hypersensitivity to zalcitabine or components of preparation. Pts w/moderate/severe peripheral neuropathy. Children <13 yrs (safety not known). **EXTREME CAUTION:** Those w/low CD4 cell counts (risk of peripheral neuropathy is greater), preexist-ing neuropathy. **CAUTIONS:** Pts w/history of pancreatitis or increased amylase, history of ethanol abuse. History of CHF, baseline cardiomyopathy, decreased renal function, liver disease. **PREGNANCY/LACTATION:** Unknown whether it crosses the placenta or is distributed in breast milk. Avoid breast-feeding in HIV-positive women. **Pregnancy Category C**.

INTERACTIONS

DRUG INTERACTIONS: Medications associated w/peripheral neuropathy may increase risk (e.g., cisplatin, disulfiram, phenytoin, vincristine). Medications causing pancreatitis may increase risk (e.g., IV pentamidine). **ALTERED LAB VALUES:** May increase SGOT (AST), SGPT (ALT), alkaline phosphatase, amylase, lipase, triglyceride concentrations. May cause leukopenia, neutropenia, eosinophilia, thrombocytopenia.

SIDE EFFECTS

OCCASIONAL (1–4%): Arthralgia (joint pain), fever, skin rash, muscle pain, ulceration of mouth/throat, nausea, diarrhea, abdominal pain, headache.

ADVERSE REACTIONS/TOXIC EFFECTS

Peripheral neuropathy occurs commonly (17–31%), characterized by numbness, tingling, burning, and pain of lower extremities. May be followed by sharp shooting pain and progress to severe continuous burning pain that may be irreversible if the drug is not discontinued in time. Pancreatitis, blood dyscrasias occur rarely.

NURSING IMPLICATIONS

BASELINE ASSESSMENT:

Offer emotional support to patient and family. Monitor CBC, triglycerides, and serum amylase levels before and during therapy.

INTERVENTION/EVALUATION:

Stop medication and notify physician immediately if signs and symptoms of peripheral neuropathy develop: numbness, tingling, burning, or shooting pains of extremities, loss of vibratory sense or ankle reflex. Although rare, be alert to impending potentially fatal pancreatitis: increasing serum amylase, rising triglycerides, nausea, vomiting, abdominal pain (withhold medication and notify physician). Assess for therapeutic response: weight gain, increased energy, decreased fatigue.

PATIENT/FAMILY TEACHING:

Not a cure for HIV; may continue to contract illnesses associated w/advanced HIV infection. Does not preclude the need to continue practices to prevent transmission of HIV. Report promptly any signs and symptoms of peripheral neuropathy or pancreatitis (see Adverse Reactions/Toxic Effects). Women of childbearing age should use contraception.

zaleplon
(Sonata)
See Supplement

zanamivir
(Relenza)
See Supplement

zidovudine
zye-**dough**-view-deen
(AZT, Retrovir)

FIXED-COMBINATION(S):
W/lamivudine, an antiviral
(Combivir)

CANADIAN AVAILABILITY:
Apo-Zidovudine, Novo-AZT, Retrovir

CLASSIFICATION

Antiviral

AVAILABILITY (Rx)

Capsules: 100 mg, 300 mg. **Syrup:** 50 mg/5 ml. **Injection:** 10 mg/ml.

PHARMACOKINETICS

Rapidly, completely absorbed from GI tract. Undergoes first-pass metabolism in liver. Widely distributed. Crosses blood-brain barrier, CSF. Primarily excreted in urine. Minimal removal by hemodialysis. Half-life: 0.8–1.2 hrs (increased in decreased renal function).

ACTION/THERAPEUTIC EFFECT

Interferes w/viral RNA-dependent DNA polymerase, an enzyme necessary for viral HIV replication, *slowing HIV replication, reducing progression of HIV infection.*

USES/UNLABELED

IV: Management of select adult pts w/symptomatic HIV infection (AIDS, advanced HIV disease). ***PO:*** Management of pts w/HIV infection having evidence of impaired immunity. HIV-infected chil-

Z

dren (>3 mos) who have HIV-related symptoms or asymptomatic w/abnormal lab values showing significant HIV-related immunosuppression. Prevents maternal–fetal HIV transmission. *Prophylaxis in occupational exposure at risk of acquiring HIV.*

STORAGE/HANDLING

Keep capsules in cool, dry place. Protect from light. After dilution, IV solution stable for 24 hrs at room temperature; 48 hrs if refrigerated. Recommend use within 8 hrs if stored at room temperature; 24 hrs if refrigerated. Do not use if particulate matter present or discoloration occurs.

PO/IV ADMINISTRATION

PO:

1. Food, milk do not affect GI absorption.
2. Space doses evenly around the clock.

IV:

1. Must dilute before administration.
2. Calculated dose added to D_5W to provide a concentration no greater than 4 mg/ml.
3. Infuse over 1 hr.

INDICATIONS/DOSAGE/ROUTES

HIV infection:
PO: Adults: 200 mg q8h or 300 mg q12h.

Usual dose for children:
PO: Children >3 mos: Initially, 180 mg/mm³ q6h up to 200 mg q6h.

Usual parenteral dosage:
IV: Adults, elderly: 1–2 mg/kg q4h around the clock.

Dosage adjustment:
Significant anemia w/o granulocytopenia may necessitate dose

interruption until some evidence of bone marrow recovery observed.

PRECAUTIONS

CONTRAINDICATIONS: Life-threatening allergies to zidovudine or components of preparation. CAUTIONS: Bone marrow compromise, renal and hepatic dysfunction, decreased hepatic blood flow. PREGNANCY/LACTATION: Unknown whether crosses placenta or is distributed in breast milk. Unknown whether fetal harm or effects on fertility can occur. **Pregnancy Category C**.

INTERACTIONS

DRUG INTERACTIONS: Bone marrow depressants, ganciclovir may increase myelosuppression. Clarithromycin may decrease concentrations. Probenecid may increase concentrations, risk of toxicity. **ALTERED LAB VALUES:** May increase mean corpuscular volume.

SIDE EFFECTS

COMMON: Headache, nausea, malaise. FREQUENT: Anorexia, dizziness. OCCASIONAL: Myopathy, diarrhea, abdominal pain, asthenia (loss of strength and energy), diarrhea, rash. RARE: Insomnia, constipation, paresthesia, dyspnea.

ADVERSE REACTIONS/TOXIC EFFECTS

Anemia (occurring most commonly after 4–6 wks of therapy) and granulocytopenia, particularly significant in those w/pretherapy low baselines, occur rarely. Nausea, vomiting, neurotoxicity (ataxia, fatigue, lethargy, nystagmus), seizures.

NURSING IMPLICATIONS

BASELINE ASSESSMENT:

Question history of allergy to zidovudine or components of

preparation. Avoid drugs that are nephrotoxic, cytotoxic, or myelosuppressive—may increase risk of toxicity. Obtain specimens for viral diagnostic tests before starting therapy (therapy may begin before results are obtained). Check hematology reports for accurate baseline.

INTERVENTION/EVALUATION:

Monitor hematology reports for anemia and granulocytopenia; check for bleeding. Assess for headache, dizziness. Determine pattern of bowel activity. Evaluate skin for acne or rash. Be alert to development of opportunistic infections, e.g., fever, chills, cough, myalgia. Assess food tolerance. Monitor I&O, renal and liver function tests. Check for insomnia.

PATIENT/FAMILY TEACHING:

Continue therapy for full length of treatment. Doses should be evenly spaced around the clock. Zidovudine does not cure AIDS or HIV disease, acts to reduce symptomatology and slow/arrest progress of disease. Avoid sexual activity; do not share needles (zidovudine does not prevent spread of infection). Do not take any medications w/o physician approval; even acetaminophen/aspirin may have serious consequence. Bleeding from gums, nose, or rectum may occur and should be reported to physician immediately. Blood counts are essential because of bleeding potential. Dental work should be done before therapy or after blood counts return to normal (often weeks after therapy has stopped). Report any new symptoms to physician.

zileuton
(Zyflo)
See Supplement
See Classification section under:
Bronchodilators

zinc acetate
(Galzin)
See Supplement

zolmitriptan
(Zomig)
See Supplement

zolpidem tartrate
zole-pih-dem
(Ambiem)

CLASSIFICATION

Sedative-hypnotic **(Schedule IV)**

AVAILABILITY (Rx)

Tablets: 5 mg, 10 mg

PHARMACOKINETICS

Rapidly absorbed from GI tract. Metabolized in liver; excreted in urine. Half-life: 1.4–4.5 hrs (increased in decreased liver function).

ACTION/*THERAPEUTIC EFFECT*

Enhances action of inhibitory neurotransmitter gamma-aminobutyric acid (GABA), *producing hypnotic effect due to CNS depression*. Interacts with GABA receptor, inducing sleep w/fewer nightly awakenings, improvement of sleep quality.

USES

Short-term treatment of insomnia. Reduces sleep-induction time, number of nocturnal awakenings; increases length of sleep, improvement of sleep quality.

PO ADMINISTRATION

1. Do not break/crush capsule form.

2. For faster sleep onset, do not give w/or immediately after a meal.

INDICATIONS/DOSAGE/ROUTES

Hypnotic:
PO: Adults: 10 mg at bedtime. **Elderly, debilitated:** 5 mg at bedtime.

PRECAUTIONS

CONTRAINDICATIONS: None significant. **CAUTIONS:** Impaired hepatic function. **PREGNANCY/LACTATION:** Unknown whether drug crosses placenta or is distributed in breast milk. **Pregnancy Category B**.

INTERACTIONS

DRUG INTERACTIONS: Potentiated effects when used w/other CNS depressants. **ALTERED LAB VALUES:** None significant.

SIDE EFFECTS

OCCASIONAL: Headache (7%). **RARE (<2%):** Drowsiness, dizziness, nausea, diarrhea, muscle pain.

ADVERSE REACTIONS/TOXIC EFFECTS

Overdosage may produce severe ataxia (clumsiness, unsteadiness), slow heartbeat, diplopia, altered vision, severe drowsiness, nausea, vomiting, difficulty breathing, unconsciousness. Abrupt withdrawal of drug after long-term use may produce weakness, facial flushing, sweating, vomiting, tremor. Tolerance/dependence may occur w/prolonged use of high doses.

NURSING IMPLICATIONS

BASELINE ASSESSMENT:

Assess B/P, pulse, respirations. Raise bed rails, provide call light. Provide environment conducive to sleep (back rub, quiet environment, low lighting).

INTERVENTION/EVALUATION:

Assess sleep pattern of pt. Evaluate for therapeutic response to insomnia: decrease in number of nocturnal awakenings, increase in length of sleep.

PATIENT/FAMILY TEACHING:

Do not abruptly withdraw medication following long-term use. Avoid alcohol, tasks that require alertness, motor skills until response to drug is established. Tolerance/dependence may occur w/prolonged use of high doses.

Drug Classification Contents

CLASSIFICATION

DRUG CLASSIFICATIONS

anesthetics: general

ACTION

Produces loss of consciousness and loss of response to all sensations including pain, touch, taste, temperature. General anesthetics can be classified as inhalation anesthetics and IV anesthetics. Inhalation anesthetics are further classified as gases and volatile liquids. IV anesthetics can be used alone or to supplement inhalation anesthetics. They decrease dosage of inhalation anesthetics and produce effects not achieved by inhalation anesthetics.

Ideally, an inhalation general anesthetic would produce unconsciousness, analgesia, muscle relaxation, and amnesia w/o side effects. Because no agent possesses all of these properties, medications are combined to achieve what inhalation anesthetics can't do alone and to reduce side effects. These medications include short-acting barbiturates (induce anesthesia), neuromuscular blocking agents (cause muscle relaxation), opioid analgesics, and nitrous oxide (provides analgesia).

Adjuncts to anesthesia are combined to enhance beneficial effects of inhalation anesthetics, reduce side effects and include:

Benzodiazepines: Reduce anxiety, enhance amnesia.
Barbiturates: Decrease anxiety, induce sedation.
Opioids: Relieve pain both preop and postop.
Anticholinergics: Decrease risk of bradycardia.
Antiemetics: Reduce nausea, vomiting.
Neuromuscular blocking agents: Cause skeletal muscle relaxation.

SIDE EFFECTS

Inhalation anesthetics: Respiratory cardiac depression (most pts require mechanical ventilation support). May increase sensitivity of heart to catecholamine stimulation (may cause dysrhythmias). Malignant hyperthermia (muscle rigidity, profound temperature increase). Aspiration of gastric fluid (may cause bronchospasm, pneumonia—prevented by use of endotracheal tube).

INTERACTIONS

Opioid analgesics may decrease the dose of inhalation anesthetic. CNS depressants may cause additive CNS depression. CNS stimulants may increase the dose of inhalation anesthetic.

NURSING IMPLICATIONS

Preop:
BASELINE ASSESSMENT: Obtain thorough history of drug use (drugs affecting cardiovascular, respiratory system may affect response to

anesthetics; accurate drug history may decrease risk of possible drug interactions), history of any disease of cardiovascular, respiratory system. Obtain baseline B/P, heart rate, respiratory rate. Ensure preop medications are administered 30–60 min before surgery.

Postop:
BASELINE ASSESSMENT: Obtain information about all medications pt received during surgery (anesthetics/adjunctive medication), which assists in anticipated time of emergence from anesthesia. EVALUATION/INTERVENTION: Position pt on side or w/head to side (decreases risk of aspiration). Monitor vital signs (B/P, pulse rate, respiratory rate) until recovery complete. Observe for cardiovascular, respiratory distress. Employ side rails or straps to prevent accidental falls. Assist in ambulation. Monitor bowel function, urine output. Assess need for opioid analgesics in management of postop pain. Assistance w/ambulation; another driver necessary upon discharge.

ANESTHETICS: GENERAL

GENERIC NAME	BRAND NAME(S)	CLASS	TYPE
desflurane	Suprane	Inhalation anesthetic	Volatile liquid
enflurane	Ethrane	Inhalation anesthetic	Volatile liquid
etomidate	Amidate	IV anesthetic	Hypnotic
halothane	Fluothane	Inhalation anesthetic	Volatile liquid
isoflurane	Forane	Inhalation anesthetic	Volatile liquid
ketamine	Ketalar	IV anesthetic	Miscellaneous
methohexital	Brevital	IV anesthetic	Barbiturate
methoxyflurane	Penthrane	Inhalation anesthetic	Volatile liquid
midazolam	Versed	IV anesthetic	Benzodiazepine
nitrous oxide	—	Inhalation anesthetic	Gas
propofol	Diprivan	IV anesthetic	Sedative-hypnotic
thiamylal	Surital	IV anesthetic	Barbiturate
thiopental	Pentothal	IV anesthetic	Barbiturate

anesthetics: local

ACTION

Blocks initiation and conduction of nerve impulses (decreases membrane permeability to sodium) that inhibit depolarization and action potential w/conduction blockade (occurs only in neurons located near site of administration). May also cause CNS depression and/or stimulation. May depress cardiac conduction, excitability and cause peripheral vasodilation. Does not cause generalized depression.

Local anesthetics can be classified based on their structure: esters or amides. Amide type have a lower incidence of allergic reaction and are metabolized by liver enzymes; esters are metabolized by enzymes in plasma.

USES

May be given topically (surface anesthesia) and by injection (local infiltration, peripheral nerve block [axillary], IV regional [Bier block], epidural, and spinal anesthesia).

Topical:

Applied to skin to relieve pain, itching, soreness to mucous membranes of nose, mouth, pharynx, larynx, trachea, bronchi, vagina, urethra.

Injection:

Local infiltration: Inject directly into tissue to be incised or stimulated mechanically.

Peripheral nerve block (axillary): Inject into/near nerves supplying surgical field, but at a site distant from surgical field.

LOCAL ANESTHETICS

GENERIC NAME	BRAND NAME(S)	TYPE	USES	ONSET	PEAK	DURATION
benzocaine	Many	Ester	Top: skin, mucous membrane	—	1 min	30–60 min
bupivacaine	Marcaine Sensorcaine	Amide	Infiltration Epidural Nerve block Spinal	5 min	—	2–4 hrs
butamben	Butesin	Ester	Top: skin	—	—	—
chloroprocaine	Nesacaine	Ester	Nerve block Epidural	6–12 min	—	15–30 min
cocaine		Ester	Top: mucous membrane	—	2–5 min	30–120 min
dibucaine	Nupercainal	Amide	Top: skin	—	<15 min	3–4 hrs
levobupivacaine	Chirocaine	Amide	Infiltration Epidural Nerve block	5 min	—	2–4 hrs
lidocaine	Xylocaine	Amide	Top: skin, mucous membrane Infiltration Nerve block	—	2–5 min	30–60 min
			IV regional Epidural Spinal	0.5–1 min	—	30–60 min
mepivacaine	Carbocaine Polocaine	Amide Infiltration	Nerve block Epidural	3–5 min	—	45–90 min
procaine	Novocain	Ester	Infiltration Nerve block	2–5 min	—	15–30 min
ropivacaine	Naropin	Amide	Epidural Nerve block Infiltration	10 min	—	2–4 hrs
tetracaine	Pontocaine	Ester	Top: skin	—	3–8 min	30–60 min
			Spinal	≤15 min	—	2–3 hrs

Top = topical.

IV regional (Bier block): Used to anesthetize limbs, injecting into distal vein of area or leg. Before administration, blood is removed from vein (apply Esmarch bandage) and tourniquet applied to limb, preventing anesthetic from entering general circulation. After administration, anesthetic diffuses from vasculature, becoming evenly distributed to all areas of occluded limb. After loosening of tourniquet, about 15–30% anesthetic is released into systemic circulation.

Epidural: Inject into epidural space (within spinal column outside dura mater). Diffusion across dura into subarachnoid space produces anesthesia of nerve roots and spinal cord.

Spinal: Inject into subarachnoid space (lumbar region below the termination of the cord).

PRECAUTIONS

CONTRAINDICATIONS: Hypersensitivity to local anesthetics. Pts w/complete heart block, severe hemorrhage, severe hypotension, shock. Local infection at site of lumbar puncture, septicemia. **CAUTIONS:** Pts w/cardiovascular function impairment, drug sensitivity. Inflammation and/or infection in region of injection. CNS disease, coagulation defects caused by anticoagulant therapy or hematologic disorders. With preparations containing a vasoconstrictor; pts w/cardiac disease, arrhythmias, hyperthyroidism, hypertension, or peripheral vascular disease.

INTERACTIONS

CNS depression–producing medications may cause additive depressant effect. Use vasoconstrictors (e.g., epinephrine) cautiously (if at all) when anesthetizing areas w/end arteries (e.g., toes, fingers).

SIDE EFFECTS

Allergic reactions ranging from dermatitis to anaphylaxis are more likely w/ester type. No cross-sensitivity between esters and amides. Cardiac depression (bradycardia, AV heart block, decreased contractility, and possibly cardiac arrest), peripheral vasodilation (may cause hypotension) can occur. CNS toxicity (stimulation followed by depression). Stimulation may cause convulsions. Depression may result in drowsiness, unconsciousness, even respiratory depression.

NURSING IMPLICATIONS

BASELINE ASSESSMENT: Resuscitative medication and equipment should be readily available. Inform pts they may experience temporary loss of sensation. **INTERVENTION/EVALUATION:** Monitor cardiovascular status, respirations, and state of consciousness closely during and after drug is administered. If ECG shows arrhythmias, prolongation of PR interval, QRS complex, inform physician immediately. Assess pulse for irregular rate, strength/weakness, bradycardia. Assess B/P for evidence of hypotension. **PATIENT/FAMILY TEACHING:** If medication used for dental procedure, avoid chewing solid foods or testing anesthetized site by biting or probing. Caution against activities that might cause unintentional harm.

CLASSIFICATION

angiotensin-converting enzyme (ACE) inhibitors

ACTION

Suppresses renin-angiotensin-aldosterone system (prevents conversion of angiotensin I to angiotensin II, a potent vasoconstrictor).

Hypertension: Inhibits activity of angiotensin I converting enzyme. Decreases conversion of angiotensin I to angiotensin II, a potent vasoconstrictor. Results in increase in plasma renin activity and decreased aldosterone secretion. Reduces peripheral vascular resistance.

CHF: Decreases peripheral vascular resistance (afterload), pulmonary capillary wedge pressure (preload), pulmonary vascular resistance. Increases cardiac output, exercise tolerance.

USES

Treatment of hypertension alone or in combination w/other antihypertensives. Adjunctive therapy for CHF (in combination w/cardiac glycosides, diuretics).

PRECAUTIONS

CONTRAINDICATIONS: History of angioedema w/previous treatment w/ACE inhibitors. **CAUTIONS:** Renal impairment, those w/sodium depletion or on diuretic therapy, dialysis, hypovolemia, coronary or cerebrovascular insufficiency. Safety in pregnancy/lactation not established.

INTERACTIONS

May increase lithium concentrations, toxicity. Hyperkalemia may occur w/potassium-sparing diuretics, potassium supplements, or potassium-containing salt substitutes. Alcohol, diuretics, hypotensive agents may increase antihypertensive effect. NSAIDs, aspirin may decrease hypotensive effect.

SIDE EFFECTS

Rash and/or urticaria, change or decrease in sense of taste, orthostatic hypotension during initial therapy. Urinary frequency. Cough, proteinuria (mostly occurs in those w/history of renal disease), dry mouth, GI distress, headache, dizziness.

TOXIC EFFECTS/ADVERSE REACTIONS

Excessive hypotension ("first-dose syncope") may occur in those w/CHF, severely salt/volume depleted. Angioedema (swelling of face/lips), hyperkalemia occur rarely. Agranulocytosis, neutropenia may be noted in those w/impaired renal function or collagen vascular disease (systemic lupus erythematosus, scleroderma). Nephrotic syndrome may be noted in those w/history of renal disease.

NURSING IMPLICATIONS

GENERAL: Use cardiac monitor for IV administration and preferably for initiation of oral therapy. BASELINE ASSESSMENT: Initial B/P, apical pulse. INTERVENTION/EVALUATION: Monitor B/P and apical pulse before giving drug and p.r.n.; notify physician before administration if B/P or pulse is not within agreed parameters. If excessive hypotension, place pt in supine position w/legs elevated. Assess extremities for edema; weigh daily; check lungs for rales. Monitor I&O. Check lab results, esp. electrolytes and drug levels. Monitor frequency, consistency of stools; prevent constipation. PATIENT/FAMILY TEACHING: Teach how to take B/P, pulse correctly. Change position slowly to prevent orthostatic hypotension. Do not take OTC cold preparations, nasal decongestants w/o consulting physician. Restrict sodium and alcohol as ordered. Do not skip dose or stop taking medication; rebound hypertension may occur.

ACE INHIBITORS

GENERIC NAME	BRAND NAME(S)	USE	DECREASE B/P ONSET (HRS)	DURATION (HRS)	RTE ADM	DOSAGE RANGE (MG/DAY)
benazepril	Lotensin	Hypertension	1	24	PO	20–80
captopril	Capoten	Hypertension	0.25	(dose related)	PO	50–450
		CHF				12.5–450
enalapril	Vasotec	Hypertension	1	24	PO	10–40
		CHF			IV	5–20
					PO	5–20
fosinopril	Monopril	Hypertension	1	24	PO	20–80
		CHF			PO	5–40
lisinopril	Prinivil	Hypertension	1	24	PO	20–40
	Zestril	CHF			PO	5–20
moexipril	Univasc	Hypertension	1	24	PO	7.5–30
perindopril	Aceon	Hypertension	1	24	PO	2–8
quinapril	Accupril	Hypertension	1	24	PO	20–80
		CHF				
ramipril	Altace	Hypertension	1	24	PO	2.5–20
		CHF			PO	1.25–5
trandolapril	Mavik	Hypertension	1	24	PO	1–4

antacids

ACTION

Act primarily in stomach to neutralize gastric acid (increase pH). The ability to increase pH depends on dose, dosage form used, presence or absence of food in stomach, and acid neutralizing capacity (ANC). ANC is the number of mEq of hydrochloric acid that can be neutralized by a particular weight or volume of antacid. There are 4 major groups of antacids: (1) aluminum compounds, (2) magnesium compounds, (3) sodium compounds, and (4) calcium compounds.

USES

Symptomatic relief of heartburn, acid indigestion; treatment of peptic ulcer disease, prevention of aspiration pneumonia before anesthesia, prophylaxis vs. stress ulceration; symptomatic relief of gastroesophageal reflux disease (GERD), gastritis, hiatal hernia. In addition, aluminum carbonate used for hyperphosphatemia; calcium carbonate for calcium deficiency states; and magnesium oxide for magnesium deficiency states.

PRECAUTIONS

CONTRAINDICATIONS: Sensitivity to any components, first trimester of pregnancy, renal dysfunction, young children. **CAUTIONS:** Specific selection of antacid should consider preexisting bowel status, components (e.g., sodium) in relation to other medical conditions. Administer with care in elderly.

INTERACTIONS

Antacids may interact with medication by increasing gastric pH (affects absorption), absorbing or binding to medications, or increasing urinary pH (affects rate of elimination). Interactions may be prevented by avoiding concurrent use and taking antacids 2 hrs before or after ingestion of other medications.

SIDE EFFECTS

Diarrhea or constipation, depending on specific drug administered.

TOXIC EFFECTS/ADVERSE REACTIONS

Aluminum compounds in large amounts may cause severe constipation, hypophosphatemia, and osteomalacia. Magnesium compounds may cause hypermagnesemia and profound diarrhea. Calcium antacids may cause acid rebound, alkalosis, and renal calculi. W/sodium compounds, risk of systemic alkalosis, sodium overload with retention, and rebound hypersecretion.

NURSING IMPLICATIONS

GENERAL: Avoid sodium-based compounds for pts on low sodium diets; calcium or magnesium compounds for pts with renal impairment. Do not give other oral medication within 1–2 hrs of antacid administration. **INTERVENTION/EVALUATION:** Monitor stools for diarrhea or constipation. Assess for relief of gastric distress. **PATIENT/FAMILY TEACHING:** For best results, take 1–3 hrs after meals. Chewable tablets should be chewed thoroughly before swallowing (may be followed by water or milk). Maintain adequate fluid intake. Eat small, frequent meals free of coffee and other caffeine products. Avoid alcohol.

ANTACIDS

BRAND NAME	ACTIVE INGREDIENT			OTHER	SODIUM CONTENT (MEQ/5 ML)	ANC
	AL(OH)₂ (MG)	MG(OH)₂ (MG)	CACO₃ (MG)			

BRAND NAME	$Al(OH)_2$ (MG)	$Mg(OH)_2$ (MG)	$CaCO_3$ (MG)	OTHER	SODIUM CONTENT (MEQ/5 ML)	ANC
Amphojel	320	—	—	—	<2.3	10
Alternagel	600	—	—	Simethicone	<2.5	16
Dialume	500	—	—	—	<1.2	10
Gelusil	200	200	—	Simethicone	0.7	12
Maalox	225	200	—	—	1.4	13.3
Maalox TC	600	300	—	Sorbitol	0.8	27.2
Mag-Ox 400	—	400	—	—	—	—
MOM	—	390	—	—	0.12	14
Mylanta	200	200	—	Simethicone	0.68	12.7
Mylanta II	400	400	—	Simethicone	1.14	25.4
Riopan Plus	—	—	—	Magaldrate Simethicone	<0.1	15
Tums	—	—	500	—	<2.0	10

ANC = acid neutralizing capacity.

antianxiety

ACTION

Benzodiazepines are the largest and most frequently prescribed group of antianxiety agents. Exact mechanism unknown; may increase the inhibiting effect of gamma-aminobutyric acid (GABA) (inhibiting nerve impulse transmission) as well as other inhibitory transmitters by binding to specific benzodiazepine receptors in various areas of the CNS.

USES

Treatment of anxiety. Additionally, some benzodiazepines are used as hypnotics, anticonvulsants to prevent delirium tremors during alcohol withdrawal and as adjunctive therapy for relaxation of skeletal muscle spasms. Midazolam, a short-acting injectable form, is used for preop sedation, relieving anxiety for short diagnostic endoscopic procedures.

PRECAUTIONS

CONTRAINDICATIONS: Hypersensitivity, renal or hepatic dysfunction, CNS depression, history of drug abuse, pregnancy, glaucoma, lactation, young children, within 14 days of MAO inhibitors, myasthenia gravis. **CAUTION:** Elderly or debilitated, pts w/COPD. Drugs should be withdrawn slowly.

INTERACTIONS

CNS depressants (e.g., alcohol, barbiturates, narcotics) may increase CNS effects of benzodiazepines (e.g., sedation).

CLASSIFICATION

ANTIANXIETY

GENERIC NAME	BRAND NAME(S)	USES	DOSAGE RANGE (MG/DAY)
alprazolam	Xanax	Anxiety Panic disorder	PO: 0.75–4
chlordiazepoxide	Librium Libritabs	Anxiety Alcohol withdrawal Preop	PO: 15–100
clonazepam	Klonopin	Anticonvulsant	PO: 1.5–20
clorazepate	Tranxene	Anxiety Alcohol withdrawal	PO: 15–60
diazepam	Valium	Anxiety Alcohol withdrawal Anticonvulsant Muscle relaxant	PO: 4–40
lorazepam	Ativan	Anxiety Preanesthetic	PO: 2–4
oxazepam	Serax	Anxiety	PO: 30–120

Dosage: oral.

SIDE EFFECTS

Drowsiness is the most common side effect; usually disappears w/continued use. Dizziness, hypotension occur frequently.

TOXIC EFFECTS/ADVERSE REACTIONS

Incidence of toxicity is very low when antianxiety drugs are taken alone. Confusion, hypersensitivity reactions, headache, stupor, paradoxical excitement, nausea and vomiting, blood dyscrasias, jaundice (hepatic dysfunction) are rare effects. These vary according to individual drug. IV administration may cause respiratory depression, apnea.

NURSING IMPLICATIONS

GENERAL: Provide restful environment and measures for comfort. Comply w/federal narcotic laws regarding Schedule IV drugs. Consider potential for abuse/dependence. For IV administration, have respiratory equipment available; keep pt recumbent. Most antianxiety drugs should not be mixed w/other drugs in a syringe. INTERVENTION/EVALUATION: Monitor B/P. Assess for therapeutic response (according to reason for use, e.g., seizure activity, anxiety, alcohol withdrawal) or paradoxical reaction. Take safety precautions for drowsiness, dizziness. PATIENT/FAMILY TEACHING: Avoid smoking; may interfere w/drug action. Do not drive or perform tasks requiring mental acuity until response to medication is controlled. Consult physician before taking other medications. Do not take alcohol. Medication must not be stopped abruptly. Inform other physicians, dentist of drug therapy.

antiarrhythmics

ACTION

Antiarrhythmics are classified according to electrophysiologic effects they produce and/or their presumed mechanism of action.

Class IA: Inhibit inward sodium current, depress phase 0 depolarization, slow conduction velocity in myocardial Purkinje fibers.

Class IB: Inhibit inward sodium current, slight change phase 0 depolarization/slows conduction velocity in Purkinje system. Effects markedly intensified when membrane depolarized or frequency of excitation is increased. Hastens repolarization.

Class IC: Marked depression phase 0, slowing impulse conduction, suppressing inward sodium current and spontaneous ventricular premature complexes.

Class II: Depress phase IV depolarization; block excessive sympathetic activity.

Class III: Prolong action potential duration and refractoriness in Purkinje and ventricular muscle fibers.

Class IV: Depress Ca^{+2}-dependent action potentials, slow conduction in AV node.

Digoxin: Decreases maximal diastolic potential and action potential duration.

Adenosine: Slows conduction time through AV node; may interrupt reentry pathways through AV node.

USES

Prevention and treatment of cardiac arrhythmias, such as premature ventricular contractions, ventricular tachycardia, premature atrial contractions, paroxysmal atrial tachycardia, atrial fibrillation and flutter.

PRECAUTIONS

CONTRAINDICATIONS: Hypersensitivity, pregnancy, lactation, children, severe bradycardia, second- or third-degree AV block, severe CHF, aortic stenosis, hypotension, cardiogenic shock, hepatic or renal dysfunction. **CAUTIONS:** Elderly generally require lowered dosage. Administer w/caution to pts w/diabetes mellitus, acute myocardial infarctions, and liver dysfunction. Have emergency cart readily available when administering agents through IV.

INTERACTIONS

Interactions are specific to each agent, which should be noted before administration. Refer to individual monographs.

SIDE EFFECTS

Hypotension, bradycardia, drowsiness, lightheadedness. Other side effects are specific to individual drug.

CLASSIFICATION

ANTIARRHYTHMICS

GENERIC NAME	BRAND NAME(S)	CLASS	ONSET	DURATION	DOSAGE RANGE
acebutolol*	Sectral	II	—	24–30 hrs	600–1,200 mg/day
adenosine	Adenocard		34 sec	1–2 min	IV: 6 mg, MR w/12 mg at 1–2 min intervals
amiodarone	Cordarone	III	1–3 wks	—	Initial: 800–1,600 mg/day for 1–3 wks Maintenance: 600–800 mg/day
bretylium	Bretylol	III	—	6–8 hrs	IV: 1–2 mg/min
digoxin*	Lanoxin		0.5–2 hrs	>24 hrs	0.125–0.375 mg/day
disopyramide	Norpace Norpace SR	IA	0.5 hr	6–7 hrs	400–800 mg/day
dofetilide	Tikosyn	III	—	—	PO: 250–1,000 mcg/day
esmolol*	Brevibloc	II	<5 min	Short	IV: 50–200 mcg/kg/min
flecainide	Tambocor	IC	—	—	200–400 mg/day
ibutilide	Corvert	III	—	—	IV: >60 kg: 1 mg over 10 min <60 kg: 0.01 mg/kg
lidocaine	Xylocaine	IB	—	0.25 hr	IV: 50–100 mg bolus, 1–4 mg/ min infusion
mexiletine	Mexitil	IB	0.5–2 hrs	8–12 hrs	600–1,200 mg/day
moricizine	Ethmozine	IA	2 hrs	10–24 hrs	600–900 mg/day
phenytoin*	Dilantin	IB	0.5–1 hr	>24 hrs	IV: 100–1,000 mg PO: 100 mg q6–12h
procainamide	Pronestyl Procan SR	IA	0.5 hr	>3 hrs 6 hrs	PO: 250–500 mg q3h SR: 250–750 mg q6h
propafenone	Rhythmol	IC	—	—	450–900 mg/day
propranolol*	Inderal	II	0.5 hr	3–5 hrs	10–30 mg 3–4x/day
quinidine	Cardioquin Quinaglute Quinidex	IA	0.5 hr	6–8 hrs 8–12 hrs	PO: 200–600 mg q2–4h SR: 300–600 mg q8h
sotalol*	Betapace	III	—	—	160–640 mg/day
tocainide	Tonocard	IB	1–2 hrs	8–12 hrs	1,200–1,800 mg/day
verapamil*	Calan Isoptin	IV	0.5 hr	6 hrs	IV: 5–10 mg

*These agents are also discussed w/other classifications.

TOXIC EFFECTS/ADVERSE REACTIONS

Visual disturbances, tinnitus or difficulty hearing, vomiting, constipation or diarrhea, headache, confusion, diaphoresis, anginal attack, rapid rhythm, cardiac arrest. Other signs specific to each drug.

NURSING IMPLICATIONS

GENERAL: Use cardiac monitor for IV administration and preferably for initiation of oral therapy. BASELINE ASSESSMENT: Initial B/P, apical pulse. INTERVENTION/EVALUATION: Monitor B/P and apical pulse before giving drug and p.r.n.; notify physician before administration if B/P or pulse is not within agreed parameters. Assess extremities for edema; weigh daily; check lungs for rales. Monitor I&O. Check lab results, esp. electrolytes and drug levels. Monitor frequency, consistency of stools; prevent constipation. PATIENT/FAMILY TEACHING: Teach how to take pulse correctly. Change position slowly to prevent ortho-static hypotension. Do not take other medications, including OTC, w/o consulting physician. Restrict sodium and alcohol as ordered.

antibiotics

ACTION

Antibiotics (antimicrobial agents) are natural or synthetic compounds that have the ability to kill or suppress the growth of microorganisms. Narrow-spectrum agents are effective against few microorganisms, whereas broad-spectrum agents are effective against a wide variety. Antimicrobial agents may also be classified based on their mechanism of action.

1. Agents that inhibit cell wall synthesis or activate enzymes that disrupt cell wall, causing a weakening in the cell wall, cell lysis, and death. Includes penicillins, cephalosporins, vancomycin, and imidazole antifungal agents.

2. Agents that act directly on cell wall, affecting permeability of cell membranes, causing leakage of intracellular substances. Includes antifungal agents amphotericin and nystatin, polymixin, and colistin.

3. Agents that bind to ribosomal subunits, altering protein synthesis and eventually causing cell death. Includes aminoglycosides.

4. Agents that affect bacterial ribosome function, altering protein synthesis and causing slow microbial growth. Does not cause cell death. Includes chloramphenicol, clindamycin, erythromycin, tetracyclines.

5. Agents that inhibit nucleic acid metabolism by binding to nucleic acid or interacting with enzymes necessary for nucleic acid synthesis. Inhibits DNA or RNA synthesis. Includes rifampin, metronidazole, quinolones (e.g., ciprofloxacin).

6. Agents that inhibit specific metabolic steps necessary for microorganisms, causing a decrease in essential cell components or synthesis of nonfunctional analogues of normal metabolites. Includes trimethoprim and sulfonamides.

7. Agents that inhibit viral DNA synthesis by binding to viral enzymes necessary for DNA synthesis, preventing viral replication. Includes acyclovir, vidarabine.

SELECTION OF ANTIMICROBIAL AGENTS

Goal of therapy is to produce a favorable therapeutic result by achieving antimicrobial action at the site of infection sufficient to inhibit the growth of the microorganism. The agent selected should be the most active against the most likely infecting organism, least likely to cause toxicity or allergic reaction. Factors to consider in selection of an antimicrobial agent include:

1. Sensitivity pattern of the infecting microorganism.

2. Location and severity of infection (may determine the route of administration).

3. Pt's ability to eliminate the drug (status of renal and liver function).

4. Pt's defense mechanisms (includes both cellular and humoral immunity).

5. Pt's age, pregnancy, genetic factors, allergy, disorder of CNS, pre-existing medical problems.

USES

Treatment of wide range of gram-positive or gram-negative bacterial infections; suppression of intestinal flora before surgery; control of acne; prophylactically to prevent rheumatic fever; prophylactically in high-risk situations (e.g., some surgical procedures or medical states) to prevent bacterial infection.

PRECAUTIONS

CONTRAINDICATIONS: Hypersensitivity to prescribed antibiotics, others in its family, or components of the drug. Some antibiotics are contraindicated in infants and children (e.g., tetracyclines, quinolones). **EXTREME CAUTION:** Pregnancy and lactation (avoid unless benefits clearly outweigh risks). **CAUTIONS:** Renal or hepatic dysfunction. Elderly and very young may be more sensitive to effects of these drugs and may require adjusted dosage. Extra care w/gastrointestinal diseases and bleeding disorders.

INTERACTIONS

Concurrent use w/other antibiotics or drugs that add to or potentiate toxic effects is to be avoided. Alcohol should not be taken w/antibiotics; several may interact w/alcohol to produce a disulfiram reaction. Antacids should be administered 2 hrs before or after oral antibiotics to prevent interference w/absorption. Refer to specific classification pages or individual monographs.

SIDE EFFECTS

Side effects most commonly associated w/antibiotics are anorexia, nausea, vomiting, and diarrhea. Some, such as tetracyclines, produce photosensitivity. Refer to individual monographs.

TOXIC EFFECTS/ADVERSE REACTIONS

Skin rash, seen most often w/penicillins and cephalosporins, is a sign of hypersensitivity. Sensitivity reactions may range from mild rash to anaphylaxis. Superinfections may result from alteration of bacterial environment. Ototoxicity and nephrotoxicity are potential adverse reactions of a number of antibiotics, esp. the aminoglycosides. Tetracyclines combine w/calcium in forming teeth and may produce discoloration. Severe diarrhea, antibiotic-associated colitis have occurred from several of the antimicrobials (clindamycin has a particular risk for this reaction).

NURSING IMPLICATIONS

GENERAL: Administer drugs on schedule to maintain blood levels.

Initiate IV solutions slowly w/close observation for sensitivity response. BASELINE ASSESSMENT: Question for history of previous drug reaction. Culture/sensitivity must be done before first dose (may give before results are obtained). Assess WBC results, temperature, pulse, respiration. INTERVENTION/EVALUATION: Monitor lab results, particularly WBC and culture/sensitivity reports. Assess for adverse reactions. PATIENT/FAMILY TEACHING: Space doses evenly. Continue therapy for full duration. Avoid alcohol, antacids, or other medication w/o consulting physician. Notify physician of diarrhea, rash, or other new symptom.

antibiotic: aminoglycosides

ACTION

Bactericidal. Transported across bacterial cell membrane, irreversibly binds to specific receptor proteins of bacterial ribosomes. Interferes w/protein synthesis, preventing cell reproduction and eventually causing cell death.

USES

Treatment of serious infections when other, less toxic agents are not effective, are contraindicated, or require adjunctive therapy (e.g., w/penicillins or cephalosporins). Used primarily in the treatment of infections caused by gram-negative microorganisms, such as those caused by *Proteus, Klebsiella, Pseudomonas, Escherichia coli, Serratia,* and *Enterobacter.* Inactive against most gram-positive microorganisms. Not well absorbed systemically from GI tract (must be administered parenterally for systemic infections). Oral agents are given to suppress intestinal bacteria.

PRECAUTIONS

CONTRAINDICATIONS: Hypersensitivity to any of the aminoglycosides; pregnancy/lactation. Not to be given orally to pts w/bowel obstruction. **CAUTIONS:** Elderly, infants, and children. Those w/dehydration or renal dysfunction must be monitored very closely. Use for pts w/Parkinson's disease or myasthenia gravis may result in further muscle weakness.

INTERACTIONS

Other aminoglycosides, nephrotoxic, ototoxic-producing medications may increase toxicity. May increase effects of neuromuscular blocking agents.

SIDE EFFECTS

Nausea or diarrhea w/oral administration. Headache, increased salivation, anorexia. Photosensitivity when administered topically.

CLASSIFICATION

AMINOGLYCOSIDES

GENERIC NAME	BRAND NAME(S)	RTE ADM	BLOOD LEVELS		DOSAGE RANGE*
			PEAK (MCG/ML)	TROUGH (MCG/ML)	
amikacin	Amikin	IM, IV	15–30	5–10	Adults: 15 mg/kg/day Children: 15 mg/kg/day
gentamicin	Garamycin Jenamicin	IM, IV, Topical Ophthalmic	4–10	1–2	Adults: 3–5 mg/kg/day Children: 6–7.5 mg/kg/day
kanamycin	Kantrex Klebcil	PO, Irrigation	—	—	PO: 8–12 g/day
neomycin	Mycifradin Neobiotic	PO, Topical Ophthalmic			PO: 1 g × 3 dose preop
netilmicin	Netromycin	IM, IV	6–12	0.5–2	Adults: 3–6.5 mg/kg/day Children: 5.5–8 mg/kg/day
streptomycin	Streptomycin	IM	—	—	Adults: 15 mg/kg/day; maximum: 1 g Children: 20–40 mg/kg/day; maximum: 1 g
tobramycin	Nebcin	IM, IV, Ophthalmic	4–10	1–2	Adults: 3–5 mg/kg/day Children: 6–7.5 mg/kg/day

*Dosage, interval based on serum drug concentration.

TOXIC EFFECTS/ADVERSE REACTIONS

Serious toxicity, primarily ototoxicity and nephrotoxicity, is a major factor in limiting the usefulness of the aminoglycosides. Ototoxicity is suggested by dizziness, vertigo, tinnitus, hearing loss. Nephrotoxicity may be signaled by proteinuria, increased BUN, oliguria. Neuromuscular blockade can occur w/high doses, resulting in weakness, shortness of breath, and even respiratory paralysis. Hypersensitivity reactions may occur. Note also that systemic effects may result from wound irrigation or topical application.

NURSING IMPLICATIONS

GENERAL: Administer on schedule to maintain blood levels. Initiate IV solutions slowly at first w/close observation for sensitivity response. BASELINE ASSESSMENT: Inquire about previous reactions to aminoglycosides. Culture/sensitivity must be done before first dose (may give before results are known). Assess WBC results, temperature, pulse, respiration. INTERVENTION/EVALUATION: Maintain good hydration and I&O. Monitor plasma concentration levels (peak and trough values) to determine continued dosage. Check WBC and culture/sensitivity results. Assess temperature, pulse, respiration, esp. rate, depth, and ease of respirations. Be alert for adverse reactions: ototoxicity, nephrotoxicity, neuromuscular blockade, allergic reaction. PATIENT/FAMILY TEACHING: Space doses evenly. Continue therapy for full duration. Avoid taking even OTC medications w/o physician direction. Notify physician in event of any hearing, visual, balance, urinary problems even after therapy is completed.

antibiotic: cephalosporins

ACTION

Cephalosporins inhibit cell wall synthesis or activate enzymes that disrupt cell wall, causing a weakening in the cell wall, cell lysis, and cell death. May be bacteriostatic or bactericidal. Most effective against rapidly dividing cells.

USES

Broad-spectrum antibiotics, which, like penicillins, may be used in a number of diseases including respiratory diseases, skin and soft tissue infection, bone/joint infections, genitourinary infections, prophylactically in some surgical procedures.

First generation cephalosporins have good activity against gram-positive organisms and moderate activity against gram-negative organisms including *Escherichia coli, Klebsiella pneumoniae, Proteus mirabilis.*

Second generation cephalosporins have increased activity against gram-negative organisms.

Third generation cephalosporins are less active against gram-positive organisms but more active against the Enterobacteriaceae w/some activity against *Pseudomonas aeruginosa.*

Fourth generation cephalosporins have good activity against gram-positive organisms (e.g., *Staphylococcus aureus*) and gram-negative organisms (e.g., *Pseudomonas aeruginosa*).

PRECAUTIONS

CONTRAINDICATIONS: Hypersensitivity to cephalosporins or penicillins. **CAUTION:** Careful monitoring is essential in bleeding disorders, gastrointestinal disease, renal and hepatic dysfunction. See individual monographs for pregnancy/lactation precautions.

INTERACTIONS

Interaction between alcohol and some of the cephalosporins (e.g., cefamandole, cefoperazone, cefotetan) may cause buildup of acetaldehyde in the blood w/disulfiramlike reaction: headache, palpitations, chest pain, hypotension, nausea, vomiting, and abdominal pain. Alcohol in any form is to be avoided up to 72 hours after drug administration. Bacteriostatic drugs may decrease effects of cephalosporins. Probenecid increases blood levels; aminoglycosides and several diuretics may increase risk of renal toxicity. Cefamandole, cefoperazone, cefotetan may increase hypoprothrombinemic effect of oral anticoagulants.

CLASSIFICATION

CEPHALOSPORINS

GENERIC NAME	BRAND NAME(S)	GENERATION	RTE ADMIN	DOSAGE RANGE
cefaclor	Ceclor	Second	PO	Adults: 250–500 mg q8h Children: 20–40 mg/kg/day
cefadroxil	Duricef Ultracef	First	PO	Adults: 1–2 g/day Children: 30 mg/kg/day
cefamandole	Mandol	Second	IM, IV	Adults: 1.5–12 g/day Children: 50–150 mg/kg/day
cefazolin	Ancef Kefzol Zolicef	First	IM, IV	Adults: 0.75–6 g/day Children: 25–100 mg/kg/day
cefdinir	Omnicef	Third	PO	Adults: 600 mg/day Children: 14 mg/kg/day
cefepime	Maxipime	Fourth	IM, IV	Adults: 1–6 g/day
cefixime	Suprax	Third	PO	Adults: 400 mg/day Children: 8 mg/kg/day
cefmetazole	Zefazone	Second	IM, IV	Adults: 4–8 g/day
cefonicid	Monocid	Second	IM, IV	Adults: 1–2 g/day
cefoperazone	Cefobid	Third	IM, IV	Adults: 2–12 g/day
cefotaxime	Claforan	Third	IM, IV	Adults: 2–12 g/day Children: 100–200 mg/kg/day
cefotetan	Cefotan	Second	IM, IV	Adults: 1–6 g/day
cefoxitin	Mefoxin	Second	IM, IV	Adults: 3–12 g/day Children: 80–160 mg/kg/day
cefpodoxime	Vantin	Second	PO	Adults: 200–800 mg/day Children: 10 mg/kg/day
cefprozil	Cefzil	Second	PO	Adults: 0.5–1 g/day Children: 30 mg/kg/day
ceftazidime	Fortaz Tazicef Tazidime	Third	IM, IV	Adults: 0.5–6 g/day Children: 90–150 mg/kg/day
ceftibuten	Cedax	Third	PO	Adults: 400 mg/day Children: 9 mg/kg/day
ceftizoxime	Cefizox	Third	IM, IV	Adults: 1–12 g/day Children: 150–200 mg/kg/day
ceftriaxone	Rocephin	Third	IM, IV	Adults: 1–4 g/day Children: 50–100 mg/kg/day
cefuroxime	Ceftin Kefurox Zinacef	Second	PO, IM, IV	Adults(PO): 0.25–1 g/day Adults (IM, IV): 2.25–9 g/day Children (PO): 250–500 mg/day Children (IM, IV): 50–100 mg/kg/day
cephalexin	Keftab Keflet	First	PO	Adults: 1–4 g/day Children: 25–100 mg/kg/day
cephalothin	Keflin Seffin	First	IM, IV	Adults: 2–12 g/day Children: 80–160 mg/kg/day
loracarbef	Lorabid	Second	PO	Adults: 200–800 mg/day Children: 15–30 mg/kg/day

SIDE EFFECTS

Mild nausea, vomiting, or diarrhea, esp. w/oral administration.

TOXIC EFFECTS/ADVERSE REACTIONS

Hypersensitivity reactions, particularly skin rash, may progress to anaphylaxis; superinfections, including antibiotic-associated colitis. Hypoprothrombinemia and thrombocytopenia may occur w/potential for hemorrhage. Nephrotoxicity may occur, esp. w/high dosages.

NURSING IMPLICATIONS

GENERAL: Administer on schedule to maintain blood levels. Initiate IV solutions slowly at first w/close observation for sensitivity response. BASELINE ASSESSMENT: Inquire about previous reactions to cephalosporins, penicillins. W/history of penicillin allergy, have emergency equipment, medications available. Culture/sensitivity must be done before first dose (may give before results are known). Assess WBC results, temperature, pulse, respiration. INTERVENTION/ASSESSMENT: Monitor WBC results, temperature, pulse, respiration. Assess for adverse reactions, esp. allergic reaction, superinfections including antibiotic-associated colitis. PATIENT/FAMILY TEACHING: Space doses evenly. Continue therapy for full duration. Avoid alcohol, antacids, or other medications w/o consulting physician. Notify physician promptly of rash or diarrhea.

antibiotic: fluoroquinolones

The fluoroquinolones include ciprofloxacin, enoxacin, levofloxacin, lomefloxacin, norfloxacin, ofloxacin, and sparfloxacin.

ACTION

Bactericidal. Inhibits DNA gyrase in susceptible microorganisms, interfering w/bacterial DNA replication and repair.

USES

Fluoroquinolones have activity against a wide range of gram-negative and gram-positive organisms. Ciprofloxacin, levofloxacin, ofloxacin, and sparfloxacin are used primarily in the treatment of lower respiratory infections, skin/skin structure, UTIs, and sexually transmitted diseases; enoxacin, lomefloxacin, and norfloxacin are used primarily in the treatment of UTIs. Ciprofloxacin, norfloxacin, and ofloxacin are also available in ophthalmic forms for treating ophthalmic infections.

PRECAUTIONS

CONTRAINDICATIONS: Hypersensitivity to fluoroquinolones or quinolone group of antibacterial agents. Do not use in children <18 yrs of age. *Ophthalmic:* vaccinia, varicella, epithelial herpes simplex, keratitis, mycobacterial infection, fungal disease of ocular structure. CAUTIONS: Concurrent theophylline or caffeine use. Pts w/CNS disorder or other factors that increase risk of seizures. Renal impairment (alterations in dosage is necessary).

INTERACTIONS

Antacids, iron preparations, sucralfate may decrease absorption. De-

CLASSIFICATION

creases clearance, may increase concentration, toxicity of theophylline. May increase effects of oral anticoagulants.

SIDE EFFECTS

FREQUENT: *Systemic:* Dizziness, lightheadedness, headache, insomnia/drowsiness, nausea, vomiting, diarrhea, stomach pain or discomfort. *Ophthalmic:* Burning, crusting in corner of eye. **OCCASIONAL:** *Systemic:* Increased sensitivity of skin to sunlight. *Ophthalmic:* Bad taste, sense of something in eye, redness of eyelids, itching eye. **RARE:** *Systemic:* Confusion, tremors, hallucinations, hypersensitivity reaction, interstitial nephritis, pain at injection site. May cause inflamed/ruptured tendons. *Ophthalmic:* Swelling of eyelid, increased sensitivity of eye to light, tearing.

TOXIC EFFECTS/ADVERSE REACTIONS

Superinfection, severe hypersensitivity reaction occur rarely. Arthropathy (joint disease w/swelling, pain, clubbing of fingers and toes, degeneration of stress-bearing portion of a joint) may occur if given to children <18 yrs. *Ophthalmic:* Sensitization may contraindicate later systemic use of fluoroquinolones.

ANTIBIOTIC: FLUOROQUINOLONES

GENERIC NAME	BRAND NAME(S)	USUAL DAILY DOSAGE
ciprofloxacin	Cipro	PO: Adults, elderly: 250–750 mg q12h
		IV: Adults, elderly: 200–400 mg q12h
	Ciloxan	Ophthalmic: Adults, elderly: 1–2 drops 4–6 times/day
enoxacin	Penetrex	PO: Adults, elderly: 200–400 mg q12h
gatifloxacin	Tequin	IV/PO: Adults, elderly: 200–400 mg/day
levofloxacin	Levaquin	PO: Adults, elderly: 250–500 mg as single daily dose
		IV: Adults, elderly: 250–500 mg as single daily dose
lomefloxacin	Maxaquin	PO: Adults, elderly: 400 mg q24h
moxifloxacin	Avelox	PO: Adults, elderly: 400 mg/day
norfloxacin	Noroxin	PO: Adults, elderly: 400 mg q12h
	Chibroxin	Ophthalmic: Adults, elderly: 1–2 drops 4 times/day
ofloxacin	Floxin	PO: Adults, elderly: 200–400 mg q12h
		IV: Adults, elderly: 200–400 mg q12h
	Ocuflox	Ophthalmic: Adults, elderly: 1–2 drops 4–6 times/day
sparfloxacin	Zagam	PO: Adults, elderly: 400 mg once, then 200 mg daily
trovafloxacin	Trovan	IV/PO: Adults: 100–300 mg/day

NURSING IMPLICATIONS

GENERAL: Administer on schedule to maintain blood levels. Initiate IV solutions slowly at first w/close observation for sensitivity response. **BASELINE ASSESSMENT:** Inquire about previous reactions to fluoroquinolones. Culture/sensitivity must be done before first dose (may give before results are known). Assess WBC results, temperature, pulse, respiration. **INTERVENTION/EVALUATION:** Maintain good hydration and I&O. Check WBC and culture/sensitivity results. Assess temperature, pulse, respirations esp. rate, depth, and ease of respirations. Be alert for adverse reaction: allergic reactions, superinfections. Check for therapeutic response, side effects.

PATIENT/FAMILY TEACHING: Space doses evenly. Continue therapy for full course. Avoid taking OTC medication w/o physician direction. Promptly notify physician of rash or diarrhea. Drink fluids liberally. Do not take antacids containing magnesium or aluminum or products containing iron or zinc simultaneously or within 4 hrs prior to or 2 hrs after dosing. Avoid excessive sunlight/artificial ultraviolet light; wear sunscreen, protective clothing. Avoid tasks requiring alertness, motor skills until response to drug is established. Notify physician of inflammation or tendon pain.

---

antibiotic: macrolides

The macrolides include azithromycin, clarithromycin, dirithromycin, and erythromycin.

ACTION

Bacteriostatic or bactericidal. Reversibly binds to the P site of the 50S ribosomal subunit of susceptible organisms, inhibiting RNA-dependent protein synthesis.

USES

Macrolides have activity primarily vs. gram-positive microorganisms and gram-negative cocci. Azithromycin and clarithromycin appear to be more potent than erythromycin. Macrolides are used in the treatment of pharyngitis/tonsillitis, sinusitis, chronic bronchitis, pneumonia, uncomplicated skin/skin structure infections.

PRECAUTIONS

CONTRAINDICATIONS: Hypersensitivity to any macrolide antibiotic. *Clarithromycin:* Pts receiving terfenadine or astemizole having preexisting cardiac abnormalities or electrolyte disturbances. **Note:** Caution with other macrolides. *Erythromycin estolate:* Preexisting liver disease. **CAUTIONS:** Hepatic and renal dysfunction.

INTERACTIONS

Azithromycin: May increase serum concentrations of carbamazepine, cyclosporine, theophylline, warfarin. Aluminum/magnesium-containing antacids may decrease concentration (give 1 hr before or 2 hrs after antacid).
Clarithromycin: May increase concentration, toxicity of astemizole, carbamazepine, cisapride, digoxin, terfenadine, theophylline. May decrease concentration of zidovudine. May increase warfarin effects. Rifampin may decrease clarithromycin concentrations.
Dirithromycin: None significant.
Erythromycin: May inhibit metabolism of carbamazepine. May decrease effects of chloramphenicol, clindamycin. May increase concentration, toxicity of cyclosporine, felodipine, lovastatin, simvastatin. Hepatotoxic medications may increase hepatotoxicity. May increase risk of cardiotoxi-

city w/cisapride, terfenadine. May increase risk of toxicity w/theophylline. May increase effect of warfarin.

SIDE EFFECTS

Azithromycin:
Occasional: Abdominal pain, nausea, vomiting, diarrhea. **Rare:** Headache, dizziness, allergic reaction, acute interstitial nephritis.

Clarithromycin:
Occasional: Abnormal taste, nausea, vomiting, diarrhea, abdominal pain, headache. **Rare:** Liver toxicity, hypersensitivity reaction, thrombycytopenia.

Dirithromycin:
Occasional: Abdominal pain, headache, nausea, diarrhea, vomiting, dyspepsia, nonspecific pain, asthenia. **Rare:** Rash, flatulence, dyspnea, pruritus, urticaria, insomnia.

Erythromycin:
Frequent: Nausea, vomiting, diarrhea, abdominal discomfort. **Occasional:** Liver toxicity, hypersensitivity reaction (skin rash, redness, itching, oral or vaginal candidiasis). **Rare:** Cardiotoxicity (QT prolongation), reversible hearing loss, pancreatitis.

TOXIC EFFECTS/ADVERSE REACTIONS

Superinfection esp. antibiotic-associated colitis may result from altered bacterial balance.

ANTIBIOTIC: MACROLIDES

GENERIC NAME	BRAND NAME(S)	USUAL DAILY DOSAGE
azithromycin	Zithromax	PO: Adults, elderly: 500 mg on day 1, 250 mg on days 2–5. Children: 10 mg/kg on day 1, 5 mg/kg on days 2–5.
clarithromycin	Biaxin	PO: Adults, elderly: 250–500 mg q12h. Children: 7.5 mg/kg q12h.
dirithromycin	Dynabec	PO: Adults, elderly, children >12 yrs: 500 mg/day as a single dose.
erythromycin	E-Mycin, Erytab, Eryc, PCE, Ilotycin, Ilosone, EES, Pediamycin, Eryped, Erythrocin	PO: Adults, elderly: 250–500 mg q6h. Children: 30–50 mg/kg/day. IV: Adults, elderly, children: 15–20 mg/kg/day. Maximum: 4 g/day.

NURSING IMPLICATIONS

GENERAL: Administer on schedule to maintain blood levels. Initiate IV solution slowly w/close observation for sensitivity response. **BASELINE ASSESSMENT:** Inquire about previous reactions to macrolides. Culture/sensitivity must be done before first dose (may give before results are known). Assess WBC results, temperature, pulse, respiration. INTERVENTION/EVALUATION: Maintain good hydration and I&O. Check WBC and culture/sensitivity results. Assess temperature, pulse, respirations esp. rate, depth, and ease of respirations. Be alert for adverse reaction: allergic reactions, superinfections. Check for therapeutic response, side effects. PATIENT/FAMILY TEACHING: Space doses evenly. Continue therapy for full course. Avoid taking OTC medication w/o physician direction. Promptly notify physician of rash or diarrhea. Drink fluids liberally.

Azithromycin: Take at least 1 hr prior to or 2 hrs after a meal. Avoid giving w/food. Avoid simultaneous administration of magnesium or aluminum-containing antacids.

Clarithromycin: May take w/o regard to meals, may take w/milk. Shake suspension well; do not refrigerate.

Dirithromycin: Take w/food or within 1 hr of eating. Do not cut, chew, crush tablets.

Erythromycin: May take w/o regard to meals.

antibiotic: penicillins

ACTION

Penicillins inhibit cell wall synthesis or activate enzymes, which disrupt cell wall, causing a weakening in the cell wall, cell lysis, and cell death. May be bacteriostatic or bactericidal. Most effective against rapidly dividing cells.

USES

Penicillins may be used to treat a large number of infections including pneumonia and other respiratory diseases, urinary tract infections, septicemia, meningitis, intra-abdominal infections, gonorrhea and syphilis, bone/joint infection.

PRECAUTIONS

CONTRAINDICATIONS: Hypersensitivity to penicillin, cephalosporins, or components. **CAUTIONS:** Extreme caution w/history of allergies, asthma; gastrointestinal disease; renal dysfunction; bleeding disorders; and (for some penicillins) hepatic dysfunction.

INTERACTIONS

Bacteriostatic antibiotics (e.g., tetracyclines) may decrease bactericidal effects of penicillins. Concurrent use w/allopurinol and ampicillin increases risk of skin rash. Pts should be advised that estrogen contraceptives may have decreased effectiveness when given w/penicillin. Anticoagulants may increase potential for bleeding w/high-dose penicillin therapy. Probenecid increases effects by interfering w/excretion.

CLASSIFICATION

SIDE EFFECTS

Mild nausea, vomiting, or diarrhea; sore tongue or mouth.

PENICILLINS

GENERIC NAME	BRAND NAME(S)	RTE ADMIN	TYPE	DOSAGE RANGE
amoxicillin	Amoxil Polymox Trimox Wymox	Broad spectrum	PO	Adults: 0.75–1.5 g/day Children: 20–40 mg/kg/day
amoxicillin/ clavulanate	Augmentin	Broad spectrum	PO	Adults: 0.75–1.5 g/day Children: 20–40 mg/kg/day
ampicillin	Omnipen Polycillin Principen	Broad spectrum	PO, IM, IV	Adults: 1–12 g/day Children: 50–200 mg/kg/day
ampicillin/ sulbactam	Unasyn	Broad spectrum	IM, IV	Adults: 6–12 g/day
bacampicillin	Spectrobid	Broad spectrum	PO	Adults: 800–1,600 mg/day Children: 25–50 mg/kg/day
carbenicillin	Geocillin	Extended spectrum	PO	Adults: 382–764 mg 4x/day
cloxacillin	Cloxapen Tegopen	Penicillinase resistant	PO	Adults: 1–2 g/day Children: 50–100 mg/kg/day
dicloxacillin	Dynapen Pathocil	Pencillinase resistant	PO	Adults: 1–2 g/day Children: 12.5–25 mg/kg/day
methicillin	Staphcillin	Penicillinase resistant	IM, IV	Adults: 4–12 g/day Children: 100–300 mg/kg/day
mezlocillin	Mezlin	Extended spectrum	IM, IV	Adults: 6–18 g/day Children: 150–300 mg/kg/day
nafcillin	Nafcil Unipen	Penicillinase resistant	PO, IM, IV	Adults (PO): 1–6 g/day Adults (IM, IV): 2–6 g/day Children (PO): 25 50 mg/kg/day Children (IM, IV): 50 mg/ kg/day
oxacillin	Bactocill Prostaphlin	Penicillinase resistant	PO, IM, IV	Adults (PO): 2–6 g/day Adults (IM, IV): 2–6 g/day Children (PO): 50 100 mg/ kg/day Children (IM, IV): 50–100 mg/ kg/day
penicillin G benzathine	Bicillin Permapen	Natural	IM	Adults: 1.2 million units/day Children: 0.3–1.2 million units/ day
penicillin G postassium	Pentids Pfizerpen	Natural	IM, IV	Adults: 2–24 million units/day Children: 100,000– 250,000 units/kg/day
penicillin G procaine	Crysticillin A.S. Wycillin	Natural	IM	Adults: 0.6–1.2 million units/day Children: 0.6–1.2 million units/ day
penicillin V potassium	Pen-Vee K V-Cillin K Veetids	Natural	PO	Adults: 0.5–2 g/day Children: 25–50 mg/kg/day

PENICILLINS *Continued*

GENERIC NAME	BRAND NAME(S)	RTE ADMIN	TYPE	DOSAGE RANGE
piperacillin	Pipracil	Extended spectrum	IM, IV	Adults: 6–18 g/day Children: 200–300 mg/kg/day
piperacillin tazobactam	Zosyn	Extended spectrum	IV	Adults: 3.375 g q6h
ticarcillin	Ticar	Extended spectrum	IM, IV	Adults: 12–24 g/day Children: 50–300 mg/kg/day
ticarcillin clavulanate	Timentin	Extended spectrum	IM, IV	Adults: 3.1 g q4–6h

Natural penicillins are very active against gram-positive cocci but ineffective against most strains of *Staphylococcus aureus* (inactivated by enzyme penicillinase).

Penicillinase-resistant penicillins are effective against penicillinase-producing *Staphylococcus aureus* but are less effective against gram-positive cocci than the natural penicillins.

Broad-spectrum penicillins are effective against gram-positive cocci and some gram-negative bacteria (e.g., *Hemophilus influenzae, Escherichia coli, Proteus mirabilis*).

Extended-spectrum penicillins are effective against *Pseudomonas aeruginosa, Enterobacter, Proteus* species, *Klebsiella,* and some other gram-negative microorganisms.

TOXIC EFFECTS/ADVERSE REACTIONS

Hypersensitivity/allergic reactions ranging from skin rashes, urticaria, itching to full anaphylaxis. Superinfections, including antibiotic-associated colitis. Neurotoxicity, hematologic effects may occur in select drugs.

NURSING IMPLICATIONS

GENERAL: Administer drugs on proper schedule to maintain blood levels. Initiate IV solutions slowly at first w/close observation for sensitivity response. BASELINE ASSESSMENT: Question for history of hypersensitivity to penicillin or cephalosporins. W/history of cephalosporin reaction, have emergency equipment, medications available. Culture/sensitivity must be done before first dose (may give before results are obtained). Assess WBC results, temperature, pulse, respiration. INTERVENTION/EVALUATION: Monitor temperature, lab results, particularly WBC and culture/sensitivity reports. Assess for adverse reactions, esp. allergic reactions, superinfection. PATIENT/FAMILY TEACHING: Space doses evenly. Continue therapy for full duration, usually 7–10 days. Avoid alcohol, antacids, or other medications w/o consulting physician. Promptly notify physician of rash or diarrhea.

CLASSIFICATION

anticholinergics

ACTION

These agents are known as anticholinergics, antimuscarinics, or parasympatholytics. Competitively block muscarinic receptors. Inhibit action of acetylcholine. Prevent stimulation of receptors by muscarinic agonists. Areas affected include:

Eye: Cause mydriasis (pupil dilation), cycloplegia (paralysis of ciliary muscle).

Heart: Increase heart rate.

Gastrointestinal: Decrease salivary secretion, gastric secretion; decrease tone and motility of gastrointestinal tract.

Respiratory: Decrease secretion of nose, mouth, pharynx, bronchi; cause relaxation of bronchi.

Urinary tract: Decrease tone, contraction of ureter and urinary bladder.

USES

Management of peptic ulcer, ophthalmic administration (produce mydriasis/cycloplegia), asthma (induce bronchodilation), antagonize reflex vagal-mediated bradycardia, Parkinson's disease, administered before general anesthetic to decrease excessive salivation/secretion of respiratory tract, spastic disorders of biliary tract, antidote/antagonize effects of anticholinesterase agents; antidote for mushroom poisoning.

PRECAUTIONS

CONTRAINDICATIONS: Hypersensitivity, glaucoma, hepatic or renal dysfunction, tachycardia, ulcerative colitis, intestinal obstruction, paralytic ileus, bladder neck obstruction, myasthenia gravis, asthma. **CAUTIONS:** Pts w/cardiac disease, elderly, infants, and young children (who are particularly susceptible to toxic effects) should be monitored closely. Drugs cross placenta and are excreted in breast milk. May inhibit lactation.

INTERACTIONS

Antacids, antidiarrheals may decrease absorption. Anticholinergics may increase effects. May decrease absorption of ketoconazole. May increase severity of gastrointestinal lesions w/potassium chloride (wax matrix).

SIDE EFFECTS

Antisalivary (dry mouth), blurred vision, urinary hesitation/retention, constipation, flushing, lightheadedness, mild tachycardia.

TOXIC EFFECTS/ADVERSE REACTIONS

CNS excitation, nausea and vomiting, hypertension, increased intraocular pressure, rash, elevated temperature, thick respiratory secretions and respiratory difficulties, impotence.

ANTICHOLINERGICS

GENERIC NAME	BRAND NAME(S)	RTE ADM	DOSAGE RANGE
atropine	Atropine	IM, IV, SubQ	Adults: 0.3–1.2 mg Children: 0.01 mg/kg
dicyclomine	Bentyl	PO, IM	Adults: PO: 80–160 mg/day; IM: 80 mg/day
glycopyrrolate	Robinul	PO, IM, IV	Adults: PO: 2–6 mg/day; IM, IV: 0.1–0.2 mg
scopolamine	Scopolamine	IM, IV, SubQ	Adults: 0.3–0.65 mg Children: 0.006 mg/kg
	Transderm Scop	Topical	Adults: 1.5 mg

NURSING IMPLICATIONS

GENERAL: For long-term therapy, change medication gradually. BASELINE ASSESSMENT: Check B/P, pulse, respirations. INTERVENTION/EVALUATION: Assess bowel activity, abdominal distention, bowel sounds. Monitor I&O, check for urination, palpate for distended bladder. Check B/P, pulse, respirations, EKG. Assess for adverse reactions, esp. in geriatric pts and those w/chronic lung conditions. PATIENT/FAMILY TEACHING: Mouthwash, cold drinks, hard candy or gum (if permitted) may be used for dry mouth. Take safety precautions w/drowsiness, blurred vision, or lightheadedness; do not drive or perform activities requiring mental acuity. Increased fluid intake to decrease viscosity of secretions, aid in bowel elimination. *Ophthalmic:* Protect eyes from light; wear sunglasses.

anticoagulants/antiplatelets/thrombolytics

ACTION

Anticoagulants: Inhibit blood coagulation by preventing the formation of new clots and extension of existing ones. *Do not dissolve formed clots.* Anticoagulants are subdivided into two common classes: *Heparin:* Directly interferes w/blood coagulation by blocking the conversion of prothrombin to thrombin and fibrinogen to fibrin. *Coumarin:* Acts indirectly to prevent synthesis in the liver of vitamin K–dependent clotting factors.

Antiplatelets: Interfere w/platelet aggregation. Effects are irreversible for life of platelet.

Thrombolytics: Act directly or indirectly on fibrinolytic system to dissolve clots (converting plasminogen to plasmin, an enzyme that digests fibrin clot).

USES

Anticoagulants: Primarily decrease risk of venous thromboembolism. *Antiplatelets:* Primarily decrease risk of arterial thromboembolism. *Thrombolytics:* Lyse existing clots.

CLASSIFICATION

Treatment and prevention of venous thromboembolism, acute myocardial infarction, acute cerebral embolism; reduces risk of acute myocardial infarction, total mortality in pts w/unstable angina; occlusion of saphenous grafts following open heart surgery; embolism in select pts w/atrial fibrillation, prosthetic heart valves, valvular heart disease, cardiomyopathy. Heparin also used for acute/chronic consumption coagulopathies (disseminated intravascular coagulation).

PRECAUTIONS

CONTRAINDICATIONS: Hypersensitivity, active bleeding, blood dyscrasias and bleeding tendencies, pregnancy. **CAUTIONS:** Renal, hepatic dysfunction; alcoholism; history of allergy.

ANTICOAGULANTS/ANTIPLATELETS/THROMBOLYTICS

GENERIC NAME	BRAND NAME(S)	CLASS	DOSAGE RANGE
abciximab	ReoPro	Antiplatelet	Adults: IV bolus: 0.25 mg/kg; IV infusion: 10 mcg/min
alteplase	Activase	Thrombolytic	Adults: IV infusion: 100 mg over 3 hrs (2 hrs for pulmonary embolism)
anagrelide	Agrylin	Antiplatelet	Adults: PO: 2–10 mg/day
anistreplase	Eminase	Thrombolytic	Adults: IV push: 30 units over 2–5 min
ardeparin	Normiflo	Anticoagulant	Adults: SubQ: 50 U/kg q12 h
aspirin	—	Antiplatelet	Adults: 81–325 mg/day
clopidogrel	Plavix	Antiplatelet	Adults: PO: 75 mg once daily
dalteparin	Fragmin	Anticoagulant	Adults: SubQ: 200 IU/kg once daily or 100 IU/kg q12h
danaparoid	Organan	Anticoagulant	Adults: SubQ: 750 units q12h
dipyridamole	Persantine	Antiplatelet	Adults: 75–100 mg 4 times/day
enoxaparin	Lovenox	Anticoagulant	Adults: 30 mg q12h
heparin	—	Anticoagulant	Adults: IV bolus: 5,000 units then IV infusion of 20,000–40,000 units/day Children: IV bolus: 50 units/kg then IV infusion of 20,000 units/m²/24 hrs
reteplase	Retavase	Thrombolytic	Adults: IV: 10 units q30min × 2 doses
streptokinase	Kabikinase Streptase	Thrombolytic	Adults: (AMI) 1.5 million units over 60 min
ticlopidine	Ticlid	Antiplatelet	Adults: 250 mg 2 times/day
urokinase	Abbokinase	Thrombolytic	Adults: IV: 4,400 IU/kg over 10 min, then 4,400 IU/kg/min for 12–24 hrs
warfarin	Coumadin	Anticoagulant	Adults: Initially, 5–10 mg/day, then 2–10 mg/day

INTERACTIONS

Anticoagulants interact with many drugs and foods. Pts should be cautioned against smoking, alcohol consumption, and use of OTC drugs. Aspirin, many NSAIDs, antihistamines, diuretics, antibiotics, estrogen contraceptives are among the drugs that affect anticoagulant action. Any medication taken with an anticoagulant should be checked for interaction. Prothrombin time (PT) may be shortened by high-fat diet or sudden increase in foods rich in vitamin K. Antidote for heparin: protamine sulfate; for coumarins: vitamin K.

SIDE EFFECTS

Not common. Local reactions w/parenteral administration. Nausea, vomiting, anorexia, and diarrhea w/oral administration.

TOXIC EFFECTS/ADVERSE REACTIONS

Minor bleeding to major hemorrhage. Thrombocytopenia and alopecia are transient and reversible. Jaundice, hepatitis, increased serum transaminase levels w/coumarin therapy. Hypersensitivity reactions are rare: fever, chills, urticaria.

NURSING IMPLICATIONS

GENERAL: Do not discontinue abruptly. Monitor coagulation test results before administration: for heparin therapy, the activated partial thromboplastin time (APTT); for coumarin therapy, the PT. Consult physician for targeted coagulation range for individual pt (generally, dosage is adjusted to keep results about 1.5–2 times control value for APTT, 1.5 times control value for PT). INTERVENTION/EVALUATION: Assess for bleeding: vital signs, bruises, overt bleeding, and blood in sputum, urine, and feces. Check for headache, abdominal or back pain. PATIENT/FAMILY TEACHING: Importance of taking drug as directed and periodic lab tests to determine response to medication. Explain how to check for bleeding signs. Carry identification indicating anticoagulant therapy. Avoid large quantities of vitamin K–rich food, such as green leafy vegetables, liver, fish, bananas, cauliflower, tomatoes (decrease effects of oral anticoagulants). Consult physician before taking other medications (including aspirin). Avoid alcohol. Avoid activities w/high risk of injury. Inform physician, dentist of anticoagulant therapy before surgical/dental procedures.

anticonvulsants

ACTION

Seizures consist of abnormal and excessive discharges from the brain. Anticonvulsants can prevent or reduce excessive discharge of neurons w/seizure foci or decrease the spread of excitation from seizure foci to normal neurons. Exact mechanism unknown. Anticonvulsants include the hydantoins, barbiturates, succinimides, oxazolidinediones, benzodiazepines, and several miscellaneous agents.

USES

Anticonvulsants are generally effective in the treatment of *absence (petit mal) seizures* (brief, abrupt loss of consciousness, some clonic motor activity ranging from eyelid blinking to jerking of entire body); *tonic-clonic (grand mal) seizures* (major convulsions, usually beginning w/spasm of all body musculature, then clonic jerking, followed by depression of all central function); and *complex partial seizures* (confused behavior, impaired consciousness, bizarre generalized EEG activity). Other types of seizures generally respond poorly to anticonvulsant therapy.

PRECAUTIONS

CONTRAINDICATIONS: Hypersensitivity, hepatic, renal, or thyroid dysfunction, alcoholism, blood dyscrasias; diabetes mellitus, cardiac disease/impairment, lactation. **CAUTIONS:** Pregnancy—risk/benefit must be weighed in relation to congenital abnormalities. Elderly, children, and debilitated.

INTERACTIONS

Drug interactions are extensive; any other medication administered should be carefully checked for interaction w/anticonvulsants. Teach pts never to take medication w/o consulting physician. Effects are increased by CNS depressants; decreased w/tricyclic antidepressants, phenothiazine antipsychotics, antacids. Refer to individual monographs.

SIDE EFFECTS

Drowsiness, sedation, mild dizziness, gingival hyperplasia, anorexia, nausea, vomiting, hyperglycemia, and glycosuria.

TOXIC EFFECTS/ADVERSE REACTIONS

Visual disturbances, unusual excitement, confusion, skin disorders. Stevens-Johnson syndrome (headache, arthralgia, skin lesions w/other symptoms), liver damage, hirsutism, blood dyscrasias, enlarged lymph glands in neck and under arms.

NURSING IMPLICATIONS

GENERAL: Status epilepticus is a life-threatening emergency that requires immediate IV medication (diazepam is the drug of choice). Never mix parenteral solutions w/other drugs or IV fluids—should be administered via slow IV push. When discontinued, gradual reduction is recommended. Provide protection against injury. INTERVENTION/EVALUATION: Monitor B/P, pulse, respirations, serum drug levels. Assess neurologic status. Identify characteristics of seizures if they occur. PATIENT/FAMILY TEACHING: Therapy is usually several years to life. Take w/food or fluids to minimize GI irritation. Important to take as directed. Do not take other medications w/o consulting physician. Avoid alcohol. Do not drive or engage in activities requiring mental acuity until physician approves (seizures and response to drug are controlled). Carry identification card/bracelet indicating anticonvulsant therapy.

ANTICONVULSANTS

GENERIC NAME	BRAND NAME(S)	CLASS	USES	DOSAGE RANGE
carbamazepine	Tegretol	Miscellaneous	Complex partial, tonic-clonic, mixed seizures, trigeminal neuralgia	Adults: 800–1,200 mg/day Children: 400–800 mg/day
clonazepam	Klonopin	Benzodiazepine	Petit mal, akinetic, myoclonic, absence	Adults: 1.5–20 mg/day Children: 0.01–0.2 mg/kg/day
clorazepate	Tranxene	Benzodiazepine	Partial seizures	Adults: 7.5–90 mg/day Children: 7.5–60 mg/day
diazepam	Valium	Benzodiazepine	Adjunctive therapy status epilepticus	Adults: PO: 4–40 mg/day; IM/IV: 5–30 mg Children: PO: 3–10 mg/day; IM/IV: 1–10 mg
ethosuximide	Zarontin	Succinimide	Absence seizures	Children: 20 mg/day
felbamate	Felbatol	Miscellaneous	Partial seizures, Lennox-Gustaut syndrome	Adults: 1,200–3,600 mg/day Children ≥14 yrs: 1,200–3,600 mg/day
fosphenytoin	Cerebyx	Hydantoin	Tonic-clonic, complex partial, autonomic seizures, status epilepticus	Status epilepticus: IV: 15–20 mg PE/kg Nonemergent: IM/IV: Initially, 10–20 mg PE/kg; then 4–6 mg PE/kg/day
gabapentum	Neurontin	Miscellaneous	Partial seizures	Adults: 900–1,800 mg/day Children >12 yrs: 900–1,800 mg/day
lamotrigine	Lamictal	Miscellaneous	Partial seizures	Adults: 100–500 mg/day
levetiracetam	Keppra	Miscellaneous	Partial	Adults: 1,000–3,000 mg/day
phenobarbital	Luminal	Barbiturate	Tonic-clonic, partial, status epilepticus	Adults: PO: 100–300 mg/day; IM/IV: 200–600 mg Children: PO: 3–5 mg/kg/day; IM/IV: 100–400 mg
phenytoin	Dilantin	Hydantoin	Tonic-clonic, complex partial, autonomic seizures, status epilepticus	Adults: PO: 300–600 mg/day; IV: 150–250 mg Status epilepticus: 15–18 mg/kg Children: PO: 4–8 mg/kg/day Status epilepticus: 10–15 mg/kg
primidone	Mysoline	Miscellaneous	Complex partial, partial, akinetic, tonic-clonic	Adults: 0.75–2 g/day Children: 10–25 mg/kg/day
tiagabine	Gabitril	Miscellaneous	Partial seizures	Adults: Initially, 4 mg; maximum: 56 mg Children: Initially, 4 mg; maximum: 32 mg
topiramate	Topamax	Miscellaneous	Partial seizures	Adults: PO: 50–400 mg/day
valproic acid	Depakene Depakote	Miscellaneous	Absence, multiple seizure types	Adults, children: 15–60 mg/kg/day
vigabatrin	Sabril	Miscellaneous	Partial seizures	Adults: 1–4 g/day
zonisamide	Zonegran	Miscellaneous	Partial seizures	Adults: 500 mg/day

CLASSIFICATION

antidepressants

ACTION

Antidepressants are classified as tricyclic, monoamine oxidase (MAO) inhibitors, or miscellaneous. Depression may be due to reduced functioning of monoamine neurotransmitters in the CNS (decreased amount and/or decreased effects at receptor sites).

Antidepressants block metabolism, increase amount/effects of monoamine neurotransmitters (e.g., norepinephrine, serotonin [5-HT]), and act at receptor sites (change responsiveness/sensitivities of both pre- and postsynaptic receptor sites).

Miscellaneous, Tricyclics: Block reuptake of neurotransmitter at presynaptic nerve endings. Potency/selectivity varies w/these agents.

MAO inhibitors: Inhibit enzyme MAO, thus interfering w/degradation of monoamine neurotransmitters.

USES

Used primarily for the treatment of depression. Imipramine is also used for childhood enuresis. Clomipramine is used only for obsessive-compulsive disorder (OCD). MAO inhibitors are rarely used as initial therapy except for pts unresponsive to other therapy or when other therapy is contraindicated.

PRECAUTIONS

CONTRAINDICATIONS: Pregnancy, lactation, children <16 yrs of age (exception: imipramine to treat enuresis in children >6 yrs of age), hypersensitivity, liver dysfunction, renal dysfunction, glaucoma, elderly, CHF. **CAUTIONS:** Never use MAO inhibitors and tricyclic antidepressants together—can result in death. Effects of antidepressants can last 2–3 wks after discontinuation.

INTERACTIONS

Tricyclic antidepressants: Alcohol, CNS depressants may increase CNS, respiratory depression, hypotensive effects. Antithyroid agents may increase risk of agranulocytosis. Phenothiazines may increase sedative, anticholinergic effects. Cimetidine may increase concentration, toxicity. May decrease effects of clonidine, guanadrel. May increase cardiac effects w/sympathomimetics. May increase risk of hypertensive crisis, hyperpyretic, convulsion w/MAO inhibitors.

MAO inhibitors: Alcohol, CNS depressants may increase CNS depressant effects. Tricyclic antidepressants, fluoxetine, trazodone may cause serotonin syndrome. May increase effect of oral hypoglycemics, insulin. B/P may increase w/buspirone. Caffeine-containing medications may increase cardiac arrhythmias, hypertension. May precipitate hypertensive crises w/carbamazepine, cyclobenzaprine, maprotiline, other MAO inhibitors. Meperidine, other opioid analgesics may produce immediate excitation, sweating, rigidity, severe hypertension or hypotension, severe respiratory distress, coma, convulsions, vascular collapse, death. May increase CNS stimulant, vasopressor effects. Tyramine, foods w/pressor amines (e.g., aged cheese) may cause sudden, severe hypertension.

ANTIDEPRESSANTS

GENERIC NAME	BRAND NAME(S)	TYPE	AMINE UPTAKE BLOCKAGE	DOSAGE RANGE (MG/DAY)
amitriptyline	Elavil Endep	Tricyclic	Norepinephrine Serotonin	PO: 40–300
amoxapine	Asendin	Tricyclic	Norepinephrine Serotonin	PO: 100–600
bupropion	Wellbutrin	Miscellaneous	—	PO: 200–450
citalopram	Celexa	Miscellaneous	Serotonin	PO: 20–40
clomipramine	Anafranil	Tricyclic	Norepinephrine Serotonin	PO: 25–250
desipramine	Norpramin Pertofrane	Tricyclic	Norepinephrine Serotonin	PO: 25–100
doxepin	Adapin Sinequan	Tricyclic	Norepinephrine Serotonin	PO: 75–300
fluoxetine	Prozac	Miscellaneous	Serotonin	PO: 20–80
fluvoxamine	Luvox	Miscellaneous	Serotonin	PO: 100–300
imipramine	Janimine Tofranil	Tricyclic	Norepinephrine Serotonin	PO: 30–300
maprotiline	Ludiomil	Miscellaneous	Norepinephrine	PO: 25–225
mirtazapine	Remeron	Miscellaneous	Norepinephrine Serotonin	PO: 5–30
nefazodone	Serzone	Miscellaneous	Serotonin Serotonin receptor	PO: 200–600
nortriptyline	Aventyl Pamelor	Tricyclic	Norepinephrine Serotonin	PO: 25–100
paroxetine	Paxil	Miscellaneous	Serotonin	PO: 20–50
phenelzine	Nardil	MAO inhibitor	—	PO: 15–90
protriptyline	Vivactil	Tricyclic	Norepinephrine Serotonin	PO: 15–60
sertraline	Zoloft	Miscellaneous	Serotonin	PO: 50–200
tranylcypromine	Parnate	MAO inhibitor	—	PO: 30–60
trazodone	Desyrel	Miscellaneous	Serotonin	PO: 50–600
venlafaxine	Effexor	Miscellaneous	Norepinephrine Serotonin	PO: 75–375

SIDE EFFECTS

Tricyclic antidepressants: Dizziness, drowsiness, dry mouth, headache, weight gain, photosensitivity. *MAO inhibitors:* Dizziness and orthostatic hypotension, blurred vision, constipation, difficulty w/urination, mild headache, weight gain, insomnia.

TOXIC EFFECTS/ADVERSE REACTIONS

Tricyclic antidepressants: Severe drowsiness, confusion, hallucinations, seizures, tachycardia or bradycardia, difficulty breathing. *MAO inhibitors:* Severe drowsiness or dizziness, hypertension or hypotension, tachycardia, difficulty sleeping, hallucinations, respiratory depression.

NURSING IMPLICATIONS

GENERAL: Closely supervise pts (potential for suicide increases when emerging from depression). Elderly should be observed carefully for increased response; small doses are usually indicated. BASELINE ASSESSMENT: Determine initial B/P. Assess pt and environment for support needed. INTERVENTION/EVALUATION: Monitor B/P. Assess mental status. Check bowel activity; avoid constipation. PATIENT/FAMILY TEACHING: Change positions slowly to avoid orthostatic hypotension. Take medication as ordered; do not stop taking or increase dosage. Avoid driving or performing tasks that require mental acuity until response to drug controlled. Extremely important to refrain from alcohol and other medications during therapy and for 2–3 wks thereafter. Omit foods rich in tyramine, such as products containing yeast, beer/wine, aged cheese (list of foods to avoid should be given); ingestion of such foods and antidepressant may cause hypertensive crisis. Inform other physicians or dentist of antidepressant therapy. Use protection from sunlight w/specific drugs. To the extent possible, drugs that cause drowsiness should be taken at bedtime, those causing insomnia should be taken in the morning.

antidiabetics

Five major groups of medication are currently available in the treatment of diabetes mellitus: insulin, sulfonylureas, alpha-glucosidase inhibitors, biguanides, and thiazolinediones.

ACTION

Insulin: A hormone synthesized and secreted by beta cells of Langerhans' islet in the pancreas. Controls storage and utilization of glucose, amino acids, and fatty acids by activated transport systems/enzymes. Inhibits breakdown of glycogen, fat, protein. Insulin lowers blood glucose by inhibiting glycogenolysis and gluconeogenesis in liver; stimulates glucose uptake by muscle, adipose tissue. Activity of insulin is initiated by binding to cell surface receptors.

Sulfonylureas: Stimulate release of insulin from beta cells; increases sensitivity of insulin to peripheral tissue. Endogenous insulin must be present for oral hypoglycemics to be effective.

Alpha-glucosidase inhibitors: Work locally in small intestine slowing carbohydrate breakdown and glucose absorption.

Biguanides: Decrease hepatic glucose output, enhances peripheral glucose uptake.

Thiazolinediones: Decrease insulin resistance.

USES

Insulin: Treatment of insulin-dependent diabetes (type I) and noninsulin-dependent diabetes (type II). Also used in acute situations such as ketoacidosis, severe infections, major surgery in otherwise noninsulin-dependent diabetics. Administered to pts receiving parenteral nutrition. Drug of choice during pregnancy.

Sulfonylureas: Controls hyperglycemia in type II diabetes not controlled by weight and diet alone. Chlorpropamide also used in adjunctive treatment of neurogenic diabetes insipidus.

Alpha-glucosidase inhibitors: Adjunct to diet to lower blood glucose in pts with noninsulin-dependent diabetes mellitus (NIDDM) whose hyperglycemia cannot be managed by diet alone.

Biguanides: Adjunct to diet to lower blood glucose in pts with noninsulin-dependent diabetes mellitus (NIDDM) whose hyperglycemia cannot be managed by diet alone.

Thiazolinediones: Adjunct in pts with NIDDM currently on insulin therapy.

INSULIN

| | **BRAND NAME(S)** | **HYPOGLYCEMIC EFFECT** | | |
		ONSET (HRS)	**PEAK (HRS)**	**DURATION (HRS)**
RAPID ACTING				
regular insulin	Humulin R Novolin R Velosulin	0.5–0.75	2–4	3–6
insulin lispro	Humalog	0.15–0.25	0.75–1	2–4
INTERMEDIATE ACTING				
lente insulin	Humulin L Novolin L	1–2.5	7–15	24
NPH	Humulin N Novolin N	1–1.5	4–12	24
LONG ACTING				
ultralente	Ultralente Humulin U	4–8	10–30	>36

PRECAUTIONS

CONTRAINDICATIONS: *Insulin:* Hypersensitivity to animal proteins (human insulin available). Hypoglycemia. *Sulfonylureas:* Hypersensitivity to sulfonamides, pregnancy, severe stress or infection, before surgical procedures, in type I insulin-dependent diabetes; hepatic or renal dysfunction; hypoglycemia; lactation. *Alpha-glucosidase inhibitors:* Hypersensitivity to drug, diabetic ketoacidosis, cirrhosis, inflammatory bowel disease, colonic ulceration, partial intestinal obstruction, chronic intestinal disease associated w/disorders of digestion or absorption. *Biguanides:* Renal disease/dysfunction, hypersensitivity to drug, acute or chronic metabolic acidosis. **CAUTION:** Elderly or debilitated pts. Renal or hepatic impairment; alcoholics; cardiac impairment.

INTERACTION

Insulin: Glucocorticoids, thiazide diuretics may increase blood glucose. Alcohol may increase insulin effect. Beta-adrenergic blockers may increase risk of hypo/hyperglycemia, mask signs of hypoglycemia, prolong period of hypoglycemia.

Sulfonylureas: May increase effects of oral anticoagulants. Chloramphenicol, MAO inhibitors, salicylates, sulfonamides may increase effects. Beta blockers may increase hypoglycemic effect, may mask signs of hypoglycemia.

Alpha-glucosidase inhibitors: Digestive enzymes, intestinal absorbents (e.g., charcoal) may decrease effect.

Biguanides: Alcohol potentiates effect on lactate metabolism. Cimetidine, furosemide, nifedipine may increase concentration. Iodinated contrast material may lead to acute renal failure, associated w/lactic acidosis.

ORAL ANTIDIABETIC AGENTS

GENERIC NAME	BRAND NAME(S)	TYPE	USUAL DAILY DOSAGE	
			INITIALLY	AVERAGE RANGE
acarbose	Precose	Alpha-glucosidase inhibitor	75 mg	150–300 mg
acetohexamide	Dymelor	Sulfonylurea	250 mg	250–1,500 mg
chlorpropamide	Diabinese	Sulfonylurea	100 mg	100–750 mg
glimepiride	Amaryl	Sulfonylurea	1–2 mg	1–4 mg
glipizide	Glucotrol	Sulfonylurea	2.5–5 mg	2.5–40 mg
glyburide	Diabeta Micronase Glynase	Sulfonylurea	1.25–5mg	1.25–20 mg
metformin	Glucophage	Biguanide	500 mg	500–2,550 mg
miglitol	Glyset	Alpha-glucosidase inhibitor	75 mg	75–300 mg
pioglitazone	Actos	Thiazolinedone	15 mg	15–45 mg
repaglinide	Prandin	Miscellaneous	—	1–16 mg/day
rosiglitazone	Avandia	Thiazolinedone	4 mg	4–8 mg
tolazamide	Tolinase	Sulfonylurea	100 mg	100–1,000 mg
tolbutamide	Orinase	Sulfonylurea	500 mg	500–3,000 mg

SIDE EFFECTS

Insulin: Hypoglycemia, local redness, swelling, itching at injection site.

Sulfonylureas: Hypoglycemia, nausea, heartburn, epigastric fullness, pruritus.

Alpha-glucosidase inhibitors: Abdominal pain, diarrhea, flatulence.

Biguanides: Watery diarrhea, abdominal pain, nausea, dyspepsia, anorexia, metallic taste.

Thiazolinedione: Infection, headache, pain, asthenia.

TOXIC EFFECTS/ADVERSE REACTIONS

Severe hypoglycemia (due to hyperinsulinism) may occur in overdose of insulin, decrease or delay of food intake, excessive exercise, or those w/brittle diabetes. *Sulfonylureas:* Urticaria or rash; mild anemia, thrombocytopenia, hepatic impairment. Diabetic ketoacidosis may result from stress, illness, omission of insulin dose, or long-term poor insulin control.

NURSING IMPLICATIONS

GENERAL: Administer per schedule; rotate insulin injection sites. Recognize peak action times (see grid) as hypoglycemic reactions may occur at these times. Provide meals on time. INTERVENTION/EVALUA-TION: Monitor blood glucose levels, food consumption. Check for hypoglycemia: cool, wet skin; tremors; dizziness; headache; anxiety; tachycardia; numbness in mouth; hunger; diplopia; restlessness, diaphoresis in sleeping pt. Check for hyperglycemia: polyuria, polyphagia, polydipsia, nausea and vomiting, dim vision, fatigue, deep rapid breathing. PATIENT/FAMILY TEACHING: Diabetes mellitus requires lifelong control. Prescribed diet is essential part of treatment; do not skip or delay meals. Weight control, exercise, hygiene (including foot care), and nonsmoking are integral part of therapy. Significance of illness, stress, and exercise on regime. Teach how to handle, administer insulin. Oral hypoglycemics should be taken 15–30 min before meal. Carry candy, sugar packets, or other sugar supplements for immediate response to hypoglycemia. Wear, carry medical alert identification. Avoid alcohol; do not take other medication w/o consulting physician. Protect skin; limit sun exposure. Select clothing, positions that do not restrict blood flow. Avoid injuries, exposure to infections. Inform dentist, physician of this medication before any treatment.

antidiarrheals

ACTION

Systemic agents: Act at smooth muscle receptors (enteric) disrupting peristaltic movements, decreasing GI motility, increasing transit time of intestinal contents.

Local agents: Adsorb toxic substances and fluids to large surface areas of particles in the preparation. Some of these agents coat and protect irritated intestinal walls. May have local anti-inflammatory action.

USES

Acute diarrhea, chronic diarrhea of inflammatory bowel disease, reduction of fluid from ileostomies.

PRECAUTIONS

CONTRAINDICATIONS: Children <2 years of age, hypersensitivity to any component. Safety not established in pregnancy, lactation. **CAUTIONS:** Young children, elderly. Not for antibiotic-associated colitis or ulcerative colitis.

INTERACTIONS

Vary according to components of individual agents. CNS depressants, anticholinergics, antihistamines increase effects of antidiarrheals.

SIDE EFFECTS

Constipation, drowsiness w/systemic agents (nausea and dry mouth w/diphenoxylate hydrochloride w/atropine sulfate).

ANTIDIARRHEALS

GENERIC NAME	BRAND NAME(S)	TYPE	FORMS	DOSAGE RANGE
bismuth subsalicylate	Pepto-Bismol	Local	Suspension Tablets	Adults: 2 tablets or 30 ml Children 9–12 yrs: 1 tablet or 15 ml Children 6–9 yrs: $2/3$ tablet or 10 ml Children 3–6 yrs: $1/3$ tablet or 5 ml
diphenoxylate (w/atropine)	Lomotil	Systemic	Liquid Tablets	Adults: 5 mg 4×/day Children: (liquid only): 0.3–0.4 mg/kg/day in 4 divided doses
kaolin (w/pectin)	Kaopectate	Local	Suspension	Adults: 60–120 ml after each BM Children 6–12 yrs: 30–60 ml Children 3–6 yrs: 15–30 ml
loperamide	Imodium	Systemic	Capsules Liquid	Adults: Initially, 4 mg; maximum: 16 mg/day Children 8–12 yrs: 2 mg 3×/day Children 5–8 yrs: 2 mg 2×/day Children 2–5 yrs: 1 mg 3×/day (liquid)

TOXIC EFFECTS/ADVERSE REACTIONS

Adverse reactions are infrequent w/proper dosage. Abdominal distention and cramps, dizziness, nausea and vomiting, drug dependence w/long-term use (atropine side effects w/diphenoxylate w/atropine).

NURSING IMPLICATIONS

GENERAL: Discontinue medication when diarrhea controlled or if abdominal distention occurs. Maintain hydration (offer 2,000–3,000 ml of fluid/day to adults). INTERVENTION/EVALUATION: Monitor stool frequency and consistency (watery, loose, soft, semisolid, solid). Check I&O and assess hydration, esp. in very young and old. PATIENT/FAMILY TEACHING: Avoid tasks that require alertness, motor skills until response to drug is established. Do not ingest alcohol or barbiturates, esp. w/drugs containing atropine. Contact physician for diarrhea that persists more than 2 days, high fever, blood in stool, or abdominal distention.

antifungals: topical

ACTION

Exact mechanism unknown. May deplete essential intracellular components by inhibiting transport of potassium, other ions into cells; alter membrane permeability resulting in loss of potassium, other cellular components.

USES

Treatment of tinea infections, cutaneous candidiasis (moniliasis) due to *Candida albicans*. Natamycin: treatment of fungal blepharitis, conjunctivitis, and keratitis.

PRECAUTIONS

CONTRAINDICATIONS: Hypersensitivity to the medication, any component of preparation. **CAUTIONS:** For external/topical use only. Avoid contact w/eyes (except natamycin). May irritate sensitized skin; discontinue if it occurs.

INTERACTIONS

None significant.

SIDE EFFECTS

OCCASIONAL: Burning, itching, stinging, erythema, pruritic rash, irritation.

TOXIC EFFECTS/ADVERSE REACTIONS

None significant.

ANTIFUNGALS: TOPICAL

GENERIC NAME	BRAND NAME(S)	AVAILABILITY
ciclopirox	Loprox	Cream
	Penlac	Lotion
clioquinol	Vioform	Cream
		Ointment
clotrimazole	Lotrimin	Cream
	Mycelex	Lotion
		Solution
econazole	Spectazole	Cream
miconazole	Micatin	Cream
	Monistat	Powder
		Spray
natamycin	Natacyn	Ophthalmic suspension
tolnaftate	NP-27	Cream
	Tinactin	Gel
		Solution
triacetin	Fungoid	Cream
		Solution
undecylenic acid	Desenex	Cream
		Ointment
		Powder

CLASSIFICATION

NURSING IMPLICATIONS

BASELINE ASSESSMENT: Assess area of infection. Question pt as to hypersensitivity history to medication. INTERVENTION/EVALUATION: Assess improvement or increased irritation, burning, itching, swelling, oozing, redness of affected area. PATIENT/FAMILY TEACHING: For external use only, avoid contact in eyes (Exception: natamycin). Cleanse skin with soap/water and dry thoroughly. If condition persists/worsens or if irritation occurs, contact physician. Use for full treatment term, even if symptoms improve. Notify physician if no improvement seen. Avoid use of occlusive dressings unless otherwise directed.

---

antiglaucoma agents

Glaucoma is a condition of the eye in which an elevation of intraocular pressure (IOP) leads to damage of the optic nerve and loss of visual fields, and ultimately blindness. Increased IOP results from decreased outflow of aqueous humor through the trabecular network. The most common type of glaucoma is primary open-angle glaucoma. Treatment is accomplished by medical, laser, or surgical management.

ACTION

Currently, seven groups of agents are used in the therapy of primary open-angle glaucoma. The goal of therapy is to reduce elevated IOP, which may be accomplished by (1) decreasing the rate of aqueous humor production, and (2) increasing the rate of outflow of aqueous humor through the trabecular meshwork or uveoscleral route.

Parasympathomimetic: Miotic: direct acting: Directly stimulates smooth muscle receptors in the eye (contracts ciliary muscle, widening the trabecular meshwork; increases aqueous fluid outflow). *Miotic: indirect (anticholinesterase inhibitor):* Inhibits enzyme cholinesterase, potentiating the action of acetylcholine. Directly stimulates smooth muscle receptors in the eye (contracts ciliary muscle, widening the trabecular meshwork; increases aqueous fluid outflow).

Sympathomimetic: Alpha/beta agonists: Stimulate both alpha and beta adrenergic receptors: increases both uveoscleral and trabecular meshwork outflow of aqueous humor. *Alpha-2 agonists:* Decrease aqueous humor production and increase uveoscleral outflow of aqueous humor.

Beta blockers: Decrease production of aqueous humor, may increase aqueous outflow.

Carbonic anhydrase inhibitors: Inhibit enzyme carbonic anhydrase (decreases formation of aqueous fluid).

Prostaglandin: Increases outflow of aqueous fluid through the uveoscleral route.

USES

Reduction of elevated IOP in pts w/open-angle glaucoma and ocular hypertension.

PRECAUTIONS

CONTRAINDICATIONS: Hypersensitivity to medication or any component of the formulation. *Sympathomimetic:* Narrow-angle or shallow-angle glaucoma. *Beta blockers:* Bronchial asthma, history of bronchial asthma, severe COPD, sinus bradycardia, second- or third-degree AV block, CHF. *Miotic: direct acting:* Conditions where constriction is undesirable (e.g., acute iritis/uveitis, some forms of secondary glaucoma). *Miotic: indirect:* Active uveal inflammation, any inflammatory disease of iris or ciliary body, glaucoma associated w/iridocyclitis. **CAUTIONS:** *Sympathomimetic:* History of hypertension, diabetes, hyperthyroidism, heart disease, cerebral arteriosclerosis, bronchial asthma. *Beta blockers:* History of diabetes, hyperthyroidism, cerebral vascular insufficiency. *Miotic: direct acting:* History of acute cardiac failure, bronchial asthma, peptic ulcer, hyperthyroidism, GI spasm, urinary tract obstruction, Parkinson's disease, recent myocardial infarction, hyper/hypotension. *Miotic: indirect:* Myasthenia gravis, narrow-angle glaucoma, bronchial asthma, GI spasm, peptic ulcer, recent myocardial infarction, epilepsy, Parkinson's disease. *Carbonic anhydrase inhibitors:* Pts w/renal or hepatic impairment.

INTERACTIONS

Sympathomimetic: Tricyclic antidepressants may increase cardiovascular effects, may decrease effects of beta blockers; digoxin, other sympathomimetics may increase risk of arrhythmias. *Beta blockers:* Systemic beta blockers may increase effects on systemic blockade; quinidine, verapamil may cause sinus bradycardia. *Miotic: direct acting:* Topical NSAIDs may decrease effect. *Miotic: indirect:* W/succinylcholine during general anesthesia, may cause respiratory and cardiovascular collapse. *Carbonic anhydrase inhibitors:* None significant. *Prostaglandin:* Eye drops containing thimerosal may cause precipitate (give w/interval of at least 5 min).

SIDE EFFECTS

Parasympathomimetic: Direct acting: Decreased vision/dark adaptation, pupil constriction, difficulty driving at night, brow ache, increased perspiration/salivation/bronchial secretions. *Indirect acting:* Same as direct acting. Additionally: cataracts, iris cysts, cystoid macular edema, corneal toxicity.

Sympathomimetic: Alpha/beta: Conjunctival pigment deposit, stinging/burning, pupil dilation, macular edema, corneal endothelium damage, hypertension, increased heart rate, arrhythmias, headache, nervousness. *Alpha-2 agonist:* Hyperemia, pruritus, lid edema, dry eye, conjunctival blanching, mydriasis, fatigue, dry mouth/nose.

Beta blockers: Burning, stinging, ocular irritation, conjunctivitis, blepharitis, keratitis, visual disturbances, brow ache.

Carbonic anhydrase inhibitors: Stinging, bitter taste, paresthesias, GI upset, altered taste, lethargy, depression, diuresis.

Prostaglandin: Redness, conjunctival irritation, iris pigmentation.

TOXIC EFFECTS/ADVERSE REACTIONS

None significant.

CLASSIFICATION

ANTIGLAUCOMA AGENTS

GENERIC NAME	BRAND NAME(S)	AVAILABILITY	USUAL DOSAGE
PARASYMPATHOMIMETIC			
Direct Acting			
carbachol	Isopto Carbachol	Solution: 0.75%, 1.5%, 2.25%, 3%	1 drop 2 times/day
pilocarpine	Isopto Carpine	Solution: 0.25%, 0.5%, 1%, 2%, 3%, 4%, 5%, 6%, 8%, 10%	1–2 drops 3–4 times/day
		Gel: 4%	0.5 inch at bedtime
	Ocusert	Insert: 20 mcg/hr, 40 mcg/hr	One insert weekly
Indirect Acting			
echothiophate	Phospholine Iodide	Solution: 0.03%, 0.06%, 0.125%, 0.25%	1 drop 2 times/day
physostigmine	Eserine	Ointment: 0.25%	Apply up to 3 times/day
demecarium	Humorsol	Solution: 0.125%, 0.25%	1–2 drops 2 times/day up to 2 times/wk
SYMPATHOMIMETIC			
Alpha/Beta			
epinephrine	Epifrin, Epinal, Glaucon	Solution: 0.5%, 1%, 2%	1 drop 1–2 times/day
dipivefrin	Propine	Solution: 0.1%	1 drop q12h
Alpha-2 agonist			
apraclonidine	Iopidine	Solution: 0.5%	1–2 drops 3 times/day
brimonidine	Alphagan	Solution: 0.2%	1–2 drops 2–3 times/day
BETA BLOCKERS			
betaxolol	Betoptic	Suspension: 0.25%	1–2 drops 2 times/day
		Solution: 0.5%	1–2 drops 2 times/day
carteolol	Ocupress	Solution: 1%	1 drop 2 times/day
levobunolol	Betagan	Solution: 0.25%, 0.5%	1 drop 1–2 times/day
metipranolol	Optipranolol	Solution: 0.3%	1 drop 2 times/day
timolol	Betimol, Timoptic	Solution: 0.25%, 0.5%	1 drop 2 times/day
	Timoptic XE	Gel: 0.25%, 0.5%	1 drop daily
CARBONIC ANHYDRASE INHIBITORS			
dorzolamide	Trusopt	Solution: 2%	1 drop 2–3 times/day
brinzolamide	Azopt	Suspension: 1%	1 drop 3 times/day
acetazolamide	Diamox	Tablets: 125 mg, 250 mg Capsules: 500 mg	250 mg to 1 g/day
methazolamide	Neptazine	Tablets: 25 mg, 50 mg	50–100 mg 2–3 times/day
dichlorphenamide	Daranide	Tablets: 50 mg	25–50 mg 1–3 times/day
PROSTAGLANDIN			
latanoprost	Xalatan	Solution: 0.005%	1 drop daily in evening

NURSING IMPLICATIONS

BASELINE ASSESSMENT: Question for hypersensitivity to medication or any component of formulation. Obtain baseline pulse, B/P. Assess physical appearance of eye and pt's perception of vision. EVALUA-TION/INTERVENTION: Evaluate therapeutic response. Assess for

systemic effects. Check B/P, pulse, respirations. PATIENT/FAMILY TEACHING: Teach proper administration of ophthalmic medication. To avoid contamination, do not touch container to any surface. Replace cap after using. Report any decrease in visual acuity, any ocular reaction. Slight stinging/burning may occur on initial instillation. Avoid allowing tip of container to contact eye or surrounding structures. If more than one topical ophthalmic drug is being used, administer at least 5 min apart.

antihistamines

ACTION

Antihistamines (H_1 antagonists) inhibit vasoconstrictor effects and vasodilator effects on endothelial cells of histamine. They block increased capillary permeability, formation of edema/wheal caused by histamine. Many antihistamines can bind to receptors in CNS causing primarily depression (decreased alertness, slowed reaction times, somnolence) but also stimulation (restless, nervousness, inability to sleep). Some may counter motion sickness.

USES

Symptomatic relief of upper respiratory allergic disorders. Allergic reactions associated w/other drugs respond to antihistamines, as do blood transfusion reactions. Used as a second-choice drug in the treatment of angioneurotic edema. Effective in treatment of acute urticaria and other dermatologic conditions. May also be used for preop sedation. Parkinson's disease and motion sickness.

PRECAUTIONS

CONTRAINDICATIONS: Hypersensitivity-cross sensitivity, infants, asthma, narrow-angle glaucoma, prostatic hypertrophy, bladder neck obstruction, CNS depression, hypertension, third trimester of pregnancy, lactation. **CAUTIONS:** Young children, elderly experience exaggerated results: Children, paradoxical excitement; elderly, heavy sedation. Care should be exercised w/cardiovascular disease, hyperthyroidism, and convulsive disorders. Safety during first and second trimester of pregnancy not established.

INTERACTIONS

Alcohol, CNS depressants may increase CNS depressant effects. Anticholinergics may increase anticholinergic effects. MAO inhibitors may increase anticholinergic, CNS depressant effects. Erythromycin, ketoconazole may increase risk of cardiotoxic effect w/astemizole, terfenadine.

CLASSIFICATION

ANTIHISTAMINES

GENERIC NAME	BRAND NAME(S)	DOSAGE RANGE
brompheniramine	Dimetane	Adults: 4 mg q4–6h
		Children 6–12 yrs: 2 mg q4–6h
cetirizine	Zyrtec	Adults: 5–20 mg/day
chlorpheniramine	Chlor-Trimeton	Adults, children >12 yrs: 4 mg q4–6h
		Children 6–12 yrs: 2 mg q4–6h
clemastine	Tavist	Adults, children >12 yrs: 1.34 mg 2×/day up to 2.68 mg 3×/day
cyproheptadine	Periactin	Adults: 4–20 mg/day
		Children 7–14 yrs: 4 mg 2–3×/day
		Children 2–7 yrs: 2 mg 2–3×/day
dexchlorpheniramine	Polaramine	Adults: 2 mg q4–6h
		Children 6–11 yrs: 1 mg q4–6h
dimenhydrinate	Dramamine	Adults, children >12 yrs: 50–100 mg q4–6h
		Children 6–12 yrs: 25–50 mg q6–8h
		Children 2–6 yrs: Up to 12.5–25 mg q6–8h
diphenhydramine	Benadryl	Adults: 25–50 mg q6–8h
		Children >10 kg: 12.5–25 mg 3–4×/day
loratidine	Claritin	Adults: 10 mg/day
		Children >12 yrs: 10 mg/day
promethazine	Phenergan	Adults: 25 mg at bedtime or 12.5 mg 3–4×/day
		Children: 25 mg at hs or 6.25 12.5 mg 3–4×/day

SIDE EFFECTS

Sedation, headache, dizziness, nervousness, restlessness, irritability, loss of appetite, palpitations, urinary retention, constipation.

TOXIC EFFECTS/ADVERSE REACTIONS

Convulsions, hallucinations, tight chest w/shortness of breath, incoordination, flushing of face, hyperthermia, CNS may demonstrate overstimulation or depression. Children are particularly susceptible to overdosage.

NURSING IMPLICATIONS

GENERAL: Take safety precautions when given concurrently w/narcotic analgesics (use side rails; assist w/ambulation). BASELINE ASSESSMENT: Determine initial B/P, temperature, pulse, respiration. INTERVENTION/EVALUATION: Monitor B/P, temperature, pulse, respiration. Assess therapeutic response to medication; be alert to adverse reactions. Check lung sounds. Maintain I&O; assess for urinary retention. Monitor bowel activity; avoid constipation. PATIENT/FAMILY TEACHING: Take oral doses w/meals. Drink 8 or more glasses of fluid/day to decrease viscosity of secretions and help prevent constipation. Do not drive or engage in activities that may be affected by sedative effects. For motion sickness, take $1/2$ to 1 hour before traveling. Avoid alcohol and other medications unless physician approves. Explain adverse reactions, need to report immediately.

antihyperlipidemics

ACTION

Hyperlipidemias are conditions in which the concentration of cholesterol or triglycerides carrying lipoprotein exceeds normal limits. These elevations can accelerate development of atherosclerosis and may lead to thrombosis or myocardial infarction. Cholesterol and triglycerides are transported in lipoproteins including chylomicrons, very low-density lipoprotein (VLDL), which transport triglycerides, low-density lipoproteins (LDL) and high-density lipoproteins (HDL), which transport cholesterol. Agents used in the treatment of hyperlipidemia include:

HMG CoA reductase inhibitors: Block synthesis of cholesterol in liver. Produce a dose-related decrease in the concentration of LDL cholesterol; decrease triglyceride concentration; increase HDL cholesterol.

Fibric acids: Reduce plasma triglycerides by decreasing concentration of VLDL. Primary effect is to increase lipoprotein lipase (promotes VLDL catabolism). May decrease hepatic synthesis/secretion of VLDL.

Bile acid sequestrants: Decrease concentration of cholesterol by lowering LDL levels. Bind bile acids in intestine causing increased fecal excretion, which causes increased production of bile acids from cholesterol.

USES

HMG CoA reductase inhibitors: Adjunctive therapy for reducing elevated total and LDL cholesterol in pts w/primary hypercholesterolemia (types IIa and IIb). *Fibric acids:* Treatment of hypertriglyceridemia in pts w/type IV and V hyperlipidemia. *Bile acid sequestrants:* Adjunctive therapy for reducing elevated serum cholesterol in pts w/primary hypercholesterolemia (types IIa and IIb).

PRECAUTIONS

CONTRAINDICATIONS: Pregnancy, lactation, hypersensitivity to drug or components, liver disease, biliary cirrhosis or obstruction, severe renal dysfunction. **CAUTIONS:** History of liver disease, substantial alcohol consumption. Safety and efficacy in children not established.

INTERACTIONS

HMG CoA reductase inhibitor: Increased risk of rhabdomyolysis, acute renal failure w/cyclosporine, erythromycin, gemfibrozil, niacin, other immunosuppressants.

Fibric acid: May increase effects of oral anticoagulants, hypoglycemics.

Bile acid sequestrants: May increase effects of anticoagulants by decreasing vitamin K. May decrease warfarin absorption. May bind, decrease absorption of digoxin, thiazides, penicillins, propranolol, tetracyclines, folic acid, thyroid hormones, other medications. Bind, decrease effect of oral vancomycin.

CLASSIFICATION

SIDE EFFECTS

GI effects usually lessen or disappear w/continued therapy: constipation, hemorrhoid irritation, diarrhea, abdominal distention, belching, nausea, vomiting. Headache, urticaria, rash. *HMG CoA reductase inhibitors:* Myalgia. Blurred vision w/lovastatin and gemfibrozil.

ANTIHYPERLIPIDEMICS

GENERIC NAME	BRAND NAME(S)	TYPE	DOSAGE RANGE
atorvastatin	Lipitor	HMG CoA reductase inhibitor	10–80 mg/day
cerivastatin	Baycol	HMG CoA reductase inhibitor	0.2–0.3 mg/day
cholestyramine	Colybar Questran	Bile acid sequestrant	4–24 g/day
colestipol	Colestid	Bile acid sequestrant	5–30 g/day
clofibrate	Atromid-S	Fibric acid	2 g/day
fenofibrate	Tricor	Fibric acid	67–201 mg/day
fluvastatin	Lescol	HMG CoA reductase inhibitor	20–40 mg/day
gemfibrozil	Lopid	Fibric acid	1,200 mg/day
lovastatin	Mevacor	HMG CoA reductase inhibitor	20–80 mg/day
pravastatin	Pravachol	HMG CoA reductase inhibitor	10–40 mg/day
simvastatin	Zocor	HMG CoA reductase inhibitor	5–40 mg/day

TOXIC EFFECTS/ADVERSE REACTIONS

Severe constipation w/fecal impaction, GI bleeding, cholelithiasis, acute appendicitis. Angina and cardiac arrhythmias have occurred w/some drugs.

NURSING IMPLICATIONS

GENERAL: Dietary corrections should be attempted before initiating drug therapy. BASELINE ASSESSMENT: Determine serum cholesterol and triglyceride levels. INTERVENTION/EVALUATION: Monitor GI effects, esp. constipation or diarrhea. Check serum cholesterol and triglyceride levels periodically. PATIENT/FAMILY TEACHING: Complete full course; do not omit or change doses. Importance of diet in therapy: Reduce fats, sugars, and cholesterol. Eat high-fiber foods (whole grain cereals, fruits, vegetables) to reduce potential for constipation. Drink several glasses of water between meals. Promptly report bleeding, constipation, or muscle pain/tenderness (esp. w/fever or malaise).

antihypertensives

ACTION

Many groups of medications are used in the treatment of hypertension. In addition to the alpha-adrenergic central agonists and peripheral antagonists and vasodilators discussed below, refer to the classifications of diuretics, beta-adrenergic blockers, calcium channel blockers, and ACE inhibitors, or individual monographs of drugs.

Alpha agonists (central action): Stimulate alpha$_2$-adrenergic receptors in cardiovascular centers of CNS, reducing sympathetic outflow and producing antihypertensive effect.

Alpha antagonists (peripheral action): Block alpha$_1$-adrenergic receptors in arterioles, veins inhibiting vasoconstriction, decreasing peripheral vascular resistance, causing a fall in B/P.

Vasodilators: Directly relax arteriolar smooth muscle, decreasing vascular resistance. Exact mechanism unknown.

USES:

Treatment of mild to severe hypertension, depending on agent selected.

PRECAUTIONS

CONTRAINDICATIONS: Hypersensitivity; severe hepatic dysfunction; pheochromocytoma; advanced renal disease; rheumatic heart disease; systemic lupus erythematosus. **CAUTIONS:** Renal impairment, children, pregnancy, lactation, elderly, angina or ischemic heart disease, after myocardial infarction.

INTERACTIONS

Diuretics, other antihypertensive agents, alcohol increase hypotensive effects. Sympathomimetics may decrease hypotensive effect. Refer to individual monographs for additional information.

SIDE EFFECTS

Specific reactions vary according to the agent given. Weakness, postural hypotension, headache, fatigue, drowsiness, nausea are common.

ANTIHYPERTENSIVES

GENERIC NAME	BRAND NAME(S)	ANTIHYPERTENSIVE EFFECT			DOSAGE RANGE
		ONSET (HRS)	PEAK (HRS)	DURATION (HRS)	
CENTRAL ACTION					
clonidine	Catapres Catapres-TTS	0.5–1	2–4	12–24	PO: 0.2–0.8 mg/day Topical: 0.1–0.6 mg/wk
guanabenz	Wytensin	1	2–4	6–12	PO: 8–32 mg/day
guanfacine	Tenex	—	1–4	24	PO: 1–3 mg/day
methyldopa	Aldomet	2	4–6	12–24	PO: 0.5–3 g/day
PERIPHERAL ACTION					
doxazosin	Cardura	—	—	—	PO: 2–16 mg/day
guanadrel	Hylorel	0.5–2	4–6	9–14	PO: 20–75 mg/day
prazosin	Minipress	2	1–3	6–12	PO: 6–20 mg/day
terazosin	Hytrin	0.25	1–2	12–24	PO: 1–20 mg/day
VASODILATORS					
hydralazine	Apresoline	0.75	0.5–2	6–8	PO: 40–300 mg/day
minoxidil	Loniten	0.5	2–3	24–72	PO: 10–40 mg/day

TOXIC EFFECTS/ADVERSE REACTIONS

Bradycardia and tachycardia; palpitations; hypersensitivity reactions; nausea, vomiting, diarrhea or constipation, arthralgia, reduced hemoglobin, leukopenia, edema. Other reactions per specific agent.

NURSING IMPLICATIONS

GENERAL: For IV administration, monitor pt carefully; place on cardiac monitor and prevent extravasation. BASELINE ASSESSMENT: Determine initial B/P and apical pulse. INTERVENTION/EVALUATION: Monitor apical pulse and B/P; check w/physician for B/P or pulse below parameters set for that pt. Check for edema of hands, feet. PATIENT/FAMILY TEACHING: Teach pt and/or family how to take B/P and pulse. Make position changes slowly (decreases orthostatic hypotension). Follow diet and control weight. Restrict sodium as indicated. Avoid alcohol. Cease smoking. Do not take other medications w/o consulting physician. Do not stop taking medication. Need for lifelong control.

antineoplastics

ACTION

Most antineoplastics inhibit cell replication by interfering w/supply of nutrients or genetic components of the cell (DNA or RNA). Some antineoplastics, referred to as cell cycle-specific (CCS), are particularly effective during a specific phase of cell reproduction (e.g., antimetabolites and plant alkaloids). Other antineoplastics, referred to as cell cycle-nonspecific, act independently of a specific phase of cell division (e.g., alkylating agents and antibiotics). Some hormones are also classified as antineoplastics. Although not cytotoxic, they act to depress cancer growth by altering the hormone environment. In addition, there are a number of miscellaneous agents acting through different mechanisms.

Alkylating agents: Highly reactive compounds forming a bond or cross-link w/DNA, and then damaging cells, likely causing cell death.

Antimetabolites: Capable of inhibiting enzymes necessary for synthesis of essential cellular components or being incorporated into DNA, disrupting DNA function.

Antibiotics: Interact w/DNA, inhibits DNA synthesis, DNA-dependent RNA synthesis; delay or inhibit mitosis.

Hormones: Noncytotoxic, inhibit proliferation by interfering at cellular membrane. May suppress lymphocytes in leukemias/lymphomas, altering hormonal balance in malignancies related to these hormones (e.g., tumors of breast).

Mitotic inhibitors: Act specifically during M (mitosis) phase of cell cycle, preventing cell division.

ANTINEOPLASTICS

GENERIC NAME	BRAND NAME(S)	TYPE	CELL CYCLE-SPECIFIC	USES
aldesleukin	Proleukin	Miscellaneous	No	Metastatic renal cell carcinoma
alitretinoin	Panretin	Miscellaneous	No	AIDS-related Kaposi's sarcoma
altretamine	Hexalen	Miscellaneous	No	Ovarian cancer
anastrozole	Arimidex	Miscellaneous	No	Advanced breast cancer
asparaginase	Elspar	Miscellaneous	No	Acute lymphocytic leukemia
BCG	TheraCys TICE BCG	Miscellaneous	No	Carcinoma in situ of urinary bladder
bexarotene	Targretin	Miscellaneous	No	Cutaneous T-cell lymphoma
bicalutamide	Casodex	Hormone	No	Metastatic prostate cancer
bleomycin	Blenoxane	Antibiotic	Yes	Squamous cell carcinoma, lymphomas, testicular carcinoma
busulfan	Myleran	Alkylating	No	Chronic myelogenous leukemia
capecitabine	Xeloda	Antimetabolite	No	Metastatic breast cancer
carboplatin	Paraplatin	Alkylating	No	Ovarian carcinoma
carmustine	BCNU	Alkylating	No	Brain tumors, multiple myeloma, Hodkin's, non-Hodgkin's lymphomas
chlorambucil	Leukeran	Alkylating	No	Chronic lymphocytic leukemia, malignant lymphomas
cisplatin	Platinol	Alkylating	No	Metastatic testicular, ovarian tumors, advanced bladder cancer
cladribine	Leustatin	Miscellaneous	No	Hairy cell leukemia
cyclophosphamide	Cytoxan	Alkylating	No	Adenocarcinoma of ovary, breast cancer, malignant lymphomas, retinoblastoma, multiple myeloma, leukemias, mycosis fungoides, neuroblastoma
cytarabine	Cytosar	Antimetabolite	Yes	Acute, chronic myelocytic leukemia, acute lymphocytic leukemia
dacarbazine	DTIC	Miscellaneous	No	Metastatic malignant melanoma, Hodgkin's disease
dactinomycin	Cosmegen	Antibiotic	No	Wilms' tumor, rhabdomyosarcoma, choriocarcinoma, testicular carcinoma, Ewing's sarcoma
daunorubicin	Cerubidine	Antibiotic	No	Acute lymphocytic, nonlymphocytic leukemia
denileukin	Ontak	Miscellaneous	No	Cutaneous T-cell lymphoma
diethylstilbestrol	Diethylstilbestrol	Hormone	No	Breast cancer, prostatic carcinoma
docetaxel	Taxotere	Miscellaneous	No	Breast cancer (local advanced/metastatic)
doxorubicin	Adriamycin Rubex	Antibiotic	No	Acute lymphoblastic leukemia, acute myeloblastic leukemia, Wilms' tumor, neuroblastoma, soft tissue and bone sarcomas, breast, ovarian carcinoma, transitional cell bladder carcinoma, thyroid carcinoma, Hodgkin's, non-Hodgkin's lymphomas, bronchogenic carcinoma, gastric carcinoma
epirubicin	Ellence	Antibiotic	No	Breast cancer
estramustine	Emcyt	Hormone	No	Carcinoma of prostate

continued

CLASSIFICATION

ANTINEOPLASTICS *Continued*

GENERIC NAME	BRAND NAME(S)	TYPE	CELL CYCLE-SPECIFIC	USES
etoposide	VePesid	Mitotic inhibitor	Yes	Refractory testicular tumor, small cell lung cancer
exemestane	Aromasin	Miscellaneous	No	Advanced breast cancer
floxuridine	FUDR	Antimetabolite	No	GI adenocarcinoma metastatic to liver
fludarabine	Fludara	Antimetabolite	No	Chronic lymphocytic leukemia
fluorouracil	Adrucil Efudex	Antimetabolite	No	Cancer of colon, rectum, breast, stomach, and pancreas
flutamide	Eulexin	Hormone	No	Metastatic prostatic carcinoma
gemcitabine	Gemzar	Miscellaneous	No	Pancreatic cancer
goserelin	Zoladex	Hormone	No	Carcinoma of prostate
hydroxy urea	Hydrea	Miscellaneous	No	Melanoma, chronic myelocytic leukemia, carcinoma of ovary
idarubicin	Idamycin	Antibiotic	No	Acute myeloid leukemia
ifosfamide	Ifex	Alkylating	No	Germ cell testicular cancer
interferon alfa-2a	Roferon-A	Miscellaneous	No	Hairy cell leukemia, AIDS-related Kaposi's sarcoma
interferon alfa-2b	Intron A	Miscellaneous	No	Hairy cell leukemia, condylomata acuminata, AIDS-related Kaposi's sarcoma
interferon alfa-n3	Alferon N	Miscellaneous	No	Condylomata acuminata
irenotecan	Camptosar	Miscellaneous	No	Metastatic cancer of colon/rectum
letrozole	Femara	Miscellaneous	No	Advanced breast cancer
leuprolide	Lupron	Hormone	No	Advanced prostatic cancer, endometriosis
levamisole	Ergamisol	Miscellaneous	No	Duke's stage C colon cancer
lomustine	CeeNu	Alkylating	No	Brain tumors, Hodgkin's disease
mechlorethamine	Mustargen	Alkylating	No	Polycythemia vera, mycosis fungoides, Hodgkin's disease, lymphosarcoma, chronic myelocytic/lymphocytic leukemia bronchogenic cancer
medroxy-progesterone	Depo-Provera	Hormone	No	Endometrial, renal carcinoma
megestrol	Megace	Hormone	No	Breast, endometrial carcinoma
melphalan	Alkeran	Alkylating	No	Multiple myeloma, ovarian carcinoma
mercaptopurine	Purinethol	Antimetabolite	Yes	Acute lymphatic myelogenous leukemia
methotrexate	Folex	Antimetabolite	Yes	Gestational choriocarcinoma, choriocarcinoma destruens, hydatiform mole, acute lymphocytic leukemia
mitomycin	Mutamycin	Antibiotic	No	Disseminated adenocarcinoma of stomach, pancreas
mitotane	Lysodren	Miscellaneous	No	Adrenal cortical carcinoma
mitoxantrone	Novantrone	Antibiotic	No	Acute nonlymphocytic leukemia
nilutamide	Nilandron	Hormone	No	Metastatic prostatic carcinoma
paclitaxol	Taxol	Miscellaneous	No	Metastatic carcinoma of ovary
pegasparagase	Oncaspar	Miscellaneous	Yes	Acute lymphoblastic leukemia
pentostatin	Nipent	Antibiotic	No	Hairy cell leukemia
plicamycin	Mithracin	Antibiotic	No	Malignant testicular tumors
porfimer	Photofrin	Miscellaneous	No	Esophageal cancer
procarbazine	Matulane	Miscellaneous	No	Hodgkin's disease
streptozocin	Zanosar	Alkylating	No	Metastatic islet cell cancer of pancreas

ANTINEOPLASTICS *Continued*

Generic Name	Brand Name(s)	Type	Cell Cycle-Specific	Uses
tamoxifen	Nolvadex	Hormone	No	Metastatic breast cancer
temozolomide	Temodar	Alkylating	No	Brain tumors
teniposide	Vumen	Mitotic inhibitor	Yes	Refractory acute lymphoblastic leukemia (ALL)
testolactone	Teslac	Hormone	No	Breast carcinoma
thioguanine	Thioguanine	Antimetabolite	Yes	Acute nonlymphocytic leukemia
thiotepa	Thiotepa	Alkylating	No	Adenocarcinoma of breast, ovary; papillary cancer of urinary bladder
topotecan	Hycamtin	Miscellaneous	No	Ovarian cancer
toremifene	Fareston	Hormone	No	Advanced breast cancer
trastuzumab	Herceptin	Miscellaneous	No	Breast cancer
tretinoin	Vesanoid	Miscellaneous	No	Acute promyelocytic leukemia
valrubicin	Valstar	Antibiotic	Yes	Bladder cancer
vinblastine	Velban	Mitotic inhibitor	Yes	Hodgkin's disease, lymphocytic lymphoma, histiocytic lymphoma, mycosis fungoides, advanced testicular carcinoma, Kaposi's sarcoma, breast cancer
vincristine	Oncovin	Mitotic inhibitor	Yes	Acute leukemia, Hodgkin's disease, non-Hodgkin's malignant lymphoma, rhabdomyosarcoma, neuroblastoma, Wilms' tumor
vinorelbine	Navelbine	Mitotic inhibitor	Yes	Metastatic breast cancer, non small cell lung cancer, ovarian cancer, Hodgkin's disease

USES

Treatment of a wide variety of cancers; may be palliative or curative. Treatment of choice in hematologic cancers. Frequently used as adjunctive therapy, e.g., w/surgery or irradiation; most effective when tumor mass has been removed or reduced by radiation. Often used in combinations to increase therapeutic results, decrease toxic effects. Certain agents may be used in nonmalignant conditions; polycythemia vera, psoriasis, rheumatoid arthritis, or immunosuppression in organ transplantation (used only in select cases that are severe and unresponsive to other forms of therapy). Refer to individual monographs.

PRECAUTIONS

CONTRAINDICATIONS: Known hypersensitivity, hepatic or renal insufficiency, severe leukopenia, thrombocytopenia, anemia, pregnancy, lactation (other per individual drug). **CAUTION:** Elderly or very young, infection, radiation therapy, use of other antineoplastics.

INTERACTIONS

Highly complex agents; therefore, check the interactions of each carefully. Anticoagulants and other bone marrow depressants (including other antineoplastics) may increase the risk of myelosuppression effects. Refer to specific monographs.

CLASSIFICATION

SIDE EFFECTS

Stomatitis, nausea and vomiting, diarrhea, alopecia w/several drugs, myelosuppression (see Toxic Effects/Adverse Reactions), hyperuricemia effects on reproduction or local tissue injury.

TOXIC EFFECTS/ADVERSE REACTIONS

Narrow margin of safety between therapeutic and toxic response. Generally proportional to dosage and length of therapy. Myelosuppression (reduction in leukocytes, lymphocytes, thrombocytes, and erythrocytes) may precipitate life-threatening hemorrhage, infection, or anemia. Extravasation at IV site. Toxicity often a major factor in continuing therapy.

NURSING IMPLICATIONS

GENERAL: Take special precautions in handling agents to protect self and others (these drugs are highly toxic and may be inhaled or absorbed through skin; also cause local tissue damage upon contact): (1) Wear gloves, perhaps gown/mask/eye protectors (NIH guidelines). (2) Avoid contaminating articles w/agents. (3) Dispose of all contaminated materials in specifically identified containers. Administer precisely according to schedule. Use strict asepsis and protect pt from infection. When platelet count drops, avoid even the slightest trauma (such as injection or rectal temperature). BASELINE ASSESSMENT: Baseline lab values for RBC/WBC, platelets, vital signs are essential. INTERVENTION/EVALUATION: Monitor laboratory results, esp. RBC, WBC, and platelet counts; promptly report significant changes. Assess for bleeding, signs of infection, anemia. Infuse IV solutions, medications carefully to prevent extravasation. Extravasation is an *emergency* (standing orders and antidote kits must be available before administration). Monitor I&O. Assess response to medication; provide interventions, e.g., mouth care to relieve stomatitis; small, frequent meals of preferred foods/antiemetics for nausea and vomiting. PATIENT/FAMILY TEACHING: Individualized nature of therapy and need for lab tests. Explain that alopecia is reversible, but new hair may have different color, texture. Assist in supporting body image. Despite possible infertility from drug, need for appropriate contraception due to risk of fetal abnormalities; inform physician immediately if pregnancy is suspected. Avoid crowds, persons w/known infections; report signs of infection at once (fever, malaise, flulike symptoms, etc.). Avoid contact w/anyone who recently received live virus vaccine; do not receive vaccinations. Promptly notify physician of bleeding, bruising, unexplained swelling.

antipsychotics

ACTION

Effects of these agents occur at all levels of the CNS. Antipsychotic mechanism unknown, but may antagonize dopamine action as a neurotransmitter in basal ganglia and limbic system. Antipsychotics may block postsynaptic dopamine receptors, inhibit dopamine release, increase dopamine turnover. These medications can be divided into the phenothiazines and nonphenothiazines (miscellaneous). In addition to their use in symptomatic treatment of psychiatric illness, some have antiemetic, antinausea, antihistamine, anticholinergic, and/or sedative effects.

USES

Antipsychotics are primarily used in managing psychotic illness (esp. those w/increased psychomotor activity). They are also used to treat manic phase of bipolar disorder, behavioral problems in children, nausea and vomiting, intractable hiccups, anxiety and agitation, as adjunct in treatment of tetanus, and to potentiate effects of narcotics.

PRECAUTIONS

CONTRAINDICATIONS: Alcoholism or other CNS depression, hepatic dysfunction, bone marrow depression, hypotension, glaucoma, cardiovascular disease, peptic ulcer, young children, hypersensitivity to any of the phenothiazines, pregnancy, lactation. **CAUTIONS:** Administer cautiously to elderly and debilitated pts; this group is more sensitive to effects and requires lower dosage. Drug should be withdrawn slowly; should be discontinued at least 48 hrs before surgery.

INTERACTIONS

Alcohol, CNS depressants may increase CNS, respiratory depression, hypotensive effects. Tricyclic antidepressants, MAO inhibitors may increase sedative, anticholinergic effects. Antithyroid agents may increase risk of agranulocytosis. Extrapyramidal symptoms (EPS) may increase w/EPS-producing medications. Hypotensives may increase hypotension. May decrease levodopa effects. Lithium may decrease absorption, produce adverse neurologic effects.

ANTIPSYCHOTICS

GENERIC NAME	BRAND NAME(S)	SEDATION	HYPOTENSION	ANTICHOLINERGIC	EPS	DOSAGE (MG/DAY)
chlorpromazine	Thorazine	High	High	Moderate	Moderate	30–800
clozapine	Clozaril	High	High	High	Low	25–900
fluphenazine	Prolixin	Low	Low	Low	High	0.5–50
haloperidol	Haldol	Low	Low	Low	High	1–100
loxapine	Loxitane	Moderate	Moderate	Low	High	20–250
mesoridazine	Serentil	High	Moderate	High	Low	30–400
molindone	Moban	Low	Low	Low	High	50–225
olanzapine	Zyprexa	Moderate	Low	Moderate	Low	5–20
perphenazine	Trilafon	Low	Low	Low	High	12–64
pimozide	Orap	Moderate	Low	Moderate	High	1–10
quetiapine	Seroquel	Moderate	Moderate	Moderate	Low	150–750
risperidone	Risperdal	Low	Low	Low	Moderate	4–6
thioridazine	Mellaril	High	High	High	Low	150–800
thiothixene	Navane	Low	Low	Low	High	6–60
trifluoperazine	Stelazine	Low	Low	Low	High	4–40

EPS = extrapyramidal symptoms.

CLASSIFICATION

SIDE EFFECTS

Orthostatic hypotension, drowsiness, blurred vision, constipation, nasal congestion, photosensitivity.

TOXIC EFFECTS/ADVERSE REACTIONS

Hyperpyrexia, depression, insomnia, convulsions, hypertension, adynamic ileus, laryngospasm, bronchospasm, urticaria, menstrual irregularities, impotence, urinary retention, blood dyscrasias, systemic lupus-like reaction, extrapyramidal reactions.

NURSING IMPLICATIONS

GENERAL: Do not mix parenteral solution w/other drugs in the same syringe; give deep IM injections. Have pt remain recumbent for at least 30 min; following parenteral dose, arise slowly and w/assistance. Avoid skin contact w/solutions (contact dermatitis). BASELINE ASSESSMENT: Determine initial B/P, pulse, respirations. Assess pt and environment for necessary supports. INTERVENTION/EVALUATION: Monitor B/P. Assess mental status, response to surroundings. Be alert to suicide potential as energy increases. Assure that oral medication is swallowed. Check bowel activity; avoid constipation. Promptly notify physician of extrapyramidal reactions (usually dose related; more frequent in female geriatric pts). PATIENT/FAMILY TEACHING: Take medication as ordered; do not stop taking or increase dosage. Do not drive or perform activities requiring motor skills until response has been controlled. Side effects usually subside after approximately 2 wks of therapy or can be eliminated/minimized by dosage adjustment. Avoid temperature extremes. Avoid alcohol, other medications. Inform other physicians, dentist of drug therapy. Change positions slowly to prevent orthostatic hypotension.

antivirals

Antiviral medications have recently expanded in number due primarily to the increased number of anti-retroviral agents available for treating patients with HIV infection and its complications. Many of the antivirals are directed toward disrupting one of the many steps in viral infection and replication. Viruses consist of either a single- or double-stranded DNA or RNA enclosed in a protein coat (capsid). Some viruses also have a lipoprotein envelope that may also contain antigenic proteins; other viruses contain enzymes that initiate viral replication inside a host cell. Viruses reproduce or replicate within cells of the host depending on metabolic processes of the host cell. They cannot reproduce independent of a host cell because viruses have no metabolic machinery of their own.

Stages of viral replication include cell entry (attachment, penetration); uncoating (release of viral genome); transcription of viral genome (transcription of viral mRNA, replication of viral genome); translation of viral proteins; post-translational modifications; assembly of virion components; release (budding). Replication cycle begins when a virion (viral particle) binds to a receptor site on the plasma membrane of a host cell. Once bound, the virus releases enzymes weakening the plasma membrane, allowing penetration of the virus. Inside the host cell, the outer coat of the virus dissolves releasing viral genetic material (viral genome), which regulates metabolic activity of the host cell by directing its own replication (synthesis of new messenger RNA [mRNA]) using host ribosomes and viral proteins. After viral nucleic acids/proteins (virion compound) are assembled to form a mature virus, it is released from the host cell (budding) for transmission to other host cells, spreading viral infection.

Viruses are DNA or RNA. DNA viruses include herpesvirus (chicken pox, shingles, herpes) and adenoviruses (conjunctivitis, sore throat). Usually DNA viruses enter the host cell nucleus where viral DNA is transcribed into mRNA of host cell by host cell mRNA polymerase; mRNA is then translated into virus-specific protein following the usual host cell mechanisms. RNA viruses include rubella (German measles), orthomyxoviruses (influenza), and paramyxoviruses (measles, mumps). RNA virus replication in the host cell relies on enzymes in the virion to synthesize its mRNA or on the viral RNA serving as its own mRNA. The mRNA is then translated into various viral proteins, including RNA polymerase that directs the synthesis of more viral mRNA. Most RNA viruses do not involve the host cell in viral replication.

One special group of RNA viruses, known as retroviruses, are responsible for diseases such as AIDS and T-cell leukemias. Retroviruses contain a reverse transcriptase enzyme activity that makes a DNA copy of the viral RNA template. This DNA copy is then integrated into the host genome and transcribed into both genome RNA and mRNA for translation into viral proteins, giving rise to new virus particles.

ACTION

Effective antivirals must inhibit virus-specific nucleic acid/protein synthesis. Possible mechanisms of action of antivirals used for non-HIV infection may include interfering with viral DNA synthesis and viral replication, inactivation of viral DNA polymerases, incorporation and termination of the growing viral DNA chain, prevention of release of viral nucleic acid into the host cell, or interference with viral penetration into cells.

Currently three classes of agents are available for the treatment of HIV infection: nucleoside analogues (reverse transcriptase inhibitors), protease inhibitors, and non-nucleoside reverse transcriptase inhibitors (NNRT).

Nucleoside analogues inhibit viral enzyme reverse transcriptase, reducing replication of cell-included HIV virus.

Protease inhibitors suppress viral replication by inhibiting protease, an enzyme responsible for cleaving viral precursor polypeptides with mature/infective virions.

NNRT inhibits catalytic reaction of reverse transcriptase that is independent of nucleoside binding.

USES

Treatment of HIV infection. Treatment of CMV retinitis in patients with AIDS, acute herpes zoster (shingles), genital herpes (recurrent), mucosal and cutaneous herpes simplex virus, chicken pox, and influenza A viral illness.

ANTIVIRALS

GENERIC NAME	BRAND NAME(S)	LABELED USES
abacavir	Ziagen	HIV infection
acyclovir	Zovirax	*Parenteral:*
		Mucosal/cutaneous HSV-1 and HSV-2
		Varicella zoster (shingles)
		Genital herpes
		Herpes simplex encephalitis
		Oral:
		Genital herpes
		Herpes zoster (shingles)
		Chicken pox (varicella)
adefovir	Preveon	HIV infection
amantadine	Symmetrel	Influenza A virus respiratory tract illness
amprenavir	Agenerase	HIV infection
cidofovir	Vistide	CMV retinitis in pts w/AIDS
delavirdine	Rescriptor	HIV infection
didanosine	Videx	HIV infection
efavirenz	Sustiva	HIV infection
famciclovir	Famvir	Acute herpes zoster (shingles)
		Genital herpes (recurrent)
fomivirsen	Vitravene	CMV retinitis
foscarnet	Foscavir	CMV retinitis
		HSV infections in immunocompromised pts
ganciclovir	Cytovene	CMV retinitis, CMV disease
indinavir	Crixivan	HIV infection
lamivudine	Epivir	HIV infection
nelfinavir	Viracept	HIV infection
nevirapine	Viramune	HIV infection
oseltamivir	Tamiflu	Influenza A and B virus
penciclovir	Denavir	Cold sores
ramantadine	Flumadine	Influenza A virus
ribavirin	Virazole	Lower respiratory infection in infants, children due to respiratory syncytial virus (RSV)
ritonavir	Norvir	HIV infection
saquinavir	Invirase	HIV infection
stavudine	Zerit	HIV infection
valacyclovir	Valtrex	Herpes zoster (shingles)
		Genital herpes (recurrent)
zalcitabine	Hivid	HIV infection
zanamivir	Relenza	Influenza A and B virus
zidovudine	Retrovir	HIV infection

PRECAUTIONS

CONTRAINDICATIONS: Hypersensitivity to any component of the product.

Note: Because of the diversity of the antivirals, refer to individual monographs for further information on cautions, side effects, adverse/toxic effects, drug interactions, etc.

NURSING IMPLICATIONS

BASELINE ASSESSMENT: Assess health history (past medical, drug history, lifestyle, type/severity of symptoms). Ask about fatigue, chills, sweating, skin color changes. Note any localized swelling, pain, tenderness in lymph node regions. Assess for pregnancy/lactation. INTERVENTION/EVALUATION: Monitor renal function, fluid status, I/O, sleep and rest patterns, altered nutrition related to nausea produced by the antivirals. Observe for therapeutic effect, signs/symptoms of improvement. Monitor for undesired clinical response/toxicity associated w/ antivirals. Review results assessing renal/hepatic function and integrity of hemopoietic system. Inspect IV infusion site carefully. PATIENT/FAMILY TEACHING: Inform pt of importance of immunization and maintaining immunization against viral infections for small children and adults at high risk of acquiring influenza. Inform pt of importance of adequate fluid intake. Call physician if condition worsens or pt experiences any toxicity with the medication. Inform of ways to control spread/recurrence of viral infections. Drug therapy for AIDS/genital herpes does not prevent transmission to others or prevent opportunistic infections.

beta-adrenergic blockers

ACTION

Beta-adrenergic blockers competitively block beta$_1$-adrenergic receptors, located primarily in myocardium, and beta$_2$-adrenergic receptors, located primarily in bronchial and vascular smooth muscle. By occupying beta-receptor sites, these agents prevent naturally occurring or administered epinephrine/norepinephrine from exerting their effects. The results are basically opposite to that of sympathetic stimulation.

Effect of beta$_1$-blockade includes slowing heart rate, decreasing cardiac output and contractility; effect of beta$_2$-blockade includes bronchoconstriction, increased airway resistance in those w/asthma or COPD. Beta blockers can affect cardiac rhythm/automaticity (decrease sinus rate, SA, AV conduction; increase refractory period in AV node). Decrease systolic and diastolic B/P; exact mechanism unknown but may block peripheral receptors, decrease sympathetic outflow from CNS, or decrease renin release from kidney. All beta blockers mask tachycardia that occurs w/hypoglycemia. When applied to the eye, reduces intraocular pressure and aqueous production.

USES

Management of hypertension, angina pectoris, arrhythmias, hypertrophic subaortic stenosis, migraine headaches, myocardial infarction (prevention), glaucoma.

PRECAUTIONS

CONTRAINDICATIONS: Severe renal or hepatic disease, history of allergy, hyperthyroidism, asthma, emphysema, CHF, cerebrovascular accident, hypotension, sinus bradycardia, pregnancy. Safety in lactation not established. **CAUTIONS:** Diabetes mellitus, elderly, peptic ulcer.

INTERACTIONS

Diuretics, other hypotensives may increase hypotensive effect. Sympathomimetics, xanthines may mutually inhibit effects. May mask symptoms of hypoglycemia, prolong hypoglycemic effect of insulin, oral hypoglycemics. NSAIDs may decrease antihypertensive effect. Cimetidine may increase concentration.

CLASSIFICATION

BETA BLOCKERS

GENERIC NAME	BRAND NAME(S)	SELECTIVITY	USES	DOSAGE RANGE
acebutolol	Sectral	Beta₁	HTN, arrhythmias	HTN: 200–1,200 mg/day Arrhythmias: 600–1,200 mg/day
atenolol	Tenormin	Beta₁	HTN, angina, MI	HTN: 50–100 mg/day Angina: 50–200 mg/day MI: 50–100 mg/day
betaxolol	Kerlone Betoptic	Beta₁	HTN, ocular HTN, glaucoma	HTN: 10–20 mg/day Ophth: 1 drop 2×/day
bisoprolol	Zebeta	Beta₁	HTN	HTN: 2.5–20 mg/day
carteolol	Cartrol	Beta₁, beta₂	HTN	HTN: 2.5–10 mg/day
carvedilol	Coreg	Beta, beta₂, alpha₁	HTN	HTN: 12.5–50 mg/day
esmolol	Brevibloc	Beta₁	Arrhythmias	Arrhythmias: 50–200 mcg/kg/min
labetalol	Normodyne Trandate	Beta₁, beta₂ Alpha₁	Hypertension	HTN: 200–400 mg/day
levobunolol	Betagan	Beta₁, beta₂	Ocular HTN, glaucoma	Ophth: 1 drop 1–2×/day
metipranolol	OptiPranolol	Beta₁, beta₂	Ocular HTN, glaucoma	Ophth: 1 drop 2×/day
metoprolol	Lopressor	Beta₁	HTN, angina, MI	HTN: 100–450 mg/day Angina: 100–400 mg/day MI: 50 mg q6h
nadolol	Corgard	Beta₁, beta₂	HTN, angina	HTN: 40–320 mg/day Angina: 40–240 mg/day
penbutolol	Levotol	Beta₁, beta₂	HTN	HTN: 10–40 mg/day
pindolol	Visken	Beta₁, beta₂	HTN	HTN: 10–60 mg/day
propranolol	Inderal	Beta₁, beta₂	HTN, angina, arrhythmias, MI, migraine, tremors	HTN: 120–640 mg/day Angina: 80–320 mg/day Arrhythmias: 10–30 mg 3–4×/day MI: 180–240 mg/day
sotalol	Betapace	Beta₁, beta₂	Arrhythmias	Arrhythmias: 160–640 mg/day
timolol	Blocadren Timoptic	Beta₁, beta₂	HTN, MI, migraine, glaucoma	HTN: 10–60 mg/day MI: 10 mg 2×/day Ophth: 1 drop 1–2×/day

HTN = hypertension; MI = myocardial infarction.

SIDE EFFECTS

Postural hypotension, lightheadedness, fatigue, weakness, reflex tachycardia.

TOXIC EFFECTS/ADVERSE REACTIONS

Severe hypotension, nausea and vomiting, bradycardia, heart block, circulatory failure.

NURSING IMPLICATIONS

GENERAL: Use cardiac monitor for IV administration and preferably for initiation of oral therapy. BASELINE ASSESSMENT: Initial B/P, apical pulse. INTERVENTION/EVALUATION: Monitor B/P and apical

pulse before giving drug; notify physician before administration if
B/P or pulse are not within agreed parameters. Assess for CHF (dyspnea, peripheral edema, jugular venous distension, increased
weight, rales in lungs, decreased urine output). Assess extremities
for peripheral circulation (warmth, color, quality of pulses). PA-
TIENT/FAMILY TEACHING: Teach how to take B/P, pulse correctly.
Change position slowly to prevent orthostatic hypotension. Do not
take OTC cold medications, nasal decongestants. Restrict sodium
and alcohol as ordered. Do not stop taking drug suddenly. Report
chest pain, fatigue, shortness of breath.

bronchodilators

ACTION

Asthma (reversible airway obstruction) is the most common breathing
disorder.

Methylxanthines: Directly relax smooth muscle of bronchial airway, pulmonary blood vessels (relieve bronchospasm, increase vital capacity).
Increase cyclic 3,5-adenosine monophosphate.

Beta$_2$-adrenergic agonists: Stimulate beta receptors in lung, relax
bronchial smooth muscle, increase vital capacity, decrease airway resistance.

Anticholinergics: Inhibit cholinergic receptors on bronchial smooth
muscle (block acetylcholine action).

Leukotriene receptor antagonist: Blocks effects of leukotriene (bronchoconstriction, inflammation, edema).

Antileukotriene: Inhibits enzyme 5-lipoxygenase, reducing production
of leukotriene, a bronchoconstrictor.

USES

Relief of bronchospasm occurring during anesthesia; in bronchial
asthma, bronchitis, or emphysema.

PRECAUTIONS

CONTRAINDICATIONS: Hypersensitivity to that agent or intolerance to
others in the classification, components of preparation. Severe renal or
hepatic dysfunction. **CAUTIONS:** Pregnancy, lactation, elderly, hepatic
disease, CHF, or other cardiac conditions that would be adversely affected by cardiac stimulation.

INTERACTIONS

Methylxanthines: Glucocorticoids may produce hypernatremia. Phenytoin, primidone, rifampin may increase metabolism. Beta blockers may
decrease effects. Cimetidine, ciprofloxacin, erythromycin, norfloxacin may
increase concentration, toxicity. Smoking may decrease concentration.

CLASSIFICATION

Beta₂-adrenergic agonists: General anesthetics may increase risk of arrhythmias. Tricyclic antidepressants, maprotiline may increase cardiovascular effects. May have mutually inhibitory effects w/beta-adrenergic blockers. May increase risk of arrhythmias w/digoxin.

Anticholinergics: None significant.

BRONCHODILATORS

GENERIC NAME	BRAND NAME(S)	ROUTE OF ADMINISTRATION	TYPE
albuterol	Proventil Ventolin	Inhalation Oral	Beta₂ agonist
aminophylline	—	Oral Intravenous	Methylxanthine
bitolterol	Tornalate	Inhalation	Beta₂ agonist
epinephrine	Adrenalin	SubQ Intravenous	Beta₂ agonist
ipratropium	Atrovent	Inhalation	Anticholinergic
isoetharine	Bronkosol	Inhalation	Beta₂ agonist
isoproterenol	Isuprel	Inhalation	Beta₂ agonist
levalbuterol	Xopenex	Inhalation	Beta₂ agonist
metaproterenol	Alupent	Inhalation	Beta₂ agonist
montelukast	Singulair	Oral	Leukotriene receptor antagonist
salmeterol	Serevent	Inhalation	Beta₂ agonist
terbutaline	Brethine Bricanyl	Inhalation Oral SubQ	Beta₂ agonist
theophylline	Aerolate Slo-Bid Slo-Phyllin Theo-24 Theo-Dur Theolair Uniphyl	Oral	Methylxanthine
zafirlukast	Accolate	Oral	Leukotriene receptor antagonist
zileuton	Zyflo	Oral	Antileukotriene

SIDE EFFECTS

Nausea, increased pulse rate, nervousness, weakness, trembling, insomnia.

TOXIC EFFECTS/ADVERSE REACTIONS

Tachycardia, irregular heartbeat, headache, nausea and vomiting, severe weakness, increased B/P.

NURSING IMPLICATIONS

GENERAL: Administer oral agents on regular schedule. Assist pt in identifying what triggered an acute bronchospasm attack. **INTERVENTION/EVALUATION:** Monitor arterial blood gases, serum levels for aminophylline, theophylline. Assess lung sounds, B/P, pulse, respirations. Encourage fluid intake to decrease viscosity of secretions. PATIENT/FAMILY TEACHING: Demonstrate correct use of inhalers. Drink 8 or more glasses of fluid/day. Avoid caffeine-containing products, e.g., coffee, tea, colas, chocolate (cause further CNS stimulation). Do not smoke. Use other medications only after consulting physician. Teach effective deep breathing and coughing. Notify physician if symptoms are not relieved or worsen. Report adverse reactions.

calcium channel blockers

ACTION

Calcium channel blockers inhibit the flow of extracellular Ca^{+2} ions across cell membrane of cardiac cells, vascular tissue. Calcium channel blockers relax arterial smooth muscle, depress the rate of sinus node pacemaker, slow AV conduction, decrease heart rate, produce negative inotropic effect (rarely seen clinically due to reflex response). All calcium channel blockers decrease coronary vascular resistance, increase coronary blood flow, reduce myocardial oxygen demand. Degree of action varies w/individual agent.

CALCIUM CHANNEL BLOCKERS

GENERIC NAME	BRAND NAME(S)	ONSET ACTION	USES	RTE ADMIN	DOSAGE RANGE
amlodipine	Norvasc	—	Angina Hypertension	PO	2.5–10 mg/day
bepridil	Vascor	1 hr	Angina	PO	200–400 mg/day
diltiazem	Cardizem Cardizem CD	30–60 min	Angina Hypertension Arrhythmias	PO, IV	PO: 120–360 mg/day IV: 20–25 mg IV bolus; 5–15 mg/hr IV infusion
felodipine	Plendil	2–5 hrs	Hypertension	PO	5–10 mg/day
isradipine	DynaCirc	2 hrs	Hypertension	PO	5–20 mg/day
nicardipine	Cardene	20 min	Angina Hypertension	PO	60–120 mg/day
nifedipine	Adalat Procardia	20 min	Angina Hypertension	SL, PO	PO: 30–120 mg/day XL: 30–60 mg/day
nimodipine	Nimotop	—	Subarachnoid hemorrhage	PO	60 mg q4h × 21 days
nisoldipine	Sular	—	Hypertension	PO	20–60 mg/day
verapamil	Calan Isoptin Verelan	30 min	Angina Hypertension Arrhythmias	PO, IV	PO: 120–480 mg/day IV: 5–10 mg, max: 10 mg/dose

SL = sublingual; XL = sustained-release.

CLASSIFICATION

USES

Treatment of essential hypertension, treatment and prophylaxis of angina pectoris (including vasospastic, chronic stable, unstable), prevent/control supraventricular tachyarrhythmias, prevent neurologic damage due to subarachnoid hemorrhage.

PRECAUTIONS

CONTRAINDICATIONS: Renal or hepatic dysfunction, heart block, hypotension, extreme bradycardia, aortic stenosis, sick-sinus syndrome, severe left ventricular dysfunction, pregnancy, lactation. **CAUTIONS:** Administer cautiously to elderly because half-life may be increased. Liver enzymes should be monitored periodically.

INTERACTIONS

Beta-adrenergic blockers may have additive effect. May increase digoxin concentration. Procainamide, quinidine may increase risk of QT interval prolongation. Carbamazepine, quinidine, theophylline may increase concentration, toxicity.

SIDE EFFECTS

Headache, nausea, dizziness or lightheadedness, hypotension, constipation.

TOXIC EFFECTS/ADVERSE REACTIONS

Peripheral edema, palpitations, bradycardia, dyspnea, wheezing w/possible pulmonary edema, severe hypotension, second- or third-degree heart block (rare). Administered IV for tachyarrhythmias, verapamil, nicardipine, diltiazem have the greatest potential for severe reactions.

NURSING IMPLICATIONS

GENERAL: Parenteral administration requires close cardiac monitoring w/emergency equipment close by. Discontinuation should be gradual. Be alert to potential for hypotension, esp. when pt is taking other antihypertensive drugs or beta-adrenergic blockers. **BASELINE ASSESSMENT:** Assess initial B/P and apical pulse. **INTERVENTION/EVALUATION:** Monitor B/P and apical pulse before administration; notify physician before giving dose if not within agreed parameters. Check frequency, consistency of stools; avoid constipation. Assess lungs for rales, extremities for peripheral edema. Check I&O. **PATIENT/FAMILY TEACHING:** Teach how to take B/P and pulse correctly. Change position slowly to avoid orthostatic hypotension. Restrict sodium as ordered. Avoid alcohol, other medications w/o consulting physician. Do not overexert when anginal pain relieved. Do not stop taking medication. Report irregular heartbeat, dizziness, shortness of breath. Angina can occur if medication is stopped abruptly.

cardiac glycosides

ACTION

Direct action on myocardium causes increased force of contraction, resulting in increased stroke volume and cardiac output. Depression of SA node, decreased conduction time through AV node, and decreased electrical impulses due to vagal stimulation slow heart rate. Improved myocardial contractility is probably due to improved transport of calcium, sodium, and potassium ions across cell membranes.

USES

CHF, atrial fibrillation, atrial flutter, paroxysmal atrial tachycardia, and treatment of cardiogenic shock w/pulmonary edema.

PRECAUTIONS

CONTRAINDICATIONS: History of hypersensitivity, digitalis toxicity, ventricular fibrillation, ventricular tachycardia (unless due to CHF), severe myocarditis. **CAUTIONS:** Renal insufficiency, hypokalemia, incomplete AV block, infants and children, elderly and debilitated pts. Safety in pregnancy, lactation not established.

INTERACTIONS

Glucocorticoids, amphotericin, potassium-depleting diuretics may increase toxicity (due to hypokalemia). Amiodarone may increase concentration, toxicity; additive effect on SA, AV nodes. Antiarrhythmics, parenteral calcium, sympathomimetics may increase risk of arrhythmias. Antidiarrheals, cholestyramine, colestipol may decrease absorption. Diltiazem, verapamil, quinidine may increase concentrations. Parenteral magnesium may cause conduction changes, heart block.

SIDE EFFECTS

The margin of safety between a therapeutic and a toxic dose is very narrow.

TOXIC EFFECTS/ADVERSE REACTIONS

Anorexia, nausea and vomiting, abdominal pain, and diarrhea occur commonly. Arrhythmias, such as premature ventricular contractions (PVCs) and bradycardia, also may signal overdosage. CNS effects are most common in elderly pts; headache, drowsiness, confusion, and visual disturbances such as halos around objects, altered color perception, blurring and flickering dots. In children arrhythmias are the most reliable sign; other effects are rarely seen.

NURSING IMPLICATIONS

GENERAL: Parenteral administration requires close cardiac monitoring. **BASELINE ASSESSMENT:** Establish initial B/P and apical pulse. **INTERVENTION/EVALUATION:** Assess apical pulse before giving each dose; withhold and notify physician if pulse below 60 or above

CLASSIFICATION

100 for adults. Measure I&O; weigh daily. Check for dependent edema; auscultate lungs for rales. Monitor potassium. PATIENT/FAMILY TEACHING: Take as prescribed; do not miss dose or take extra dose. Teach pt/family to take pulse and report pulse outside parameters determined by physician. Restrict sodium and alcohol as ordered. Cease smoking. Avoid OTC cold preparations, nasal decongestants, coffee, tea, colas, chocolates (stimulants).

cholinergic agonists/anticholinesterase

ACTION

CHOLINERGIC AGONISTS: Referred to as muscarinics or parasympathetics and consist of two basic drug groups: choline esters and cholinomimetic alkaloids. Primary action mimics actions of acetylcholine at postganglionic parasympathetic nerves. Primary properties include the following: *Cardiovascular system:* Vasodilation, decreased cardiac rate, decreased conduction in SA, AV nodes, decreased force of myocardial contraction. *Gastrointestinal:* Increased tone, motility of GI smooth muscle, increased secretory activity of GI tract. *Urinary tract:* Increased contraction of detrusor muscle of urinary bladder, resulting in micturition. *Eye:* Miosis, contraction of ciliary muscle.

ANTICHOLINESTERASE (anti-ChE), also known as cholinesterase inhibitors: Inactivates cholinesterase, which prevents acetylcholine breakdown causing acetylcholine to accumulate at cholinergic receptor sites. These agents can be considered indirect-acting cholinergic agonists. Primary properties include action of cholinergic agonists just noted. *Skeletal neuromuscular junction:* Effects are dose dependent. At therapeutic doses, increases force of skeletal muscle contraction; at toxic doses, reduces muscle strength.

USES

Paralytic ileus and atony of urinary bladder. Treatment of primary, and some secondary, glaucoma. Myasthenia gravis (weakness, marked fatigue of skeletal muscle). Terminates, reverses effects of neuromuscular blocking agents.

PRECAUTIONS

CONTRAINDICATIONS: Intestinal or urinary tract obstructions, known hypersensitivity, pregnancy, lactation, acute peptic ulcer, hyperthyroidism, peritonitis, bronchial asthma. **CAUTIONS:** Have atropine readily available in case of cholinergic crisis.

INTERACTIONS

Given with other cholinergics—increased effects w/greater potential for toxicity. Ganglionic blocking agents, used concurrently with cholinergics, may produce significant fall in B/P. Anticholinergics antagonize effects of cholinergics.

SIDE EFFECTS

Increased urinary frequency, salivation, belching, nausea, dizziness. Side effects infrequent, more likely w/subcutaneous injection or high doses.

TOXIC EFFECTS/ADVERSE REACTIONS

Overdose (cholinergic crisis): Abdominal cramps, diarrhea, excessive salivation, diaphoresis, muscle weakness, respiratory difficulty. Requires immediate treatment.

CHOLINERGIC AGONISTS

GENERIC NAME	BRAND NAME(S)	TYPE	USE	DOSAGE RANGE
acetylcholine	Miochol	Cholinergic	Miotic	Ophth: 0.5–2 ml
bethanechol	Urecholine	Cholinergic	Nonobstructive urinary retention	PO: 10–50 mg 3–4×/day SubQ: 2.5–5 mg 3–4×/day
carbachol	Carbachol	Cholinergic	Miotic	Ophth: 0.5 ml
			Glaucoma	Ophth: 1–2 drops up to 4×/day
demecarium	Humorsol	Anti-ChE	Glaucoma	Ophth: 1–2 drops 2×/day to 2 drops/wk
echothiophate	Phospholine	Anti-ChE	Glaucoma	Ophth: 1 drop qOd to 2×/day
edrophonium	Tensilon	Anti-ChE	Dx, myasthenia gravis Reverse tubocurarine	IV: 10 mg in 30–45 secs; max: 40 mg
isoflurophate	Floropryl	Anti-ChE	Glaucoma	Ophth ointment: q8–72h
neostigmine	Prostigmin	Anti-ChE	Dx/tx, myasthenia gravis Antidote Neuromuscular blocker	PO: 15–375 mg/day SubQ, IM: 0.5 mg; 0.01–0.04 mg/kg IV: 0.5–2 mg
physostigmine	Eserine	Anti-ChE	Glaucoma Antidote	Ophth: 1–2 drops up to 4×/day IM, IV: 0.5–2 mg
pilocarpine	Isopto Carpine Ocusert	Cholinergic	Glaucoma	Ophth: 1–2 drops up to 6×/day Every 7 days
pyridostigmine	Mestinon	Anti-ChE	Tx, myasthenia gravis Reverse tubocurarine	PO: 60–1,500 mg/day IM: 0.5–1.5 mg/kg IV: 0.1–0.25 mg/kg

NURSING IMPLICATIONS

GENERAL: Have atropine readily available in case of cholinergic crisis. BASELINE ASSESSMENT: Check pulse, respirations. INTERVENTION/EVALUATION: Monitor pulse, respiration; be alert for signs/symptoms of cholinergic crisis. Assess for therapeutic results: (1) In abdominal distention or paralytic ileus, listen for bowel sounds, check passing of flatus or stool, measure abdomen for decreased distention. (2) For urinary retention, palpate bladder and check for urination. Implement measures that support urination, e.g., running water, pouring warm water over perineum, privacy. If urina-

CLASSIFICATION

tion does not occur, determine whether catheterization is needed. Determine cause of urinary retention, e.g., trauma from surgical manipulation or narcotics given for pain. (3) For myasthenia gravis, observe for improved muscle tone and subsequently greater activity, less fatigue. PATIENT/FAMILY TEACHING: Explain purpose of medication. Increased salivation is to be expected. Call for assistance to bathroom after subcutaneous injection.

corticosteroids

ACTION

Synthesized by adrenal cortex, the corticosteroids can be divided into glucocorticoids (hepatic glycogen deposition) and mineralocorticoids (sodium retention). Corticosteroids have numerous effects including the following: *Carbohydrate, protein metabolism:* Increase glucose formation, decrease peripheral utilization, enhance glycogen storage, increase gluconeogenesis (transformation of protein to glucose). *Lipid metabolism:* Redistribute body fat, lipolysis of triglyceride of adipose tissue. *Electrolyte/water balance:* Enhance sodium reabsorption, potassium excretion, increase extracellular volume. *Formed elements:* Increase hemoglobin, red blood cell count, decrease number of lymphocytes, eosinophils, monocytes, basophils, increase polymorphonuclear leukocytes. *Anti-inflammatory:* Inhibit anti-inflammatory process (edema, capillary dilatation, migration of leukocytes into inflamed area, phagocytic activity). *Immunosuppression:* Inhibit early steps in immunity.

USES

Replacement therapy in adrenal insufficiency, including Addison's disease. Symptomatic treatment of multiorgan disease/conditions. Rheumatoid and osteo arthritis, severe psoriasis, ulcerative colitis, lupus erythematosus, anaphylactic shock, status asthmaticus, organ transplant.

PRECAUTIONS

CONTRAINDICATIONS: Hypersensitivity; peptic ulcer, tuberculosis, or any suspected infection; blood clotting disorders; severe renal or hepatic impairment; CHF or hypertension, lactation. **CAUTIONS:** Cautious administration in children, geriatric, and postmenopausal pts. Safe use during pregnancy has not been established.

INTERACTIONS

Amphotericin may increase hypokalemia. May decrease effect of oral hypoglycemics, insulin, diuretics, potassium supplements. May increase digoxin toxicity (due to hypokalemia). Hepatic enzyme inducers may decrease effect. Live virus vaccines may potentiate virus replication, increase vaccine side effects, decrease pt's antibody response to vaccine.

CORTICOSTEROIDS

GENERIC NAME	BRAND NAME(S)	RTE ADMIN
alclometasone	Acolvate	Topical
amcinonide	Cyclocort	Topical
beclomethasone	Beclovent, Vanceril Beconase, Vancenase	Inhalation, intranasal
betamethasone	Celestone, Diprosone Uticort, Valisone	Topical, oral, IV, intralesional, intra-articular
budesonide	Rhinocort	Intranasal
clobetasol	Temovate	Topical
cortisone	Cortone	Topical, oral
desonide	Tridesilone	Topical
desoximetasone	Topicort	Topical
dexamethasone	Decadron	Topical, oral, IM, IV, ophthalmic, intranasal, inhalation
fludrocortisone	Florinef	Oral
flunisolide	Aerobid, Nasalide	Inhalation, intranasal
fluocinolone	Synalar, Synemol	Topical
fluorometholone	FML	Ophthalmic
flurandrenolide	Cordran	Topical
fluticasone	Cutivate, Flonase	Topical, intranasal
halcinonide	Halog	Topical
halobetasol	Ultravate	Topical
hydrocortisone	Cort-Dome, Cortef, Hydrocortone, Solu-Cortef	Topical, oral, IM, IV, SubQ, rectal
methylprednisolone	Medrol, Solu-Medrol	Oral, IM, IV
mometasone	Elocon	Topical
prednicarbate	Dermatop	Topical
prednisolone	Delta-Cortef, Hydeltra, Hydeltrasol	Oral, IM, IV, intralesional, intra-articular
prednisone	Deltasone, Meticorten, Orasone	Oral
rimexolone	Vexol	Ophthalmic
triamcinolone	Azmacort, Kenalog, Nasacort	Oral, inhalation, intranasal

SIDE EFFECTS

Rarely cause side effects w/short-term high dose or replacement therapy. Sodium/water retention, increased appetite.

TOXIC EFFECTS/ADVERSE REACTIONS

Long-term therapy causes numerous adverse reactions; peptic ulcer and steroid diabetes are the most serious. Osteoporosis, petechiae, hirsutism, acne, menstrual irregularities. Cushing-like symptoms (moon face, excess fat deposits of trunk, neck, and shoulders w/buffalo hump, wasting of arms and legs). Edema, hypertension. May have depression, personality change, and insomnia; cataracts or glaucoma, delayed healing, suppressed immune response.

NURSING IMPLICATIONS

GENERAL: Take precautions to avoid infection; recognize that these agents mask signs and symptoms of developing illness. Administer oral drugs w/food or milk in early morning in a single dose. Withdraw medication slowly. BASELINE ASSESSMENT: Determine initial B/P, temperature, pulse, respiration, weight, blood glucose, electrolytes, EKG and TB skin test results. INTERVENTION/EVALUATION: Monitor B/P, temperature, pulse, respiration, daily weight, I&O, blood glucose, and electrolytes (esp. potassium and calcium). Be alert for signs and symptoms of hypokalemia, hypocalcemia. Check dependent areas for edema. Assess for mood, personality change. PATIENT/FAMILY TEACHING: Follow-up visits and lab tests are essential. Carry identification of drug and dose, physician name and phone number. Do not change dose/schedule or stop taking drug; must taper off gradually under medical supervision. Report severe symptoms (visual disturbances or severe gastric distress) to physician immediately. Promptly report sudden weight gain or swelling, sore throat, fever, or other signs of infection. Wounds may heal slowly. Avoid crowds, persons w/known infections. Do not receive vaccinations. Do not take aspirin or any other medication w/o consulting physician. Give instructions for diet (usually sodium restricted w/high vitamin D, protein, and potassium). Inform dentist or other physicians of glucocorticoid therapy now or within past 12 mos. Do not overuse joint that was injected for symptomatic relief. For topical application, apply after shower for best absorption; do not cover; avoid sunlight on treated area.

corticosteroids: topical

ACTION

Diffuses across cell membranes, forms complexes w/cytoplasm. Complexes stimulate protein synthesis of inhibitory enzymes responsible for anti-inflammatory effects (e.g., inhibit edema, erythema, pruritus, capillary dilation, phagocytic activity).

Topical corticosteroids can be classified based on potency:

Low: Modest anti-inflammatory effect, safest for chronic application, facial and intertriginous application, w/occlusion, for infants/young children.

Medium: For moderate inflammatory conditions (e.g., chronic eczematous dermatoses). May use for facial and intertriginous application for only limited time.

High: For more severe inflammatory conditions (e.g., lichen simplex chronicus, psoriasis). May use for facial and intertriginous application for short time only. Used in areas of thickened skin due to chronic conditions.

Very high: Alternative to systemic therapy for local effect (e.g., chronic lesions caused by psoriasis). Increased risk of skin atrophy. Used for short periods on small areas. Avoid occlusive dressings.

CORTICOSTEROIDS: TOPICAL

GENERIC NAME	BRAND NAME(S)	POTENCY	DOSAGE FORMS
alclometasone	Aclovate	Low	Cream, ointment
amcinonide	Cyclocort	High	Cream, ointment, lotion
betamethasone benzoate	Uticort	Medium	Cream, lotion, gel
betamethasone dipropionate	Diprosone Maxivate	High	Ointment, cream, lotion, aerosol
betamethasone dipropionate (augmented)	Diprolene	Very high	Ointment, cream, gel, lotion
betamethasone valerate	Valisone	High	Ointment, cream, lotion
clobetasol	Temovate	Very high	Ointment, cream
desonide	Tridesilon	Low	Ointment, cream, lotion
desoximetasone	Topicort	High	Ointment, cream, gel
dexamethasone	Decadron	Medium	Cream
flucinonide	Lidex	High	Cream, ointment, solution, gel
fluocinolone	Synalar	High	Ointment, cream, solution
flurandrenolide	Cordran	Medium	Ointment, cream, lotion
fluticasone	Cutivate	Medium	Ointment, cream
halcinonide	Halog	High	Ointment, cream, solution
halobetasol	Ultravate	Very high	Ointment, cream
hydrocortisone	Cort-Dome Hytone	Medium	Ointment, cream, lotion, gel
mometasone	Elocon	Medium	Ointment, cream, lotion
prednicarbate	Dermatop	—	Cream
triamcinolone	Aristocort Kenalog	Medium	Ointment, cream, lotion

USES

Provides relief of inflammation/pruritus associated w/corticosteroid-responsive disorders: e.g., contact dermatitis, eczema, insect bite reactions, first- and second-degree localized burns/sunburn.

PRECAUTIONS

CONTRAINDICATIONS: Hypersensitivity to corticosteroids. Do not use on preexisting skin atrophy, infection at treatment site w/o antibiotics, herpes simplex. Treatment of rosacea, perioral dermatitis or acne. Prolonged use (may cause glaucoma, cataracts). **CAUTIONS:** Use smallest therapeutic dose for children (chronic use may interfere w/growth and development). Local irritation: discontinue. Skin infection: treat w/appropriate antifungal or antibacterial agent.

INTERACTIONS

None significant.

SIDE EFFECTS

Contact dermatitis (burning/itching of skin). Painful, red, itchy, pus-containing blisters; thinning of skin w/easy bruising. Dryness, irritation, skin redness or scaling of skin lesions, skin rash.

CLASSIFICATION

TOXIC EFFECTS/ADVERSE REACTIONS

None significant.

NURSING IMPLICATIONS

BASELINE ASSESSMENT: Question for hypersensitivity to corticosteroid. Establish baseline assessment of skin disorder. **INTERVENTION/EVALUATION:** Assess involved area for therapeutic response or irritation. **PATIENT/FAMILY TEACHING:** Apply after shower or bath for best absorption; rub thin film gently into affected area. Do not cover; do not use tight diapers, plastic pants, or coverings. Do not apply to weepy, denuded areas. Do not expose treated areas to sunlight (severe sunburn may occur). Use only for prescribed area and no longer than ordered. Report adverse local reactions. Avoid contact w/eyes.

diuretics

ACTION

Diuretics act to increase the excretion of water/sodium and other electrolytes via the kidneys. Exact mechanism of antihypertensive effect unknown; may be due to reduced plasma volume or decreased peripheral vascular resistance. Subclassifications of diuretics are based on their mechanism and site of action.

Thiazides: Act at the cortical diluting segment of nephron, block reabsorption of Na, Cl, and water; promote excretion of Na, Cl, K, and water.

Loop: Act primarily at the thick ascending limb of Henle's loop to inhibit Na, Cl, and water absorption.

Potassium-sparing: Spironolactone blocks aldosterone action on distal nephron (causes K retention, Na excretion). Triamterene, amiloride act on distal nephron, decreasing Na reuptake, reducing K secretion.

Osmotic: Elevate osmolarity of glomerular filtrate preventing reabsorption of water, increased excretion of Na, Cl.

USES

Thiazides: Management of edema resulting from a number of causes (e.g., CHF, hepatic cirrhosis); hypertension either alone or in combination w/other antihypertensives.

Loop: Management of edema associated w/CHF, cirrhosis of liver, and renal disease. Furosemide used in treatment of hypertension alone or in combination w/other antihypertensives.

Potassium-sparing: Adjunctive treatment w/thiazides, loop diuretics in treatment of CHF and hypertension.

Osmotics: Reduction of intraocular pressure for ophthalmic surgery, edema, elevated intracranial pressure, and facilitating excretion of toxic substances.

DIURETICS

GENERIC NAME	BRAND NAME(S)	TYPE	DIURETIC EFFECT ONSET	PEAK	DURATION	DOSAGE RANGE
amiloride	Midamor	K-sparing	2 hrs	6–10 hrs	24 hrs	HTN: 5–20 mg/day Edema: 5–20 mg/day
bumetanide	Bumex	Loop	0.5–1 hr	1–2 hrs	4–6 hrs	Edema: 0.5–10 mg/day
chlorothiazide	Diuril	Thiazide	1–2 hrs	4 hrs	6–12 hrs	HTN: 0.5–2 g/day Edema: 0.5–2 g 1–2x/day
chlorthalidone	Hygroton	Thiazide	2 hrs	2–6 hrs	24–72 hrs	HTN: 25–100 mg/day Edema: 50–200 mg/day
ethacrynic acid	Edecrin	Loop	0.5 hrs	2 hrs	6–8 hrs	Edema: 50–200 mg/day
furosemide	Lasix	Loop	1 hr	1–2 hrs	6–8 hrs	HTN: 40 mg 2x/day Edema: up to 600 mg/day
glycerin	Glycerin	Osmotic	10–30 min	1–1.5 hrs	4–5 hrs	Edema: 1–1.5 g/kg
hydrochloro-thiazide	Esidrix Hydro-Diuril Oretic	Thiazide	2 hrs	4–6 hrs	6–12 hrs	HTN: 25–100 mg/day Edema: 25–200 mg/day
indapamide	Lozol	Thiazide	1–2 hrs	2 hrs	Up to 36 hrs	HTN: 2.5–5 mg/day Edema: 2.5–5 mg/day
mannitol	Mannitol	Osmotic	0.5–1 hr	1 hr	6–8 hrs	Edema: 50–200 g/day
metolazone	Diulo Zaroxolyn	Thiazide	1 hr	2 hrs	12–24 hrs	HTN: 2.5–5 mg/day Edema: 5–20 mg/day
spironolactone	Aldactone	K-sparing	24–48 hrs	48–72 hrs	48–72 hrs	HTN: 50–100 mg/day Edema: 25–200 mg/day
torsemide	Demadex	Loop	10–60 min	1–2 hrs	6–8 hrs	HTN: 5–10 mg/day Edema: 10–200 mg/day
triamterene	Dyrenium	K-sparing	2–4 hrs	6–8 hrs	12–16 hrs	HTN: up to 300 mg/day Edema: up to 300 mg/day

HTN = hypertension.

PRECAUTIONS

CONTRAINDICATIONS: Severe hepatic or renal dysfunction. Hypersensitivity to the drug (sensitivity to sulfonamides when giving thiazides). Potassium-sparing diuretics should not be given in hyperkalemia; osmotics are contraindicated in intracranial bleeding. Dehydration, pregnancy, infants and children, lactation. **CAUTIONS:** Administer cautiously to elderly, pts w/diabetes mellitus, gout or hyperuricemia, history of lupus erythematosus (may cause exacerbation).

INTERACTIONS

Thiazides: Cholestyramine, colestipol may decrease absorption, effects. May increase digoxin toxicity (due to hypokalemia). May increase lithium toxicity.

Loop: Amphotericin, ototoxic, nephrotoxic agents may increase toxicity. May decrease effect of anticoagulants, heparin. Hypokalemia-causing agents may increase hypokalemia. May increase risk of lithium toxicity.

Potassium-sparing: May decrease anticoagulants, heparin effects.

CLASSIFICATION

NSAIDs may decrease antihypertensive effect. ACE inhibitors (e.g., captopril), potassium-containing medications, potassium supplements may increase potassium. May increase digoxin, lithium toxicity.

SIDE EFFECTS

Orthostatic hypotension, dizziness, anorexia or nausea, headache, lethargy.

TOXIC EFFECTS/ADVERSE REACTIONS

Unusual weakness, heaviness of legs, weak pulse indicate electrolyte (potassium) imbalance. Dehydration; hyperkalemia w/potassium-sparing diuretics; tinnitus and hearing loss w/loop diuretics; hypotension. Hypersensitivity reactions rarely. Impotence, GI bleeding.

NURSING IMPLICATIONS

GENERAL: If possible, administer dose in morning to avoid disturbing sleep w/urination. Provide assistance to bathroom, if needed; be sure pts confined to bed have call light handy. INTERVENTION/ EVALUATION: Monitor I&O, weight. Check B/P and apical pulse, potassium levels. Assess for edema of dependent areas. Auscultate lungs for rales. PATIENT/FAMILY TEACHING: Medication will cause increased urination. Consult physician regarding alcohol and other medications. Eat foods high in potassium such as whole grains (cereals), legumes, meat, bananas, apricots, orange juice, potatoes (white, sweet), raisins (except w/potassium-sparing diuretics).

---

fertility agents

Infertility is defined as a decreased ability to reproduce as opposed to sterility, the inability to reproduce. Infertility may be due to reproduction dysfunction of the male, female, or both. In order to make an accurate diagnosis of the cause of infertility, a variety of tests may be performed: semen analysis, determining basal body temperature patterns, measuring estrogen and progesterone levels, endometrial biopsy and fallopian tube patency. The more accurate the diagnosis, the better chance of treating infertility successfully.

FEMALE INFERTILITY

Female infertility can be due to disruption of any phase of the reproductive process. The most critical phases include follicular maturation, ovulation, transport of the ovum through the fallopian tubes, fertilization of the ovum, nidation and growth/development of the conceptus. Causes of infertility include the following:

Anovulation, failure of follicular maturation: Absence of adequate hormonal stimulation; ovarian follicles do not ripen and ovulation will not occur.

Unfavorable cervical mucus: Normally the cervical glands secrete large volumes of thin, watery mucus, but if the mucus is unfavorable (scant or thick or sticky), sperm is unable to pass through to the uterus.

Hyperprolactinemia: Excessive prolactin secretion may cause amenorrhea, galactorrhea, and infertility.

Luteal phase defect: Progesterone secretion by the corpus luteum is insufficient to maintain endometrial integrity.

Endometriosis: Endometrial tissue is implanted in abnormal locations (e.g., uterine wall, ovary, extragenital sites).

Androgen excess: May decrease fertility (the most common condition is polycystic ovary).

MALE INFERTILITY

Male infertility is due to decreased density or motility of sperm or semen of abnormal volume or quality. The most obvious manifestation of male infertility is impotence (inability to achieve erection). Whereas in female infertility, an identifiable endocrine disorder can be found, most cases of male infertility are not associated with an identifiable endocrine disorder.

MEDICATIONS TREATING INFERTILITY

The majority of medications used in treating infertility are directed at improving female reproductive function. These medications can improve maturation of ovarian follicles, ovulation, produce a favorable cervical mucus, control endometriosis, and reduce excessive prolactin levels.

Clomiphene (Clomid, Serophene)
Action: Blocks receptors for estrogen. The hypothalamus stimulates the anterior pituitary to increase secretion of luteinizing hormone (LH) and follicle-stimulating hormone (FSH), which then stimulate the ovary, promoting follicular maturation and ovulation.
Uses: Promotes follicular maturation and ovulation in selected infertile women.
Adverse Effects: Hot flushes, nausea, abdominal discomfort, bloating, breast engorgement. Multiple births occur in 8–10% of pregnancies. Excessive stimulation may produce ovarian enlargement. May induce luteal phase defect.

Menotropins (Humegon, Pergonal)
Action: Gonadotropic agent w/follicle-stimulating hormone (FSH) and luteinizing hormone (LH) actions. Promotes ovarian follicular growth and maturation in women; stimulates spermatogenesis in men.
Uses: Treatment of infertility: in conjunction w/chorionic gonadotropin (HCG) to stimulate ovulation and pregnancy in women w/secondary ovarian dysfunction and to stimulate spermatogenesis in men w/primary or secondary hypogonadotropic hypogonadism.
Adverse Effects: Pain, rash, swelling, irritation at injection site. Mild to moderate ovarian enlargement w/abdominal distention and pain. Ovarian enlargement occurring rapidly may be accompanied by ascites, pleural effusion, and pain. Additionally, menotropins may produce spontaneous abortion and multiple births (20% of pregnancies).

DRUGS FOR INFERTILITY

GENERIC NAME	BRAND NAME	DOSAGE
bromocriptine	Parlodel	PO: Initially 0.5–2.5 mg/day increased by 2.5 mg every 3–7 days. Range: 2.5–15 mg/day.
clomiphene	Clomid Serophene	PO: Initially, 50 mg/day for 5 days (start any time in patients who have had no recent uterine bleeding). If progestin-induced bleeding is planned, or spontaneous uterine bleeding occurs prior to therapy, start on or about the 5th day of cycle. If ovulation has not occurred, administer a 2nd course at 100 mg/day for 5 days starting as early as 30 days after the previous course. Three courses are an adequate therapeutic trial.
danazol	Danocrine	PO: 200–300 mg 2 ×/day
follitropin	Gonal-F	SC: 75–150 IU/day
ganirelix	Antagon	SQ: 250 mcg/day
gonadorelin	Lutrepulse	Pump via indwelling catheter 5 mcg q90 min SC/IV: 100 mcg as single injection
human chorionic gonadotropin	Pergonal Profasai	IM: 5,000–10,000 units 24 hrs after last dose of menotropins
menotropins	Pergonal	IM: 75 IU FSH/75 IU LH daily for 7–12 days. Follow with 10,000 HCG 1 day after last dose of menotropins (if estrogen levels >150 mcg/24 hrs, not advised to give HCG). May repeat course at least twice. If no response, increase FSH/LH to 150 IU daily. May repeat twice.
nafarelin	Synarel	Intranasal: 200 mcg (one spray) in morning and evening alternating nostrils
urofollitropin	Fertinex	SC: 75–150 IU/day

Gonadorelin (Factrel, Lutrepulse)

Action: Stimulates synthesis, release of luteinizing hormone (LH) and follicle-stimulating hormone (FSH) from the anterior pituitary. Stimulates release of gonadotropin-releasing hormone from the hypothalamus.

Uses: Induction of ovulation in women with primary hypothalamic amenorrhea; promotes follicular maturation and ovulation.

Adverse Effects: Ovarian hyperstimulation. Inflammation, infection, mild phlebitis, hematoma at catheter site (if administration via an indwelling IV catheter). Multiple births (12% of pregnancies).

Human Chorionic Gonadotropin (HCG) (APL, Pregnyl, Profasai HP)

Action: Similar in structure and identical in action to luteinizing hormone (LH). Stimulates production of progesterone by the corpus luteum causing maturation of the corpus luteum and triggers ovulation in women with normally functioning ovaries.

Uses: Induction of ovulation and pregnancy in women with secondary anovulation (after pretreatment with menotropin).

Adverse Effects: Ovarian hyperstimulation. May provoke rupture of ovarian cysts. Multiple births may be induced. Edema, pain at injection site, and CNS effects (headache, irritability, restlessness, fatigue).

Bromocriptine (Parlodel)

Action: Directly inhibits prolactin release from the anterior pituitary. Stimulates presynaptic and postsynaptic dopamine receptors.

Uses: Treatment of hyperprolactinemia conditions (amenorrhea with or without galactorrhea, prolactin secreting adenomas, infertility).
Adverse Effects: Nausea, headache, dizziness, fatigue, abdominal cramps.

Danazol (Danocrine)

Action: Inhibits several enzymes required for synthesis of ovarian hormones, suppresses secretion of LH and FSH, and acts directly on the implant to block ovarian hormone receptors. Atrophies ectopic endometrial tissue.
Uses: Treatment of endometriosis and associated infertility.
Adverse Effects: May induce virilization (acne, deepening of the voice, growth of facial hair). May cause edema, liver dysfunction.

Nafarelin (Synarel)

Action: Indirectly suppresses ovarian hormone production (LH and FSH).
Uses: Management of endometriosis, including pain relief and reduction of endometriotic lesions.
Adverse Effects: Hot flushes, vaginal dryness, decreased libido, mood changes, headache, nasal irritation, decreased bone density.

H₂ antagonists

ACTION

Inhibit gastric acid secretion by interfering w/histamine at the histamine H₂ receptors in parietal cells. Also inhibits acid secretion caused by gastrin. Inhibition occurs w/basal (fasting), nocturnal, food-stimulated, or fundic distention secretion. H₂ antagonists decrease both the volume and H₂ concentration of gastric juices.

USES

Short-term treatment of duodenal ulcer, active benign gastric ulcer; maintenance therapy of duodenal ulcer; pathologic hypersecretory conditions (e.g., Zollinger-Ellison syndrome); gastroesophageal reflux disease; and prevention of upper GI bleeding in critically ill pts.

PRECAUTIONS

CONTRAINDICATIONS: Cross-sensitivity. Pregnancy and lactation; children. **CAUTIONS:** Elderly pts and those w/reduced renal or hepatic function.

INTERACTIONS

Note: Interactions more likely to occur w/cimetidine.
Antacids may decrease absorption (avoid use within ½–1 hr). May decrease ketoconazole absorption (give at least 2 hrs after). May decrease metabolism, increase concentration of oral anticoagulants, tricyclic antidepressants, oral hypoglycemics, metoprolol, metronidazole, phenytoin, propranolol, theophylline, calcium channel blockers, cyclosporine, lidocaine.

CLASSIFICATION

H₂ ANTAGONISTS

GENERIC NAME	BRAND NAME(S)	RTE ADMIN	USE: DOSAGE
cimetidine	Tagamet	PO, IM, IV, IV infusion	Tx duodenal ulcer: 800 mg/hs, 400 mg 2×/day, 300 mg 4×/day
			Maintenance duodenal ulcer: 400 mg/hs
			Tx gastric ulcer: 800 mg/hs; 300 mg 4×/day
			GERD: 1,600 mg/day
			Hypersecretory conditions: 1,200–2,400 mg/day
			Prevents upper GI bleeding: 50 mg/hr as IV infusion
famotidine	Pepcid	PO, IV	Tx duodenal ulcer: 40 mg/day
			Maintenance duodenal ulcer: 20 mg/day
			Tx gastric ulcer: 40 mg/day
			GERD: 40–80 mg/day
			Hypersecretory conditions: 80–640 mg/day
nizatidine	Axid	PO	Tx duodenal ulcer: 300 mg/day
			Maintenance duodenal ulcer: 150 mg/day
ranitidine	Zantac	PO, IM, IV, IV infusion	Tx duodenal ulcer: 300 mg/day
			Maintenance duodenal ulcer: 150 mg/day
			Tx gastric ulcer: 300 mg/day
			GERD: 300 mg/day
			Hypersecretory conditions: 0.3–6 g/day

GERD = gastroesophageal reflux disease; Tx = treatment; hs = bedtime.

SIDE EFFECTS

Dizziness, headache, muscle cramps, rash, diarrhea or constipation. Confusion, esp. in elderly, debilitated, those w/renal or hepatic dysfunction.

TOXIC EFFECTS/ADVERSE REACTIONS

Unusual weakness or tiredness (may suggest blood dyscrasias), bradycardia or tachycardia, unusual bleeding; decreased sexual ability—esp. w/Zollinger-Ellison syndrome.

NURSING IMPLICATIONS

GENERAL: Administer oral agents w/meals and at bedtime for maximal effects. Antacids should not be taken within 1 hr of histamine receptor antagonists. Infuse IV solution slowly. BASELINE ASSESSMENT: Determine baselines for B/P, pulse. INTERVENTION/EVALUATION: Assess for abdominal pain, discomfort. Monitor B/P, pulse (esp. w/IV route). Check stools and emesis for blood. Assess for confusion, esp. in elderly, debilitated, and those w/renal or hepatic dysfunction. PATIENT/FAMILY TEACHING: Avoid alcohol, aspirin, spicy foods, and other foods known to cause distress. Need to cease smoking. Importance of completing therapy. Notify physician of abdominal or epigastric pain, blood in stool or emesis, dark tarry stools.

hematinic preparations

ACTION

Iron supplements are provided to assure adequate supplies for the formation of hemoglobin, which is needed for erythropoiesis and O_2 transport.

USES

Prevention or treatment of iron deficiency resulting from improper diet, pregnancy, impairment of absorption, or prolonged blood loss.

PRECAUTIONS

CONTRAINDICATIONS: Peptic ulcers, anemias caused by other factors, multiple blood transfusions, ulcerative colitis, cirrhosis, hypersensitivity to agent, hepatitis. **CAUTIONS:** Pts w/allergy, rheumatoid arthritis.

IRON PREPARATIONS

GENERIC NAME	BRAND NAME(S)	IRON (%)	DOSE PROVIDING 100 MG IRON
ferrous fumarate	Feostat	33	300
ferrous gluconate	Fergon	11.6	860
ferrous sulfate	Mol-Iron	20	500
	Fer-In-Sol liquid		
	Feosol liquid		
ferrous sulfate exsiccated	Fer-In-Sol caps	30	330
	Feosol tabs/caps		
	Slow FE		

INTERACTIONS

Antacids, cimetidine, tetracycline may decrease iron absorption; iron may decrease absorption of methyldopa, quinolones, tetracycline.

SIDE EFFECTS

Nausea, vomiting, diarrhea or constipation, heartburn, hypersensitivity reactions: rash, urticaria, pruritus.

TOXIC EFFECTS/ADVERSE REACTIONS

Severe gastrointestinal effects, anaphylactic reactions, fever, chills, arthralgia, hypotension, local abscess at IM injection site.

NURSING IMPLICATIONS

GENERAL: Give oral iron on empty stomach, w/food to reduce gastrointestinal symptoms. Provide straw w/oral liquid form to avoid tooth discoloration. INTERVENTION/EVALUATION: Laboratory results (hemoglobin, blood counts). Assess skin color, esp. at nail beds, earlobes, sublingual areas. Check for fatigue, increased respi-

CLASSIFICATION

rations (low hemoglobin may cause hypoxia). PATIENT/FAMILY TEACHING: Stools will be discolored (dark green or black). Importance of balanced diet; identify foods high in iron: egg yolks, dried fruits, meats (esp. organ meats), whole grains, and dark green leafy vegetables.

hormones

Functions of the body are regulated by two major control systems: the nervous system and endocrine (hormone) system. Together, they maintain homeostasis and control different metabolic functions in the body.

Hormones are concerned with control of different metabolic functions in the body (e.g., rates of chemical reactions in cells, transporting substances through cell membranes, cellular metabolism [growth/secretions]). By definition, a hormone is a chemical substance secreted into body fluids by cells and has control over other cells in the body. Hormones can be local or general. *Local hormones* have specific local effects (e.g., acetylcholine, which is secreted at parasympathetic and skeletal nerve endings). *General hormones* are mostly secreted by specific endocrine glands (e.g., epinephrine/norepinephrine are secreted by the adrenal medulla in response to sympathetic stimulation), transported in the blood to all parts of the body causing many different reactions. Some general hormones affect all or almost all cells of the body (e.g., thyroid hormone from the thyroid gland increases the rate of most chemical reactions in almost all cells of the body); other general hormones affect only specific tissue (e.g., ovarian hormones are specific to female sex organs and secondary sexual characteristics of the female).

ACTION

Endocrine hormones almost never directly act intracellularly affecting chemical reactions. They first combine with hormone receptors either on the cell surface or inside the cell (cell cytoplasm or nucleus). The combination of hormone and receptors alters the function of the receptor, and the receptor is the direct cause of the hormone effects. Altered receptor function may include the following: *Altered cell permeability,* which causes a change in protein structure of the receptor usually opening or closing a channel for one or more ions. The movement of these ions causes the effect of the hormone. *Activation of intracellular enzymes* immediately inside the cell membrane: e.g., hormone combines with receptor that then becomes the activated enzyme adenyl cyclase, which causes formation of cAMP. **Note:** Camp has effects inside the cell. It is not the hormone but cAMP causing these effects.

Regulation of hormone secretion is controlled by internal control system, the negative feedback system:

Endocrine gland oversecretes
Hormone exerts more and more of its effect

Target organ performs its function

Too much function in turn feeds back to endocrine gland to decrease secretory rate

The endocrine system contains many glands and hormones. A summary of the important glands and their hormones secreted are as follows:

The pituitary gland (hypophysis) is a small gland found in the sella turcica at the base of the brain. The pituitary is divided into two portions physiologically: the anterior pituitary (adenohypophysis) and the posterior pituitary (neurohypophysis). Six important hormones are secreted from the anterior pituitary and two from the posterior pituitary.

Anterior pituitary hormones:
  Growth hormone
  Adrenocorticotropin (corticotropin)
  Thyroid-stimulating hormone (thyrotropin)
  Follicle-stimulating hormone (FSH)
  Luteinizing hormone (LH)
  Prolactin

Posterior pituitary hormones:
  Antidiuretic hormone (vasopressin)
  Oxytocin

Almost all secretions of the pituitary hormones are controlled by hormonal or nervous signals from the hypothalamus. The hypothalamus is a center of information concerned with the well-being of the body, which in turn is used to control secretions of the important pituitary hormones just listed. Secretions from the posterior pituitary are controlled by nerve signals originating in the hypothalamus; anterior pituitary hormones are controlled by hormones secreted within the hypothalamus. These hormones are as follows:

Thyrotropin releasing hormone (TRH) releasing thyroid-stimulating hormone

Corticotropin-releasing hormone (CRH) releasing adrenocorticotropin

Growth hormone–releasing hormone (GHRH) releasing growth hormone and growth hormone inhibitory hormone (GHIH) (also same as somatostatin)

Gonadotropin-releasing hormone (GnRH) releasing the two gonadotropic hormones LH and FSH

Prolactin inhibitory factor (PIF) causing inhibition of prolactin and prolactin-releasing factor

ANTERIOR PITUITARY HORMONES

All anterior pituitary hormones (except growth hormone) have as their principal effect stimulating target glands.

Growth Hormone (GH)

Growth hormone affects almost all tissues of the body. GH (somatropin) causes growth in almost all tissues of the body (increases cell size, increases mitosis with increased number of cells, and differentiates certain types of cells). Metabolic effects include increased rate of protein synthesis, mobilization of fatty acids from adipose tissue, decreased rate of glucose utilization.

THYROID-STIMULATING HORMONE (TSH)

Thyroid-stimulating hormone controls secretion of the thyroid hormones. The thyroid gland is located immediately below the larynx on either side of and anterior to the trachea and secretes two significant hormones, thyroxine (T4) and tri-iodothyroxine (T3), which have a profound effect on increasing the metabolic rate of the body. The thyroid gland also secretes calcitonin, an important hormone for calcium metabolism. Calcitonin promotes deposition of calcium in the bones, which decreases calcium concentration in the extracellular fluid.

ADRENOCORTICOTROPIN

Adrenocorticotropin causes the adrenal cortex to secrete adrenocortical hormones. The adrenal glands lie at the superior poles of the two kidneys. Each gland is composed of two distinct parts, the adrenal medulla and cortex. The adrenal medulla, related to the sympathetic nervous system, secretes the hormones epinephrine and norepinephrine. When stimulated, they cause constriction of blood vessels, increased activity of the heart, inhibitory effects on the GI tract, and dilation of the pupils. The adrenal cortex secretes corticosteroids, of which there are two major types: mineralocorticoids and glucocorticoids. Aldosterone, the principal mineralocorticoid, primarily affects electrolytes of the extracellular fluids. Cortisol, the principal glucocorticoid, affects glucose, protein, and fat metabolism.

LUTEINIZING HORMONE (LH)

Luteinizing hormone plays an important role in ovulation and causes secretion of female sex hormones by the ovaries and testosterone by the testes.

FOLLICLE-STIMULATING HORMONE (FSH)

Follicle-stimulating hormone causes growth of follicles in the ovaries prior to ovulation and promotes formation of sperm in the testes.

Ovarian sex hormones are estrogens and progestins. Estradiol is the most important estrogen; progesterone, the most important progestin.

Estrogens mainly promote proliferation and growth of specific cells in the body and are responsible for development of most of the secondary sex characteristics. Primarily cause cellular proliferation and growth of tissues of sex organs/other tissue related to reproduction. Ovaries, fallopian tubes, uterus, vagina increase in size. Estrogen initiates growth of breast and milk-producing apparatus, external appearance.

Progesterone stimulates secretion of the uterine endometrium during the latter half of the female sexual cycle, preparing the uterus for implantation of the fertilized ovum. Decreases the frequency of uterine contractions (helps prevent expulsion of the implanted ovum). Progesterone promotes development of breasts, causing alveolar cells to proliferate, enlarge, and become secretory in nature.

Testosterone is secreted by the testes and formed by the interstitial cells of Leydig. Testosterone production increases under the stimulus of the anterior pituitary gonadotropic hormones. It is responsible for distinguishing characteristics of the masculine body (stimulates the growth of male sex organs and promotes the development of male secondary sex characteristics: e.g., distribution of body hair, effect on voice, protein formation, and muscular development).

PROLACTIN

Prolactin promotes the development of breasts and secretion of milk.

POSTERIOR PITUITARY HORMONES

ANTIDIURETIC HORMONE (ADH) (VASOPRESSIN)

Antidiuretic hormone can cause antidiuresis (decreased excretion of water by the kidneys). In the presence of ADH the permeability of the renal collecting ducts and tubules to water increases, which allows water to be absorbed, conserving water in the body. ADH in higher concentrations is a very potent vasoconstrictor, constricting arterioles everywhere in the body, increasing B/P.

OXYTOCIN

Oxytocin contracts the uterus during the birthing process, esp. toward the end of the pregnancy, helping to expel the baby. Oxytocin also contracts myoepithelial cells in the breasts, causing milk to be expressed from the alveoli into the ducts so the baby can obtain it by suckling.

PANCREAS

The pancreas is composed of two tissue types: (1) acini (secretes digestive juices in the duodenum) and (2) islets of Langerhans (secrete insulin/glucagon directly into the blood). The islets of Langerhans contain three cells: alpha, beta, delta. Alpha cells secrete glucagon, beta cells secrete insulin, and delta cells secrete somatostatin.

Insulin promotes glucose entry into most cells, thus controlling the rate of metabolism of most carbohydrates. Also insulin affects fat metabolism.

Glucagon effects are opposite insulin, the most important of which is increasing blood glucose concentration by releasing it from the liver into the circulating body fluids.

Somatostatin (same chemical as secreted by the hypothalamus) has multiple inhibitory effects: depresses secretion of insulin and glucagon, decreases GI motility, decreases secretions/absorption of the GI tract.

CLASSIFICATION

human immunodeficiency virus (HIV) infection

Acquired immunodeficiency syndrome (AIDS) was first recognized in 1981. Initially described in healthy, young homosexual men. AIDS was characterized by profound immunologic deficits, multiple opportunistic infections, and malignant neoplasms.

AIDS is caused by a retrovirus, human immunodeficiency virus (HIV). There are two types of HIV: HIV-1 and HIV-2, with HIV-1 the most common in the United States. Infection with HIV causes progressive deterioration in cell-mediated immunity, the most severe form resulting in AIDS. Although there is no cure for HIV infection, many advances in our understanding of the replication cycles of the HIV virus, therapies designed to inhibit this retrovirus, and therapies to overcome the many opportunistic infections associated with this virus have given renewed hope that controlling the progression of HIV may be possible and AIDS may be treated as a chronic disease.

HIV is a retrovirus primarily infecting CD4+ T-helper cells. After binding to a CD4 receptor protein, the virus enters the cell, is uncoated, and with the help of the enzyme reverse transcriptase (RT), the viral RNA is transcribed into a complementary DNA, which in turn is incorporated into the genome (complete gene complement) of the CD4+ T-cell. HIV replication is a continuous process without a period of latency.

HIV infection causes a wide range of immunologic abnormalities; the most important is a decrease in the number of CD4+ T cells. By definition, AIDS includes all HIV-infected adolescents and adults having a CD4 count below 200/mm^3 (normal: CD4 >1,000 cells/mm^3) regardless of symptoms or one of the AIDS-related opportunistic infections, regardless of CD4 count.

TRANSMISSION/GOALS OF THERAPY

HIV infection occurs through contact with infected blood and contaminated body fluids. Contact may occur through sexual intercourse (hetero- and homosexual), sharing blood-contaminated needles by injection drug users, infection of infants through pregnancy and during delivery and by breast feeding, via a needle stick injury or splashing of skin or mucous membranes, and through receipt of infected blood products or organs.

The goal in managing HIV/AIDS is to delay disease progression and to minimize associated opportunistic infections and malignancies. Therapy should prolong survival and improve quality of life. This is undertaken by initiating antiretroviral therapy, being aggressive in offering prophylaxis/treatment of opportunistic infections, and intensive nutritional therapy/supportive care.

ANTIRETROVIRAL AGENTS

As of April 1997, there are 11 antiretroviral agents classified as nucleoside analogues, non-nucleoside analogues, and protease inhibitors. Nucleoside and non-nucleoside analogues act by inhibiting HIV RT, which is responsible for viral replication early in the virus life cycle. Protease inhibitors block protease, an enzyme required for viral replication late in the virus life cycle.

Usually combinations of these agents may be most effective in suppressing viral replication. Several different combinations are currently being used, but the most effective combination is still unclear at this time. For more information about these agents, refer to the individual monographs.

ANTIRETROVIRAL AGENTS FOR TREATMENT OF HIV INFECTION

GENERIC NAME	BRAND NAME(s)	AVAILABILITY	DOSAGE
NUCLEOSIDE ANALOGUES:			
abacavir	Ziagen	—	300 mg 2 times/day
didanosine (ddI)	Videx	Tablets	(>60 kg): 200 mg 2 times/day
			(<60 kg): 125 mg 2 times/day
		Oral solution	(>60 kg): 250 mg 2 times/day
			(<60 kg): 167 mg 2 times/day
lamivudine (3TC)	Epivir	Tablets	Adults: 150 mg 2 times/day
		Oral solution	Children (3 mos–12 yrs): 4 mg/kg 2 times/day
stavudine (d4T)	Zerit	Capsules	(>60 kg): 40 mg 2 times/day (20 mg 2 times/day if peripheral neuropathy occurs)
zalcitabine (ddC)	Hivid	Tablets	(>60 kg): 0.75 mg 3 times/day
			(<60 kg): 0.375 mg 3 times/day
zidovudine (ZDV)	Retrovir	Capsules Tablets	500–600 mg/day (100 mg 5 times/day or 200 mg 3 times/day or 300 mg 2 times/day (Decrease to 100 mg 3 times/day if anemia, headache, nausea, insomnia)
NUCLEOTIDE ANALOGUES			
adefovir	Preveon	—	120 mg daily (w/L-carnitine)
NON-NUCLEOTIDE ANALOGUES			
delavirdine (DLV)	Rescriptor	Tablets	200 mg 3 times/day for 14 days, then 400 mg 3 times/day if no rash
efavirenz	Sustiva	Capsules	Adults: 600 mg/day
			Children: 10–15 kg: 200 mg; 15–20 kg: 250 mg; 20–25 kg: 300 mg; 25–32.5 kg: 350 mg; 32.5–40 kg: 400 mg; > 40 kg: 600 mg
nevirapine (NVP)	Viramune	Tablets	200 mg daily for 14 days, then 200 mg 2 times/day if no rash
PROTEASE INHIBITORS			
amprenavir	Agenerase	Capsules	Adults: 1,200 mg 2 times/day
		Oral solution	Children: 20 mg/kg twice daily or 15 mg/kg 3 times/day
indinavir	Crixivan	Capsules	800 mg every 8 hrs (adjust dosage in liver disease)
nelfinavir	Viracept	Tablets	Adults: 750 mg q8h
		Oral powder	Children: 20–25 mg/kg q8h
ritonavir	Norvir	Capsules	300 mg 2 times/day for 1 day, then 400 mg 2 times/day for 2 days, then 500 mg 2 times/day for 1 day, then 600 mg 2 times/day
		Oral solution	
saquinavir	Invirase	Capsules	600 mg 3 times/day

OPPORTUNISTIC INFECTIONS AND NEOPLASMS

Once the CD4 count drops to <200/mm³, many opportunistic infections develop. The lower the CD4 count, the greater the risk and number of infections. In most instances, with all the microorganisms, there is breakthrough and progression. There are no cures, and lifelong treatment is required to prevent recurrence of infections.

Candida: Fungal infection. Symptoms: patches of inflammation with or without ulceration. May cause difficulty swallowing, nausea, sternal pain. Women: thick vaginal discharge/pruritus. Diagnosis by KOH-scraping from mucous membranes.

Cryptococcus: Fungal infection. Symptoms: fever, malaise, headache, cough, GI disturbances. May localize in CNS (meningitis, encephalitis), memory loss, confusion. Diagnosis by culture of cerebrospinal fluid (CSF).

Cytomegalovirus: Symptoms: painless, progressive loss of vision, sometimes complicated by retinal detachment. In the GI tract, causes nausea, vomiting, weight loss. Diagnosis by fundoscopic examination.

Herpes Simplex: HSV-1 and HSV-2. Symptoms: orolabial, genital, anorectal (pain, itching, painful defecation), mucocutaneous lesions, esophagitis; less common: encephalitis. Diagnosis by viral culture.

Histoplasma: Fungal infection. Symptoms: often asymptomatic, may cause flulike symptoms, high fever, weight loss, liver and spleen enlargement. Diagnosis by fungal cultures.

Kaposi's Sarcoma: Symptoms: red-blue blotches or nodules ranging in size from a few millimeters to several centimeters in diameter. The lesion may bleed. Nodules may appear in the mouth or in the viscera. Diagnosis by biopsy.

Mycobacterium avium complex (MAC): Symptoms: high spiking fevers, diarrhea, night sweats, malaise, weight loss, anemia, neutropenia. Diagnosis by blood cultures or biopsy of liver, bone marrow, and lymph nodes.

Pneumocystis carnii pneumonia (PCP): Symptoms: fever, dyspnea, tachypnea with or without rales or rhonchi, and nonproductive or mildly productive cough, chills, sweats. Diagnosis by special stains of bronchial washings or open lung biopsy.

THERAPIES FOR COMMON OPPORTUNISTIC INFECTIONS

CLINICAL DISEASE	PROPHYLACTIC AGENTS	AGENTS FOR ACUTE INFECTION	
Candida	clotrimazole troches fluconazole ketoconazole nystatin	Oral:	clotrimazole nystatin
		Esophageal:	fluconazole ketoconazole
Cryptococcus	fluconazole	amphotericin w/or w/o flucytosine, followed by fluconazole	
Cytomegalovirus	oral ganciclovir	ganciclovir (IV) foscarnet	
Herpes simplex	oral acyclovir	oral acyclovir	
Histoplasma	—	amphotericin itraconazole	
Kaposi's sarcoma	—	individualized:	bleomycin doxorubicin etoposide interferon a vinblastine vincristine
Mycobacterium avium complex	azithromycin clarithromycin rifabutin	clarithromycin + ethambutol (may add rifampin) clofazime ciprofloxacin	
Pneumocystic carnii pneumonia	trimethoprim-sulfa-methoxazole dapsone pentamidine (aerosol)	trimethoprim-sulfamethoxazole pentamidine IV atovaquone (mild cases)	
Salmonella	—	ciprofloxacin trimethoprim-sulfamethoxazole	
Toxoplasma gondii	trimethoprim-sulfa-methoxazole dapsone + pyrimethamine	pyrimethamine + sulfadiazine + folinic acid	
Tuberculosis	isoniazid rifampin	isoniazid + rifampin + pyrazinamide + ethambutol or streptomycin	

Salmonella: Symptoms: fever, chills, night sweats. Diagnosis by blood cultures.

Toxoplasma gondii: Primarily infects the brain and eye. Symptoms: fever, headache, seizures, focal neurologic abnormalities and mental status changes. Diagnosis is presumptive or based on CT or MRI.

Tuberculosis (mycobacterium): Symptoms: Cough, fever, sweating, malaise, fatigue, weight loss, nonpleuritic chest pain, dyspnea. Diagnosis by TB smear, culture.

immunizations

DIPHTHERIA AND TETANUS TOXOID, PERTUSSIS VACCINE (DTP)

INDICATIONS

Immunization vs. diphtheria, tetanus, and pertussis (whooping cough).

DOSAGE

Note: Diphtheria and tetanus toxoid for pediatric use (DT) indicated for immunization of infants and children 6 wks up to 7 yrs when there is a contraindication to pertussis vaccine (acute infection or febrile illness, occurrence of any neurologic symptoms following administration of DPT for use, history of seizures, any evolving or changing disorder affecting the CNS). If no contraindication, diphtheria/tetanus/pertussis is preferred.

IM: Children >2 mos and <7 yrs: 0.5 ml at 2, 4, and 6 mos. The fourth dose of DTP may be administered as early as 12 mos, provided at least 6 mos have elapsed since the 3rd dose. Combined DTP-Hib products may be used when administered simultaneously. Diphtheria and tetanus toxoids and acellular pertussis vaccine (DTaP) can be used for the 4th and/or 5th dose of DTP in children 15 mos. If 4th dose given after 4th birthday, a booster (5th) dose is not necessary.

CONTRAINDICATIONS

Evolving or changing CNS disorders, progressive encephalopathy, uncontrolled epilepsy, severe febrile illness.

ADVERSE EFFECTS

Mild to moderate swelling, tenderness, redness, pain or lump at injection site. Fever 100.4–102.2° F.

DIPHTHERIA AND TETANUS TOXOID

INDICATIONS

Immunization against diphtheria and tetanus.

CLASSIFICATION

DOSAGE

Note: Diphtheria and tetanus toxoid for pediatric use (DT) indicated for immunization of infants and children 6 wks up to 7 yrs when there is a contraindication to pertussis vaccine (acute infection or febrile illness, occurrence of any neurologic symptoms following administration of DPT for use, history of seizures, any evolving or changing disorder affecting the CNS). If no contraindication, diphtheria/tetanus/pertussis is preferred.

IM: Children >6 wks to 1 yr: 0.5 ml at 4–8 wk intervals for a total of 3 doses. A 4th dose of 0.5 ml given 6–12 mos after 3rd dose. A booster (5th) dose given at 4–6 yrs of age.

IM: Children 1–7 yrs: 0.5 ml followed by 0.5 ml 4–8 wks later. A 3rd 0.5 ml dose given 6–12 mos after the 2nd dose. A booster (4th) dose given at 4–6 yrs unless the 3rd dose given after the 4th birthday; then the 4th dose is not necessary.

IM: Adults, adolescents: (Note: Use DT for adult use): 0.5 ml followed by 0.5 ml 4–8 wks later. A 3rd dose of 0.5 ml given 6–12 mos after the 2nd. A booster dose of 0.5 ml given every 10 yrs thereafter.

CONTRAINDICATIONS

Acute infection, febrile illness, tetanus infection, sensitivity to tetanus/diphtheria.

ADVERSE EFFECTS

Redness, hard lump at injection site, induration. *Adults:* Axillary lymphadenopathy, chills, headache, hypotension, muscle aches. *Pediatrics:* Fever under 103° F, swelling/pain/tenderness at injection site, anorexia, drowsiness, vomiting, persistent crying.

HAEMOPHILUS INFLUENZAE TYPE B CONJUGATE VACCINE

INDICATIONS

Routine immunization of children against invasive disease caused by *H. influenzae* type b (bacterial meningitis, epiglottis, sepsis, septic arthritis, osteomyelitis, pericarditis, pneumonia).

DOSAGE

Note: Three haemophilus b conjugate vaccines are available for use in infants: (1) Hib oligosaccaride conjugate vaccine (HbOC) HibTITER, (2) Hib polysaccharide conjugate vaccine (PRP-T) ActHIB and OmniHIB, and (3) Hib polysaccharide conjugate vaccine (PRP-OMP) PedvaxHIB. Children who have received PRP-OMP at 2 and 4 mos do not require a dose at 6 mos. Following the primary infant Hib conjugate vaccine series, any Hib conjugate vaccine may be administered as a booster dose at age 12–15 mos. PRP-D (ProHIBit) is licensed only for use >15 mos.

IM: Infants: 0.5 ml at 2, 4 and 6 mos, booster at age 12–15 mos.

CONTRAINDICATIONS

Acute or febrile illness.

ADVERSE EFFECTS

Erythema at injection site, induration, fever, diarrhea, vomiting, irritability, lethargy, anorexia.

HEPATITIS B VACCINE

INDICATIONS

Immunization against infection caused by all known subtypes hepatitis B virus for persons of all ages esp. those at increased risk of infection (e.g., health-care workers who may be exposed via blood or pts' specimens, household and sexual contacts of hepatitis B carriers, dialysis, renal failure pts, hematology/oncology units, infants born of HBsAg-positive mothers whether HBsAg positive or negative, military personnel, persons at increased risk due to sexual practices).

DOSAGE

Children of HBsAg-negative mothers:
IM: Recombivax HB: 2.5 mcg, Engerix-B: 10 mcg: Birth, 2nd dose between 1–4 mos (provided at least 1 mo elapsed since receiving the first dose); 3rd dose between 6 and 18 mos.

Children of HBsAg-positive mothers:
Note: Hepatitis B immune globulin (HBIG) given within 12 hrs of birth.
IM: Recombivax HB: 5 mcg, Engerix-B: 10 mcg: Birth, 2nd dose 1–2 mos, and 3rd dose at 6 mos.

Children of HbsAg status unknown:
IM: Recombivax HB: 5 mcg, Engerix-B: 10 mcg: Birth, 2nd dose at 1 mo, and 3rd dose at 6 mos.
Note: Adolescents who have not received 3 doses of hepatitis B should initiate or complete series at 11–12 yrs, the 2nd dose at least 1 mo after the 1st dose, the 3rd dose at least 4 mos after the 1st and 2 mos after the 2nd dose.

Adolescents, adults:
Recombivax HB:
IM: 11–19 yrs: 0.5 ml (5 mcg) initially, 1 and 6 mos after initial dose; **20 yrs or greater:** 1 ml (10 mcg) initially, then 1 and 6 mos after initial dose.

Engerix-B:
IM: >11 yrs: 1 ml (20 mcg) initially, then 1 and 6 mos after initial dose.

CONTRAINDICATIONS

Sensitivity to hepatitis B vaccine, allergy to yeast, severely compromised cardiopulmonary status, moderate to severe illness w/ or w/o fever, immune deficiency conditions.

CLASSIFICATION

ADVERSE EFFECTS

Soreness at injection site, fatigue, fever, headache, vertigo, induration, redness, swelling, pain, itching, ecchymoses, tenderness at injection site.

HEPATITIS B IMMUNE GLOBULIN (HBIG)

INDICATIONS

Postexposure prophylaxis for hepatitis B infection. Provides passive immunization following exposure to hepatitis B virus and for infants born to mothers who are hepatitis B surface antigen positive (HBsAg-positive).

DOSAGE

Infants of HBsAg-positive mothers:
IM: 0.5 ml within 12 hrs of birth.

Postexposure prophylaxis:
IM: Adults: 0.06 ml/kg (usually 3–5 ml) within 24 hrs if possible after exposure. Begin hepatitis B vaccine as soon as possible but within 7 days of exposure.

ADVERSE REACTIONS

Local pain, tenderness, urticaria.

INFLUENZAE VIRUS VACCINE

INDICATIONS

Annual vaccination for adults w/chronic cardiovascular/pulmonary diseases, metabolic disease, nursing home residents, health-care workers dealing w/high-risk pts, healthy adults >65 yrs, children w/chronic metabolic or cardiopulmonary disease.

DOSAGE

IM: Adults, elderly, children >9 yrs: 0.5 ml as single dose. **Children 3–9 yrs:** 0.5 ml one or two times (1 mo apart). **Children 6–35 mos:** 0.25 ml one or two times (1 mo apart). **Note:** Give two doses to children <9 yrs when receiving vaccine for first time.

CONTRAINDICATIONS

History of allergy to eggs. Defer immunization in presence of acute respiratory disease or other active infection or febrile illness.

ADVERSE EFFECTS

Tenderness, redness, induration at injection site, low-grade fever, malaise.

MEASLES VACCINE, LIVE

INDICATIONS

Active immunization against measles (rubeola) in persons 15 mos or older, infants 12–15 mos in high-risk areas or traveling outside the United States. A second dose is recommended.

DOSAGE

SubQ: Adults, children ≥15 mos: 0.5 ml into outer aspect of upper arm. Usually given as MMR (Measles, Mumps, Rubella) for most vaccinations at age 15 mos.
Note: The second dose of MMR vaccine may be given at any time provided 1 mo has elapsed since the first dose. Monovalent measles vaccine may be given as early as 6 mos but two doses of trivalent vaccine still to be given w/first at age 15 mos.

CONTRAINDICATIONS

Immunosuppressed pts, pregnant women, history of egg allergy, hypersensitivity to neomycin (contained in product). Any febrile respiratory infection or other active febrile infection. Active untreated TB. Pts w/blood dyscrasias, leukemia, lymphomas, malignant neoplasms affecting bone marrow or lymphatic system.

ADVERSE EFFECTS

Febrile reaction (rarely above 39.4° C), transient rash, burning, stinging at injection site.

MUMPS VIRUS VACCINE, LIVE

INDICATIONS

Active immunity against mumps in persons ≥12 mos of age.

DOSAGE

SubQ: Adults, children >12 mos: 0.5 ml into outer aspect of upper arm. Usually given as MMR for most vaccinations at age 15 mos.
Note: The second dose of MMR may be given at any time provided at least 1 mo has elapsed since the first dose. Those born after 1/1/57 should receive two trivalent doses (MMR).

CONTRAINDICATIONS

Immunosuppressed pts, pregnant women, history of egg allergy, hypersensitivity to neomycin (contained in product). Any febrile respiratory infection or other active febrile infection. Active untreated TB. Pts w/blood dyscrasias, leukemia, lymphomas, malignant neoplasms affecting bone marrow or lymphatic system.

ADVERSE EFFECTS

Febrile reaction (rarely above 39.4° C), transient rash, burning, stinging at injection site.

CLASSIFICATION

PERTUSSIS
See Diphtheria and Tetanus Toxoid, Pertussis Vaccine (DTP)

PNEUMOCOCCAL VACCINE, POLYVALENT

INDICATIONS

Immunization against pneumococcal pneumonia/bacteremia caused by types of pneumococci in vaccine. Indicated in pts at increased risk of pneumococcal disease: immunocompromised (e.g., Hodgkin's disease, renal failure, HIV infection), pts w/splenic dysfunction or anatomic asplenia, chronic cardiovascular or pulmonary disease, alcoholism, elderly (esp. institutionalized).

DOSAGE

IM/SubQ: Adults, children ≥2 yrs: 0.5 ml as single dose.

CONTRAINDICATION

Hypersensitivity, previous immunization w/any polyvalent pneumococcal vaccine.

ADVERSE EFFECTS

Erythema, hard lump, swelling, soreness at injection site, swollen glands, arthralgia, myalgia, asthenia, fever, skin rash.

POLIO VACCINE, LIVE, ORAL

INDICATIONS

Prevention of poliomyelitis caused by poliovirus 1, 2, 3. Immunization recommended for all children and young adults up to 18 yrs.

DOSAGE

Note: Polio vaccine live oral (OPV) is recommended for routine childhood vaccination. Inactivated poliovirus vaccine (IPV) is recommended for individuals with altered immunocompetence. For primary immunization, IPV should be given w/minimum interval of 4 wks between 1st and 2nd doses and 6 mos between 2nd and 3rd doses.
PO: Infants: Three doses of 0.5 ml. First dose at 6–12 wks of age, 2nd dose 8 wks after 1st dose, 3rd dose 8–12 mos after 2nd dose. **Older children:** First 2 doses 8 wks apart, 3rd dose 6–12 mos following the 2nd dose. Fourth dose given upon entering elementary school (not required if 3rd dose given on or after 4th birthday).

CONTRAINDICATIONS

Pts or household members w/immunosuppression (e.g., leukemia, lymphoma, lowered resistance to infection from steroid therapy). Defer in presence of any acute illness, vomiting, diarrhea, and in pts w/advanced debilitated disease (inactivated poliovirus vaccine recommended).

ADVERSE EFFECTS

No immediate effect seen with oral administration.

RECOMMENDATIONS FOR IMMUNIZATION OF INFANTS/CHILDREN

	BIRTH	1 MO	2 MOS	4 MOS	6 MOS	12 MOS	15 MOS	18 MOS	4–6 YRS
Diphtheria[1,2]			X	X	X			X	X
Tetanus[1,2]			X	X	X			X	X
Pertussis[1,2]			X	X	X			X	X
Measles[3]							X		X
Mumps[3]							X		X
Rubella[3]							X		X
Haemophilus[4]			X	X	X		X		
HibTITER									
ProHIBit							X		
PedvaxHIB			X	X		X			
Hepatitis B	X	X			X				
HBsAg-negative[5] mothers									
HBsAg-positive mothers	X	X			X				
Poliovirus			X	X				X	X
varicella						X			

[1]Usually given as diphtheria and tetanus toxoid combined w/pertussis vaccine.

[2]Booster given at 10 yr intervals to maintain immunity.

[3]Usually given as combined measles, mumps, rubella (MMR) vaccine.

[4]Dosage schedule dependent on vaccine formulation and manufacturer used.

[5]See monograph for alternate schedule.

RH$_O$(D) IMMUNE GLOBULIN (RDIG)

INDICATIONS

Suppresses immune response of nonsensitized Rh$_o$(D) negative pts who receive Rh$_o$(D) positive blood due to fetomaternal hemorrhage, abdominal trauma, amniocentesis, abortion, or full-term delivery. RDIG prevents future chance of erythroblastosis fetalis in subsequent pregnancies with an Rh$_o$(D) positive fetus.

DOSAGE

Term delivery:
IM: 300 mcg within 72 hrs.

After amniocentesis, miscarriage, abortion, ectopic pregnancy >13 wks:
IM: 300 mcg one time.

Before delivery:
IM: 300 mcg at 28 wks, 300 mcg within 72 hrs of delivery.

Transfusion accident:
IM: Dependent on volume of packed red cells or whole blood transfused.

Termination of pregnancy (<13 wks):
IM: 50 mcg within 72 hrs.
Note: Do not give to individuals that are positive $Rh_o(D)$ and Du antigens or those w/anti-$Rh_o(D)$ antibodies.

ADVERSE EFFECTS

Fever, injection site tenderness.

RUBELLA VIRUS VACCINE, LIVE (GERMAN MEASLES)

INDICATIONS

Active immunization against rubella (German measles). Intended to reduce occurrence of congenital rubella syndrome among offspring or women contracting rubella during pregnancy. Indicated for children ≥12 mos w/o evidence of wild virus infection, women of childbearing potential for whom serologic testing unavailable (up to 45 yrs of age), those at substantial risk for exposure.

DOSAGE

SubQ: Adults, children at age 15 mos: 0.5 ml into outer aspect of upper arm. Usually given as MMR for most vaccinations at 15 mos.
Note: Second dose of MMR may be given at any time provided at least 1 mo has elapsed since the first dose.

CONTRAINDICATIONS

Immunosuppressed pts, pregnant women, history of egg allergy, hypersensitivity to neomycin (contained in product). Any febrile respiratory infection or other active febrile infection. Active untreated TB. Pts w/blood dyscrasias, leukemia, lymphomas, malignant neoplasms affecting bone marrow or lymphatic system.

ADVERSE EFFECTS

Increase w/age of pt. Lymphadenopathy, skin rash, urticaria, fever, malaise, sore throat, headache, myalgia, paresthesia of extremities.

TETANUS TOXOID ADSORBED (TTA)

INDICATION

Active immunity against tetanus (esp. military personnel, farm/utility workers, those working w/horses, firefighters, occupations that render liable to even minor lacerations/abrasions).

DOSAGE

Also see Diphtheria/Tetanus/Pertussis and Diphtheria/Tetanus.

IM: **Adults, adolescents:** 0.5 ml at initial visit, 2nd dose 4–8 wks after 1st dose, 3rd dose 6–12 mos after 2nd dose. Booster dose every 10 yrs.

CONTRAINDICATIONS

Acute respiratory infection or other active infection except for emergency booster doses.

ADVERSE EFFECTS

Local reactions at injection site (warmth, redness, induration, hard lump, pain, tenderness, itching, swelling), chills, fever, skin rash.

VARICELLA VIRUS VACCINE

INDICATIONS

Vaccination against varicella (chicken pox).

DOSAGE

SubQ: **Adults, children >12 yrs:** 1st dose 0.5 ml, then 2nd dose 4–8 wks later. **Children (1–12 yrs):** Single 0.5 ml dose at any time after 12 mos of age.

CONTRAINDICATIONS

Hypersensitivity to any component of vaccine. History of allergy to neomycin. Pts w/blood dyscrasias, leukemia, lymphoma, other malignant neoplasms affecting bone marrow or lymphatic system. Pts immunosuppressed, active untreated tuberculosis, any febrile respiratory illness or active febrile infection, pregnancy.

ADVERSE EFFECTS

Pain, redness at injection site, rash, fever.

laxatives

ACTION

Laxatives ease or stimulate defecation. Mechanisms by which this is accomplished include (1) attracting, retaining fluid in colonic contents due to hydrophilic or osmotic properties; (2) acting directly or indirectly on mucosa to decrease absorption of water and NaCl; or (3) increasing intestinal motility, decreasing absorption of water and NaCl by virtue of decreased transit time.

Bulk-forming: Acts primarily in small/large intestine. Retains water in stool, may bind water, ions in colonic lumen (soften feces, increase bulk); may increase colonic bacteria growth (increases fecal mass). Produces soft stool in 1–3 days.

CLASSIFICATION

LAXATIVES

GENERIC NAME	BRAND NAME(S)	TYPE	DOSAGE RANGE
bisacodyl	Dulcolax	Stimulant	Adults (PO): 10–15 mg; (Rectal): 10 mg Children >6 yrs (PO): 5–10 mg Children <2 yrs (Rectal): 5 mg
cascara	Cascara	Stimulant	Adults: 1 tablet or 5 ml
castor oil	Castor Oil	Stimulant	Adults: 15–60 ml Children (6–12 yrs): 5–15 ml
docusate CA	Surfak	Surfactant	Adults: 240 mg/day Children >6 yrs: 50–150 mg/day
docusate K	Dialose	Surfactant	Adults: 100–300 mg/day Children >6 yrs: 100 mg at hs
docusate Na	Colace	Surfactant	Adults: 50–500 mg/day Children (6–12 yrs): 40–120 mg; (3–6 yrs): 20–60 mg; (<3 yrs): 10–40 mg
lactulose	Cephulac	Osmotic	Adults: 30–45 ml 3–4×/day Children: 40–90 ml/day in divided doses Infants: 2.5–10 ml/day in divided doses
magnesium citrate	Citro-Nesia	Saline	Adults: 240 ml as needed Children: 120 ml as needed
magnesium hydroxide	MOM	Saline	Adults: 30–60 ml/day Children: 5–30 ml/day
magnesium sulfate	Epsom Salt	Saline	Adults: 10–15 g in glass water Children: 5–10 g in glass water
methylcellulose	Citrucel	Bulk-forming	Adults: 5–20 ml liquid 3×/day or 1 tablespoonful 1–3×/day (mix w/water, other fluid)
mineral oil	Mineral Oil	Lubricant	Adults: 5–45 ml Children: 5–20 ml
phenolpthalein	Modane	Stimulant	Adults: 60–194 mg at hs
poycarbophil	Mitrolan	Bulk-forming	Adults: 1 g 4×/day; maximum: 6 g/day Children (6–12 yrs): 500 mg 1–3×/day; maximum: 3 g/day Children (3–6 yrs): 500 mg 2×/day; maximum: 2 g/day
psyllium	Metamucil	Bulk-forming	Adults: 1 tsp 1–3×/day (mix w/water, other fluid)
senna	Senokot	Stimulant	Adults: 2–8 tablets/day Children: 1–4 tablets/day

hs = bedtime.

Castor oil: Acts in small intestine. Reduces absorption of fluid, electrolytes; stimulates intestinal peristalsis. Produces watery stool in 2–6 hrs.

Lactulose: Acts in colon. Similar to saline laxatives. Osmotic action may be enhanced in distal ileum/colon by bacterial metabolism to lactate, other organic acids. This decrease in pH increases motility, secretion. Produces soft stool in 1–3 days.

Saline: Acts in small/large intestine, colon (sodium phosphate). Poorly, slowly absorbed, causes hormone cholecystokinin release from duodenum (stimulates fluid secretion, motility), possesses osmotic properties, produces watery stool in 2–6 hrs (low doses produce semifluid stool in 6–12 hrs).

Stimulant: Acts in colon. Enhances accumulation of water/electrolytes in colonic lumen, enhances intestinal motility. May act directly on intestinal mucosa. Produces semifluid stool in 6–12 hrs (**Note:** Bisacodyl suppository acts in 15–60 min).

Surfactants: Act in small and large intestines. Hydrate and soften stools by their surfactant action facilitating penetration of fat and water into stool. Produce soft stool in 1–3 days.

USES

Short-term treatment of constipation; evacuate colon before rectal/bowel examination; prevent straining (e.g., after anorectal surgery, myocardial infarction); reduce painful elimination (e.g., episiotomy, hemorrhoids, anorectal lesions); modify effluent from ileostomy, colostomy; prevent fecal impaction; remove ingested poisons.

PRECAUTIONS

CONTRAINDICATIONS: Acute surgical abdomen, abdominal pain, intestinal obstruction or perforation, fecal impaction, undiagnosed rectal bleeding, young children. **CAUTIONS:** Select laxative carefully for diabetics and pts on sodium-restricted diet. (No saline laxative.) Avoid overuse/abuse.

INTERACTIONS

Cholinergics increase effects; anticholinergics and CNS depressants decrease effects. Mineral oil impairs absorption of vitamins A, D, E, and K. Antacids decrease laxative action of bisacodyl tablets. Laxative may decrease absorption of other drugs by increasing rate of passage.

SIDE EFFECTS

Cramping, frequent liquid stools, nausea, weakness, perianal irritation.

TOXIC EFFECTS/ADVERSE REACTIONS

Incidence rare. Severe diarrhea may cause dehydration and electrolyte imbalance. Fluid retention with saline laxative may cause edema and electrolyte imbalance. *Bulk-forming laxative:* Allergic reaction, impaction.

NURSING IMPLICATIONS

GENERAL: Give w/at least 8 oz of water and provide 6–8 glasses of water that day (unless pt on water restriction). Most laxatives should be given on an empty stomach at bedtime to provide morning evacuation. Provide call light and assistance as indicated. **BASELINE ASSESSMENT:** Results of laxative. **PATIENT/FAMILY TEACHING:** Avoid chronic use. Stress value of high-fiber diet, fluid intake, exercise, and regular bowel habits.

neuromuscular blockers

ACTION

Interrupt nerve impulse transmission at skeletal neuromuscular junction and/or autonomic ganglia (these receptors are called "nicotinic-cholinergic"). Further classified by whether or not they cause depolarization of motor end plate (nondepolarizing vs. depolarizing). Combine w/nicotinic-cholinergic receptor at postjunctional membrane blocking competitive transmitter action of acetylcholine. When administered, motor weakness gives way to total flaccid paralysis. Cause relaxation of skeletal muscle. Can produce decreased B/P due to release of histamine and to partial ganglionic blockade. Lack CNS effects—do not diminish consciousness or pain perception.

USES

Adjuvant in surgical anesthesia to obtain relaxation of skeletal muscle (esp. abdominal wall) for surgery (allows lighter level of anesthesia, valuable in orthopedic procedures). Neuromuscular blocking agents of short duration often used to facilitate intubation w/endotracheal tube; facilitates laryngoscopy, bronchoscopy, and esophagoscopy in combination w/general anesthetics. Provide muscle relaxation in pts undergoing mechanical ventilation, muscle relaxation in diagnosis of myasthenia gravis. Prevent convulsive movements during electroconvulsive therapy.

PRECAUTIONS

CONTRAINDICATIONS: Contraindicated during pregnancy, lactation, hypersensitivity to drug or components, pts who have own or family history of malignant hyperthermia. Use w/extreme caution, if at all, in pts w/myasthenia gravis. **CAUTIONS:** During cesarean delivery (potential respiratory depression in neonate); caution and reduced dosage during delivery when magnesium sulfate has been administered to pregnant woman (potentiates effects). Cautious use in pts w/hepatic, renal, or pulmonary impairment; respiratory depression; geriatric or debilitated pts.

INTERACTIONS

General anesthetics, antibiotics (esp. aminoglycosides) may increase effects. Anticholinesterase inhibitors (e.g., neostigmine) may decrease effects.

SIDE EFFECTS

Prolonged apnea, residual muscle weakness, hypersensitivity reactions. Many drugs also cause hypotension, wheezing and bronchospasm, cardiac disturbances, flushing, urticaria, pruritus.

TOXIC EFFECTS/ADVERSE REACTIONS

Malignant hyperthermia is rare, but often fatal (esp. w/halothane or succinylcholine). Severely compromised respiratory function; respiratory paralysis.

NEUROMUSCULAR BLOCKING AGENTS

GENERIC NAME	BRAND NAME(S)	TYPE	USES
atracurium	Tracrium	Nondepolarizing	Endotracheal intubation Surgery Mechanical ventilation
cisatracurium	Nimbex	Nondepolarizing	Endotracheal intubation Mechanical ventilation Surgery
doxacurium	Nuromax	Nondepolarizing	Endotracheal intubation Surgery
mivacurium	Mivacron	Nondepolarizing	Surgery Mechanical ventilation Endotracheal intubation
pancuronium	Pavulon	Nondepolarizing	Surgery Mechanical ventilation
pipecuronium	Arduan	Nondepolarizing	Endotracheal intubation Surgery
rapacuronium	Raplon	Nondepolarizing	Surgery
rocuronium	Zemuron	Nondepolarizing	Endotracheal intubation Surgery Mechanical ventilation
succinylcholine	Anectine Quelicin	Depolarizing	Endotracheal intubation Surgery Mechanical ventilation ECT
tubocurarine	Tubocurarine	Nondepolarizing	Surgery Mechanical ventilation ECT Dx: Myasthenia gravis
vecuronium	Norcuron	Nondepolarizing	Endotracheal intubation Surgery Mechanical ventilation

ECT = electroconvulsive therapy; Dx = diagnosis.

NURSING IMPLICATIONS

GENERAL: Have equipment and personnel immediately available to intubate pt and provide mechanical ventilation, including use of positive pressure oxygen. Have anticholinesterase reversal agents immediately available. Drugs do not alter consciousness; pt may be conscious but unable to move, breathe. INTERVENTION/EVALUATION: Continuously monitor B/P, pulse, EKG. PATIENT/FAMILY TEACHING: Explain to conscious pt, family that muscle tone will return. Provide emotional support and monitor respirations carefully during recovery period.

nitrates
ACTION

Relax most smooth muscles, including arteries and veins. Effect is primarily on veins (decrease left/right ventricular end-diastolic pressure). In angina, nitrates decrease myocardial work and O_2 requirements (decrease preload by venodilation and afterload by arteriodilation). Nitrates also appear to redistribute blood flow to ischemic myocardial areas improving perfusion w/o increase in coronary blood flow.

NITRATES

GENERIC NAME	RTE ADMIN	BRAND NAME(S)	CARDIOVASCULAR EFFECT		DOSAGE RANGE
			ONSET	DURATION	
erythrityl	PO	Cardilate	5–30 min	3–6 hrs	5–10 mg before event, up to 100 mg/day
isosorbide	SL	Isordil Sorbitrate	2–5 min	1–3 hrs	2.5–10 mg q2–3h
	PO	Isordil Sorbitrate	20–40 min	4–6 hrs	10–40 mg q6h
	SR	Dilatrate-SR Isordil Sorbitrate	up to 4 hrs	6–8 hrs	40–80 mg q8–12 h
nitroglycerin	SL	Nitrostat	1–3 min	30–60 min	0.3–0.6 mg to 3×/ 15 min
	SR	Nitrobid Nitroglyn	20–45 min	3–8 hrs	2.5 mg 3–4×/day up to 26 mg 3–4×/day
	Trans	Minitran Nitro-Dur Nitrodisc Transderm-Nitro	30–60 min	Up to 24 hrs	0.2–0.4 mg/hr up to 0.8 mg/hr
	Top	Nitrol	30–60 min	2–12 hrs	1–2 in q8h up to 4–5 in q4h
pentaerythritol	PO	Duotrate Peritrate	PO: 20–60 min SR: 30 min	5 hrs up to 12 hrs	PO: 10–20 mg 3–4×/ day up to 40 mg 4×/day SR: 1 cap/tab q12h

SL = sublingual; SR = sustained release; Trans = transdermal; Top = topical.

USES

Sublingual: Acute relief of angina pectoris.

Oral, topical: Long-term prophylactic treatment of angina pectoris.

Intravenous: Adjunctive treatment in CHF associated w/acute myocardial infarction. Produces controlled hypotension during surgical procedures; controls B/P in perioperative hypertension, angina unresponsive to organic nitrates or beta blockers.

PRECAUTIONS

CONTRAINDICATIONS: Hypersensitivity, hypotension, severe anemia, head trauma or cerebral hemorrhage, renal or hepatic dysfunction, closed-angle glaucoma, pregnancy, lactation. **CAUTIONS:** Acute MI, hepatic or renal dysfunction, blood volume decrease from diuretics, systolic B/P below 90 mm Hg. Chronic administration may lead to tolerance.

INTERACTIONS

Alcohol, antihypertensives, vasodilators may increase risk of orthostatic hypotension.

SIDE EFFECTS

Headache, hypotension, dizziness, palpitations, skin or mucous membrane sensitivity to nitrites/nitrates.

TOXIC EFFECTS/ADVERSE REACTIONS

Severe headache, significant hypotension, difficulty breathing, chest pain, hypersensitivity reactions.

NURSING IMPLICATIONS

GENERAL: IV infusion of nitroglycerin requires special administration set and precise flow rate. BASELINE ASSESSMENT: Record onset, type (sharp, dull, squeezing), radiation, location, intensity, and duration of anginal pain and precipitating factors (exertion, emotional stress). Obtain baseline B/P and apical pulse. INTERVENTION/EVALUATION: Monitor B/P and apical pulse (withhold and notify physician if systolic B/P below 90 mm Hg). Continuous cardiac monitoring is indicated for unrelieved, acute episodes. Assess for relief of anginal pain. Check for local irritation when given dermally or sublingually. PATIENT/FAMILY TEACHING: Avoid high-caffeine foods/fluids, such as coffee, colas, chocolate, tea (increased risk of anginal attacks). Do not take alcohol (can cause hypotensive, shocklike state) or other drugs w/o physician approval. Identify precipitating factors. Take sublingual tablets sitting or lying down for anginal relief; may repeat every 5 min, up to 3 tablets in 15 min. If no relief, have ambulance transport to hospital. Do not change brands; discard expired drugs. Notify physician of severe or persistent headache.

nonsteroidal anti-inflammatory drugs (NSAIDs)

ACTION

Exact mechanism for anti-inflammatory, analgesic, antipyretic effects unknown. Inhibition of enzyme cyclooxygenase, the enzyme responsible for prostaglandin synthesis, appears to be a major mechanism of action. May inhibit other mediators of inflammation (e.g., leukotrienes). Direct action on hypothalamus heat-regulating center may contribute to antipyretic effect.

NSAIDS

GENERIC NAME	BRAND NAME(S)	USE: DOSAGE RANGE
aspirin	many	Aches/pains: 325–650 mg q4h prn
		Arthritis: 3.2–6 g/day
		Juvenile rheumatoid arthritis: 60–110 mg/kg/day
		Acute rheumatic fever: Adults: 5–8 g/day; Children: 100 mg/kg/day ×14 days; then, 75 mg/kg/day ×4–6 wks
		Transient ischemic attacks: 1,300 mg/day
		Myocardial infarction prophylaxis: 81–325 mg/day
		Analgesic/antipyretic (children): up to 60–80 mg/kg/day or 10–15 mg/kg/dose q4h
bromfenac	Duract	Pain: 25 mg q6–8h prn
choline salicylate	Arthropan	Arthritis/pain/fever: 870 mg (5 ml) q3–4h up to 6×/day
diclofenac	Voltaren	Arthritis: 100–200 mg/day
diflunisal	Dolobid	Arthritis: 0.5–1 g/day
		Pain: 1 g, then 0.5 g q8–12h
etodolac	Lodine	Arthritis: 600–800 mg/day
		Pain: 200–400 mg q6–8h; max: 1200 mg/day
fenoprofen	Nalfon	Arthritis: 300–600 mg 3–4×/day
		Pain: 200 mg q4–6h prn
flurbiprofen	Ansaid	Arthritis: 200–300 mg/day
ibuprofen	Motrin	Arthritis: 1.2–3.2 g/day
		Pain: 400 mg q4–6h prn
		Fever: 200 mg q4–6h prn
		Primary dysmenorrhea: 400 mg q4h prn
		Juvenile arthritis: 30–40 mg/kg/day
indomethacin	Indocin	Arthritis: 50–200 mg/day
		Bursitis/tendonitis: 75–150 mg/day
		Gouty arthritis: 150 mg/day
ketoprofen	Orudis	Arthritis: 150–300 mg/day
		Pain/primary dysmenorrhea: 25–50 mg q6–8h as needed
ketorolac	Toradol	Pain: PO: 10 mg q4–6h prn; max: 40 mg/day; IM/IV: 60–120 mg/day
magnesium salicylate	Magan	Arthritis/pain/fever: 3.6–4.8 g/day in 3–4 divided doses
meclofenamate	Meclomen	Arthritis: 200–400 mg/day
		Pain: 50 mg q4–6h prn
		Primary dysmenorrhea: 100 mg 3×/day
nabumetone	Relafen	Arthritis: 1–2 g/day
naproxen	Anaprox	Arthritis: 250–550 mg/day
	Naprosyn	Pain/1° dysmenorrhea/bursitis/tendonitis: 500 mg, then 250 mg q6–8h
		Juvenile arthritis: 10 mg/kg in 2 divided doses
		Gouty arthritis: 750 mg, then 250 mg q8h
oxaprozin	Daypro	Arthritis: 600–1,800 mg/day
piroxicam	Feldene	Arthritis: 20 mg/day
sodium salicylate	Sodium Salicylate	Arthritis/pain/fever: 325–650 mg q4h prn
sulindac	Clinoril	Arthritis: 300 mg/day
		Acute gouty arthritis/painful shoulder: 400 mg/day
tolmetin	Tolectin	Arthritis: 600–1,800 mg/day
		Juvenile arthritis: 15–30 mg/kg/day

1° = primary; prn= as circumstances may require.

USES

Provides symptomatic relief from *pain/inflammation* in the treatment of musculoskeletal disorders (e.g., rheumatoid arthritis, osteoarthritis, ankylosing spondylitis); *analgesic* for low to moderate pain; *reduces fever* (many agents not suited for routine/prolonged therapy due to toxicity). By virtue of its action on platelet function, aspirin is used in treatment or prophylaxis of diseases associated w/hypercoagulability (reduces risk of stroke/heart attack).

PRECAUTIONS

CONTRAINDICATIONS: Aspirin sensitivity or allergy to other components; pregnancy; lactation; children <14 yrs of age, gastrointestinal disorders. **CAUTIONS:** Renal or hepatic dysfunctions, cardiac or hypertensive disorders, severe infections, elderly, coagulation defects, otic disease.

INTERACTIONS

Salicylates: Antacids, NSAIDs may increase risk of GI effects (e.g., ulceration). Urinary alkalinizers, antacids increase excretion. Anticoagulants, heparin, thrombolytics increase risk of bleeding. Large doses may increase insulin, oral hypoglycemic effects. Valproic acid, platelet aggregation inhibitors may increase risk of bleeding. May increase toxicity of methotrexate, zidovudine. Ototoxic medications, vancomycin may increase ototoxicity. May decrease effect of probenecid, sulfinpyrazone.

NSAIDs: May increase effects of oral anticoagulants, heparin, thrombolytics. May decrease effect of antihypertensives, diuretics. Salicylates, aspirin may increase risk of GI side effects, bleeding. Bone marrow depressants may increase risk of hematologic reactions. May increase methotrexate toxicity. Probenecid may increase concentration.

SIDE EFFECTS

Gastrointestinal upset, dizziness, headache, constipation or diarrhea. *Ophthalmic:* Burning, stinging on instillation, keratitis, elevated intraocular pressure.

TOXIC EFFECTS/ADVERSE REACTIONS

Hypersensitivity reactions, including skin rash or urticaria. Renal or hepatic toxicity, bone marrow suppression, bleeding, esp. of gastrointestinal tract. Tinnitus and hearing disturbances. Reactions vary by individual drug.

NURSING IMPLICATIONS

GENERAL: Check for aspirin sensitivity (cross-sensitivity). Administer on schedule to maintain blood levels. Provide rest, positioning, and other comfort measures for pain relief. BASELINE ASSESSMENT: Assess pain (type, location, intensity). Check temperature, pulse, respirations. INTERVENTION/EVALUATION: Assess pain, therapeutic response (decreased temperature, pain relief, improved mobility). PATIENT/FAMILY TEACHING: Take w/meals or on empty stomach, as

CLASSIFICATION

indicated by individual drug; however, all drugs may be taken w/food, if necessary, to reduce GI side effects. Avoid alcohol and consult physician about other medications. Refrain from driving or other activities requiring motor response until certain no dizziness present. Inform other physicians or dentist of drug therapy.

nutrition: enteral

Enteral nutrition (EN), also known as tube feedings, provides food/nutrients via GI tract using special formulas, techniques of delivery, and equipment. All routes of enteral nutrition consist of placement of a tube through which liquid formula is infused.

INDICATIONS

Tube feedings are used in pts w/major trauma, burns, undergoing radiation and/or chemotherapy, w/liver failure, severe renal impairment, w/physical or neurologic impairment, preop and postop to promote anabolism, prevent cachexia, malnutrition.

ROUTES OF ENTERAL NUTRITION DELIVERY

Nasogastric (NG):
INDICATIONS: Most common for short-term feeding in pts unable or unwilling to consume adequate nutrition by mouth. Requires at least partially functioning GI tract. **ADVANTAGES:** Does not require surgical intervention and is fairly easily inserted. Allows full use of digestive tract. Decreases chance hyperosmolar solutions may cause distention, nausea, vomiting. **DISADVANTAGES:** Temporary. May be easily pulled out during routine nursing care. Has potential for pulmonary aspiration of gastric contents, risk of reflux esophagitis, regurgitation.

Nasoduodenal (ND), nasojejunal (NJ):
INDICATIONS: Pts unable or unwilling to consume adequate nutrition by mouth. Requires at least partially functioning GI tract. **ADVANTAGES:** Does not require surgical intervention and is fairly easily inserted. Preferred for pts at risk of aspiration. Valuable for pts w/gastroparesis. **DISADVANTAGES:** Temporary. May be pulled out during routine nursing care. May be dislodged by coughing, vomiting. Small lumen size increases risk of clogging when medication is given through them, more susceptible to rupturing when using infusion device. Must be radiographed for placement, frequently extubated.

Gastrostomy:
INDICATIONS: Pts w/esophageal obstruction or impaired swallowing, pts in whom NG, ND, or NJ not feasible, or when long-term feeding indicated. **ADVANTAGES:** Permanent feeding access. Tubing has larger bore allowing noncontinuous (bolus) feeding (300–400 ml over 30–60 min q3–6h). May be inserted endoscopically using local anesthetic (procedure called percutaneous endoscopic gastrostomy [PEG]).

ENTERAL FORMULAS

PRODUCT	DESCRIPTION	CAL/ML	OSMOLALITY (mOsm/kg)	PROTEIN G/L	CHO G/L	FAT G/L
Advera	HIV infection AIDS	1.3	—	60	216	22.8
Alitraq	Metabolic stress Impaired GI function	1.0	575	52.5	165	15.5
Compleat	Tube feeding	1.1	450	43	130	43
Ensure Plus	Nutrient-dense oral supplement	1.5	690	54.9	199	53.2
Glucerna	Glucose intolerance	1.0	375	41.8	93.7	55.7
Isocal HN	Low residue	1.06	—	43.9	122	45.2
Jevity	Tube feeding w/fiber	1.06	310	44.4	151	36.7
Nepro	Renal dialysis	2.0	635	69.9	212	94.4
Osmolite HN	Low residue	1.06	300	44.4	139	36.7
Pediasure	Children 1–6 yrs	1.0	310	30.0	110	49.9
Perative	Metabolic stress	1.3	425	66.6	176	36.9
Pulmocare	Pulmonary	1.5	465	62.6	106	92
Suplena	Predialysis	2.0	615	30.0	254	95.4
Sustacal	Complete balanced nutrition	1.0	650	61.2	139	23.2
Traumacal	Multiple trauma, major burns	1.5	490	82.3	144	68.4
Travasorb HN	Elemental diet	—	560	15.0	58.3	4.5
Twocal HN	Nutrient dense oral supplement	2.0	690	83.7	216	90.3
Vital HN	Elemental diet	1.0	500	41.7	185	10.8

DISADVANTAGES: Requires surgery, may be inserted in conjunction w/other surgery or endoscopically (see Advantages). Stoma care required. Tube may be inadvertently dislodged. Risk of aspiration, peritonitis, cellulitis, leakage of gastric contents.

Jejunostomy:
INDICATIONS: Pts w/stomach or duodenal obstruction, impaired gastric motility, pts in whom NG, ND, or NJ not feasible, or when long-term feeding indicated. **ADVANTAGES:** Allows early postop feeding (small-bowel function is least affected by surgery). Risk of aspiration reduced. Rarely pulled out inadvertently. **DISADVANTAGES:** Requires surgery (laparotomy). Stoma care required. Risk of intraperitoneal leakage. Can be dislodged easily.

INITIATING ENTERAL NUTRITION

With continuous feeding, initiation of isotonic (about 300 mOsm/L) or moderately hypertonic feeding (up to 495 mOsm/L) can be given full strength usually at a slow rate (30–50 ml/hr) and gradually increased (25 ml/hr q6–24h). Formulas w/osmolality of >500 mOsm/L are generally started at half strength and gradually increased in rate, then concentration. Tolerance increased if the rate and concentration are not increased simultaneously.

SELECTION OF FORMULAS

Protein: Has many important physiologic roles and is the primary source of nitrogen in the body. Provides 4 kcal/g protein. Sources of protein in enteral feedings: sodium caseinate, calcium caseinate, soy protein, dipeptides.

Carbohydrate (CHO): Provides energy for the body and heat to maintain body temperature. Provides 3.4 kcal/g carbohydrate. Sources of carbohydrate (CHO) in enteral feedings: corn syrup, cornstarch, maltodextrin, lactose, sucrose, glucose.

Fat: Provides concentrated source of energy. Referred to as "kilocalorie dense" or "protein sparing." Provides 9 kcal/g fat. Sources of fat in enteral feedings: corn oil, safflower oil, medium chain triglycerides.

Electrolytes, vitamins, trace elements: Contained in formulas (not found in specialized products for renal and hepatic insufficiency).

All products containing protein, fat, carbohydrate, vitamin, electrolytes, trace elements are nutritionally complete and designed to be used by pts for long periods.

COMPLICATIONS

MECHANICAL: Usually associated w/some aspect of the feeding tube.

Aspiration pneumonia: Caused by delayed gastric emptying, gastroparesis, gastroesophageal reflux, or decreased gag reflex. May be prevented or treated by reducing infusion rate, using lower fat formula, feeding beyond pylorus, checking residuals, using small-bore feeding tubes, elevating head of bed 30–45° during and for 30–60 min after intermittent feeding, and regularly checking tube placement.

Esophageal, mucosal, pharyngeal irritation, otitis: Caused by using large-bore NG tube. Prevented by use of small bore whenever possible.

Irritation, leakage at ostomy site: Caused by drainage of digestive juices from site. Prevented by close attention to skin/stoma care.

Tube, lumen obstruction: Caused by thickened formula residue, formation of formula-medication complexes. Prevented by frequently irrigating tube w/clear water (also before and after giving formulas/medication), avoiding instilling medication if possible.

GASTROINTESTINAL: Usually associated w/formula, rate of delivery, unsanitary handling of solutions or delivery system.

Diarrhea: Caused by low-residue formulas, rapid delivery, use of hyperosmolar formula, hypoalbuminemia, malabsorption, microbial contamination, or rapid GI transit rate. Prevented by using fiber-supplemented formulas, decreasing rate of delivery, using dilute formula and gradually increasing strength.

Cramping, gas, abdominal distention: Caused by nutrient malabsorption, rapid delivery of refrigerated formula. Prevented by delivering formula by continuous methods, giving formulas at room temperature, decreasing rate of delivery.

Nausea, vomiting: Caused by rapid delivery of formula, gastric retention. Prevented by reducing rate of delivery, using dilute formulas, selecting low-fat formulas.

Constipation: Caused by inadequate fluid intake, reduced bulk, inactivity. Prevented by supplementing fluid intake, using fiber-supplemented formula, encouraging ambulation.

METABOLIC: Fluid/electrolyte status should be monitored. Refer to monitoring section. Additionally, the very young and very old are at greater risk in developing complications such as dehydration or over-hydration.

MONITORING

Daily: Estimate nutrient intake, fluid intake/output, weight of pt, clinical observations.

Weekly: Electrolytes (potassium, sodium, magnesium, calcium, phosphorus), blood glucose, BUN, creatinine, liver function tests (e.g., SGOT [AST], alkaline phosphatase), 24 hour urea and creatinine excretion, total iron binding capacity (TIBC) or serum transferrin, triglycerides, cholesterol.

Monthly: Serum albumin.

Other: Urine glucose, acetone (when blood glucose >250), vital signs (temperature, respirations, pulse, B/P) q8h.

nutrition: parenteral

Parenteral nutrition (PN), also known as total parenteral nutrition (TPN) or hyperalimentation (HAL), provides required nutrients to pts by IV route of administration. The goal of PN is to maintain or restore nutritional status caused by disease, injury, or inability to consume nutrients by other means.

INDICATIONS

Conditions when pt is unable to use alimentary tract via oral, gastrostomy, or jejunostomy routes. Impaired absorption of protein caused by obstruction, inflammation, or antineoplastic therapy. Bowel rest necessary because of GI surgery or ileus, fistulas, or anastomotic leaks. Conditions w/increased metabolic requirements (e.g., burns, infection, trauma). Preserve tissue reserves as in acute renal failure. Inadequate nutrition from tube feeding methods.

COMPONENTS OF PN

In order to meet IV nutritional requirements six essential categories in PN are needed for tissue synthesis and energy balance.

Protein: In the form of crystalline amino acids (CAA), primarily used for protein synthesis. Several products are designed to meet specific needs for pts w/renal failure (e.g., NephrAmine), liver disease (e.g., HepatAmine), stress/trauma (e.g., Aminosyn HBC), use in neonates and pediatrics (e.g., Aminosyn PF, TrophAmine). Calories: 4 kcal/g protein.

Energy: In the form of dextrose, available in concentrations of 5–70%. Dextrose <10% may be given peripherally; concentrations >10% must be given centrally. Calories: 3.4 kcal/g dextrose.

IV fat emulsion: Available in the form of 10 or 20% concentrations. Provides a concentrated source of energy/calories (9 kcal/g fat) and is a source of essential fatty acids. May be administered peripherally or centrally.

Electrolytes: Major electrolytes (calcium, magnesium, potassium, sodium; also acetate, chloride, phosphate). Doses of electrolytes are individualized, based on many factors (e.g., kidney and/or liver function, fluid status).

Vitamins: Essential components in maintaining metabolism and cellular function; widely used in PN.

Trace elements: Necessary in long-term PN administration. Trace elements include zinc, copper, chromium, manganese, selenium, molybdenum, and iodine.

Miscellaneous: Additives include insulin, albumin, heparin, and histamine$_2$ blockers (e.g., cimetidine, rantidine, famotidine). Other medication may be included, but compatibility for admixture should be checked on an individual basis.

ROUTE OF ADMINISTRATION

PN is administered via either peripheral or central vein.

Peripheral: Usually involves 2–3 L/day of 5–10% dextrose w/3–5% amino acid solution along w/IV fat emulsion. Electrolytes, vitamins, trace elements added according to pt needs. Peripheral solutions provide about 2,000 kcal/day and 60–90 g protein/day. **ADVANTAGES:** Lower risks vs. central mode of administration. **DISADVANTAGES:** Peripheral veins may not be suitable (esp. in pts w/illness of long duration); more susceptible to phlebitis (due to osmolalities >600 mOsm/L); veins may be viable only 1–2 wks; large volumes of fluid are needed to meet nutritional requirements, which may be contraindicated in many pts.

Central: Usually utilizes hypertonic dextrose (concentration range of 15–35%) and amino acid solution of 3–7% w/IV fat emulsion. Electrolytes, vitamins, trace elements added according to pt needs. Central solutions provide 2,000–4,000 kcal/day. Must be given through large central vein w/high blood flow allowing rapid dilution avoiding phlebitis/thrombosis (usually through percutaneous insertion of catheter into subclavian vein then advancement of catheter to superior vena cava). **ADVANTAGES:** Allows more alternatives/flexibility in establishing regimens; allows ability to provide full nutritional requirements w/o need of daily fat emulsion; useful in pts who are fluid restricted (increased concentration), pts needing large nutritional requirements (e.g., trauma, malignancy), or for whom PN indicated >7–10 days. **DISADVANTAGES:** Risk w/insertion, use, maintenance of central line; increased risk of infection, catheter-induced trauma, and metabolic changes.

MONITORING

May vary slightly from institution to institution.

Baseline: CBC, platelet count, prothrombin time, weight, body length/head circumference (in infants), electrolytes, glucose, BUN, creatinine, uric acid, total protein, cholesterol, triglycerides, bilirubin, alkaline phosphatase, LDH, SGOT (AST), albumin, other tests as needed.

Daily: Weight, vital signs (TPR), nutritional intake (kcal, protein, fat), electrolytes (potassium, sodium chloride), glucose (serum, urine), acetone, BUN, osmolarity, other tests as needed.

2–3 times/week: CBC, coagulation studies (PT, PTT), creatinine, calcium, magnesium, phosphorus, acid-base status, other tests as needed.

Weekly: Nitrogen balance, total protein, albumin, prealbumin, transferrin, liver function tests (SGOT [AST], SGPT [ALT]), alkaline phosphatase, LDH, bilirubin, Hgb, uric acid, cholesterol, triglycerides, other tests as needed.

COMPLICATIONS

Mechanical: Malfunction in system for IV delivery (e.g., pump failure, problems w/lines, tubing, administration sets, catheter). Pneumothorax, catheter misdirection, arterial puncture, bleeding, hematoma formation may occur w/catheter placement.

Infectious: Infections (pts often more susceptible to infections), catheter sepsis (e.g., fever, shaking chills, glucose intolerance) where no other site of infection identified.

Metabolic: Includes hyperglycemia, elevated cholesterol and triglycerides, abnormal liver function tests.

Fluid, electrolyte, acid-base disturbances: May alter potassium, sodium, phosphate, magnesium levels.

Nutritional: Clinical effects seen may be due to lack of adequate vitamins, trace elements, essential fatty acids.

opioid analgesics

ACTION

Opioids refer to all drugs, natural and synthetic, having actions similar to morphine and to receptors combining w/these agents. Three opioid receptors have been identified: mu, kappa, and delta. Morphinelike opioid agonists act primarily at mu receptors; and opioids w/mixed action are agonists at some receptors, antagonists/weak agonists at other receptors.

Morphinelike: Major effects are on the CNS (produce analgesia, drowsiness, mood changes, mental clouding, analgesia w/o loss of consciousness, nausea and vomiting) and gastrointestinal tract (decrease HCl secretion, diminish biliary, pancreatic, and intestinal secretions; diminish propulsive peristalsis). Also affects respiration (depressed) and cardiovascular system (peripheral vasodilation, decrease peripheral resistance, inhibit baroreceptor reflexes).

Opioids w/mixed action: After binding to receptor, may produce no effect or only limited action. Produce analgesia, euphoria, respiratory and physical depression, have lower abuse potential, may produce withdrawal symptoms in pts w/opioid dependence.

USES

Relief of moderate to severe pain associated w/surgical procedures, myocardial infarction, burns, cancer, or other conditions. May be used as an adjunct to anesthesia, either as a preop medication or intraoperatively as a supplement to anesthesia. Also used for obstetrical analgesia. Codeine and hydrocodone have an antitussive effect. Opium tinctures, such as paregoric, are used for severe diarrhea. Methadone relieves severe pain but is used primarily as part of heroin detoxification.

OPIOID ANALGESICS

GENERIC (BRAND) NAMES	EQUIANALGESIC TO 10 MG IM MORPHINE	TYPE	ANALGESIC EFFECT ONSET	PEAK	DURATION	DOSAGE RANGE
Alfentanil (Alfenta)	—	Agonist	Immediate	—	—	—
buprenorphine (Buprenex)	IM: 0.3 mg	Mixed	15 min	1 hr	6 hrs	IM, IV: 0.3 mg q6h prn
butorphanol (Stadol)	IM: 2 mg	Mixed	<10 min	0.5–1 hr	2–4 hrs	IM: 2 mg q3–4h prn IV: 1 mg q3–4h prn
codeine	PO: 200 mg IM: 120 mg	Agonist	10–30 min	0.5–1 hr	4–6 hrs	PO, SubQ, IM: Adults: 15–60 mg q4–6h prn Children: 0.5 mg/ kg q4–6h prn
dezocine (Dalgan)	IM: 10 mg	Mixed	15–30 min	30–150 min	2–4 hrs	IM: 5–20 mg q3–6h prn IV: 2.5–10 mg q2–4h prn
fentanyl (Sublimaze)	IM: 0.1 mg	Agonist	7–8 min	—	1–2 hrs	—
hydrocodone	—	Agonist	—	—	4–8 hrs	—
hydromorphone (Dilaudid)	PO: 7.5 mg IM: 1.5 mg	Agonist	15–30 min	0.5–1 hr	4–5 hrs	PO: 2 mg q4–6h prn SubQ, IM: 1–2 mg q4–6h prn Rectal: 3 mg q6–8h prn
levorphanol (Levo-dromoran)	IM: 2 mg	Agonist	0.5–1.5 hrs	0.5–1 hr	6–8 hrs	SubQ: 2–3 mg q4h prn
meperidine (Demerol)	PO: 300 mg IM: 75 mg	Agonist	10–45 min	0.5–1 hr	2–4 hrs	PO, IM, SubQ: Adults: 50–150 mg q3–4h prn Children: 1–1.8 mg/kg q3–4h prn
methadone (Dolophine)	PO: 20 mg IM: 10 mg	Agonist	30–60 min	0.5–1 hr	4–6 hrs	IM, SubQ, PO: 2.5–10 mg q4h prn
morphine (Roxanol, MS Contin)	PO: 60 mg	Agonist	15–60 min	0.5–1 hr	3–7 hrs	PO: 10–30 mg q4h prn IM: 5–20 mg q4h prn
nalbuphine (Nubain)	IM: 10 mg	Mixed	2–15 min	0.5–1 hr	3–6 hrs	SubQ, IM, IV: 10 mg q3–6h prn

OPIOID ANALGESICS *Continued*

GENERIC (BRAND) NAMES	EQUIANALGESIC TO 10 MG IM MORPHINE	TYPE	ANALGESIC EFFECT			DOSAGE RANGE
			ONSET	PEAK	DURATION	
oxycodone (Roxicodone)	PO: 30 mg	Agonist	15–30 min	1 hr	4–6 hrs	PO: 5 mg or 5 ml q6h prn
oxymorphone (Numorphan)	IM: 1 mg RTL: 10 mg	Agonist	5–10 min	0.5–1 hr	3–6 hrs	SubQ, IM: 1–1.5 mg q4h prn Rectal: 5 mg q4h prn
pentazocine (Talwin)	PO: 180 mg IM: 60 mg	Mixed	PO: 15–30 min	1–3 hrs	3 hrs	PO: 50–100 mg q3–4h prn
			IM: 15–20 min	15–60 min	3 hrs	IM, SubQ, IV: 30 mg
			IV: 2–3 min	—	3 hrs	q3–4 h prn
propoxyphene (Darvon)	—	Agonist	30–60 min	2–2.5 hrs	4–6 hrs	PO: 100 mg q4h prn
remifentanil (Ultiva)	—	Agonist	<1 min	2–3 min	5 min	IV infusion: 0.025–0.2 mcg/kg/min
sufentanil (Sufenta)	IM: 0.02 mg	Agonist	1.3–3 hrs	—	—	IV: 1–2 mcg/kg

PRECAUTIONS

CONTRAINDICATIONS: Hypersensitivity, pregnancy or lactation, infants, diarrhea caused by poisoning, respiratory depression, asthma, emphysema, convulsive disorders, severe renal or hepatic dysfunction, prostatic hypertrophy, acute ulcerative colitis, increased intracranial pressure. **CAUTIONS:** Pediatric, geriatric, and debilitated pts may be more susceptible to effects. Caution when using for obstetrical analgesia to prevent respiratory depression in neonate. Respiratory depression is a concern in the severely obese. Care when administered to pts in shock or w/reduced blood volume.

INTERACTIONS

Any of the CNS depressants, including alcohol, potentiate effects. Combination w/MAO inhibitors or administration within 14 days of MAO inhibitors may potentiate effects of either agent. Death has resulted from interactions of the above. There is increased muscle relaxation and respiratory depression w/skeletal muscle relaxants. A few of the narcotics have both agonist and antagonist actions; when administered to pts who have been receiving or abusing narcotics, withdrawal symptoms may develop. Narcotic antagonists are given to reverse respiratory depression of narcotic analgesics.

SIDE EFFECTS

Lightheadedness, dizziness, orthostatic hypotension, drowsiness, constipation.

CLASSIFICATION

TOXIC EFFECTS/ADVERSE REACTIONS

Respiratory depression, which can lead to respiratory arrest; brady-cardia; hypotension; urinary retention/oliguria; CNS depression w/slurred speech, dulled mental responses, or stupor. May have converse excitation reaction w/euphoria and tremors. Hypersensitivity may be evidenced by rash, itching, sneezing. Tolerance, physical and/or psychological dependence may develop.

NURSING IMPLICATIONS

GENERAL: When administering intravenously, dilute and give slowly to prevent severe CNS depression and possible cardiac arrest. Give narcotic before pain is intense to break the pain cycle. Maintain appropriate records (most of these are schedule II drugs). BASELINE ASSESSMENT: Determine initial B/P, pulse, respirations. Assess pain for type, location, intensity. INTERVENTION/EVALUATION: Assess response to pain medication. Monitor B/P, pulse, respirations. Maintain I&O; be alert to decreased urination. Avoid constipation. PATIENT/FAMILY TEACHING: Do not smoke (may cause hypoxemia, respiratory depression). Physical and/or mental abilities may be impaired. Do not ambulate w/o assistance; do not drive or engage in activities requiring mental acuity. Refrain from alcohol or other medications. Drug dependence is not likely for short-term medical purposes.

opioid antagonists

ACTION

Prevents/reverses effects of mu receptor opioid agonists (e.g., increases respiration, reverses sedative effect).

USES

Primarily used to reverse respiratory depression induced by narcotic overdosage. Naloxone is the drug of choice for reversal of respiratory depression.

PRECAUTIONS

CONTRAINDICATIONS: Respiratory depression due to other than narcotic analgesics, hypersensitivity, narcotic dependency, pregnancy, lactation, severe hepatic dysfunction. CAUTION: Obstetric and surgical pts should be monitored carefully for bleeding. Care in pts w/cardiac irritability.

INTERACTIONS

Reverses opioid effects. Causes withdrawal symptoms in narcotic-dependent pts.

OPIOID ANTAGONISTS

GENERIC NAME	BRAND NAME(S)	USUAL DOSAGE
nalmefene	Revex	IV/IM/SC: titrated individually
naloxone	Narcan	IV/IM/SC: Adults: 0.4–2 mg
		Children: 0.01 mg/kg
naltrexone	ReVia	PO: 50 mg/day or 100 mg qOd

SIDE EFFECTS

Reduces or eliminates analgesia. Nausea, vomiting, increase in sweating.

TOXIC EFFECTS/ADVERSE REACTIONS

Hypertension, tachycardia. Withdrawal symptoms when administered to pts dependent on narcotics; general achiness, runny nose, restlessness and irritability, insomnia, anorexia, nausea, and vomiting.

NURSING IMPLICATIONS

GENERAL: Have resuscitative equipment immediately available, as well as the antagonist agent. INTERVENTION/EVALUATION: Monitor respirations carefully after antagonist is given (naloxone is not as long acting as some narcotics and dose may have to be repeated). Check B/P and pulse. Be alert to return of pain when narcotic action is reversed. May cause withdrawal symptoms in narcotic-dependent pts.

oral contraceptives

ACTION

Oral contraceptives include estrogen-progestin combinations and progestin-only products. The combinations in turn may be monophasic, biphasic, or triphasic.

Progestin only: Exact mechanism of pregnancy prevention is unknown but may alter cervical mucus, exert a progestational effect on the endometrium rendering the endometrium hostile to implantation by a fertilized ovum, and suppress ovulation.

Estrogen-progestin combination: Suppresses the gonadotropins, follicle-stimulating hormone (FSH) and luteinizing hormone (LH), also alters the genital tract (cervical mucus inhibiting sperm penetration and endometrium reducing likelihood of implantation).

USES

Prevention of pregnancy.

PRECAUTIONS

CONTRAINDICATIONS: Thrombophlebitis, thromboembolic disorders, or a history of deep vein thrombophlebitis, cerebral vascular disease,

CLASSIFICATION

myocardial infarction, coronary artery disease, known or suspected breast carcinoma or estrogen-dependent neoplasms, carcinoma of endometrium, hepatic adenomas/carcinoma; past/present angina pectoris; undiagnosed abnormal genital bleeding; known or suspected pregnancy; cholestatic jaundice of pregnancy/jaundice w/prior pill use. **CAUTIONS:** History of cigarette smoking (increased risk of cardiovascular side effects from oral contraceptives), lipidemias, history of depression, convulsive disorders, migraine syndrome, asthma, cardiac, liver, or renal impairment, obesity, diabetes mellitus, hypertension.

INTERACTIONS

May increase therapeutic effect, concentration, or toxicity w/tricyclic antidepressants, benzodiazepines, beta-blocking agents, corticosteroids, theophylline. May decrease therapeutic effect of salicylates (increases clearance). Griseofulvin, penicillins, tetracyclines may decrease effect of oral contraceptives. Barbiturates, hydantoins, rifampin may increase hepatic metabolism, decrease oral contraceptive effect.

SIDE EFFECTS

FREQUENT: Breakthrough bleeding, nausea, vomiting. **OCCASIONAL:** Spotting, altered menstrual flow, amenorrhea, vaginal candidiasis, breast tenderness, enlargement, abdominal cramps, bloating, rash, edema, weight change, cholestatic jaundice, migraines, mental depression.

TOXIC EFFECTS/ADVERSE REACTIONS

Thrombophlebitis, venous thrombosis, pulmonary embolism, coronary thrombosis, myocardial infarction, cerebral hemorrhage, hypertension, cerebral thrombosis, arterial thromboembolism, congenital anomalies.

ORAL CONTRACEPTIVES

MONOPHASIC		
BRAND NAME(S)	**ESTROGEN (MCG)**	**PROGESTIN (MG)**
Genora 1/50 Nelova 1/50M Norethin 1/50M Norinyl 1+50 Ortho-Novum 1/50	50 mestranol	1 norethindrone
Ovcon-50	50 ethinyl estradiol	1 norethindrone
Demulen 1/50	50 ethinyl estradiol	1 ethynodiol diacetate
Ovral	50 ethinyl estradiol	0.5 norgestrel
Genora 1/35 Nelova 1/35E Norethin 1/35E Norinyl 1+35 Ortho-Novum 1/35	35 ethinyl estradiol	1 norethindrone
Brevicon Genora 0.5/35 Modicon Nelova 0.5/35E	35 ethinyl estradiol	0.5 norethindrone

ORAL CONTRACEPTIVES *Continued*

MONOPHASIC

BRAND NAME(S)	ESTROGEN (MCG)	PROGESTIN (MG)
Ovcon-35	35 ethinyl estradiol	0.4 norethindrone
Ortho-Cyclen	35 ethinyl estradiol	0.25 norgeestimate
Demulen 1/35	35 ethinyl estradial	1 ethynodiol diacetate
Loestrin 21 1.5/30 Loestrin Fe 1.5/30	30 ethinyl estradio	1.5 norethindrone acetate
Lo/Ovral	30 ethinyl estradiol	0.3 norgestrel
Desogen Ortho-Cept	30 ethinyl estradiol	0.15 desogestrel
Levlen Levora Nordette	30 ethinyl estradiol	0.15 levonorgestrel
Loestrin 21 1/20	20 ethinyl estradiol	1 norethindrone acetate

BIPHASIC

	PHASE 1	PHASE 2
Jenest-28	0.5 mg norethindrone 35 mcg ethinyl estradiol	1 mg norethindrone 35 mcg ethinyl estradiol
Nelova 10/11	0.5 mg norethindrone 35 mcg ethinyl estradiol	1 mg norethindrone 35 mcg ethinyl estradiol
Ortho-Novum 10/11	0.5 mg norethindrone 35 mcg ethinyl estradiol	1 mg norethindrone 35 mcg ethinyl estradiol

TRIPHASIC

	PHASE 1	PHASE 2	PHASE 3
Estrastep	1 mg norethindrone 20 mcg ethinyl estradiol	1 mg norethindrone 30 mcg ethinyl estradiol	1 mg norethindrone 35 mcg ethinyl estradiol
Tri-Norinyl	0.5 mg norethindrone 35 mcg ethinyl estradiol	1 mg norethindrone 35 mcg ethinyl estradiol	0.5 mg norethindrone 35 mcg ethinyl estradiol
OrthoNovum 7/7/7	0.5 mg norethindrone 35 mcg ethinyl estradiol	0.75 mg norethindrone 35 mcg ethinyl estradiol	1 mg norethindrone 35 mcg ethinyl estradiol
Tri-Levlen Triphasil	0.05 mg levonorgestrel 30 mcg ethinyl estradiol	0.075 mg levonorgestrel 40 mcg ethinyl estradiol	0.125 mg levonorgestrel 30 mcg ethinyl estradiol
Ortho Tri-Cyclen	0.18 mg norgestimate 35 mcg ethinyl estradiol	0.215 mg norgestimate 35 mcg ethinyl estradiol	0.25 mg norgestimate 35 mcg ethinyl estradiol

PROGESTIN ONLY

Micronor Nor Q D	0.35 mg norethindrone
Ovrette	0.075 mg norgestrel

NURSING IMPLICATIONS

BASELINE ASSESSMENT: Take complete medical and family history before initiating therapy. B/P, exam of breasts, abdomen and pelvic organs, PAP smear. Assess total and HDL cholesterol. INTERVEN-TION/EVALUATION: Monitor B/P, total and HDL cholesterol, breast, abdomen, and pelvic organ exams. Be alert to earliest symptoms of thromboembolic and thrombotic disorders. PATIENT/FAMILY TEACHING: Patient package insert available w/product. Take as directed at intervals not exceeding 24 hrs (take at same time each day) w/meals or at bedtime. May cause breakthrough bleeding/spotting; notify physician if bleeding occurs in more than one cycle or lasts longer than a few days. Oral contraceptive do not protect against HIV and other sexually transmitted diseases. Use additional birth control method until after the first week of administration in initial cycle or entire cycle if vomiting/diarrhea occurs.

oxytocics

ACTION

Oxytocics (Pitocin, Syntocinon) stimulate frequency/force of contraction of uterine smooth muscle. Responsiveness of uterus increases closer to term. Stimulates breast (contracting of myoepithelial cells surrounding mammary gland) to release milk.

USES

To induce, augment labor when maternal or fetal medical need exists; control of postpartum hemorrhage; cause uterine contraction after cesarean section or during other uterine surgery; induce therapeutic abortion.

PRECAUTIONS

CONTRAINDICATIONS: Hypersensitivity, cephalopelvic disproportions, unfavorable fetal position, fetal distress when delivery is not immediate, prolapsed cord or indication for surgical intervention. Methylergonovine should not be given to hypertensive pts or in toxemia or pregnancy. Ergonovine is used for postpartum hemorrhage and is contraindicated for labor induction. CAUTIONS: Pts >35 yrs of age; heart disease, hypertension; renal or hepatic dysfunction; sepsis.

INTERACTIONS

Caudal block anesthetics, vasopressors may increase pressor effects. Other oxytocics may cause uterine hypertonus, uterine rupture, or cervical lacerations.

SIDE EFFECTS

Nausea or vomiting.

TOXIC EFFECTS/ADVERSE REACTIONS

Arrhythmias, increased bleeding, uterine hypertonicity, hypotension, water intoxication, anaphylactic reaction. Fetus may develop bradycardia, hypoxia and experience trauma from too rapid birth. Peripheral ischemia, severe hypertension w/ergonovine, methylergonovine.

NURSING IMPLICATIONS

GENERAL: Regulate infusions precisely. BASELINE ASSESSMENT: Determine initial maternal B/P, pulse, fetal heart rate. INTERVENTION/EVALUATION: Monitor fetal heart rate, maternal B/P and pulse, uterine contractions (duration, strength, frequency) every 15 min. Notify physician of contractions that exceed 1 min, occur more frequently than every 2 min, or stop. Maintain careful I&O; be alert to potential water intoxication. For postpartum hemorrhage: Check uterus for firmness, amount of vaginal bleeding, vital signs. Evaluate extremities for warmth, color, movement, pain. PATIENT/FAMILY TEACHING: Keep pt, family informed of labor progress. Postpartum: Avoid smoking (added vasoconstriction).

sedative-hypnotics

ACTION

Sedatives decrease activity, moderate excitement, and have calming effects. Hypnotics produce drowsiness, enhance onset/maintenance of sleep (resembling natural sleep). Benzodiazepines are the most widely used agents (largely replace barbiturates): greater safety, lower incidence of drug dependence. Benzodiazepines potentiate gamma-aminobutyric acid, which inhibits impulse transmission in the CNS reticular formation in brain. Benzodiazepines decrease sleep latency, number of awakenings, and time spent in awake stage of sleep; increase total sleep time. Schedule IV drugs. See individual monographs for barbiturates.

USES

Treatment of insomnia, e.g., difficulty falling asleep initially, frequent awakening, awakening too early. For preop sedation.

PRECAUTIONS

CONTRAINDICATIONS: Hypersensitivity. Respiratory depression; respiratory diseases, porphyria, severe renal or hepatic dysfunction, history of alcohol or drug abuse, pregnancy, lactation, children. **CAUTIONS:** Elderly are more sensitive to adverse effects.

INTERACTIONS

Alcohol, narcotic analgesics, and other CNS depressants cause further CNS depressive effects. Combination w/CNS depressants should be avoided when possible.

CLASSIFICATION

SIDE EFFECTS

Drowsiness, dizziness, hangover, rebound insomnia due to altered REM, non-REM sleep stages.

TOXIC EFFECTS/ADVERSE REACTIONS

Hypersensitivity reactions: rash, urticaria. Confusion, extreme drowsiness, diarrhea. Paradoxical excitation may occur, particularly in the elderly. Overdose: respiratory depression, pulmonary edema, tachycardia and palpitations, marked hypotension, renal and hepatic damage, anoxia, cardiac collapse may proceed to coma and death. Potential for drug abuse and dependence, esp. w/barbiturates.

NURSING IMPLICATIONS

GENERAL: Provide environment conducive to sleep and pain relief. Put side rails up, lower bed, and put call light within reach. Assist in identifying cause of insomnia and encourage pt not to depend on medication. Comply w/federal narcotic laws regarding schedule IV drugs. Consider potential for abuse, dependence. Narcotics may need to be reduced when given w/hypnotics. BASELINE ASSESSMENT: Determine initial B/P, pulse, respirations, and sleep pattern. INTERVENTION/EVALUATION: Assure that pt has swallowed oral medication. Assess response to medication, sleep pattern. Monitor B/P, pulse, and respirations. PATIENT/FAMILY TEACHING: Instruct pt not to smoke or get up alone after taking hypnotic. Drowsiness may continue into next day; avoid driving or activities requiring mental acuity until response to drug controlled. Avoid alcohol. Consult physician before taking other medications. Take only as directed; do not increase dosage or abruptly discontinue (possible rebound insomnia).

HYPNOTICS

GENERIC NAME	BRAND NAME(S)	DOSAGE RANGE
estazolam	ProSom	Adults: 1–2 mg before bedtime
		Elderly, debilitated: 0.5–1 mg at bedtime
flurazepam	Dalmane	Adults: 15–30 mg before bedtime
		Elderly, debilitated: Initially, 15 mg, then based on pt response
quazepam	Doral	Adults: Initially, 15 mg, may decrease to 7.5 mg in some pts
		Elderly, debilitated: Initially, 15 mg, then attempt to decrease dose after 1–2 nights
temazepam	Restoril	Adults: 15–30 mg before bedtime
		Elderly, debilitated: Initially, 15 mg, then based on pt response
triazolam	Halcion	Adults: 0.125–0.5 mg before bedtime
		Elderly, debilitated: Initially, 0.125 mg until response determined. Range: 0.125–0.25 mg
zaleplon	Sonata	Adults: 5–20 mg
		Elderly: 5–10 mg
zolpidem	Ambien	Adults: 10 mg immediately before bedtime
		Elderly: 5 mg immediately before bedtime.

skeletal muscle relaxants

ACTION

Centrally acting muscle relaxants: Exact mechanism unknown. May act in CNS at various levels to depress polysynaptic reflexes; sedative effect may be responsible for relaxation of muscle spasm.

Baclofen and diazepam: May mimic actions of gamma-aminobutyric acid on spinal neurons; do not directly affect skeletal muscles.

Dantrolene: Acts directly on skeletal muscle relieving spasticity.

SKELETAL MUSCLE RELAXANTS

GENERIC NAME	BRAND NAME(S)	DOSAGE RANGE
baclofen	Lioresal	Adults: 40–80 mg/day
carisoprodol	Rela Soma	Adults: 350 mg 4×/day
chlorzoxazone	Parafon Forte DSC	Adults: 250–750 mg 3–4×/day Children: 125–500 mg 3–4×/day
cyclobenzaprine	Flexeril	Adults: 10 mg 3×/day
dantrolene	Dantrium	Adults: 25 mg/day initially; gradually increase to 400 mg/day or less
diazepam	Valium	Adults: 2–10 mg 3–4×/day Elderly: 2–2.5 mg initially; gradually increase Children: 1–2.5 mg 3–4×/day
methocarbamol	Robaxin	Adults: 500–1,000 mg 4×/day
orphenadrine	Norflex	Adults: 100 mg morning and evening

USES

Central acting muscle relaxants: Adjunct to rest, physical therapy for relief of discomfort associated w/acute, painful musculoskeletal disorders, i.e., local spasms from muscle injury.

Baclofen, dantrolene, diazepam: Treatment of spasticity characterized by heightened muscle tone, spasm, loss of dexterity caused by multiple sclerosis, cerebral palsy, spinal cord lesions, stroke.

PRECAUTIONS

CONTRAINDICATIONS: Pregnancy, lactation, cross-sensitivity, CNS depression, renal or hepatic dysfunction, children <12 yrs of age. According to specific drug. **CAUTIONS:** Cautious use in pts w/cardiac disease; history of allergy, epilepsy.

INTERACTIONS

Alcohol, narcotic analgesics, sedatives, hypnotics, and other CNS depressants may increase CNS effects (e.g., drowsiness, dizziness, fatigue).

SIDE EFFECTS

Drowsiness, orthostatic hypotension, w/dizziness and lightheaded-

CLASSIFICATION

ness, nausea or vomiting, stomach cramps, headache, constipation, blurred vision.

TOXIC EFFECTS/ADVERSE REACTIONS

Hypersensitivity reactions. Severe hypotension, tachycardia, blood dyscrasias, GI bleeding, unusual muscle weakness, hepatotoxicity.

NURSING IMPLICATIONS

Provide supportive measures, e.g., bed rest, positioning, exercise, moist heat as indicated. Withdraw drugs slowly. BASELINE ASSESSMENT: Determine degree of immobility. Assess pain (type, location, intensity). INTERVENTION/EVALUATION: Monitor B/P, pulse, respirations. Assess for therapeutic response (increased mobility and decreased pain). PATIENT/FAMILY TEACHING: Administer on schedule to maintain blood levels. Avoid alcohol and consult physician before taking other medications. Do not drive or engage in activities requiring mental acuity (drowsiness, dizziness). Prolonged use may cause dependence.

sympathomimetics

ACTION

Sympathetic nervous system (SNS) is involved in maintaining homeostasis (involved in regulation of heart rate, force of cardiac contractions, B/P, bronchial airway tone, carbohydrate, fatty acid metabolism). The SNS is mediated by neurotransmitters (primarily norepinephrine, epinephrine, and dopamine), which act on adrenergic receptors. These receptors include $beta_1$, $beta_2$, $alpha_1$, $alpha_2$, and dopaminergic. Sympathomimetics differ widely in their actions based on their specificity to affect these receptors. Actions expected by stimulating these receptors include the following:

$Alpha_1$: Mydriasis, constriction of arterioles, veins.

$Alpha_2$: Inhibits transmitter release.

$Beta_1$: Increases rate, force of contraction, conduction velocity of heart, releases renin from kidney.

$Beta_2$: Dilates arterioles, bronchi, relaxes uterus.

Dopamine: Dilates kidney vasculature.

USES

Stimulation of alpha_1-receptors: Induces vasoconstriction primarily in skin and mucous membranes; nasal decongestion; combines w/local anesthetics to delay anesthetic absorption; increases B/P in certain hypotensive states; produces mydriasis, facilitating eye exams, ocular surgery.

Stimulation of alpha_2-receptors: No therapeutic use.

Stimulation of beta_1-receptors: Treatment of cardiac arrest (not primary); treatment of heart failure, shock, AV block (temporary only).

Stimulation of beta₂-receptors: Treatment of asthma; delays premature labor.

Stimulation of dopamine receptors: Treatment of shock.

PRECAUTIONS

CONTRAINDICATIONS: Hyperthyroidism, hypertension, cardiovascular disease, narrow-angle glaucoma, Parkinson's disease, psychoneuroses, hypersensitivity. **CAUTIONS:** Diabetes mellitus, urinary tract obstructions, elderly, debilitated, infants and children. See individual monograph for pregnancy, lactation precautions.

SYMPATHOMIMETICS

GENERIC NAME	BRAND NAME(S)	RECEPTOR SPECIFICITY	PRIMARY CLINICAL USE
albuterol	Proventil Ventolin	Beta₂	Bronchodilator
bitolterol	Tornalate	Beta₂	Bronchodilator
dobutamine	Dobutrex	Beta₁ Beta₂ Alpha₁	Inotropic support in pts w/cardiac decompensation
dopamine	Intropin	Beta₁ Alpha₁ Dopaminergic	Cardiogenic, septic shock Pressor agent
epinephrine	Adrenalin Sus-phrine	Beta₁ Beta₂ Alpha₁	Allergic reaction Bronchodilator Local vasoconstriction (w/anesthetics)
isoetharine	Bronkosol	Beta₂	Bronchodilator
isoproterenol	Isuprel	Beta₁ Beta₂	Heart rate stimulator in bradycardia, heart block Vasopressor in shock Bronchodilator
metaproterenol	Alupent	Beta₂	Bronchodilator
metaraminol	Aramine	Beta₁ Alpha₁	Pressor in acute hypotensive states
norepinephrine	Levophed	Beta₁ Alpha₁	Pressor in acute hypotensive states
phenylephrine	Neo-synephrine	Alpha₁	Arterial vasoconstrictor Nasal decongestant Mydriatic
ritodrine	Yutopar	Beta₂	Arrest premature labor
terbutaline	Brethine Bricanyl	Beta₂	Bronchodilator

CLASSIFICATION

INTERACTIONS

Monoamine oxidase (MAO) inhibitors are contraindicated; in combination w/adrenergics, potentiated effects can cause hypertensive crisis, intracranial hemorrhage, and death. Effects of MAO inhibitors may last 3 wks after discontinuation. General anesthetics may increase risk of arrhythmias. Tricyclic antidepressants, maprotiline may increase cardiovascular effects. Norepinephrine may decrease effect of methyldopa. May have mutually inhibitory effects w/beta-adrenergic blockers. May increase risk of arrhythmias w/digoxin. Ergonovine, oxytocin may increase vasoconstriction. Numerous agents interact with adrenergics; review each monograph individually.

SIDE EFFECTS

Palpitations, nervousness, restlessness, sweating, difficulty urinating, headache.

TOXIC EFFECTS/ADVERSE REACTIONS

Nausea and vomiting, tachycardia, pale/cold skin, difficulty breathing, significant increase or decrease in B/P. *Rare:* Chest pain and irregular heartbeat.

NURSING IMPLICATIONS

GENERAL: Immediately obtain IV access in cardiac arrest or other emergency. When infusions indicated, pt should be in intensive care unit w/cardiac monitor. Infuse titrate carefully; use infusion pumps for accurate delivery. INTERVENTION/EVALUATION: Monitor vital signs frequently, blood gases, electrolytes, renal and hepatic function results. Assess multiorgan response. PATIENT/FAMILY TEACHING: Measures to prevent recurrence when given for asthma, COPD such as avoidance of respiratory infection, prevention of allergen exposure, increased hydration.

thyroid

ACTION

Thyroid hormone (T_4 [thyroxine] and T_3 [triiodothyroxine]) are essential for normal growth, development, and energy metabolism. *Promotes growth/development:* Controls DNA transcription and protein synthesis. Necessary in development of nervous system. *Stimulates energy use:* Increases basal metabolic rate (increases O_2 consumption, heat production). *Cardiovascular:* Stimulates heart by increased rate, force of contraction, cardiac output.

USES

Treatment of primary or secondary hypothyroidism, myxedema, cretinism, or simple goiter.

PRECAUTIONS

CONTRAINDICATIONS: Hyperthyroidism, myocardial infarction, thyrotoxicosis, nephrosis, hypoadrenalism. **CAUTIONS:** Use with care in pts who have hypertension, cardiac disease, renal insufficiency, diabetes mellitus, or are on anticoagulant therapy.

THYROID

Generic Name	Brand Name(s)	T_4:T_3 Ratio	Dosage Equivalent
levothyroxine	Synthroid	T_4 only	50–60 mcg
liothyronine	Cytomel	T_3 only	15–37.7 mcg
liotrix	Thyrolar	4:1	50–60 mcg T_4 12.5–15 mcg T_3
thyroid	Thyroid	2.5:1	65 mg

INTERACTIONS

May alter oral anticoagulant effects. Cholestyramine, colestipol may decrease absorption. Sympathomimetics may increase effects, coronary insufficiency.

SIDE EFFECTS

Most reactions are due to excessive dosage w/signs, symptoms of hyperthyroidism: weight loss, palpitations, increased appetite, tremors, nervousness, tachycardia, increased B/P, headache, insomnia, menstrual irregularities.

TOXIC EFFECTS/ADVERSE REACTIONS

Hypersensitivity reactions; cardiac arrhythmias, possibly death due to cardiac failure.

NURSING IMPLICATIONS

Children need very close monitoring; dosage needs to be higher for growing child. BASELINE ASSESSMENT: Check B/P and pulse, weight. INTERVENTION/EVALUATION: Monitor pulse for rate, rhythm; notify physician of pulse above 100/min or irregular. Check weight daily; assess food intake. Observe for tremors, nervousness, insomnia. PATIENT/FAMILY TEACHING: Do not stop taking medication; generally lifelong therapy. Take medication at the same time each day, preferably in the morning. Teach correct method of taking pulse; check pulse before taking medication, esp. when dosage adjusted. Notify physician of resting pulse that is markedly increased, irregular, 100/min or above. Important to remain under medical supervision, have periodic lab tests. Children may have reversible hair loss, increased aggressiveness during first few months of therapy. Do not take other medications w/o consulting physician. Notify physician promptly of chest pain, weight loss, tremors, insomnia.

CLASSIFICATION

vitamins

Vitamins are organic substances required for growth, reproduction, and maintaining health and are obtained from food or supplementation in small quantities (vitamins cannot be synthesized by the body or the rate of synthesis is too slow/inadequate to meet metabolic needs). Vitamins are essential for energy transformation and regulation of metabolic processes. They are catalysts for all reactions using proteins, fats, carbohydrates for energy, growth, and cell maintenance.

Vitamins are divided into two major groups: water soluble and fat soluble. Water-soluble vitamins include vitamin C (ascorbic acid), B-1 (thiamine), B-2 (riboflavin), niacin, B-6 (pyridoxine), folic acid, B-12 (cyanocobalamin). Water-soluble vitamins act as co-enzymes for almost every cellular reaction in the body. B-complex vitamins differ from one another in both structure and function but are grouped together because they first were isolated from the same source (yeast and liver). Fat-soluble vitamins include vitamin A, D, E, and K. They are soluble in lipids and are usually absorbed into the lymphatic system of the small intestine and then into the general circulation. Absorption is facilitated by bile. These vitamins are stored in the body tissue when excessive quantities are consumed. May be toxic when taken in large doses (see sections on individual vitamins).

WATER-SOLUBLE VITAMINS

ASCORBIC ACID (VITAMIN C)

Function: Co-factor in a number of reactions by transferring electrons to enzymes that provide reducing equivalents (collagen synthesis, conversion of folic acid to folinic acid, microsomal drug metabolism); promotes absorption of iron. At tissue level, required for collagen production, other compounds that compose the intercellular matrix that binds cells together.
Symptoms of Deficiency: Scurvy: loosening of teeth, gingivitis, anemia, poor wound healing, hemorrhage into muscle/joints, ecchymosis, faulty bone/teeth development, malaise, weakness.
Food Source: Citrus fruits and juices (esp. orange and lemon), tomatoes, potatoes, strawberries, cabbage greens, green/red peppers, broccoli, spinach.

THIAMINE (VITAMIN B-1)

Function: Co-enzyme for metabolism of carbohydrate, important biochemical conversion cycles.
Symptoms of Deficiency: Nervous system (dry beriberi): peripheral neuritis, gradual loss of muscle strength, personality disturbances, depression, lack of initiative, poor memory, wrist-foot drop. Cardiovascular (wet beriberi): dyspnea on exertion, palpitations, tachycardia, abnormal EKG, high output cardiac failure, fluid accumulation in legs.
Food Source: Pork, peanuts, asparagus, whole grain cereal, beef, beans, fresh peas.

RIBOFLAVIN (VITAMIN B-2)

Function: Consists of two co-enzymes that are involved in the metabolism of a wide variety of respiratory flavoproteins.
Symptoms of Deficiency: Sore throat, angular stomatitis (cracks in skin at corners of mouth), glossitis, cheilosis (red denuded lips), seborrheic dermatitis of face, dermatitis over trunk/extremities, anemia, neuropathy,

corneal vasculization, cataract formation, eyes become light sensitive, easily fatigued, blurred vision, itching.

Food Sources: Meats, chicken, eggs, milk, fish, grain, cereal, broccoli, asparagus, spinach.

NIACIN (NICOTINIC ACID)

Function: Active form of niacin is nicotinic acid, a constituent of co-enzymes NAD and NADP, which are vital in metabolism for a wide variety of proteins that catalyze oxidation-reduction reactions essential for tissue respiration.

Symptoms of Deficiency: Pellagra. Symptoms include dermatitis (erythematous eruptions similar to sunburn appearing on back of hands then forehead, feet, and head), digestive tract (stomatitis, enteritis, diarrhea), and CNS (headache, dizziness, insomnia, depression, impaired memory, delusions, hallucinations, dementia).

Food Source: Liver, chicken, yeast, peanuts, cereal bran, fish, cold cereals, whole grains, green vegetables.

PYRIDOXINE (VITAMIN B-6)

Function: Co-enzyme (active form pyridoxal phosphate) in metabolism of amino acids and proteins. A co-factor for more than 60 enzymes.

Symptoms of Deficiency: Skin: seborrheic-like skin lesions about the eyes, nose, mouth with glossitis and stomatitis. Nervous system: convulsive seizures, peripheral neuritis, dulling of mentation.

Food Source: Milk, soybeans, whole grain cereals, meats, bananas, avocados, potatoes, nuts, lentils.

FOLIC ACID

Function: Co-enzyme with important role in synthesis of purine and pyrimidine bases in RNA and DNA; maintenance of normal levels of mature red cells.

Symptoms of Deficiency: Megaloblastic anemia, glossitis, diarrhea, poor growth, frequent infections, depression, mental confusion, irritability, forgetfulness.

Food Source: Green leafy vegetables, liver, lean beef, fish, legumes, whole grains, veal, eggs.

CYANOCOBALAMIN (VITAMIN B-12)

Function: Active co-enzyme essential for cell growth and replication. Essential factor in synthesis of DNA. Involved in fat, protein, carbohydrate metabolism. Primarily active in bone marrow, CNS, and GI tract.

Symptoms of Deficiency: Pernicious or megaloblastic anemia, peripheral neuropathy (tingling/numbness of hands/feet), unsteadiness, decreased deep tendon reflexes, confusion, moodiness, loss of memory, loss of central vision, delusions, hallucinations, glossitis, dementia, mental confusion.

Source: Primary source are certain microorganisms that synthesize B-12. Found in animal protein (meats, oysters, clams) and small amounts in root nodules of legumes and selected vegetables/fruit.

CLASSIFICATION

FAT-SOLUBLE VITAMINS

VITAMIN A (RETINOIDS/CAROTENOIDS)

Function: Essential role in the function of the retina. Necessary for growth and differentiation of epithelial tissue. Required for growth of bone, reproduction, and embryonic development. Enhances immune function, may protect against development of certain malignancies.

Symptoms of Deficiency: Skin lesion, night blindness, keratomalacia (desiccation, ulceration, xerosis of cornea), increased respiratory infections, keratinization and drying of epidermis, urinary calculi, impairment of spermatogenesis, degeneration of testes, abortion, diarrhea, impaired taste/smell/hearing.

Toxicity: Dry, pruritic skin, skin desquamation, dermatitis, loss of body hair, fissures of lips, pain/tenderness of bone, hyperostosis, throbbing headache, peripheral edema, fatigue, irritability, increased intracranial pressure, bulging fontanelles, brittle nails, night sweats, insomnia, restlessness.

Food Source: Liver, butter, cheese, whole milk, egg yolk, fish, yellow or green fruits/vegetables.

VITAMIN D (CALCIFEROL)

Function: Positive regulator of calcium and phosphate homeostasis (facilitates absorption by small intestine, interacts w/parathyroid to enhance mobilization from bone, decrease excretion by kidney). Necessary for proper formation of skeleton and mineral homeostasis.

Symptoms of Deficiency: Children: Rickets: failure to mineralize newly formed bone and cartilage matrix causing a defect in growing, weight bearing causing deformities. *Adults:* Osteomalacia: extreme bone pain/tenderness, muscle weakness.

Toxicity: Anorexia, nausea, vomiting, diarrhea, polyuria, muscle weakness, headache, irreversible renal failure, soft tissue calcification, hypercalcemia, weight loss, hypertension, constipation, vague aches/stiffness.

Food Source: Milk, margarine, liver, butter, egg yolk. Synthesized in skin from endogenous or dietary cholesterol on exposure to sunlight.

VITAMIN E (TOCOPHEROL)

Function: Antioxidant (may protect essential cell components from oxidation); protects red blood cells from hemolysis. High dose *may* protect against heart disease.

Symptoms of Deficiency: Red blood cell hemolysis, abnormal fat deposits; may cause hemolytic anemia in infants (edema, reticulocytosis, thrombocytosis).

Toxicity: May cause increased serum lipids and cholesterol, erythrocyte hemolysis.

Food Source: Fresh greens, vegetable oil, nuts, whole grains, margarine (made from plant oils), wheat germ.

VITAMIN K (MENADIONE, PHYTONADIONE)

Function: Necessary for synthesis of several factors required for clotting of blood: prothrombin, and factors VII, IX, X.

VITAMIN-DIETARY ALLOWANCES

AGE (YRS)	FAT SOLUBLE				C MG	WATER SOLUBLE					
	A MCG	D MCG	E MG	K MCG		B-1 MG	B-2 MG	Niacin MG	B-6 MG	Folic Acid MCG	B-12 MCG
0.0–0.5	375	7.5	3	5	30	0.3	0.4	5	0.3	25	0.3
0.5–1.0	375	10	4	10	35	0.4	0.5	6	0.6	35	0.5
1–3	400	10	6	15	40	0.7	0.8	9	1.0	50	0.7
4–6	500	10	7	20	45	0.9	1.1	12	1.1	75	1.0
7–10	700	10	7	30	45	1.0	1.2	13	1.4	100	1.4
MALES:											
11–14	1,000	10	10	45	50	1.3	1.5	17	1.7	150	2.0
15–18	1,000	10	10	65	60	1.5	1.8	20	2.0	200	2.0
19–24	1,000	10	10	70	60	1.5	1.7	19	2.0	200	2.0
25–50	1,000	5	10	80	60	1.5	1.7	19	2.0	200	2.0
51+	1,000	5	10	80	60	1.2	1.4	15	2.0	200	2.0
FEMALES:											
11–14	800	10	8	45	50	1.1	1.3	15	1.4	150	2.0
15–18	800	10	8	55	60	1.1	1.3	15	1.5	180	2.0
19–24	800	10	8	60	60	1.1	1.3	15	1.6	180	2.0
25–50	800	5	8	65	60	1.0	1.3	15	1.6	180	2.0
51+	800	5	8	65	60	1.0	1.2	13	1.6	180	2.0
PREGNANT	800	10	10	65	70	1.5	1.6	17	2.2	400	2.2
BREAST-FEEDING:											
1st 6 mos	1,300	10	12	65	95	1.6	1.8	20	2.1	280	2.6
2nd 6 mos	1,200	10	11	65	90	1.6	1.7	20	2.1	260	2.6

CLASSIFICATION

Symptoms of Deficiency: Increased tendency to bleed (ecchymosis, epistaxis, hematuria, GI bleeding, postop hemorrhage).

Toxicity: Hypersensitivity reaction: flushing, dyspnea, chest pain, cardiovascular collapse. Produces hemolytic anemia, hyperbilirubinemia, kernicterus in newborn.

Food Source: Green leafy vegetables, cauliflower, cabbage, egg yolk, liver.

Appendixes

Appendix A
THERAPEUTIC AND TOXIC BLOOD LEVELS

Note: 1 mg (milligram) = 1,000 mcg (microgram) = 1,000,000 ng (nanogram)

GENERIC NAME	BRAND NAME(S)	THERAPEUTIC LEVEL	TOXIC LEVEL
acetaminophen	Tylenol	10–30 mcg/ml	>200 mcg/ml
amikacin	Amikin	Peak: 15–30 mcg/ml	>30 mcg/ml
		Trough: 5–10 mcg/ml	>10 mcg/ml
amiodarone	Cordarone	1–2.5 mcg/ml	not established
amitriptylline	Elavil	120–250 ng/ml	>500 ng/ml
carbamazepine	Tegretol	4–12 mcg/ml	>12 mcg/ml
chloramphenicol	Chloromycetin	10–25 mcg/ml	>25 mcg/ml
chlordiazepoxide	Librium	1–3 mcg/ml	>5 mcg/ml
chlorpromazine	Thorazine	50–300 ng/ml	>750 ng/ml
clonazepam	Klonopin	10–80 ng/ml	>100 ng/ml
clonidine	Catapres	1–2 ng/ml	not established
clorazepate	Tranxene	0.12–1.5 mcg/ml	>5 mcg/ml
cyclosporine	Sandimmune	100–400 ng/ml	>400 ng/ml
desipramine	Norpramin	50–300 ng/ml	>400 ng/ml
diazepam	Valium	0.5–2 mcg/ml	>3 mcg/ml
digoxin	Lanoxin	0.5–2 ng/ml	>2 ng/ml
disopyramide	Norpace	2–5 mcg/ml	>5 mcg/ml
doxepine	Sinequan	30–250 ng/ml	>300 ng/ml
ethosuximide	Zarontin	40–100 mcg/ml	>100 mcg/ml
flecainide	Tambocor	0.2–1 mcg/ml	>1 mcg/ml
flurazepam	Dalmane	30–120 ng/ml	>500 ng/ml
gentamicin	Garamycin	Peak: 4–10 mcg/ml	>10 mcg/ml
		Trough: 1–2 mcg/ml	>2 mcg/ml
haloperidol	Haldol	3–20 ng/ml	>20 ng/ml
imipramine	Tofranil	125–300 ng/ml	>500 ng/ml
lidocaine	Xylocaine	1.5–5 mcg/ml	>5 mcg/ml
lithium	Lithane	0.5–1.3 mEq/L	>1.5 mEq/L
lorazepam	Ativan	50–240 ng/ml	not established
meperidine	Demerol	100–550 ng/ml	>1,000 ng/ml
N-acetylprocainamide		5–30 mcg/ml	>30 mcg/ml
netilmicin	Netromycin	Peak: 6–12 mcg/ml	>12 mcg/ml
		Trough: 0.5–2 mcg/ml	>2 mcg/ml
nortriptyline	Pamelor	50–140 ng/ml	>300 ng/ml
oxazepam	Serax	0.2–1.4 mcg/ml	not established
phenobarbital	Luminal	15–40 mcg/ml	>40 mcg/ml
phenytoin	Dilantin	10–20 mcg/ml	>20 mcg/ml
primidone	Mysoline	5–12 mcg/ml	>12 mcg/ml
procainamide	Procan	4–10 mcg/ml	>10 mcg/ml

GENERIC NAME	BRAND NAME(S)	THERAPEUTIC LEVEL	TOXIC LEVEL
propoxyphene	Darvon	100–400 ng/ml	>500 ng/ml
quinidine		2–5 mcg/ml	>5 mcg/ml
salicylates		50–300 mcg/ml	>300 mcg/ml
secobarbital	Seconal	1–5 mcg/ml	>5 mcg/ml
theophylline	Theo-Dur	8–20 mcg/ml	>20 mcg/ml
thioridazine	Mellaril	0.2–2.6 mcg/ml	not established
tobramycin	Nebcin	Peak: 4–10 mcg/ml	>10 mcg/ml
		Trough: 1–2 mcg/ml	>2 mcg/ml
tocainide	Tambocor	4–10 mcg/ml	not established
valproic acid	Depakote	50–100 mcg/ml	>100 mcg/ml
vancomycin	Vancocin	Peak: 25–40 mcg/ml	>40 mcg/ml
		Trough: 5–10 mcg/ml	>10 mcg/ml
verapamil	Calan/Isoptin	100–600 ng/ml	not established

Appendix B
CALCULATION OF DOSES

Frequently, dosages ordered do not correspond exactly to what is available and must therefore be calculated.

Ratio/proportions: Most important in setting up this calculation is that the units of measure are the same on both sides of the equation.

Problem: Pt A is to receive 65 mg of a medication only available in an 80 mg/2 ml vial. What volume (ml) needs to be administered to the pt?

STEP 1: Set up ratio.

$$\frac{80}{2\ ml} = \frac{65}{x(ml)}$$

STEP 2: Cross multiply.

$$(80\ mg)(x\ ml) = (65\ mg)(2\ ml)$$
$$80\ x = 130$$

STEP 3: Divide each side of equation by number with x.

$$\frac{80\ x}{80} = \frac{130}{80}$$

STEP 4: Volume to be administered for correct dose.

$$x = 130/80\ or\ 1.625\ ml$$

Calculations in micrograms/kilogram per minute: Frequently, medications given by IV infusion are ordered as micrograms/kilogram per minute.

Problem: 63-year-old pt (weight 165 lbs) is to receive Medication A at a rate of 8 micrograms/kilogram per minute (mcg/kg/min). Given a solution containing Medication A in a concentration of 500 mg/250 ml, at what rate (ml/hr) would you infuse this medication?

STEP 1: Convert to same units. In this problem, the dose is expressed in mcg/kg; therefore convert pt weight to kg (1 kg = 2.2 lbs) and drug concentration to mcg (1 mg = 1,000 mcg).

$$165\ lbs \times \frac{1\ kg}{2.2\ lbs} = \frac{165\ kg}{2.2} = 75\ kg$$

$$\frac{500\ mg}{250\ ml}\ or\ \frac{2\ mg}{ml} \times \frac{1,000\ mcg}{1\ mg} = \frac{2,000\ mcg}{1\ ml}\ or\ \frac{1\ ml}{2,000\ mcg}$$

STEP 2: Number of micrograms per minute (ml/min).

$$\frac{8\ \text{mcg}}{\text{kg}} \times 75\ \text{kg(pt wt)} = \frac{600\ \text{mcg}}{1\ \text{min}} \quad \text{or} \quad \frac{1\ \text{min}}{600\ \text{mcg}}$$

STEP 3: Number of milliliters per minute (ml/min).

$$\frac{600\ \text{mcg}}{1\ \text{min}} \times \frac{1\ \text{ml}}{2{,}000\ \text{mcg}} = \frac{600\text{(ml)}}{2{,}000\text{(min)}} = \frac{0.3\ \text{ml}}{\text{min}}$$

STEP 4: Number of milliliters per hour (ml/hr).

$$\frac{0.3\ \text{ml}}{\text{min}} \times \frac{60\ \text{min}}{1\ \text{hr}} = \frac{18\ \text{ml}}{\text{hr}}$$

STEP 5: If the number of drops per minute (gtts/min) were desired, and if the IV set delivered 60 drops per milliliter (gtts/ml) (varies with IV set, information provided by manufacturer), then:

$$\frac{0.3\ \text{ml}}{\text{min}} \times \frac{60\ \text{drops}}{\text{ml}} = \frac{18\ \text{drops}}{\text{min}}$$

Appendix C
CONTROLLED DRUGS (United States)

Schedule I: Medications having no legal medical use. These substances may be used for research purposes with proper registration (e.g., heroin, LSD).

Schedule II: Medications having a legitimate medical use but are characterized by a very high abuse potential and/or potential for severe physical and psychic dependency. Emergency telephone orders for limited quantities of these drugs are authorized, but the prescriber must provide a written, signed prescription order (e.g., morphine, amphetamines).

Schedule III: Medications having significant abuse potential (less than Schedule II). Telephone orders are permitted (e.g., opiates in combination with other substances such as acetaminophen).

Schedule IV: Medications having a low abuse potential. Telephone orders are permitted (e.g., benzodiazepines, propoxyphene).

Schedule V: Medications having the lowest abuse potential of the controlled substances. Some Schedule V products may be available without a prescription (e.g., certain cough preparations containing limited amounts of an opiate).

Appendix D
NORMAL LABORATORY VALUES

HEMATOLOGY/COAGULATION

TEST	SPECIMEN	NORMAL RANGE
Activated partial thromboplastin time (APTT)	Whole blood	25–35 secs
Erythrocyte count (RBC count)	Whole blood	M: 4.3–5.7 million cells/mm^3 F: 3.8–5.1 million cells/mm^3
Hematocrit (HCT, Hct)	Whole blood	M: 39–49% F: 35–45%
Hemoglobin (Hb, Hgb)	Whole blood	M: 13.5–17.5 g/dl F: 12.0–16.0 g/dl
Leucocyte count (WBC count)	Whole blood	4.5–11.0 thousand cells/mm^3
Leucocyte differential count	Whole blood	
Basophils		0–0.75%
Eosinophils		1–3%
Lymphocytes		23–33%
Monocytes		3–7%
Neutrophils—bands		3–5%
Neutrophils—segmented		54–62%
Mean corpuscular hemoglobin (MCH)	Whole blood	26–34 pg/cell
Mean corpuscular hemoglobin concentration (MCHC)	Whole blood	31–37% Hb/cell
Mean corpuscular volume (MCV)	Whole blood	80–100 fL
Partial thromboplastin time (PTT)	Whole blood	60–85 secs
Platelet count (thrombocyte count)	Whole blood	150–450 thousand/mm^3
Prothrombin time (PT)	Whole blood	11–13.5 secs
RBC count (see Erythrocyte count)		

SERUM/URINE VALUES

TEST	SPECIMEN	NORMAL RANGE
Alanine aminotransferase (ALT, SGPT)	Serum	0–55 units/L
Albumin	Serum	3.5–5 g/dl
Alkaline phosphatase	Serum	M: 53–128 units/L F: 42–98 units/L
Anion gap	Plasma or serum	5–14 mEq/L
Aspartate aminotransferase (AST, SGOT)	Serum	0–50 units/L

continued

APPENDIX

TEST	SPECIMEN	NORMAL RANGE
Bilirubin (conjugated direct)	Serum	0–0.4 mg/dl
Bilirubin (total)	Serum	0.2–1.2 mg/dl
Calcium (total)	Serum	8.4–10.2 mg/dl
Carbon dioxide (CO_2) total	Plasma or serum	20–34 mEq/L
Chloride	Plasma or serum	96–112 mEq/L
Cholesterol (total)	Plasma or serum	<200 mg/dl
C-Reactive protein	Serum	68–8200 ng/ml
Creatine kinase (CK)	Serum	M: 38–174 units/L
		F: 26–140 units/L
Creatine kinase isoenzymes	Serum	Fraction of total: <0.04–0.06
Creatinine	Plasma or serum	M: 0.7–1.3 mg/dl
		F: 0.6–1.1 mg/dl
Creatinine clearance	Plasma or serum and urine	M: 90–139 ml/min/1.73m²
		F: 80–125 ml/min/1.73m²
Free thyroxine index (FTI)	Serum	1.1–4.8
Glucose	Serum	Adults: 70–105 mg/dl
		>60 yrs: 80–115 mg/dl
Hemoglobin A_{1c}	Whole blood	5.6–7.5% of total Hgb
Homovanillic acid (HVA)	Urine, 24 hr	1.4–8.8 mg/day
17-Hydroxycorticosteroids (17-OHCS)	Urine, 24 hr	M: 3–10 mg/day
		F: 2–8 mg/day
Iron	Serum	M: 65–175 mcg/dl
		F: 50–170 mcg/dl
Iron binding capacity, total (TIBC)	Serum	250–450 mcg/dl
Lactate dehydrogenase (LDH)	Serum	0–250 units/L
Magnesium	Serum	1.3–2.3 mg/dl
Oxygen (PO_2)	Whole blood, arterial	83–100 mm Hg
Oxygen saturation	Whole blood, arterial	95–98%
pH	Whole blood, arterial	7.35–7.45
Phosphorus, inorganic	Serum	2.7–4.5 mg/dl
Potassium	Serum	3.5–5.1 mEq/L
Protein (total)	Serum	6–8.5 g/dl
Sodium	Plasma or serum	136–146 mEq/L
Specific gravity	Urine	1.002–1.030
Thyrotropin (hTSH)	Plasma or serum	2–10 mcgU/ml
Thyroxine (T_4) total	Serum	5–12 mcg/dl
Triglycerides (TG)	Serum, after 12 hr fast	20–190 mg/dl
Triiodothyronine resin uptake test (T_3RU)	Serum	22–37%
Urea nitrogen	Plasma or serum	7–25 mg/dl
Urea nitrogen/creatinine ratio	Serum	12/1–20/1
Uric acid	Serum	M: 3.5–7.2 mg/dl
		F: 2.6–6 mg/dl
Vanillylmandelic acid (VMA)	Urine, 24 hr	2–7 mg/day

Appendix E
FDA PREGNANCY CATEGORIES

Note: Medications should be used during pregnancy only if clearly needed.

A: Adequate and well-controlled studies have failed to show a risk to the fetus in the first trimester of pregnancy (also, no evidence of risk has been seen in later trimesters).

B: Animal reproduction studies have failed to show a risk to the fetus, and there are no adequate/well-controlled studies in pregnant women.

C: Animal reproduction studies have shown an adverse effect on the fetus, and there are no adequate/well-controlled studies in humans. However, the benefits may warrant use of the drug in pregnant women despite potential risks.

D: There is positive evidence of human fetal risk based on data from investigational or marketing experience or from studies in humans, but the potential benefits may warrant use of the drug despite potential risks (e.g., use in life-threatening situations in which other medications cannot be used or are ineffective).

X: Animal or human studies have shown fetal abnormalities, and/or there is evidence of human fetal risk based on adverse reaction data from investigational or marketing experience where the risks in using the medication clearly outweigh potential benefits.

Appendix F

SIGNS AND SYMPTOMS OF TOXIC EFFECTS/ADVERSE REACTIONS

HYPOGLYCEMIA (excessive insulin):
Tremulousness, cold/clammy skin, mental confusion, rapid/shallow respirations, unusual fatigue, hunger, drowsiness, anxiety, headache, muscular incoordination, paresthesia of tongue/mouth/lips, hallucinations, increased pulse/blood pressure, tachycardia, seizures, coma.

HYPERGLYCEMIA (insufficient insulin):
Hot/flushed/dry skin, fruity breath odor, excessive urination (polyuria), excessive thirst (polydipsia), acute fatigue, air hunger, deep/labored respirations, mental changes, restlessness, nausea, polyphagia (excessive appetite).

HYPOKALEMIA (serum potassium level <3.5 mEq/L):
Weakness/paresthesia of extremities, muscle cramps, nausea, vomiting, diarrhea, hypoactive bowel sounds, absent bowel sounds (paralytic ileus), abdominal distention, weak/irregular pulse, postural hypotension, difficulty breathing, disorientation, irritability.

HYPERKALEMIA (serum potassium level >5.0 mEq/L):
Diarrhea, muscle weakness, heaviness of legs, paresthesia of tongue/hands/feet, slow/irregular pulse, decreased blood pressure, abdominal cramps, oliguria/anuria, respiratory difficulty, cardiac abnormalities.

HYPONATREMIA (plasma Na level <130 mEq/L):
Abdominal cramping, nausea, vomiting, diarrhea, cold/clammy skin, poor skin turgor, tremulousness, muscle weakness, leg cramps, increased pulse rate, irritability, apprehension, hypotension, headache.

HYPERNATREMIA (plasma Na level >150 mEq/L):
Hot/flushed/dry skin, dry mucous membranes, fever, extreme thirst, dry/rough/red tongue, edema, restlessness, postural hypotension, oliguria.

DEHYDRATION:
Poor skin turgor, dry mucous membranes, thirst, flushed/dry skin, sunken eye sockets/darkening of skin under eyes (adults), sunken fontanelle (infants), rapid respirations, increased pulse rate, longitudinal furrows in tongue, decreased blood pressure, postural hypotension, oliguria/anuria, urine specific gravity greater than 1.030.

SUPERINFECTION:
Fever, diarrhea, ulceration (white patches) on mucous membranes of mouth, inflammation of tongue (glossitis), black furry tongue, anogenital itching, vaginal itching/discharge.

STOMATITIS:
Redness/burning of oral mucous membranes, inflammation of gums (gingivitis), inflammation of tongue (glossitis), difficulty swallowing, ulceration of oral mucosa.

CONGESTIVE HEART FAILURE:
Dyspnea, cough, distended neck veins, fatigue with exertion, orthopnea, cool extremities, nail bed cyanosis, peripheral edema, weight gain, rales at base of lungs, wheezing, rust-colored/brown-tinged sputum.

BONE MARROW DEPRESSION (IMMUNOSUPPRESSION):
Fever, chills, sore throat, increased pulse rate, cloudy/foul smelling urine, urgency/burning/increased frequency of urination, white blood cells/bacteria in urine, redness/irritation of oral mucous membranes, redness/swelling/draining at injection sites/cuts, easy bruising/bleeding, perineal/rectal pain, vaginal/rectal discharge.

Appendix G

RATES OF INTERMITTENT IV (PIGGYBACK) ADMINISTRATION

GENERIC NAME	BRAND NAME(S)	COMPATIBILITY 0.9% NaCl	COMPATIBILITY 5% DEXTROSE	USUAL INFUSION TIME
acyclovir	Zovirax	Yes	Yes	At least 1 hr
amikacin	Amkin	Yes	Yes	Adults, children: 30–60 min Infants: 1–2 hrs
amphotericin	Fungizone	No	Yes	2–6 hrs
ampicillin	Polycillin	Yes	Yes	15–30 min
ampicillin/sulbactam	Unasyn	Yes	Yes	15–30 min
aztreonam	Azactam	Yes	Yes	20–60 min
cefamandole	Mandol	Yes	Yes	15–30 min
cefazolin	Ancef Kefzol	Yes	Yes	15–30 min
cefmetazole	Zefazone	Yes		10–60 min
cefonicid	Monocid	Yes	Yes	20–30 min
cefoperazone	Cefobid	Yes	Yes	15–30 min
cefotaxime	Claforan	Yes	Yes	20–30 min
cefotetan	Cefotan	Yes	Yes	20–30 min
cefoxitin	Mefoxin	Yes	Yes	15–30 min
ceftazidime	Fortaz Tazidime	Yes	Yes	15–30 min
ceftizoxime	Cefizox	Yes	Yes	15–30 min
ceftriaxone	Rocephin	Yes	Yes	Adults: 15–30 min Children: 10–30 min
cefuroxime	Zinacef	Yes	Yes	15–60 min
cephalothin	Keflin	Yes	Yes	15–30 min
chloramphenicol	Chloromycetin	Yes	Yes	15–30 min
cimetidine	Tagamet	Yes	Yes	15–20 min
ciprofloxacin	Cipro	Yes	Yes	60 min
clindamycin	Cleocin	Yes	Yes	300–600 mg: 10–20 min 900 mg–1.2 g: 30–40 min
doxycycline	Vibramycin	Yes	Yes	1–4 hrs
erythromycin	Erythrocin	Yes	Yes	20–60 min
famotidine	Pepcid	Yes	Yes	15–30 min
fluconazole	Diflucan	—	Yes	200 mg/hr
gentamicin	Garamycin	Yes	Yes	30–120 min
glanciclovir	Cytovene	Yes	Yes	1 hr
granisetron	Kytril	Yes	Yes	5 min
hydrocortisone	Solu-Cortef	Yes	Yes	15–30 min
imipenem cilastatin	Primaxin	Yes	Yes	250–500 mg: 20–30 min 1 g: 40–60 min

GENERIC NAME	BRAND NAME(S)	COMPATIBILITY		USUAL INFUSION TIME
		0.9% NaCl	5% Dextrose	
methicillin	Staphcillin	Yes	Yes	30–120 min
methylprednisolone	Solu-Medrol	Yes	Yes	15–30 min
metoclopramide	Reglan	Yes	Yes	15–30 min
metronidazole	Flagyl	Yes	Yes	30 min
mezlocillin	Mezlin	Yes	Yes	30 min
miconazole	Monistat IV	Yes	Yes	30–60 min
minocycline	Minocin	Yes	Yes	6 hrs
nafcillin	Nafcil Unipen	Yes	Yes	30–60 min
netilmicin	Netromycin	Yes	Yes	30–120 min
ofloxacin	Floxin	Yes	Yes	60 min
ondansetron	Zofran	Yes	Yes	15 min
penicillin G	Pfizerpen	Yes	Yes	Adults: 1–2 hrs Children: 15–30 min
pentamidine	PentAM 300	Yes	Yes	At least 1 hour
piperacillin	Pipracil	Yes	Yes	30 min
piperacillin/ tazobactam	Zosyn	Yes	Yes	30 min
ranitidine	Zantac	Yes	Yes	15–20 min
rifampin	Rifadin	Yes	Yes	100 mg/30 min 500 mg/3 hrs
ticarcillin	Ticar	Yes	Yes	Adults: 30–120 min Neonates: 10–20 min
ticarcillin/clavulanate	Timentin	Yes	Yes	30 min
tobramycin	Nebcin	Yes	Yes	20–60 min
trimethoprim/ sulfamethoxazole	Bactrim, Septra	No	Yes	60–90 min
vancomycin	Vancocin	Yes	Yes	At least 1 h
vidarabine	Vira-A	Yes	Yes	12–24 hrs
zidovudine	Retrovir	—	Yes	Over 60 min

Note: Compatibility information of medications to large-volume parenterals or admixture with other medications is beyond the scope of this chart. Refer inquiries to the Pharmacy Department or Drug Information Centers.

APPENDIX

Appendix H
THE PRESCRIPTION

The prescription should be written legibly and in ink with only one prescription per order blank. Medications are prescribed by either generic name or brand name and should always use the metric system when designating the amount, strength, and/or volume.

A prescription follows a definite pattern. These are the major components:

1. Date: Date when the prescription is written (controlled drugs have federal law stipulating how long after issuing the prescription it can be filled).
2. Name, address, age of patient: Avoids possible confusion w/medications intended for someone else and enables the pharmacist to monitor the dose.
3. Rx: latin symbol for "take thou."
4. Medication: Name, strength (dose): avoid abbreviations.
5. Directions for pharmacist: How many or how much to dispense.
6. Directions for the patient: Always write precisely the amount to be taken, the exact time of day and frequency of the dose, route of administration. Directions should also include a reminder as to the intended purpose of the medication (e.g., "for relief of pain" or "for control of blood pressure"). Avoid terms such as "take as directed" or "take as necessary."
7. Refills: The number of refills should be indicated. Do not use "refill as needed."
8. Signature: Sign the bottom of the prescription with appropriate professional degree.

Sample Prescriptions:

June 1, 1997

John Doe, Age 7
817 Woodhaven Dr
Sumwear, FL 33333

Rx	Amoxicillin Oral Suspension 250 mg/5 ml
	Dispense 150 ml
Sig:	Take 5 ml orally at 7 AM, 3 PM, and 9 PM daily for 10 days for infection.

Do not refill

Prescriber

Prescriber's Address

Appendix I
DIALYSIS OF MEDICATIONS

Medication removal by dialysis is important because the extent of dialysis determines whether supplemental dosing of medication is needed during or following dialysis. The extent to which a medication is removed by dialysis depends on physical-chemical characteristics of the medications (e.g., size, protein binding, water solubility).

GENERIC NAME	BRAND NAME	REMOVED BY HEMODIALYSIS
Abciximab	ReoPro	—
Acarbose	Precose	—
Acebutolol	Sectral	Yes
Acetaminophen	Tylenol	Yes
Acetazolamide	Diamox	No
Acyclovir	Zovirax	Yes
Adenosine	Adenocard	—
Albuterol	Ventolin	No
Aldesleukin	Proleukin	—
Alendronate	Fosamax	—
Allopurinol	Zyloprim	Yes
Alprazolam	Xanax	No
Alteplase	Activase	No
Amantadine	Symmetrel	No
Amifostine	Ethyol	—
Amikacin	Amikin	Yes
Amiodarone	Cordarone	No
Amitriptyline	Elavil	No
Amlodipine	Norvasc	No
Amoxapine	Asendin	No
Amoxicillin	Polymox	Yes
Amphotericin	Fungizone	No
Amphotericin Lipid	—	No
Ampicillin	Polycillin	Yes
Anastrozole	Arimedex	—
Anistreplase	Eminase	No
Aprotinin	Trasylol	No
Asparaginase	Elspar	No
Aspirin	Ecotrin	Yes
Astemizole	Hismanal	No
Atenolol	Tenormin	Yes
Atovaquone	Mepron	No
Azathioprine	Imuran	Yes
Azithromycin	Zithromax	—
Aztreonam	Azactam	Yes

APPENDIX

continued

GENERIC NAME	BRAND NAME	REMOVED BY HEMODIALYSIS
Baclofen	Lioresal	—
Benazepril	Lotensin	No
Bepridil	Bepadin	No
Betaxolol	Kerlone	No
Bicalutamide	Casodex	No
Bisoprolol	Zebeta	No
Bleomycin	Blenoxane	No
Bretylium	Bretylol	Yes
Bumetanide	Bumex	No
Bupropion	Wellbutrin	No
Buspirone	BuSpar	No
Busulfan	Myleran	No
Butorphanol	Stadol	No
Cabidopa/levodopa	Sinemet	—
Captopril	Capoten	Yes
Carbamazepine	Tegretol	No
Carboplatin	Paraplatin	Yes
Carmustine	BiCNU	No
Carteolol	Cartrol	—
Carvedilol	Coreg	No
Cefaclor	Ceclor	Yes
Cefadroxil	Duricef	Yes
Cefazolin	Ancef	Yes
Cefepine	Maxipime	Yes
Cefixime	Suprax	No
Cefmetazole	Zefazone	Yes
Cefonicid	Monocid	No
Cefoperazone	Cefobid	No
Cefotaxime	Claforan	Yes
Cefoxitin	Mefoxin	Yes
Cefpodoxine	Vantin	Yes
Cefprozil	Cefzil	Yes
Ceftazidime	Fortaz	Yes
Ceftibuten	Cedax	Yes
Ceftizoxime	Cefizox	Yes
Ceftriaxone	Rocephin	No
Cefuroxime	Zinacef	Yes
Cephalexin	Keflex	Yes
Cetirizine	Zyrtec	No
Chlorambucil	Leukeran	No
Chloramphenicol	Chloromycetin	No
Chlordiazepoxide	Librium	No
Chorpromazine	Thorazine	No
Chlorpropamide	Diabinese	No
Chlorthalidone	Hygroton	No
Cidofovir	Vistide	—
Cilastatin	—	Yes

GENERIC NAME	BRAND NAME	REMOVED BY HEMODIALYSIS
Cimetidine	Tagamet	No
Ciprofloxacin	Cipro	No
Cisapride	Propulsid	No
Cisplatin	Platinol	Yes
Cladribine	Leustatin	—
Clarithromycin	Biaxin	No
Clavulanic acid	—	Yes
Clindamycin	Cleocin	No
Clonazepam	Klonopin	No
Clonidine	Catapres	No
Clorazepate	Tranxene	No
Cloxacillin	Tegopen	No
Clozapine	Clozaril	No
Codeine	—	No
Colchicine	—	No
Cortisone	Cortone	No
Cyclophosphamide	Cytoxan	Yes
Cyclosporine	Sandimmune	No
Cytarabine	Cytosar	—
Dacarbazine	DTIC	—
Dactinomycin	Cosmegen	No
Daunorubicin	Cerubidine	—
Deferoxamine	Desferal	Yes
Desipramine	Norpramin	No
Dexamethasone	Decadron	No
Dexrazoxane	Zinecard	—
Dezocine	Dalgan	—
Diazepam	Valium	No
Diclofenac	Voltaren	No
Dicloxacillin	Dynapen	No
Didanosine	Videx	Yes
Diflunisal	Dolobid	No
Digoxin	Lanoxin	No
Diltiazem	Cardizem	No
Diphenhydramine	Benadryl	No
Dipyridamole	Persantine	No
Dirithromycin	Dyanbac	No
Disopyramide	Norpace	Yes
Doxazosin	Cardura	No
Doxepin	Sinequan	No
Doxorubicin	Adriamycin	No
Doxycycline	Vibramycin	No
Dronabinol	Marinol	No
Enalapril	Vasotec	Yes
Enoxacin	Penetrex	No
Enoxaparin	Lovenox	No

continued

GENERIC NAME	BRAND NAME	REMOVED BY HEMODIALYSIS
Epoetin alfa	Epogen	No
Epoprostenol	Flolan	—
Erythromycin	Eryc-C	No
Esmolol	Brevibloc	Yes
Ethacrynic acid	Edecrin	No
Ethambutol	Myambutol	Yes
Ethinyl estradiol	Estinyl	—
Ethosuximide	Zarontin	Yes
Etodolac	Lodine	No
Etoposide	Vepesid	No
Famciclovir	Famvir	—
Famotidine	Pepcid	No
Felodipine	Plendil	No
Fenoprofen	Nalfon	No
Fentanyl	Duragesic	—
Filgrastim	Neupogen	No
Finasteride	Proscar	No
Flecainide	Tambocor	No
Floxuridine	FUDR	—
Fluconazole	Diflucan	Yes
Fludarabine	Fludara	—
Flumazenil	Romazicon	—
Fluorouracil	—	Yes
Fluoxetine	Prozac	No
Flurazepam	Dalmane	No
Fluriprofen	Ansaid	—
Flutamide	Eulexin	No
Fluvastatin	Lescol	No
Foscarnet	Foscavir	Yes
Fosinopril	Monopril	No
Furosemide	Lasix	No
Gabapentin	Neurontin	Yes
Gallium	Ganite	—
Ganciclovir	Cytovene	Yes
Gemfibrozil	Lopid	No
Gentamicin	Garamycin	Yes
Glimepiride	Amaryl	No
Glipizide	Glucotrol	No
Glyburide	Micronase/Diabeta	No
Granisetron	Kytril	—
Guanabenz	Wytensin	No
Guanadrel	Hylorel	—
Guanfacine	Tenex	No
Haloperidol	Haldol	No
Heparin	—	No

GENERIC NAME	BRAND NAME	REMOVED BY HEMODIALYSIS
Hydralazine	Apresoline	No
Hydrochlorothiazide	Hydrodiuril	No
Hydrocodone	Vicodin	—
Hydrocortisone	Cortef	No
Hydromorphone	Dilaudid	—
Hydroxyurea	Hydrea	—
Hydroxyzine	Vistaril	No
Ibuprofen	Motrin	No
Ibutilide	Corvert	—
Idarubicin	Idamycin	No
Imipenem	Primaxin	Yes
Imipramine	Tofranil	No
Indapamide	Lozol	No
Indinavir	Crixivan	—
Indomethacin	Indocin	No
Insulin	—	No
Interferons	—	No
Isoniazid	—	Yes
Isoproterenol	Isuprel	—
Isosorbide dinitrate	Isordil	No
Isosorbide mononitrate	ISMO	Yes
Isradipine	Dynacric	No
Itraconazole	Sporanex	No
Ketoconazole	Nizoral	No
Ketoprofen	Orudis	No
Ketorolac	Toradol	No
Labetalol	Trandate/Normodyne	No
Lamivudine	Epivir	—
Lamotrigine	Lamictal	No
Lansoprazole	Prevacid	No
Levamisole	Ergamsol	—
Levorphanol	Levo-Dromoran	—
Lidocaine	Xylocaine	No
Lisinopril	Prinivil/Zestril	Yes
Lithium	Lithane	Yes
Lomefloxacin	Maxaquin	No
Lomustine	CeeNU	No
Loperamide	Imodium	No
Loracarbef	Lorabid	Yes
Loratadine	Claritin	No
Lorazepam	Ativan	No
Losartan	Cozaar	No
Lovastatin	Mevacor	No
Loxapine	Loxitane	—

continued

APPENDIX

GENERIC NAME	BRAND NAME	REMOVED BY HEMODIALYSIS
Mannitol	—	Yes
Maprotiline	Ludiomil	No
Mechlorethamine	Mustargen	—
Melphalan	Alkeran	No
Meperidine	Demerol	No
Mercaptopurine	Purinethol	Yes
Meropenem	Merrem	Yes
Mesalamine	Asacol/Pentasa	No
Mesna	Mesnex	—
Mesoridazine	Serentil	No
Metaproterenol	Alupent	—
Metformin	Glucophage	Yes
Methadone	Dolophine	No
Methicillin	Staphcillin	No
Methotrexate	Folex	Yes
Methyldopa	Aldomet	Yes
Methylphenidate	Ritalin	No
Methylprednisolone	Medrol	Yes
Metoclopramide	Reglan	No
Metolazone	Zaroxolyn	No
Metoprolol	Lopressor	No
Metronidazole	Flagyl	Yes
Mexiletine	Mexitil	Yes
Mezlocillin	Mezlin	Yes
Miconazole	Monistat	No
Midazolam	Versed	No
Minocycline	Minocin	No
Minoxidil	Loniten	Yes
Misoprostol	Cytotec	No
Mitomycin	Mutamycin	—
Mitoxantrone	Novantrone	No
Moexipril	Univasc	—
Molindone	Moban	—
Moricizine	Ethmozine	No
Morphine	—	—
Muromonab-CD3	Orthoclone	No
Mycophenolate	CellCept	No
Nabumetone	Relafen	No
Nadolol	Corgard	Yes
Nafcillin	Unipen	No
Nalmefene	Revex	—
Naloxone	Narcan	—
Naproxen	Naprosyn	No
Netilmicin	Netromycin	Yes
Nevirapine	Virammune	—
Nicardipine	Cardene	No
Nicotinic acid	—	—

GENERIC NAME	BRAND NAME	REMOVED BY HEMODIALYSIS
Nifedipine	Adalat/Procardia	No
Nilutamide	Nilandron	—
Nimodipine	Nimotop	No
Nisoldipine	Sular	No
Nitrofurantoin	Macrodantin	Yes
Nitroglycerin	—	No
Nitroprusside	Nipride	Yes
Nizatidine	Axid	No
Norfloxacin	Noroxin	No
Nortriptyline	Pamelor	No
Octreotide	Sandostatin	—
Ofloxacin	Floxin	No
Olsalazine	Dipentum	No
Omeprazole	Prilosec	No
Ondansetron	Zofran	No
Oxacillin	Prostaphlin	No
Oxaprozin	DayPro	No
Oxazepam	Serax	No
Oxycodone	Roxicodone	—
Paclitaxel	Taxol	No
Pamidronate	Aredia	—
Paroxetine	Paxil	No
Pegaspargase	Oncaspar	No
Pemoline	Cylert	Yes
Penbutolol	Levatol	No
Penicillamine	Cuprimine	—
Penicillin G	Pentids	Yes
Pentamidine	Pentam-300	No
Pentazocine	Talwin	Yes
Pentostatin	Nipent	—
Pentoxifylline	Trental	No
Pergolide	Permax	No
Perphenazine	Trilafon	No
Phenobarbital	Luminal	Yes
Phenytoin	Dilantin	No
Pindolol	Visken	—
Piperacillin	Piperacil	Yes
Piroxicam	Feldene	No
Plicamycin	Mithracin	—
Pravastatin	Pravachol	—
Prazosin	Minipress	No
Prednisone	—	No
Primidone	Mysoline	Yes
Procainamide	Procan	Yes
Procarbazine	Matulane	—
Prochlorperazine	Compazine	No

continued

APPENDIX

GENERIC NAME	BRAND NAME	REMOVED BY HEMODIALYSIS
Promethazine	Phenergan	No
Propafenone	Rythmol	No
Propoxyphene	Darvon	No
Propranolol	Inderal	No
Protriptyline	Vivactil	No
Pseudoephedrine	Sudafed	No
Quazepam	Doral	No
Quinapril	Accupril	No
Quinidine	—	No
Quinine	—	Yes
Ramipril	Altace	Yes
Ranitidine	Zantac	No
Rifabutin	Mycobutin	No
Rifampin	Rifadin	No
Rimantidine	Flumadine	No
Risperidone	Risperdal	—
Ritonavir	Norvir	No
Roxatidine	Roxid	Yes
Salsalate	Disalcid	Yes
Sargramostim	Leukine	—
Selegiline	Eldepryl	—
Sertraline	Zoloft	No
Simvastatin	Zocor	No
Sotalol	Betapace	Yes
Spironolactone	Aldactone	No
Stavudine	Zerit	—
Streptomycin	—	Yes
Streptozocin	Zanosar	—
Sucralfate	Carafate	No
Sulbactam	—	Yes
Sulfamethoxazole	—	Yes
Sulindac	Clinoril	No
Sumatriptan	Imitrex	—
Tacrine	Cognex	No
Tacrolimus	Prograf	No
Tamoxifen	Nolvadex	—
Tazobactam	—	Yes
Temazepam	Restoril	No
Teniposide	Vumon	No
Terazosin	Hytrin	No
Terbutaline	Brethine	—
Terfenadine	Seldane	No
Theophylline	TheoDur	Yes
Thioguanine	—	—

GENERIC NAME	BRAND NAME	REMOVED BY HEMODIALYSIS
Thioridazine	Mellaril	No
Thiotepa	—	—
Thiothixene	Navane	No
Ticarcillin	Ticar	Yes
Ticlopidine	Ticlid	No
Timolol	Blocadren	No
Tobramycin	Nebcin	Yes
Tocainide	Tonocard	Yes
Tolazamide	Tolinase	No
Tolbutamide	Orinase	No
Tolmetin	Tolectin	No
Torsemide	Demedex	No
Tramadol	Ultram	No
Tranylcypromine	Parnate	—
Trazodone	Desyrel	No
Tretinoin	Vesanoid	—
Triamterene	Dyrenium	No
Triazolam	Halcion	No
Trifluoperazine	Stelazine	No
Trimethoprim	Trimpex	Yes
Trimetrexate	Neutrexin	No
Ursodiol	Actigall	No
Valacyclovir	Valtrex	Yes
Valproic acid	Depakote	No
Vancomycin	Vancocin	No
Venlafaxine	Effexor	No
Verapamil	Calan	No
Vinblastine	Velban	No
Vincristine	Oncovin	No
Warfarin	Coumadin	No
Zalcitabine	Hivid	—
Zidovudine	Retrovir	No
Zolpidem	Ambien	No

APPENDIX J
TECHNIQUES OF MEDICATION ADMINISTRATION

Ophthalmic:

EYE DROPS:

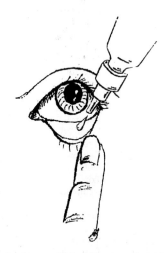

1. Wash hands.
2. Instruct patient to lie down or tilt head backward and look up.
3. Gently pull lower eyelid down until a pocket (pouch) is formed between eye and lower lid (conjunctival sac).
4. Hold dropper above pocket. Without touching tip of eye dropper to eyelid or conjunctival sac, place prescribed number of drops into the center pocket *(placing drops directly onto eye may cause a sudden squeezing of eyelid, with subsequent loss of solution)*. Continue to hold the eyelid for a moment after the drops are applied *(allows medication to distribute along entire conjunctival sac)*.
5. Instruct patient to close eyes gently so medication will not be squeezed out of sac.
6. Apply gentle finger pressure to the lacrimal sac at the inner canthus (bridge of the nose, inside corner of the eye) for 1–2 min *(promotes absorption, minimizes drainage into nose and throat, lessens risk of systemic absorption)*.
7. Remove excess solution around eye with a tissue.
8. Wash hands immediately to remove medication on hands. Never rinse eye dropper.

EYE OINTMENT:

1. Wash hands.
2. Instruct patient to lie down or tilt head backward and look up.

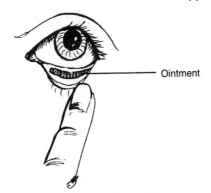

Ointment

3. Gently pull lower eyelid down until a pocket (pouch) is formed between eye and lower lid (conjunctival sac).
4. Hold applicator tube above pocket. Without touching the applicator
   tip to eyelid or conjunctival sac, place prescribed amount of ointment ($^1/_4$–$^1/_2$ inch) into the center pocket *(placing ointment directly
   onto eye may cause discomfort)*.
5. Instruct patient to close eye for 1–2 min, rolling eyeball in all directions *(increases contact area of drug to eye)*.
6. Inform patient of temporary blurring of vision. If possible, apply
   ointment just before bedtime.
7. Wash hands immediately to remove medication on hands. Never
   rinse tube applicator.

Otic:

1. Ear drops should be at body temperature (wrap hand around bottle
   to warm contents). *Body temperature instillation prevents startling of
   patient.*
2. Instruct patient to lie down with head turned so affected ear is upright *(allows medication to drip into ear)*.
3. Instill prescribed number of drops toward the canal wall, not directly
   on eardrum.

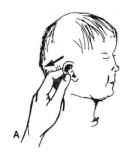

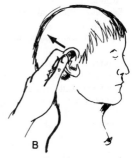

A

B

4. To promote correct placement of ear drops, pull the auricle down and posterior in children (A) and pull the auricle up and posterior in adults (B).

Nasal:

NOSE DROPS AND SPRAYS:

1. Instruct patient to blow nose to clear nasal passages as much as possible.
2. Tilt head slightly forward if instilling nasal spray, slightly backward if instilling nasal drops.
3. Insert spray tip into 1 nostril, pointing toward inflamed nasal passages, away from nasal septum.
4. Spray or drop medication into 1 nostril while holding other nostril closed and concurrently inspire through nose to permit medication as high into nasal passages as possible.
5. Discard unused nasal solution after 3 mos.

Inhalation:

AEROSOL (MULTIDOSE INHALERS):

1. Shake container well before each use.
2. Exhale slowly and as completely as possible through the mouth.
3. Place mouthpiece fully into mouth, holding inhaler upright, and close lips fully around mouthpiece.
4. Inhale deeply and slowly through the mouth while depressing the top of the canister with the middle finger.
5. Hold breath as long as possible before exhaling slowly and gently.
6. When two puffs are prescribed, wait 2 min and shake container again before inhaling a second puff *(allows for deeper bronchial penetration)*.
7. Rinse mouth w/water immediately after inhalation *(prevents mouth and throat dryness)*.

Sublingual:

1. Administer while seated.
2. Dissolve sublingual tablet under tongue (do not chew or swallow tablet).
3. Do not swallow saliva until tablet is dissolved.

Topical:

1. Gently cleanse area prior to application.
2. Use occlusive dressings only as ordered.
3. Without touching applicator tip to skin, apply sparingly; gently rub into area thoroughly unless ordered otherwise.

4. When using aerosol, spray area for 3 secs from 15 cm distance; avoid inhalation.

Transdermal:

1. Apply transdermal patch to clean, dry, hairless skin on upper arm or body (not below knee or elbow).
2. Rotate sites *(prevents skin irritation).*
3. Do not trim patch to adjust dose.

Rectal:

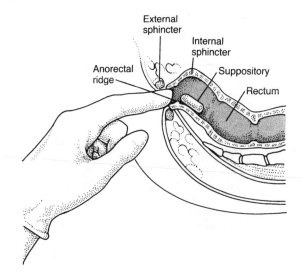

External sphincter

Internal sphincter

Anorectal ridge

Suppository

Rectum

1. Instruct patient to lie in left lateral Sims' position.
2. Moisten suppository with cold water or water-soluble lubricant.
3. Instruct patient to slowly exhale *(relaxes anal sphincter)* while inserting suppository well up into rectum.
4. Inform patient as to length of time (20–30 min) before desire for defecation occurs or <60 min for systemic absorption to occur, depending on purpose for suppository.

SubQ:

1. Use 25–27 gauge, $\frac{1}{2}$–$\frac{5}{8}$ inch needle; 1–3 ml. Angle of insertion depends on body size: 90° if patient is obese. If patient is very thin, gather the skin at the area of needle insertion and administer also

APPENDIX

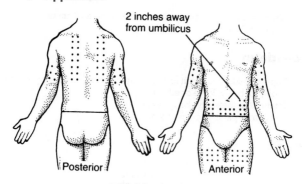

2 inches away
from umbilicus

Posterior

Anterior

SubQ injection sites

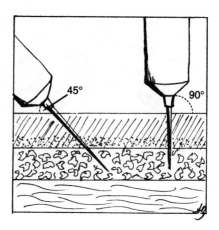

45°

90°

at a 90° angle. A 45° angle may be used in a patient with average weight.

2. Cleanse area to be injected with circular motion.
3. Avoid areas of bony prominence, major nerves, blood vessels.
4. Aspirate syringe before injecting *(to avoid intra-arterial administration),* except insulin, heparin.
5. Inject slowly; remove needle quickly.

IM:

INJECTION SITES:

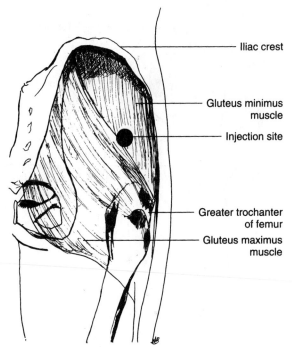

- Iliac crest
- Gluteus minimus muscle
- Injection site
- Greater trochanter of femur
- Gluteus maximus muscle

Dorsogluteal (upper outer quadrant)

1. Use this site if volume to be injected is 1–3 ml. Use 18–23 gauge, 1.25–3 in needle. Needle should be long enough to reach the middle of the muscle.
2. Do not use this site in children <2 yrs old or in those who are emaciated. Patient should be in prone position.
3. Using 90° angle, flatten the skin area using the middle and index finger and inject between them.

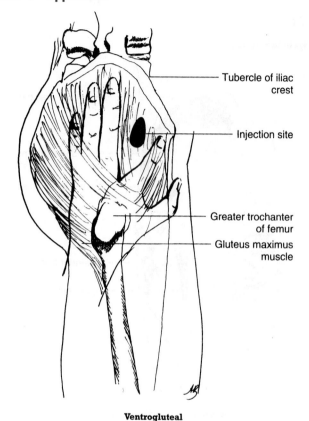

Tubercle of iliac
crest

Injection site

Greater trochanter
of femur

Gluteus maximus
muscle

Ventrogluteal

1. Use this site if volume to be injected is 1–5 ml. Use 20–23 gauge,
    1.25–2.5 in needle. Needle should be long enough to reach the mid-
    dle of the muscle.
2. Preferred site for adults, children >7 mos. Patient should be in
    supine lateral position.
3. Using 90° angle, flatten the skin area using the middle and index fin-
    ger and inject between them.

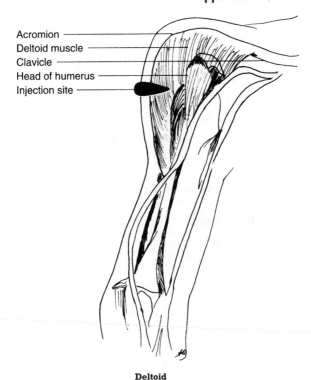

Acromion
Deltoid muscle
Clavicle
Head of humerus
Injection site

Deltoid

1. Use this site if volume to be injected is 0.5–1 ml. Use 23–25 gauge, $1/8$–$1\,1/2$ in needle. Needle should be long enough to reach the middle of the muscle.
2. Patient may be in prone, sitting, supine, or standing position.
3. Using 90° angle or angled slightly toward acromion, flatten the skin area using the thumb and index finger and inject between them.

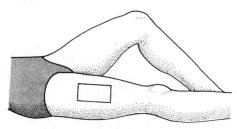

Anterolateral thigh

1. Anterolateral thigh is site of choice for infants and children <7 mos. Use 22–25 gauge, ⅝–1 in needle.
2. Patient may be in supine or sitting position. Using 90° angle, flatten the skin area using the thumb and index finger and inject between them.

Z-Track Technique:

1. Draw up medication with one needle, and use new needle for injection *(minimizes skin staining)*.
2. Administer deep IM in upper outer quadrant of buttock only (dorsogluteal site).
3. Displace the skin lateral to the injection site before inserting the needle.
4. Withdraw the needle before releasing the skin.

IV:

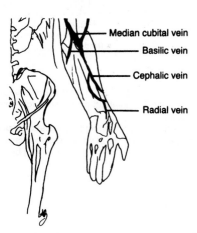

Median cubital vein
Basilic vein
Cephalic vein
Radial vein

1. Medication may be given as direct IV, intermittent (piggyback), or continuous infusion.
2. Ensure that medication is compatible with solution being infused (see IV compatibility chart in this drug handbook).

3. Do not use if precipitate is present or discoloration occurs.
4. Check IV site frequently for correct infusion rate, evidence of infiltration, extravasation.

INTRAVENOUS MEDICATIONS ARE ADMINISTERED BY THE FOLLOWING:

a. Continuous infusing solution.
b. Piggyback (intermittent infusion).
c. Volume control setup (medication contained in a chamber between the IV solution bag and the patient).
d. Bolus dose (a single dose of medication given through an infusion line or heparin lock). Sometimes this is referred to as an IV push.

ADDING MEDICATION TO A NEWLY PRESCRIBED IV BAG:

1. Remove the plastic cover from the IV bag.
2. Cleanse rubber port with an alcohol swab.
3. Insert the needle into the center of the rubber port.
4. Inject the medication.
5. Withdraw the syringe from the port.
6. Gently rotate the container to mix the solution.
7. Label the IV including the date, time, medication, and dosage. It should be placed so it is easily read when hanging.
8. Spike the IV tubing and prime the tubing.

HANGING AN IV PIGGYBACK (IVPB):

1. When using the piggyback method, lower the primary bag at least 6 inches below the piggyback bag.
2. Set the pump as a secondary infusion when entering the rate of infusion and volume to be infused.
3. Most piggyback medications contain 50–100 cc and usually infuse in 20 to 60 minutes, although larger-volume bags will take longer.

ADMINISTERING IV MEDICATIONS THROUGH A VOLUME CONTROL SETUP (BURETROL):

1. Insert the spike of the volume control set (Buretrol, Soluset, Pediatrol) into the primary solution container.
2. Open the upper clamp on the volume control set and allow sufficient fluid into volume control chamber.
3. Fill the volume control device with 30 cc of fluid by opening the clamp between the primary solution and the volume control device.

ADMINISTERING AN IV BOLUS DOSE:

1. If an existing IV is infusing, stop the infusion by pinching the tubing above the port.
2. Insert the needle into the port and aspirate to observe for a blood return.
3. If the IV is infusing properly with no signs of infiltration or inflammation, it should be patent.
4. Blood indicates that the intravenous line is in the vein.
5. Inject the medication at the prescribed rate.
6. Remove the needle and regulate the IV as prescribed.

APPENDIX K
NOMOGRAM FOR THE DETERMINATION OF BODY SURFACE AREA OF CHILDREN AND ADULTS

To determine the surface area, find the height of the person and the weight on the appropriate scales, and then connect these points with a straight edge. The point at which this line intersects with the line of the surface area scale indicates the surface area of the patient in square meters.

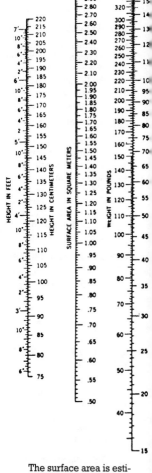

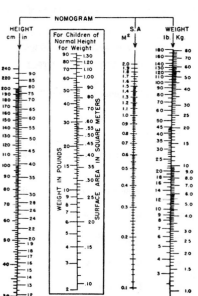

The surface area is estimated by a straight line connecting the height of the patient with his or her weight intersecting the surface area line. If the patient is of average size, the surface area can be estimated from weight alone (see boxed scale in diagram).

APPENDIX L
HERBAL THERAPIES

The use of herbal therapies is on the increase in the United States. In 1990, an estimated 1 in 3 Americans used at least one form of alternative medicine (of which herbal therapy is part). By 1997, over $12 billion was spent in the United States for vitamins and minerals, herbals, sports supplements or specialty supplements (e.g., glucosamine).

Because of the rise in the use of herbal therapy in the United States, the following is presented to provide some basic information on some of the more popular herbs. Please note this is not an all-inclusive list, which is beyond the scope of this handbook.

NAME	PURPORTED BENEFIT	INTERACTIONS	PRECAUTIONS
DHEA	Slows aging, boosts energy, controls weight.	None	Side effects: May increase risk of breast/prostate cancer. Women may develop acne, hair growth on face/body.
Echinacea	Prevents/treats colds, flu, bacterial and fungal infections. An immune system stimulator. Aid to wound healing.	May interfere with immunosuppressive therapy.	Not to be used w/weakened immune system (e.g., HIV/AIDS, tuberculosis, multiple sclerosis). Habitual or continued use may cause immune system suppression (should only be taken for 2–3 mos or alternating schedule of q2–3wks).
Feverfew	Relieves migraine. Treatment of fever, headache, menstrual-irregularities.	May increase bleeding time w/aspirin, dipyridamole, warfarin.	Side effects: headache, mouth ulcers. Should be avoided in pregnancy (stimulates menstruation), nursing mother, infants <2 yrs of age.
Garlic	Reduces cholesterol, LDL, triglycerides, increases HDL, lowers B/P, inhibits platelet aggregation. May also possess antibacterial, antiviral, antithrombotic activity.	May increase bleeding time w/aspirin, dipyridamole, warfarin.	Side effects: taste, offensive odor. Large doses may cause heartburn, flatulence, other GI distress.
Ginger	Relieves nausea, effective treatment for motion sickness, anti-inflammatory for arthritis, nausea/vomiting associated w/pregnancy. Possesses ability to lower platelet aggregation; antithrombotic properties.	None	Avoid during pregnancy when bleeding is a concern. Large overdose could potentially depress the CNS, cause cardiac arrhythmias.

(continued)

APPENDIX

Name	Purported Benefit	Interactions	Precautions
Ginko	Boosts mental prowess by improving memory. Sharpens concentration, pt may think more clearly. Overcomes sexual dysfunction occurring w/SSRI antidepressants. May be able to slow progress of Alzheimer's, improve intermittent claudication.	May increase bleeding time w/aspirin, dipyridamole, warfarin.	Avoid in pt taking blood thinners or those hypersensitive to poison ivy, cashews, mangos. Side effects: GI disturbances, headache, dizziness, vertigo.
Ginseng	Boosts energy, sexual stamina; decreases stress, effects of aging.	May affect platelet adhesiveness/blood coagulation. Use caution w/anticoagulants. May increase hypoglycemia w/insulin.	Avoid in pts receiving anticoagulants, medications that increase B/P. Side effects: breast tenderness, nervousness, headache, increased B/P, abnormal vaginal bleeding.
Kava kava	Reduces stress, muscle relaxant, relieves anxiety, induces sleep and counters fatigue.	Increases CNS depression w/alcohol, sedatives.	Side effects: GI disturbances, temporary discoloration of skin, hair, nails. Do not use in pregnancy, lactation, endogenous depression. High doses cause muscle weakness. Chronic use may cause scaly skin resembling psoriasis (reversible). Causes pupil diation affecting vision (avoid driving,.operating heavy machinery).
St. John's wort	Relieves mild to moderate depression, heals wounds.	May cause "seratonin syndrome" (confusion, agitation, chills, fever, sweating, diarrhea, nausea, muscle spasms or twitching), hyperreflexia, tremor w/antidepressants, yohimbe.	Store in cool, dry place (excess heat/light will alter contents). Side effects: dizziness, dry mouth, increased sensitivity to sunlight. Report symptoms of "serotonin syndrome."
Ma Huang (Ephedra)	Controls weight, boosts energy. Treatment of colds, allergies, appetite suppressant.	Increases toxicity w/beta blockers, MAOIs, caffeine, theophylline, decongestants, St. John's wort.	Linked to high B/P, headache, seizures. Can cause confusion, insomnia, dizziness, sweating, fever, nausea, vomiting.

NAME	PURPORTED BENEFIT	INTERACTIONS	PRECAUTIONS
Melatonin	Aids sleep, prevents jet lag.	Decreases effects of antidepressants.	Side effects: headache, confusion, fatigue. Does not lengthen total sleep time.
Saw Palmetto	Eases symptoms of large prostate (frequency, dysuria, nocturia).	None	Side effects: upset stomach, headache, erectile dysfunction. Does not reduce size of enlarged prostate. Obtain baseline PSA levels before initiating. High doses can cause diarrhea.
Valerian	Aids sleep, relieves restlessness and nervousness. Does not decrease night awakenings.	None	Side effects: heart palpitations, upset stomach, headache, excitability, uneasiness. May cause increased morning drowsiness.
Yohimbe	Male aphrodisiac. Used to treat impotence, erectile dysfunction, orthostatic hypotension.	Decreases effects of antidepressants, antihypertensives, St. John's wort.	High doses linked to weakness, paralysis.

INDEX

Generic names appear in lower case boldface type. U.S. trade names are in regular type, Canadian trade names appear in capital letters, and classifications are in lower case italics.

New Drug Supplement

abacavir

Aceon (see perindopril)

Aciphex (see rabeprazole)

acitretin

Acthrel (see corticorelin)

Actonel (see risedronate)

Actos (see pioglitazone)

adapalene

adefovir

Agenerase (see amprenavir)

Aggrastat (see tirobifan)

Agrylin (see anagrelide)

Alamast (see pemirolast)

albendazole

Albenza (see albendazole)

Aldara (see imiquimod)

alitretinoin

Alphagan (see brimonidine)

Amerge (see naratriptan)

aminolevulinic acid (ALA)

amlexanox

amprenavir

anagrelide

Antagon (see ganirelix)

anti-thymocyte globulin

Anzemet (see dolasetron)

apraclonidine

Apthasol (see amlexanox)

Arava (see leflunomide)

ardeparin

Aricept (see donepezil)

Aromasin (see exemestane)

Astelin (see azelastine)

Atacand (see candesartan)

Atgam (see anti-thymocyte)

atorvastatin

Avandia (see rosiglitazone)

Avapro (see irbesartan)

Avelox (see moxifloxacin)

azelastine

Azopt (see brinzolamide)

balsalazide

basiliximab

Baycol (see cerivastatin)

becaplermin

bexarotene

brimonidine

brinzolamide

butenafine

cabergoline

calfactant

candesartan

capecitabine

cefdinir

Celebrex (see celecoxib)

Celexa (see citalopram)

celecoxib

Cerezyme (see imiglucerase)

cerivastatin

cilostazol

citalopram

clopidogrel

coagulation factor VIIa

Colazide (see balsalazide)

Comtan (see entacapone)

Condylox (see podofilox)

Copaxone (see glatiramer)

Corlopam (see fenoldopam)

corticorelin

Curosurf (see poractant)

Cystagon (see cysteamine)

cysteamine

daclizumab

danaparoid

delavirdine

denileukin

Dermatop (see prednicarbate)

Detrol (see tolterodine)

dexmedetomidine

Differin (see adapalene)

Diovan (see valsartan)

dofetilide

dolasetron

donepezil

dorzolamide

Dostinex (see cabergoline)

doxercalciferol

efavirenz

Ellence (see epirubicin)

Elmiron (see pentosan)

Emadine (see emedastine)

emedastine

Enbrel (see etanercept)

entacapone

epirubicin

eprosartan

eptifibatide

etanercept

Evista (see raloxifene)

exemestane

Fareston (see toremifene)

Femara (see letrozole)

fenofibrate

fenoldopam

Ferrlecit (see sodium ferric gluconate complex)

Flomax (see tamsulosin)

follitropin alpha

fomivirsen sodium

fosfomycin

Gabritril (see tiabagine)

Galzin (see zinc acetate)

ganirelix

gatifloxacin

Geref (see sermorelin)

glatiramer

Glyset (see miglitol)

Gonal-f (see follitropin alpha)

Havrix (see hepatitis A vaccine)

Hectorol (see doxercalciferol)

hepatitis A vaccine

hepatitis B immune globulin

Herceptin (see trastuzumab)

Hyalgan (see hyaluronate sodium)

hyaluronate sodium

imiglucerase

imiquimod

Infasurf (see calfactant)

Infergen (see interferon alfacon-1)

infliximab

INOmax (see nitric oxide)

interferon alfacon-1

interferon alfa-n1

Intergrillin (see eptifibatide)

Iopidine (see apraclonidine)

irbesartan

ivermectin

Keppra (see levetiracetam)

ketotifen

leflunomide

lepirudin

letrozole

Levaquin (see levofloxacin)

levetiracetam

levofloxacin

Levulan Kerastick (see aminole-vulinic acid)

Lipitor (see atorvastatin)

Lotemax (see loteprednol)

loteprednol

Maxalt (see rizatriptan)

Mentax (see butenafine)

mequinol/tretinoin

Meridia (see sibutramine)

Micardis (see telmisartan)

midodrine

miglitol

Mirapex (see pramipexole)

modafinil

montelukast

Monurol (see fosfomycin)

moxifloxacin

Nabi-HB (see hepatitis B immune globulin)

nalmefene

naratriptan

nelfinavir

Neumega (see oprelvekin)

nitric oxide

Normiflo (see ardeparin)

NovoSeven (see coagulation factor VIIa)

olopatadine

Omnicef (see cefdinir)

Ontak (see denileukin)

oprelvekin

Organan (see danaparoid)

orlistat

oseltamivir

palivizumab

Panretin (see alitretinoin)

pantoprazole

paricalcitol

Patanol (see olopatadine)

pemirolast

pentosan

perindopril

pioglitazone

Plavix (see clopidogrel)

Pletal (see cilastazol)

podofilox

poractant

pramipexole

Prandin (see repaglinide)

Precedex (see dexmedetomidine)

prednicarbate

Preveon (see adefovir)

Priftin (see rifapentine)

ProAmatine (see midodrine)

Protonix

Provigil (see modafinil)

quetiapine

rabeprazole

raloxifene

Rapamune (see sirolimus)

Refludan (see lepirudin)

Regranex (see becaplermin)

Relenza (see zanamivir)

Remicade (see infliximab)

Renagel (see sevelamer)

repaglinide

Requip (see ropinirole)

Rescriptor (see delavirdine)

Respigam (see respiratory syncytial immune globulin)

respiratory syncytial immune globulin

Retavase (see reteplase)

reteplase

Revex (see nalmefene)

Rho(D) immune globulin IV (human)

rifapentine

risedronate

Rituxan (see rituximab)

rituximab

rizatriptan

rofecoxib

ropinirole

rosiglitazone

Sabril (see vigabatrin)

sacrosidase

Sclerosol (see talc)

scopolamine

sermorelin

Seroquel (see quetiapine)

sevelamer

sibutramine

sildenafil

Simulect (see basiliximab)

Singulair (see montelukast)

sirolimus

Skelid (see tiludronate)

sodium ferric gluconate complex

Solage (see mequinol/tretinoin)

Sonata (see zaleplon)

Soriatane (see acitretin)

sparfloxacin

abacavir

ah-bah-**kay**-veer
(Ziagen)

CLASSIFICATION

Antiviral

AVAILABILITY (Rx)

Tablets: 300 mg. **Oral Solution:** 20 mg/ml.

ACTION/*THERAPEUTIC EFFECT*

Inhibits HIV reverse transcriptase via viral DNA chain termination. Also inhibits RNA and DNA-dependent DNA polymerase, an enzyme necessary for viral HIV replication, *slowing HIV replication and reducing progression of HIV infection.*

USES

Treatment of HIV infection in adults and children >3 months.

INDICATIONS/DOSAGE/ROUTES

HIV infection:
PO: Adults: 300 mg 2 times/day. **Children:** 8 mg/kg 2 times/day. **Maximum:** 600 mg/day.

SIDE EFFECTS

OCCASIONAL: Hypersensitivity reaction (fever, dyspnea, cough, pharyngitis, GI symptoms, malaise, rash). **RARE:** Hypotension, respiratory distress.

acitretin

ah-sa-**tree**-tin
(Soriatane)

CLASSIFICATION

Antipsoriatic

AVAILABILITY (Rx)

Capsules: 10 mg, 25 mg

ACTION/*THERAPEUTIC EFFECT*

Exact mechanism unknown. May modulate factors influencing epidermal proliferation, regulate RNA/DNA synthesis, control glycoprotein formation, or govern immune response. *Regulates keratinocyte growth and differentiation.*

USES

Treatment of severe recalcitrant psoriasis (reduces severity of scaling, erythema, and epidural induration and percentage of body surface involvement).

INDICATIONS/DOSAGE/ROUTES

Psoriasis:
PO: Adults, elderly: 25–50 mg/day. **Range:** 10–75 mg/day. **Children:** 0.4–0.5 mg/kg/day. **Maximum:** 1 mg/kg/day.

SIDE EFFECTS

FREQUENT (>10%): Drying of eyes, nose, lips, skin; cheilitis; desquamation of palms, soles. Alopecia, nail abnormalities, pruritus, fatigue. **OCCASIONAL (1–10%):** Nausea, headache, sweating, chills, sensation of cold. **Note:** Contraindicated in pregnancy.

adapalene

ah-**dap**-ah-leen
(Differin)

CLASSIFICATION

Antiacne

AVAILABILITY (Rx)

Gel: 0.1%

ACTION/*THERAPEUTIC EFFECT*

Binds to retinoic acid receptors

in cell nuclei modulating cell differentiation, keratinization. Possesses anti-inflammatory, comedolytic properties. *Normalizes differentiation of follicular epithelial cells, reduces microcomedome formation.*

USES

Topical treatment of acne vulgaris.

INDICATIONS/DOSAGE/ROUTES

Acne vulgaris:
Topical: Adults, children >12 yrs: Apply to affected area once daily at bedtime after washing.

SIDE EFFECTS

FREQUENT (10–40%): Erythema, scaling, dryness, pruritus, burning. OCCASIONAL (1–5%): Skin irritation, stinging, sunburn, acne flares.

adefovir

add-eh-**foe**-veer
(Preveon)

CLASSIFICATION

Antiviral

AVAILABILITY (Rx)

Tablets: 120 mg

ACTION/THERAPEUTIC EFFECT

Inhibits HIV reverse transcriptase via viral DNA chain termination. Inhibits RNA- and DNA-dependent DNA polymerase, an enzyme necessary for viral HIV replication, *slowing HIV replication and reducing progression of HIV infection.*

USES

Treatment of HIV infection.

INDICATIONS/DOSAGE/ROUTES

HIV infection:
PO: Adults: 120 mg/day.

SIDE EFFECTS

FREQUENT (30%): Mild to moderate nephrotoxicity (dose-related). OCCASIONAL: Nausea, diarrhea, asthenia, increased aminotransferase activity.

albendazole

all-**ben**-dah-zole
(Albenza)

CLASSIFICATION

Anthelmintic

AVAILABILITY (Rx)

Tablets: 200 mg

ACTION/THERAPEUTIC EFFECT

Vermicidal. Degrades parasite cytoplasmic microtubules, irreversibly blocks cholinesterase secretion, glucose uptake in helminth and larvae (depletes glycogen, decreases ATP production, depletes energy). *Immobilizes and kills worms.*

USES

Treatment of parenchymal neurocysticercosis caused by active lesions caused by larval forms of pork tapeworm, *Taenia solium.* Treatment of cystic hydatid disease of liver, lung, and peritoneum caused by larval form of dog tapeworm, *Echinococcus granulosus.*

INDICATIONS/DOSAGE/ROUTES

Neurocysticercosis:
PO: Adults, elderly, >60 kg: 400

mg 2 times/day; **<60 kg:** 15 mg/kg/day. Continue for 28 days, rest 14 days, repeat cycle 3 times.

Cystic hydatid:
PO: Adults, elderly, >60 kg: 400 mg 2 times/day; **<60 kg:** 15 mg/ kg/day. Continue for 8–30 days.

SIDE EFFECTS

FREQUENT (3–10%): *Neurocysticercosis:* Nausea, vomiting, headache. *Hydatid:* Abnormal liver function tests, abdominal pain, nausea, vomiting. **OCCASIONAL (1–3%):** *Neurocysticercosis:* Increased intracranial pressure, meningeal signs. *Hydatid:* Headache, dizziness, alopecia, fever.

alitretinoin

al-**lee**-tret-ih-nown
(Panretin)

CLASSIFICATION

Antineoplastic: Retinoid

AVAILABILITY (Rx)

Gel: 0.1%

ACTION / *THERAPEUTIC EFFECT*

Binds to and activates all known retinoid receptors. Once activated, receptors act as transcription factors, regulating expression of genes that control cellular differentiation, proliferation. *Inhibits growth of Kaposi's sarcoma cells.*

USES / *UNLABELED*

Topical treatment of cutaneous lesions in pts w/AIDS-related Kaposi's sarcoma. *Breast, cervical, ovarian, prostatic carcinomas, myelodysplastic syndrome, psoriasis.*

INDICATIONS/DOSAGE/ROUTES

Kaposi's sarcoma:
Topical: Adults: Initially, apply 2 times/day to lesions. May increase to 3–4 times/day. Allow gel to dry 3–5 mins before covering w/clothing.

SIDE EFFECTS

FREQUENT (>5%): Rash (erythema, scaling, irritation, redness, dermatitis), burning pain, itching, exfoliative dermatitis (flaking, peeling, desquamation, exfoliation), stinging, tingling, swelling, inflammation.

aminolevulinic acid (ALA)

ah-**mean**-oh-lev-you-lin-ick
(Levulan Kerastick)

CLASSIFICATION

Photochemotherapy

AVAILABILLITY (Rx)

Topical Solution: 20% (354 mg ALA)

ACTION / *THERAPEUTIC EFFECT*

ALA is a metabolic precursor of protoporphyrin IX (PpIX), which is a photosensitizer. ALA, when provided to the cell, results in accumulation of PpIX, which is converted into heme. When exposed to light of appropirate wavelength and energy, PpIX produces a photodynamic reaction, a cytotoxic process. *Photosensitization of actinic (solar) keratosis lesions occurs (ALA plus illumination w/BLU-U is the basis for ALA photodynamic therapy [PDT].)*

USES / *UNLABELED*

Treatment of nonhyperkeratotic actinic keratoses of the face/scalp.

Barrett's esophagus, Bowen's disease, epidermodysplasia verruciformis, nevus sebaceus, mycosis fungoides, oral leukoplakia, multifocal superficial transitional cell carcinoma of upper urinary tract, squamous cell carcinoma, Kaposi's sarcoma.

INDICATIONS/DOSAGE/ROUTES

Actinic keratosis:
Topical: Adults: One application of ALA and one dose of illumination/treatment site per 8-wk treatment session. Photodynamic therapy is a 2-stage process: apply ALA, followed 14–18 hrs later by illumination w/blue light using Blue Light Photodynamic Therapy Illuminator (BLU-U).

SIDE EFFECTS

FREQUENT: Scaling, crusting (64–71%), itching (14–25%), hypo/hyperpigmentation (22–36%), wheal/flare (7%), skin disorder NOS (5–12%). **OCCASIONAL (1–4%):** Ulceration, bleeding, hemorrhage, edema, pain, tenderness, vasculation, scabbing.

amlexanox

am-**lecks**-ah-knocks
(Apthasol)

CLASSIFICATION

Antiallergic/anti-inflammatory

AVAILABILITY (Rx)

Oral Paste: 5%

ACTION/*THERAPEUTIC EFFECT*

Exact mechanism unknown. Has antiallergic and anti-inflammatory properties. Appears to inhibit formation and/or release of inflammatory mediators (e.g., histamine) from mast cells, neutrophils, mono-

nuclear cells. *Alleviates signs/symptoms of aphthous ulcers.*

USES

Treatment of signs/symptoms of aphthous ulcers in pts with normal immune system.

INDICATIONS/DOSAGE/ROUTES

Aphthous ulcers:
Topical: Adults, elderly: Administer 1/4 inch directly to ulcers 4 times/day (after meals and at bedtime), following oral hygiene.

SIDE EFFECTS

OCCASIONAL: Stinging, burning at administration site; nausea, diarrhea, vomiting, transient pain.

amprenavir

am-**prenn**-ah-veer
(Agenerase)

CLASSIFICATION

Antiviral: Protease inhibitor

AVAILABILITY (Rx)

Capsules: 50 mg, 150 mg. **Oral Solution:** 15 mg/ml.

ACTION/*THERAPEUTIC EFFECT*

Inhibits HIV-1 protease by binding to active site of HIV-1 protease. Prevents processing of viral precursors. *Formation of immature noninfectious viral particles. Impairment of HIV viral replication and proliferation.*

USES

Treatment of HIV-1 infection in combination w/other antiretroviral agents.

INDICATIONS/DOSAGE/ROUTES

HIV-1 infection:
PO: Adults, children 13–16 yrs: *Capsules:* 1,200 mg 2 times/day.

Children 4–12 yrs, 13–16 yrs <50 kg: 20 mg/kg 2 times/day or 15 mg/kg 3 times/day. **Maximum:** 2,400 mg/day. *Oral solution:* Children 4–12 yrs, 13–16 yrs <50 kg: 22.5 mg/day (1.5 ml/kg) 2 times/day or 17 mg/kg (1.1 ml/kg) 3 times/day. **Maximum:** 2,800 mg/day.

SIDE EFFECTS

FREQUENT: Nausea (73%), vomiting (29%), diarrhea (33%), oral paresthesia (26%), depression (15%), rash (25%). **OCCASIONAL (5–10%):** Paresthesia (peripheral), taste disorders.

anagrelide

an-ah-**gree**-lide
(Agrylin)

CLASSIFICATION

Antiplatelet

AVAILABILITY (Rx)

Capsules: 0.5 mg, 1 mg

ACTION/ *THERAPEUTIC EFFECT*

Prevents platelet shape changes caused by platelet-aggregating agents. *Inhibits platelet aggregation.*

USES

Treatment of essential thrombocythemia, reducing elevated platelet count and risk of thrombosis. Thromobocythemia due to myeloproliferative disorders.

INDICATIONS/DOSAGE/ROUTES

Thrombocythemia:
PO: Adults, elderly: Initially, 0.5 mg 4 times/day or 1 mg 2 times/day. Adjust dose to lowest effective dose. Increase by ≤0.5 mg/day in any 1 week. **Maximum:** 10 mg/day or 2.5 mg/dose.

SIDE EFFECTS

FREQUENT (>10%): Palpitations, diarrhea, abdominal pain, nausea, gas, headache, bloating, edema, asthenia, pain, dizziness, dyspnea, fullness in chest. **OCCASIONAL (5–10%):** Tachycardia, chest pain, vomiting, loss of appetite, dyspepsia, rash.

anti-thymocyte globulin

an-tie-**thigh**-mow-site
(Atgam)

CLASSIFICATION

Biologic response modifier: Immunosuppressant

AVAILABILITY (Rx)

Injection: 50 mg/ml amps

ACTION/ *THERAPEUTIC EFFECT*

A lymphocyte-selective immunosuppressant; reduces number of circulating thymus-dependent lymphocytes (T-lymphocytes), altering function of T-lymphocytes, which are responsible for cell-mediated and humoral immunity. Stimulates release of hematopoietic growth factors. *Allows increase in graft survival rate.*

USES/ *UNLABELED*

Management of allograft rejection in renal transplant pts, increasing frequency of resolution of acute rejection period. Treatment of moderate to severe aplastic anemia in pts not suited for bone marrow transplants. *Immunosuppressant in liver, bone marrow, heart transplants, treatment of multiple sclerosis, myasthenia gravis, pure red cell aplasia, scleroderma.*

INDICATIONS/DOSAGE/ROUTES

Renal allograft recipients:
IV infusion: Adults: 10–30 mg/kg/day. **Children:** 5–25 mg/kg/day. *Delay of onset of rejection:* 15 mg/kg/day for 14 days, then 15 mg/kg/day every other day for 14 days. Give first dose within 24 hrs before or after transplant. *Treatment of rejection:* 10–15 mg/kg/day for 14 days. May continue with alternate day therapy up to 21 doses.

Aplastic anemia:
IV infusion: Adults: 10–20 mg/kg/day for 8–14 days. May continue alternate day therapy up to 21 doses.

SIDE EFFECTS

FREQUENT: Fever (51%), thrombocytopenia (30%), rashes (2%), chills (16%), leukopenia (14%), systemic infection (13%). **OCCASIONAL (5–10%):** Abnormal renal function tests, serum sickness-like symptoms, dyspnea, apnea, arthralgia, chest/back/flank pain, nausea, vomiting, diarrhea, phlebitis.

apraclonidine

aye-prah-**clon**-ih-deen
(Iopidine)

CLASSIFICATION

Antiglaucoma

AVAILABILITY (Rx)

Ophthalmic Solution: 0.5%, 1%

ACTION/*THERAPEUTIC EFFECT*

Stimulates alpha-adrenergic system reducing formation of aqueous humor. *Reduces elevated intraocular pressure (IOP).*

USES

At 0.5% strength: Short-term adjunctive therapy in glaucoma to decrease IOP. *At 1%:* Controls/prevents postsurgical increased IOP following trabeculoplasty or iridotomy.

INDICATIONS/DOSAGE/ROUTES

Glaucoma:
Ophthalmic: Adults, elderly: 1–2 drops 3 times/day.

SIDE EFFECTS

FREQUENT (4–13%): Hyperemia, pruritus, tearing, lid edema, foreign body sensation, blurred vision, dry eye. **OCCASIONAL (1–3%):** Dry mouth, asthenia, headache, dry nose, altered taste.

ardeparin

ar-deh-**pear**-inn
(Normiflo)

CLASSIFICATION

Anticoagulant

AVAILABILITY (Rx)

Injection: 5,000 U/0.5 ml, 10,000 U/0.5 ml

ACTION/*THERAPEUTIC EFFECT*

Antithrombin, in presence of low molecular weight heparin, *produces anticoagulation* by inhibition of factor Xa. Ardeparin causes less inactivation of thrombin, inhibition of platelets, and bleeding than standard heparin. Does not significantly influence bleeding time, prothrombin time (PT), activated partial thromboplastin time (APTT).

USES/*UNLABELED*

Prevents deep vein thrombosis (DVT) following knee replacement surgery. *Treatment of unstable angina/MI.*

INDICATIONS/DOSAGE/ROUTES

Prevention of DVT:
SC: Adults, elderly: 50 U/kg q12hrs.

SIDE EFFECTS

OCCASIONAL (>2%): Bleeding, hemorrhage, hematoma at injection site, anemia, nausea, fever, constipation. **RARE (<2%):** Vomiting, itching, rash, confusion.

atorvastatin

aye-**tore**-vah-stah-tin
(Lipitor)

CLASSIFICATION

Antihyperlipidemic

AVAILABILITY (Rx)

Tablets: 10 mg, 20 mg, 40 mg

ACTION/ *THERAPEUTIC EFFECT*

Inhibits HMG-CoA reductase, the enzyme that catalyzes the early step in cholesterol synthesis. *Decreases LDL, cholesterol, VLDL, plasma triglycerides. Increases HDL cholesterol concentration.*

USES

Adjunct to diet to reduce elevated total cholesterol, LDL, triglyceride levels in patients w/primary hypercholesterolemia and mixed dyslipidemia. Increases HDL-C in primary hypercholesterolemia/ mixed dyslipidemia.

INDICATIONS/DOSAGE/ROUTES

Hypercholesterol/ hypertriglycerides:
PO: Adults, elderly: Initially, 10 mg/day. **Range:** 10–80 mg/day. **Maximum:** 80 mg/day.

SIDE EFFECTS

OCCASIONAL (1–10%): Headache, pain, diarrhea, flatulence, constipation, indigestion. **RARE (<1%):** Nausea, insomnia.

azelastine

aye-zeh-**las**-teen
(Astelin)

CLASSIFICATION

Antihistamine

AVAILABILITY (Rx)

Nasal Spray

ACTION/ *THERAPEUTIC EFFECT*

Prevents activation of basophils, mast cells, eosinophils, macrophages, and monocytes; blocks synthesis, release, or target receptors of several mediators of immediate inflammatory response (e.g., histamine); regulates late-phase allergic responses by inhibition of leukotriene-mediated and T-cell responses. *Relieves rhinitis.*

USES

Treatment of symptoms of seasonal allergic rhinitis (e.g., rhinorrhea, sneezing, nasal pruritus).

INDICATIONS/DOSAGE/ROUTES

Seasonal allergic rhinitis:
Intranasal: Adults, elderly, children >12 yrs: 1–2 sprays to each nostril 2 times/day.

SIDE EFFECTS

FREQUENT: Headache (20%), bitter taste (15%), somnolence (11.5%). **OCCASIONAL:** Nasal burning, pharyngitis, dry mouth, paroxysmal sneezing, nausea, rhinitis, fatigue, dizziness, epistaxis.

balsalazide

ball-**sall**-ah-zide
(Colazide)

CLASSIFICATION

GI anti-inflammatory agent

AVAILABILITY (Rx)

ACTION/ *THERAPEUTIC EFFECT*

Must be converted to 5-aminos-alicylic acid to be effective. Action may include changes in intestinal microflora, altered prostaglandin production, inhibition of function of natural killer cells, mast cells, neutrophils, macrophages, *diminishing inflammatory effect in colon.*

USES

Treatment of ulcerative colitis.

INDICATIONS/DOSAGE/ROUTES

Ulcerative colitis:
PO: Adults, elderly: 1–2.25 g 2–3 times/day.

SIDE EFFECTS

OCCASIONAL: Nausea, headache, diarrhea, abdominal pain, flatus, constipation.

basiliximab

bay-zul-**ix**-ah-mab
(Simulect)

CLASSIFICATION

Immunosuppressive

AVAILABILITY (Rx)

Powder for Injection: 20 mg

ACTION/ *THERAPEUTIC EFFECT*

Binds and blocks interleukin-2 receptor chains found on surface of activated T-lymphocytes, *inhibiting lymphocytic activity, thereby preventing cellular immune response involved in allograft rejection.*

USES

Adjunct w/cyclosporine, corticosteroids in the prophylaxis of acute organ rejection in patients receiving renal trasnplant.

INDICATIONS/DOSAGE/ROUTES

Prophylaxis of organ rejection:
IV: Adults, elderly: Two doses of 20 mg each in reconstituted volume of 50 ml given as IV infusion over 20–30 min. Give first dose of 20 mg within 2 hrs before transplant surgery and the second dose of 20 mg 4 days after transplant. Children: 12 mg/m^2 as above.

SIDE EFFECTS

FREQUENT (>10%): GI disturbances, constipation, diarrhea, dyspepsia, CNS (headache, tremor, dizziness, insomnia), respiratory infection, dysuria, acne, leg/back pain, peripheral edema, hypertension. OCCASIONAL (3–10%): Angina, neuropathy, abdominal distention, tachycardia, rash, hypotension, urinary disturbances (hematuria, frequent micturation, genital edema), joint pain, increased hair growth, muscle pain.

becaplermin

beh-**cap**-lear-min
(Regranex)

CLASSIFICATION

Growth factor

AVAILABILITY (Rx)

Gel: 0.003%, 0.01%

ACTION/*THERAPEUTIC EFFECT*

Platelet-derived growth factor that *stimulates body to grow new tissue* to heal open wounds.

USES

Treatment of lower-extremity diabetic neuropathic ulcers extending into subcutaneous tissue or beyond.

INDICATIONS/DOSAGE/ROUTES

Ulcers:
Topical: Adults, elderly: Apply once daily (spread evenly, covered w/saline-moistened gauze dressing). After 12 hrs, rinse ulcer, recover with saline gauze.

SIDE EFFECTS

No known side effects noted. Note: Side effects not significantly different from placebo in one study.

---

bexarotene

becks-**aye**-row-teen
(Targretin)

CLASSIFICATION

Antineoplastic

AVAILABILITY (Rx)

Capsules. Soft gelatin: 75 mg.

ACTION/*THERAPEUTIC EFFECT*

A selective agonist at retinoid X receptors, which are involved in process of apoptosis (natural process in which body rids itself of unwanted cells). *Shown to inhibit some tumor cell lines of hematopoietic and squamous cell origin.*

USES/*UNLABELED*

Treatment of cutaneous T-cell lymphoma (CTCL) in pts refractory to at least one prior systemic therapy. *Treatment of diabetes mellitus, head, neck, lung, renal cell carcinomas, Kaposi's sarcoma.*

INDICATIONS/DOSAGE/ROUTES

CTCL:
PO: Adults: 300 mg/m^2/day. If no response and initial dose well tolerated, may be increased to 400 mg/m^2/day.

SIDE EFFECTS

FREQUENT: Lipid abnormalities (79%), hypothyroidism (29%), leukopenia (17%). **OCCASIONAL (<10%):** Diarrhea, fatigue, headache, abnormal liver function tests, rash, itching, pancreatitis.

---

brimonidine

bri-**moe**-nih-deen
(Alphagan)

CLASSIFICATION

Antiglaucoma

AVAILABILITY (Rx)

Ophthalmic Solution: 0.2%

ACTION/*THERAPEUTIC EFFECT*

Alpha-2 adrenergic agonist that reduces aqueous humor and increases uveoscleral outflow. *Reduces intraocular pressure (IOP).*

USES

Lowers IOP in patients w/open-angle glaucoma or ocular hypertension.

INDICATIONS/DOSAGE/ROUTES

Usual ophthalmic dosage:
Ophthalmic: Adults, elderly: 1 drop to affected eye(s) 3 times/day (approximately 8 hrs apart).

SIDE EFFECTS

FREQUENT (10–30%): Oral dryness, ocular hyperemia, burning, stinging, headache, fatigue, foreign body sensation, ocular pruritus/allergic reaction. **OCCASIONAL (3–9%):** Corneal staining, photophobia, eyelid erythema, ocular pain/dryness, tearing, eyelid edema, dizziness, asthenia, conjunctival blanching, muscular pain, abnormal vision. **RARE (1–3%):** Lid crusting, conjunctival hemorrhage/discharge, nasal dryness, abnormal taste.

brinzolamide

Brin-**zoll**-ah-mide
(Azopt)

CLASSIFICATION

Glaucoma agent

AVAILABILITY (Rx)

Ophthalmic Suspension: 1%

ACTION/*THERAPEUTIC EFFECT*

Inhibits carbonic anhydrase, an enzyme, decreasing aqueous humor secretion, *reducing intraocular pressure (IOP).*

USES

Treatment of elevated intraocular pressure (IOP) in pts w/ocular hypertension or open-angle glaucoma.

INDICATIONS/DOSAGE/ROUTES

Elevated intraocular pressure (IOP):
Ophthalmic: Adults, elderly: Apply 1 drop into affected eye 3 times/day.

SIDE EFFECTS

FREQUENT (5–10%): Blurred vision; bitter, sour, or unusual taste.

OCCASIONAL (1–5%): Blepharitis, dermatitis, dry eye, foreign body sensation, headache, hyperemia, eye discharge/discomfort, itching eyes, rhinitis. **RARE (<1%):** Allergic reaction, dry mouth, tearing, lid margin crusting, eye fatigue.

butenafine

beu-**ten**-ah-feen
(Mentax)

CLASSIFICATION

Antifungal: topical

AVAILABILITY (Rx)

Cream: 1%

ACTION/*THERAPEUTIC EFFECT*

Inhibits epoxidation of squalene, blocking biosynthesis of ergosterol, essential for fungal cell membranes. Fungicidal. *Relieves athlete's foot.*

USES

Treatment of interdigital tinea pedis (athlete's foot) due to *E. Floccosum, T. Mentagrophytes,* or *T. Rubrum.*

INDICATIONS/DOSAGE/ROUTES

Tinea pedis:
Topical: Adults, elderly, children >12 yrs: Apply to affected area and immediately surrounding skin daily for 4 wks.

SIDE EFFECTS

OCCASIONAL (2%): Contact dermatitis, burning/stinging, worsening of the condition. **RARE (<2%):** Erythema, irritation, itching.

cabergoline

cab-**err**-go-leen
(Dostinex)

CLASSIFICATION

Antihyperprolactemic

AVAILABILITY (Rx)

Tablets: 0.5 mg

ACTION/*THERAPEUTIC EFFECT*

Agonist at dopamine D2 receptors suppressing prolactin secretion. *Shrinks prolactinomas, restores gonadal function.*

USES

Treatment of hyperprolactemic disorders, either idiopathic or due to pituitary adenomas.

INDICATIONS/DOSAGE/ROUTES

Hyperprolactemia:
PO: Adults, elderly: 0.5 mg 2 times/week.

SIDE EFFECTS

FREQUENT: Nausea (29%). **OCCASIONAL (5–20%):** Headache, vomiting, vertigo, dizziness, dyspepsia, orthostatic hypotension, constipation.

calfactant

cal-**fact**-tant
(Infasurf)

CLASSIFICATION

Lung surfactant

AVAILABILITY (Rx)

Intratracheal Suspension: 35 mg/ml vials

ACTION/*THERAPEUTIC EFFECT*

Modifies alveolar surface tension, stabilizing the alveoli, *restoring surface activity to infant lungs, improving lung compliance and respiratory gas exchange.*

USES

Prevention of respiratory distress syndrome (RDS) in premature infants <29 wks of gestational age and for treatment of premature infants <72 hrs of age who develop RDS and require endotracheal intubation.

INDICATIONS/DOSAGE/ROUTES

Respiratory distress syndrome (RDS):
Endotracheal: Infant: Instill 3 ml/kg of birth weight as soon as possible after birth, administered as 2 doses of 1.5 ml/kg. Repeat doses of 3 ml/kg of birth weight, up to a total of 3 doses, 12 hrs apart.

SIDE EFFECTS

FREQUENT: Cyanosis (65%), airway obstruction (39%), bradycardia (34%), reflux of surfactant into endotracheal tube (21%), requirement of manual ventilation (16%). **OCCASIONAL (3%):** Reintubation.

candesartan

can-deh-**sar**-tan
(Atacand)

CLASSIFICATION

Angiotensin II receptor antagonist

AVAILABILITY (Rx)

Tablets: 4 mg, 8 mg, 16 mg, 32 mg

ACTION/*THERAPEUTIC EFFECT*

Potent vasodilator, an angiotensin II receptor antagonist, blocks vasoconstrictor and aldosterone-secreting effects of angiotensin II, inhibiting the binding of angiotensin II to the AT1 receptors. *Produces vasodilation, decreased peripheral resistance, decreased B/P.*

USES/*UNLABELED*

Treatment of hypertension alone or in combination with other antihypertensives. *Treatment of heart failure.*

INDICATIONS/DOSAGE/ROUTES

Note: If antihypertensive effect using once daily is inadequate, a twice-daily regimen at the same total daily dose or an increase in dose may provide therapeutic response. May be given concurrently w/other antihypertensives. If B/P is not controlled by candesartan alone, a diuretic may be added.

Hypertension:
PO: Adults, elderly, mildly impaired renal or hepatic function: Initially, 16 mg once daily in pts who are not volume depleted. Can be given once or twice daily w/total daily doses ranging from 8 to 32 mg. Give lower dose in pts treated w/diuretics, severe impaired renal function.

SIDE EFFECTS

OCCASIONAL (3–6%): Upper respiratory infection, dizziness, back and leg pain. **RARE (1–2%):** Pharyngitis, rhinitis, headache, fatigue, diarrhea, nausea, dry cough, peripheral edema.

capecitabine

cap-eh-**site**-ah-bean
(Xeloda)

CLASSIFICATION

Antineoplastic: metabolite

AVAILABILITY (Rx)

Tablets: 150 mg, 500 mg

ACTION/*THERAPEUTIC EFFECT*

Enzymatically converted to 5-fluorouracil. Inhibits enzymes necessary for synthesis of essential cellular components, *interfering with DNA synthesis, RNA processing, and protein synthesis.*

USES

Treatment of metastatic breast cancer resistant to other therapy.

INDICATIONS/DOSAGE/ROUTES

Metastatic breast cancer:
PO: Adults, elderly: Initially, 2,500 mg/m^2/day in two equally divided doses approximately 12 hrs apart for 2 wks. Follow with a 1 wk rest period given as 3 wk cycles.

SIDE EFFECTS

FREQUENT (>5%): Diarrhea, nausea, vomiting, stomatitis, hand and foot syndrome (palmar-plantar erythema, paresthesia, tingling, swelling, blistering, desquamation), fatigue, anorexia, dermatitis, GI irritation. **OCCASIONAL (<5%):** Constipation, dyspepsia, nail disorder, headache, dizziness, insomnia, dehydration, eye irritation, pyrexia, edema, myalgia, limb pain, blood dyscrasias (neutropenia, thrombocytopenia, anemia, lymphopenia).

cefdinir

cef-dih-near
(Omnicef)

CLASSIFICATION

Antibiotic: third-generation cephalosporin

AVAILABILITY (Rx)

Capsules: 300 mg. **Oral Suspension:** 125 mg/5 ml.

ACTION/*THERAPEUTIC EFFECT*

Bactericidal. Binds to bacterial membranes, inhibiting bacterial cell wall synthesis.

USES

Adults: Treatment of community-acquired pneumonia, acute exacerbation of chronic bronchitis. *Adults/children:* Treatment of acute bacterial sinusitis, pharyngitis, tonsillitis, uncomplicated skin/skin structure infections. *Children:* Treatment of acute bacterial otitis media.

INDICATIONS/DOSAGE/ROUTES

Usual adult dosage:
PO: 600 mg/day as single dose or in 2 divided doses.

Usual pediatric dosage:
PO: 14 mg/kg/day as single dose or in 2 divided doses.

SIDE EFFECTS

FREQUENT (Adult): Diarrhea, vaginal moniliasis, nausea, headache, abdominal pain, vaginitis. **Note:** Side effects in the pediatric population not known at time of writing.

celecoxib

seal-ee-**cox**-ib
(Celebrex)

CLASSIFICATION

Cyclo-oxygenase-2 inhibitor

AVAILABILITY (Rx)

Capsules: 100 mg, 200 mg

ACTION/*THERAPEUTIC EFFECT*

Selectively inhibits cyclo-oxygenase-2 (required for synthesis of prostaglandins and thromboxane that cause pain and inflammation). *Produces anti-inflammatory and analgesic effects.*

USES

Treatment of osteoarthritis, rheumatoid arthritis. Adjunct in pts w/familial adenomatous polyposis (FAP).

INDICATIONS/DOSAGE/ROUTES

Osteoarthritis:
PO: Adults, elderly: 200 mg/day as single dose or 100 mg 2 times/day.

Rheumatoid arthritis:
PO: Adults, elderly: 100–200 mg 2 times/day.

FAP:
PO: Adults: 200 mg 2 times/day.

SIDE EFFECTS

FREQUENT (>5%): Diarrhea, dyspepsia, headache (16%), upper respiratory tract infection. **OCCASIONAL (1–5%):** Abdominal pain, flatus, nausea, back pain, peripheral edema, dizziness, pharyngitis, rhinitis, rash.

cerivastatin

ser-**ee**-vah-stah-tin
(Baycol)

CLASSIFICATION

Antihyperlipidemic

AVAILABILITY (Rx)

Tablets: 0.2 mg, 0.3 mg, 0.4 mg

ACTION/*THERAPEUTIC EFFECT*

Inhibits HMG-CoA reductase, the enzyme that catalyzes the early step in cholesterol synthesis. *Decreases LDL, cholesterol, VLDL, plasma triglycerides. Increases HDL cholesterol concentrations.*

USES

Reduction of elevated total/LDL cholesterol, triglycerides, apolipoprotein in pts w/hyperlipidemia.

INDICATIONS/DOSAGE/ROUTES

Hyperlipidemia:
PO: Adults, elderly: Initially, 0.3 mg once daily in the evening (0.2 mg in pts with significant renal impairment (creatinine clearance <60 ml/min).

SIDE EFFECTS

OCCASIONAL (1–5%): Rhinitis, pharyngitis, headache.

---

cilostazol

sigh-**low**-tah-zoll
(Pletal)

CLASSIFICATION

Antiplatelet, vasodilator

AVAILABILITY (Rx)

Tablets: 100 mg

ACTION/*THERAPEUTIC EFFECT*

Inhibits platelet aggregation, direct arterial vasodilator, *improving walking distance in pts w/intermittent claudication.*

USES

Treatment of symptomatic intermittent claudication.

INDICATIONS/DOSAGE/ROUTES

Intermittent claudication:
PO: Adults, elderly: 100 mg 2 times/day (take at least $1/2$ hr before or 2 hrs after breakfast and dinner). **Note:** Do not take w/grapefruit juice.

SIDE EFFECTS

OCCASIONAL: Headache, diarrhea, abnormal stools, dizziness, palpitations, increased heart rate.

---

citalopram

sigh-**tail**-oh-pram
(Celexa)

CLASSIFICATION

Antidepressant

AVAILABILITY (Rx)

Tablets: 20 mg, 40 mg. **Oral Solution:** 10 mg/5 ml.

ACTION/*THERAPEUTIC EFFECT*

Blocks uptake of the neurotransmitter serotonin at CNS neuronal presynaptic membranes, increasing availability at postsynaptic receptor sites. *Results in enhancement of postsynaptic activity, producing antidepressant effect.*

USES

Treatment of major depressive disorder.

INDICATIONS/DOSAGE/ROUTES

Depression:
PO: Adults: Initially, 20 mg once daily in the morning or evening. Dosage may be increased in increments of 20 mg at intervals of no less than 1 wk. **Maximum:** 40 mg/day. **Elderly, impaired hepatic function:** 20 mg/day. May titrate to 40 mg/day only for nonresponding pts.

SIDE EFFECTS

FREQUENT: Sexual dysfunction (e.g., decreased libido, impotence), drowsiness, dry mouth, nausea, insomnia. **OCCASIONAL:** Blurred vision, loss of memory, apathy, confusion, difficulty breathing, fever, increased urination, skin rash/itching, abdominal pain, decreased appetite, anxiety, muscle pain, diarrhea, dizziness, increased sweating, trembling, or shakiness, vomiting.

clopidogrel

klo-**pie**-dough-grill
(Plavix)

CLASSIFICATON

Antithrombotic

AVAILABILITY (Rx)

Tablets: 75 mg

ACTION/THERAPEUTIC EFFECT

Inhibits binding of ADP to its platelet receptor, preventing ADP-mediated activation of glycoprotein IIb/IIIa complex, *inhibiting platelet aggregation.*

USES

Reduction of myocardial infarction (MI), stroke, vascular death in pts w/atherosclerosis documented by recent stroke, MI, or established peripheral arterial disease.

INDICATIONS/DOSAGE/ROUTES

Inhibition of platelet aggregation:
PO: Adults, elderly: 75 mg once daily.

SIDE EFFECTS

FREQUENT: Skin disorders (15.8%), upper respiratory tract infections (8.7%), chest pain (8.3%), flu-like symptoms (7.5%), pain (6.4%), headache (7.6%), dizziness (6.2%), arthralgia (6.3%). OCCASIONAL (3–5%): Fatigue, edema, hypertension, abdominal pain, dyspepsia, diarrhea, nausea, epistaxis, dyspnea, rhinitis, bronchitis, cough, rash.

coagulation factor VIIa

(NovoSeven)

CLASSIFICATION

Antihemophilic agent

AVAILABILITY (Rx)

Powder for Injection: 1.2 mg, 4.8 mg/vials

ACTION/THERAPEUTIC EFFECT

Activates extrinsic pathway of coagulation cascade (activates factor X to Xa and IX to IXa). Factor Xa w/other factors converts prothrombin to thrombin, which leads to conversion of fibrinogen to fibrin, *inducing local hemostasis.*

USE

Treatment of bleeding episodes in hemophilia A or B patients.

INDICATIONS/DOSAGE/ROUTES

Bleeding:
IV bolus: 90 mcg/kg q2hrs until hemostasis achieved or treatment judged to be inadequate. Range: 35–120 mcg/kg.

SIDE EFFECTS

FREQUENT (5–15%): Fever, hemorrhage, hemarthrosis, fibrinogen plasma decreased, hypertension. OCCASIONAL (<5%): Allergic reaction, coagulation disorder, edema, fibrinolysis increased, headache, hypotension, injection site reaction, pain, decreased prothrombin, pruritus, rash, vomiting.

corticorelin

core-tih-co-**ree**-lynn
(Acthrel)

CLASSIFICATION

Diagnostic aid

AVAILABILITY (Rx)

Injection: 100 mcg lyophylized cake

ACTION / THERAPEUTIC EFFECT

Unknown.

USES

Differentiates pituitary and ectopic production of adrenocorticotropin hormone (ACTH) in patients w/ACTH-dependent Cushing's syndrome.

INDICATIONS / DOSAGE / ROUTES

Differential Dx Cushing syndrome:
IV Infusion: Adults: 1 mcg/kg over 30–60 seconds.

SIDE EFFECTS

OCCASIONAL (16%): Flushing of face, neck, upper chest.

cysteamine bitartrate

sis-**tea**-ah-mean
(Cystagon)

CLASSIFICATION

Urinary tract: Cystine depletor

AVAILABILITY (Rx)

Capsules: 50 mg, 150 mg

ACTION / THERAPEUTIC EFFECT

Cystine-depleting agent, *lowering cystine content of cells in pts w/cystinosis (an autosomal reces-sive inborn error of metabolism:* abnormal transport of cystine out of lysosomes). Nephropathic form (accumulation of cystine, crystal formation) may lead to organ damage (esp. kidney, producing end stage renal failure).

USES

Management of nephropathic cystinosis in adults and children.

INDICATIONS / DOSAGE / ROUTES

Nephropathic cystinosis:
PO: Adults, elderly, children: Initially: maintenance dose gradually increased over 4–6 wks. **Maintenance: Adults, children >12 yrs, >49.5 kg:** 2 g/day in 4 divided doses. **Children (up to 12 yrs):** 1.3 g/m^2/day given in 4 divided doses. **Note:** Do not give intact capsule to children 6 yrs or less. Sprinkle capsule over food.

SIDE EFFECTS

FREQUENT (5–35%): Vomiting, anorexia, fever, diarrhea, lethargy, rash. **OCCASIONAL (1–5%):** Nausea, abdominal pain, dyspepsia, ataxia, confusion, dizziness, nervousness.

daclizumab

day-**cly**-zu-mab
(Zenapax)

CLASSIFICATION

Monoclonal antibody–immunosuppressive

AVAILABILITY (Rx)

Injection: 25 mg/5 ml

ACTION / THERAPEUTIC EFFECT

Binds to and inhibits interleukin-2–mediated lymphocyte activation (critical pathway in cellular immune response involved in allograft rejection), *preventing organ rejection.*

USES

Prophylaxis of acute organ rejection in pts receiving renal transplants.

INDICATIONS/DOSAGE/ROUTES

IV: Adults, children: 1 mg/kg over 15 min. First dose no more than 24 hrs before transplantation, then q14 days for total of 5 doses.

SIDE EFFECTS

OCCASIONAL (>2%): Constipation, nausea, diarrhea, vomiting, abdominal pain, edema, headache, dizziness, fever, pain, fatigue, insomnia, weakness, arthralgia, myalgia, increased sweating.

---

danaparoid

dan-ah-**pair**-oiyd
(Organan)

CLASSIFICATION

Heparinoid (low molecular weight)

AVAILABILITY (Rx)

Injection: 750 units/0.6 ml amps

ACTION/*THERAPEUTIC EFFECT*

Possesses greater antithrombotic activity than anticoagulant activity. Binds to antithrombin III to inactivate factor Xa; activates heparin cofactor II. *Produces anticoagulation.*

USES

Prevention of deep vein thrombosis (DVT) in elective hip surgery.

INDICATIONS/DOSAGE/ROUTES

Prevention of DVT:
SubQ: Adults, elderly: 750 units q12h until risk of DVT has diminished.

SIDE EFFECTS

FREQUENT: Hemorrhage (45%) [serious bleeding: 0–6%], fever (22%), nausea (14%), constipation (11%). **OCCASIONAL:** Pain at injection site, rash, pruritus, peripheral edema, insomnia.

---

delavirdine

dell-ah-**veer**-deen
(Rescriptor)

CLASSIFICATION

Antiviral

AVAILABILITY (Rx)

Tablets: 100 mg, 200 mg

ACTION/*THERAPEUTIC EFFECT*

Inhibits catalytic reaction of HIV reverse transcriptase that is independent of nucleoside binding. *Interrupts HIV replication, slows progression of HIV infection.*

USES

Treatment of HIV infection (in combination with other antivirals).

INDICATIONS/DOSAGE/ROUTES

HIV Infection:
PO: Adults: 200–400 mg 3 times/day on empty stomach.

SIDE EFFECTS

FREQUENT (>2%): Rash. **OCCASIONAL (<2%):** Headache, nausea, diarrhea, fatigue, increased liver enzymes.

denileukin
den-ee-**lew**-kin
(Ontak)

CLASSIFICATION

Biologic response modifier: Antineoplastic

AVAILABILITY (Rx)

Solution for Injection: 150 mcg/ml

ACTION/ *THERAPEUTIC EFFECT*

A cytotoxic fusion protein that targets cells expressing inter-leukin-2 (IL-2) receptors. After binding to IL-2 receptor, directs cytocidal action to malignant cuta-neous T-cell lymphoma (CTCL) cells, *causing inhibition of protein synthesis and cell death.*

USES

Treatment of persistent or recur-rent CTCL whose malignant cells express the CD 25 component of the IL-2 receptor.

INDICATIONS/DOSAGE/ROUTES

CTCL:
IV infusion: Adults: 9 or 18 mcg/kg/day for 5 consecutive days every 21 days. Infuse over at least 15 mins.

SIDE EFFECTS

FREQUENT (>25%): Flu-like symptoms, acute hypersensitivity reactions, nausea, vomiting, infec-tions, vascular leak syndrome characterized by hypotension, edema, hypoalbuminemia, dysp-nea, rash. Asthenia, diarrhea. **OC-CASIONAL (10–25%):** Chest pain, vasodilation, decreased weight, myalgia, rhinitis, pruritus.

dexmedetomidine
decks-mead-eh-**tome**-ih-deen
Precedex)

CLASSIFICATION

Sedative

AVAILABILITY (Rx)

Injection: 100 mcg/ml

ACTION/ *THERAPEUTIC EFFECT*

Selective alpha-2 adrenoceptor agonist.

USES

Sedation of initially intubated and mechanically ventilated adults during treatment in intensive care setting.

INDICATIONS/DOSAGE/ROUTES

Sedation:
IV infusion: Adults: Loading dose of 1 mcg/kg over 10 mins followed by maintenance dose of 0.2–0.7 mcg/kg/hr. Can be continuously infused in mechanically ventilated pt before, during, after extubation. **Note:** Must be diluted with 0.9% NaCl prior to use.

SIDE EFFECTS

FREQUENT: Hypotension (30%), nausea (11%). **OCCASIONAL (<10%):** Bradycardia, atrial fibril-lation, hypoxia, anemia, pain, pleural effusion, pulmonary edema, leukocytosis.

doftilide
doe-**fet**-ill-ide
Tikosyn)

CLASSIFICATION

Anti-arrhythmic: Class III

AVAILABILITY (Rx)

Capsules: 125 mcg, 250 mcg, 500 mcg

ACTION/*THERAPEUTIC EFFECT*

A selective potassium-channel blocker; prolongs repolarization w/o affecting conduction velocity by blocking one or more time-dependent potassium currents. No effect on sodium channels, adrenergic alpha, beta receptors. *Terminates re-entrant tachyarrhythmias, preventing reinduction.*

USES

Maintenance and conversion of normal sinus rhythm (NSR) in pts w/highly symptomatic atrial fibrillation/atrial flutter.

INDICATIONS/DOSAGE/ROUTES

Anti-arrhythmias:
PO: Adults, elderly: Individualized using a seven-step dosing algorithm dependent upon calculated creatinine clearance and QT measurements.

SIDE EFFECTS

OCCASIONAL (<5%): Increased flatulence, loose stools, mild headaches, ventricular tachycardia, most notably torsade de pointes.

---

dolasetron

doe-lah-**sea**-tron
(Anzemet)

CLASSIFICATION

Antiemetic

AVAILABILITY (Rx)

Tablets: 100 mg. Injection: 20 mg/ml.

ACTION/*THERAPEUTIC EFFECT*

Exhibits selective 5-HT3 receptor antagonism for *preventing nausea/vomiting associated w/cancer chemotherapy.* Action may be central (CTZ) or peripheral (vagus nerve terminal).

USES

Prevention of nausea/vomiting associated w/emetogenic cancer chemotherapy, post-operative nausea/vomiting. *(Injection):* Treatment of postoperative nausea/vomiting.

INDICATIONS/DOSAGE/ROUTES

Prevention of cancer chemotherapy-induced nausea/vomiting:
IV: Adults, children (2–16 yrs): 1.8 mg/kg 30 min prior to chemotherapy. **Maximum:** 100 mg for children.
PO: Adults: 100 mg within 1 hr of chemotherapy. Children (2–16 yrs): 1.8 mg/kg within 1 hr of chemotherapy. Maximum: 100 mg.

Treatment/prevention of postoperative nausea/vomiting:
IV: Adults: 12.5 mg. Children (2–16 yrs): 0.35 mg/kg. Maximum: 12.5 mg. (Give approximately 15 min before cessation of anesthesia or as soon as nausea/vomiting present.)
PO: Adults: 100 mg. Children (2–16 yrs.): 1.2 mg/kg. Maximum: 100 mg within 2 hrs of surgery.

SIDE EFFECTS

FREQUENT (6–20%): Headache, diarrhea, fever, fatigue.

---

donepezil

doe-**nep**-ah-zill
(Aricept)

CLASSIFICATION

Cholinergic

AVAILABILITY (Rx)

Tablets: 5 mg, 10 mg

ACTION/ *THERAPEUTIC EFFECT*

Enhances cholinergic function by increasing concentration of acetylcholine by reversible inhibition of its hydrolysis by acetylcholinesterase. *Slows progression of Alzheimer's disease.*

USES

Treatment of mild to moderate Alzheimer's disease.

INDICATIONS/DOSAGE/ROUTES

Alzheimer's disease:
PO: Adults, elderly: 5–10 mg/day as a single dose.

SIDE EFFECTS

FREQUENT (5–10%): Nausea, diarrhea, vomiting, insomnia, muscle cramps, fatigue, anorexia, dizziness. **OCCASIONAL (1–5%):** Headache, pain, syncope, ecchymosis, decreased weight, arthritis, depression, increased urination.

dorzolamide

door-**zoll**-ah-mide
(Trusopt)

CLASSIFICATION

Carbonic anhydrase inhibitor

AVAILABILITY (Rx)

Ophthalmic Solution: 2%

ACTION/ *THERAPEUTIC EFFECT*

Inhibits carbonic anhydrase in ciliary processes of eye, decreasing secretion of aqueous humor. Exact mechanism unknown. May slow formation of bicarbonate ions, reducing sodium and fluid transport. *Decreases intraocular pressure (IOP).*

USES

Treatment of elevated IOP in pts with ocular hypertension or open-angle glaucoma.

INDICATIONS/DOSAGE/ROUTES

Reduction of IOP:
Ophthalmic: Adults, elderly: 1 drop in affected eye 3 times/day.

SIDE EFFECTS

FREQUENT (10–33%): Ocular burning, stinging, discomfort immediately after administration; bitter taste; superficial punctate keratitis; ocular allergic reactions. **OCCASIONAL (10%):** Blurred vision, tearing, dryness, photophobia, headache, nausea, asthenia/fatigue.

doxercalciferol

docks-er-cal-**siff**-err-all
(Hectorol)

CLASSIFICATION

Vitamin D analog: Calcium modifier

AVAILABILITY (Rx)

Capsules: 2.5 mcg

ACTION/ *THERAPEUTIC EFFECT*

Pro-hormone of vitamin D; once activated in the liver *increases intestinal absorption of dietary calcium and renal tubular reabsorption of urinary calcium.* Modulates bone formation/resorption in conjunction w/parathyroid hormone (PTH).

USES

Reduces elevated serum or plasma PTH concentration in management of secondary hyper-parathyroidism in pts w/chronic renal failure undergoing dialysis.

INDICATIONS/DOSAGE/ROUTES

Hyperparathyroidism:
PO: Adults, elderly: 10 mcg 3 times/wk at time of dialysis (before, during, or after) w/o regard to meals. If PTH not lowered by 50% and fails to reach target range of 150–300 pg/ml, may increase dose at 8-wk intervals. **Maximum:** 60 mcg/wk divided into 3 doses at time of dialysis.

SIDE EFFECTS

OCCASIONAL (2–5%): Edema, headache, malaise, nausea, vomiting, dizziness, dyspnea, pruritus, constipation, sleep disorders, hypercalcemia, hyperphosphatemia.

efavirenz

eh-fah-**vir**-enz
(Sustiva)

CLASSIFICATION

Antiviral

AVAILABILITY (Rx)

Capsules: 50 mg, 100 mg, 200 mg

ACTION/*THERAPEUTIC EFFECT*

Inhibits activity of HIV reverse transcriptase (RT) of human immunodeficiency virus type 1 (HIV-1). *Interrupts HIV replication, slowing progression of HIV infection.*

USES

Treatment of HIV infection in combination with other appropriate anti-retroviral agents.

INDICATIONS/DOSAGE/ROUTES

HIV infection:
PO: Adults, elderly: 600 mg once daily in combination. Bedtime dosing is recommended during first 2–4 wks (due to temporary nervous system side effects). **Children >3 yrs, 88 lbs:** 600 mg once daily; **71.5–88 lbs:** 400 mg once daily; **55–71.5 lbs:** 350 mg once daily; **44–55 lbs:** 300 mg once daily; **33–44 lbs:** 250 mg once daily; **22–33 lbs:** 200 mg once daily.

SIDE EFFECTS

FREQUENT (>28%): Dizziness, abnormal dreaming, insomnia, confusion, abnormal thinking, impaired concentration, amnesia, agitation, depersonalization, hallucinations, euphoria. OCCASIONAL (<28%): Maculopapular rash, mild to moderate degree, nausea, fatigue, headache, diarrhea, fever, cough.

emedastine

em-eh-**das**-teen
(Emadine)

CLASSIFICATION

Antiallergic

AVAILABILITY (Rx)

Ophthalmic Solution: 0.05%

ACTION/*THERAPEUTIC EFFECT*

Selective H_2 receptor antagonist. Blocks histamine release from mast cells. *Reduces symptoms of allergic conjunctivitis.*

USES

Treatment of signs/symptoms of allergic rhinitis, conjunctivitis.

INDICATIONS/DOSAGE/ROUTES

Usual ophthalmic dosage:
Adults: 1–2 drops 2 times/day.

SIDE EFFECTS

FREQUENT: Headache (7%). **OC-CASIONAL (<5%):** Burning/stinging, dry eyes, foreign body sensation, hyperemia, keratitis, lid edema, pruritus, asthenia, cold syndrome, pharyngitis, rhinitis, sinusitis, taste perversion.

entacapone

en-tah-cah-**pone**
(Comtan)

CLASSIFICATION

Anti-Parkinson agent

AVAILABILITY (Rx)

Tablets: 200 mg

ACTION/*THERAPEUTIC EFFECT*

Inhibits enzyme COMT, potentiating dopamine activity. *Increases duration of action of levodopa doses,* decreasing daily levodopa requirements.

USES

In conjunction w/levodopa, improves quality of life in pts w/Parkinson's disease.

INDICATIONS/DOSAGE/ROUTES

Parkinson's disease:
PO: Adults, elderly: 200 mg/day.

SIDE EFFECTS

FREQUENT: Dyskinesia, hyperkinesia, nausea, urine discoloration (dark yellow or orange), diarrhea, abdominal pain, vomiting, dizziness, orthostatic hypotension, falls, shortness of breath, ataxia, fatigue, constipation, hallucinations.

epirubicin

eh-pea-**rew**-bih-sin
(Ellence)

CLASSIFICATION

Antineoplastic

AVAILABILITY (Rx)

Injection: 2 mg/ml single-use vial

ACTION/*THERAPEUTIC EFFECT*

Exact mechanism unknown but may include formation of a complex w/DNA by intercalation of its planar rings w/consequent inhibition of DNA, RNA, protein synthesis; inhibits DNA helicase activity, preventing enzymatic separation of double-stranded DNA and interfering w/replication and transcription. *Possesses antiproliferative and cytotoxic activity.*

USES/*UNLABELED*

Component of adjuvant therapy in pts w/evidence of axillary node tumor involvement following resection of primary breast cancer. *Lung, ovarian carcinoma, non-Hodgkin's lymphoma, sarcomas.*

INDICATIONS/DOSAGE/ROUTES

Breast cancer:
IV infusion: Adults: (In combination w/5-FU and Cytoxan). Initially, 100–120 mg/m^2 in repeated cycles of 3–4 wks. Total dose may be given day 1 of each cycle or divided equally on days 1 and 8 of each cycle.
Note: Dosage adjustment for pts

w/bone marrow, liver dysfunction, and hematologic toxicities.

SIDE EFFECTS

Note: Irreversible damage to heart muscle may occur. Risk increased w/total cumulative dose in excess of 900 mg/m^2.
FREQUENT: Nausea, diarrhea, vomiting, stomatitis, hair loss, mouth sores, myelosuppression.
OCCASIONAL: Anorexia, infection, conjunctivitis, rash, pruritus.

eprosartan

ee-pro-**sar**-tan
(Teveten)

CLASSIFICATION

Angiotensin II receptor antagonist

AVAILABILITY (Rx)

Tablets: 200 mg

ACTION/ *THERAPEUTIC EFFECT*

Potent vasodilator. An angiotensin II receptor (type AT1) antagonist: blocks vasoconstrictor and aldosterone-secreting effects of angiotensin II, inhibiting the binding of angiotensin II to the AT1 receptors, *causing vasodilation, decreased peripheral resistance, decrease in B/P.*

USES

Treatment of hypertension.

INDICATIONS/DOSAGE/ROUTES

Hypertension:
PO: Adults, elderly: Initially, 200 mg/day. **Range:** 400–600 mg/day.

SIDE EFFECTS

OCCASIONAL: Cough, upper respiratory infection, dizziness, diarrhea. **RARE:** Back pain, sinusitis, dyspepsia, insomnia.

eptifibatide

ep-tih-**fye**-bah-tide
(Integrilin)

CLASSIFICATION

Antiplatelet, antithrombotic

AVAILABILITY (Rx)

Injection: 0.75 mg/ml, 2 mg/ml

ACTION/ *THERAPEUTIC EFFECT*

Produces rapid inhibition of platelet aggregation by preventing binding of fibrinogen to receptor sites on platelets. *Prevents closure of treated coronary arteries. Prevents acute cardiac ischemic complications.*

USES

Treatment of pts w/acute coronary syndrome (ACS), including those managed medically and those undergoing percutaneous coronary intervention (PCI).

INDICATIONS/DOSAGE/ROUTES

Adjunct PCI:
IV Bolus/IV Infusion: Adults, elderly: 135 mcg/kg bolus over 1–2 min, then infusion of 0.5 mcg/kg/min for 20–24 hrs

ACS:
IV Bolus/IV Infusion: Adults, elderly: 180 mcg/kg bolus then 2 mcg/kg/min until discharge or CABG, up to 72 hrs.

SIDE EFFECTS

FREQUENT (>5%): Bleeding, GI bleeding, hematuria, hematemesis. **OCCASIONAL (1–5%):** Hypotension. **RARE (<1%):** Stroke, anaphylactic shock.

etanercept

ee-**tan**-er-cept
(Enbrel)

CLASSIFICATION

Anti-arthritic

AVAILABILITY (Rx)

Powder for Injection: 25 mg

ACTION/*THERAPEUTIC EFFECT*

Binds to tumor necrosis factor (TNF), blocking its interaction with cell surface receptors (TNFR). (TNF is involved in inflammatory and immune responses; elevated TNF is found in synovial fluid of rheumatoid arthritis patients.)

USES

Reduction of signs and symptoms of moderate to severe active rheumatoid arthritis (RA).

INDICATIONS/ROUTES/DOSAGE

Rheumatoid arthritis:
SubQ: Adults, elderly: 25 mg twice weekly. **Children (4–17 yrs):** 0.4 mg/kg twice weekly. **Maximum:** 25 mg/dose.

SIDE EFFECTS

FREQUENT (>16%): Injection-site reaction (erythema, itching, pain, swelling), abdominal pain, vomiting (incidence higher in children), infection, including upper respiratory tract. **OCCASIONAL (4–16%):** Headache, rhinitis, dizziness, pharyngitis, cough, asthenia, dyspepsia. **RARE (<4%):** Sinusitis, allergic reactions, heart failure, hypertension, hypotension, pancreatitis, GI hemorrhage, dyspnea.

exemestane

x-eh-**mess**-tane
(Aromasin)

CLASSIFICATION

Antineoplastic: Hormone

AVAILABILITY (Rx)

Tablets: 25 mg

ACTION/*THERAPEUTIC EFFECT*

An irreversible, steroidal aromatase inactivator (aromatase is the principal enzyme that converts androgens to estrogens in both pre- and postmenopausal women); acts as false substrate for aromatase enzyme; binds irreversibly to active site of enzyme, causing its inactivation. *Significantly lowers circulating estrogen concentration in postmenopausal women.*

USES/*UNLABELED*

Treatment of advanced breast cancer in postmenopausal women whose disease has progressed following tamoxifen therapy. *Prevention of prostate cancer.*

INDICATIONS/DOSAGE/ROUTES

Breast cancer:
PO: Adults, elderly: 25 mg once daily after a meal.

SIDE EFFECTS

FREQUENT (10–25%): Depression, insomnia, anxiety, nausea, dyspnea, fatigue, hot flashes, pain. **OCCASIONAL (2–10%):** Headache, dizziness, vomiting, constipation, anorexia, diarrhea, increased appetite, cough, edema, flu-like symptoms, fever, weakness, confusion, arthralgia, pain (abdominal, back, skeletal), infection, dyspepsia, pharyngitis, rhinitis, alopecia.

fenofibrate

fen-oh-**figh**-brate
(Tricor)

CLASSIFICATION

Antihyperlipidemic

AVAILABILITY (Rx)

Capsules: 67 mg

ACTION/*THERAPEUTIC EFFECT*

Reduces very low-density lipoprotein (VLDL) and stimulates the catabolism of triglyceride-rich lipoprotein. *Decreases plasma triglycerides, cholesterol.* Reduces serum uric acid levels *by increasing urinary excretion of uric acid.*

USES

Adjunct to diet therapy in adult pts w/very high elevations of serum triglyceride levels who are at risk of pancreatitis and who do not respond adequately to a determined dietary effort to control triglyceride levels.

INDICATIONS/DOSAGE/ROUTES

Hyperlipidemia:
PO: Adults, renal function impairment (Ccr <50 ml/min): Initially, 67 mg/day w/meals. **Maximum:** 3 capsules (201 mg)/day. **Elderly:** Limit dosage to 67 mg/day.

SIDE EFFECTS

FREQUENT (4–8%): Pain, rash, headache, asthenia/fatigue, flu syndrome, dyspepsia, nausea, vomiting, rhinitis. OCCASIONAL (2–3%): Diarrhea, abdominal pain, constipation, flatulence, arthralgia, decreased libido, dizziness, pruritus. RARE (<2%): Increased appetite, insomnia, polyuria, cough, blurred vision, eye floater, earache, pancre-atitis, hepatitis, thrombocytopenia, agranulocytosis.

fenoldopam

phen-**ole**-doe-pam
(Corlopam)

CLASSIFICATION

Antihypertensive

AVAILABILITY (Rx)

Injection: 10 mg/ml ampule.

ACTION/*THERAPEUTIC EFFECT*

Dopamine reception agonist, *decreasing B/P.* Rapid-acting vasodilator.

USES

Short-term (up to 48 hrs) management of severe hypertension.

INDICATIONS/DOSAGE/ROUTES

Hypertension:
IV Infusion (continuous): Adults: 0.01–0.3 mcg/kg/min (without use of bolus injection). **Must be diluted.**

SIDE EFFECTS

FREQUENT: Headache (4–8%), flushing (3%), nausea (3–5%), hypotension (2%). OCCASIONAL (0–2%): Injection site reactions, vomiting, diarrhea, constipation, dizziness. **Note:** Avoid beta blockers (may cause unexpected hypotension).

follitropin alpha

fole-ee-**trow**-pin
(Gonal-F)

CLASSIFICATION

Gonadotropin

AVAILABILITY (Rx)

Powder for Injection: 75 IU, 150 IU

ACTION/*THERAPEUTIC EFFECT*

Human follicle-stimulating hormone, *stimulation of ovarian follicular growth.*

USES

Ovulation stimulation, follicle stimulation.

INDICATIONS/DOSAGE/ROUTES

Ovulation induction:
SubQ: Adults: 75 IU/day. Incremental dosage adjustment up to 37.5 IU/day may be considered after 14 days; similar adjustments if needed every 7 days thereafter.

Follicle stimulation:
SubQ: Adults: 150 IU/day (until sufficient follicular development is attained, usually not to exceed 10 days).

SIDE EFFECTS

OCCASIONAL: Ovarian hyperstimulation, adnexal torsion, mild to moderate ovarian enlargement, abdominal pain, ovarian cysts, nausea, vomiting, diarrhea, abdominal cramps, pain, rash, swelling or irritation at injection site.

ACTION/*THERAPEUTIC EFFECT*

Inhibits protein synthesis. *Prevents human cytomegalovirus (CMV) replication.*

USES

Treatment of cytomegalovirus (CMV) retinitis in pts w/acquired immunodeficiency syndrome (AIDS).

INDICATIONS/DOSAGE/ROUTES

Cytomegalovirus (CMV) retinitis:
Intravitreal (Ophthalmic): Adults, elderly: 330 mcg (0.05 ml/eye) as a single intravitreal injection every other week for 2 doses. Maintenance: 330 mcg (0.05 ml/eye) once every 4 weeks.

SIDE EFFECTS

FREQUENT (25%): Ocular inflammation (uveitis), including iritis and vitritis. OCCASIONAL (5–20%): Abnormal vision, blurred vision, cataract, decreased visual acuity, eye pain, floaters, photophobia, abdominal pain, asthenia, diarrhea, fever, headache, nausea, rash, sinusitis, vomiting, increased intraocular pressure (IOP), conjunctival bleeding, retinal detachment, retinal edema, retinal pigment changes, abnormal liver function. RARE (2–5%): Conjunctivitis, decreased peripheral vision, eye irritation, application site reaction.

fomvirsen sodium

foam-ih-**vir**-sen
(Vitravene)

CLASSIFICATION

Antiviral

AVAILABILITY (Rx)

Injection: 6.6 mg/ml

fosfomycin

foss-foe-**my**-sin
(Monurol)

CLASSIFICATION

Antibiotic

AVAILABILITY (Rx)

Powder: 3 g

ACTION/*THERAPEUTIC EFFECT*

Inhibits the synthesis of peptido-glycan, the initial step in bacterial cell wall synthesis. *Antibacterial.*

USES

Single-dose treatment for un-complicated urinary tract infections (UTI) in women.

INDICATIONS/DOSAGE/ROUTES

UTI:
PO: Adults, elderly: 3 g mixed in water as a single dose.

SIDE EFFECTS

OCCASIONAL (1–10%): Diarrhea, nausea, vomiting, epigastric discomfort, anorexia, headache, dizziness, fatigue, drowsiness.

ganirelix
gan-ih-**rea**-licks
(Antagon)

CLASSIFICATION

Gonadotropin-releasing hormone (GnRH) antagonist

AVAILABILITY (Rx)

Injection: 250 mcg/0.5 ml syringe

ACTION/*THERAPEUTIC EFFECT*

An analog of naturally occurring gonadotropin-releasing hormone, ganirelix is a GnRH antagonist. Competitively blocks GnRH receptors, inducing rapid, reversible suppression of gonadotropin (FSH and LH) secretion. *Prevents LH surges associated w/ovarian stimulation, improving implantation and pregnancy rates.*

USES

Prevention of premature LH surges in women undergoing ovarian hyperstimulation.

INDICATIONS/DOSAGE/ROUTES

Prevention of LH surges:
SubQ: Adults: 250 mcg daily during early–mid-follicular phase of menstrual cycle; continue until adequate follicular response achieved. (Begin FSH on day 2 or 3 of menstrual cycle, ganirelix on day 7 or 8; discontinue and start hCG when adequate follicular response achieved.)

SIDE EFFECTS

OCCASIONAL (1–5%): Headache, abdominal pain, ovarian hyperstimulation syndrome, vaginal bleeding, nausea, injection site reaction.

gatifloxacin
gat-ih-**flocks**-ah-sin
(Tequin)

CLASSIFICATION

Anti-infective: Quinolone

AVAILABILITY (Rx)

Tablets: 200 mg, 400 mg. **Injection:** 200 mg, 400 mg vials.

ACTION/*THERAPEUTIC EFFECT*

Inhibits DNA enzyme in susceptible micro-organisms, *interfering w/bacterial DNA replication.* Bactericidal.

USES

Treatment of community-acquired pneumonia (CAP), sinusitis, acute bacterial exacerbation of chronic bronchitis, urinary tract infections (UTI), gonorrhea.

INDICATIONS/DOSAGE/ROUTES

CAP:
PO/IV: Adults, elderly: 400 mg/day for 7–14 days.

Acute bacterial exacerbation of chronic bronchitis:
PO/IV: Adults, elderly: 400 mg/day for 7–10 days.

Sinusitis:
PO/IV: Adults, elderly: 400 mg/day for 10 days.

UTI:
PO/IV: Adults, elderly: 200 mg 2 times/day for 7 days.

Gonorrhea:
PO: Adults: 400 mg as single dose.

SIDE EFFECTS

FREQUENT (5–10%): Nausea.
OCCASIONAL (1–5%): Diarrhea, headache, dizziness, vaginitis.

glatiramer
glah-**tie**-rah-mir
(Copaxone)

CLASSIFICATION

Neurologic agent

AVAILABILITY (Rx)

Injection: 20 mg/ml

ACTION/*THERAPEUTIC EFFECT*

Exact mechanism unknown. May act as a decoy to locally generated autoantibodies that are thus neutralized before causing tissue damage. *Relieves symptoms of multiple sclerosis.*

USES

Treatment of relapsing, remitting multiple sclerosis.

INDICATIONS/DOSAGE/ROUTES

Multiple sclerosis:
SubQ: Adults, elderly: 20 mg once daily.

SIDE EFFECTS

FREQUENT (>20%): Flushing, chest pain, palpitations, anxiety, dyspnea, urticaria, constriction of the throat, injection site reaction, flulike symptoms.

hepatitis A vaccine
(Havrix, Vaqta)

USES

Active immunization of persons >2yrs against disease caused by hepatitis A virus.

DOSAGE

IM: Adults (>18 yrs): Havrix: 1440 ELU, Vaqta: 50 U. Children (2–18 yrs): Havrix: 720 ELU, Vaqta: 25 U. Booster shot varies from 6 to 18 months (provides persistent antibody concentration).

CONTRAINDICATIONS

Hypersensitivity to any component of the vaccine.

SIDE EFFECTS

OCCASIONAL (1–10%): Injection site soreness, pain, tenderness, induration, redness, swelling, fatigue, fever, malaise, nausea, anorexia, headache.

hepaptis B immune globulin (Human)
(Nabi-HB)

CLASSIFICATION

Immunization agent

AVAILABILITY (Rx)

Injection: 5 ml vial

ACTION/*THERAPEUTIC EFFECT*

Immune globulin of inactivated hepatitis B virus, *providing passive immunization against hepatitis B virus.*

USES

Treatment of acute exposure to blood containing hepatitis B surface antigen (HbsAg), prenatal exposure of infants born to HbsAg-positive mothers, sexual exposure to HbsAg-positive partners, household exposure to those w/acute hepatitis B virus infection.

INDICATIONS/DOSAGE/ROUTES

Acute exposure:
IM: 0.06 ml/kg, ideally within 24 hrs.
Infants born to HbsAg-positive mothers:
IM: 0.5 ml, ideally within 12 hrs of birth.
Sexual exposure:
IM: 0.06 ml/kg within 14 days of last sexual contact or if sexual contact is to continue.
Household exposure:
IM: 0.5 ml.

SIDE EFFECTS

FREQUENT: Headache (26%), local pain (12%). **OCCASIONAL (5%):** Malaise, nausea, myalgia.

hyaluronate sodium
hi-al-**your**-on-ate
(Hyalgan, Synvisc)

CLASSIFICATON

Hyaluronic acid derivative

AVAILABILITY (Rx)

Solution: 20 mg/2 ml, 16 mg/2 ml

ACTION/*THERAPEUTIC EFFECT*

Naturally occurring; maintains viscosity of synovial fluid, supports lubricating/shock-absorbing properties of auricular cartilage.

USES

Treatment of pain associated with osteoarthritis of the knee.

INDICATIONS/DOSAGE/ROUTES

Osteoarthritis:
INTRA-ARTICULAR: Adults: *Hyalgan:* 5 injections/treatment cycle. Synvisc: 3 injections/treatment cycle.

SIDE EFFECTS

OCCASIONAL: *Hyalgan* (7–23%): Injection-site pain, skin reaction (ecchymosis, rash), pruritus, headache. *Synvisc* (1–3%): Knee pain/swelling, rash, pruritus, calf cramps, muscle pain.

imiglucerase
im-ih-**gloo**-sir-ace
(Cerezyme)

CLASSIFICATION

Enzyme

AVAILABILITY (Rx)

Powder for Injection: 200 units

ACTION/*THERAPEUTIC EFFECT*

Analogue of enzyme beta-glucocerebrosidase, which catalyzes hydrolysis of glycolipid glucocerebroside to glucose and ceramide. *Minimizes conditions (e.g., anemia, bone disease) associated w/Gaucher's disease.*

USES

Treatment of Gaucher's disease (characterized by deficiency of beta-glucocerebrosidase activity) results in accumulation of glucocerebrosidase in tissue macrophages becoming engorged. Secondary hematologic sequelae include severe anemia, thrombocytopenia, progressive hepatosplenomegaly, skeletal complications.

INDICATIONS/DOSAGE/ROUTES

Gaucher's disease:
IV Infusion (over 1–2 hrs): Adults, elderly, children: Initially, 2.5 units/kg 3 times/wk up to 60 units/kg/wk. **Maintenance:** Progressive reduction in dosage while monitoring pt response.

SIDE EFFECTS

FREQUENT (3%): Headache. **OCCASIONAL (1–3%):** Nausea, abdominal discomfort, dizziness, pruritus, rash, small decrease in B/P or urinary frequency.

imiquimod
im-**ee**-kwee-mod
(Aldara)

CLASSIFICATION

Immune response modifier

AVAILABILITY (Rx)

Cream: 5%

ACTION/*THERAPEUTIC EFFECT*

Mechanism unknown.

USES

Treatment of external genital and perianal warts/condyloma acuminata in adults.

INDICATIONS/DOSAGE/ROUTES

Warts/condyloma acuminata:
PO: Adults: Apply 3 times/wk before normal sleeping hours; leave on skin 6–10 hrs. Remove following treatment period. Continue therapy for maximum of 16 weeks.

SIDE EFFECTS

FREQUENT: Local skin reactions: erythema (61%), itching (32%), burning (26%), erosion (30%), excoriation /flaking (20%), fungal infections (women) 11%. **OCCASIONAL (3–8%):** Pain, induration, ulceration, scabbing, soreness, headache, flulike symptoms.

infliximab
inn-**flicks**-ih-mab
(Remicade)

CLASSIFICATION

Monoclonal antibody

AVAILABILITY (Rx)

Injection

ACTION/*THERAPEUTIC EFFECT*

Blocks tumor necrosis factor, slowing inflammation.

USES

Treatment of Crohn's disease, rheumatoid arthritis in combination w/methotrexate.

INDICATIONS/DOSAGE/ROUTES

Crohn's disease:
IV Infusion: Adults, elderly: 5 mg/kg.

Rheumatoid arthritis:
IV Infusion: Adults, elderly: 3 mg/kg; repeat at 2 and 6 wks then q8wks.

SIDE EFFECTS

FREQUENT (10–25%): Headache, nausea, upper respiratory tract infection, abdominal pain, fatigue, fever. **OCCASIONAL (5–10%):** Pain, vomiting, dizziness, rash, pharyngitis.

interferon alfacon-1

inn-ter-**fear**-on
(Infergen)

CLASSIFICATION

Antiviral

AVAILABILITY (Rx)

Injection: 15 mcg vials, 9 mcg vials

ACTION/*THERAPEUTIC EFFECT*

Stimulates immune system, *inhibiting hepatitis C virus.*

USES

Treatment of chronic hepatitis C viral (HCV) infections in patients w/compensated liver disease who have anti-HCV serum antibodies and/or presence of HCV RNA.

INDICATIONS/DOSAGE/ROUTES

Hepatits C:
SubQ: Adults: 9 mcg 3 times/wk for 24 weeks. May increase to 15 mcg in patients tolerating 9 mcg dose and not responding adequately. **Note:** At least 48 hrs should elapse between doses.

SIDE EFFECTS

FREQUENT (>50%): Headache, fatigue, fever, depression.

interferon alfa-n1

inn-ter-**fear**-on
(Wellferon)

CLASSIFICATION

Interferon

AVAILABILITY (Rx)

Injection

ACTION/*THERAPEUTIC EFFECT*

Stimulates immune system, *inhibiting hepatitis C virus.*

USE

Treatment of chronic hepatitis C in adults w/o decompensated liver disease.

INDICATIONS/DOSAGE/ROUTES

Chronic hepatitis C:
IM/SC: Adults: 3 million units 3 times/wk for 12 mos. Reduce dose by 50% if pt cannot tolerate until symptoms resolve.

SIDE EFFECTS

FREQUENT: Asthenia (62%), headache (52%), fever (43%). **OCCASIONAL (5%):** Neutropenia, hyperglycemia, thrombocytopenia, increased creatinine, thyroid test abnormalities.

irbesartan

ir-beh-**sar**-tan
(Avapro)

CLASSIFICATION

Angiotensin II receptor antagonist

AVAILABILITY (Rx)

Tablets: 75 mg, 150 mg, 300 mg

ACTION/*THERAPEUTIC EFFECT*

Potent vasodilator. An angiotensin II receptor (type AT1) antagonist: blocks vasoconstrictor and aldosterone-secreting effects of angiotensin II, inhibiting the binding of angiotensin II to the AT1 receptors, *causing vasodilation, decreased peripheral resistance, decrease in B/P.*

USES

Treatment of hypertension alone or in combination with other antihypertensives.

INDICATIONS/DOSAGE/ROUTES

Hypertension:
PO: Adults: Initially, 150 mg once daily. May increase up to 300 mg once daily.

SIDE EFFECTS

OCCASIONAL: Upper respiratory infections (9%), fatigue (4%), diarrhea (3%).

ivermectin

eye-ver-**meck**-tin
(Stromectol)

CLASSIFICATION

Antihelmintic

AVAILABILITY (Rx)

Tablets: 6 mg.

ACTION/*THERAPEUTIC EFFECT*

Selectively binds to chloride ion channels in invertebrate nerve/muscle cells, increasing permeability to chloride ions. *Causes paralysis/death of parasite.*

USES

Treatment of intestinal strongyloidiasis and onchocerciasis.

INDICATIONS/DOSAGE/ROUTES

Strongyloidiasis:
PO: Adults: 200 mcg/kg as a single dose.

Onchocerciasis:
PO: Adults: 150 mcg/kg as single dose at 3–12 month intervals.

SIDE EFFECTS

OCCASIONAL: *(strongyloidiasis):* Dizziness (2.8%), pruritus (2.8%), diarrhea (1.8%); nausea (1.8%). *(onchocerciasis):* Tachycardia (3.5%), peripheral edema (3.2%), facial edema (1.2%), orthostatic hypotension (1.1%).

ketotifen

key-**tow**-tih-fen
(Zaditor)

CLASSIFICATION

Antiallergic

AVAILABILITY (Rx)

Ophthalmic Solution: 0.025%

ACTION/*THERAPEUTIC EFFECT*

Selective histamine H1-antagonist and mast cell stabilizer, suppresses release of mediators from cells involved in hypersensitivity reactions, decreases chemotoxis and activation of eosinophils. *Reduces symptoms of allergic conjunctivitis.*

USES

Temporary relief of itching of the eye due to allergic conjunctivitis.

INDICATIONS/DOSAGE/ROUTES

Allergic conjunctivitis:
Ophthalmic: Adults, elderly, children >3 yrs: 1 drop in affected eye q8–12 hrs.

SIDE EFFECTS

FREQUENT (10–25%): Conjunctival infection, headache, rhinitis. **OCCASIONAL (1–5%):** Allergic reaction, burning, stinging, eyelid disorder, flu-like syndrome, keratitis, mydriasis, ocular discharge/pain, pharyngitis, photophobia, rash, xerophthalmia.

leflunomide

lee-**flew**-no-mide
(Arava)

CLASSIFICATION

Immunomodulatory agent

AVAILABILITY (Rx)

Tablets: 10 mg, 20 mg

ACTION/*THERAPEUTIC EFFECT*

Attenuates the immune response exhibited in rheumatoid synovium. Hinders proliferation of lymphocytes. *Possesses anti-inflammatory action, reducing signs and symptoms of rheumatoid arthritis and retarding structural damage.*

USES

Treatment of active rheumatoid arthritis.

INDICATIONS/DOSAGE/ROUTES

Rheumatoid arthritis:
PO: Adults, elderly: Initially, 100 mg daily for 3 days, then 10–20 mg/day.

SIDE EFFECTS

FREQUENT (10–20%): Diarrhea, respiratory tract infections, hair loss, rash, nausea. **RARE:** Transient thrombocytopenia, leukopenia.

lepirudin

leh-**pier**-ruh-din
(Refludan)

CLASSIFICATION

Anticoagulant

AVAILABILITY (Rx)

Powder for Injection: 50 mg

ACTION/*THERAPEUTIC EFFECT*

Inhibits thrombogenic action of thrombin, *producing an increase in activated partial thromboplastin time (APTT).* Action independent of antithrombin II and not inhibited by platelet factor 4.

USES

Anticoagulant in pts w/heparin-induced thrombocytopenia and associated thromboembolic disease to prevent further thromboembolic complications.

INDICATIONS/DOSAGE/ROUTES

Note: Give initial dose as soon as possible after surgery but not more than 24 hrs after surgery.

Anticoagulant:
IV/IV Infusion: Adults, elderly: 0.2–0.4 mg/kg, IV slowly over 15–20 sec, followed by IV infusion of 0.15 mg/kg/hr for 2–10 days or longer.

SIDE EFFECTS

FREQUENT (>10%): Bleeding complications (e.g., bleeding from puncture sites/wound), hematoma. **OCCASIONAL (1–10%):** Allergic reaction (rash, itching), unusual tiredness, blood in urine, GI/rectal bleeding, nosebleed, vaginal bleeding, fever, swelling of feet or lower legs, pneumonia.

letrozole

leh-troe-zoll
(Femara)

CLASSIFICATION

Aromatase inhibitor

AVAILABILITY (Rx)

Tablets: 2.5 mg

ACTION/*THERAPEUTIC EFFECT*

Suppresses estrogen biosynthesis in peripheral tissue and cancer tissue by inhibiting enzyme aromatase.

USES

Treatment of advanced breast cancer in postmenopausal women whose disease progressed after antiestrogen therapy.

INDICATIONS/DOSAGE/ROUTES

Breast cancer:
PO: Adults, elderly: 2.5 mg daily. Continue until tumor progression is evident.

SIDE EFFECTS

FREQUENT: Musculoskeletal effects: skeletal pain, back, arm, leg pain (21%); nausea (13%), headache (9%), fatigue (8%), constipation (8%), arthralgia (8%), vomiting (7%), dyspnea (7%).

levetiracetam

leave-ty-rah-**see**-tam
(Keppra)

CLASSIFICATION

Anticonvulsant

AVAILABILITY (Rx)

Tablets: 250 mg, 500 mg, 750 mg

ACTION/*THERAPEUTIC EFFECT*

Exact mechanism unknown at time of writing. Unrelated to other anticonvulsants.

USES

Adjunctive therapy in treatment of partial onset seizures in adults w/epilepsy.

INDICATIONS/DOSAGE/ROUTES

Partial onset seizures:
PO: Adults, elderly: Initially, 500 mg q12hrs. May increase by 1,000 mg/day every 2 wks. **Maximum:** 3,000 mg/day.

Dosage in renal impairment:

CREATININE CLEARANCE (ML/MIN)	DOSAGE
80	500–1500 mg q12hrs
50–80	500–1000 mg q12hrs
30–50	250–750 mg q12hrs
<30	250–500 mg q12hrs
ESRD using dialysis	500–1000 mg q12hrs (following dialysis, a 250–500 mg supplemental dose is recommended.

SIDE EFFECTS

FREQUENT (10–15%): Somnolence, asthenia, headache, infection. **OCCASIONAL (3–10%):** Dizziness, pharyngitis, pain, depression, nervousness, vertigo, rhinitis, anorexia. **RARE (<3%):** Amnesia, anxiety, emotional lability, increased cough, sinusitis, anorexia, diplopia.

levofloxacin

lee-voe-**flocks**-ah-sin
(Levaquin)

CLASSIFICATION

Antibiotic: fluoroquinolones

AVAILABILITY (Rx)

Tablets: 250 mg, 500 mg. **Injection:** 500 mg/20 ml vials.

ACTION / *THERAPEUTIC EFFECT*

Inhibits DNA enzyme in susceptible microorganisms, *interfering w/bacterial DNA replication.* Bactericidal.

USES

Treatment of respiratory infections including pneumonia, bronchitis, sinusitis. Treatment of skin, skin structure, kidney, and urinary tract infections.

INDICATIONS/DOSAGE/ROUTES

Usual dosage:
PO/IV: Adults, elderly: 250–500 mg/day as a single dose for 7–14 days.

SIDE EFFECTS

FREQUENT (2–5%): Dizziness, lightheadedness, headache, insomnia/drowsiness, nausea, vomiting, diarrhea, stomach pain/discomfort. **OCCASIONAL (<2%):** Increased sensitivity of skin to sunlight.

---

loteprednol

low-teh-**pred**-noll
(Lotemax)

CLASSIFICATION

Glucocorticoid

AVAILABILITY (Rx)

Ophthalmic Suspension: 0.2%, 0.5%

ACTION / *THERAPEUTIC EFFECT*

Inhibits accumulation of inflammatory cells at inflammation sites, phagocytosis, lysosomal enzyme release and synthesis and/or release of mediators of inflammation. *Prevents/suppresses cell and tissue immune reactions, inflammatory process.*

USES

Treatment of seasonal allergic conjunctivitis, giant papillary conjunctivitis, ureitis.

INDICATIONS/DOSAGE/ROUTES

Usual ophthalmic dosage:
Adults: 1 drop 4 times/day for 4–6 weeks.

SIDE EFFECTS

FREQUENT: Blurred vision. **OCCASIONAL:** Decreased vision, watering of eyes, eye pain, nausea, vomiting, burning, stinging, redness of eyes.
Note: Metabolized by enzymes in the eye, minimizing systemic adverse effects.

---

mequinol/tretinoin

meh-**kwin**-oll/tret-**inn**-won
(Solage)

CLASSIFICATION

Depigmenting agent

AVAILABILITY RX)

Topical Solution

ACTION / *THERAPEUTIC EFFECT*

Exact mechanism unknown.

USES

Adjunct to a comprehensive skin care and sun avoidance program in treatment of solar lentigines (SL).

INDICATIONS/DOSAGE/ROUTES

SL:
Topical: Adults: Apply twice daily (morning and evening at least 8 hrs apart).

SIDE EFFECTS

FREQUENT: Erythema (49%), burning, stinging, tingling (26%), desquamation (14%), pruritus (12%). **OCCASIONAL:** Hypopigmentation (7%).

midodrine

my-doe-dreen
(ProAmatine)

CLASSIFICATION

Vasopressor

AVAILABILITY (Rx)

Tablets: 2.5 mg, 5 mg

ACTION/*THERAPEUTIC EFFECT*

Prodrug forms active metabolite desglymidodrine, which is an alpha-1 agonist activating alpha receptors of arteriolar and venous vasculature. *Increases vascular tone, B/P.*

USES

Treatment of symptomatic orthostatic hypotension.

INDICATIONS/DOSAGE/ROUTES

Orthostatic hypotension:
PO: Adults, elderly: 10 mg 3 times/day. Give during day when patient is upright (upon arising, midday, late afternoon not later than 6 PM).

SIDE EFFECTS

FREQUENT (7–20%): Paresthesia, piloerection, pruritus, dysuria, supine hypertension. **OCCASIONAL (1–7%):** Pain, rash, chills, headache, facial flushing, confusion, dry mouth, anxiety.

miglitol

mig-lih-toll
(Glyset)

CLASSIFICATION

Antidiabetic

AVAILABILITY (Rx)

Tablets: 25 mg, 50 mg

ACTION/*THERAPEUTIC EFFECT*

An oral alpha-glucosidase inhibitor that delays the digestion of ingested carbohydrates into simple sugars such as glucose. *Produces smaller rise in blood glucose concentration following meals.*

USES

Treatment of type II noninsulin-dependent diabetes mellitus.

INDICATIONS/DOSAGE/ROUTES

Antidiabetic:
PO: Adults, elderly: Initially, 25 mg 3 times/day (w/first bite of each main meal). **Maintenance:** 50 mg 3 times/day. **Maximum:** 100 mg 3 times/day.

SIDE EFFECTS

FREQUENT (10–40%): Flatulence, soft stools, diarrhea, abdominal pain. **OCCASIONAL (5%):** Rash.

modafinil

moe-**dah**-fin-ill
(Provigil)

CLASSIFICATION

Alpha-1 agonist: neurologic agent

AVAILABILITY (Rx)

Tablets: 100 mg, 200 mg

ACTION/*THERAPEUTIC EFFECT*

Binds to dopamine re-uptake carrier site, increasing alpha activity and decreasing delta, theta, and beta activity. *Reduces the number of daytime sleepiness episodes and the duration of total daytime sleep time.*

USES

Treatment of excessive daytime sleepiness associated w/narcolepsy and other sleep disorders.

INDICATIONS/DOSAGE/ROUTES

Narcolepsy, sleep disorders:
PO: Adults, elderly: 200 mg/day in the morning; decrease dose to 100 mg/day in pts w/severe liver impairment.

SIDE EFFECTS

Appear to be dose-related: dry mouth, dry eyes, nausea, insomnia, sweating, headache, dizziness, hot flushes, hypersalivation, anorexia, anxiety, bad temper, choking, dysphoria, euphoria, increased B/P, fatigue, weight gain, sexual hyperactivity.

montelukast

mon-**tee**-leu-cast
(Singulair)

CLASSIFICATION

Anti-asthmatic (leukotriene receptor antagonist)

AVAILABILITY (Rx)

Tablets: 10 mg. **Tablets, chewable:** 5 mg.

ACTION/*THERAPEUTIC EFFECT*

A leukotirene receptor antagonist; inhibits airway edema, smooth muscle contraction, altered cellular activity associated w/inflammatory process. *Relieves signs and symptoms of bronchial asthma.*

USES

Prophylaxis and chronic treatment of asthma. Not for use in reversal of bronchospasm in acute asthma attacks, status asthmaticus, exercise-induced bronchospasm.

INDICATIONS/DOSAGE/ROUTES

Asthma:
PO: Adults, children >14 yrs: 10 mg/day. **Children: 6–14 yrs:** 5 mg/day.

SIDE EFFECTS

Adults, adolescents >15 yrs: FREQUENT (18%): Headache. OCCASIONAL (4%): Influenza. RARE (2–3%): Abdominal pain, cough, dyspepsia, dizziness, fatigue, dental pain. *Children 6–14 yrs:* RARE (<2%): Diarrhea, laryngitis, pharyngitis, nausea, otitis media, sinusitis, viral infection.

moxifloxacin

mock-ih-**flocks**-ah-sin
(Avelox)

CLASSIFICATION

Anti-infective: Quinolone

AVAILABILITY (Rx)

Tablets: 400 mg

ACTION/*THERAPEUTIC EFFECT*

Inhibits DNA enzyme in susceptible micro-organisms, *interfering w/bacterial DNA replication.* Bactericidal.

USES

Treatment of community-acquired pneumonia (CAP), sinusitis, acute bacterial exacerbation of chronic bronchitis.

INDICATIONS/DOSAGE/ROUTES

Sinusitis, CAP:
PO: Adults, elderly: 400 mg/day for 10 days.
Chronic bronchitis:
PO: Adults, elderly: 400 mg/day for 5 days.

SIDE EFFECTS

FREQUENT (5–10%): Nausea, diarrhea. **OCCASIONAL (1–5%):** Dizziness, headache, abdominal pain, vomiting, altered taste, dyspepsia.

nalmefene

nal-meh-feen
(Revex)

CLASSIFICATION

Antidote

AVAILABILITY (Rx)

Injection: 100 mcg/ml, 1 mg/ml

ACTION/ THERAPEUTIC EFFECT

An opioid antagonist, *prevents/reverses effects of opioids (respiratory depression, sedation, hypotension).*

USES

Complete/partial reversal of opioid drug effects; management of known or suspected opioid overdose.

INDICATIONS/DOSAGE/ROUTES

Postop pts:
IV/IM/SubQ: Adults: Initially, 0.25 mcg/kg followed by additional 0.25 mcg doses at 2 to 5 min intervals until desired response. Cumulative doses >1 mcg/kg do not provide additional therapeutic effect.

Known/suspected overdose:
IV/IM/SubQ: Adults: Initially, 0.5 mg/70 kg. May give 1 mg/70 kg in 2–5 min. If physical opioid dependence suspected, initial dose is 0.1 mg/70 kg.

SIDE EFFECTS

FREQUENT (5–20%): Nausea, vomiting, tachycardia, hypertension. **OCCASIONAL (1–5%):** Postop pain, fever, dizziness, headache, chills, hypotension, vasodilation.

naratriptan

nar-ah-**trip**-tan
(Amerge)

CLASSIFICATION

Antimigraine

AVAILABILITY (Rx)

Tablets: 2.5 mg

ACTION/ THERAPEUTIC EFFECT

Binds selectively to vascular receptors, producing a vasoconstrictive effect on cranial blood vessels, *producing relief of migraine headaches.*

USES

Acute treatment of migraine headaches with or without aura.

INDICATIONS/DOSAGE/ROUTES

Migraine headaches:
PO: Adults: 2.5 mg.

SIDE EFFECTS

FREQUENT: Tingling (4–8%), nasal discomfort (5–7%). **OCCASIONAL (2–4%):** Weakness, warm/hot sensation, flushing, sense of tightness.

nelfinavir

nell-**fine**-ah-veer
(Viracept)

CLASSIFICATION

Antiviral

AVAILABILITY (Rx)

Tablets: 250 mg. **Oral Powder:** 50 mg/g powder.

ACTION/*THERAPEUTIC EFFECT*

Supresses HIV protease, the enzyme necessary for the formation of infectious HIV inhibiting the activity of the enzyme. *Results in formation of immature noninfectious viral particles rather than HIV replication.*

USES

Treatment of HIV infection when antiretroviral therapy is warranted.

INDICATIONS/DOSAGE/ROUTES

HIV Infection:
PO: Adults: 750 mg q8h or 1,250 mg q12h with food. **Children:** 20–25 mg/kg/dose q8h.

SIDE EFFECTS

FREQUENT (>5%): Mild diarrhea. **OCCASIONAL (1–5%):** Nausea, abdominal pain, rash, flatulence.

---

nitric oxide
(INOmax)

CLASSIFICATION

Respiratory gas

AVAILABILITY (Rx)

Inhalation Gas: 100 ppm, 800 ppm

ACTION/*THERAPEUTIC EFFECT*

Nitric oxide is produced by many cells in the body. Relaxes vascular smooth muscle, producing pulmonary vasodilation. *Improves oxygenation and reduces need for extracorporeal membrane oxygenation.*

USES

Treatment of term and near-term neonates w/respiratory failure associated w/clinical or echocardiographic evidence of pulmonary hypertension.

INDICATIONS/DOSAGE/ROUTES

Respiratory failure:
Inhalation: Neonates: 20 ppm for up to 14 days.

SIDE EFFECTS

FREQUENT: Hypotension (13%), withdrawal syndrome (12%), atelectasis (9%). **OCCASIONAL (6–8%):** Hematuria, hyperglycemia, sepsis, infection, cellulitis, stridor.

---

olopatadine
owe-low-**pay**-tah-deen
(Patanol)

CLASSIFICATION

Antiallergic

AVAILABILITY (Rx)

Ophthalmic Solution: 0.1%

ACTION/*THERAPEUTIC EFFECT*

Selective H_1 receptor antagonist. Blocks histamine release from mast cells. *Reduces symptoms of allergic conjunctivitis.*

USES

Temporary prevention of itching of the eye due to allergic conjunctivitis.

INDICATIONS/DOSAGE/ROUTES

Allergic conjunctivitis:
Ophthalmic: Adults, elderly, children >3 yrs: 1–2 drops in affected eye(s) q5–8 hrs.

SIDE EFFECTS

FREQUENT: Headache (7%), burning/stinging. **OCCASIONAL:** Dry eye, foreign body sensation, hyperemia, keratitis, lid edema, pruritus, asthenia, cold syndrome, pharyngitis, rhinitis, sinusitis, altered taste.

oprelvekin
oh-prel-vee-kinn
(Neumega)

CLASSIFICATION
Platelet growth factor

AVAILABILITY (Rx)
Injection: 5 mg

ACTION/*THERAPEUTIC EFFECT*
Stimulates the production of blood platelets (essential in the blood-clotting process).

USES
Prevents severe thrombocytopenia; reduces need for platelet tranfusions following myelosuppression chemotherapy in pts with nonmyeloid malignancies.

INDICATIONS/DOSAGE/ROUTES
Prevention of thrombocytopenia:
SubQ: Adults: 50 mcg/kg once daily. **Children:** 75–100 mcg/kg once daily. Continue for 14–28 days or until platelet count reaches 50,000 cell/mcl after its nadir.

SIDE EFFECTS
FREQUENT: Edema (59%), neutropenic fever (48%), headache (41%), fever (36%), rash (25%), tachycardia (20%), vasodilation (19%), nausea/vomiting (77%), diarrhea (43%), dizziness (38%), insomnia (33%), dyspnea (48%), rhinitis (42%), increased cough (29%), pharyngitis (25%).

orlistat
or-lih-stat
(Xenical)

CLASSIFICATION
Weight loss agent

AVAILABILITY (Rx)
Capsules: 120 mg

ACTION/*THERAPEUTIC EFFECT*
Irreversible lipase inhibitor, *decreasing amount of ingested dietary fat absorbed and increasing fecal fat excretion.*

USES
Treatment of obesity.

INDICATIONS/DOSAGE/ROUTES
Obesity:
PO: Adults: 120 mg 3 times/day.

SIDE EFFECTS
FREQUENT (>70%): Gastrointestinal complaints (loose bowel movements, oily-appearing stools, abdominal cramps, fecal incontinence, nausea).

oseltamivir
oh-sell-**tam**-ih-veer
(Tamiflu)

CLASSIFICATION
Antiviral

AVAILABILITY (Rx)
Capsules: 75 mg

ACTION/*THERAPEUTIC EFFECT*
Pro-drug hydrolyzed to active ingredient. Selective inhibitor of influenza virus neuraminidase, an enzyme essential for viral replication. Acts against both influenza A and B viruses. *Suppresses spread of infection within respiratory system, reduces duration of clinical symptoms.*

USES
Symptomatic treatment of un-

complicated acute illness caused by influenza A or B virus in adults symptomatic no longer than 2 days.

INDICATIONS/DOSAGE/ROUTES

Influenza:
PO: Adults, elderly: 75 mg 2 times/day for 5 days.

SIDE EFFECTS

OCCASIONAL (>1%): Nausea, vomiting, bronchitis, insomnia, vertigo.

palivizumab

pal-**iv**-ih-zoo-mab
(Synagis)

CLASSIFICATION

Monoclonal antibody

AVAILABILITY (Rx)

Lyophilized Injection: 100 mg

ACTION/*THERAPEUTIC EFFECT*

Exhibits neutralizing activity against respiratory syncytial virus (RSV) in infants, *inhibiting RSV replication in the lower respiratory tract.*

USES

Prevention of serious lower respiratory tract disease caused by RSV in pediatric pts at high risk for RSV disease.

INDICATIONS/DOSAGE/ROUTES

Respiratory syncytial virus (RSV) prevention:
IM: Children: 15 mg/kg once/mo.

SIDE EFFECTS

FREQUENT (20–50%): Upper respiratory tract infection, otitis media, rhinitis, rash. OCCASIONAL

(2–10%): Pain, hernia, increased AST, pharyngitis. RARE (<2%): Cough, diarrhea, vomiting, injection-site reaction, flu syndrome.

pantoprazole

pan-tow-**pray**-zoll
(Protonix)

CLASSIFICATION

Gastric acid pump inhibitor

AVAILABILITY (Rx)

Tablets: 40 mg. Injection: 40 mg.

ACTION/*THERAPEUTIC EFFECT*

Converted to active metabolite that irreversibly binds to and inhibits H+/K+ ATPase (an enzyme on surface of gastric parietal cells). Inhibits hydrogen ion transport into gastric lumen. *Increases gastric pH, reducing gastric acid production.*

USES

Treatment of gastric, duodenal ulcers, gastro-esophageal reflux disease (GERD), *H. pylori* (in combination with antibacterial agents).

INDICATIONS/DOSAGE/ROUTES

Gastric, duodenal ulcers, GERD, H. pylori:
PO/IV: Adults, elderly: 40 mg/day.

SIDE EFFECTS

OCCASIONAL (<2%): Diarrhea, headache, dizziness, pruritus, skin rash.

paricalcitol

pear-ee-**kal**-cih-toll
(Zemplar)

CLASSIFICATION

Vitamin D analog

AVAILABILITY (Rx)

Injection: 0.005 mg/ml (5 mcg/ml)

ACTION

A vitamin D analog. Reduces parathyroid hormone levels. Exact mechanism unknown.

USES

Treatment and prevention of secondary hyperparathyroidism associated w/chronic renal failure.

INDICATIONS/DOSAGE/ROUTES

Hyperparathyroidism:
IV: Adults, elderly: 0.04 mcg/kg to 0.1 mcg/kg (2.8–7 mcg) no more than every other day at any time during dialysis.

SIDE EFFECTS

FREQUENT (5–15%): Chills, fever, flu-like symptoms, sepsis, GI bleeding, nausea, vomiting, edema, lightheadedness, pneumonia. **OCCASIONAL (1–5%):** Palpitations, dry mouth.

---

pemirolast

pem-ee-**row**-last
(Alamast)

CLASSIFICATION

Antiallergic

AVAILABILITY (Rx)

Ophthalmic Solution: 0.1%

ACTION/*THERAPEUTIC EFFECT*

Prevents activation, release of mediators of inflammation (e.g., mast cells). *Reduces symptoms of allergic conjunctivitis.*

USES

Prevention of itchy eyes due to allergic conjuntivitis.

INDICATIONS/DOSAGE/ROUTES

Allergic conjunctivitis:
Ophthalmic: Adults, elderly: 1–2 drops 3–4 times/day.

SIDE EFFECTS

FREQUENT: Transient stinging, burning, instillation discomfort. **OCCASIONAL:** Ocular itching, blurred vision, tearing, headache.

---

pentosan

pen-toe-san
(Elmiron)

CLASSIFICATION

Urinary tract analgesic

AVAILABILITY (Rx)

Capsules: 100 mg

ACTION/*THERAPEUTIC EFFECT*

Appears to adhere to bladder wall mucosal membrane, may act as a buffering agent to control cell permeability preventing irritating solutes in the urine. Has anticoagulant/fibrinolytic effects. *Relieves bladder pain.*

USES

Relief of bladder pain/discomfort associated with interstitial cystitis.

INDICATIONS/DOSAGE/ROUTES

Interstitial cystitis:
PO: Adults, elderly: 100 mg 3 times/day.

SIDE EFFECTS

FREQUENT (3–5%): Alopecia, diarrhea, nausea, headache, rash, abdominal pain, dyspepsia. **OCCASIONAL (1–2%):** Dizziness, depression, increased liver function tests.

perindopril

per-**inn**-doe-prill
(Aceon)

CLASSIFICATION

Angiotensin-converting enzyme (ACE) inhibitor

AVAILABILITY (Rx)

Tablets: 2 mg, 4 mg, 8 mg

ACTION / *THERAPEUTIC EFFECT*

Suppresses renin-angiotensin-aldosterone system (prevents conversion of angiotensin I to angiotensin II, a potent vasoconstrictor; may also inhibit angiotensin II at local vascular and renal sites). *Reduces peripheral arterial resistance, B/P.*

USES / *UNLABELED*

Management of hypertension (HTN) alone or in combination w/other classes of antihypertensives (e.g., thiazides). *Management of heart failure.*

INDICATIONS / DOSAGE / ROUTES

HTN:
PO: Adults, elderly: 2–8 mg/day as single dose or in 2 divided doses. **Maximum:** 16 mg/day.

SIDE EFFECTS

OCCASIONAL (1–5%): Cough, back pain, sinusitus, viral infection, upper extremity pain, dyspepsia, fever, proteinuria, palpitations, hyperkalemia, angioneurotic edema, hypotension, dizziness, fatigue, syncope, azotemia.

pioglitazone

pie-oh-**glit**-ah-zone
(Actos)

CLASSIFICATION

Antidiabetic

AVAILABILITY (Rx)

Tablets: 15 mg, 30 mg, 45 mg

ACTION / *THERAPEUTIC EFFECT*

Increases glucose consumption, facilitates glucose entry to target cells, reduces glucose production by improving insulin sensitivity in pts w/insulin resistance. *Reduces plasma glucose, triglycerides, insulin levels in pts w/hyperinsulinemia; improves fasting, postprandial hyperglycemia, hyperinsulinemia.*

USES

Monotherapy or in combination w/sulfonylurea, metformin, or insulin as adjunct to diet and exercise in pts w/type 2 diabetes mellitus.

INDICATIONS / DOSAGE / ROUTES

Diabetes mellitus, monotherapy:
PO: Adults, elderly: 15–30 mg/day. **Maximum:** 45 mg/day.

Diabetes mellitus, combination:
PO: Adults, elderly: 15–30 mg/day.

SIDE EFFECTS

FREQUENT (5–15%): Headache, myalgia, pharyngitis, sinusitis, tooth disorder, upper respiratory tract infection, sore throat, increased weight, edema, anemia.

podofilox

poe-doe-**fie**-locks
(Condylox)

CLASSIFICATION

Antimitotic

AVAILABILITY (Rx)

Topical Gel: 0.5%. **Topical Solution:** 0.5%.

ACTION/ *THERAPEUTIC EFFECT*

Exact mechanism of action unknown. *Causes necrosis of visible wart tissue.*

USES

Gel: Treatment of anogenital warts. *Solution:* Treatment of external warts.

INDICATIONS/DOSAGE/ROUTES

Anogenital warts:
Topical: Adults: Apply twice daily to warts w/applicator tip or finger.

External warts:
Topical: Adults: Apply morning and evening (q12 hrs) w/cotton-tipped applicator.

SIDE EFFECTS

FREQUENT (50–80%): Burning, pain, inflammation, erosion, itching.

collapse at resting pressure. Deficiency of surfactant results in respiratory distress syndrome (RDS). Poractant compensates for surfactant deficiency, *restoring surface activity to lungs of infants.*

USES/ *UNLABELED*

Treatment (rescue) of RDS in premature infants. *Prophylaxis for RDS, adult RDS due to viral pneumonia, following near-drowning, HIV-infected infants w/PCP.*

INDICATIONS/DOSAGE/ROUTES

RDS:
Endotracheal: Infants: Initially, 2.5 ml/kg birth weight (BW). Up to 2 subsequent doses of 1.25 ml/kg BW at 12 hr intervals. **Maximum:** 5 ml/kg.

SIDE EFFECTS

FREQUENT: Pneumonia (17%), septicemia (14%), bronchopulmonary dysplasia (18%), intracranial hemorrhage (51%), patent ductus arteriosus (60%), pneumothorax (21%), pulmonary interstitial emphysema (21%).

poractant

pour-**act**-tant
(Curosurf)

CLASSIFICATION

Lung surfactant

AVAILABILITY (Rx)

Intratracheal Suspension: 1.5 ml, 3 ml

ACTION/ *THERAPEUTIC EFFECT*

Endogenous surfactant reduces surface tension of alvioli during ventilation, stabilizes alveoli against

pramipexole

pram-ih-**pecks**-all
(Mirapex)

CLASSIFICATION

Dopamine agonist

AVAILABILITY (Rx)

Tablets: 0.125 mg, 0.25 mg, 1 mg, 1.5 mg

ACTION/ *THERAPEUTIC EFFECT*

Stimulation of dopamine receptors in the striatum.

USES

Treatment of signs/symptoms of idiopathic Parkinson's disease.

INDICATIONS/DOSAGE/ROUTES

Parkinson's disease:
PO: Adults, elderly: Initially, 0.375 mg/day in 3 divided doses. Gradually increase dose. **Maintenance:** 1.5–4.5 mg/day in equally divided doses 3 times/day. Dosage is decreased in pts with renal impairment.

SIDE EFFECTS

FREQUENT: Nausea (28%), dizziness (25%), somnolence (22%), postural hypotension (53%), dyskinesias (47%), extrapyramidal symptoms (28%), hallucinations (9%), constipation (14%).

prednicarbate
pred-nih-**car**-bate
(Dermatop)

CLASSIFICATION

Corticosteroid: Topical

AVAILABILITY (Rx)

Cream: 0.1%

ACTION/*THERAPEUTIC EFFECT*

Diffuses across cell membranes forming complexes w/cytoplasm. Complexes stimulate protein synthesis of inhibitory enzymes responsible for anti-inflammatory effects. *Inhibits edema, erythema, pruritus, capillary dilation, phagocytic activity.*

USES

Provides relief of inflammation/pruritus associated w/corticosteroid-responsive disorders.

INDICATIONS/DOSAGE/ROUTES

Usual topical dosage:
Adults, elderly: Apply sparingly 2–4 times/day.

SIDE EFFECTS

FREQUENT: Contact dermatitis (burning/itching of skin); painful, red, itchy, pus-containing blisters; thinning of skin w/easy bruising; dryness, irritation, skin redness or scaling of skin lesions, skin rash.

quetiapine
kwe-**tie**-ah-peen
(Seroquel)

CLASSIFICAITON

Antipsychotic

AVAILABILITY (Rx)

Tablets: 25 mg, 100 mg, 200 mg

ACTION/*THERAPEUTIC EFFECT*

Exact mechanism unknown. Interacts with multiple neurotransmitter receptors, including serotonin, dopamine, and histamine.

USES

Management of manifestations of psychotic disorders.

INDICATIONS/DOSAGE/ROUTES

Psychotic disorders:
PO: Adults: Initially, 25 mg 2 times/day, then 25–50 mg 2–3 times on second and third days, up to 300–400 mg/day by the fourth day.

SIDE EFFECTS

FREQUENT: Headache (19%), somnolence (18%), dizziness (10%), agitation (20%), insomnia (19%), dry mouth (8%), postural hypotension (5%).

rabeprazole

ray-beh-**pray**-zoll
(Aciphex)

CLASSIFICATION

Gastric acid pump inhibitor

AVAILABILITY (Rx)

Tablets: 20 mg.

ACTION/ *THERAPEUTIC EFFECT*

Converted to active metabolite that binds to and inhibits H+/K+ ATPase (an enzyme on surface of gastric parietal cells). This action is partially reversible. Inhibits hydrogen ion transport into gastric lumen. *Increases gastric pH, reducing gastric acid production.*

USES

Treatment of duodenal ulcers, gastro-esophageal reflux disease (GERD), hypersecretory syndromes.

INDICATIONS/DOSAGE/ROUTES

Duodenal ulcers, GERD:
PO: Adults, elderly: 20 mg/day.
Hypersecretory syndromes:
PO: Adults, elderly: Initially, 60 mg/day. May increase up to 60 mg 2 times/day.

SIDE EFFECTS

OCCASIONAL (<3%): Headache, nausea, dizziness, rash, diarrhea, malaise, skin eruptions.

raloxifene

rah-**locks**-ih-feen
(Evista)

CLASSIFICATION

Selective estrogen receptor modulator

AVAILABILITY (Rx)

Tablets: 60 mg

ACTION/ *THERAPEUTIC EFFECT*

Increases bone density, lowers LDL and total cholesterol. *Prevents bone loss and lowers cholesterol without stimulating the endometrium.*

USES

Prevention and treatment of osteoporosis in postmenopausal women.

INDICATIONS/DOSAGE/ROUTES

Prevention/treatment osteoporosis:
PO: Adults: 60 mg once daily.

SIDE EFFECTS

FREQUENT: Infection (15%), flu syndrome (14.6%), hot flashes (24%), nausea (8%), increased weight (8.8%), arthralgia (10.7%), sinusitis (10.3%). **OCCASIONAL (3–8%):** Chest pain, fever, migraine, depression, insomnia, rash, sweating, dyspepsia, vomiting, peripheral edema, myalgia, leg cramps, arthritis, increased cough, pneumonia, laryngitis.

repaglinide

reh-**pah**-glih-nide
(Prandin)

CLASSIFICATION

Antidiabetic

AVAILABILITY (Rx)

Tablets: 0.5 mg, 1 mg, 2 mg

ACTION/ *THERAPEUTIC EFFECT*

Stimulates insulin secretion from beta cells of pancreas. Action is glucose dependent.

USES

Treatment of type-2 diabetes mellitus as monotherapy or in combination w/metformin (Glucophage).

INDICATIONS/DOSAGE/ROUTES

Diabetes mellitus:
PO: Adults, elderly: 0.5–4 mg 2–4 times/day. Take each dose w/meals up to 30 min before meals. **Maximum:** 16 mg/day.

SIDE EFFECTS

FREQUENT: Respiratory tract infections (10–16%), hypoglycemia (16–31%), headache (9–11%). **OCCASIONAL:** Sinusitis, rhinitis, bronchitis, nausea, diarrhea, vomiting, constipation, dyspepsia, back pain, arthralgia.

respiratory syncytial immune globulin
(Respigam)

CLASSIFICATION

Immune serum

AVAILABILITY (Rx)

Injection: 2,500 mcg RSV immune globulin

ACTION/*THERAPEUTIC EFFECT*

High concentration of neutralizing and protective antibodies specific for respiratory syncytial virus (RSV).

USES

Prevents serious lower respiratory tract infections caused by RSV in children <24 months w/bronchopulmonary dysplasia or history of premature birth.

INDICATIONS/DOSAGE/ROUTES

RSV:
IV Infusion: Children (<24 months): 750 mg/kg (15 ml/kg). Initially, 1.5 ml/kg/hr for first 15 min; increase to 3 ml/kg/hr for next 15 min, then 6 ml/kg/hr for remainder of infusion. Administer monthly for total of 5 doses beginning in September or October.

SIDE EFFECTS

OCCASIONAL: Fever (6%), respiratory distress (2%), vomiting (2%), wheezing (2%). **RARE (<1%):** Diarrhea, rales, fluid overload, rash, tachycardia, hypertension, hypoxia, gastroenteritis, injection site inflammation.

reteplase
rhet-eh-place
(Retavase)

CLASSIFICATION

Thrombolytic

AVAILABILITY (Rx)

Powder for Injection: 10.8 units (18.8 mg)

ACTION/*THERAPEUTIC EFFECT*

Directly activates the conversion of plasminogen to plasmin. Additionally, reteplase is a fibrin-specific agent. *Lyses clots.*

USES

Management of acute myocardial infarction (AMI) for improvement of ventricular function following AMI, reducing incidence of CHF and mortality associated with AMI.

INDICATIONS/DOSAGE/ROUTES

AMI:
IV Bolus: Adults, elderly: 10 units over 2 min, then repeat 10 units 30

min after initiation of first bolus injection.

SIDE EFFECTS

FREQUENT (4–50%): Bleeding at superficial sites (injection sites, catheter insertion sites, venous cutdowns). **OCCASIONAL (2–10%):** Internal bleeding involving the gastrointestinal, genitourinary, and respiratory tracts; retroperitoneum. **RARE (<2%):** Arrhythmias.

Rh$_o$(D) immune globulin IV (human)

(WinRho SD)

CLASSIFICATION

Immune serum

AVAILABILITY (Rx)

Injection: 600 IU (120 mcg), 1,500 IU (300 mcg)

ACTION/*THERAPEUTIC EFFECT*

Gamma globulin (IgG) fraction containing antibodies to Rh$_o$(D) antigen negative individuals. *Increases platelets in idiopathic thrombocytopenic purpura (ITP).* Exact mechanism unknown.

USES

Pregnancy/other obstetric conditions: Suppresses Rh isoimmunization in nonsensitized Rh$_o$(D) antigen-negative women, reduces hemolytic disease in Rh$_o$(D)-positive fetus in present and future pregnancies. *Transfusion:* Suppresses isoimmunization transfusion w/Rh$_o$(D) antigen-positive RBCs or blood components containing Rh$_o$(D)-positive RBCs. Treatment of nonsplenectomized Rh$_o$(D) antigen-positive children w/chronic or acute ITP, adults w/chronic ITP, or children and adults w/ITP secondary to HIV infection in clinical conditions to prevent excessive hemorrhage.

INDICATIONS/DOSAGE/ROUTES

Pregnancy:
IV/IM: Adults: 1,500 IU (300 mcg) at 28 wks gestation. Give at 12 wk intervals if administered early in pregnancy, 600 IU (120 mcg) as soon as possible after delivery of confirmed Rh$_o$(D) antigen-positive baby, and within 72 hrs of delivery.

Other obstetric conditions:
IV/IM: Adults: 600 IU (120 mcg) immediately after abortion, amniocentesis, or other manipulations late in pregnancy (after 34 wks gestation) associated w/increased risk of Rh isoimmunization. Give within 72 hrs after the event. Administer 1,500 IU (300 mcg) immediately after amniocentesis before 34 wks gestation or after chorionic villus sampling. Repeat every 12 wks during the pregnancy. In case of threatened abortion, give as soon as possible.

Transfusion:
Note: Within 72 hrs after exposure of incompatible blood transfusion or massive fetal hemorrhage.
IV: Adults: 3,000 IU (600 mcg) q8h until total dose given.
IM: Adults: 6,000 IU (1,200 mcg) q12h until total dose given.

ITP:
IV/IM: Adults, children: Initially, 250 IU (50 mcg)/kg. If Hgb <10 g/dl, give 125–200 IU (25–40 mcg)/kg. Additional doses give 125–300 IU (25–60 mcg)/kg.

SIDE EFFECTS

OCCASIONAL (1–7%): *Rh isoimmunization suppression:* Discomfort, slight swelling at injection site, slight elevation of temperature. *ITP:* Headache, chills, fever.

---

rifapentine
rif-ah-**pen**-teen
(Priftin)

CLASSIFICATION

Anti-tuberculosis agent

AVAILABILITY (Rx)

Tablets: 150 mg

ACTION/*THERAPEUTIC EFFECT*

Inhibits DNA-dependent RNA polymerase in *m. tuberculosis.* Interferes w/bacterial RNA synthesis, preventing attachment of enzyme to DNA, thereby blocking RNA transcription. *Bactericidal activity.*

USES

Treatment of pulmonary tuberculosis in combination w/at least one other anti-tuberculosis medication.

INDICATIONS/DOSAGE/ROUTES

Note: Use only w/another anti-tuberculosis agent.

Tuberculosis:
PO: Adults, elderly: *Intensive phase:* 600 mg 2 times/wk for 2 mos (interval no less than 3 days). *Continuation phase:* 600 mg weekly for 4 mos.

SIDE EFFECTS

FREQUENT (>1%): Hyperuricemia, increased ALT, AST, neutropenia, pyruria, proteinuria, hematuria, lymphopenia, arthralgia, pain, nausea, vomiting, headache, dyspepsia, hypertension, dizziness, diarrhea, hemoptysis.

---

risedronate
rize-droe-nate
(Actonel)

CLASSIFICATION

Calcium regulator

AVAILABILITY (Rx)

Tablets: 30 mg

ACTION/*THERAPEUTIC EFFECT*

Binds to bone hydroxyapatite and inhibits osteoclasts. *Reduces bone turnover and bone resorption.*

USES

Treatment of Pagetis disease of bone (osteitis deformans).

INDICATIONS/DOSAGE/ROUTES

Note: Must take w/6–8 oz water 30 min before first food or drink of the day. Avoid lying down for at least 30 min after taking.
Paget's disease:
PO: Adults, elderly: 30 mg/day for 2 mos. Retreatment may occur after 2 mo post-treatment observation period.

SIDE EFFECTS

OCCASIONAL: Diarrhea, abdominal pain, headache, arthralgia, rash.

---

rituximab
rye-**tucks**-ih-mab
(Rituxan)

CLASSIFICATION

Monoclonal antibody

AVAILABILITY (Rx)

Injection: 10 mg/ml

ACTION/ *THERAPEUTIC EFFECT*

Binds to malignant cells, allowing immune system to recognize and eliminate these cells. *Reduces tumor size.*

USES

Treatment of relapsed or refractory low-grade or follicular B-cell non-Hodgkins' lymphoma.

INDICATIONS/DOSAGE/ROUTES

Non-Hodgkins' lymphoma:
IV Infusion: Adults: 375 mg/m² given once weekly for 4 weeks.

SIDE EFFECTS

FREQUENT: Fever (49%), chills (32%), headache (14%), asthenia (16%), angioedema (13%), hypotension (10%), nausea (18%), rash/pruritus (10%). **OCCASION-AL (<10%):** Myalgia, dizziness, abdominal pain, throat irritation, vomiting, neutropenia, rhinitis, bronchospasm, urticaria.

rizatriptan

rise-ah-**trip**-tan
(Maxalt)

CLASSIFICATION

Antimigraine

AVAILABILITY (Rx)

Tablets: 5 mg, 10 mg

ACTION/ *THERAPEUTIC EFFECT*

Binds selectively to vascular receptors, producing a vasoconstrictive effect on cranial blood vessels, *producing relief of migraine headaches.*

USES

Acute treatment of migraine headaches with or without aura.

INDICATIONS/DOSAGE/ROUTES

Migraine headaches:
PO: Adults: 5–10 mg.

SIDE EFFECTS

FREQUENT (4–8%): Tingling, nasal discomfort. **OCCASIONAL (2–4%):** Weakness, warm/hot sensation, flushing, tightness feeling.

rofecoxib

row-feh-**cox**-ib
(Vioxx)

CLASSIFICATION

Cyclo-oxygenase-2 inhibitor

AVAILABILITY (Rx)

Tablets: 12.5 mg, 25 mg. **Oral Suspension:** 12.5 mg/5 ml, 25 mg/5 ml.

ACTION/ *THERAPEUTIC EFFECT*

Selectively inhibits cyclo-oxygenase-2 (required for synthesis of prostaglandins and thromboxane that cause pain and inflammation). *Produces anti-inflammatory and analgesic effects.*

USES

Relief of signs/symptoms of osteoarthritis, management of acute pain in adults, treatment of primary dysmenorrhea.

INDICATIONS/DOSAGE/ROUTES

Osteoarthritis:
PO: Adults, elderly: 12.5–25 mg/day as single daily dose.
Acute pain, dysmenorrhea:
PO: Adults, elderly: 50 mg/day as single daily dose.

SIDE EFFECTS

FREQUENT (5–10%): Upper respiratory tract infection, diarrhea, nausea. **OCCASIONAL (1–5%):** Abdominal pain, fatigue, dizziness, flu-like symptoms, edema, hypertension, dyspepsia, heartburn, sinusitis, headache, urinary tract infection, bronchitis.

ropinirole

row-**pin**-ih-roll
(Requip)

CLASSIFICATION

Dopamine agonist

AVAILABILITY (Rx)

Tablets: 0.25 mg, 0.5 mg, 1 mg, 2 mg, 4 mg, 5 mg

ACTION/*THERAPEUTIC EFFECT*

Stimulation of dopamine receptors in the striatum.

USES

Treatment of signs/symptoms of idiopathic Parkinson's disease.

INDICATIONS/DOSAGE/ROUTES

Parkinson's disease:
PO: Adults, elderly: Initially, 0.25 mg 3 times/day. Titrate dose weekly up to maximum of 24 mg/day.

SIDE EFFECTS

FREQUENT: Fatigue (11%), pain (8%), edema (7%), syncope (12%), dizziness/somnolence (40%), nausea (60%), vomiting (12%), dyspepsia (10%). **OCCASIONAL (6%):** Increased sweating, asthenia, orthostatic hypotension, pharyngitis, abdominal discomfort (5%). Dry mouth, hypertension, hallucinations, confusion, urinary tract infections.

rosiglitazone

row-see-**glit**-ah-zone
(Avandia)

CLASSIFICATION

Antidiabetic

AVAILABILITY (Rx)

Tablets: 2 mg, 4 mg, 8 mg

ACTION/*THERAPEUTIC EFFECT*

Increases glucose consumption, facilitates glucose entry to target cells, reduces glucose production by improving insulin sensitivity in pts w/insulin resistance. *Reduces plasma glucose, triglycerides, insulin levels in pts w/hyperinsulinemia; improves fasting, postprandial hyperglycemia, hyperinsulinemia.*

USES

Monotherapy or in combination w/metformin as adjunct to diet and exercise in pts w/type 2 diabetes mellitus.

INDICATIONS/DOSAGE/ROUTES

Diabetes mellitus, monotherapy, combination therapy:
PO: Adults, elderly: Initially, 4 mg/day as single or divided doses. May increase to 8 mg/day.

SIDE EFFECTS

FREQUENT (>5%): Headache, upper respiratory tract infection. **OCCASIONAL (1–5%):** Anemia, diarrhea, back pain, edema, fatigue, sinusitis.

sacrosidase

sack-row-**sigh**-daze
(Sucraid)

CLASSIFICATION

Enzyme

AVAILABILITY (Rx)

Oral Solution: 8,500 IU/ml. Oral Powder.

ACTION / *THERAPEUTIC EFFECT*

Hydrolyzes sucrose into glucose and fructose (w/o enzymes, sucrose cannot be absorbed; and its persistent presence in intestinal lumen leads to osmotic retention of water, resulting in loose stools). *Absorbed sucrose prevents excessive gas, bloating, abdominal cramps, nausea, vomiting.*

USES

Oral replacement therapy for genetically determined sucrase deficiency (part of congenital-isomaltase deficiency).

INDICATIONS / DOSAGE / ROUTES

Sucrase deficiency:
PO: Infants: 1–2 ml (or 1–2 scoops of powder) diluted in 2–4 oz water, milk, or infant formula taken w/each meal or snack. **DO NOT HEAT SOLUTIONS CONTAINING SACROSIDASE.** Discard bottles of sacrosidase 4 wks after opening due to bacterial growth potential.

SIDE EFFECTS

FREQUENT (5–10%): Abdominal pain, vomiting. OCCASIONAL (1–5%): Diarrhea.

scopolamine
sko-**poll**-ah-meen
(Trans-Derm Scop)

CLASSIFICATION

Anticholinergic

AVAILABILITY (Rx)

Tablets: 0.4 mg. **Transdermal System:** 1.5 mg.

ACTION / *THERAPEUTIC EFFECT*

Reduces excitability of labyrinthine receptors, depressing conduction in vestibular cerebellar pathway, preventing nausea/vomiting induced by motion.

INDICATIONS / DOSAGE / ROUTES

Prevention of motion sickness:
PO: Adults: 1–2 tablets an hour before travel provide effect for several hours.
Transdermal: Adults: 1 system q72 hrs.

SIDE EFFECTS

FREQUENT (>15%): Dry mouth, drowsiness, blurred vision. RARE (1–5%): Dizziness, restlessness, hallucinations, confusion, difficulty urinating, rash.

sermorelin
sir-moe-**real**-inn
(Geref)

CLASSIFICATION

Growth hormone

AVAILABILITY (Rx)

Powder for Injection

ACTION / *THERAPEUTIC EFFECT*

Directly stimulates pituitary gland to release growth hormone, *increasing plasma growth hormone concentration.*

USES

Treatment of idiopathic growth hormone deficiency in children w/growth failure. Diagnostic aid to evaluate pituitary gland's ability to secrete growth hormone.

INDICATIONS/DOSAGE/ROUTES

Growth hormone deficiency:
SC: Children: 0.03 mg/kg once daily at bedtime. Discontinue when epiphyses are fused.

SIDE EFFECTS

OCCASIONAL: Pain, swelling, redness at injection site, facial flushing, nausea, headache, vomiting, altered taste, chest tightness.

---

sevelamer

seh-**vell**-ah-mur
(Renagel)

CLASSIFICATION

Urinary tract agent

AVAILABILITY (Rx)

Capsules: 403 mg

ACTION/*THERAPEUTIC EFFECT*

Binds/removes dietary phosphorus in GI tract and eliminates phosphorus through normal digestive process. *Decreases incidence of hypercalcemic episodes in pts receiving calcium acetate treatment.*

USES

Reduction of serum phosphorous in pts w/end-stage renal disease (ESRD).

INDICATIONS/DOSAGE/ROUTES

Hyperphosphatemia:
PO: Adults, elderly: 2–4 capsules w/each meal depending on severity of hyperphosphatemia.

SIDE EFFECTS

FREQUENT (11–20%): Infection, pain, hypotension, diarrhea, dyspepsia, vomiting. **OCCASIONAL (1–10%):** Headache, hypertension, thrombosis, increased coughing.

---

sibutramine

sigh-**bew**-trah-meen
(Meridia)

CLASSIFICATION

Anorectic

AVAILABILITY (Rx)

Capsules: 5 mg, 10 mg, 15 mg

ACTION/*THERAPEUTIC EFFECT*

Inhibits reuptake of serotonin (enhancing satiety) and norepinephrine (raises metabolic rate) centrally. Induces and maintains weight loss.

USES

Management of obesity, including weight loss and maintenance of weight loss, when used in conjunction with a reduced-calorie diet.

INDICATIONS/DOSAGE/ROUTES

Weight loss:
PO: Adults: Initially, 10 mg/day. May increase up to 15 mg/day. **Maximum:** 20 mg/day.

SIDE EFFECTS

FREQUENT: Dry mouth (18%), constipation (11%), insomnia (11%). **OCCASIONAL:** Headache, dizziness, increase in blood pressure/heart rate, nervousness.

---

sildenafil

sill-**den**-ah-fill
(Viagra)

CLASSIFICATION

Cardiovascular agent

AVAILABILITY (Rx)

Tablets: 25 mg, 50 mg, 100 mg

ACTION/*THERAPEUTIC EFFECT*

Inhibits type V cyclic GMP, a specific phosphodiesterase, the predominant isoenzyme in human corpus cavernosum in the penis. *Relaxes smooth muscle, increases blood flow, facilitates having an erection.*

USES

Treatment of male erectile dysfunction.

INDICATIONS/DOSAGE/ROUTES

Erectile dysfunction:
PO: Adults: 50 mg (½–4 hrs prior to sexual activity). **Range:** 25–100 mg.

SIDE EFFECTS

OCCASIONAL (1–3%): Mild headache, myalgia, dyspepsia, flushed sensation, blue-green color perception.

sirolimus

sigh-row-**lie**-mus
(Rapamune)

CLASSIFICATION

Immunosuppressant

AVAILABILITY (Rx)

Oral Solution: 1 mg/ml

ACTION/*THERAPEUTIC EFFECT*

Inhibits T-lymphocyte proliferation induced by stimulation of cell surface receptors, mitogens, alloantigens, lymphokines. Prevents activation of enzyme TOR, a key regulatory kinase in cell cycle progression. *Inhibits T and B cell proliferation (essential components of immune response).*

USES

Prophylaxis of organ rejection in pts after renal transplants in combination w/cyclosporine and corticosteroids.

INDICATIONS/DOSAGE/ROUTES

Prophylaxis of organ rejection:
PO: Adults: Loading dose: 6 mg.
Maintenance: 2 mg/day.
Children ≥13 yrs <40 kg: 3 mg/m^2 loading dose; then, 1 mg/m^2/day.

SIDE EFFECTS

OCCASIONAL: Hypercholesterolemia, hyperlipidemia, hypertension, rash. (**High dose 5 mg/day):** Anemia, arthralgia, diarrhea, hypokalemia, thrombocytopenia.

sodium ferric gluconate complex

(Ferrlecit)

CLASSIFICATION

Hematinic

AVAILABILITY (Rx)

Ampules: 12.5 mg/ml elemental iron

ACTION/*THERAPEUTIC EFFECT*

Repletes total body content of iron.

USES

Treatment of iron-deficiency anemia in pts undergoing chronic hemodialysis who are receiving supplemental erythropoietin therapy.

INDICATIONS/DOSAGE/ROUTES

Note: Initially, a 25 mg test dose is

diluted in 50 ml 0.9% NaCl and given over 60 mins.
IV infusion: Adults, elderly: 125 mg in 100 ml 0.9% NaCl infused over 1 hr. Minimum cumulative dose 1 g elemental iron given over 8 sessions at sequential dialysis treatment. (May be given during dialysis session itself.)

SIDE EFFECTS

FREQUENT (>3%): Flushing, hypotension, hypersensitivity reaction. **OCCASIONAL (1–3%):** Injection site reaction, pain, headache, abdominal pain, chills, flu-like syndrome, dizziness, leg cramps, dyspnea, nausea, vomiting, diarrhea, myalgia, pruritus, edema.

sparfloxacin

spar-**flocks**-ah-sin
(Zagam)

CLASSIFICATION

Antibiotic: fluoroquinolone

AVAILABILITY (Rx)

Tablets: 200 mg

ACTION/*THERAPEUTIC EFFECT*

Inhibits DNA enzyme in susceptible microorganisms, *interfering w/bacterial DNA replication.* Bactericidal.

USES

Treatment of community-acquired pneumonia, acute bacterial exacerbations of chronic bronchitis, acute maxillary sinusitis, skin infections, complicated UTI.

INDICATIONS/DOSAGE/ROUTES

Usual dosage:
PO: Adults, elderly: Initially, 400

mg on day 1, then 200 mg once daily for total of 10 days.

SIDE EFFECTS

FREQUENT: Photosensitivity (8%), diarrhea, 4.6%), nausea (4.3%), headache (4.2%). **OCCASIONAL:** Dyspepsia (2.3%), dizziness (2%), insomnia (1.9%), abdominal pain (1.8%), dysgeusia (1.4%).

talc

(Sclerosol)

AVAILABILITY (Rx)

Aerosol Spray Intrapleural: 4 g

ACTION/*THERAPEUTIC EFFECT*

Obliterates the pleural space and prevents reaccumulation of pleural fluid through induction of an inflammatory reaction.

USES

Remedy for cancer pts suffering from pleural effusions.

INDICATIONS/DOSAGE/ROUTES

Pleural effusions:
Aerosol: Adults: 8 g as single treatment.

SIDE EFFECTS

No side effects reported.

tamsulosin

tam-sul-**owe**-sin
(Flomax)

CLASSIFICATION

Antihypertensive

AVAILABILITY (Rx)

Capsule: 0.4 mg

ACTION/*THERAPEUTIC EFFECT*

Prostate selective alpha-1 antagonist, targeting receptors around bladder neck and prostate capsule, resulting in *relaxation of problem organs, improvement in urinary flow, symptoms of prostate hyperplasia.*

USES

Treatment of signs and symptoms of benign prostatic hyperplasia (BPH). Not approved for treatment of hypertension.

INDICATIONS/DOSAGE/ROUTES

BPH:
PO: Adults: 0.4 mg once daily (approximately 30 minutes after same meal each day).

SIDE EFFECTS

FREQUENT: Headache (19.3%), dizziness (14.9%), rhinitis (13.1%), abnormal ejaculation (8.4%). **OCCASIONAL (2–3%):** Nausea, stomach discomfort, bitter taste.

---

tazarotene

tay-zah-**row**-teen
(Tazorac)

CLASSIFICATION

Antipsoriatic

AVAILABILITY (Rx)

Gel: 0.05%, 0.1%

ACTION/*THERAPEUTIC EFFECT*

Modulates differentiation and proliferation of epithelial tissue; binds selectively to retinoic acid receptors. *Restores normal differentiation of the epidermis and reduction in epidermal inflammation.*

USES

Treatment of stable plaque psoriasis in pts with at least 20% body surface area involvement. Treatment of mild to moderate facial acne.

INDICATIONS/DOSAGE/ROUTES

Psoriasis:
Topical: Adults: Thin film applied once daily in the evening; only cover the lesions, and area should be dry before application.

Acne:
Topical: Adults: Thin film applied to affected areas once daily in the evening, after face is gently cleansed and dried.

SIDE EFFECTS

FREQUENT (10–30%): Acne: Desquamation, burning or stinging, dry skin, itching, erythema. *Psoriasis:* Itching, burning or stinging, erythema, worsening of psoriasis, irritation, skin pain. **OCCASIONAL (1–10%):** *Acne:* Irritation, skin pain, fissuring, localized edema, skin discoloration. *Psoriasis:* Rash, desquamation, contact dermatitis, skin inflammation, fissuring, bleeding, dry skin.

---

telmisartan

tell-my-**sar**-tan
(Micardis)

CLASSIFICATION

Angiotensin II receptor antagonist

AVAILABILITY (Rx)

Tablets: 40 mg, 80 mg

ACTION/*THERAPEUTIC EFFECT*

Potent vasodilator, an angiotensin II receptor antagonist. Blocks vasoconstrictor and aldosterone-secreting effects of angiotensin II. Inhibits the binding of angiotensin II to the AT1 receptors, *producing vasodilation, decreased peripheral resistance, decreased B/P.*

USES/*UNLABELED*

Treatment of hypertension alone or in combination with other antihypertensives. *Treatment of heart failure.*

INDICATIONS/DOSAGE/ROUTES

Hypertension:
PO: Adults, elderly: Initially, 40 mg/day. **Range:** 20–80 mg/day.

SIDE EFFECTS

OCCASIONAL (3–7%): Diarrhea, pain (back, leg), upper respiratory tract infection, sinusitis. **RARE (1%):** Dizziness, headache, fatigue, anxiety, nausea, vomiting, dyspepsia, abdominal pain muscle pain, cough, hypertension, rhinitis.

temozolomide

teh-moe-**zoll**-oh-mide
(Temodar)

CLASSIFICATION

Antineoplastic: Alkylating agent

AVAILABILITY (Rx)

Capsules: 5 mg, 20 mg, 100 mg, 250 mg

ACTION/*THERAPEUTIC EFFECT*

Pro-drug, converted to highly active cytotoxic metabolite. Cytotoxic effect associated w/methylation of DNA. *DNA replication inhibited, causing cell death.*

USES

Treatment of refractory anaplas-

tic astrocytoma in adults whose disease has relapsed after initial therapy w/other agents.

INDICATIONS/DOSAGE/ROUTES

Anaplastic astrocytoma:
PO: Adults: Initially, 150 mg/m^2 daily for 5 consecutive days of a 28 day treatment cycle. If myelosuppression is not severe on day 22, dose may increase to 200 mg/m^2 and repeated at 4 wk intervals.

SIDE EFFECTS

FREQUENT: Nausea (53%), vomiting (42%), headache (41%), fatigue (34%), constipation (33%).

thalidomide

thah-**lid**-owe-mide
(Thalomid)

CLASSIFICATION

Immunosuppressive

AVAILABILITY (Rx)

Capsules: 50 mg

ACTION/*THERAPEUTIC EFFECT*

Exact mechanism unknown. Has sedative, anti-inflammatory, and immunosuppressive activity. Action may be due to selective inhibition of the production of tumor necrosis factor alpha.

USES/*UNLABELED*

Treatment of leprosy. *Wasting syndrome of HIV or cancer, recurrent aphthous ulcers in HIV pts, multiple myeloma, Crohn's disease.*

INDICATONS/DOSAGE/ROUTES

AIDS-related muscle wasting:
PO: Adults: 100–200 mg daily.

SIDE EFFECTS

FREQUENT: Drowsiness, dizziness, mood changes, constipation, xerostimia, peripheral neuropathy. **OCCASIONAL:** Increased appetite, weight gain, headache, loss of libido, edema of face and limbs, nausea, hair loss, dry skin, skin rash, hypothyroidism.

tiagabine

tie-**ag**-ah-bean
(Gabitril)

CLASSIFICATION

Anticonvulsant

AVAILABILITY (Rx)

Tablets: 4 mg, 12 mg, 16 mg, 20 mg

ACTION/*THERAPEUTIC EFFECT*

Blocks reuptake of GABA, the major inhibitory neurotransmitter in the CNS, increasing GABA levels, *inhibiting seizures.*

USES

Adjunctive therapy for treatment of partial seizures.

INDICATIONS/DOSAGE/ROUTES

Partial seizures:
PO: Adults: Initially, 4 mg once daily. May increase by 4–8 mg/day at weekly intervals. **Maximum:** 56 mg/day. **Children (12–18 yrs):** Initially, 4 mg once daily, may increase by 4 mg at week 2 and by 4–8 mg/week thereafter. **Maximum:** 32 mg/day.

SIDE EFFECTS

FREQUENT: Dizziness (34%), asthenia (20%), somnolence (25%), nervousness (15%), confusion (13%), headache (23%), infection (23%), tremor (20%). **OCCASIONAL:** Nausea, diarrhea, stomach pain, trouble concentrating, weakness.

tiludronate

tie-**lew**-dro-nate
(Skelid)

CLASSIFICATION

Bone resorption inhibitor, calcium regulator

AVAILABILITY (Rx)

Tablets: 200 mg

ACTION/*THERAPEUTIC EFFECT*

Inhibits functioning osteoclasts through disruption of cytoskeletal ring structure and inhibition of osteoclastic proton pump. *Inhibits bone resorption.*

USES

Treatment of Paget's disease of bone (osteitis deformans).

INDICATIONS/DOSAGE/ROUTES

Paget's disease:
PO: Adults: 400 mg once daily for 3 mos. Must take with 6–8 oz plain water. Do not take within 2 hrs of food intake. Avoid taking aspirin, calcium supplements, mineral supplements, and antacids within 2 hrs of taking tiludronate.

SIDE EFFECTS

FREQUENT: Nausea (9.3%), diarrhea (9.3%), generalized body pain (21.3%), back pain (8%), headache (6.7%). **OCCASIONAL:** Rash (2.7%), dyspepsia (5.3%), vomiting (4%), rhinitis (5.3%), sinusitis (5.3%), dizziness (4%).

tirobifan

tie-**row**-bih-fan
(Aggrastat)

CLASSIFICATION

Antiplatelet, antithrombotic

AVAILABILITY (Rx)

Injection Premix: 25 mg/500 ml (50 mcg/ml). **Vial:** 250 mcg/ml.

ACTION/*THERAPEUTIC EFFECT*

Produces rapid inhibition of platelet aggregation by preventing binding of fibrinogen to receptor sites on platelets. *Prevents closure of treated coronary arteries. Prevents acute cardiac ischemic complications.*

USES

Treatment of pts w/acute coronary syndrome (ACS), including those managed medically and those undergoing percutaneous coronary intervention (PCI).

INDICATIONS/DOSAGE/ROUTES

Note: Must dilute to concentration of 50 mcg/ml in sodium chloride or 5% dextrose. Give w/aspirin/heparin (may give heparin through same IV catheter).

Adjunct PCI:
IV: Adults, elderly: 0.4 mg/kg/min for 30 min then continued at 0.1 mg/kg/min through procedure and for 12–24 hrs following procedure.

SIDE EFFECTS

FREQUENT (5–15%): Minor bleeding. **OCCASIONAL (1–5%):** Major bleeding.

tizanidine

tih-**zan**-ih-deen
(Zanaflex)

CLASSIFICATION

Muscle relaxant

AVAILABILITY (Rx)

Tablets: 4 mg

ACTION/*THERAPEUTIC EFFECT*

Prevents release of excitatory amino acids that inhibit spinal motor neurons mediated by alpha-2 adrenergic agonism. *Reduces muscle tone.*

USES

Treatment of muscle spasticity (abnormal increase in voluntary muscle tone, producing painful muscle spasms, stiffness, rigidity).

INDICATIONS/DOSAGE/ROUTES

Muscle spasticity:
PO: Adults, elderly: Initially 4 mg, gradually increased in 2–4 mg increments and repeated q6–8h. **Maximum:** 3 doses/day or 36 mg total in 24 hrs.

SIDE EFFECTS

FREQUENT (3–10%): Drowsiness, sedation, dry mouth (48%), fatigue, muscle weakness, mild hypotension, GI disturbances, nervousness, dizziness **(16%)**, elevated liver function tests.

tolcapone

toll-cah-pone
(Tasmar)

CLASSIFICATION

Anti-Parkinson

AVAILABILITY (Rx)

Tablets: 100 mg, 200 mg

ACTION/*THERAPEUTIC EFFECT*

Inhibits enzyme COMT, thus potentiating dopamine activity. Increases duration of action of levodopa doses, thus decreasing daily levodopa requirements.

USES

In conjunction w/levodopa, to improve quality of life in pts with Parkinson's disease.

INDICATIONS/DOSAGE/ROUTES

Parkinson's disease:
PO: Adults, elderly: 100 mg 3 times/day. **Maximum:** 200 mg 3 times/day.

SIDE EFFECTS

OCCASIONAL (5–10%): Nausea (30%)/vomiting, dyspepsia, abdominal pain, orthostatic hypotension, sedation, headache.

tolterodine
toll-**tear**-oh-dine
(Detrol)

CLASSIFICATION

Muscarinic receptor antagonist

AVAILABILITY (Rx)

Tablets: 1 mg, 2 mg

ACTION/*THERAPEUTIC EFFECT*

Binds to muscarinic receptor primarily in urinary bladder, antagonizing muscarinic activity. Significantly *reduces frequency of micturition, number of incontinent episodes. Increased average urine volume voided.*

USES

Treatment of overactive bladder w/symptoms of urinary frequency, urgency, or urge incontinence.

INDICATIONS/DOSAGE/ROUTES

Overactive bladder:
PO: Adults, elderly: Initially, 2 mg 2 times/day, then lowered dose based on response, tolerability. **Decreased liver function, medications inhibiting cytochrome P450 (e.g., erythromycin):** 1 mg 2 times/day.

SIDE EFFECTS

FREQUENT: Dry mouth. **OCCASIONAL:** Dyspepsia, headache, constipation, dry eyes, dizziness, blurring of near vision, slowing urinary stream, inability to urinate.

topiramate
toe-**pie**-rah-mate
(Topamax)

CLASSIFICATION

Anticonvulsant

AVAILABILITY (Rx)

Tablets: 25 mg, 100 mg, 200 mg. **Sprinkle Capsules:** 15 mg, 25 mg, 50 mg.

ACTION/*THERAPEUTIC EFFECT*

Blocks repetitive sustained firing of neurons, *decreasing seizure frequency.* May decrease rapid neuronal firing by inhibiting sodium or calcium channels. May potentiate inhibitory action of GABA, inhibit release of excitatory amino acids, or block action of glutamate.

USES/*UNLABELED*

Adjunctive therapy for adults, children (2–16 yrs) w/partial onset or primary generalized tonic-clonic seizures. *Lennow-Gastaut syndrome.*

INDICATIONS/DOSAGE/ROUTES

Partial onset/generalized tonic-clonic seizures:
PO: Adults, elderly: 50 mg/day; increase by 50 mg/day at weekly intervals. **Maximum:** 400 mg/day.

Children (2–16 yrs): Initailly, 25 mg at hs, increase q1–2 wks in increments of 1–3 mg/kg/day up to 5–9 mg/kg/day.

SIDE EFFECTS

FREQUENT: Somnolence (30%), psychomotor slowing (17%), speech disorders (17%), fatigue (11%). **OCCASIONAL:** Difficulty concentrating (8%), nephrolithiasis (1.5%).

toremifene

tore-mih-feen
(Fareston)

CLASSIFICATION

Antineoplastic

AVAILABILITY (Rx)

Tablets: 60 mg

ACTION/ THERAPEUTIC EFFECT

Interacts w/estrogen receptors to serve as an antiestrogen, depleting cytosolic estrogen receptors, resulting in *cytostatic effects on tumor growth.*

USES

Treatment of advanced breast cancer in postmenopausal women w/estrogen receptor-positive disease.

INDICATIONS/DOSAGE/ROUTES

Breast cancer:
PO: Adults: 60 mg daily until disease progression is observed.

SIDE EFFECTS

FREQUENT: Nausea (14%), hot flashes (35%), sweating (20%), dizziness (9%), vaginal discharge (13%). **OCCASIONAL:** Anxiety, tremors, irritability, bone pain, insomnia, lethargy, headache, fatigue, skin rash, abdominal pain, weight gain, edema, vaginal bleeding.

trastuzumab

traz-**two**-zoo-mab
(Herceptin)

CLASSIFICATION

Monoclonal antibody, antineoplastic

AVAILABILITY (Rx)

Lyophilized Powder: 440 mg

ACTION/ *THERAPEUTIC EFFECT*

Inhibits proliferation of human tumor cells that overexpress HER-2 (HER-2 protein overexpression is seen in 25–30% of primary breast cancer pts). Mediates antibody-dependent cellular cytotoxicity.

USES

Treatment of metastatic breast cancer pts whose tumors overexpress HER-2 protein and who have received one or more chemotherapy regimens. May be used w/paclitaxel without previous treatment for metastatic disease.

INDICATIONS/DOSAGE/ROUTES

Note: Do not give as IV bolus or IV push. Dextrose solutions should NOT be used.
Breast cancer:
IV Infusion: Adults, elderly: Initially, 4 mg/kg as 90 min infusion, then weekly infusion of 2 mg/kg as 30 min infusion.

SIDE EFFECTS

FREQUENT (>20%): Pain, asthenia, fever, chills, headache, abdominal pain, back pain, infection, nausea, diarrhea, vomiting, cough, dyspnea. **OCCASIONAL (5–15%):** Tachycardia, CHF, flu-like symptoms, anorexia, edema, bone pain, arthralgia, insomnia, dizziness, paresthesia, depression, rhinitis, pharyngitis, sinusitus. **RARE (<5%):** Allergic reaction, anemia, leukopenia, neuropathy, herpes simplex.

trovafloxacin

tro-vah-**flocks**-ah-sin
(Trovan)

CLASSIFICATION

Anti-infective: Quinolone

AVAILABILITY (Rx)

Tablets: 100 mg, 200 mg. **Injection:** 200 mg, 300 mg vials.

ACTION/ *THERAPEUTIC EFFECT*

Bactericidal. Inhibits DNA gyrase in susceptible microorganisms, interfering w/bacterial DNA replication and repair.

USES

Activity against gram negative, gram positive, atypical organisms and efficacy against anaerobic organisms. Treatment of acute bacterial exacerbations of chronic bronchitis, acute sinusitis, pneumonia, intra-abdominal, gynecological, pelvic, urinary tract, skin/skin structure infections, surgical prophylaxis.

INDICATIONS/DOSAGE/ROUTES

Usual dosage:
IV/PO: Adults: 100–300 mg/day as single dose for 7–14 days.

SIDE EFFECTS

FREQUENT: Dizziness (2–11%), lightheadedness (1–4%), nausea (4–8%), headache (1–5%), vomiting (1–3%), diarrhea (2%). **OCCASIONAL:** Abdominal pain, rash, vaginitis, pruritus.

valrubicin

val-**rue**-bih-sin
(Valstar)

CLASSIFICATION

Antineoplastic

AVAILABILITY (Rx)

Solution for Intravesical Instillation: 40 mg/ml

ACTION/ *THERAPEUTIC EFFECT*

Following intracellular penetration, inhibits incorporation of nucleosides into nucleic acids. *Causes chromosomal damage, arresting cell cycle in G2 phase, interfering w/DNA.*

USES

Intravesical therapy of BCG-refractory carcinoma in situ of urinary bladder in pts for whom cystectomy is unacceptable.

INDICATIONS/DOSAGE/ROUTES

Note: Not for IM/IV use.

Bladder cancer:
Intravesical: Adults, elderly: 800 mg once weekly for 6 wks.

SIDE EFFECTS

Local reaction: **FREQUENT (>10%):** Local bladder symptoms, urinary frequency, dysuria, urinary urgency, hematuria, bladder pain, cystitis, bladder spasms. **OCCASIONAL (<10%):** Nocturia, local burning, urethral pain, pelvic pain, gross hematuria.

Systemic: **FREQUENT (5–15%):** Abdominal pain, nausea, urinary tract infection. **OCCASIONAL (2–5%):** Diarrhea, vomiting, urinary retention, microscopic hematuria, asthenia, headache, malaise, back pain, chest pain, dizziness, rash, anemia, fever, vasodilation.

RARE (1%): Flatus, peripheral edema, increased glucose, pneumonia, myalgia.

valsartan

val-**sar**-tan
(Diovan)

CLASSIFICATION

Angiotensin II inhibitor

AVAILABILITY (Rx)

Capsules: 80 mg, 160 mg

ACTION/*THERAPEUTIC EFFECT*

High affinity/selectivity for angiotensin receptor subtype 1 (AT-1). Blocks vasoconstrictor and aldosterone secreting effects of angiotensin II by inhibiting the binding of angiotensin II to AT-1 receptors *causing vasodilation, decreased peripheral resistance, decrease in B/P.*

USES

First-line treatment of hypertension, used alone or with other antihypertensives.

INDICATIONS/DOSAGE/ROUTES

Hypertension:
PO: **Adults, elderly:** Initially, 80 mg/day. **Range:** 80–320 mg/day.

SIDE EFFECTS

OCCASIONAL (1–3%): Cough, upper respiratory infection, dizziness, diarrhea. RARE (<1%): Back pain, sinusitis, dyspepsia, insomnia.

vigabatrin

vye-gah-**bay**-trin
(Sabril)

CLASSIFICATION

Anticonvulsant

AVAILABILITY (Rx)

Tablets

ACTION/*THERAPEUTIC EFFECT*

Irreversibly inhibits GABA transaminase (the primary enzyme responsible for metabolizing GABA), increasing GABA levels in brain, *preventing seizure activity.*

USES

Add-on therapy in treatment of refractory complex partial seizures.

INDICATIONS/DOSAGE/ROUTES

Partial seizures:
PO: **Adults:** 1–4 g/day in divided doses. **Children:** 50–150 mg/kg/day in divided doses.

SIDE EFFECTS

FREQUENT: Drowsiness, fatigue, abdominal pain, loss of appetite, dizziness, headache, poor concentration, irritability. OCCASIONAL: Nervousness, weight gain, gastrointestinal upset.

zaleplon

zall-eh-plon
(Sonata)

CLASSIFICATION

Sedative hypnotic **(Schedule IV)**

AVAILABILITY (Rx)

Capsules: 5 mg, 10 mg

ACTION/*THERAPEUTIC EFFECT*

Selectively binds to the benzodiazepine-1 receptor (omega-1), which is involved in sedation. Has little effect on normal stages of sleep and few, if any, anxiolytic, anticonvulsant, muscle relaxant properties. *Produces hypnotic effect.*

USES

Short-term treatment of insomnia.

INDICATIONS/DOSAGE/ROUTES

Insomnia:
PO: Adults: 10 mg/day. **Elderly:** 5 mg/day.

SIDE EFFECTS

FREQUENT (5–10%): Abdominal pain, asthenia, headache (28%), nausea, myalgia, dizziness. **OCCASIONAL (1–5%):** Fever, dyspepsia, amnesia, paresthesia, tremor, eye pain, dysmenorrhea. **RARE (<1%):** Malaise, photosensitivity, anorexia, edema, anxiety, vertigo, altered vision, ear pain.

zanamivir

zah-**nah**-mih-veer
(Relenza)

CLASSIFICATION

Antiviral

AVAILABILITY (Rx)

Powder for Oral Inhalation: 5 mg/inhalation

ACTION/*THERAPEUTIC EFFECT*

Selective inhibitor of influenza virus neuraminidase, an enzyme essential for viral replication. Activity against both influenza A and B viruses. *Suppresses spread of infection within respiratory system, reduces duration of clinical symptoms.*

USES

Symptomatic treatment of uncomplicated acute illness caused by influenza A or B virus in adults symptomatic no longer than 2 days.

INDICATIONS/DOSAGE/ROUTES

Influenza:
Oral inhalation: Adults, children >12 yrs: 2 inhalations twice daily (approximately 12 hrs apart) for 5 days initiated within 2 days of onset of symptoms.

SIDE EFFECTS

OCCASIONAL (1.5–3%): Sinusitis, diarrhea, nausea, bronchitis, cough, ear, nose, throat infection, headache, vomiting, dizziness.

zileuton

zye-**lew**-ton
(Zyflo)

CLASSIFICATION

Lipooxygenase inhibitor

AVAILABILITY (Rx)

Tablets: 300 mg, 600 mg

ACTION/*THERAPEUTIC EFFECT*

Inhibits 5-lipoxygenase, the enzyme responsible for producing inflammatory leukotriene products. Prevents formation of leukotrienes (leukotrienes induce bronchoconstrictor response, enhance vascular permeability, stimulate mucus secretion). *Improves airway function, symptoms of asthma.*

USES

Long-term treatment of asthma in patients also taking beta-agonist medication.

INDICATIONS/DOSAGE/ROUTES

Asthma:
PO: Adults, elderly: 600 mg 4

times/day (w/meals and at bedtime).

SIDE EFFECTS

FREQUENT: Headache (25%), dyspepsia (8%), unspecified pain (8%). **OCCASIONAL:** Nausea (6%), abdominal pain (5%), altered liver function tests (4.6%).

---

zinc acetate
(Galzin)

CLASSIFICATION

Electrolyte

AVAILABILITY (Rx)

Capsules: 25 mg, 50 mg

ACTION/*THERAPEUTIC EFFECT*

Zinc induces synthesis of intestinal metallothionein, a metal-binding protein present in intestinal mucosa. Binds copper, *reducing copper accumulation (decreases hepatic/neurologic toxicity).*

USES

Maintenance treatment for pts with Wilson's disease initially treated with a chelating agent.

INDICATIONS/DOSAGE/ROUTES

Wilson's disease:
PO: Adults, children: Initially, 25 mg 3 times/day. May increase up to 50 mg 3 times/day. Each dose should be separated from food/beverages (except water) by 1 hr.

SIDE EFFECTS

FREQUENT (10%): Gastric irritation. **OCCASIONAL (1–10%):** Elevation of alkaline phosphatase, amylase, lipase, sharp, severe stomach pain, upset stomach, mild heartburn.

---

zolmitriptan
zoll-mih-**trip**-tan
(Zomig)

CLASSIFICATION

Antimigraine

AVAILABILITY (Rx)

Tablets: 2.5 mg, 5 mg

ACTION/*THERAPEUTIC EFFECT*

Produces cranial vasoconstriction, inhibits release of neuropeptides (which produce inflammation of cerebral blood vessels). *Produces symptom relief of migraines.*

USES

Acute treatment of migraine with or without an aura in adults.

INDICATIONS/DOSAGE/ROUTES

Migraines:
PO: Adults: Initially, 2.5 mg or lower. If headache returns, may repeat dose in 2 hrs. Do not exceed 10 mg/24 hrs.

SIDE EFFECTS

FREQUENT: Asthenia (3–9%), nausea (4–9%), dizziness (6–10%), somnolence (5–8%), paresthesia (5–9%), tingling (7–9%), warm/hot sensation (5–7%), pain (3–10%), weakness (4–11%). **OCCASIONAL (1–3%):** Myalgia, sweating, chest pain/pressure, palpitations.

SAUNDERS NURSING DRUG HANDBOOK AND PHARMACOLOGY REVIEW SOFTWARE 2001

About this software

Welcome to the **Saunders Nursing Drug Handbook and Pharmacology Review**. This software presents the most commonly used drugs in a database that resembles the **Saunders Nursing Drug Handbook**. You can view about 200 drugs on screen, print the drug information in its entirety, or customize the information to create your own drug cards. The software also offers a review of pharmacology using drugs in the database. By selecting the NCLEX-Test Mode, you can respond to true NCLEX-style questions, randomly generated from a pool of questions. After a review or exam session, you can print out your results and create drug flash cards for further review.

W.B. Saunders Company
A Harcourt Health Sciences Company

System Requirements

80486 with 4Mb of RAM (Pentium with 8 Mb RAM recommended)
VGA (16 color) graphics (SVGA recommended)
3 Mb hard disc available
Windows 95 and above
2x tray-loaded CD-ROM drive

Software Support

For technical software support, call 1 800 692-9010
Monday – Friday, 9:00 a.m. – 5:00 p.m. Central Time.
Fax: 1 314 579-3316
E-mail: **technical.support@harcourt.com**

This program has been produced for Windows 95 and above, single users only.

Brief Instructions

This CD will only work when placed into tray-loaded CD-ROM drives.

- Center the CD in your computer's CD-ROM drive tray. (It will fit!)
- Double click "My Computer."
- Double click on the icon that represents your CD-ROM drive. This will cause a new window to open.
- Double click the "setup.exe" icon in the new window.
- Follow the on-screen instructions.